Textbook of Veterinary Physiology

Third Edition

James G. Cunningham, DVM, PhD

Associate Professor
Departments of Physiology and Small Animal Clinical Sciences
College of Veterinary Medicine
Michigan State University
East Lansing, Michigan

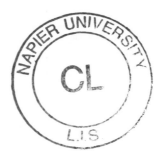

W.B. SAUNDERS COMPANY
An Imprint of Elsevier Science
Philadelphia   London   New York   St. Louis   Sydney   Toronto

W.B. SAUNDERS COMPANY

An Imprint of Elsevier Science

The Curtis Center
Independence Square West
Philadelphia, Pennsylvania 19106

Library of Congress Cataloging-in-Publication Data

Textbook of veterinary physiology / [edited by] James G. Cunningham—3rd ed.

p.   cm.

ISBN 0–7216–8994–9

1. Veterinary physiology.   I. Title: Veterinary
   physiology.   II. Cunningham, James G.

SF768.T49 2002   636.089'2—dc21

DNLM/DLC   2001020597

Acquisitions Editor: Raymond R. Kersey
Developmental Editor: Denise LeMelledo
Project Manager: Mimi McGinnis
Manuscript Editor: Anne Ostroff
Production Manager: Mary B. Stermel
Illustration Specialist: Rita Martello
Book Designer: Lynn Foulk

TEXTBOOK OF VETERINARY PHYSIOLOGY   ISBN 0–7216–8994–9

Printed in the United States of America.

Last digit is the print number: 9   8   7   6   5   4   3   2

This book is dedicated to
veterinary students throughout the world,
because it is these students who give
pleasure, meaning, and value
to our teaching.

CONTRIBUTORS

Steven P. Brinsko, DVM, MS, PhD
Diplomate, American College of Theriogenologists;
Assistant Professor of Theriogenology, Department
of Large Animal Medicine and Surgery, Texas A&M
University, College Station, Texas
REPRODUCTIVE PHYSIOLOGY OF THE MALE
(Chapter 39)

James G. Cunningham, DVM, PhD
Associate Professor, Departments of Physiology and
Small Animal Clinical Sciences, College of Veterinary
Medicine, Michigan State University, East Lansing,
Michigan
NEUROPHYSIOLOGY (Chapters 2 to 16)

Autumn P. Davidson, DVM
Diplomate, American College of Veterinary Internal
Medicine (Internal Medicine); Associate Clinical
Professor, Department of Medicine and
Epidemiology, School of Veterinary Medicine,
University of California at Davis; Director,
Veterinary Clinic, Guide Dogs for the Blind, Inc., San
Rafael, California
REPRODUCTION AND LACTATION (Chapters 34 to 38)

Deborah Greco, DVM, PhD
Diplomate, American College of Veterinary Internal
Medicine (Internal Medicine); Associate Professor,
Department of Clinical Sciences, College of
Veterinary Medicine and Biological Sciences,
Colorado State University, Fort Collins, Colorado
ENDOCRINOLOGY (Chapters 32 and 33)

Steven R. Heidemann, PhD
Professor, Departments of Physiology and of
Microbiology, College of Osteopathic Medicine,
Michigan State University, East Lansing, Michigan
THE CELL (Chapter 1)

Thomas Herdt, DVM
Diplomate, American College of Veterinary Internal
Medicine (Internal Medicine) and American College
of Veterinary Nutrition; Professor, Department of
Large Animal Clinical Sciences and of the Animal
Health Diagnostic Laboratory, and Chief, Nutrition
Section, Animal Health Diagnostic Laboratory,
College of Veterinary Medicine, Michigan State
University, East Lansing, Michigan
GASTROINTESTINAL PHYSIOLOGY AND METABOLISM
(Chapters 26 to 31)

N. Edward Robinson, BVetMED, PhD, MRCVS
Professor, Department of Physiology, and Matilda R.
Wilson Professor, Department of Large Animal
Clinical Sciences, College of Veterinary Medicine,
Michigan State University, East Lansing, Michigan
RESPIRATORY FUNCTION (Chapters 44 to 49)
HOMEOSTASIS (Chapters 50 to 52)

George H. Stabenfeldt, DVM, PhD (Deceased)
Professor, Department of Reproduction, School of
Veterinary Medicine, University of California at
Davis, Davis, California
ENDOCRINOLOGY (Chapters 32 and 33)
REPRODUCTION AND LACTATION (Chapters 34 to 38)

Robert B. Stephenson, PhD
Associate Professor, Department of Physiology,
College of Osteopathic Medicine, Michigan State
University, East Lansing, Michigan
CARDIOVASCULAR PHYSIOLOGY (Chapters 17 to 25)

Jill W. Verlander, DVM
Diplomate, American College of Veterinary Internal
Medicine (Internal Medicine); Associate Scientist,
Department of Medicine, and Director, College of
Medicine Electron Microscopy Care Facility,
University of Florida College of Medicine,
Gainesville, Florida
RENAL PHYSIOLOGY (Chapters 40 to 43)

PREFACE

Physiology is the study of the normal functions of the body: the study of the body's various molecules, cells, and organ systems and the interrelationships among them. Because the study of medicine is the study of the abnormal functions of the body, it is essential to understand normal physiology if one is to understand the mechanisms of disease. For this reason, physiology and other important sciences basic to medicine are introduced first in the veterinary curriculum.

Physiology is a vast subject, and veterinary students are too busy to learn all that is known about it. We have, therefore, made an effort to limit the concepts presented in this book to those germane to the practice of veterinary medicine. All of the authors are either physiologists and also veterinarians or physiologists who have had extensive discussions about content with veterinary clinicians.

This book is designed for first-year veterinary students. Its goal is to introduce the student to the principles and concepts of physiology that are pertinent to the practice of veterinary medicine. Other goals are to introduce the reader to physiopathology and clinical problem-solving techniques and to help the reader understand the relationship between physiology and the practice of veterinary medicine.

This book is designed to be as student friendly as possible. New concepts in the text are introduced by a declarative statement designed to summarize the essential point. This format also helps the reader survey the chapter or review for an examination. These declarative statements are also listed at the beginning of the chapter as an outline.

Chapters include one or more Clinical Correlations at the end. These are designed to show the reader how knowledge of physiology is applied to the diagnosis and treatment of veterinary patients. They also provide the student with an additional way to think through the principles and concepts presented, and they can serve as a basis for classroom case discussions.

In most chapters, several practice questions and answers are included as another method for students to review the book's content. The brief bibliography for each chapter is designed to lead the reader to more advanced textbooks, assuming that most veterinary students are too busy to read original literature. I welcome suggestions of ways to improve this book in subsequent editions.

I particularly want to thank the book's medical illustrator, Ms. Deborah Moulton, who created all the new illustrations for this third edition. I also want to thank Dr. Bari Olivier for his help in developing the Clinical Correlations in the cardiovascular physiology chapters. And last, I want to thank the several classes of veterinary students at Michigan State University who have made constructive suggestions for improvements in this third edition of the book.

Jim Cunningham

CONTENTS

SECTION I
THE CELL

Steven R. Heidemann

CHAPTER 1   **The molecular and cellular bases of physiologic regulation**   2
Clinical Correlations:
Peripheral edema, 28

SECTION II
NEUROPHYSIOLOGY

James G. Cunningham

CHAPTER 2   **Introduction to the neuromuscular system**   32

CHAPTER 3   **The neuron**   34
Clinical Correlations:
Hypoglycemia, 39

CHAPTER 4   **The neuromuscular synapse**   41
Clinical Correlations:
Myasthenia gravis, 43

CHAPTER 5   **The physiology of muscle**   44

CHAPTER 6   **The concept of a reflex**   51

CHAPTER 7   **Skeletal muscle stretch receptors**   53
Clinical Correlations:
Femoral nerve mononeuropathy, 56

CHAPTER 8   **The concept of lower and upper motor neurons and their malfunction**   58
Clinical Correlations:
Lower motor neuron disease, 59

CHAPTER 9   **The brain's control of posture and locomotion**   62
Clinical Correlations:
Focal lesion of the motor cortex, 69

CHAPTER 10   **The vestibular system**   70
Clinical Correlations:
Vestibular syndrome, 73

CHAPTER 11   **The cerebellum**   75
Clinical Correlations:
Cerebellar hypoplasia, 78

CHAPTER 12   **The autonomic nervous system and adrenal medulla**   80
Clinical Correlations:
Horner's syndrome, 86

CHAPTER 13   **The visual system**   87
Clinical Correlations:
Homonymous hemianopia, 92

CHAPTER 14   **Cerebrospinal fluid and the blood-brain barrier**   94
Clinical Correlations:
Increased intracranial pressure, 96

CHAPTER 15   **The electroencephalogram and sensory evoked potentials**   98
Clinical Correlations:
Brain tumor, 103

CHAPTER 16   **Hearing**   104
Clinical Correlations:
Congenital deafness, 106

SECTION III
CARDIOVASCULAR PHYSIOLOGY

Robert B. Stephenson

CHAPTER 17   **Overview of cardiovascular function**   110
Clinical Correlations:
Colic and endotoxic shock in a horse secondary to *Strongylus* parasitism, 121

CHAPTER 18   **Electrical activity of the heart**   123
Clinical Correlations:
Third-degree atrioventricular block, 140

CHAPTER 19 **The electrocardiogram** 142
Clinical Correlations:
Dilative cardiomyopathy with
paroxysmal atrial tachycardia, 151

CHAPTER 20 **The heart as a pump** 154
Clinical Correlations:
Pulmonic stenosis, 166

CHAPTER 21 **The systemic and pulmonary circulations** 169
Clinical Correlations:
Canine heartworm disease with
pulmonary embolism, 179

CHAPTER 22 **Capillaries and fluid exchange** 181
Clinical Correlations:
Acute protein-losing enteropathy
in a horse, 190

CHAPTER 23 **Local control of blood flow** 192
Clinical Correlations:
Patent ductus arteriosus, 197

CHAPTER 24 **Neural and hormonal control of blood pressure and blood volume** 199
Clinical Correlations:
Intraoperative hemorrhage, 207

CHAPTER 25 **Integrated cardiovascular responses** 209
Clinical Correlations:
Exercise intolerance secondary to
congestive heart failure, 217

SECTION IV
GASTROINTESTINAL PHYSIOLOGY AND METABOLISM

Thomas Herdt

CHAPTER 26 **Regulation of gastrointestinal function** 222

CHAPTER 27 **Movements of the gastrointestinal tract** 230
Clinical Correlations:
Equine rabies, 243

CHAPTER 28 **Secretions of the digestive tract** 245

CHAPTER 29 **Digestion and absorption: the nonfermentative processes** 254
Clinical Correlations:
Calf diarrhea with dehydration and
acidosis, 278
Juvenile pancreatic atrophy, 278

CHAPTER 30 **Digestion: the fermentative processes** 280
Clinical Correlations:
Grain engorgement toxemia, 302
Impaction colic, 302

CHAPTER 31 **Postabsorptive nutrient utilization** 304
Clinical Correlations:
Hepatic lipidosis in a cat, 321

SECTION V
ENDOCRINOLOGY

Deborah Greco, George H. Stabenfeldt

CHAPTER 32 **The endocrine system** 324
Clinical Correlations:
Equine Cushing's disease, 338

CHAPTER 33 **Endocrine glands and their function** 341
Clinical Correlations:
Diabetes mellitus, 371

SECTION VI
REPRODUCTION AND LACTATION

George H. Stabenfeldt, Autumn P. Davidson
Chapter 39 by Steven P. Brinsko

CHAPTER 34 **Control of gonadal and gamete development** 374
Clinical Correlations:
Androgen insensitivity, 380

CHAPTER 35 **Control of ovulation and the corpus luteum** 382
Clinical Correlations:
Persistent luteal phase in the
mare, 387

CHAPTER 36 **Reproductive cycles** 389
Clinical Correlations:
Sexual attractiveness in the spayed
bitch, 396

CHAPTER 37 **Pregnancy and parturition** 398
Clinical Correlations:
Prolonged gestation, 404

CHAPTER 38 **The mammary gland** 406
Clinical Correlations:
Neonatal isoerythrolysis, 419

CHAPTER 39 **Reproductive physiology of the male** 421
Clinical Correlations:
Infertility in a stallion, 427

SECTION VII
RENAL PHYSIOLOGY

Jill W. Verlander

CHAPTER 40 **Glomerular filtration** 430
Clinical Correlations:
Chronic renal failure, 437
Glomerulonephritis, 438

CHAPTER 41 **Solute reabsorption** 439
Clinical Correlations:
Glycosuria, 449
Hypoadrenocorticism, 449

CHAPTER 42 **Water balance** 452
Clinical Correlations:
Diabetes insipidus, 457
Chronic renal insufficiency, 457

CHAPTER 43 **Acid-base balance** 459
Clinical Correlations:
Respiratory acidosis with renal
compensation, 465
Metabolic alkalosis with paradoxic
aciduria, 465

SECTION VIII
RESPIRATORY FUNCTION

N. Edward Robinson

CHAPTER 44 **Overview of respiratory function: ventilation of the lung** 468
Clinical Correlations:
Lung fibrosis in the dog, 476
Chronic airway disease in the
horse, 477

CHAPTER 45 **Pulmonary blood flow** 479
Clinical Correlations:
Brisket disease in a heifer, 484

CHAPTER 46 **Gas exchange** 486
Clinical Correlations:
Hypoventilation in a bulldog, 491
Hypoxemia in an anesthetized
Clydesdale horse, 492

CHAPTER 47 **Gas transport in the blood** 494
Clinical Correlations:
Flea infestation in a cat, 499
Atrial fibrillation in a horse, 499

CHAPTER 48 **Control of ventilation** 501
Clinical Correlations:
Hypoxemia with hyperventilation in
an 8-month-old Samoyed, 505
Hypoventilation in an anesthetized
Saint Bernard, 506

CHAPTER 49 **Nonrespiratory functions of the lung** 508
Clinical Correlations:
Pleuritis in a thoroughbred
horse, 512
Mitral insufficiency in a dog, 513

SECTION IX
HOMEOSTASIS

N. Edward Robinson

CHAPTER 50 **Fetal and neonatal oxygen transport** 516
Clinical Correlations:
Patent ductus arteriosus in a
Pomeranian, 520

CHAPTER 51 **Acid-base homeostasis** 522
Clinical Correlations:
Upper airway obstruction in a Boston
terrier, 529
Torsion of the abomasum in a
cow, 529
Neonatal diarrhea in a foal, 530

CHAPTER 52 **Thermoregulation** 533
Clinical Correlations:
Influenza in pigs, 543
Heat stroke in a Boston terrier, 543

Index 545

NOTICE

Veterinary Medicine is an ever-changing field. Standard safety precautions must be followed, but as new research and clinical experience broaden our knowledge, changes in treatment and drug therapy may become necessary or appropriate. Readers are advised to check the most current product information provided by the manufacturer of each drug to be administered to verify the recommended dose, the method and duration of administration, and contraindications. It is the responsibility of the treating veterinarian, relying on experience and knowledge of the animal, to determine dosages and the best treatment for each individual animal. Neither the publisher nor the editor assumes any liability for any injury and/or damage to animals, persons, or property arising from this publication.

THE PUBLISHER

THE CELL

Steven R. Heidemann

The molecular and cellular bases of physiologic regulation

1 All physiologic change is mediated by proteins

2 Protein function depends on protein shape and shape changes

3 A series of enzymatic reactions converts tyrosine into the signaling molecules dopamine, norepinephrine, and epinephrine

4 Muscle contraction and its initiation and cessation depend on the binding specificity and allosteric properties of proteins

5 Biologic membranes are a mosaic of proteins embedded in a phospholipid bilayer

Transport

1 Only small, uncharged molecules and oily molecules can penetrate biomembranes without the aid of proteins

2 Molecules move spontaneously from regions of high free energy to regions of lower free energy

3 Important transport equations summarize the contributions of the various driving forces

4 Starling's hypothesis relates fluid flow across the capillaries to hydrostatic pressure and osmotic pressure

5 Membrane proteins that serve the triple functions of selective transport, catalysis, and coupling can pump ions/molecules to regions of higher free energy

6 Many membrane proteins selectively facilitate the transport of ions/molecules from high to low electrochemical potential

7 Passive transport of K^+ across the plasma membrane creates an electrical potential

8 Spatial organization of active and passive transport proteins enables material to pass completely through the cell

9 Membrane fusion allows for a combination of compartmentalization and transport of material

Information transmission and transduction

1 Cell signaling often occurs via a long sequence of molecular cause and effect

2 External signaling molecules bind to receptors on the surface of cells, causing a "second message" to be sent to the cytoplasm of the cell

3 Specific physiologic information is inherent in the receptor-ligand complex, not in the hormone/neurotransmitter molecule

4 Ca^{2+} transport across plasma and intracellular membranes is an important second messenger

5 Cyclic AMP is produced by activation of a membrane-bound enzyme in response to hormone/neurotransmitter binding to receptors

6 The receptor-mediated hydrolysis of a rare phospholipid of the plasma membrane produces two different second messengers with different actions

7 Steroid hormones interact with receptors within the cell, not with cell surface receptors

Physiology is the study of the regulation of change within organisms—in this case, higher animals. Our understanding of physiology has changed dramatically since the 1980s as a result of insight into the molecular basis of biologic regulation. This chapter summarizes (and simplifies!) our current understanding of the molecular and cellular basis of that regulation. Most of the principles in this chapter apply to all animal cells. The approach taken is that of functional molecular anatomy; that is, the molecular structure of the cell is examined with particular emphasis on the physiologic function, in the intact animal, of the molecules and supramolecular structures responsible for the function. Only the aspects of cell function that

illuminate the medical physiology of the higher animals are discussed. (The reader is referred to the list of texts at the end of this chapter for more complete coverage of the cell.) Some review of basic concepts and vocabulary is presented. However, the discussion assumes that the reader is familiar with the cell and its constituent molecules as presented in courses in general biology and undergraduate biochemistry.

All physiologic change is mediated by proteins

All physiologic change is mediated by a single class of polymeric macromolecules (large molecules): the proteins. Protein function can be subdivided into a number of categories: catalysis, reaction coupling, transport, structure, and signaling.

Catalysis is the ability to markedly increase the rate of a chemical reaction without altering the equilibrium of the reaction. Most biochemical reactions occur at a physiologically useful rate only because of protein catalysts called *enzymes*. Examples of enzymatic catalysis in the synthesis of a class of physiologic regulator molecules, catecholamines, are given later in the chapter.

In *reaction coupling,* two reactions are joined together with the transfer of energy. Energy from a spontaneous reaction (similar to water flowing downhill) is funneled to a nonspontaneous reaction (e.g., sawing wood) so that the sum of the two reactions is spontaneous; that is, the energy liberated by the "downhill" reaction is used to drive the "uphill" reaction. This is the basic function of a motor: the "downhill" burning of gasoline is coupled with the "uphill" movement of the car. The ability of proteins to couple spontaneous and nonspontaneous reactions allows cells to be chemical motors, using chemical energy to perform various jobs of work. One such job of work, the contraction of striated muscle, is discussed later with particular emphasis on the proteins involved.

Proteins provide a pathway for the *transport* of most molecules and all ions into and out of the cell. Transport and transport proteins are discussed more fully after a discussion of the lipid bilayer membrane, the major obstacle to transport.

Proteins that form filaments and that glue cells to each other and to their environment are responsible for the *structure and organization of cells and of multicellular assemblies* (the tissues and organs of animals). The internal structure of the muscle cell, as well as its ability to do work, is governed by the properties of the muscle proteins discussed later.

At its most basic, *signaling* requires only a controlled change or difference. Human signaling occurs through open and closed electric circuits (telegraphy), puffs of smoke in the air, and complex black marks on a contrasting background (numbers and letters). As is discussed next, a fundamental property of proteins is the ability to change shape. The cell can use changes of protein shape directly to send signals, and the function of some proteins is purely informational; that is, the only thing a protein does by changing shape is transmit or transduce information. Information can be defined as "any difference that makes a difference," or, more simply, any difference that regulates something. Catalysis, coupling, transport, structural, and signaling functions can be combined on individual protein molecules. As will become apparent, such multifunctional proteins carry out many important physiologic functions. Also important is the fact that a change in one or more of these protein functions can be used to carry information, to serve as a signal within the cell. So in addition to proteins that exclusively carry information, changes in enzymatic activity or ion transport can "make a differ-

ence," transmitting information and triggering an appropriate response.

Protein function depends on protein shape and shape changes

Protein function is founded on two molecular characteristics: (1) proteins can bind to other molecules very specifically and (2) proteins change shape, which in turn alters their binding properties and their function. The binding specificity of protein is the result of their complex three-dimensional structure. Grooves or indentations on the surface of protein molecules, called *binding sites,* permit specific interactions with a molecule of a complementary shape, called the *ligand.* This complementary shape mechanism that underlies binding is similar to the shape interaction between a lock and key.

Several aspects of the lock-and-key analogy are worth noting. Like a lock, only a small part of the protein is engaged in binding. The binding is very specific, and small changes in the shape of the binding site (keyhole) or the shape of the ligand (key) can cause major changes in protein (lock) behavior. Like the lock and key, the complementary shape interaction serves a recognition function; only molecules with the right shape affect protein function. This recognition function plays a primary role in information transfer. The protein recognizes a particular signal by binding to it, thus changing the shape and thus the function of the protein. Unlike the majority of locks, however, proteins frequently have multiple binding sites for multiple ligands.

Thus, the three-dimensional shape of a protein, its *conformation,* determines protein function. A major force that stabilizes protein conformation is the *hydrophobic interaction.* Oily, hydrophobic ("water-fearing") amino acids tend to congregate in the middle of a protein away from water, whereas *hydrophilic* ("water-loving") amino acids tend to be found on the outer surface of the protein, interacting with the abundant cellular water. The hydrophobic interaction is also important in stabilizing the interaction of proteins with the lipids of biologic membranes, as is discussed shortly. Protein shape is also stabilized by *hydrogen bonding* between the amino acids that compose the protein and by the hydrophobic and hydrophilic properties of the constituent amino acids. Hydrogen bonds also stabilize the positions of polar amino acid pairs in the polypeptide (protein) chain.

The same weak forces responsible for protein conformation are used to hold the ligand in the protein-binding site. The position of the ligand in the binding site is stabilized by hydrogen bonds between the polar groups of the ligand and polar amino acid side groups that line the binding site, just as hydrogen bonds within the polypeptide chain stabilize the shape of the polypeptide. Precisely because the same forces are responsible for the shape of the protein and for its binding properties, shape influences binding, and in turn, binding can influence protein shape. The ability of proteins to change shape is called *allostery* (Greek for "other shape").

Allosteric changes in protein conformation arise in four general ways, as summarized in Figure 1–1. One way (see Fig. 1–1*A*), just mentioned, is that most proteins change shape depending on which ligands are bound at particular binding sites. The sequence of specific ligand binding → protein shape change → change in protein-binding properties and protein function → this change regulates something is a common molecular mechanism underlying physiologic control. This method involves no alteration in the covalent structure of the protein.

A second method of producing conformational change, however, occurs as a result of the covalent modification of one or more of the amino acid side groups of the protein (see Fig. 1–1*B*). By far the most common such change is the covalent addition of a phosphate group to the hydroxyl (—OH) group on the side chain of serine, threonine, or tyrosine residues in the protein. Because the phosphate group is highly charged, phosphorylation of a protein alters hydrogen bonding and other electrostatic interactions within the protein chain, altering its conformation and functional properties.

In a third method, some physiologically important proteins change shape in response to the electrical field surrounding the protein (see Fig. 1–1*C*). These respond to a voltage change by altering the position of charged amino acids, thus altering protein shape.

The fourth method of protein shape change is the least well understood (not shown). Some proteins change shape in response to mechanical forces. Although this is not surprising, insofar as all solids and solid-like substances change shape at least slightly in response to force, we know relatively little about mechanosensitive proteins. The best example is a protein involved in the very early events of hearing that changes its transport of ions in response to the mechanical stimulation of sound (small changes of air pressure in waves).

The significance of binding specificity and allostery can be better appreciated with two examples of their roles in physiologic function. The first example is the role of enzymes in the synthesis of three small, structurally similar, nonprotein signaling molecules. This example shows how binding specificity is important in catalytic function and how allostery underlies the regulation of the synthesis. The second example is more complex: the role of proteins in the contraction of muscle. The contraction of muscle shows how proteins can exploit the basic properties of specific binding and allosteric shape change to do more than one job of work at the same time; muscle proteins serve a structural role, serve a catalytic function, and couple the "downhill" hydrolysis of adeno-

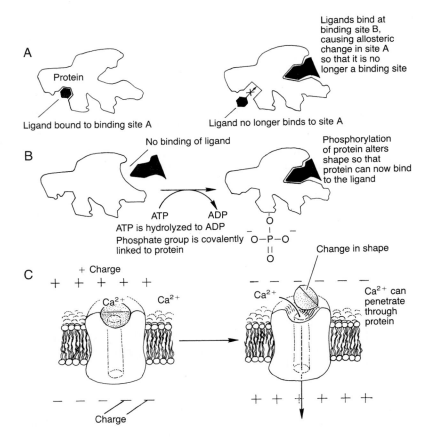

FIGURE 1–1. Three common mechanisms of allosteric shape change in proteins. *A,* Ligand binding. Ligand binding to an allosteric site (site B) on a protein changes the protein's conformation such that binding site A is altered; ligand no longer binds at site A because of the binding event at site B. *B,* Phosphorylation. Addition of a phosphate group to a serine, threonine, or tyrosine residue of a protein alters the protein's conformation, changing its binding characteristics. Shown here is a hypothetical example in which phosphorylation activates an otherwise inactive protein. Some proteins inactivate by this mechanism. *C,* Voltage-dependent proteins. The conformation of some proteins, particularly ion channels, is altered by the electrical field surrounding the protein. Shown here is the opening (activation) of a voltage-dependent, gated Ca^{2+} channel when the membrane depolarizes.

sine triphosphate (ATP) to do mechanical work, the "uphill" lifting of weight.

A series of enzymatic reactions converts tyrosine into the signaling molecules dopamine, norepinephrine, and epinephrine

Figure 1–2 is a diagram of the series of reactions by which the amino acid tyrosine is converted into three different signaling molecules: dopamine, a brain neurotransmitter; norepinephrine, a neurotransmitter of the peripheral autonomic nervous system; and epinephrine, an autonomic neurotransmitter and hormone. Dopamine, norepinephrine, and epinephrine share a similar structure. All contain a phenyl (benzene) ring with two hydroxyl groups (i.e., catechol) and an amine group (hence, catecholamines). They are among the large number of molecules that function as neurotransmitters; that is, the electrically coded information sent along nerve cells causes the release of a chemical, the neurotransmitter, at the terminal of the neuron, which is next to a target cell such as another nerve, a muscle, or an endocrine cell. The electrically encoded information of the nerve is transmitted to the target cell through the binding of the neurotransmitter to proteins on the surface of the target cell. Obviously, proper neurotransmitter synthesis is crucial to nervous function and physiologic regulation.

In the first step of catecholamine biosynthesis, tyrosine binds to the enzyme tyrosine hydroxylase, which catalyzes the addition of another hydroxyl group to the phenyl group to form dihydroxyphenylalanine, nearly always called *dopa*. This hydroxyl group alters the enzyme/ligand interaction; the key no longer fits the keyhole. Dopa is released from the tyrosine hydroxylase and then is bound by another enzyme, L-aromatic amino acid decarboxylase. As the name implies, this enzyme catalyzes the removal of the carboxyl group, converting dopa to dopamine. Dopamine is converted into norepinephrine through the activity of dopamine hydroxylase, which adds yet another hydroxyl group, this time to the two-carbon tail of dopamine. Finally, the addition of a methyl group to the amino nitrogen by phenylethanolamine N-methyltransferase gives rise to epinephrine (also called adrenaline). Note the binding specificity of the enzymes: although the catecholamine structures are all similar to each another, different enzymes bind each one (e.g., epinephrine does not bind to dopamine hydroxylase).

The allosteric properties of one enzyme in this pathway provide an example of physiologic regulation. Certain hormones and neurotransmitters cause the phosphorylation of tyrosine hydroxylase, the first enzyme in the pathway, increasing its activity. In other words, phosphorylation of the enzyme increases the rate at which it catalyzes the conversion of tyrosine to dopa. Because this step is the slowest in the pathway, an increase in the activity of this protein increases the net rate of synthesis of all the catecholamines. Regulated decreases in the rate of catecholamine synthesis are achieved via a different allosteric mechanism: the binding of end products to the enzyme. Dopamine, norepinephrine, and epinephrine can all bind to tyrosine hydroxylase at a site different than the site for tyrosine. These binding events inhibit the enzymatic activity. The inhibition of the pathway by its own end products makes this a classical case of allosteric control called *end product inhibition*. Many substances regulate their own synthesis by inhibiting an initial enzyme in the pathway. If the cell has sufficient end product, these products inhibit further synthesis by allosteric changes in the enzyme. This is an example of the following sequence: specific binding → protein shape change → change in protein binding properties and protein function → this change regulates something: in this case, the synthesis of neurotransmitters.

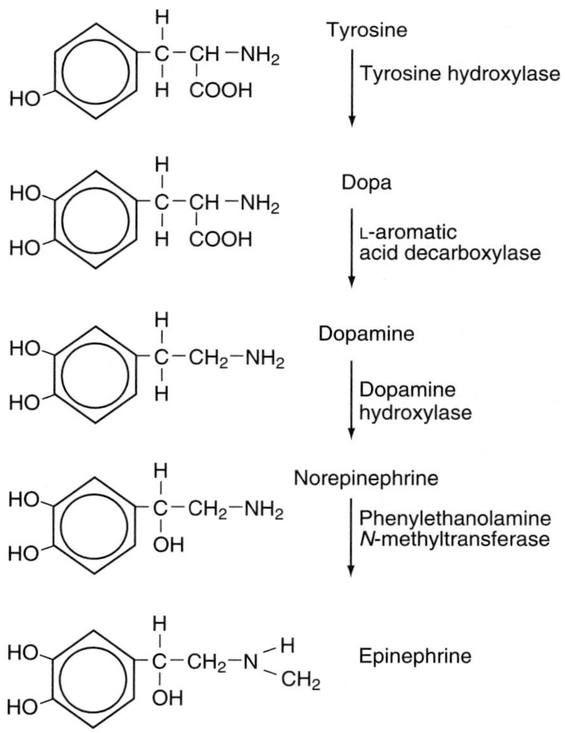

FIGURE 1–2. Epinephrine biosynthetic pathway. The amino acid tyrosine is metabolized to the neurotransmitters dopamine, norepinephrine, and epinephrine. The diagram shows the names and structural formulae for each compound in the path and the names of the enzymes that catalyze each reaction.

Muscle contraction and its initiation and cessation depend on the binding specificity and allosteric properties of proteins

There are three types of muscle tissue in vertebrates: skeletal muscle, which is responsible for the ability of the animal to move; cardiac muscle, a muscle type found only in the heart but structurally similar to skeletal muscle; and smooth muscle, which surrounds hollow organs such as blood vessels, gut, and uterus. All three produce tensile force by contracting and shortening the length of the muscle, and all muscle contraction occurs through the binding and allosteric properties of two proteins: actin and myosin. Starting and stopping the contraction process depend on two additional proteins in skeletal and cardiac muscle: troponin and tropomyosin. Contraction initiation and cessation in smooth muscle depend on a different system with different proteins and are discussed later in this chapter.

Myosin is a large protein that is shaped rather like a two-headed golf club. The elongated tail of the myosin molecule corresponds to the shaft of the golf club, and there are two knobs at one end of the tail that, like golf clubs, are called *heads*. Myosin tails bind specifically to other myosin tails, forming bipolar aggregates called *thick filaments* (Fig. 1–3). Myosin heads specifically bind ATP and another muscle protein, *actin*. Actin binds to itself to form long, thin filaments that are called *thin filaments* in muscle and *microfilaments* or *F-actin* (filamentous actin) in other cell types (see Fig. 1–3). Actin filaments play an important architectural role in all animal cells. Although actin is best understood in muscle cells, all animal cells depend on actin filaments for their shape and for their capacity to migrate in their environment. Actin filaments can be

"woven" in various ways to produce different structures such as rope-like bundles and cloth-like networks. These actin bundles and actin networks are used to support the cell in particular shapes, like ropes holding up the woven cloth of a tent.

In muscle, the interaction of myosin, ATP, and actin to produce contraction and force is shown in Figure 1–4.

Step A: ATP binds to a myosin head; in this conformation myosin has little ability to bind to actin.

Step B: An enzymatic activity associated with the myosin head (an ATPase) rapidly causes a partial hydrolysis of ATP to adenosine diphosphate (ADP) and inorganic phosphate (Pi), both of which stay bound to the myosin. With ADP and Pi bound, myosin has a slightly different shape that binds avidly to nearby actin filaments.

Step C: When myosin binds to actin, called *crossbridging,* the myosin head couples the complete hydrolysis of ATP to a forceful flexing of the myosin head. This allosteric change causes the actin filament to slide past the thick filament. This sliding puts the actin filament under tension, which in turn causes the muscle to contract (shorten) against the load of the muscle (i.e., lifting a weight or pumping out blood). *All muscle contraction depends on the sliding of actin and myosin filaments.* This same allosteric change of myosin also alters myosin binding properties so that it releases the ADP and Pi.

Step D: The binding of a new ATP molecule to the myosin head again causes myosin to change shape; the head unflexes and loses its affinity for actin, releasing the cross-bridge, and the cycle can start over. Rigor mortis of dead animals is caused by a lack of new ATP to bind to myosin heads. In the absence of ATP, myosin heads remain in step C (i.e., bound to actin). The muscle is stiff because it is completely cross-bridged together.

The actomyosin motor uses the binding and allosteric properties of proteins to (1) create structural filaments capable of withstanding and transmitting mechanical force, (2) catalyze the hydrolysis of ATP, and (3) couple the "downhill" ATP hydrolysis to the "uphill" contraction to produce force. For just the one protein, myosin, there are a number of examples of the characteristic sequence described earlier: specific binding → protein shape change → change in protein's binding properties and protein function → this change makes a difference.

This system of contractile proteins requires some control so that, for example, the heart beats rhythmically and skeletal muscle contraction is coordinated. At the organismal level, skeletal and cardiac muscle contraction is primarily under control by electrical stimulation from nerves or other electrically active cells (see Chapter 5). The transmission of electrical

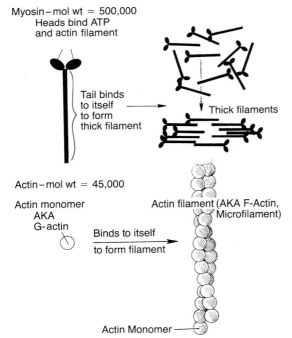

Myosin – mol wt = 500,000
Heads bind ATP and actin filament

Tail binds to itself to form thick filament

Thick filaments

Actin – mol wt = 45,000

Actin monomer AKA G-actin

Binds to itself to form filament

Actin filament (AKA F-Actin, Microfilament)

Actin Monomer

FIGURE 1–3. The assembly of myosin and actin to form filamentous structure. Myosin tails aggregate with one another to form a thick filament, a substructure of striated muscle. Actin monomers (G-actin) are a single polypeptide chain forming a globular protein that can bind to other actin monomers to form actin filament, also called microfilaments. The actin filament is the basic structure of striated muscle thin filaments; thin filaments have troponin and tropomyosin as part of their structure also.

The Power Stroke of Actomyosin

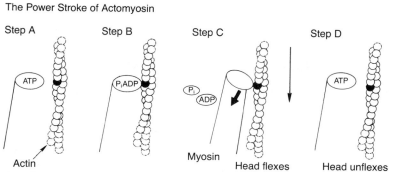

FIGURE 1–4.   The power stroke of actomyosin. *A,* The myosin head has bound to ATP. In this conformation, myosin has little affinity to bind to actin. *B,* ATP is partially hydrolyzed to ADP and Pi; the hydrolysis is partial because the products remain bound to the myosin head. The change in what is bound to the myosin (ADP and Pi, not ATP) has the conformation of myosin so that it binds to actin with high affinity. *C,* Hydrolysis is complete, myosin releases ADP and Pi. This change in what is bound at the myosin head causes an allosteric change in the head; it flexes. Because the myosin head is still bound to the thin filament, the flexion causes the thin filament to slide past the thick filament. *D,* A new ATP molecule binds to the myosin head; as for step A, myosin had little affinity for actin in this state, and the head releases from the thin filament and unflexes.

excitation to the actomyosin system is called *excitation-contraction coupling. Excitation-contraction coupling in all types of muscle depends on changes in intracellular* Ca^{2+} *concentration.* In skeletal and cardiac muscle, but not smooth muscle, two additional thin filament proteins, *troponin* and *tropomyosin,* are required for this coupling. (Excitation-contraction coupling for smooth muscle is discussed later in this chapter.) In striated muscles, troponin binds to tropomyosin and to Ca^{2+}. Tropomyosin is a long, thin protein that binds in the groove of the actin filament in such a way that its positions, high in the groove or snuggled down deep in the groove, allow or prevent the myosin head access to the thin filament (Fig. 1–5). Excitation-contraction coupling of striated muscle works as follows:

Step A: Electrical excitation of a striated muscle cell causes an increase in the intracellular concentration of Ca^{2+}.

Step B: The additional Ca^{2+} binds to troponin, causing an allosteric change in troponin.

Step C: Because Ca^{2+} is bound to troponin, which in turn is bound to tropomyosin, the Ca^{2+}-induced change in troponin conformation is transmitted to the tropomyosin molecule. When troponin binds Ca^{2+}, tropomyosin changes its binding to actin in such a way that it exposes the actin site for myosin cross-bridging. (Tropomyosin snuggles down deeper in its actin groove, revealing actin to the myosin head.) As long as tropo-

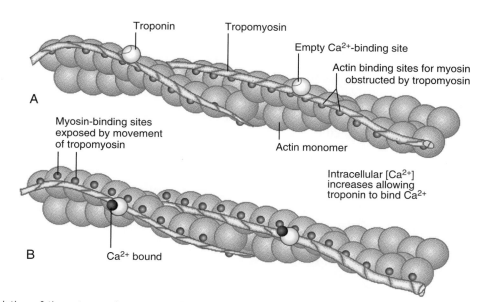

FIGURE 1–5.   Regulation of the actomyosin ATPase and *striated* muscle contraction by Ca^{2+}. *A,* In the absence of high concentrations of Ca^{2+}, tropomyosin sits in the groove of the actin filament to obstruct the binding sites on actin for myosin. *B,* In the presence of higher Ca^{2+} concentrations, the ion binds to troponin, causing an allosteric change in the interaction of troponin with tropomyosin. This allosteric change, in turn, changes the interaction of tropomyosin with the actin filament to expose the myosin-binding sites on actin.

nin binds Ca^{2+}, the muscle contracts according to the actomyosin cycle outlined earlier.

Step D: When the Ca^{2+} concentration drops to normal, however, troponin no longer binds Ca^{2+}. This causes tropomyosin to move up in the thin filament groove so that it again blocks the myosin-binding sites on actin. Myosin heads can no longer cross-bridge, and muscle contraction stops.

As with the actomyosin force generation itself, its regulation also shows many examples of the specific binding function. The specific binding of Ca^{2+} to troponin is a purely informational use of protein binding and shape change; that is, troponin has no catalytic, transport, or structural function but transmits the "on" signal to the next protein. The binding of tropomyosin to actin serves not only a regulatory role but also a structural role; the actin filament is stabilized by tropomyosin, making it less likely to disassemble into actin subunits. The change in the binding geometry of tropomyosin that directly regulates myosin access to actin is a good example of the importance of allosteric change and the following sequence: specific binding (troponin to tropomyosin) → protein (tropomyosin) shape change → change in protein's binding properties (tropomyosin to actin) → a difference in the position of tropomyosin, which in turn regulates the actomyosin motor.

Biologic membranes are a mosaic of proteins embedded in a phospholipid bilayer

Before continuing the discussion of the cellular basis of physiologic control, an additional basic structure must be introduced. This is the phospholipid bilayer of the biomembranes of cells. Phospholipids are molecules that have two long tails of hydrophobic fatty acids and a head that contains a charged, hydrophilic phosphate group. Under appropriate aqueous conditions, these molecules spontaneously form an organized membrane structure, roughly similar to the film of a soap bubble. This filmy layer is composed of two layers (a bilayer) of phospholipid molecules. In both

layers, the hydrophilic heads point outward to hydrogen bond with water, and the oily, fatty acid tails point inward, toward one another and away from the water. Proteins embedded in this lipid bilayer, called *intrinsic membrane proteins* or just *membrane proteins*, produce the *fluid mosaic* structure of biomembranes shown in Figure 1–6. All biologic membranes share this fluid mosaic structure, whether the membrane is the outer plasma membrane that separates cytoplasm from extracellular fluid or the membrane that surrounds intracellular membranous organelles such as endoplasmic reticulum or lysosomes. It is called a "fluid mosaic" because of the mosaic of proteins among phospholipids and because the phospholipid layer is fluid; proteins can move around and diffuse within the plane of the bilayer "like icebergs floating in a phospholipid sea" (the apt phrase of S. J. Singer, one of the originators of the model).

Biologic membranes are another crucial molecular structure that underlies physiologic control. The basic fluid mosaic structure serves four broad functions: (1) compartmentalization, (2) selective transport, (3) information processing and transmission, and (4) organization of biochemical reactions in space.

Compartmentalization is the ability to separate and segregate different regions by composition and function. For example, the lysosome is a membranous organelle within cells that contains hydrolytic (digestive) enzymes that have the potential to digest the cell. Indeed, this organelle was called the "suicide sac" by its discoverer, C. DeDuve. The lysosomal membrane compartmentalizes these potentially harmful enzymes, segregating them from the bulk cytoplasm. The rigor mortis, mentioned earlier, that begins shortly after death is transitory because on death, the lysosomes begin to break open, releasing their enzymes, and the actomyosin cross-bridges are eventually digested apart.

Clearly, the membrane cannot keep a compartment perfectly sealed; material must enter and leave the cell and its internal compartments. *Selective transport* is caused in part by the properties of the phospholipid bilayer but mostly by transport proteins embedded in the membrane. These proteins are characteristically selective in their transport functions; for example, the protein that is the specialized ion channel underlying

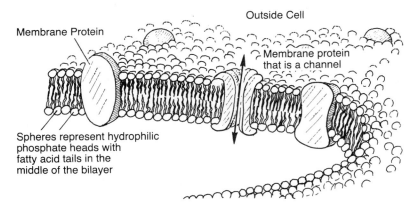

Outside Cell

Membrane Protein

Membrane protein that is a channel

Spheres represent hydrophilic phosphate heads with fatty acid tails in the middle of the bilayer

FIGURE 1–6. The fluid mosaic model for biomembranes. Biomembranes consist of a lipid bilayer in which membrane proteins are embedded.

neuronal signaling is 15 times more permeable to Na^+ than to K^+. Transport is a major topic of cell physiology and is discussed in more detail later.

If the cells of an organism are to respond to external changes, they must receive information about the state of the outside world. Just as higher animals have sensory organs—eyes, ears, nose, and so forth—arrayed on the outside surface of the body, so, too, do cells have most of their information processing and transmission apparatus on their external surfaces. These are intrinsic membrane proteins of the plasma membrane that serve the purely informational function discussed earlier.

At first glance, it might seem odd that a fluid membrane could provide spatial organization for biochemical reactions. However, returning to the "icebergs on a phospholipid sea" analogy, random collisions are much more likely for material in the two-dimensional membrane surface than for material moving through the three-dimensional volume of the cytoplasm. (If the Titanic had been able to dive or fly, it would have had additional ways to avoid its iceberg!) This much larger collision probability is exploited by the cell in a number of physiologic processes. Membranes can also be fenced off into distinct regions across which there is limited diffusion of membrane proteins. For example, certain cells in the kidney have two membrane regions that are quite distinct with respect to transport proteins, which is important in the regulation of salt and water balance by the animal.

━ TRANSPORT

━ Only small, uncharged molecules and oily molecules can penetrate biomembranes without the aid of proteins

Charged particles (ions) do not pass through a pure phospholipid bilayer because of the inner, hydrophobic region of bilayer. Polar molecules (molecules with no net charge but with electrical imbalances) with a molecular weight of more than about 100 D are also unable to pass readily through a pure lipid bilayer, thus excluding all sugar molecules (monosaccharides), amino acids, nucleosides, and their polymers: polysaccharides, proteins, and nucleic acids. On the other hand, some crucially important polar molecules, such as water and urea, are small enough to pass through the lipid bilayer. Small, moderate-size, and large molecules that are soluble in oily solvents readily pass through a pure lipid bilayer. Physiologically important molecules in this class include O_2, N_2, and the steroid hormones (see Chapters 32 and 46). However, many toxic, synthetic molecules, such as insecticides, are also in this category.

━ Molecules move spontaneously from regions of high free energy to regions of lower free energy

The majority of biochemicals do not pass readily through a phospholipid bilayer. Transport of this molecular majority requires a protein pathway across the biomembrane. Also needed is a force that causes movement along the pathway. Before elaborating on membrane proteins as pathways through the lipid bilayer, the energy factors that drive the transport are considered.

We are all familiar with the fact that objects fall spontaneously as a result of gravity. This is a manifestation of the principle that movement occurs to minimize the potential energy of the object. Indeed, all change in the universe (at scales greater than the subatomic particles) occurs to minimize the potential energy, also called the *free energy,* of the system. The movement of molecules is strongly affected by forces such as concentration, pressure (both part of chemical potential), and voltage (electrical potential). Molecules move spontaneously from a region of higher concentration to one of lower concentration, from higher to lower pressure, and from higher to lower electrical potential. Each of these factors—concentration, pressure, and electrical potential—is a source of free energy. The transport of a molecule does not depend necessarily on any one factor; rather, the sum of all of the free energy contributions is the determinant of transport. The sum of all of the free energy contributions on a substance is usually expressed on a per-mole basis as the *electrochemical potential.* The electrochemical potential is the free energy of the substance, from all sources, per mole of the substance.

For spontaneous transport to occur, there must be a difference in the electrochemical potential of the substance between two regions. The two regions are usually two compartments separated by a membrane. This difference in electrochemical potential is called the *driving force.* Typically, students have little difficulty understanding the direction of spontaneous flow as long as only one factor contributes to the electrochemical potential: pressure, or concentration, or voltage. However, understanding physiologic transport, both across cells and across tissues, requires an understanding of the contribution of each factor to the driving force. For example, the flow of fluid from the capillaries of the vascular system depends on the balance between both the hydrostatic pressure difference and the concentration difference of solutes (osmotic pressure) across the capillary. Similarly, movement of Na^+ and K^+ (ions) across the plasma membrane of nerve cells depends on the driving forces contributed by both voltage differences and ion concentration differences across the membrane.

Material moves spontaneously from regions of high electrochemical potential to regions of low electrochemical potential. Such transport is called *diffusion* or *passive transport.* Net movement of material (diffusion) stops when the electrochemical difference between regions equals zero. The state at which the free energy or the electrochemical potential difference is zero is called *equilibrium.* Equilibrium means balance, not equality. Equilibrium is reached when the free energy (electrochemical potential) is balanced; the value on one side is the same as the other. In most cases, the sources of the free energies on the two sides never becomes equal; the concentrations, the pressures, and the voltages remain different, but their differences balance out so that the sum of the free energy differences is zero.

Equilibrium is a particularly important concept because it describes the state toward which change occurs if no work is put into the system. Once the system reaches equilibrium, no further net change occurs unless some work is done on the system. The words "net change" are important. Molecules at equilibrium still move and exchange places, but as much goes in one direction as in the other, so there is no net flow of material.

If the cell requires material to move from low to high electrochemical potential (i.e., in the direction away from equilibrium), thus increasing the difference in free energy between two regions, then some driving force, some work, most be provided by some other decrease in free energy. This type of transport is *active transport*. Active transport uses proteins that combine transport and reaction coupling functions; the protein couples the "uphill" movement of material to a "downhill" reaction such as ATP hydrolysis.

Important transport equations summarize the contributions of the various driving forces

It is worthwhile to develop some quantitative aspects of transport, beginning with simple examples and developing equations for the effect of more than one driving force. These equations can be seen as summaries of the physical laws. In most cases, the equations describe phenomena with which people have experience by living in a technologic society. In these equations, c stands for concentration, V for volume, P for pressure, and so forth. These are common enough concepts. It is important to think about these equations in real-life terms, not as abstract symbols.

One of these equations relates a hydrostatic (pressure) driving force for water movement that just balances a driving force as a result of a chemical potential difference. Recall that *osmosis* is the movement of water across a semipermeable membrane in response to the difference in the electrochemical potential of water on the two sides of the membrane (Fig. 1–7). The chemical potential of water is lower in 1 L of water in which 2 mmol of NaCl is dissolved than in 1 L of water in which 1 mmol of NaCl is dissolved. If these two solutions are separated by a pure lipid bilayer, Na^+ and Cl^- ions cannot move to equilibrate the concentration. Rather, the freely permeable water moves from the side with the higher water potential (low concentration of solute) to the side with the lower water potential (higher concentration of solute). Thus, *water follows solute* (a good summary of osmosis), and this water movement dilutes the 2-mmol solution. However, water movement never produces equal concentrations of salt. Rather, another driving force appears as the water moves. The hydrostatic pressure of water increases on the side to which the water moves, increasing the electrochemical potential of the water on that side. Net water movement stops when the increase in water potential from hydrostatic pressure exactly balances the decrease in water potential from the dissolved salt, so that the electrochemical potential becomes equal on both sides of the membrane.

The initial potential difference of water in Figure 1–7 is caused by the difference in the concentration of material dissolved in the water. A proper explanation of why the water in a solution has a lower chemical potential than pure water (and why water in a concentrated solution has a lower potential than in a dilute solution) is beyond the scope of this chapter. However, readers familiar with the concept of

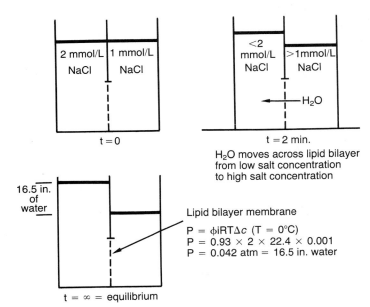

t = 0

t = 2 min.

H₂O moves across lipid bilayer from low salt concentration to high salt concentration

2 mmol/L NaCl | 1 mmol/L NaCl

<2 mmol/L NaCl | >1mmol/L NaCl

—H₂O

16.5 in. of water

Lipid bilayer membrane

$P = \phi iRT\Delta c$ (T = 0°C)
$P = 0.93 \times 2 \times 22.4 \times 0.001$
$P = 0.042$ atm = 16.5 in. water

t = ∞ = equilibrium

FIGURE 1–7. Osmosis. At time (t) = 0, two compartments are separated by a lipid bilayer membrane (no transport proteins) that contains salt solutions of differing concentrations. At t = 2 minutes, the salt ions cannot move across the membrane to equilibrate their concentration, but water can move. Water moves from the region of higher water potential (low salt) to the region of lower water potential (high salt). Water continues to pass the lipid bilayer until at t = equilibrium; the difference in the height of water between the two sides creates a difference in pressure that is equal but opposite to the difference in the water potential between the two sides. That is, the free energy difference due to differing salt concentrations is equilibrated by an equal but opposite free energy difference due to pressure.

entropy will realize that the disorder of a system increases with the introduction of different particles into a pure substance and with the number of different particles that are introduced. An analogy would be that a canister with mixed sugar and salt is more disordered, therefore at higher entropy, than a canister with only pure salt or pure sugar. Also, the disorder of the system increases as more sugar is added to salt (up to 50:50); a pinch of sugar in a canister of salt only slightly increases the disorder. Because an increase in entropy causes a decrease in free energy, the free energy of a solution is decreased as the mole fraction of solute increases.

Osmosis is important to cells and tissues because in general, water can move freely across them, whereas much of the dissolved material cannot. Given a concentration difference of some nonpermeable substances, van't Hoff's equation relates how much water pressure is required to bring the system to equilibrium (the free energy contributed by a pressure difference across the membrane that exactly balances an opposing free energy contribution as a result of a concentration difference):

$$\Pi = iRT\Delta c,$$

where Π is osmotic pressure, the driving force for water movement expressed as an equivalent hydrostatic pressure in atmospheres (1 atm = 15.2 lb/in² = 760 mm Hg) (osmotic pressure is symbolized by Π to distinguish it from other types of pressure terms); i is the number of ions formed by dissociating solutes (2 for NaCl, 3 for $CaCl_2$, and so forth); R is the gas constant (0.082 L atm/mol degree); T is temperature on the Kelvin scale (0°C = 273°K) (RT is a measure of the free energy of 1 mol of material because of its temperature; at 0°C, RT = 22.4 L atm/mol); and Δc is the difference in the molar concentration of the *impermeable* substance across the membrane

This equation summarizes a balance of driving forces; Π amount of hydrostatic (osmotic) pressure is the same driving force as a particular concentration difference, Δc. The osmotic pressure depends only on the concentration difference of the substance; no other property of the substance need be taken into account. Those phenomena that depend only on concentration, such as osmotic pressure, freezing point depression, and boiling point elevation, are called *colligative properties*. Van't Hoff's law is strictly true only for ideal solutions that are approximated in our less-than-ideal world only by very dilute solutions. Real solutions require a "fudge factor" called the *osmotic coefficient,* symbolized by ϕ. The osmotic coefficient can be looked up in a table and then plugged into the equation as follows:

$$\Pi = \phi iRT\Delta c$$

The term ϕic for a given substance represents the osmotically effective concentration of that substance and is often called the *osmolar* or *osmotic concentration,* measured in osm/L. In general, the osmolar concentration of a substance is approximated by the usual concentration times the number of ions formed by the

substance; the osmotic coefficient provides a small correction. The osmolarity of a 100-mmol NaCl solution (0.1 mol) is 0.93 (ϕ for NaCl) × 2 (NaCl → Na^+ + Cl^-) × 0.1 mol = 0.186 osm = 186 mOsm.

This equation summarizes a phenomenon crucial for physiologic function. The greater the concentration difference of an impermeable substance across a membrane, the greater is the tendency for water to move to the side of high concentration (water follows solute). Indeed, if you plug some numbers into this equation, you may be surprised at the large pressures required to balance modest concentration differences. For example, an NaCl concentration difference of 0.1 mol (5.8 g/L) is equilibrated by a pressure (4.2 atm) equal to a column of water 141 feet high (divers must be wary of "the bends" when ascending from depths of more than 70 feet). The importance of this is that a small concentration difference can produce a strong force for moving water. The body makes effective use of this to transport water in many tissues: ions/molecules are transported into or out of a compartment → water follows by osmosis.

▬ Starling's hypothesis relates fluid flow across the capillaries to hydrostatic pressure and osmotic pressure

An excellent practical example of how a balance of driving forces is responsible for the flow of water and permeable substances across a semipermeable membrane is the movement of water and ions across the single layer of cells (endothelial cells) that compose blood capillaries. The single cell layer composes, in effect, a semipermeable membrane with transport qualities different from those of a simple lipid bilayer membrane. The junctions between cells have holes large enough for small molecules and ions to diffuse between compartments. Only large molecules, most importantly proteins, are unable to move through the holes. The difference in protein concentration between the blood and the water solution surrounding tissue cells, called the *extracellular fluid* or *interstitial fluid,* creates an osmotic pressure for the movement of water with all of its dissolved small molecules and ions. This osmotic pressure resulting from dissolved proteins has a special name: *colloid osmotic pressure* or *oncotic pressure.* Protein is more concentrated in the blood than in the interstitial fluid, producing an oncotic pressure of about 0.02 to 0.03 atm (15 to 25 mm Hg), driving water into the capillary. On the basis of this driving force alone, one would expect the capillaries to fill up with water, thus dehydrating the tissue spaces. However, the heart is a pump that exerts a true hydrostatic pressure on the blood, tending to drive the water (and other permeable molecules) out of the capillaries. The net driving force is the algebraic sum of the oncotic pressure difference and hydrostatic pressure difference between the capillaries and the interstitial fluid:

$$\text{net driving force in capillary} = (P_c - P_i) - (\pi_c - \pi_i),$$

where P_c is hydrostatic pressure in the capillary, P_i is hydrostatic pressure in the interstitial space (usually near 0), π_c is oncotic pressure of blood plasma in capillary (approximately 28 mm Hg), and π_i is oncotic pressure of interstitial fluid (approximately 5 mm Hg but depends on the particular tissue).

This equation has enormous relevance to the function of the circulatory system. On the arterial end of capillaries, the hydrostatic pressure (P_c) is high, about 35 mm Hg. By plugging this number into the equation along with the others, the net pressure in the capillary is 12 mm Hg; fluid is being driven out of the capillary on the arterial side (*capillary filtration*). The flow of fluid through the resistance of the capillary causes a decline in pressure so that the hydrostatic pressure on the venous side is low (P_c = 15 mm Hg). The oncotic pressures have not changed, so the net driving force on the venous side is −8 mm Hg; there is a net absorption of fluid into the capillary on the venous side (*capillary reabsorption*). This arrangement achieves a major function of the circulatory system; in this way, the fluid of the blood circulates among the cells and then is recycled back into the circulatory system.

Pathologic alterations in this system emphasize the physiologic importance of balance of driving forces for transport. Chronic liver disease occurs with some frequency in horses and dogs, among other mammals. The liver is compromised in its ability to synthesize and secrete a major blood protein, serum albumin. The decline in the concentration of serum albumin lowers the oncotic pressure of the blood. As a result, there is more force to drive fluid out of the capillaries on the arterial side and less driving force for net absorption of fluid on the venous side of capillaries. This causes the tissue spaces of the diseased animals to fill with fluid, a painful and visually obvious symptom called *edema*. The clinical correlation at the end of the chapter provides another example of edema in which increased hydrostatic pressure in the veins and capillaries causes increased capillary filtration and less capillary reabsorption.

— Membrane proteins that serve the triple functions of selective transport, catalysis, and coupling can pump ions/molecules to regions of higher free energy

Van't Hoff's law and Starling's hypothesis dealt with passive transport (i.e., movement of material in the direction of lower electrochemical potential). However, the cell moves many ions/molecules against their electrochemical potential; that is, this selective transport requires the expenditure of energy by the cell. Transport in a direction requiring an expenditure of energy (i.e., input of work) is called *active transport*. Active transport depends on intrinsic membrane proteins that use specific binding and allostery to achieve the dual functions of selective transport and reaction coupling. Many, but by no means all, active transport proteins obtain the energy for transport from ATP

TABLE 1–1. Concentrations of various substances in the intracellular, extracellular, and plasma fluids

	Concentration (mmol/L)		
	INTRACELLULAR	EXTRACELLULAR	BLOOD PLASMA
Na$^+$	15	140	142
K$^+$	150	5	4
Ca^{2+}	0.0001	1	2.5
Mg^{2+}	12	1.5	1.5
Cl$^-$	10	110	103
HCO$_3^-$	10	30	27
Phosphate	40	2	1
Glucose	1	5.6	5.6
Protein	4.0	0.2	2.5

hydrolysis; these proteins must also function as enzymes (ATPases).

An important example of active transport is the Na$^+$,K$^+$ pump (also known as Na$^+$,K$^+$-ATPase). This intrinsic membrane protein consists of four polypeptide chains (two α and two β) and has a molecular mass of approximately 300,000 D. This molecule catalyzes the hydrolysis of ATP and couples the hydrolysis energy to the movement of Na$^+$ out of the cell and K$^+$ into the cell. This ion pump creates and maintains a considerable concentration gradient across the cell membrane for both ions (for ionic concentrations in cell, plasma, and extracellular fluid, see Table 1–1). Figure 1–8 shows the current understanding of the structure of this protein and outlines the cycle of binding and conformational changes that underlie its transport function. The Na$^+$,K$^+$-ATPase pumps three Na$^+$ *out of* the cell and two K$^+$ *into* the

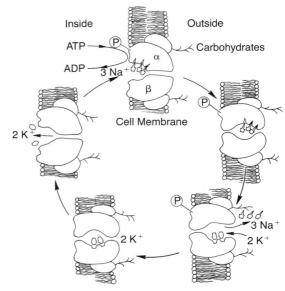

FIGURE 1–8. A hypothetical transport cycle for Na$^+$,K$^+$-ATPase. Changes in the conformation of this transport protein driven by ATP hydrolysis and ion-binding events cause three Na$^+$ ions to be moved out of the cell against a concentration gradient and two K$^+$ ions to be moved into the cell, also against a concentration gradient, for each ATP hydrolyzed. (Redrawn from a diagram by Dr. Seth Hootman.)

cell for each ATP hydrolyzed. These directions of ion pumping cause a high Na$^+$ concentration outside the cell and a low concentration inside, whereas K$^+$ concentration is high inside and low outside the cell. The different directions of pumping for the two ions depend on differing binding specificity of the pump protein in the two conformational states. The ability of the protein to couple this transport to the enzymatic breakdown of ATP allows the transport to occur against the concentration gradients, from lower to higher electrochemical potentials for both ions. In the particular case of the Na$^+$,K$^+$ pump, the number of transported electrical charges is asymmetric; three positive charges leave for each two positive charges that enter. This asymmetry of electrical charge transport means that the Na$^+$,K$^+$ pump is *electrogenic,* making a minor contribution to the electrical potential (voltage) across cell membranes, as is discussed more fully later.

Many different intrinsic membrane proteins actively transport a wide variety of ions/molecules against the electrochemical gradient of the transported molecules. Many, like the Na$^+$,K$^+$ pump, couple the energy-requiring "uphill" transport with the "downhill" hydrolysis of ATP. However, any potential source of free energy can be coupled to the energy-requiring transport. Indeed, the gradient of Na$^+$ set up by the Na$^+$,K$^+$ pump is itself used frequently as a source of energy; that is, the "downhill" flow of Na$^+$ from outside the cell to the inside is a spontaneous reaction whose energy can be coupled to some "uphill" reaction (Fig. 1–9). For example, the transport of glucose and many amino acids from the food mass in the small intestines into the cells that line the

gut is an active transport process and requires a Na$^+$ concentration gradient. Transport proteins in the plasma membrane of intestinal epithelial cells couple the spontaneous diffusion of Na$^+$ into the cell to the inward, energy-requiring transport of the sugar or amino acids. These nutrients are at a higher concentration inside the cell than outside, so they must be actively transported into the cell at the expense of the energy stored in the Na$^+$ electrochemical gradient. In other words, the energy from the "downhill" diffusion of Na$^+$ into the cell is coupled to the "uphill" transport of the nutrient into the cell. Such active transport coupled to Na$^+$ diffusion across the cell membrane is called *secondary active transport* because of its dependence on the Na$^+$ concentration gradient established by the primary active transport of the Na$^+$,K$^+$ pump.

Examples of transport can be referred to in a number of ways. Our examples have been instances in which two ions/molecules must be transported together or not at all, and such transport is called *cotransport.* Cotransport can involve one process of passive transport (diffusion) with an active transport process, as in the two examples in the preceding paragraph; it can involve two active transport processes, like the Na$^+$,K$^+$-ATPase; or it can involve two diffusion processes. In the first case, the need for cotransport is energetic; the flow of one ion is needed to drive the other. In the two latter cases, the need for cotransport is a restriction based on the binding properties of the transport protein; it cannot bind one without the other. Cotransport proteins that transport both substances in the same direction are called *symports* or *symporters.* The Na$^+$/glucose cotransporter in

FIGURE 1–9. Secondary active transport as exemplified by uptake of nutrients by gut epithelia. Nutrients such as glucose and amino acids must be actively transported from relatively low concentration in the gut lumen toward higher concentrations within the cells lining the gut. This active transport process uses the concentration gradient of Na$^+$ ions set up by Na$^+$,K$^+$-ATPase (see Fig. 1–8) as the source of energy for the active transport process. In other words, the energy released by the passive diffusion of Na$^+$ into the cell along its concentration gradient is coupled to the energy-requiring transport of glucose or amino acids against their concentration gradients. Thus, the secondary active transport protein both serves a transport function and couples the "downhill" transport of Na$^+$ to the "uphill" transport of nutrients. There are many such secondary active transport processes in the body. For example, the same mechanism shown here is used to reabsorb nutrients from blood filtrate in the kidney.

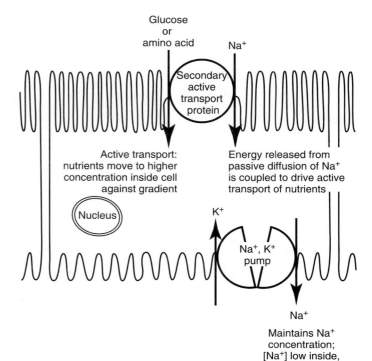

the gut is a symport. Cotransport proteins that transport the two substances in opposite directions, like Na^+,K^+-ATPase, are called *antiports* or *antiporters*. Parenthetically, proteins that transport just a single ion or molecule are called *uniports* or *uniporters*.

Many membrane proteins selectively facilitate the transport of ions/molecules from high to low electrochemical potential

The movement of ions and of medium and large polar molecules requires a protein molecule to serve as a pathway through the obstruction of the phospholipid bilayer. If the movement of the substance is in the natural direction of its electrochemical gradient (movement from high to low), the transport process is called *facilitated diffusion*. The membrane proteins that mediate this transport process through the phos-

pholipid bilayer are *channels* or *carriers* (Fig. 1–10). These are distinguished by the extent to which the protein interacts with the transported substance.

Carriers (see Fig. 1–10A) bind the transported substance in the lock-and-key manner, so there is a site-specific binding of the transported substance to the transport protein. Carrier-mediated transport is typically much slower than channel-mediated diffusion because of the relatively slow binding and unbinding processes. The Na^+,K^+ pump and the Na^+/glucose symport are both examples of carriers.

Channels can be thought of as protein donuts embedded in the phospholipid bilayer. The hole in the donut is a pore in the membrane through which small ions such as Na^+, K^+, Ca^{2+}, Cl^-, and H^+ are transported. Although most channels transport ions, a class of channels called *aquaporins* are channels for water flow. (Although water will flow through a pure lipid bilayer, this transport is too slow for some functions. Kidney cells, for example, are particularly rich

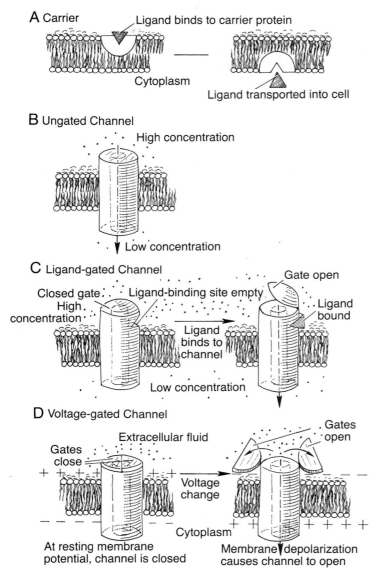

A Carrier — Ligand binds to carrier protein — Cytoplasm — Ligand transported into cell

B Ungated Channel — High concentration — Low concentration

C Ligand-gated Channel — Closed gate — High concentration — Ligand-binding site empty — Gate open — Ligand bound — Ligand binds to channel — Low concentration

D Voltage-gated Channel — Extracellular fluid — Gates close — Gates open — Voltage change — Cytoplasm — At resting membrane potential, channel is closed — Membrane depolarization causes channel to open

FIGURE 1–10. Types of transport proteins mediating facilitated diffusion. In all cases, the ion moves from a region of high potential (shown here as high concentration) to a region of low potential. *A,* Carriers. In a few instances, material is carried by a transport protein that binds tightly to the material, and the complex moves through the lipid bilayer. *B,* Leak channels. These channels are thought not to open and close as do gated channels and so support a small but persistent leak of a particular ion through the pore. Although their existence was long postulated, distinct, ungated leak channels have only recently been identified and isolated, as opposed to leaks through normally gated channels. Selectivity of these and other channels is based on the size of the pore and the weak interactions of ions with the atoms lining the pore. *C,* Ligand-gated channels. The transport protein again forms a pore through the membrane. In the case of gated channels, access of the ion to the pore is controlled by a gate, a substructure of the transport protein that can open and close the pore. In ligand-gated channels, the opening and closing of the gate is controlled by the binding of a ligand to the channel. *D,* Voltage-gated channels are similar to ligand-gated channels except that the opening and closing of the gate is controlled by the electrical field around the channel.

in aquaporins, which are required for the water balance function of the kidney.) For all channels, the pore size and the interaction of the transported material with the amino acid side groups lining the pore allow membrane channels to be selective. Only specific molecules or ions can move through a particular channel. The movement of material through channels is nearly as rapid as simple diffusion through a water-filled space of the same area as the channel pore.

The plasma membranes of most cells have passive leaks of ions, particularly K^+. These ionic leaks are typically ascribed to *leak channels* that are open at all times (see Fig. 1–10B). However, most ion channels open or close in response to signals; these latter types are called *gated channels*. The opening and closing of the gates are examples of the allosteric property of proteins. The same signals responsible for allosteric changes in general—ligand binding, phosphorylation, and voltage differences—also control the opening and closing of gated channels, as shown in Figure 1–10. (Because mechanically gated channels are so poorly understood, these are not discussed here.)

Channels that open in response to ligand binding are called *ligand-gated channels* (see Fig. 1–10C). The nicotinic acetylcholine receptor is a ligand-gated channel found in skeletal muscle membrane directly beneath incoming neurons (nerve cells). This channel is found also in the membrane of neurons in autonomic ganglia and in the brain. As the name implies, the nicotinic acetylcholine receptor binds to the drug nicotine and the neurotransmitter acetylcholine. In both cases, the channel opens in response to ligand binding.

This nicotinic acetylcholine channel plays a key role in transmitting electrical stimulation from neurons to skeletal muscle cells. Briefly, motor neurons release the neurotransmitter acetylcholine in response to the electrical signal coming down the neuron. This acetylcholine binds to and opens the ligand-gated channel on the skeletal muscle. The influx of Na^+ into the muscle cell initiates an electrical response in the muscle, causing the release of Ca^{2+} (through gated channels in the endoplasmic reticulum), in turn causing contraction. (This brief account of neuromuscular transmission, presented only to provide orientation to the function of acetylcholine channel, is expanded in Chapters 4 and 5.) In the case of the nicotinic acetylcholine receptor/channel, the specific binding and allosteric properties of the protein serve the dual functions of selective transport across the membrane and information reception and transmission to the muscle cell.

Channels that open in response to voltage changes across the membrane are called *voltage-gated* or *voltage-dependent channels* (see Fig. 1–10D). This type of channel is in large part responsible for the ability of the neurons to transmit information along their length and to release neurotransmitters. All voltage-gated channels have a range of membrane potentials that cause them to open; this is the *activation* range of the channel. The minimum membrane potential that causes opening is the *threshold* of the channel. The

activation range and threshold vary from channel to channel, depending on the conformation of the protein and the electrical properties of the amino acid side groups that form the gate of the channel. In addition to an open and closed configuration, many voltage-dependent channels have a third conformation, called *inactivated*. Like the closed configuration, the inactivated conformation prohibits the diffusion of ions through the channel. Unlike the closed configuration, it does not open immediately in response to changes in membrane potential. Inactivation can be regarded as an enforced rest period for the channel. Voltage-dependent channels that do not inactivate have only open and closed conformations, and they take up one or the other conformation, depending on the membrane potential.

In the discussion of protein function, it was pointed out that any of the functions of proteins could be used to transmit information if a difference in the protein function changed the cell. Gated channels, both ligand and voltage gated, are ideal candidates for information transmission because they change their function: opening and closing, permitting or stopping transport. Indeed, the sole physiologic function of the nicotinic acetylcholine receptor/channel, described earlier, is the transmission of information: turning the chemical stimulation by the neuron of the muscle into electrical stimulation (see discussion below) of the muscle membrane, leading to muscle contraction.

Passive transport of K^+ across the plasma membrane creates an electrical potential

As just discussed, gated ion channels can convert chemical information into electrical information. Electrical signaling in the animal body is the result of electrical imbalances maintained across the plasma membrane of virtually all cells: cells maintain an electrical potential difference across their plasma membrane. In other words, the cell membrane is a battery; if one attaches electrodes to the two ends of a battery or to the inside and outside of a cell, one finds a voltage difference between the two ends or sides. If one provides a path for electrical charges to move—a metal wire containing free electrons in the case of a battery, or a membrane channel through which ions can move in the case of the cell—an electrical current flows from higher to lower electrical potential. The diversity of battery-powered devices in our society suggests how many ways this electrical potential can be exploited. The physiology of animals also exploits the baseline electrical potential across the plasma membrane, called the *resting membrane potential*. The word "resting" is added to distinguish the baseline potential from the instantaneous values of membrane potential during the passage of membrane currents.

The resting membrane potential is the indirect result of the concentration gradients of ions across the plasma membrane caused by the activity of the

Na$^+$,K$^+$-ATPase. In part, this membrane potential is a result of the asymmetry in numbers of ions pumped by the Na$^+$,K$^+$-ATPase. However, most of the membrane potential is caused by the passive flow of K$^+$ through K$^+$ *leak channels* in response to the concentration gradient of K$^+$ (high inside, low outside). This concentration gradient sets up an electrical driving force (voltage) that exactly balances the concentration driving force. The concentration of K$^+$ inside a mammalian cell is about 150 mmol; outside in the interstitial fluid, it is about 5 mmol. As a result, K$^+$ tends to diffuse from the cytoplasm through the leak channel to the interstitial fluid. However, when K$^+$ alone leaves the cytoplasm without an accompanying negative ion, it causes an electrical imbalance. The exit of K$^+$ ions leaves the inside of the cell with negative charges not neutralized by positive potassium ions, and the interstitial fluid now has positive K$^+$ ions not balanced by negative charges. The cell is building an electrical potential difference across the plasma membrane with the cytoplasm being negative relative to the interstitial fluid.

This electrical potential driving force increases until it balances the concentration driving force for K$^+$. This situation is analogous to osmosis: the concentration-driven flow of water across a semipermeable membrane creates a different driving force (pressure) that eventually balances the concentration driving force. Similarly for the resting membrane potential, the concentration-driven flow of K$^+$ across the semipermeable membrane (semipermeable in the sense that negative ions do not accompany the K$^+$) creates a different driving force (an electrical voltage) that eventually balances the concentration force. As in the case of osmosis, an equation is used to relate the size of the concentration gradient to the size of the electrical potential that provides an exact balance. This equation is called the *Nernst equation*:

$$E_X = RT/zF \ln([X_{outside}]/[X_{inside}]),$$

where E_X is the equilibrium potential for ion X, RT is the gas constant multiplied by the absolute temperature, z is the electrical valence for the ion ($+1$ for Na$^+$ and K$^+$, -1 for Cl$^-$, and so forth), F is the Faraday constant (the number of coulombs of electrical charge in a mole of ions: 96,500 coulombs/mol), and $[X]$ is concentration of ion X.

A simpler form of this equation can be written by taking advantage of the fact that R and F are constants, T is nearly constant under physiologic conditions, and the natural log (ln) of a number is 2.3 times the common log (log$_{10}$):

$$E_X = -60 \text{ mV}/z \log([X_{inside}]/[X_{outside}]),$$

where mV indicates millivolts.

Because the state of balance between the electrical driving force and the concentration driving force is equilibrium, the value of the electrical potential is called the *equilibrium potential* of the ion. Given the concentrations above for K$^+$ inside (150 mmol) and outside (5 mmol) the cell, the equilibrium potential for K$^+$ is

$$
\begin{aligned}
E_{K^+} &= -60 \text{ mV}/+1 \times \log 150/5 \\
&= -60 \text{ mV} \log 30 \\
&= -60 \text{ mV} \times 1.47 \\
&= -88.2 \text{ mV}.
\end{aligned}
$$

Indeed, the measured resting membrane potential across a human muscle cell is -90 mV.

A number of aspects of this important equation are worth discussing. If the equilibrium potential for a particular ion is the same as the measured membrane potential, the net driving force for the ion is zero. In this case, there is no net movement even in the presence of wide open channels to provide a path through the membrane. However, for any gradient of a specific ion, if the measured membrane potential is *not* the equilibrium potential of that ion, there is a driving force for the transport of that ion. In other words, when the membrane potential is anything other than the equilibrium potential, that ion will flow across the membrane if an appropriate channel is open. Thus, the equilibrium potential for an ion provides a "baseline" for comparison with the actual membrane potential to determine whether an ion will tend to move across the plasma membrane. If the measured membrane potential has the same sign but is larger in magnitude than the equilibrium potential, the ion flows in the direction of the electrical potential. If the sign is the same but the magnitude is lower, the concentration driving force determines the direction of flow of the ion. If the measured potential is opposite in sign to that of the equilibrium potential, both electrical and concentration forces are acting on the ion in the same direction. Flows of ions across the plasma membrane (electrical currents) in response to the balance of force between concentration and voltage produce the electrical changes in neurons that underlie the nervous system, as discussed in Chapter 3.

It would be reasonable, but incorrect, to assume that the transport of ions required to set up the electrical potential measurably alters the concentration gradient. This is untrue because of the large amount of energy required to separate electrical charges. The separation of charge arising from the transport of a few ions balances the energy of quite substantial concentration gradients. Indeed, so few ions move that they cannot be measured by chemical means. Thus, electrical, not chemical, measurements are used routinely to assess the transport of ions in cells. The measurable voltage changes caused by immeasurably small concentration changes of ions also means that the electrical phenomena at the membrane persist for many hours, even if the Na$^+$,K$^+$-ATPase is inactivated by a toxin. In other words, an existing concentration gradient of K$^+$ would require hours to dissipate at the rate of K$^+$ leakage characteristic of the plasma membrane. Using the membrane battery analogy, the Na$^+$,K$^+$-ATPase is a battery recharger. A portable radio does not require the minute-to-minute services of a battery recharger. Sufficient energy is stored in the battery to operate the radio for an appreciable period, although the battery recharger is needed ultimately. Similarly, sufficient energy is stored in the K^+ concentration gradient to maintain the membrane potential for a period of time. The Na^+,K^+-ATPase is not required on a minute-to-minute basis, although it is needed ultimately to maintain the concentration gradient on which the resting membrane potential depends.

Spatial organization of active and passive transport proteins enables material to pass completely through the cell

Although macromolecules and biomembranes clearly underlie physiologic function, many phenomena of the intact animal emerge that are not initially apparent as a simple sum of parts. One interesting example is the spatial organization of plasma membrane transport proteins so that ions move across the cell from one extracellular fluid compartment to another. This *transcellular transport* is important in the kidney (see Chapter 40). The plasma membrane of the epithelial cells in the proximal tubules of the kidney contains two distinct regions. The *apical* membrane regions face the lumen of the tubule and the fluid that will become urine, and the *basolateral* regions are near the capillaries and the blood. The apical surface contains ungated, leak channels for Na^+, whereas the basolateral surface contains Na^+,K^+-ATPase molecules. The membrane proteins in one region are prevented from diffusing into the other by membrane structures called *tight junctions*. Na^+ diffuses into the cell on the apical surface from the urine-like fluid driven by both the concentration gradient and the resting membrane potential. Once inside the cell, the Na^+ is pumped out the basolateral surface, essentially into the blood, by the Na^+,K^+-ATPase. This allows the kidney to reabsorb and thus conserve Na^+. As long as the Na^+,K^+-ATPase remains restricted to the basolateral surface and the passive channel to the apical membrane, Na^+ can move through the cell from the urine-like fluid in the tubule to the blood in the capillaries. If either protein should lose its spatial restriction, Na^+ would be transported into and out of the cell on the same surface, merely consuming ATP with no net transport of Na^+ from lumen to capillary.

Membrane fusion allows for a combination of compartmentalization and transport of material

Impermeable molecules can be transported across the cell membrane as carriers or channels by means other than membrane proteins. This method involves use of the membrane as a carrier compartment. The lipid bilayer of biologic membranes shares a basic similarity of structure with soap bubbles. As with soap bubbles, small vesicles of biomembrane (essentially membrane bubbles) can fuse to form larger membrane

surfaces. A large membrane surface can also pinch off (requiring the fusion of two membrane surfaces) into small vesicles. When these processes occur at the plasma membrane, they are called *exocytosis* and *endocytosis,* respectively (Fig. 1–11). When these processes occur at internal membrane sites, the process is referred to as *membrane fusion,* regardless of the direction. Membrane fusion underlies a good deal of membrane vesicle traffic around the cell. This traffic creates intracellular vesicles, renews plasma membrane by adding newly synthesized membrane, and transports material within the cell and across the plasma membrane. Because the transport is compartmentalized within a membrane bubble, the transported material can be targeted specifically to one or another region of the cell. Also, changes to the "cargo" can occur within a particular membrane compartment, as is shown in the example of cholesterol transport.

Exocytosis and endocytosis are crucial in the transport of cholesterol (Fig. 1–12). Cholesterol is an essential lipid component of many animal biomembranes; the plasma membrane lipids of animals is composed of about 15% cholesterol and 60% phospholipids. Cholesterol is also the starting material for the synthesis of the entire group of hormones called *steroids* (see Chapter 32). Cholesterol can be synthesized by

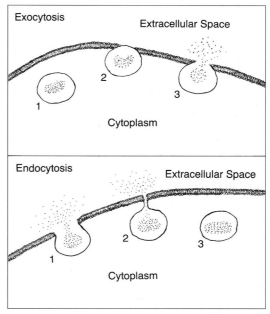

FIGURE 1–11. Two membrane fusion processes: exocytosis and endocytosis. *Top,* In exocytosis, a membrane-bound vesicle from the cytoplasm (1) makes contact and fuses with the plasma membrane (2). As the vesicle membrane becomes continuous with the plasma membrane, the contents of the vesicle are released to the extracellular space (3). *Bottom,* In endocytosis, some material from the extracellular space is surrounded by plasma membrane (1), which continues to invaginate until the edges are able to fuse (2), thus pinches off a vesicle from the plasma membrane (3). Membrane fusion can occur between any two compartments within cells separated by lipid bilayer membrane, not only between the cytoplasm and extracellular space as shown here.

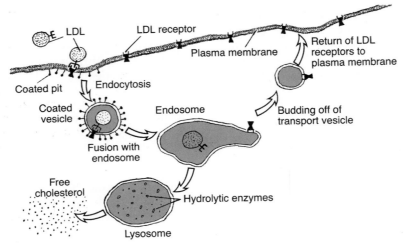

FIGURE 1–12. Processes of membrane fusion involved in cholesterol uptake by cells. Starting at the left, a low-density lipoprotein (LDL)-containing cholesterol binds to an LDL receptor protein of the plasma membrane and undergoes endocytosis, forming an endosome. The receptor is detached from its LDL ligand in the endosome. The LDL portion of the endosome fuses with a lysosome to digest the LDL and produce free cholesterol, while the receptor-containing portion of the endosome pinches off a vesicle to return to the plasma membrane, thus recycling the receptor. (Redrawn from Alberts B, Bray D, Johnson A, et al: Molecular Biology of the Cell. New York: Garland, 1983.)

animals and is also absorbed by meat-eating animals from their diet. Because cholesterol is soluble in oil, it passes from food through the plasma membrane without protein mediation into the cells of the gut lining. However, transport of dietary cholesterol through the circulatory system requires that cholesterol molecules form a complex with a protein molecule to form low-density lipoprotein (LDL). To take up cholesterol from the circulation, cells bind the LDL to intrinsic membrane proteins that act as LDL receptors, as shown in Figure 1–12. The receptor/LDL complex then diffuses in the plane of the membrane into specific regions to form coated pits. The coated pit is taken into the cytoplasm via endocytosis. In addition to the transport function, *receptor-mediated endocytosis* functions to concentrate extracellular material before internalization. The coated pit is not taken into the cell until it has collected the LDL from a far larger volume of extracellular fluid than the cell could "drink." The membrane vesicles formed by this endocytosis fuse subsequently to become an *endosome.* The endosome compartment becomes acidic, which causes dissociation of the LDL and the receptor. Through unknown means, the endosome then is able to further separate and to compartmentalize the receptor from the LDL. Membrane vesicles containing the now vacated LDL receptors return to the plasma membrane and fuse via exocytosis. The LDL receptor is recycled to the plasma membrane to pick up more LDL. Experimental evidence suggests that a single LDL receptor molecule can cycle between the plasma membrane and endosomal vesicles more than 100 times before losing its activity. Meanwhile, the LDL moiety is segregated to another endosomal vesicle, which fuses with the lysosome. The lysosome contains hydrolytic enzymes, thus allowing the internalized LDL to be digested. The cholesterol is now avail-

able to the cell for steroid synthesis or incorporation into membrane.

Other molecules also are recycled via endocytosis. For example, released catecholamine neurotransmitters (discussed earlier) are recycled back via endocytosis into the neuron that released them, saving the neuron the effort of manufacturing new neurotransmitters. Not all molecules that undergo endocytosis are recycled. Many are broken down after their endosome fuses with a lysosome. Indeed, as described later, this is one method of regulating receptor number on the plasma membrane.

INFORMATION TRANSMISSION AND TRANSDUCTION

Cell signaling usually occurs via a long sequence of molecular cause and effect

One of the areas of most rapid progress in cellular physiology has been understanding of the mechanism by which extracellular signals, such as hormones, growth factors, and neurotransmitters, alter cellular function, which in turn alters tissue, organ, and animal function. At the molecular level, nearly all chemical signaling shares a common "strategy" of mechanism: signals are sent as a long chain of chemical cause-and-effect interactions transmitted between many sequential chemical steps. Indeed, chemical signaling pathways are structured like the whimsical "machines" in the cartoons of Rube Goldberg, who was a famous American newspaper cartoonist in the first decades of the 20th century. Figure 1–13 shows his 1928 illustration of an outlandish contraption (a "Rube Goldberg device") to serve as an automatic

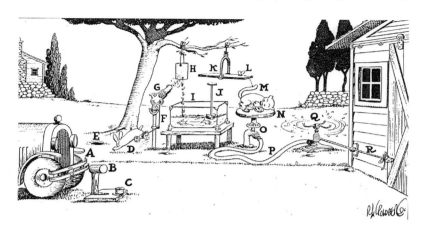

FIGURE 1–13. A Rube Goldberg device (garage door opener, circa 1928) as an analogy for the complex cause-and-effect sequence characteristic of cellular chemical signaling. Automobile (A) drives into driveway, causing hammer (B) to ignite toy cap (C), frightening rabbit (D) into its burrow (E) and causing a pistol (G) to fire and so forth, ultimately leading to the opening of the garage door (R). As explained in the text, this whimsical "machine" serves as an analogy for chemical signaling within cells because of the multiple control elements, their connection as a cause-and-effect sequence, and the use of household items, similar to the use of evolutionarily conserved proteins of cells in signaling.

garage door opener, realistic versions of which had not yet been invented. The automobile (A) drives in, causing hammer (B) to ignite a toy cap gun (C), which frightens rabbit (D) with string (F) tied to its leg, thus firing pistol (G) and so forth until a connection to a rotating water sprinkler causes the carriage-house door to slide open (overhead doors also had not yet been invented). Although much of the humor of this parody of a machine is lost on us (our attitudes about machines have changed markedly since Goldberg's heyday), Rube Goldberg's devices are a surprisingly useful analogy to the overall mechanism of cellular chemical signaling.

Just as the garage door opener of Figure 1–13 depends on a series of sequential cause-and-effect interactions, so does chemical signaling occur through a series of cause-and-effect changes in protein shape and binding. Just as the complex events of Goldberg's device are linked to signal and to actuate garage door opening, so is a cascade of changes in protein shape and function linked to signal and actuate physiologic events. Our earlier example of muscle contraction nicely illustrates such a pathway of cause and effect and the analogy to Rube Goldberg devices. Electrical excitation (A) of a muscle cell increases intracellular Ca^{2+} concentration (B), causing Ca^{2+} to bind to troponin (C). This in turn alters the binding of tropomyosin (D) to actin (E), allowing the myosin heads (F) to bind to actin, thus leading to cross-bridging (G) and hydrolysis of ATP and contraction.

As this example indicates, the sequence of cause and effect for both chemical signaling and Rube Goldberg devices is complex. Both involve many different elements, no single one of which can be identified as *the* controller; all of the elements are involved in control. Importantly, this creates multiple sites for regulation and for therapeutic drug action. Just as increasing the caliber of the pistol in the garage door opener would change the response time for opening, so could a drug that bound to an element in the middle of a signaling pathway in a cell increase or decrease the final physiologic change in response to, for example, a particular hormone. Also related to the complexity is that the chain of cause and effect is not obvious; the particular sequence that connects a particular signal

(epinephrine binding to a receptor on heart muscle) to a particular outcome (increased cardiac output) must be memorized. However, once the sequence is understood, it can be predicted from the state of one element in the chain what should happen next. Finally, Rube Goldberg devices were cobbled together from reasonably common household items, such as the bucket, fish tank, sprinkler, and even pistols. Similarly, the elements of chemical signaling pathways are often highly conserved, and the same molecules or same basic types of molecules are used in a wide variety of different stimulus-response pathways.

External signaling molecules bind to receptors on the surface of cells, causing a "second message" to be sent to the cytoplasm of the cell

The LDL receptor discussed earlier (see Fig. 1–12) is involved in the transport of material into cells, but most other *receptors* are intrinsic proteins of the plasma membrane whose task is to transmit and transduce information to the cell from the extracellular environment. Receptors distinguish among the large number of external signaling molecules (various hormones, neurotransmitters, growth factors, and so forth) through the usual protein mechanism of highly specific binding. As shown in Figure 1–14, binding of the hormone/neurotransmitter to the receptor causes an allosteric change in the receptor conformation, which in turn can (1) open (or, less commonly, close) a ligand-gated channel or (2) activate (or, less commonly, inactivate) a ligand-dependent enzyme activity. The receptor molecule may itself be the enzyme or channel, as in the case of the acetylcholine receptor discussed earlier. Frequently, as shown in Figure 1–14, the receptor is a distinct protein that then activates the channel or enzyme. Figure 1–14 is a simplified view of such an information transduction system that shows the diffusion of the receptor in the plane of the membrane and its collision with and activation of membrane channels or membrane-associated enzymes. Activation occurs only if the receptor is in the hormone/neurotransmitter-bound shape (i.e., activa-

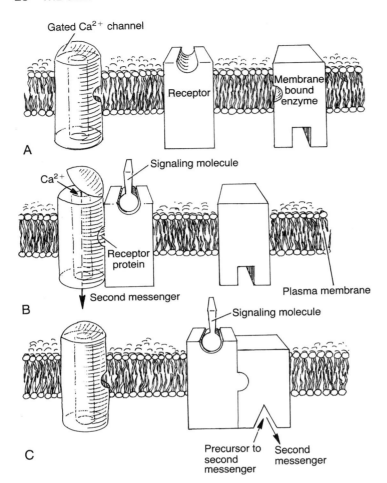

FIGURE 1–14. A simplified diagram of receptor-mediated information transduction via second messengers. *A,* The plasma membrane of virtually all animal cells contains receptors, receptor-mediated ion channels, and receptor-mediated enzymes. *B,* A signaling molecule, such as a neurotransmitter (the first message), binds to its receptor, altering the affinity of the receptor for a gated Ca^{2+} channel. The binding of the neurotransmitter/receptor complex changes the conformation of the gated channel, opening the gate and permitting the inward diffusion of Ca^{2+}. The increased cytoplasmic Ca^{2+} is the second messenger that stimulates a change in cytoplasmic physiology appropriate for the signaling molecule. *C,* A signaling molecule, such as a hormone (the first message), binds to its membrane receptor, altering the affinity of the receptor for a membrane-associated enzyme. The binding of the hormone/receptor complex causes an allosteric change in the enzyme, activating its enzymatic activity. This activity synthesizes a molecule, which acts as a second messenger, stimulating a cytoplasmic response appropriate for the hormone.

tion requires the hormone/receptor complex) (see Fig. 1–14). The signal carried by the hormone/neurotransmitter is communicated to the cell through a series of "differences that make a difference." As shown later, there are more steps in this series than shown in Figure 1–14.

After binding of the external signal to the receptor, the ensuing change in ion channel or enzyme function can alter the membrane potential or cause certain ions/molecules to change their concentration in the cytoplasm. Those ions/molecules that are linked to receptor-ligand binding are called *second messengers.* A second messenger is an ion or a molecule that carries the information *within* the cytoplasm of a cell in response to a signal on the outside surface of a cell (the first message), such as the binding of a hormone or neurotransmitter, or to an electrical event. One of the major advances in understanding of the molecular basis of physiologic signaling is the realization that there are only a few second messenger systems within animals cells. These are (1) changes in Ca^{2+} concentration within the cytoplasm as a result of transport of Ca^{2+} through gated channels; (2) changes in the concentration *cyclic AMP* (cAMP), a special hydrolytic breakdown product of ATP; and (3) increases in the concentration of inositol triphosphate in the cytoplasm and increases in the concentration of diacyl-glycerol in the plasma membrane, both as a result of the breakdown of a rare membrane phospholipid, *phosphotidyl inositol-4,5-bisphosphate* (PIP$_2$).

There are many more different hormones, neurotransmitters, and growth factors than there are second messengers. This means that several receptor-mediated events are converted into the same intracellular signal. How does the cell sort out this information? Different cells respond differently to the same second messenger ion/molecule as a result of the specialized function and makeup of that cell (the differentiated state it achieved during the development of the animal). Muscle cells respond differently to an increase in Ca^{2+} concentration ($[Ca^{2+}]$) than do nerve cells because the two cells have different proteins that are responsible for their specialized tasks. In other words, muscle-specific proteins respond differently than do neuron-specific proteins to an increase in Ca^{2+}.

Specific physiologic information is inherent in the receptor-ligand complex, not the hormone/neurotransmitter molecule

Before a more detailed discussion of the three second messenger systems, it is useful to elaborate on some important points about the nature and regulation of the information transfer between the external signal molecule and receptor. Further reading in this book provides ample evidence that the same hormone and, in particular, neurotransmitter molecule can bind to different receptors. These different receptor-binding events send different information to the cell from the same external signal molecule. For example, acetylcholine is bound by two different receptors: the nicotinic ion channel (described earlier) and the muscarinic receptor, which is not an ion channel and sends completely different information to the cell. The hormone/neurotransmitter itself does not contain any specific information; rather, it is a simple signal, like the ringing of a telephone. One must answer the telephone to obtain the information. The information content of the hormone/neurotransmitter is contained in the three-dimensional shape of the receptor molecule. The change in the shape of the receptor on binding of the hormone/neurotransmitter is the specific message to the cell.

Cells can make themselves more or less sensitive to the signal of the hormone/neurotransmitter. For example, most cells respond to a prolonged period of exposure to a hormone/neurotransmitter by reducing their sensitivity to that molecule. One way is to internalize the receptors via endocytosis, to fuse the endosome with a lysosome, and to digest the receptor. Typically, receptor number is decreased via endocytosis in response to a sustained high concentration of ligand. This is called *down-regulation* of the receptor. This process allows the cell to adapt to high ligand concentrations; receptor-ligand interaction is a true chemical equilibrium. The proportion of receptor-ligand complexes, which determines physiologic response, depends on the concentration of both receptors and ligands. In the presence of a high ligand concentration, a decrease in receptor number returns the binding equilibrium to the normal proportion of bound/unbound receptors. This allows the cell to respond to increases and decreases in ligand even at high concentrations of ligand. Another way of regulating the response to a hormone/neurotransmitter is to alter the binding function of the receptor (e.g., through phosphorylation), so that its affinity for the ligand is reduced (*desensitization*) or increased (*hypersensitization*).

Ca²⁺ transport across plasma and intracellular membranes is an important second messenger

The transport of Ca^{2+} ions through gated channels across the plasma membrane and across intracellular membranes (e.g., endoplasmic reticulum) is a major second messenger system for physiologic information transfer. The available evidence suggests that the major role of Ca^{2+} *within* cells is as a physiologic signal. In the extracellular compartment, the major physiologic function of Ca^{2+} is as the principal mineral of bone. One example of Ca^{2+} as a second messenger,

the role of Ca^{2+} in regulation of the actomyosin ATPase of muscle, has been discussed. Ca^{2+} is an excellent ion for use as a second messenger, because the cytoplasmic concentration of Ca^{2+} is extremely low, about 10^{-7} mol/L in a resting cell. Increases in intracellular $[Ca^{2+}]$ can be (1) detected easily because the background noise is so low and (2) achieved easily because the $[Ca^{2+}]$ in the extracellular fluid and in some cellular compartments, such as the endoplasmic reticulum and mitochondria, is 10^4 times higher than that in the cytoplasm (see Table 1–1). Thus, there is an enormous driving force for Ca^{2+} into the cytoplasm under most conditions.

Increased Ca^{2+} concentration in the cytoplasm alters cellular function by binding to any of several Ca^{2+}-binding proteins that serve as control proteins. Troponin is one Ca^{2+}-binding protein that has already been mentioned. In a review of the example of striated muscle contraction from the point of view of Ca^{2+}, Ca^{2+} (second messenger) diffuses through gated channels in the endoplasmic reticulum (sarcoplasmic reticulum) of muscle in response to electrical events (first message) on the plasma membrane of the muscle cell. The diffusion of Ca^{2+} from the concentrated storehouse of the sarcoplasmic reticulum increases $[Ca^{2+}]$ in the cytoplasm of the muscle cell, where it binds to troponin. On the binding of Ca^{2+}, troponin changes its interaction with tropomyosin, which now moves to allow myosin heads access to the actin of the thin filament. The actomyosin ATPase is activated and muscle contraction ensues.

Calmodulin is a Ca^{2+}-binding protein that plays an important control function in nearly all animal cells. Like troponin, calmodulin binds Ca^{2+} when the cytoplasmic $[Ca^{2+}]$ increases. The Ca^{2+}/calmodulin complex activates a large number of different cellular processes. In most cases, but not all, the Ca^{2+}/calmodulin complex binds to and activates an enzyme. One such enzyme, a protein kinase, is involved in the excitation-contraction coupling in smooth muscle (Fig. 1–15), which was not discussed earlier with the striated muscle types. Protein kinases in general catalyze the hydrolysis of ATP and couple it to the simultaneous phosphorylation of other proteins:

$$\text{protein} + \text{ATP} \xrightarrow[\text{protein kinase}]{\text{Ca}^{2+}\text{-calmodulin-dependent}} \text{protein phosphate} + \text{ADP}$$

In the case of smooth muscle, the particular protein kinase is *myosin kinase*, which, as its name implies, specifically phosphorylates myosin. This phosphorylation increases the affinity of the myosin heads for actin filaments, thus allowing cross-bridging to actin. On formation of the cross-bridge, myosin strokes past the thin filament, producing filament sliding, contraction, and force production by smooth muscle. Cessation of contraction is achieved through cleavage of the phosphate from the myosin by another enzyme: *myosin phosphatase*.

Thus, the initiation of smooth muscle contraction involves a Rube Goldberg sequence in which environmental stimulation of a smooth muscle cell causes an

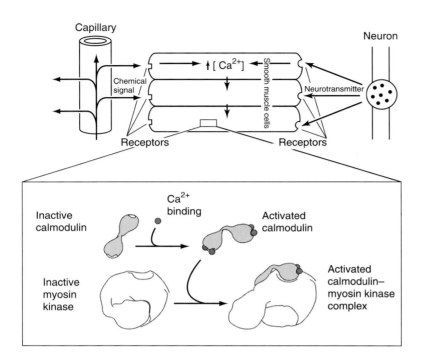

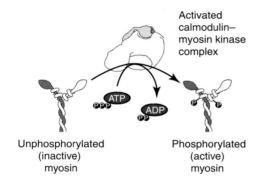

Unphosphorylated
(inactive)
myosin

Phosphorylated
(active)
myosin

Phosphorylated myosin catalyzes
cross-bridge cycling/ ATP hydrolysis

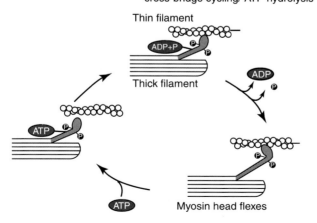

FIGURE 1–15. The role of Ca^{2+} and calmodulin in the regulation of smooth muscle contraction. Smooth muscle regulation is more complex than that of striated muscle, and the account here is a simplification. Smooth muscle can be stimulated to contract by a variety of stimuli, including neural signals and soluble chemical signals, as shown here. These external signals all stimulate increased intracellular $[Ca^{2+}]$, which leads to smooth muscle contraction. In the presence of increased intracellular $[Ca^{2+}]$, the Ca^{2+} ions bind to calmodulin, activating it by causing a conformational change. In smooth muscle cytoplasm, the activated Ca^{2+}/calmodulin complex activates myosin kinase, which, as its name implies, now catalyzes the phosphorylation of myosin. Phosphorylated, activated myosin in turn catalyzes actin-dependent ATP hydrolysis (cross-bridge cycling). Thus, smooth muscle contraction is thick filament regulated, because changes in myosin activate cross-bridging, whereas striated muscle contraction is thin filament controlled, because changes in troponin and tropomyosin of the thin filament activate cross-bridging.

increase in intracellular [Ca^{2+}], the second messenger. This in turn leads to a cascade of cause and effect. Increased intracellular [Ca^{2+}] causes calmodulin to bind Ca^{2+}. The Ca^{2+}/calmodulin complex activates the myosin kinase. This enzyme phosphorylates the myosin head, allowing it to cross-bridge to actin. Cross-bridging leads to actomyosin activation, causing filament sliding that is observed as muscle contraction at the tissue level.

Cyclic AMP is produced by activation of a membrane-bound enzyme in response to hormone/neurotransmitter binding to receptors

Changes in membrane-associated enzyme activity are important mechanisms of information transmission across the cell membrane. Binding of a signaling molecule to receptors on the extracellular face of the plasma membrane changes the activity of an enzyme located on the cytoplasmic face. The enzyme catalyzes a breakdown reaction; one or more of the breakdown products released into the cytoplasm are second messengers. One important such second messenger system, and the first to have been discovered, is the hydrolytic breakdown of ATP to cyclic adenosine-3',5'-monophosphate (cAMP) by the enzyme adenyl cyclase. cAMP is the second messenger, and adenyl cyclase is turned on or off as a result of the binding of various hormones and neurotransmitters to cell surface receptors.

As summarized in Figure 1–16, three distinct membrane proteins interact to produce cAMP: (1) any of several receptors, (2) a regulatory protein that binds guanosine triphosphate (GTP) (called the *G protein*), and (3) the catalytic protein that actually hydrolyzes ATP to cAMP. Their interaction provides an example of the ability of biomembranes to organize biochemical reactions in space. The likelihood of the three proteins colliding and thus being able to interact is much greater in the two-dimensional "phospholipid sea" than in the three-dimensional cytoplasm.

A large number of different hormones/neurotransmitters that bind to different membrane receptors use cAMP to transmit information across the membrane. Receptors and their hormones/neurotransmitters that use cAMP as their second messenger include β-*adrenergic receptors* that bind epinephrine or norepinephrine, increasing cAMP production and providing important regulation to nearly all tissues. The starvation message carried by the binding of *glucagon* to its receptor (see Chapter 32) is carried to the cytoplasm by an increase in cAMP. *Antidiuretic hormone* (ADH) binding to its receptors in kidney cells uses cAMP to regulate urine production (see Chapter 41). A number of therapeutic drugs bind to these same receptors and mimic or prevent the physiologic action of the hormone/neurotransmitter that normally binds to the receptor.

After ligand binding, the receptor-ligand complex is able to bind to and activate the regulatory G protein

(see Fig. 1–16B). The G protein in turn changes shape and binds to the catalytic subunit, altering its shape and regulating its ability to bind ATP, and hydrolyzes the catalytic subunit to cAMP (see Fig. 1–16C). There are two types of G proteins in the adenyl cyclase system. The G_s (s for stimulatory) activates the catalytic subunit; this is the G protein shown in Figure 1–16. A different G protein, G_i, inhibits adenyl cyclase when activated. Some diseases are the result of the binding of bacterial toxins to the G proteins. Cholera symptoms result in part from the binding of the toxin of the bacterium *Vibrio cholera* to G_s and the irreversible activation of G_s, which in turn irreversibly activates the catalytic subunit. Pertussis (whooping cough) toxin binds irreversibly to and activates G_i, thus inactivating the enzymatic activity.

As suggested by the inhibitory G protein, regulated decreases in cAMP concentrations are an important part of the cAMP second messenger system. There are two mechanisms for such decreases: decreased rate of cAMP production or increased elimination of cAMP after formation. The former is achieved through the inhibition by G_i of the catalytic subunit. Certain inhibitory receptors specifically interact with G_i. Opium and drugs derived from it, such as codeine and morphine, are examples of signaling molecules that bind to inhibitory receptors, activate G_i, and inhibit the production of cAMP. Other examples are norepinephrine and epinephrine, which act through α_2-adrenergic receptors. Recall that these same neurotransmitters activated adenyl cyclase when bound to β-adrenergic receptors. This is another example of the principle that the receptor-ligand complex contains the information, not the hormone/neurotransmitter itself. The elimination of cAMP after formation is regulated by the enzyme *cyclic nucleotide phosphodiesterase*. This enzyme hydrolyzes the 3' ester bond of the phosphate to the sugar to produce "plain" 5' AMP. Like myosin kinase (discussed earlier), phosphodiesterase is a Ca^{2+}/calmodulin-activated enzyme, so in many cells the activities of the Ca^{2+} and cAMP second messenger systems antagonize one another.

The increase or decrease in cAMP concentrations affects cell function through the interaction of cAMP with a particular protein kinase. This protein kinase is called *cAMP-dependent protein kinase*, or *protein kinase A*. This protein kinase is distinct from the Ca^{2+}/calmodulin-dependent protein kinase discussed earlier, but the basic outline of action is similar. Protein kinase A is activated by the binding of cAMP. The higher the concentration of cAMP in a cell, the greater is the number of active protein kinase A molecules. The activated kinase binds to proteins and ATP, hydrolyzing the ATP and phosphorylating the protein. As several examples have shown, this phosphorylation alters the activity of the target protein, altering its particular characteristic function: catalysis, transport, coupling, and so forth.

Mammals respond to a stressful stimulus by increasing the force and rate of heart contraction, among other physiologic effects. This increase in force

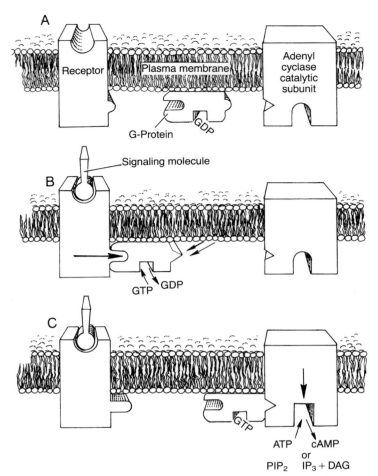

FIGURE 1–16. Receptor-mediated information transduction by the plasma membrane involves a regulatory G protein for many second messengers. Shown here is the classical example of adenyl cyclase, although phosphotidyl inositol-4,5-bisphosphate (PIP$_2$) and some ion channels are similarly regulated. *A,* Membrane receptor and enzyme similar those in Figure 1–12 are shown along with the G protein. The G protein has three binding sites: one for the hormone/receptor complex, one for guanosine triphosphate (GTP) and guanosine diphosphate (GDP), and one for the catalytic protein of adenyl cyclase. *B,* Binding of the signaling molecule stimulates an allosteric change in the receptor protein *(single arrow),* allowing it to bind to the G protein. The binding of the receptor complex stimulates an allosteric change in the G protein such that GDP is released and GTP is bound by the G$_s$ protein. In turn, the binding of GTP causes an allosteric change in the G protein *(double arrows),* allowing it to bind to the catalytic subunit. *C,* The binding of the GTP/G protein to the catalytic subunit causes an allosteric change in the catalytic subunit such that ATP can now bind to its active site and be hydrolyzed to cAMP. If the catalytic subunit were phospholipase C, its activation would permit the hydrolysis of PIP$_2$ to inositol-1,4,5-trisphosphate (IP$_3$) and diacylglycerol (DAG), as shown in Figure 1–17.

demonstrates the role of cAMP as a second messenger and is yet another example of physiologic Rube Goldberg devices based on allosteric changes in proteins. The stressful stimulus causes the adrenal medulla to release epinephrine to the blood, and sympathetic nerves release norepinephrine to the heart. Both catecholamines bind to β-adrenergic receptors on the cardiac muscle cells. The receptor/ligand interaction stimulates adenyl cyclase by way of G$_s$, increasing intracellular [cAMP] and thus increasing protein kinase A activity. Protein kinase A phosphorylates a number of substrates in the cardiac muscle cells; among these are voltage-dependent Ca^{2+} channels in the plasma membrane. In the phosphorylated state, these channels remain open somewhat longer in response to membrane potentials above threshold. Consequently, more Ca^{2+} enters the cell for a given electrical stimulation than at lower levels of cAMP. The increase in Ca^{2+} allows more troponin to bind Ca^{2+}; more tropomyosin moves out of the way of myosin heads, causing more cross-bridging and more force production. (Rube Goldberg would have loved modern physiology!)

Another cyclic nucleotide, cyclic guanosine monophosphate (cGMP) also serves as a second messenger but is not nearly as widely used as cAMP. cGMP is the second messenger in the rod cells of the retina that underlies vision and causes relaxation of some vascular smooth muscle, including that responsible for penile erection (i.e., blood flow into the corpus cavernosum). For example, the drug sildenafil (Viagra) inhibits the breakdown of cGMP by a cyclic nucleotide phosphodiesterase, thus increasing blood flow to the penis and aiding in erection, but this occurs only if neural signals (i.e., sexual stimulation) have stimulated cGMP production in the first place. This is a good example of how the multistep pathway of cell signaling provides multiple potential sites for appropriate therapeutic intervention: a drug that simply stimulated cGMP production would cause inappropriate erections, whereas inhibition of its breakdown aids timely erections. Although used mostly by men, sildenafil is occasionally used for stallions to aid them in "covering" a mare.

The receptor-mediated hydrolysis of a rare phospholipid of the plasma membrane produces two different second messengers with different actions

The most recently discovered second messenger system differs from either Ca^{2+} or cAMP in that *two* distinct second messenger molecules are produced as a result of enzymatic activation by a single receptor-ligand complex. Phosphotidyl inositol is a membrane phospholipid that can accept additional phosphate groups by reaction with the —OH groups on the inositol (Fig. 1–17). PIP_2 is the membrane phospholipid that is broken down to produce two important second messengers. PIP_2 is hydrolyzed to *diacylglycerol* (DAG) and *inositol-1,4,5-trisphosphate* (IP_3) by a receptor-mediated enzyme called phospholipase C, or phosphoinositidase. Although many distinct processes are controlled through the PIP_2 pathway, it plays a particularly important role in the control of growth and of receptor-mediated secretion. The effect of the action of acetylcholine through muscarinic receptors (*not* the nicotinic receptor/ion channel of the nerve-muscle synapse) is often transmitted and transduced through activation of the PIP_2 pathway.

The events involved in the receptor-mediated production of IP_3 and DAG from PIP_2 are rather similar to those in the production of cAMP. The membrane system appears to consist of three distinct intrinsic membrane proteins: (1) any of several different receptors, including the muscarinic acetylcholine receptor and the receptors for some growth factors; (2) a regulatory GTP-binding protein, similar but not identical to G_s of the cAMP pathway; and (3) the hydrolytic enzyme phospholipase C (or phosphoinositidase). A hormone/neurotransmitter or growth factor binds to the receptor, forming a receptor-ligand complex. This complex activates the G protein, which in turn activates the hydrolytic enzyme. Only a stimulatory G activity for phosphoinositidase is known; there is no evidence for an inhibitory G activity in this system.

The activation of the hydrolytic enzyme increases the concentration of IP_3, which is water soluble and so diffuses through the cytoplasm. IP_3 binds to and opens ligand-gated Ca^{2+} channels in the endoplasmic reticulum. This releases Ca^{2+} from that high $[Ca^{2+}]$ compartment into the cytoplasm. Ca^{2+} thus becomes, in a manner of speaking, the third messenger in this system, although this term is not in widespread use. The ensuing increase in intracellular $[Ca^{2+}]$ affects cellular function via the same mechanisms outlined earlier for Ca^{2+} as a second messenger (e.g., binding to calmodulin; the Ca^{2+}/calmodulin complex in turn activates various enzyme activities). In receptor-mediated secretion, for example, the binding of acetylcholine to muscarinic receptors in the pancreas (the organ that secretes digestive enzymes) causes an increase in PIP_2 breakdown and an increase in cytoplasmic IP_3. The IP_3 opens ligand-gated Ca^{2+} channels in the endoplasmic reticulum, and intracellular $[Ca^{2+}]$ increases. The process then becomes somewhat similar to that of smooth muscle contraction. Calmodulin binds Ca^{2+} and the complex activates a protein kinase. Rather than activating myosin, however, as for smooth muscle, activation of this protein kinase causes exocytosis of secretory vesicles (membrane bubbles full of secretory product) with the plasma membrane, releasing

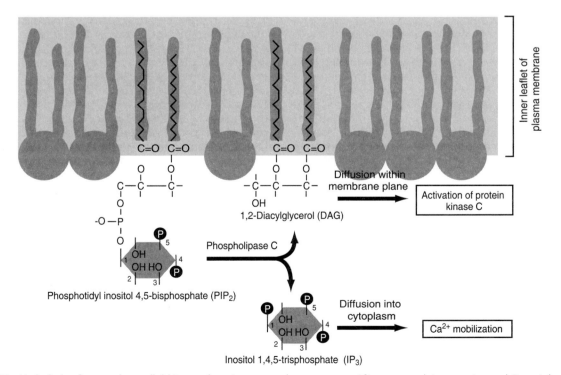

FIGURE 1–17. Hydrolysis of a membrane lipid to produce two second messengers. After appropriate receptor and G-protein activation, the rare membrane phospholipid shown to the left, phosphotidyl inositol-4,5-bisphosphate (PIP_2), is hydrolyzed into two separate second messengers by phospholipase C. The phosphate "head" of the PIP_2 molecule is cleaved to produce the soluble messenger inositol-1,4,5-trisphosphate (IP_3), which mobilizes intracellular Ca^{2+}, as well as the lipidic messenger diacylglycerol (DAG), which remains in the membrane and activates protein kinase C.

the enzymes into an extracellular space that is contiguous with the gut.

DAG is also produced at the activation of phospholipase C, but it is not at all water-soluble. DAG diffuses in the plasma membrane, binding to and activating a membrane-associated protein kinase, protein kinase C (PKC). PKC is not an intrinsic membrane protein, and it can bind reversibly to the cytoplasmic face of the plasma membrane. PKC phosphorylates other proteins and changes their activity. Because of the membrane-bound character of the enzyme, most evidence indicates that PKC phosphorylates membrane proteins such as receptors and ion channels, regulating their function. In the case of the secretory response to some hormone/neurotransmitter stimulus, PKC generally acts separately but additively with IP_3 to produce the response. However, much interest focuses on longer-term effects of PKC activation, particularly its role in growth control and cancer. A class of chemicals long known to promote the onset of cancer, phorbol esters, are potent substitutions for DAG in the activation of PKC. Also, overproduction of PKC by tissue culture cells induced through genetic engineering methods causes a loss of growth control by the cells. This effect is consistent with the evidence that the receptors for some growth factors (extracellular polypeptides that act as cell division hormones) act through the PIP_2 pathway.

Steroid hormones interact with receptors within the cell, not with cell surface receptors

Recall that steroid hormones are soluble in oily solvents and are able to diffuse through the lipid bilayer without the mediation of transport proteins. Thyroid hormones are also lipophilic and diffuse through the lipid bilayer. Consequently, the receptors for steroid and thyroid hormones are soluble proteins within the target cell. The lipid-soluble hormone diffuses from the blood into the cell and binds to its receptor, and the hormone/receptor complex is, as in previous examples, the physiologically active entity that ultimately triggers a cellular response. Because the signaling molecule itself can get into the cell, steroids and thyroid hormones do not require a second messenger; the hormone/receptor complex is itself active within the cytoplasm (Fig. 1–18). Steroid and thyroid hormones have a wide variety of physiologic effects, including sexual development, control of reproduction, control of growth and metabolism, and salt and water balance.

These effects are produced when the expression of particular genes is turned on by the binding of the hormone/receptor complex to specific regions of the DNA of the cell. In other words, these hormones regulate which genes will be transcribed into RNA, which in turn determines whether and how much protein is synthesized by a cell. A well-studied example of this mechanism with some relevance to veterinary medicine is the action of estrogen on the repro-

ductive tracts of female chickens (see Fig. 1–18). Estrogen is the principal female sex hormone of birds and mammals, and, of course, hens lay eggs whose embryo and yolk are surrounded by an "egg white." The principal protein of egg white is ovalbumin, which is secreted by the epithelial cells of the avian oviduct as the ovum slides by. Thus, one of the targets of estrogen in female chickens is oviduct epithelial cells. Estrogen enters the cytoplasm of these cells and binds to its receptor, reasonably enough called the *estrogen receptor*. The hormone/receptor complex, but not the ligand-free receptor, is able to mediate estrogen-specific, essentially female-specific, gene transcription. The estrogen receptor complex binds to a sequence of DNA, called a *estrogen response element*, that controls the transcription of a neighboring gene, for ovalbumin in this case. In other cells of the female, binding of the estrogen receptor to the estrogen response elements of other genes would cause these other female-specific genes to be transcribed and ultimately expressed as a protein (e.g., the proteins in the yolk of the egg). Different steroids bind to different receptors (e.g., the male sex hormone testosterone binds to the testosterone receptor), which bind to different response elements, leading to different genes being expressed (e.g., male-specific gene expression).

Steroid hormone receptors, like other multifunctional proteins, are regarded as examples of larger subsets of regulatory elements. Because steroid hormone receptors both bind the extracellular signaling molecule and function in the nucleus directly, steroid hormones are among the regulatory proteins called *nuclear receptors*, which distinguishes them from plasma membrane receptors. Other extracellular signals, acting through other similar nuclear receptors, include thyroid hormones (see Chapter 33) and vitamin A (retinoic acid) signaling. From the standpoint of molecular biology, steroid hormone receptors are one type among many regulatory proteins that serve as *transcription factors*. In other words, their regulatory function in the cell is to transduce signals of various kinds into differential gene expression. All transcription factors participate in some way with enabling (or disabling) transcription of genes into messenger RNA by binding, directly or indirectly, to regulatory regions of DNA. The binding of the transcription factor to its response region of DNA in turn then stimulates (or inhibits) RNA polymerase activity along the adjacent DNA sequence. This DNA sequence then is copied into messenger RNA, to be translated into protein. Transcription factors play a crucial role in the gene expression that underlies the physiologic and developmental responses that are dependent on having new or different proteins produced by the cell. This includes control of cell division (and therefore cancers), control of cell specialization (and therefore breed-specific birth defects), and, as the estrogen-receptor example indicates, sexual differentiation and function. Like all other proteins, the binding function of transcription factors is based on their shape. The estrogen receptor, for example, binds to DNA by a part of the protein shaped into "fingers" by a zinc

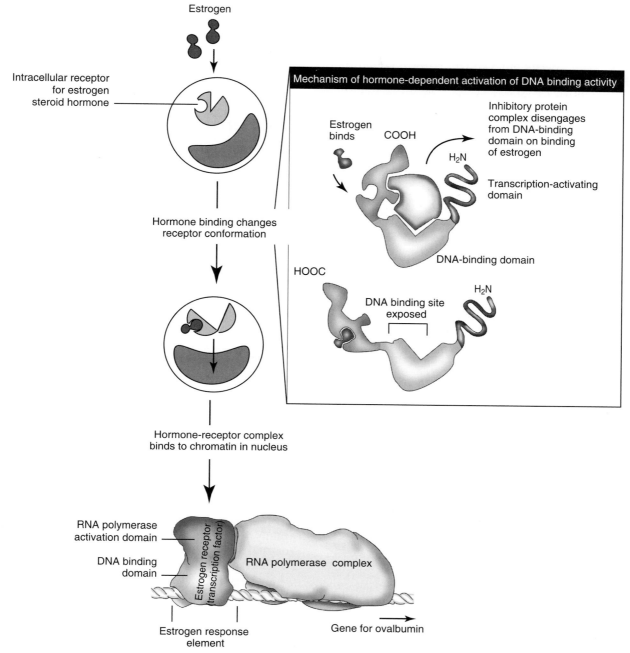

Estrogen

Intracellular receptor for estrogen steroid hormone

Hormone binding changes receptor conformation

Hormone-receptor complex binds to chromatin in nucleus

Mechanism of hormone-dependent activation of DNA binding activity

Estrogen binds

COOH

Inhibitory protein complex disengages from DNA-binding domain on binding of estrogen

H_2N

Transcription-activating domain

DNA-binding domain

HOOC

DNA binding site exposed

H_2N

RNA polymerase activation domain

DNA binding domain

Estrogen receptor (transcription factor)

RNA polymerase complex

Estrogen response element

Gene for ovalbumin

FIGURE 1–18. Steroid hormone action as illustrated by control of ovalbumin expression by estrogen in hens. The steroid hormone estrogen penetrates the lipid bilayer passively because of the oil solubility of the steroid. Inside the cell, the estrogen binds to a cytoplasmic receptor, namely, the estrogen receptor. The binding of estrogen to its receptor causes the receptor protein to change conformation, which in turn changes the DNA-binding activity of the receptor. The hormone/receptor complex enters the nucleus and binds to regulatory sequences of DNA, the estrogen-response element. This binding, in turn, activates RNA polymerase. This initiates transcription of the ovalbumin gene, an estrogen-responsive gene, to produce messenger RNA (mRNA), which is ultimately translated into the ovalbumin protein for secretion.

ion. These "zinc fingers," also found in many other transcription factors, fit into the grooves of the double helix of DNA at the response region.

Differential gene expression and its regulation have historically been pursued primarily by molecular biologists, but they are rapidly gaining importance in physiology and will do so soon in veterinary medicine. Humankind will have fewer scruples about controlling gene expression in domestic animals than in their own species. Indeed, it seems possible that understanding control of gene expression will prove more important to veterinary medical students in the near term than for human medical students.

CLINICAL CORRELATION

Peripheral edema

History You examine a 2-year-old cow that has been grazing on a poor-quality pasture. The owner states that she seems to have a poor appetite, walks slowly, and stands apart from the rest of the herd. She has developed swelling beneath the skin of her brisket and ventral thorax.

Clinical examination On clinical examination, you find a listless cow standing in a pasture littered with various metal objects. Examination of the cardiovascular system reveals distended jugular veins and abnormal heart sounds characterized by irregular sloshing sounds throughout the cardiac cycle that drastically muffle the first and second heart sounds. Subcutaneous edema (swelling) can be seen throughout the chest and abdomen but most prominently in the dependent ventral areas of the thorax. Pushing on these swollen areas leaves a dent (pitting edema).

Comment This is a characteristic history of a cow with *hardware disease.* The cow, grazing on a pasture littered with metal debris, swallows nails, wire, and so forth. Because these objects are heavier than the feed, they drop into the reticulum, a stomach chamber located just caudal to the diaphragm and heart. With the contractions of the reticulum, a metal object migrates through the reticular wall, diaphragm, and pericardium, leading to an inflammatory response in the pericardium (pericarditis). An inflammatory exudate fills the pericardial sac; it muffles the heart sounds, and if gas is present in the exudate, a sloshing sound may be heard on auscultation. As this exudative fluid fills the pericardial sac, it limits the pumping efficiency of the heart by limiting its filling during diastole and by obstructing venous return to the heart (see Chapter 20). The result is backward failure of the heart that causes increased hydrostatic pressure in the veins and capillaries. As the capillary hydrostatic pressure rises, capillary filtration is favored over reabsorption, and water leaves the capillary and accumulates in the interstitial space. This accumulated interstitial fluid, primarily as the result of increased capillary filtration, is seen clinically as edema. The other common cause of edema is decreased capillary colloidal osmotic pressure from low serum protein. However, this does not usually play a part in hardware disease.

Treatment Treatment includes surgical removal of the foreign object or objects and antibiotic treatment for the pericarditis. However, in such an advanced case as mentioned here, treatment often is not completely successful.

Bibliography

Alberts B, Bray D, Johnson A, et al: Essential Cell Biology, New York: Garland Publishing, 1997.
Lodish H, Berk A, Zipursky SL, et al: Molecular Cell Biology, 4th ed. San Francisco: WH Freeman, 2000.
Miller RJ: G proteins flex their muscle. Trends Neurosci 11:3–6, 1988.
Schramm M, Selinger Z: Message transmission: Receptor controlled adenylate cyclase system. Science 225:1350–1356, 1984.

PRACTICE QUESTIONS

1. Increasing the extracellular [K^+] will
   a. have no effect on the resting membrane potential.
   b. cause the resting membrane potential to decrease (i.e., cause the inside to become less negative with respect to the outside).
   c. cause the resting membrane potential to increase (i.e., cause the inside to become more negative with respect to the outside).
   d. increase the concentration potential for K^+ across the plasma membrane.
   e. require the Na^+,K^+ pump to work harder to pump K^+.

2. G proteins are similar to receptors in that both
   a. bind extracellular signaling molecules.
   b. interact directly with adenyl cyclase catalytic subunits.
   c. have activated and inactivated states dependent on ligand binding.
   d. are extracellular protein molecules.
   e. directly activate a protein kinase activity.

3. Which of the following statements concerning intracellular Ca^{2+} is *false*?
   a. It is a second messenger for hormones and neurotransmitters.
   b. It is responsible for excitation-contraction coupling in smooth muscle.
   c. An increase in its concentration in a nerve terminal stimulates the release of a neurotransmitter.
   d. It activates protein kinase A.
   e. Its concentration is increased in the presence of IP_3.

4. If, in a particular capillary bed, the plasma oncotic pressure were to increase and hydrostatic pressure remained constant
   a. more blood plasma would filter from the capillaries.
   b. the transport effect would be similar to decreasing hydrostatic pressure.
   c. one would suspect a deficiency in blood protein levels.
   d. one would suspect an increase in extracellular fluid protein concentrations.
   e. fluid reabsorption on the venous side of the capillary bed would decline.

5. Substance X is found to be at a much higher concentration on the outside of a cell than in the cytoplasm, yet no transport of X from the extracellular fluid to the cytoplasm occurs. Which of the following statements is *inconsistent* with this state of affairs?

   a. Substance X has the same electrochemical potential outside and inside the cell.

   b. Substance X is large, is poorly soluble in oil, and has no transport proteins in the membrane.

   c. Substance X is an ion, and the measured membrane potential is the equilibrium potential calculated by the Nernst equation.

   d. Substance X is a steroid molecule.

   e. Substance X is actively transported from the cell to the extracellular fluid.

PRACTICE ANSWERS

1. b   2. c   3. d   4. b   5. d

NEUROPHYSIOLOGY

James G. Cunningham

2

Introduction to the neuromuscular system

1 The neuron is the major functional unit of the nervous system

2 The mammalian nervous system is divided into two subsections: the central nervous system and the peripheral nervous system

The nervous system is the first multicellular system described in this book because it is one of the major coordinating systems of the body and because many concepts that concern the nervous system must be clarified in order to understand other systems of the body.

Because most clinical signs in veterinary neurology involve abnormal movement (e.g., seizures, paralysis), the physiology of posture and locomotion is emphasized in the following chapters. Veterinary ophthalmology has become an extensive subspecialty; therefore, the physiology of vision is also emphasized. Understanding the autonomic nervous system is essential for understanding much pharmacology and the reflex control of many of the body's most critical functions. Similarly, understanding the blood-brain barrier and the cerebrospinal fluid system is essential to understanding the results of the diagnostic cerebrospinal fluid tap and the homeostasis of the central nervous system (CNS). The electroencephalogram and sensory evoked potentials are described because of their emerging clinical importance in veterinary medicine. Because of space limitations, only the basic physiologic concepts essential to understanding the mechanisms of disease and the practice of veterinary medicine are emphasized. For a more expansive study of neuromuscular physiology, the reader may refer to the texts mentioned in the bibliography.

THE NEURON IS THE MAJOR FUNCTIONAL UNIT OF THE NERVOUS SYSTEM

The major functional unit of the nervous system is the neuron, or nerve cell, a cell type whose shape varies considerably with its location in the nervous system. Nearly all neurons have an information-receiving area of the cell membrane, usually called the *dendrite;* a cell body containing the organelle for most cell metabolic activity; an information-transmitting

extension of the cell membrane, called an *axon;* and a presynaptic terminal to the axon.

The other cell type in the nervous system is the glial (from the Greek word for "glue") cell, thought originally to play largely a structural role. Glial cells do not produce action potentials, but there is growing evidence that they may play important roles in producing myelin for the nervous system, in producing growth factors for developing neurons, and in buffering extracellular concentrations of potassium and neurotransmitters.

THE MAMMALIAN NERVOUS SYSTEM IS DIVIDED INTO TWO SUBSECTIONS: THE CENTRAL NERVOUS SYSTEM AND THE PERIPHERAL NERVOUS SYSTEM

The CNS is divided into the brain and spinal cord (Table 2–1). A series of protective bones surround the entire CNS. The brain is surrounded by the skull, and the spinal cord is surrounded by a series of cervical, thoracic, and lumbar vertebrae and ligaments. These vertebrae are aligned so that they form a functional

TABLE 2–1. **Organization of the nervous system**

Central nervous system
Brain
Spinal cord
Peripheral nervous system
Efferent (motor)
Somatic-skeletal muscle
Autonomic-cardiac muscle
Smooth muscle
Exocrine gland
Afferent (sensory)
Somatic
Visceral

canal or conduit through which the spinal cord passes; some degree of flexion is possible between vertebrae.

The peripheral nervous system is divided into motor (efferent) and sensory (afferent) subsystems. Within the motor peripheral nerves are (1) somatic motor neurons, which carry action potential commands from the CNS to synaptic junctions at skeletal muscles, and (2) the autonomic nervous system's motor neurons, which carry action potentials through an intermediate synapse to synapses at smooth muscle, cardiac muscle, and some exocrine glands. Sensory peripheral nerves bring action potential messages to the CNS from peripheral receptors. These receptors are responsible for transducing some environmental energy (e.g., light, sound, stretch of a muscle) into action potentials that travel to the CNS and for encoding the intensity of this energy's stimulation of the receptor by increasing the frequency of action potentials as the intensity of stimulation increases. Sensory nerves carrying action potentials from receptors such as the photoreceptors of the eye, auditory receptors of the ear, or stretch receptors of the skeletal muscle are classified as somatic sensory peripheral nerves. Receptors located within visceral organs of the chest and abdomen send action potentials to the CNS along visceral sensory peripheral nerves.

Within the spinal canal, sensory and motor peripheral nerves are separated; sensory nerves enter the spinal cord through the dorsal nerve roots, whereas the motor nerves exit the spinal cord through the ventral roots (Fig. 2–1).

The entire CNS is surrounded by three protective layers called *meninges*: the *pia mater, arachnoid,* and *dura mater* (see Fig. 2–1). The innermost layer, lying next to the CNS, is the pia mater, which is a single layer of fibroblast cells joined to the outer edge of the brain and spinal cord. The middle layer, the arachnoid, so named because it looks like a spider's web, is a thin layer of fibroblast cells that traps cerebrospinal fluid between it and the pia mater (in the subarachnoid space). The outermost meningeal layer is the dura mater, which is a much thicker layer of fibroblast cells that protect the CNS. Within the brain cavity of the skull, the dura mater is often fused with the inner surface of the bone.

Cerebrospinal fluid is a clear, colorless fluid found within the subarachnoid space, the central canal of

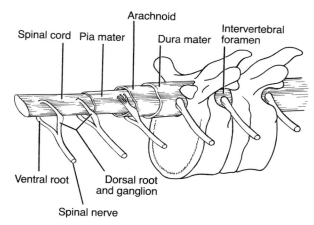

FIGURE 2–1. The spinal cord and the three layers of the meninges within the vertebral canal. Sensory action potentials enter the spinal cord along axons in the dorsal roots. Motor action potentials exit the spinal cord along axons in the ventral roots. (Redrawn from Gardner E: Fundamentals of Neurology, 3rd ed. Philadelphia: WB Saunders, 1959.)

the spinal cord, and the ventricular system of the brain (see Chapter 14). It is produced primarily in the ventricles of the brain, flows down a pressure gradient from the ventricles to the subarachnoid space, and from this space passes into the venous system. It is a dynamic fluid, being replaced several times daily. Cerebrospinal fluid serves as a shock absorber for the CNS during abrupt body movement.

The brain can be divided approximately into a lower brain and an upper brain. The lower brain consists of the medulla, pons, mesencephalon, diencephalon, cerebellum, and basal ganglia and is responsible for much subconscious coordination, such as the control of blood pressure, respiratory rate, and equilibrium. The upper brain consists of the cerebral cortex and is responsible for much conscious activity. Some more detailed anatomy of the brain is presented later as necessary for understanding of the physiology of posture and locomotion.

Bibliography

Guyton AC, Hall JE: Textbook of Medical Physiology, 10th ed. Philadelphia: WB Saunders, 2000, pp 512–527.
Haines DE: Fundamental Neuroscience. New York: Churchill Livingstone, 1997, pp 1–9.
Kandel ER, Schwartz JH, Jessell TM (eds): Principles of Neural Science, 4th ed. New York: McGraw-Hill, 2000, pp 5–18.

The neuron

1 Neurons have four distinct anatomic regions
2 Nerve cell membranes contain a resting electrical membrane potential
3 The resting membrane potential is the result of three major determinants

4 The resting membrane potential can be changed by synaptic signals from a presynaptic cell
5 Action potentials begin at the axon's initial segment and spread down the entire length of the axon

There are two classes of cells in the nervous system: the neuron (or nerve cell) and the neuroglial cell (or glial cell). The neuron is the basic functional unit of the nervous system. The large number of neurons and their interconnections account for the complexity of the nervous system. There are approximately 10 billion neurons in the average vertebrate nervous system, far more neurons in a nervous system than people on Earth, and 10 to 50 times more glial cells, the cells that provide firmness and structure for the central nervous system. The numbers of cells in the nervous system are huge, but knowing that they all have common elements makes it easier to understand them.

▬ NEURONS HAVE FOUR DISTINCT ANATOMIC REGIONS

A typical neuron has four morphologically defined regions (Fig. 3–1): the *dendrites*, the *cell body* (also called the *soma* or *perikaryon*), the *axon*, and the *presynaptic terminals* to the axon. These four anatomic regions are important in four major electrical and chemical responsibilities of neurons: receiving signals from the axons of neighboring neurons (on dendrites), integrating these often-opposing signals (on the cell body), transmitting action potential impulses some distance along the axon, and signaling an adjacent cell at the presynaptic terminal. Three organelles are common in nerve cell bodies: the nucleus; the endoplasmic reticulum, upon which secretory and membrane proteins are synthesized; and the Golgi apparatus, which carries out the processing of secretory and membrane components. The cell body usually gives rise to several branch-like extensions, called *dendrites*, whose surface area and extent far exceed those of the cell body. The dendrites serve as the major receptive apparatus of the neuron, receiving signals from neighboring neurons. The cell body also gives rise to the

axon, a tubular process that is often long (over 1 m in some large animals). The axon is the conducting unit of the neuron, transmitting an electrical impulse (the action potential) from its initial segment at the cell body to the other end of the axon at the presynaptic terminal. Axons lack ribosomes and therefore cannot synthesize proteins. Instead, macromolecules are synthesized in the cell body and are carried along the axon to the presynaptic terminals by a process called *axoplasmic transport.* Large axons are surrounded by a fatty insulating coating called *myelin.* In the peripheral nervous system, myelin is formed by Schwann cells, specialized glial cells that wrap around the axon much like toilet paper wrapped around a broomstick. The myelin sheath is interrupted at regular intervals by spaces called *nodes of Ranvier.*

Axons branch near their ends into several specialized endings called *presynaptic terminals.* These presynaptic terminals transmit a chemical signal to an adjacent cell, usually another nerve cell or a muscle cell. The site of contact of the presynaptic terminal with the adjacent cell is called the *synapse.* It is formed by the presynaptic terminal of one cell (presynaptic cell), the receptive surface of the adjacent cell (postsynaptic cell), and the space between these two cells (the *synaptic cleft).* The presynaptic terminals of an axon usually contact the receptive surface of an adjacent nerve or muscle cell, usually on the nerve cell's dendrites, but sometimes this contact is made on the cell body or, occasionally, on the terminal end of another cell's axon (for presynaptic inhibition). Presynaptic terminals contain *synaptic vesicles* that contain a chemical transmitter before its release into the synaptic cleft.

▬ NERVE CELL MEMBRANES CONTAIN A RESTING ELECTRICAL MEMBRANE POTENTIAL

Nerve cells, like other cells of the body, have an electrical charge that can be measured across their

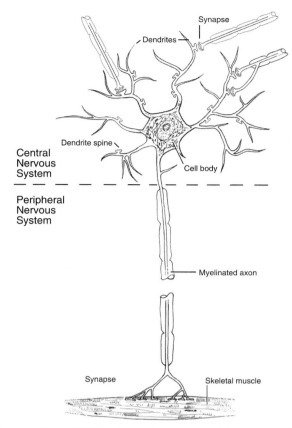

FIGURE 3-1. A typical neuron has four functionally important regions. The dendrites receive signals from neighboring neurons, the cell body integrates these signals, the axon transmits action potentials some distance along the cell, and the presynaptic terminal signals adjacent cells.

outer cell membrane (*resting membrane potential*). However, the electrical membrane potential in nerve and muscle cells is unique in that its magnitude can be changed as the result of synaptic signaling from neighboring cells or within a receptor as a response to transduction of some environmental energy. When the membrane potential of a nerve or muscle is reduced sufficiently, a further and dramatic change in the membrane potential, called an *action potential,* occurs; this action potential spreads along the entire length of the nerve axon.

The origins of the resting electrical membrane potential are complicated, particularly in a quantitative way. In qualitative terms, however, the resting membrane potential is the result of the differential separation of charged ions, especially Na^+ and K^+, across the membrane and the resting membrane's differential permeability to these ions diffusing back down their concentration gradients (see also Chapter 1). Even though the net concentration of positively and negatively charged ions is similar in the intracellular and extracellular fluids, an excess of positively charged cations accumulates immediately outside the cell membrane, and an excess of negatively charged anions accumulates immediately inside the cell membrane (Fig. 3–2). This makes the inside of the cell

negatively charged with regard to the outside of the cell. The magnitude of the resulting electrical difference across the membrane varies from cell to cell, ranging from about 40 to 75 mV, and is commonly about 70 mV in mammalian nerve cells. Because the extracellular fluid is arbitrarily considered to be 0 mV, the resting membrane potential is −70 mV, more negative on the inside than on the outside.

THE RESTING MEMBRANE POTENTIAL IS THE RESULT OF THREE MAJOR DETERMINANTS

Three major factors cause the resting membrane potential.

1. The Na^+,K^+ pump. Cell membranes have an energy-dependent pump that pumps Na^+ ions out of the cell and draws K^+ ions into the cell against their concentration gradients. The pump itself generates some of the resting membrane potential, because it pushes three molecules of Na^+ out for every two molecules of K^+ drawn into the cell, thus concentrating positively charged cations outside the cell.

2. Differential permeability of the membrane to diffusion of ions. The resting membrane is much more permeable to K^+ ions than to Na^+ ions. Therefore, positively charged K^+ cations are allowed to diffuse out of the cell through nongated leak channels back down their concentration gradient until the resulting electrical membrane potential reaches an equilibrium with the driving force of the K^+ concentration gradient. This further contributes to the buildup of positive charges immediately outside the membrane. The resting membrane is almost completely impermeable to Na^+ ions; therefore, once pumped out of the cell, Na^+ cannot diffuse back into the cell, even though both the electrical and concentration gradients for Na^+ would drive Na^+ ions back into the cell if the sodium channels in the resting membrane were open. (See Chapter 1 for a more complete discussion of ion channels.)

3. Negatively charged anions trapped in the cell. Many intracellular anions are macromolecules synthesized within the neuron and are too big to get back out through the cell's plasma membrane. Therefore, they are trapped within the cell and attracted to the inner surface of the membrane by the accumulated positive charges just outside the cell.

These three determinants—the Na^+,K^+ pump, the differentially permeable membrane, and the trapped intracellular anions—are the primary source of the resting membrane potential. The magnitude of this potential can be predicted by the Nernst and Goldman equations, and the reader is referred to Chapter 1 and to the bibliography for a more quantitative understanding of the resting membrane potential.

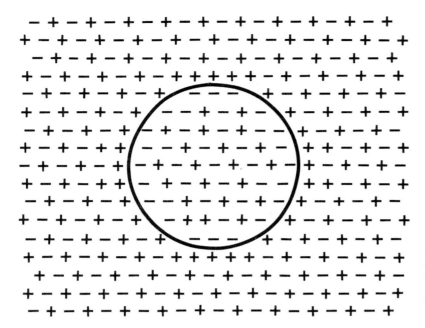

Figure 3–2. The concentrations of positively and negatively charged ions are similar in both the intracellular and extracellular spaces. However, more positively charged ions accumulate immediately outside the cell membrane, and more negatively charged ions accumulate immediately inside the nerve membrane.

There are a number of important clinical implications of this discussion of the resting membrane potential. The Na^+,K^+ pump requires energy in the form of adenosine triphosphate (ATP), which is derived from the intracellular metabolism of glucose and oxygen. Because the neuron cannot store either glucose or oxygen, anything that deprives the nervous system of either substrate leads to serious clinical neurologic deficits. Fortunately, hormones and other forces normally maintain serum glucose and oxygen levels within narrow limits. Because Na^+ and K^+ are the primary ions determining the resting membrane potential (in most cells, Cl^- ions align themselves passively along the membrane as a result of the charge established by Na^+ and K^+), it is essential that serum levels of Na^+ and K^+ be regulated carefully. The endocrine system (Chapter 33) and kidney (Chapter 41) maintain serum Na^+ and K^+ levels within narrow limits. Anything altering serum levels of either ion beyond normal limits also leads to potentially severe neurologic deficits.

THE RESTING MEMBRANE POTENTIAL CAN BE CHANGED BY SYNAPTIC SIGNALS FROM A PRESYNAPTIC CELL

Although most cells of the body have a resting membrane potential, nerve and muscle cells are unique in that their membrane potential can be altered by a synaptic signal from an adjacent cell. Even though there are billions of synapses in the nervous system, there are basically only two ways that a presynaptic signal can alter the postsynaptic electrical potential: decreasing or increasing its magnitude. Whether a synapse results in a decreased or an increased postsynaptic potential depends on the nature of the chemical transmitter in the presynaptic vesicle and on the nature of the receptor to that chemical transmitter in the postsynaptic membrane.

If a chemical synaptic transmission leads to a reduction in the postsynaptic membrane potential in comparison with the resting level (e.g., from -75 to -55 mV), the postsynaptic potential change is said to be an *excitatory postsynaptic potential* (EPSP) (Fig. 3–3A). It is called *excitatory* because each such synaptic transmission increases the chances that an action potential will originate at the initial segment of the nerve's axon. When the magnitude of the membrane potential is reduced to a smaller quantity (e.g., from -75 to -55 mV) by an EPSP, the membrane is said to be *depolarized* or, more accurately, *hypopolarized*. Hypopolarization of the postsynaptic membrane results from the interaction of the chemical transmitter from the presynaptic nerve and its appropriate receptor on the postsynaptic membrane. This interaction causes ligand-gated Na^+ channels to open, thus allowing Na^+ ions to diffuse into the neuron down both the concentration and the electrical gradients of sodium. Because the presynaptic chemical transmitter is destroyed quickly at the postsynaptic membrane, this postsynaptic potential change is transient, lasting only a few milliseconds. The magnitude of the change in this postsynaptic potential is greatest at the synapse. Although the hypopolarization spreads over the nerve cell membrane, it decreases with the distance from the originating synapse, much as the waves created by throwing a stone into a lake decrease in size with the distance from the place where the stone fell.

If instead the presynaptic neurotransmitter's interaction with the postsynaptic receptor results in further opening of the membrane's K^+ channels, then K^+ ions diffuse out of the cell even faster than usual, and an increase *(hyperpolarization)* in the postsynaptic

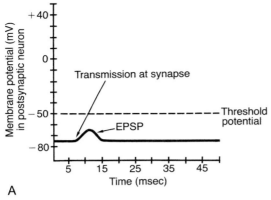
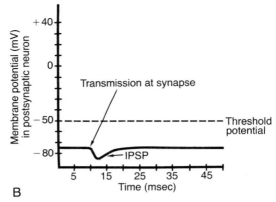

A   B

FIGURE 3–3. Postsynaptic potentials. *A,* An excitatory postsynaptic potential (EPSP) resulting from an excitatory presynaptic transmitter drives the membrane potential toward threshold. *B,* An inhibitory postsynaptic potential (IPSP) resulting from an inhibitory presynaptic transmitter drives the membrane potential away from threshold.

membrane potential is the result. Such hyperpolarization of the postsynaptic membrane is called an *inhibitory postsynaptic potential* (IPSP) (see Fig. 3–3*B*), because each such transmission makes it less likely that an action potential will result at the axon's initial segment. Like EPSPs, IPSPs spread over the neuron's membrane, and the hyperpolarization decreases with the distance from the originating synapse.

ACTION POTENTIALS BEGIN AT THE AXON'S INITIAL SEGMENT AND SPREAD DOWN THE ENTIRE LENGTH OF THE AXON

Both EPSPs and IPSPs are the result, on the postsynaptic membrane, of an action potential and synaptic transmission from a presynaptic cell. However, these postsynaptic potentials decrease in magnitude as they spread along the postsynaptic cell membrane. Because many nerve and muscle cells are long, the cell needs a mechanism for sending an electrical signal from its information-receiving end on the postsynaptic dendritic and soma membrane to the information-transmitting zone at the end of the often-lengthy axon. This is accomplished by an explosive event called an *action potential,* a regenerative electrical signal that begins at the axon's initial segment, results from competing EPSP and IPSP forces, and spreads down the length of the axon without decreasing in magnitude.

At the axon's initial segment, the arriving EPSPs and IPSPs are averaged. If only a few EPSPs arrive at the axon's initial segment, its membrane potential is not reduced sufficiently to reach its *threshold potential* and cause an action potential. However, if a lot more EPSPs than IPSPs arrive, the initial segment's membrane potential is lowered to its threshold potential, and an action potential is created. This action potential is the result of the sequential opening of voltage-gated membrane channels first to sodium and shortly thereafter to potassium (see Chapter 1).

The action potential is characterized by explosive changes in the membrane potential: First, there occurs a dramatic and swift depolarization of the membrane potential in which the inside of the cell actually becomes more positively charged than the outside, followed by a more gradual repolarization of the membrane. The depolarization phase of the action potential is caused by the extensive opening of voltage-gated Na^+ channels and the consequent influx of Na^+ ions. As the action potential's depolarization phase continues, the Na^+ channels close gradually and the K^+ channels open gradually, allowing even more K^+ ions to exit. This brings depolarization to a halt and allows repolarization to occur. As repolarization continues, the membrane potential returns temporarily beyond its resting level to a hyperpolarized state and then eventually returns to its resting state. The whole action potential takes about 1 to 2 msec in most nerves but longer in many muscle cells. Figure 3–4 illustrates this sequence of events.

An analogy may be helpful for understanding these

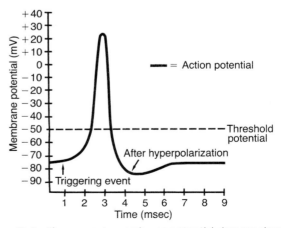

FIGURE 3–4. The neuron's membrane potential changes dramatically during an action potential. It depolarizes first well beyond threshold and then repolarizes again to its original resting potential. (Redrawn from Sherwood L: Human Physiology: From Cells to Systems. St. Paul: Wadsworth, 1989, p 95.)

difficult concepts. Imagine the resting nerve membrane as a toilet. Like the nerve, the toilet has stored potential energy by filling its water tank. (The nerve has done so by generating the resting membrane potential.) If the handle of the toilet is pushed down only briefly, some water runs into the toilet, but the flush cycle is not initiated. (This is much like an EPSP without the action potential.) However, if the handle is held down long enough, a critical threshold is reached, the flush cycle is triggered, and it must run its course, including the refilling of the tank, before another flush cycle can be started. The action potential is like this flush cycle. It is triggered once a critical hypopolarization threshold is reached. It must run its course, including reestablishing the resting membrane potential, before another action potential can be initiated. Because the flush cycle takes a finite amount of time, only a limited number of flush cycles could be completed in an hour, even if the toilet were flushed

again each time the tank refilled. Similarly, because the action potential also has a finite duration, there is a limit to the number of action potentials per second that can be generated on a nerve.

The action potential spreads from its origin at the initial segment down the axon. The dramatic action potential depolarization of the initial segment's membrane causes voltage-gated Na^+ channels to open in the immediately adjacent axon membrane. This causes an action potential to develop there, which triggers a similar cycle in its adjacent membrane, and so on down the axon. In this way an action potential spreads from the axon's initial segment down to the presynaptic terminal at the axon's far end (Fig. 3–5).

The speed with which the action potential is conducted down the axon varies. In a small unmyelinated axon, the conduction velocity is relatively slow (e.g., 0.5 m/second); conduction velocities of greater than 70 m/second (so that a distance nearly as long

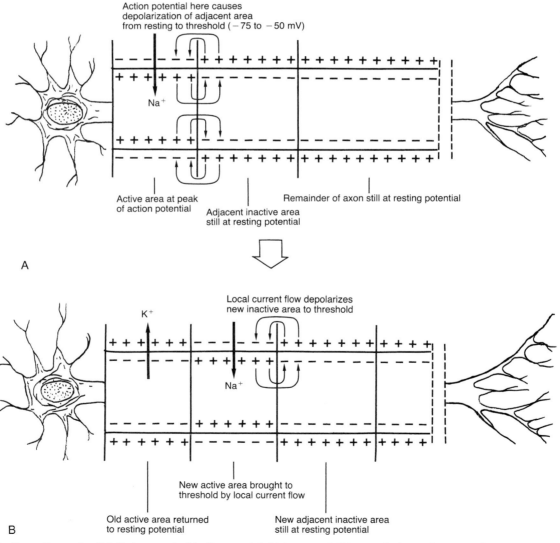

FIGURE 3–5. The action potential, first generated in the axon's initial segment *(A)*, spreads down the unmyelinated axon by triggering an action potential in the immediately adjacent membrane *(B)*. (Redrawn from Sherwood L: Human Physiology: From Cells to Systems. St. Paul: Wadsworth, 1989, p 99.)

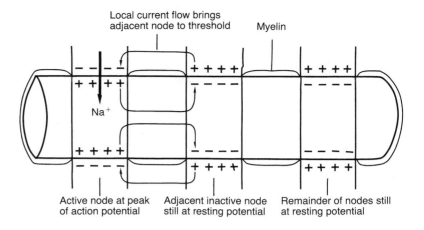

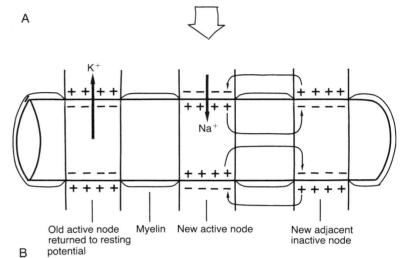

FIGURE 3–6. Saltatory conduction of action potentials in myelinated axons (A and B) is faster than action potential conduction in unmyelinated axons, because the action potential functionally jumps from node to node. (Adapted from Sherwood L: Human Physiology: From Cells to Systems. St. Paul: Wadsworth, 1989, p 102.)

as a football field is traveled in 1 second), however, are known to occur in large myelinated nerve axons. This occurs because the action potential functionally jumps from node to node (saltatory conduction) as a result of the influence of the myelin and the greater concentration of voltage-gated Na^+ channels at the nodes of Ranvier (Fig. 3–6).

CLINICAL CORRELATIONS

Hypoglycemia

History You examine an 8-year-old boxer dog whose owner complains that the dog experiences seizures, weakness, and confusion near the time he is fed.

Clinical examination The findings of the dog's physical examination, including his neurologic examination, were within normal limits. His fasting serum glucose level, however, was 29 mg/dL (normal is 70 to 110 mg/dL), and the ratio between serum insulin and serum glucose levels was markedly elevated.

Comment Neurons are dependent primarily on oxygen and glucose as metabolites for ATP energy production, and neurons cannot store appreciable quantities of glucose. ATP is needed for maintenance of the normal electrical membrane potential. Deprived of adequate glucose, and hence ATP, the brain malfunctions, commonly with seizures, weakness, and confusion. In this animal, these signs were more common at the time of feeding because insulin's release is stimulated either by eating or psychologically in anticipation of eating.

In this case, the ratio of insulin to glucose is elevated, probably because of an insulin-secreting tumor of the pancreas. Because insulin facilitates glucose transport through cell membranes, too much insulin results in the transfer of too much serum glucose to the cytoplasm of other cells of the body, thus depriving the brain's neurons of this essential metabolite.

Treatment Insulinomas can usually be found and removed from the pancreas surgically. However, there is a high rate of metastasis with this tumor, which means that other tumor sites may remain, in the liver and elsewhere, to overproduce insulin.

Bibliography

Guyton AC, Hall JE: Textbook of Medical Physiology, 10th ed. Philadelphia: WB Saunders, 2000, pp 52–66.

Haines DE: Fundamental Neuroscience. New York: Churchill Livingstone, 1997, pp 31–50.

Kandel ER, Schwartz JH, Jessell TM (eds): Principles of Neural Science, 4th ed. New York: McGraw-Hill, 2000, pp 67–174.

PRACTICE QUESTIONS

1. In treating critically ill patients with intravenous fluids, which two ions are most important to the nerve membrane potential?
   a. Na^+ and Cl^-.
   b. K^+ and Cl^-.
   c. Ca^{2+} and Cl^-.
   d. K^+ and Ca^{2+}.
   e. Na^+ and K^+.

2. The energy required by the Na^+,K^+ nerve membrane pump is derived from ATP. In the neuron, this energy results from the nearly exclusive metabolism of oxygen and
   a. amino acids.
   b. fatty acids.
   c. glucose.
   d. glycogen.
   e. proteins.

3. If the frequency of IPSPs on a nerve membrane decreases while the frequency of EPSPs remains the same, what will happen to the action potentials on the nerve cell membrane?
   a. Frequency of action potentials increases.
   b. Frequency of action potentials decreases.
   c. Frequency of action potentials remains unchanged.

   d. Action potentials would be eliminated.
   e. Action potentials would be conducted with increased velocity.

4. During an excitatory postsynaptic potential in a nerve membrane, which of the following is the most important ion flow?
   a. Sodium ions diffuse out of the cell.
   b. Sodium ions diffuse into the cell.
   c. Potassium ions diffuse out of the cell.
   d. Potassium ions diffuse into the cell.
   e. None of the above.

5. Choose the *incorrect* statement below:
   a. Conduction velocity of action potentials is slower in myelinated than in unmyelinated nerves.
   b. Conduction velocity of action potentials is faster in myelinated than in unmyelinated nerves.
   c. In saltatory conduction of action potentials, the action potential jumps from node to node (nodes of Ranvier).
   d. Action potentials are of equal magnitude at the beginning and at the end of an axon.

PRACTICE ANSWERS

1. e   2. c   3. a   4. b   5. a

4

The neuromuscular synapse

1 The anatomy of the neuromuscular synapse is specialized for one-way communication

2 An action potential on the presynaptic nerve triggers an action potential on the muscle through the release of acetylcholine

Nerves communicate with each other and with other cells of the body, such as muscle and secretory cells. Such communication occurs between cells at specialized junctions called *synapses* (from the Greek word for "junction" or "to bind tightly"). Synaptic transmission between cells can be either electrical or chemical. At electrical synapses, ionic current flows between presynaptic and postsynaptic cells as the mediator for transmission. More commonly, synaptic transmission is mediated by a chemical messenger. Released from the presynaptic cell by the arriving action potential, this chemical messenger diffuses to the postsynaptic cell membrane, where it binds with a receptor, thus initiating the postsynaptic potential change. The best understood of these chemical synapses is the synapse between a motor neuron and a skeletal muscle cell: the neuromuscular synapse. This is the synapse discussed in this chapter. Other synapses are discussed in subsequent chapters.

━ THE ANATOMY OF THE NEUROMUSCULAR SYNAPSE IS SPECIALIZED FOR ONE-WAY COMMUNICATION

The motor neuron (later to be called the *lower motor neuron*) comes into close apposition with the skeletal muscle cell at a specialized junction called the *neuromuscular synapse* (Fig. 4–1). This synapse has a *presynaptic* (nerve) side; a narrow space between the nerve and muscle, called the *synaptic cleft*; and a *postsynaptic* (muscle) side.

The presynaptic side of the synapse is made up of the terminal portion of the motor neuron, whose axon extends from the central nervous system to the muscle cell in order to signal muscular contraction. This synaptic, transmitting end of the axon contains a large number of synaptic vesicles that contain the chemical transmitter substance—in this case, acetylcholine. These vesicles are clustered around an active zone of the presynaptic membrane, adjacent to the postsynaptic junctional folds. The presynaptic nerve terminal also contains mitochondria, which is an indication of

the active metabolism that takes place in the nerve cytoplasm while acetylcholine is synthesized before it is absorbed into the synaptic vesicles.

The presynaptic (nerve) and postsynaptic (muscle) cell membranes are separated by a narrow space, the synaptic cleft, that is 20 to 30 nm wide. The cleft contains extracellular fluid and a basal lamina of spongy reticular fibers.

The postsynaptic cell membrane has several specialized features that facilitate synaptic transmission. The membrane has a series of invaginations, called *junctional folds,* that increase the surface area of the postsynaptic membrane. Receptors to the acetylcholine neurotransmitter are located on the postsynaptic membrane at the mouth of these junctional folds.

Because the neurotransmitter is found only on the presynaptic nerve side of the synapse, transmission can go only from nerve to muscle, not in the reverse direction.

━ AN ACTION POTENTIAL ON THE PRESYNAPTIC NERVE TRIGGERS AN ACTION POTENTIAL ON THE MUSCLE THROUGH THE RELEASE OF ACETYLCHOLINE

The function of the neuromuscular synapse is to transmit an action potential message unidirectionally between a motor nerve and a skeletal muscle cell with a frequency and a speed established by the nervous system. The arrival of an action potential along the motor nerve triggers the release of the acetylcholine transmitter, which then binds with receptors on the postsynaptic muscle cell membrane, resulting in the genesis of an action potential along the muscle cell.

An action potential on a motor nerve arises at its initial axon segment and then spreads along the entire axon, eventually arriving at its terminal, presynaptic end (see Chapter 3). As the action potential arrives at the presynaptic membrane, the wave of depolarization opens voltage-gated Ca^{2+} channels, and in the presence of sufficient extracellular Ca^{2+}, Ca^{2+} diffuses

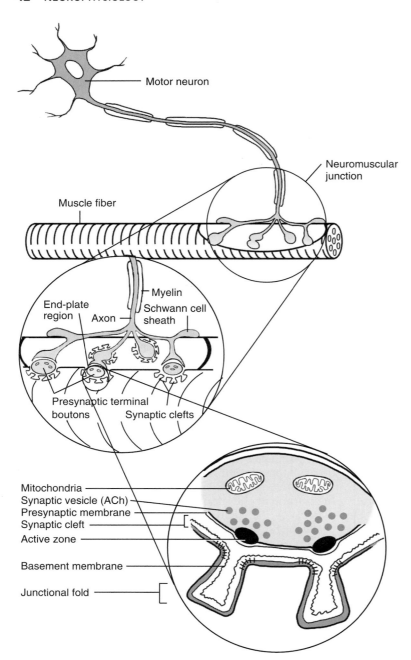

Motor neuron

Neuromuscular junction

Muscle fiber

Myelin

End-plate region

Axon

Schwann cell sheath

Presynaptic terminal boutons

Synaptic clefts

Mitochondria

Synaptic vesicle (ACh)

Presynaptic membrane

Synaptic cleft

Active zone

Basement membrane

Junctional fold

FIGURE 4–1. The neuromuscular synapse has a *presynaptic* (nerve) side, a narrow space between the nerve and muscle called the *synaptic cleft*, and a *postsynaptic* (muscle) side.

into the presynaptic nerve cytoplasm. This increase in the intracellular Ca^{2+} level somehow causes many of the acetylcholine-containing synaptic vesicles to fuse with the presynaptic membrane, open, and release their acetylcholine into the synaptic cleft. After transmitter release, the vesicle membrane is recycled back into the presynaptic nerve cytoplasm to be refilled with acetylcholine from the cytoplasm.

Acetylcholine then diffuses across the synaptic cleft. Arriving at the postsynaptic membrane, acetylcholine binds with a transmitter-specific receptor, which controls ligand-gated ion channels in the postsynaptic muscle membrane (see Chapter 1).

As acetylcholine binds with its postsynaptic receptor, ligand-gated ion channels are opened, and a net

quantity of Na^+ ions diffuses into the muscle cell, causing depolarization of the postsynaptic muscle cell membrane. This depolarization opens voltage-gated Na^+ channels deep within the junctional folds and leads to the generation of an action potential on the muscle cell membrane (see Chapter 3). Acetylcholine is allowed to bind with its receptor only briefly before it is destroyed by the enzyme acetylcholinesterase. This enzyme, anchored to the basement membrane, inactivates acetylcholine by cleaving it into acetyl and choline molecules. Because the neurotransmitter is destroyed soon after its binding with the muscle membrane receptor, and because more transmitter is not available to attach to the receptors in sufficient quantities until another nerve action potential occurs, there is an approximately 1:1 ratio between action potentials on the nerve and muscle cell membranes.

As seen in the next chapter, action potentials on the muscle cell membrane lead to contraction, or mechanical shortening, of the muscle cell. When this contraction is combined with the shortening of many muscle cells, movement of the body occurs.

CLINICAL CORRELATIONS

Myasthenia gravis

History   You examine a 5-year-old female German shepherd whose owner states that the dog becomes progressively weaker with exercise. The owner also states that recently, just after eating, the dog has begun to vomit food in formed, cylinder-shaped boluses.

Clinical examination   All abnormalities found on physical examination were referable to the neuromuscular system. After resting, the dog's neurologic examination findings were within normal limits. But with even moderate exercise, the dog became progressively weaker, particularly in the front legs. Intravenous injection of an acetylcholinesterase inhibitor, edrophonium (Tensilon), eliminated all clinical signs of weakness. Radiographs of the chest revealed an enlarged esophagus and thymus.

Comment   The history, enlarged esophagus, and response to an acetylcholinesterase inhibitor confirm the diagnosis of myasthenia gravis (grave muscle weakness). This is caused by a failure of transmission at the neuromuscular synapse. This transmission failure is caused by antibodies produced by the body against its own acetylcholine receptors. Receptors complexed with these abnormal antibodies cannot cause the depolarization of the postsynaptic membrane in the time acetylcholine normally has to work at the synapse. Antibodies also alter the junctional folds and number of acetylcholine receptors available to bind with the transmitter. Acetylcholinesterase inhibitors allow acetylcholine to work longer at the synapse, facilitating normal transmission.

The large amount of skeletal muscle in the dog's esophagus explains its enlargement from paralysis. These patients often vomit formed boluses of food shortly after eating.

Myasthenia gravis is often associated with mediastinal masses, usually of the thymus, which may be a source of either the antireceptor antibodies or the antigen.

Treatment   Spontaneous remissions are common. Until then, oral daily acetylcholinesterase inhibitors are given. Surgical removal of mediastinal masses may also be necessary.

Bibliography

Guyton AC, Hall JE: Textbook of Medical Physiology, 10th ed. Philadelphia: WB Saunders, 2000, pp 512–527.
Haines DE: Fundamental Neuroscience. New York: Churchill Livingstone, 1997, pp 51–64.
Kandel ER, Schwartz JH, Jessell TM (eds): Principles of Neural Science, 4th ed. New York: McGraw-Hill, 2000, pp 175–316.

PRACTICE QUESTIONS

1. At the somatic neuromuscular synapse, Ca^{2+} ions are necessary for
   a. binding the transmitter with the postsynaptic receptor.
   b. facilitating diffusion of the transmitter to the postsynaptic membrane.
   c. splitting the transmitter in the cleft, thus deactivating the transmitter.
   d. fusing the presynaptic vesicle with the presynaptic membrane, thus releasing the transmitter.
   e. metabolizing the transmitter within the presynaptic vesicle.

2. A drug that would prevent the release of acetylcholine at the neuromuscular synaptic junction would cause what, if any, clinical signs?
   a. Convulsions and excess muscle contractions.
   b. Paralysis.
   c. No effect on an animal's movement.

3. The neurotransmitter between the motor neuron and the extrafusal skeletal muscle fiber is
   a. norepinephrine.
   b. acetylcholine.
   c. epinephrine.
   d. gamma-aminobutyric acid.
   e. dopamine.

4. You examine a dog that can walk briefly but tires quickly and, after a few minutes of walking, is unable to rise until she rests for several minutes. She is bright, alert, and responsive. Neurologic examination after the dog has rested is essentially within normal limits. The intravenous infusion of an acetylcholinesterase-inhibiting drug eliminates the clinical signs of fatigue. Where is the most likely location for this dog's abnormality?
   a. Brain.
   b. Neuromuscular junction.
   c. Thoracolumbar spinal cord.
   d. Lower motor neurons to one or both front legs.
   e. Lower motor neurons to one or both hind legs.

5. Several drugs compete with acetylcholine for the postsynaptic receptor at the neuromuscular junction. If you overdosed your patient with one of these competitive drugs, what would the antidote have to do at the synapse?
   a. Decrease the release of acetylcholine.
   b. Decrease the effectiveness of acetylcholinesterase.
   c. Decrease the synaptic Ca^{2+} level.
   d. Increase the postsynaptic membrane potential.
   e. None of the above.

PRACTICE ANSWERS

1. d   2. b   3. b   4. b   5. b

5

The physiology of muscle

1 All movement is the result of contraction of skeletal muscle across a movable joint

2 There are several levels of organization in any skeletal muscle

3 Action potentials on the sarcolemma spread to the interior of the cell along the transverse tubules

4 The sliding of actin along the myosin molecule results in physical shortening of the sarcomere

5 The action potential on the sarcolemma is coupled to the contraction mechanism through the release of Ca^{2+} from the sarcoplasmic reticulum

6 Muscles change their strength of contraction by varying the number of active motor units

7 The electromyogram is the clinical measurement of the electrical behavior within a skeletal muscle

8 Most skeletal muscle fibers can be classified as either fast-contracting or slow-contracting fibers

9 The structure of cardiac and smooth muscle differs from that of skeletal muscle

10 The role of Ca^{2+} ions in excitation-contraction coupling in cardiac and smooth muscle differs from that in skeletal muscle

There are three types of muscle in the body: skeletal, cardiac, and smooth muscle. Skeletal muscle makes up about 40% of the body, and smooth muscle and cardiac muscle make up nearly 10% more. Because most veterinary patients with disease of the neuromuscular system exhibit abnormalities of movement, it is important to understand how skeletal muscle functions and how it is controlled by the nervous system. Abnormalities of cardiac muscle and smooth muscle feature prominently in many other clinical disorders and also in pharmacologic mechanisms.

This chapter explains the physiology of skeletal muscle. Brief comparisons with cardiac and smooth muscle are also made. Cardiac muscle is mentioned more extensively in chapters on the cardiovascular system, and the role of smooth muscle in other body systems is mentioned numerous times throughout this book.

ALL MOVEMENT IS THE RESULT OF CONTRACTION OF SKELETAL MUSCLE ACROSS A MOVABLE JOINT

All body movement is the result of contraction of skeletal muscle. Skeletal muscle consists of a central fleshy contractile muscle "belly" and two tendons, one on each end of the muscle. The muscle and its tendons are arranged in the body so that they originate on one bone and insert on a different bone while spanning a joint. As the muscle contracts, shortening the distance between the origin and insertion tendons, the bones move with regard to each other, bending at

the joint (Fig. 5–1). When activated by the motor nerve, a skeletal muscle can only shorten. Most joints have one or more muscles on both sides, either to decrease its angle (flexion) or to increase its angle (extension). All movement performed by an animal is the result of contraction of skeletal muscle across a movable joint. It is therefore important to understand the anatomy and physiology of skeletal muscle before the discussion of how the nervous system choreographs the contraction of groups of muscle cells in order to perform purposeful movement.

THERE ARE SEVERAL LEVELS OF ORGANIZATION IN ANY SKELETAL MUSCLE

Figure 5–2 illustrates the several levels of organization in a typical skeletal muscle. Each muscle belly seen during dissection is made up of differing numbers of muscle cells (usually called *muscle fibers*) that span the several inches between the origin and insertion tendons. They range between 10 and 80 μm in diameter and contain multiple mitochondria and other intracellular organelles. The outer limiting membrane is called the *sarcolemma*. It consists of a true cell membrane, called the *plasma membrane,* and an outer polysaccharide layer that attaches to the tendons at the cells' extremities. Each muscle cell is innervated by only one nerve ending, located near the middle of the fiber.

Each muscle fiber is made up of successively smaller subunits (see Fig. 5–2). Muscle fibers each contain several hundred to several thousand *myofibrils*

Located between sarcoplasmic reticula, but perpendicular to the long axis of the muscle fiber, are the *transverse tubules* (see Fig. 5–3). These tubules traverse the diameter of the muscle cell from one side of the sarcolemma to the other, much like piercing a sausage with a nail perpendicular to the long axis of the sausage. These tubules are filled with extracellular fluid. They are important because they allow the muscle cells' action potential to be transmitted to the interior of the cell.

ACTION POTENTIALS ON THE SARCOLEMMA SPREAD TO THE INTERIOR OF THE CELL ALONG THE TRANSVERSE TUBULES

Skeletal muscle cells have a resting membrane potential like that of nerve, a membrane potential that can be excited by synaptic transmission at the neuromuscular junction (see Chapter 4). It is at the neuromuscular junction that action potentials are generated. Once an action potential is generated at the synapse near the center of the muscle fiber, it spreads in both directions along the length of the fiber by mechanisms similar to action potential spread in unmyelinated nerve axons. In contrast to those on axons, however, action potentials on the sarcolemma are also transmitted to the interior of the cell along the transverse tubules. This allows the action potential to reach the sarcoplasmic reticulum even in the innermost regions of the muscle fiber. The consequences of the action potential's arrival at the sarcoplasmic reticulum are discussed later when the coupling of excitation (the action potential) with contraction (shortening) of the sarcomeres is examined.

THE SLIDING OF ACTIN ALONG THE MYOSIN MOLECULE RESULTS IN PHYSICAL SHORTENING OF THE SARCOMERE

Figure 5–4 illustrates the sarcomere in the relaxed state and in its shorter, contracted state. The sarcomere is changed from its relaxed state to the shorter, contracted state when Ca^{2+} ions become available to the sarcomere. In the presence of Ca^{2+} ions and a sufficient source of adenosine triphosphate (ATP), actin and myosin molecules slide over one another, thus shortening the sarcomere. Because each myofibril is made up of a series of repeating and connected sarcomeres, the net result is the physical shortening of the distance between the two ends of the muscle. A detailed molecular explanation of this sliding filament mechanism of sarcomere shortening is not available, but several portions of the process have been established. At several points along the actin molecule, there are active sites that chemically interact with the head of the myosin molecule. In the absence of Ca^{2+} ions, these sites are either inhibited or covered by the tropomyosin molecules in their helix. But in the presence of Ca^{2+}, which binds with troponin, the

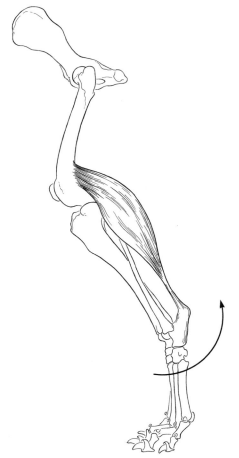

FIGURE 5–1. All noticeable movement is the result of contraction (shortening) of a skeletal muscle attached across a movable joint.

arranged in parallel along its length, like a handful of spaghetti. Each myofibril is made up of a series of repeating *sarcomeres,* the basic contractile unit of the muscle fiber.

The sarcomere has a disk at each end called the *Z disk.* The sarcomere contains four types of large, polymerized protein molecules responsible for muscular contraction. (A fifth, *titan,* appears to contribute to the elastic properties of the muscle.) Numerous thin protein filaments, called *actin,* are attached to the Z disks and extend toward the center of the sarcomere like parallel fingers pointing at each other. Each actin filament consists of two strands of actin protein and two strands of *tropomyosin* protein wound together as a helix. Also located intermittently along the tropomyosin molecules are globular protein molecules called *troponin,* which have an affinity for Ca^{2+} ions. Suspended between the actin filaments are thicker *myosin* protein filaments. Myosin also consists of protein helixes and contains intermittent cross-bridges that interact with actin to shorten the sarcomere (see also Chapter 1).

Located in parallel to the myofibrils are numerous long endoplasmic reticula called the *sarcoplasmic reticula* in muscle cells (Fig. 5–3). They sequester Ca^{2+} ions in relaxed muscle.

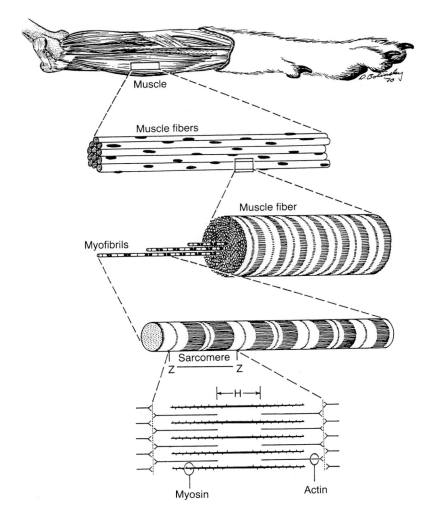

Muscle

Muscle fibers

Muscle fiber

Myofibrils

Sarcomere

Z — Z

|← H →|

Myosin

Actin

FIGURE 5–2. There are several levels of organization in a typical skeletal muscle. "H" and "Z" are letters assigned to stripes seen during microscopic examination of skeletal muscle.

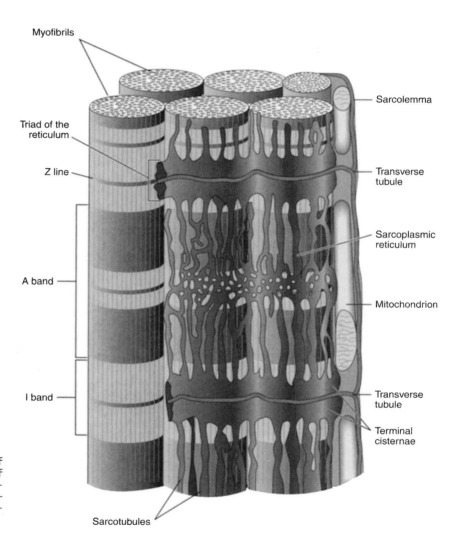

Myofibrils

Sarcolemma

Triad of the
reticulum

Z line

Transverse
tubule

A band

Sarcoplasmic
reticulum

Mitochondrion

I band

Transverse
tubule

Terminal
cisternae

Sarcotubules

FIGURE 5–3. A three-dimensional diagram of
skeletal muscle showing the juxtaposition of
myofibrils, transverse tubules, and sarcoplasmic reticula. (From Guyton AC, Hall JE: Textbook of Medical Physiology, 10th ed. Philadelphia: WB Saunders, 2000, p 84.)

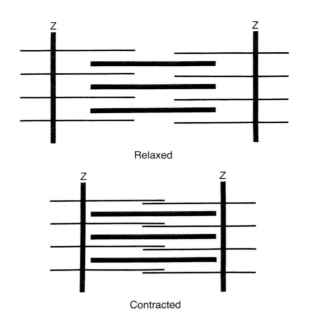

FIGURE 5–4. The sliding of actin along the myosin molecule results in the physical shortening (contraction) of the sarcomere.

tropomyosin molecule is in some way changed so that these active actin sites are freed to react with the myosin molecules. In some poorly understood way, these reactions cause actin and myosin to "walk along" each other in order to shorten the sarcomere. In the absence of Ca^{2+}, this "walk-along" bonding no longer occurs, and relaxation results.

▬ THE ACTION POTENTIAL ON THE SARCOLEMMA IS COUPLED TO THE CONTRACTION MECHANISM THROUGH THE RELEASE OF Ca^{2+} FROM THE SARCOPLASMIC RETICULUM

At rest, Ca^{2+} ions are pumped out of the sarcoplasmic fluid and into the sarcoplasmic reticulum by an energy-dependent pump. This leaves too low a concentration of Ca^{2+} in the sarcomere to allow contraction. However, as an action potential spreads along the cell surface and into the muscle fiber along the transverse tubules, it arrives eventually in the neighborhood of the sarcoplasmic reticulum. The arrival of the action potential at the sarcoplasmic reticulum causes the release of Ca^{2+} ions, which diffuse down their concentration gradient out of the sarcoplasmic reticulum and into the fluid bathing the sarcomere. These Ca^{2+} ions then trigger contraction. As the action potential passes, Ca^{2+} is pumped again into the sarcoplasmic reticulum, and relaxation results. This cycle is known as *excitation-contraction coupling.*

▬ MUSCLES CHANGE THEIR STRENGTH OF CONTRACTION BY VARYING THE NUMBER OF ACTIVE MOTOR UNITS

A *motor unit* is defined as one α motor neuron and all the extrafusal muscle fibers that it innervates. Even

though each muscle fiber is innervated by only one neuron, each motor neuron's axon branches as it reaches the muscle and innervates several muscle fibers. The ratio of nerve to muscle fiber varies with the function of the muscle. For example, large antigravity muscles (see Chapter 9) such as the quadriceps femoris and gastrocnemius muscles have several hundred muscle fibers innervated by each motor nerve. Muscles requiring little strength but discrete control, such as the muscles that control the position of the eyes, may have fewer than 10 muscle fibers for each motor axon.

The nervous system can call on a muscle to contract with greater force primarily by increasing the number of motor units that contract at any one time (called *spatial summation*). The force of contraction can also be increased by increasing the frequency of contraction within a motor unit (called *temporal summation*). A muscle contracts by gradually increasing and then decreasing the number of active motor units. As seen in Chapter 9, this choreography is the responsibility of the central nervous system.

In skeletal muscle, the nervous system can command some percentage of motor units (although not the same motor units) to contract all the time, thus continually shortening the distance between the origin and insertion tendon. When contraction of a whole muscle belly occurs without relaxation, the muscle is said to be in *tetany*. Tetanization of cardiac muscle would be fatal, because heart muscle must relax to allow cardiac filling before it contracts to pump out the blood. Later (Chapter 18), it is shown how cardiac muscle prevents tetany.

▬ THE ELECTROMYOGRAM IS THE CLINICAL MEASUREMENT OF THE ELECTRICAL BEHAVIOR WITHIN A SKELETAL MUSCLE

As an action potential spreads along a muscle fiber, a small portion of the electrical current generated spreads away from the fiber, even to the overlying skin. Electrodes placed on the skin or inserted into the muscle belly can record a summated electrical potential when the muscle contracts. Such a measurement, when printed or displayed on an oscilloscope, is called an *electromyogram* and is for skeletal muscle what the electrocardiogram is for cardiac muscle. The electromyogram is useful for trying to determine whether weakness or paralysis is caused by disease in the skeletal muscle, neuromuscular junction, motor neuron, or central nervous system.

▬ MOST SKELETAL MUSCLE FIBERS CAN BE CLASSIFIED AS EITHER FAST-CONTRACTING OR SLOW-CONTRACTING FIBERS

Skeletal muscle fibers with short contraction times are sometimes called *fast-twitch fibers.* They tend to be larger, have extensive sarcoplasmic reticulum for rapid release of Ca^{2+} ions, and have less extensive blood and mitochondrial supplies, because aerobic metabolism is less important. Fast-twitch fibers are well adapted for jumping, sprinting, and other brief, powerful movements.

In contrast, *slow-twitch fibers* are smaller muscle fibers, have a rich blood and mitochondrial supply, and have a great deal of myoglobin, an iron-containing and oxygen-storing protein similar to hemoglobin. These fibers rely more heavily on oxidative metabolism and are better adapted for the continual contraction of antigravity extensor muscles.

Because slow-twitch muscles have more myoglobin, they are sometimes called *red muscle*; fast-twitch fibers are called *white muscle*. Usually, a muscle belly is made up of a blend of these two types, the proportions varying in accordance with the muscle's use. This blend can be changed somewhat with exercise, such as in an athlete training for a different type of sports event.

THE STRUCTURE OF CARDIAC AND SMOOTH MUSCLE DIFFERS FROM THAT OF SKELETAL MUSCLE

Like skeletal muscle, *cardiac muscle* is striated and contains sarcoplasmic reticulum and myofibrils; the fundamental contractile component is formed by actin and myosin subunits. Cardiac muscle also contains transverse tubules, but cardiac muscle differs from skeletal muscle in some important ways. Cardiac muscle cells are shorter than those of skeletal muscle and are connected to each other through end-to-end *intercalated disks*. Action potentials can spread from one cardiac muscle cell to another across these intercalated disks without the need for any nerve transmission or chemical transmitter. In fact, as explained in Chapter 18, action potentials arise spontaneously in specialized cardiac muscle cells and then spread throughout a large population of cardiac muscle cells as if they were a functional syncytium. The frequency of such action potentials and the force of the resulting contraction are influenced by the autonomic nervous system, but such innervation is not necessary for action potential genesis.

Smooth muscle cells are much smaller and shorter than skeletal muscle cells. They do not contain transverse tubules, presumably because their actin and myosin molecules are close enough to the outer cell membrane to be influenced directly by the sarcolemma's action potential and the transmembrane diffusion of Ca^{2+} ions.

Some smooth muscle cell tissues, usually called *visceral smooth muscle*, have gap junctions between cells and operate like a functional syncytium with cell-to-cell action potential transmission much as in cardiac muscle. This type of smooth muscle is described more fully in Chapter 27. Another type of smooth muscle cell tissue, usually called *multiunit smooth muscle*, has completely separate muscle cells, each of which receives autonomic innervation.

Multiunit smooth muscle can be found, for example, in the iris and ciliary body of the eye, where precise control of muscular contraction is needed. Visceral smooth muscle is abundant in the gastrointestinal tract and other organs of the thoracic and abdominal cavities.

THE ROLE OF Ca^{2+} IONS IN EXCITATION-CONTRACTION COUPLING IN CARDIAC AND SMOOTH MUSCLE DIFFERS FROM THAT IN SKELETAL MUSCLE

Contraction of both cardiac and smooth muscle cells results from the sliding together of actin and myosin protein filaments, just as in skeletal muscle. This sliding of actin over myosin requires ATP and does not occur unless Ca^{2+} ions are present, again as in skeletal muscle. But the origins of the intracytoplasmic Ca^{2+} ions that permit contraction differ. In skeletal muscle, Ca^{2+} is sequestered in the sarcoplasmic reticulum. With the arrival of the action potential along the sarcolemma and transverse tubule, Ca^{2+} is released from the sarcoplasmic reticulum and diffuses out into the cytoplasm, where it triggers contraction. With the passage of the action potential, Ca^{2+} is pumped back into the sarcoplasmic reticulum, and the muscle relaxes. In skeletal muscle, little if any extracellular Ca^{2+} is needed for contraction. However, in cardiac and smooth muscle, both extracellular and sarcoplasmic reticulum Ca^{2+} ions are important in triggering contraction. Both muscle types contain sarcoplasmic reticulum with sequestered Ca^{2+}, although they are not as well developed in smooth muscle. With the arrival of the action potential along the cell membrane (and the T tubules in cardiac muscle), slow channels are opened to Ca^{2+}, allowing the influx of extracellular Ca^{2+} ions. This second source of Ca^{2+} supplements the sarcoplasmic reticulum Ca^{2+} in triggering contraction. If drugs called *calcium channel blockers* are used to block the entry of extracellular Ca^{2+} ions, the force of contraction is reduced. Once the action potential has passed, muscle relaxation is accomplished by pumping cytoplasmic Ca^{2+} back into the sarcoplasmic reticulum and through the sarcolemma into the extracellular space.

Bibliography

Guyton AC, Hall JE: Textbook of Medical Physiology, 10th ed. Philadelphia: WB Saunders, 2000, pp 80–86.
Kandel ER, Schwartz JH, Jessell TM (eds): Principles of Neural Science, 4th ed. New York: McGraw-Hill, 2000, pp 674–712.

PRACTICE QUESTIONS

1. The number of extrafusal muscle fibers in each motor unit would be lowest in which of the following muscles?
   a. Quadriceps.
   b. Triceps.
   c. Gluteal muscles.

d. Muscles for moving the human fingers.

e. Muscles for wagging the canine tail.

2. Action potentials in skeletal muscle cells trigger the release from the sarcoplasmic reticulum of what ion critical to the muscle's contractile process?

a. Ca^{2+}.

b. Na^+.

c. K^+.

d. Cl^-.

e. HCO_3^-.

3. A gross skeletal muscle belly can be made (by the central nervous system) to contract more forcefully by

a. causing more of its motor units to contract simultaneously.

b. increasing the amount of acetylcholine released during each neuromuscular synaptic transmission.

c. increasing the frequency of action potentials in the α motor neuron's axon.

d. both a and c.

e. both b and c.

4. Choose the *incorrect* statement below:

a. The muscle fiber and nerve cell membranes are similar because they both have a resting membrane potential.

b. A whole muscle, such as the gastrocnemius muscle, can be made to contract more forcefully by increasing the number of motor units contracting.

c. The muscle membrane's transverse tubular system transmits the action potential to the interior of the cell.

d. The muscle cell membrane transmits action potentials by saltatory conduction.

e. The shortening of a skeletal muscle during contraction is due to the sliding together of actin and myosin filaments.

5. Which of the following is *not* a part of a motor unit?

a. The α motor neuron.

b. The neuromuscular synapse.

c. Extrafusal muscle fibers.

d. The sarcomere.

e. The intrafusal muscle fiber (see Chapter 7).

PRACTICE ANSWERS

1. d   2. a   3. d   4. d   5. e

6

The concept of a reflex

1 A reflex arc contains five fundamental components

2 Reflex arcs are either segmental or intersegmental

3 Reflexes are widespread in the nervous system and underlie a major portion of the neurologic examination of a patient

The reflex arc is fundamental to the physiology of posture and locomotion as well as to the clinical examination of the nervous system. The word *reflex* comes from the Latin word *reflectere*, which means "to bend backward." A reflex arc, in a sense, is reflected off the central nervous system (CNS). A reflex can be defined as an involuntary, qualitatively unvarying response of the nervous system to a stimulus. The anatomy and function of a reflex arc are programmed genetically and are fully developed at birth.

▬ A REFLEX ARC CONTAINS FIVE FUNDAMENTAL COMPONENTS

All reflex arcs contain five basic components (Fig. 6–1). If any one of these five components malfunctions, the reflex response is altered.

1. All reflex arcs begin with a *receptor*. Receptors vary widely within the body, but all share a common function: they transduce some environmental energy and convert that energy into action potentials along a sensory nerve. For example, receptors of the retina transduce light; those in the skin transduce heat, cold, pressure, and other cutaneous stimuli; muscle spindle receptors transduce stretch. Many other types of receptors also transduce some particular form of environmental energy. In transduction, action potentials are generated along sensory nerves at a frequency proportional to the intensity of the energy transduced. This proportionality between the intensity with which the receptor is stimulated and the frequency of the resulting sensory nerve action potentials is called *frequency coding* and is how the receptor communicates to the CNS the intensity of light, heat, stretch, and so forth that it has transduced.

2. The next component in a reflex arc is a *sensory nerve* (afferent nerve). These nerves carry action potentials from the receptor to the CNS. They enter the spinal cord by way of the dorsal roots.

3. The third component of a reflex arc is a *synapse*

in the CNS. Actually, for most reflex arcs, more than one synapse occurs. However, a few reflex arcs, such as those that come from the muscle spindle, are monosynaptic.

4. The fourth component is a *motor nerve* (efferent nerve), which carries action potentials from the CNS to the target (effector) organ. Motor nerves leaving the spinal cord depart by way of the ventral roots.

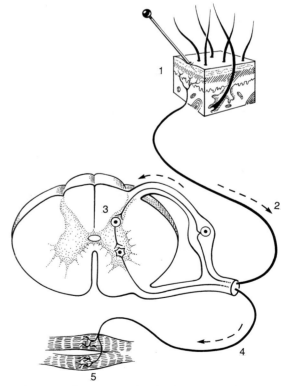

FIGURE 6–1. A reflex arc contains five fundamental components: *(1)* a receptor, *(2)* a sensory neuron, *(3)* one or more synapses in the central nervous system, *(4)* a motor neuron, and *(5)* a target organ, usually a muscle. (From De Lahunta A [ed]: Veterinary Neuroanatomy and Clinical Neurology. Philadelphia: WB Saunders, 1983, p 60.)

5. The last component is some *target organ* (effector organ) that causes the reflex response. This is usually a muscle, such as the skeletal muscle fibers of the quadriceps muscle of the leg, in the case of the knee jerk (muscle stretch) reflex, or the smooth muscle of the iris, in the case of the pupillary light reflex.

— REFLEX ARCS ARE EITHER SEGMENTAL OR INTERSEGMENTAL

A *segmental reflex* is a reflex in which the reflex arc passes through only a small segment of the CNS. The muscle stretch reflex and the pupillary light reflex are examples of segmental reflexes, because they use only a small segment of either the spinal cord or the brainstem. In an *intersegmental reflex,* multiple segments of the CNS are used. Conscious proprioception response is a good example of this type, because sensory action potentials may enter as far away as the lumbar spinal cord and yet travel all the way to the cerebral cortex before the motor response is generated. The motor response returns along roughly the same intersegmental route.

— REFLEXES ARE WIDESPREAD IN THE NERVOUS SYSTEM AND UNDERLIE A MAJOR PORTION OF THE NEUROLOGIC EXAMINATION OF A PATIENT

Reflex arcs are ubiquitous in the nervous system and are the basis of much of an animal's subconscious response to its environment. Much of a veterinarian's clinical examination of the nervous system involves evoking reflex responses, such as the pupillary light reflex, muscle stretch (knee jerk) reflex, and flexor reflex.

If any of these five components malfunctions, the expected reflex response does not occur. It is important to know the general anatomy, physiology, and expected normal clinical response of the common reflexes in order to perform a neurologic examination so that lesions can be localized. Several such reflexes are discussed in some detail in subsequent chapters of this book.

Bibliography

Guyton AC, Hall JE: Textbook of Medical Physiology, 10th ed. Philadelphia: WB Saunders, 2000, pp 622–633.

Kandel ER, Schwartz JH, Jessell TM (eds): Principles of Neural Science, 4th ed. New York: McGraw-Hill, 2000, pp 713–736.

PRACTICE QUESTIONS

1. Which of the following is *not* a necessary part of a reflex arc?
   a. Receptor.
   b. Sensory (afferent) nerve.
   c. Internuncial (connector) nerve.
   d. Motor nerve.
   e. Target (responding) organ.

2. Which of the following is *not* a function of a receptor?
   a. Transduction of light into action potentials by the retina.
   b. Transduction of sound into action potentials by the cochlea.
   c. Transduction of action potentials from the motor neuron into physical shortening by skeletal muscle.
   d. Transduction of painful stimuli into action potentials by free nerve endings of the skin.

3. When the intensity with which a receptor is stimulated is increased, what happens to the frequency of action potentials along the sensory nerve from that receptor?
   a. Increases.
   b. Decreases.
   c. No change.

4. Which of the following is *not* an example of a segmental reflex?
   a. Muscle stretch reflex.
   b. Pupillary light reflex.
   c. Conscious proprioception reflex.

5. An intersegmental reflex arc is one in which
   a. no receptor is present.
   b. axons in the arc traverse many segments of the CNS.
   c. neurons are unmyelinated.
   d. only smooth muscle is the target organ.

PRACTICE ANSWERS

1. c 2. c 3. a 4. c 5. b

CHAPTER 7

Skeletal muscle stretch receptors

1 The muscle spindle stretch receptor is an encapsulated, specialized group of muscle fibers with separate motor and sensory innervations

2 The muscle spindle conveys information about muscle length to the central nervous system

3 Action potentials along the spindle sensory nerve lead in a reflexive manner to contraction of the extrafusal muscles

4 The central nervous system can control spindle sensitivity directly through the γ motor neurons

5 The Golgi tendon organ is a stretch receptor located in the tendons of the muscle and senses tension in the tendon

Movement, characteristic of all animals, is one of the qualities that distinguish animals from plants. An animal's movement must oppose gravity and should be purposeful. Such movement, the end product of skeletal muscle contraction, is initiated and coordinated by the central nervous system (CNS) through its control of the motor unit (see Chapter 5). In order for the CNS to control the appropriateness of body movement, it must assess the effect of gravity on the many muscles of the body, and it must detect any discrepancy between the movement it intends to command and the movement that actually occurs. Once such discrepancies are detected, appropriate adjustments can be made.

In this context, it should not be surprising that two important receptor systems have evolved in the skeletal muscles of mammals to detect the result of a muscle's attempt to carry out a CNS command and to assess the effect of gravity on the body. These two receptors are the *muscle spindle* and the *Golgi tendon organ* (Fig. 7–1). The muscle spindles, arranged in

parallel to the contracting skeletal muscle fibers, provide information about muscle length. The Golgi tendon organ, arranged in series with the contracting skeletal muscle fibers, detects muscle tension. The anatomy and physiology of these two receptor systems are discussed in this chapter. How the CNS uses the information gathered from these receptors to coordinate posture and locomotion is discussed in Chapter 9.

— THE MUSCLE SPINDLE STRETCH RECEPTOR IS AN ENCAPSULATED, SPECIALIZED GROUP OF MUSCLE FIBERS WITH SEPARATE MOTOR AND SENSORY INNERVATIONS

The muscle spindle is an encapsulated group of several slender and specialized skeletal muscle fibers (Fig. 7–2). Because their capsule is spindle-shaped (or fusiform), these muscle fibers are called *intrafusal*

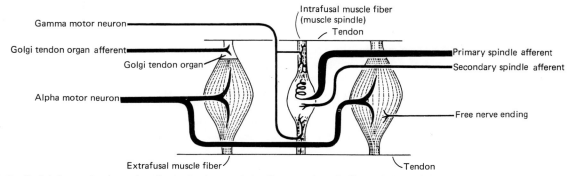

FIGURE 7–1. Skeletal muscles have two important receptors: the muscle spindle and the Golgi tendon organ. The intrafusal muscle fibers (muscle spindle) are arranged in parallel with the extrafusal muscle fibers; the Golgi tendon organ is in series with the extrafusal fibers. (From Kandel ER, Schwartz JH: Principles of Neural Science, 2nd ed. New York: Elsevier Science Publishing, 1985.)

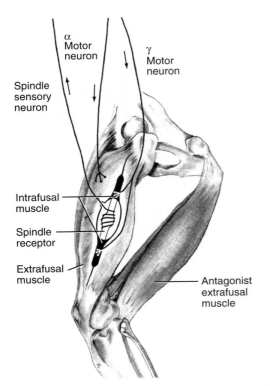

α Motor neuron

γ Motor neuron

Spindle sensory neuron

Intrafusal muscle

Spindle receptor

Extrafusal muscle

Antagonist extrafusal muscle

FIGURE 7–2. The muscle spindle receptor is an encapsulated group of specialized skeletal muscle fibers with a separate set of motor and sensory nerves. The muscle spindle detects and sends to the central nervous system information about muscle length and changes in muscle length.

muscle fibers, and the receptor is called the muscle spindle. They are too few, small, and weak to contribute much to the shortening of a gross muscle, but their contraction has a dramatic effect on the receptor. The muscle fibers that cause physical shortening of the muscle (the majority of muscle fibers in a muscle belly) are called *extrafusal muscle fibers.* Extrafusal muscle fibers span the length of the gross muscle from origin to insertion tendon. Intrafusal muscle fibers and their capsules are much shorter (about 4 to 10 mm long) but are functionally connected to both tendons through the connective tissue of the muscle.

Intrafusal muscle fibers have contractile proteins at their polar ends but none in their middle (equatorial) region. Therefore, their polar ends can contract, but their equatorial region, which is fluid filled, cannot. The spindle sensory (afferent) nerve arises from this equatorial region and carries action potentials from the spindle to the CNS by way of the peripheral nerves. The contractile, polar regions of the intrafusal muscle are innervated by their own separate motor nerves, called γ *motor neurons.* Extrafusal muscle fibers—the muscle fibers that cause the physical shortening of the muscle—receive a different nerve supply within the motor unit; these nerves are called α *motor neurons.* With few exceptions, γ motor neurons go only to intrafusal muscle fibers and α motor neurons go only to the extrafusal muscle fibers.

There are two subtly different types of intrafusal

fibers—spindle sensory neurons and γ motor neurons within the spindle—but their functional difference in detecting muscle length is not important enough to mention here.

THE MUSCLE SPINDLE CONVEYS INFORMATION ABOUT MUSCLE LENGTH TO THE CENTRAL NERVOUS SYSTEM

The only way in which action potentials can be generated along the spindle sensory nerve is by stretching (lengthening) the equatorial segment of the intrafusal muscle fiber. As this equatorial segment is lengthened, stretch-sensitive ion channels open, leading to membrane depolarization, and action potentials are generated. However, this equatorial segment can be lengthened in two ways. First, because spindle receptors lie parallel to the extrafusal fibers and are functionally connected to both the origin and insertion tendons (see Fig. 7–1), anything that would cause lengthening of the whole muscle would also stretch the equatorial region of the spindle's intrafusal muscle fiber. A change in body position as a result of gravity is an example of movement that would usually cause extensor muscle lengthening. The second way in which the intrafusal muscle's equatorial region can be lengthened is by the contraction of the polar ends of the intrafusal muscle itself: something it does in response to γ motor nerve stimulation.

Regardless of which way the intrafusal muscle's central region is lengthened, action potentials are generated along the spindle sensory nerve in direct proportion to the amount of lengthening of the middle of the intrafusal muscle. These sensory nerves can detect not only a change in length during the dynamic phase of muscle lengthening but also the steady-state length of the muscle as the animal holds the joint still.

ACTION POTENTIALS ALONG THE SPINDLE SENSORY NERVE LEAD IN A REFLEXIVE MANNER TO CONTRACTION OF THE EXTRAFUSAL MUSCLES

Action potentials are generated on the spindle sensory nerve at a frequency proportional to the degree of lengthening of the spindle's equatorial region. They are transmitted to the CNS, where they make an excitatory, monosynaptic connection with the α motor neurons that return to the extrafusal fibers of the same muscle (Fig. 7–3). This leads to contraction of the extrafusal motor units in that muscle, which in turn results in a shortening of the muscle spindle's equatorial region. This shuts off the action potentials from the spindle receptor. (The cycle is a classic negative feedback system.)

This reflex can be elicited in any animal or human by striking the patellar tendon, which is the insertion tendon of the quadriceps muscle, with a blunt object. Because this tendon goes over a "pulley" (the patella), hitting this tendon results in a longitudinal stretch of

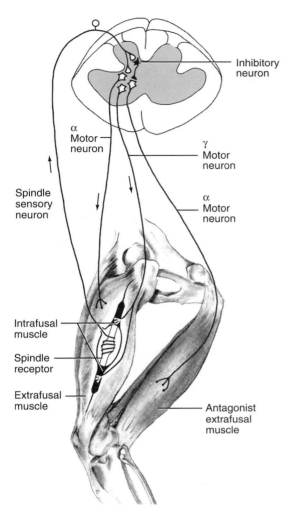

FIGURE 7-3. The muscle spindle stretch reflex (illustrated here as the "knee jerk reflex") begins when the spindle receptor is stretched. This causes action potentials on the receptor's sensory neurons, which in turn cause excitatory postsynaptic potentials on the α motor neurons returning to the extrafusal muscle fibers of that same muscle. Action potentials on the α motor neurons cause extrafusal muscle fibers to contract, and the knee extends ("jerks"). Through an inhibitory interneuron, the α motor neurons to the antagonist muscles are also inhibited.

the whole quadriceps muscle, thus also stretching the muscle spindles. Action potentials from the spindle receptor go to the lumbar spinal cord, by way of the dorsal roots, and cause excitatory postsynaptic potentials (EPSPs) on the motor neurons of the motor units that return to the quadriceps muscle. This causes contraction of the quadriceps muscle and an extension of the knee joint, which is an example of the *muscle stretch reflex,* or *myotatic reflex.* When it is applied to the quadriceps muscle, it is called the *knee jerk reflex,* but the mechanisms are present in all muscles. However, this is the muscle from which it is easiest to evoke the stretch reflex, because it is one of the few whose tendon goes over a sesamoid pulley before inserting on the next bone. Because of the pulley under the tendon, a lateral deflection of the tendon, as from a reflex hammer, results in a longitu-

dinal stretch of the muscle; hence, the reflex. Hitting other tendons only moves the muscle belly laterally and does not easily result in the stretch reflex. Therefore, in the clinical neurologic examination of most animals, the knee jerk reflex is the most commonly evoked muscle stretch reflex.

Of course, this system has not evolved to teach veterinarians and physicians to use a reflex hammer. Among other things, it allows the CNS to know when the muscle is stretched by change in body position. Later, many other functions of the muscle spindles are described.

THE CENTRAL NERVOUS SYSTEM CAN CONTROL SPINDLE SENSITIVITY DIRECTLY THROUGH THE γ MOTOR NEURONS

As mentioned earlier, contraction of the extrafusal muscle fibers is controlled by the larger α motor neurons; intrafusal muscle fibers are controlled by the smaller γ motor neurons. The γ motor neurons innervate the intrafusal muscle fibers at their polar ends, the regions containing contractile protein. Action potentials on the γ motor neurons cause shortening of the polar regions of the spindle's intrafusal muscles, but not the equatorial region, because this middle section is devoid of contractile protein. Instead, the equatorial portion stretches.

The significance of γ innervation to the intrafusal muscle fibers is much debated, but there are many probable functions for this unique motor innervation of a receptor. As the gross muscle shortens because of extrafusal muscle contraction, simultaneous contraction of the intrafusal fibers, caused by γ motor nerve stimulation, allows the spindle receptor to remain sensitive to sudden stretches of the gross muscle over the entire range of its length. The CNS can initiate contraction of the extrafusal fibers in a reflexive manner by way of the γ motor neurons through what is known as the γ *loop.* The γ loop consists, in sequence, of the γ motor nerve; the intrafusal muscle fiber, including the equatorial receptor portion; the spindle sensory nerve with its monosynaptic excitatory synapse; the α motor neuron back to the same muscle; and the extrafusal muscle fibers. Chapter 9 describes how simultaneous coactivation of both the α and γ motor neurons allows the brain to test the initial load on a muscle and to test whether the amount of contraction intended by the brain was what actually occurred. It is because of these many important roles of the muscle spindle in posture and locomotion that they have been emphasized here.

THE GOLGI TENDON ORGAN IS A STRETCH RECEPTOR LOCATED IN THE TENDONS OF THE MUSCLE AND SENSES TENSION IN THE TENDON

Each Golgi tendon organ is a slender capsule within the tendon in series with 15 to 20 extrafusal skeletal

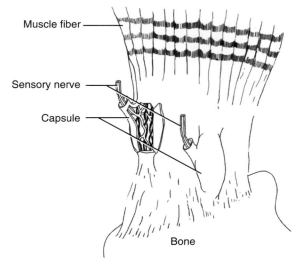

FIGURE 7–4. The Golgi tendon organ is a stretch receptor located in the tendons of skeletal muscle. It detects tension in the tendon and sends information about this tension to the central nervous system.

muscle fibers (Fig. 7–4). Each tendon organ has an afferent sensory nerve that carries action potentials to the CNS. The Golgi tendon organ has no motor innervation.

As mentioned, the Golgi tendon organ is in series with the extrafusal fibers; therefore, when the fibers contract, the tendon organ is stretched, and action potentials are generated and sent to the CNS along the sensory nerve at a frequency proportional to the tension developed by the muscle. In contrast, the muscle spindle is arranged in parallel with the extrafusal muscle fibers, and when they contract, the spindle reduces its action potential frequency.

When action potentials along the spindle sensory nerve reach the CNS, as mentioned earlier, they cause reflex EPSP stimulation to the α motor neurons returning to the same muscle. Action potentials along the sensory nerves from the Golgi tendon organ have the opposite effect: they cause inhibitory postsynaptic potentials (IPSPs) on the α motor neuron, leading to a reduced extrafusal muscle fiber contraction.

These two skeletal muscle stretch receptors provide the CNS with vital information about muscle length (the spindle) and muscle tension (the Golgi tendon organ). Such information is essential if the CNS is to adequately coordinate posture and locomotion.

CLINICAL CORRELATIONS

Femoral nerve mononeuropathy

History You examine an 8-year-old male golden retriever. The owner complains that the dog cannot bear weight on his right rear leg.

Clinical Examination Physical examination deficits are limited to the right rear leg, where you find that the quadriceps femoris muscles of this leg are much smaller than those of the left rear leg. The dog cannot bear weight on the right rear leg because the right quadriceps femoris muscles are paralyzed. When you tap on the left patellar tendon with a reflex hammer, the knee briskly extends (the knee jerk or muscle stretch reflex). However, when you tap on the right patellar tendon, no movement occurs.

Comment The quadriceps femoris muscle group is one of the major antigravity muscle groups of the leg causing the stifle joint (knee joint) to extend. The paralysis in this animal's quadriceps muscle is the reason why he cannot bear weight on the leg. The small size of the right quadriceps muscle is caused by atrophy, or muscle wasting, which in turn is caused by the loss of the α motor neuron to the extrafusal muscle fibers in the quadriceps muscle belly (see Chapter 8). This would also cause a loss of the muscle stretch reflex, because even though the spindle sensed the stretch of the muscle belly caused by either gravity or the reflex hammer, the α motor neuron returning to the quadriceps muscle is unable to signal the muscle to contract, hence completing the reflex arc. This syndrome could occur if the femoral nerve is damaged by a tumor or trauma. If the pathologic lesion were in the peripheral nerve rather than only in the ventral roots, then there would likely be some sensory loss in addition to the motor deficits.

Treatment This is a femoral nerve mononeuropathy. Its treatment would depend on the cause of the nerve damage (e.g., trauma, neoplasia, inflammation).

Bibliography

Guyton AC, Hall JE: Textbook of Medical Physiology, 10th ed. Philadelphia: WB Saunders, 2000, pp 622–633.
Haines DE: Fundamental Neuroscience. New York: Churchill Livingstone, 1997, pp 335–346.
Kandel ER, Schwartz JH, Jessell TM (eds): Principles of Neural Science, 4th ed. New York: McGraw-Hill, 2000, pp 713–736.

PRACTICE QUESTIONS

1. As the distance between the origin and insertion tendons is increased (the muscle is stretched), what happens to the frequency of action potentials along the sensory nerve from the muscle spindle in that muscle?
    a. Increases.
    b. Decreases.
    c. Does not change.

2. Activation of the Golgi tendon organ leads to
    a. EPSPs to the α motor neuron that returns to that muscle.
    b. EPSPs to the α motor neuron innervating the antagonist muscle.
    c. EPSPs to the γ motor neuron innervating the antagonist muscle.
    d. IPSPs to the α motor neuron that returns to that muscle.
    e. IPSPs to the γ motor neuron innervating that antagonist muscle.

3. The muscle spindle receptor in skeletal muscle can be stimulated to generate action potentials by

a. contraction of the extrafusal fiber.
b. contraction of the intrafusal fiber.
c. passive stretch of the whole muscle.
d. stimulation of the γ motor neuron.
e. b, c, and d.

4. Which of the following situations will *not* lead to action potentials on the sensory nerve coming from the muscle spindle?

a. Contractions of the extrafusal muscle fibers in the muscle antagonistic to the muscle in which the spindle is being recorded.
b. Contraction of the intrafusal muscle fibers within the recorded spindle.
c. Contraction of the extrafusal muscle fibers in the muscle in which the spindle is being recorded.
d. Passive stretch of the muscle in which the spindle is being recorded.

e. Stimulation of the γ motor neuron to the muscle in which the spindle is being recorded.

5. Which of the following is *not* a component of the γ loop to an extensor muscle?

a. The α motor neuron to the extensor muscle.
b. The γ motor neuron to the extensor muscle.
c. The muscle spindle in the extensor muscle.
d. The extrafusal muscle fiber of the extensor fiber.
e. The α motor nerve of the antagonistic flexor muscle.

PRACTICE ANSWERS

1. a   2. d   3. e   4. c   5. e

8

The concept of lower and upper motor neurons and their malfunction

1 The lower motor neuron is classically defined as the α motor neuron

2 Disease of lower motor neurons causes stereotypical clinical signs

3 Upper motor neurons are in the central nervous system

4 Signs of upper motor neuron disease differ from those of lower motor neuron disease

The majority of veterinary patients with neurologic disease display some abnormality of posture and locomotion; the abnormalities span a range from weakness or paralysis to spasticity, rigidity, and convulsions. The goal of the diagnostic process is deciding where such a patient's lesion is located and what the lesion is. Central to diagnostic logic in neurology is deciding whether the patient's lesion is located in the lower motor neurons or the upper motor neurons. (The two other possible locations of lesions causing movement disorders are the neuromuscular junction and skeletal muscle.) This chapter defines lower and upper motor neurons, because these concepts are useful in understanding the physiology of posture and locomotion and are essential in locating pathologic processes in the nervous system.

Malfunctions of these two neuron populations are also described briefly.

THE LOWER MOTOR NEURON IS CLASSICALLY DEFINED AS THE α MOTOR NEURON

The concept of a lower motor neuron is decades old in neurology. The α motor neuron is classically defined as a neuron whose cell body and dendrites are located in the central nervous system and whose axon extends out through the peripheral nerves to synapse with the extrafusal skeletal muscle fibers. This is the final common pathway through which the central nervous system channels commands to the extrafusal skeletal muscle. This definition predates the discovery of γ motor neurons, which innervate muscle spindles, and some authors would include γ motor neurons in

the definition of lower motor neurons. Yet all the clinical signs caused by lower motor neuron disease can be explained by the loss of the α motor neuron.

DISEASE OF LOWER MOTOR NEURONS CAUSES STEREOTYPICAL CLINICAL SIGNS

Regardless of the pathologic basis for disease of lower motor neurons, a stereotypical set of clinical signs results in the skeletal muscles they innervate.

1. *Paralysis.* Disease of the α motor neurons usually prevents the nerve's action potentials from reaching the neuromuscular junction. Therefore, despite the brain's intention to command the muscle to contract, the message cannot get to the muscle, and paralysis is the result. In fact, such paralysis is usually so complete that the adjective *flaccid* is used to describe the paralysis in which no muscle contraction occurs.

2. *Atrophy.* Atrophy means the shrinking or wasting of skeletal muscle mass distal to the lower motor neuron lesion. This occurs within days of the injury to the nerve. The origins of this atrophy are the subject of controversy. Some physiologists believe that nerves produce nutrients transmitted across the synapse and needed for the muscle's health. Lack of such nutrients, as a result of the loss of the lower motor neuron, would then lead to atrophy. (The word *atrophy* comes from the Greek word meaning "without food," so Greek philosophers may have been particularly farsighted in choosing this term.) However, other physiologists now believe that it is

simply a matter of the frequency with which the muscle is stimulated, because denervation atrophy can be reduced by electrical stimulation of the muscle itself.

3. *Loss of segmental and intersegmental reflexes.* Segmental and intersegmental reflexes (see Chapter 6) require the α motor neuron in the reflex arc in order for the reflex response to occur. Hence, such reflexes as the muscle stretch reflex, toe-pinch withdrawal (nociceptive) reflex, and conscious proprioception do not occur, because the motor nerve portion of the arc is gone.

Because diseases of the motor nerve occur often in a mixed peripheral nerve that also contains sensory nerve axons, there may be loss of sensory modalities. This sensory loss is not, strictly speaking, a sign of lower motor neuron loss.

UPPER MOTOR NEURONS ARE IN THE CENTRAL NERVOUS SYSTEM

Upper motor neurons are all the neurons of the central nervous system that influence the lower motor neuron. In the next chapter, upper motor neurons are subdivided into three subsystems: the pyramidal system, the extrapyramidal system, and the cerebellum. For now, upper motor neurons may be thought of as multineuronal systems beginning in the brain but sending axons down the spinal cord or into the brainstem to synapse with the lower motor neurons.

SIGNS OF UPPER MOTOR NEURON DISEASE DIFFER FROM THOSE OF LOWER MOTOR NEURON DISEASE

Lesions of upper motor neurons cause clinical signs that are significantly different from those produced by lower motor neuron disease.

1. *Inappropriate movement.* In contrast to the inevitable paralysis resulting from lower motor neuron disease, lesions of upper motor neurons cause a variety of movement disorders, depending on the location of the lesion. Spinal cord disease usually causes various degrees of weakness below the lesion, whereas disease of the brain may cause seizures, rigidity, circling gaits, inability of the animal to know the position of limbs (proprioceptive deficits), and other inappropriate movements. A more precise description of this general category is presented in the Chapters 9, 10, and 11 on the brain's control of posture and locomotion, on the vestibular apparatus, and on the cerebellum.

2. *No atrophy.* Because the lower motor neuron is intact, the muscle does not atrophy. (Modest disuse atrophy may develop much later.)

3. *Retained segmental reflexes.* Because the neuronal circuit or the segmental reflex arc (see Chapter 6) is not interrupted in upper motor neuron disease, reflexes such as the muscle stretch and toe-pinch withdrawal reflexes are retained, whereas in lower motor neuron disease, all reflexes are lost.

The following clinical correlations illustrate common examples of lower and upper motor neuron disease. Before reading Chapter 9, the reader should understand these concepts and why these dogs have the clinical signs they do.

CLINICAL CORRELATIONS

Lower motor neuron disease

History A 2-year-old male German short-haired pointer dog was admitted to the local veterinary clinic. His vaccinations were current, and there was no history of contributing prior illness.

A few days before admission, the dog had had a fight with a skunk. For 48 hours before admission, an ascending paralysis developed, characterized first by weakness, and then by the lack of voluntary movement, of first the back legs and then the front legs. No barking was noticed during the illness. He was able to control his bladder and bowel and to move his head.

Clinical Examination On admission, the dog was unable to bear weight on any of his four legs. Other than an elevated respiratory rate, physical examination deficits were limited to the nervous system. He was able to eat, drink, and move his head. A dense paralysis was noted in all legs, and no motor response to a toe pinch or tapping of the quadriceps tendon could be elicited. There was widespread atrophy of the muscles of all four legs, as well as those of the thorax and abdomen. The dog did seem to be aware of painful stimuli. There were no cranial nerve deficits. Results of routine blood cell counts and serum chemistry results were within normal limits.

Comment Generalized atrophy, paralysis, and loss of segmental reflexes indicate widespread, bilateral loss of lower motor neuron function. Fortunately, the disease has spared the muscles of the head and the diaphragm, although the elevated respiratory rate indicates an attempt to compensate for paralysis of some of the respiratory muscles. A clinical diagnosis of polyradiculoneuritis (or coonhound paralysis) was made. This disease is often preceded by the bite of another animal. Pathologic changes are found predominantly in the ventral roots of the spinal cord where the axons of the lower motor neurons leave the spinal cord. The dorsal roots are usually spared; hence this dog's apparent ability to feel pain. The clinical signs are those of widespread lower motor neuron disease. The syndrome resembles Guillain-Barré syndrome in humans, and both syndromes have been suggested to be autoimmune in origin.

Treatment Animals with this form of paralysis usually recover spontaneously. Good nursing care is essential during the illness. A respirator may be necessary temporarily if respiratory paralysis occurs.

Upper motor neuron disease

History   A 5-year-old male dachshund is brought to a local veterinary clinic. His vaccination history is current, and he has had no contributing past medical or surgical illnesses. Two days before his admission he seemed to be in pain. Throughout the next day he became progressively weak in his hind legs.

Clinical Examination   Physical examination abnormalities were limited to the nervous system. The dog was bright, alert, responsive, and able to bear weight normally on his front legs. However, he was weak and unsteady on his hind legs. No atrophy was apparent. All cranial nerve reflexes were normal, as were the spinal segmental reflexes of both front and hind legs. Intersegmental responses were normal in the front legs but absent in the hind legs. (Such responses include conscious proprioception of a paw's being placed upside down while the animal's weight is supported. Normally an animal realizes the paw is in an unusual position and returns the paw to the correct, pads-down position. Failure to do this promptly indicates a lesion somewhere along the sensory or motor routing for this response. This routing includes the peripheral nerves for that limb, the spinal cord rostral to that limb on the same side, and the contralateral side of the brain.) Results of a complete blood cell count and serum chemistry analysis were within normal limits.

Comment   The absence of atrophy and the retention of segmental reflexes in the affected limbs indicate that the lower motor neurons, neuromuscular junction, and skeletal muscle are normal and that this is an upper motor neuron disease. Because only the hind limbs are affected by weakness and proprioceptive deficits, the cervical spinal cord and brain must be normal, as motor commands to the front legs are transmitted reliably. Therefore, the lesion must be between the front and hind limbs. This is a typical history and a typical clinical presentation for a dog with a herniated intervertebral disk.

Treatment   Treatment and prognosis depend on the severity of the spinal cord trauma. Medical management is aimed at reducing edema, vasospasm, and other metabolic consequences of the disease that make the damage to the spinal cord worse. When surgery is indicated by the severity of the trauma, its goal is to relieve spinal cord compression. With appropriate medical and surgical management, many dogs recover useful spinal function.

Bibliography

Kandel ER, Schwartz JH, Jessell TM (eds): Principles of Neural Science, 4th ed. New York: McGraw-Hill, 2000, pp 695–712.

PRACTICE QUESTIONS

1. You examine a dog that is unable to stand and bear weight on the right rear leg. The right rear leg is much smaller in diameter than the left rear leg. Pinching the toe on the left rear leg results in withdrawal of the left rear leg, but pinching the toe on the right rear leg results in no movement of the right rear leg. Conscious proprioception response to the left rear leg is normal but to the right rear leg is absent. Where is this dog's pathologic lesion?
   a. Lower motor neuron to the right rear leg.
   b. Lower motor neuron to the left rear leg.
   c. Upper motor neuron to the right rear leg.
   d. Upper motor neuron to the left rear leg.
   e. Neuromuscular synapse of the right rear leg.

2. You examine a dog that is bright, alert, and responsive. She can stand and bear weight on both her front legs, but she cannot stand or bear any weight on her back legs. Her knee-jerk and toe-pinch withdrawal reflexes are normal in all four legs. There is no atrophy. A conscious proprioception response is normal in the front legs but absent in both rear legs. Injecting acetylcholinesterase-inhibiting drugs causes no change in the clinical signs. Where is the dog's pathologic lesion?
   a. Brain.
   b. Cervical spinal cord (spinal cord of the neck).
   c. Spinal cord between the front and rear legs (thoracolumbar spinal cord).
   d. Lower motor neurons to the rear legs.
   e. Neuromuscular junction.

3. You examine a dog that is bright, alert, and responsive but unable to stand on any of his four legs. Toe-pinch and knee-jerk local (segmental) reflexes are normal in all four legs. There is no atrophy. A conscious proprioception response is absent in all four legs. Injecting an acetylcholinesterase-inhibiting drug does not change the clinical signs. Where is this dog's pathologic lesion?
   a. Brain.
   b. Cervical spinal cord (spinal cord in the neck).
   c. Spinal cord between the front and rear legs (thoracolumbar spinal cord).
   d. Lower motor neurons to all four legs.
   e. Neuromuscular junction.

4. You are presented with a horse that is unable to stand or support any weight on his hind legs. You electrically stimulate both the sciatic and femoral nerves with a sufficient stimulus, but neither stimulation results in muscular contraction. However, direct stimulation of both the gastrocnemius and quadriceps femoris muscles of the rear leg results in muscular contraction. From these observations, what do you logically conclude to be the location of this horse's pathologic lesion?
   a. Upper motor neurons to the rear legs.
   b. Lower motor neurons to the rear legs.
   c. Neuromuscular synapses of the rear legs.
   d. Muscles of the rear legs.
   e. Either b or c.

5. You examine a cat that cannot bear weight on her hind legs. She is bright, alert, and responsive. Atrophy is present in the back legs. Cranial nerve reflexes are within normal limits, as are segmental reflexes and conscious proprioception to the front legs. Knee-jerk and toe-pinch withdrawal reflexes are absent in

the hind legs. What is the most likely location for this cat's pathologic lesion?

a. Brain.
b. Cervical spinal cord.
c. Thoracolumbar spinal cord.
d. Lower motor neurons to the front legs.
e. Lower motor neurons to the hind legs.

PRACTICE ANSWERS

1. a   2. c   3. b   4. e   5. e

9

The brain's control of posture and locomotion

1   The central nervous system can be divided into six anatomic regions
2   The pyramidal system consists of two major axon pathways descending from the cerebral cortex
3   Pyramidal system axons originate from particular regions of the cerebral cortex
4   The pyramidal system initiates voluntary, discrete, often learned movements
5   Pyramidal system axons influence both α and γ lower motor neurons
6   Lesions in the pyramidal system cause contralateral weakness and loss of proprioception

7   The extrapyramidal system has three major tracts descending from the brainstem to influence spinal lower motor neurons
8   The extrapyramidal system maintains postural muscle tone in proximal, antigravity extensor muscles
9   The role of the basal ganglia is poorly understood
10   The cerebral cortex plays a role in extrapyramidal system function
11   Clinical syndromes resulting from extrapyramidal system lesions may include either rhythmic or nonrhythmic movement disorders

Movement can be divided into two general forms. The first is a largely learned, voluntary, conscious, and skilled form, usually mediated by flexor muscles. The second is characterized by a postural, antigravity muscle tone that is generally subconscious, involuntary, and the result of extensor muscle contraction. The skilled, flexor-mediated movement results from fairly discrete contraction of a few muscle groups, many of which are distal to the spinal column. Standing is always opposed by gravity. Hence, postural muscle tone must result from continuing contraction of larger groups of extensor antigravity muscles, many of which are located closer to the spinal column.

Unlike the sensory system, which transforms physical energy into neural information, the motor system transforms neural information into physical energy. All movement is the result of the contraction of varying numbers of extrafusal skeletal muscle fibers within varying numbers of motor units. These extrafusal muscle fibers do not contract until commanded to do so by the α lower motor neuron. The α motor neuron, in turn, does not send such an action potential command until signaled to do so by descending upper motor neurons from the brain or from incoming sensory nerves in a reflex arc. Hence, the α motor neuron is the final common neural pathway by which the brain can initiate the extrafusal muscle contractions that result in both voluntary and antigravity movements.

Initiating the learned, skilled, voluntary movement is largely the responsibility of a subgroup of upper motor neurons called the *pyramidal system.* Initiating antigravity, postural extensor muscle tone is the responsibility of the upper motor neurons that constitute the *extrapyramidal system.* A third subgroup of upper motor neurons, those of the *cerebellum,* helps coordinate movement initiated by either the pyramidal or the extrapyramidal system. It constantly compares the intended movement with the actual movement and makes appropriate adjustments. The cerebellum is discussed in Chapter 11. Before discussion of the pyramidal and extrapyramidal systems, however, some general principles of neuroanatomy must first be mentioned.

THE CENTRAL NERVOUS SYSTEM CAN BE DIVIDED INTO SIX ANATOMIC REGIONS

The central nervous system (CNS) has an axial organization: the phylogenetically oldest part (the spinal cord) is caudal, and the newest portions (the cerebral cortex) are rostral. The CNS can be divided into six major regions (Fig. 9–1):

1. The *spinal cord* is the most caudal region in the CNS. As mentioned in Chapter 2, it receives action potentials along sensory dorsal root axons from receptors in the skin, muscles, tendons, joints, and visceral organs. It contains the cell bodies and dendrites of

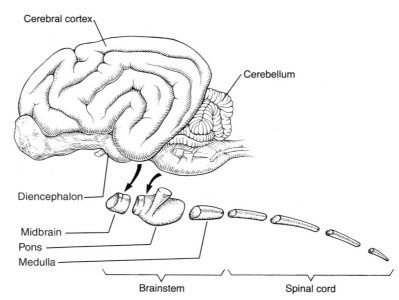

FIGURE 9–1. The central nervous system (CNS) has an axial organization in which the phylogenetically oldest part (the spinal cord) is caudal and the newest part (the cerebral cortex) is rostral. The CNS can be divided into six major regions: the spinal cord, the medulla, the pons, the midbrain, the diencephalon, and the cerebral hemispheres.

the lower motor neurons whose axons exit through the ventral roots to reach skeletal muscles. The spinal cord also contains axons carrying sensory information to the brain and motor commands from the brain to the lower motor neurons. The spinal cord is continued rostrally as the *brainstem,* which consists of the next three major regions of the CNS.

2. The *medulla* is the most rostral extension of the spinal cord, resembling it in many ways. It also contains several cranial nerve motor nuclei and centers for controlling the respiratory and cardiovascular systems.

3. The *pons* lies rostral to the medulla and contains the cell bodies of large numbers of neurons in a two-neuron chain that relays information from the cerebral cortex to the *cerebellum.* The cerebellum is not a part of the brainstem but is usually described along with the pons because of its position dorsal to the pons in the posterior fossa. The cerebellum is important in coordination of movement and motor learning.

4. The *midbrain* lies rostral to the pons and is important in eye movement and subconscious postural control. Each region of the brainstem contains axon tracts carrying action potentials back and forth between the spinal cord and the rostral portion of the brain. The brainstem also contains the *reticular formation,* a net-like complex of many small neurons that regulates consciousness and modifies spinal reflexes.

5. The *diencephalon* contains the *thalamus,* a relay station for sensory systems projecting into the cerebral cortex, and the *hypothalamus,* which regulates the autonomic nervous system and hormone secretion of the pituitary gland.

6. The *cerebral hemispheres* are made up of the cerebral cortex and the basal ganglia. Collectively called the *cerebrum,* these structures are associated with higher motor and sensory functions and with consciousness.

The CNS surrounds a system of interconnected cav-

ities called *ventricles* that contain cerebrospinal fluid (see Chapter 14).

The sensory, motor, and consciousness systems of the brain have several distinct pathways arranged in parallel. For instance, both the visual and the auditory system have separate, parallel systems, and the motor system has the parallel pyramidal and extrapyramidal tracts. Each of these pathways contains synaptic relay stations along its routes and is usually topographically organized. Most pathways are crossed for unknown reasons.

Keeping these principles in mind allows a better understanding of the anatomy and function of the pyramidal and extrapyramidal systems. It also helps in appreciating the complexity of this remarkable evolutionary biologic achievement.

THE PYRAMIDAL SYSTEM CONSISTS OF TWO MAJOR AXON PATHWAYS DESCENDING FROM THE CEREBRAL CORTEX

All axons within the pyramidal system originate from neurons located in the fifth of the six histologic layers of the cerebral cortex. These pyramidal upper motor neuron axons then extend to terminations in two different regions of the CNS. Like most axon tracts within the CNS, they are named for their sites of origin and termination.

The longest of the two pyramidal system tracts, the *corticospinal tract,* begins in the cerebral cortex and ends in the contralateral (opposite) side of the spinal cord (Fig. 9–2). Along its route, it descends from the cerebral cortex through the internal capsule, diencephalon, mesencephalon, and pons. At the point where it reaches to the medulla oblongata, about 90% of corticospinal tract axons cross to the opposite side of the nervous system and continue descending to

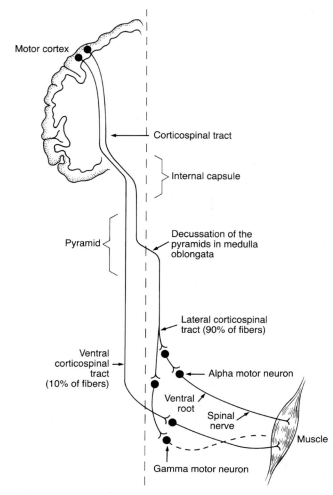

FIGURE 9–2. The corticospinal tract begins in the cerebral cortex and ends in the contralateral side of the spinal cord to influence both α and γ lower motor neurons.

An additional set of axon tracts, a companion to the pyramidal system's descending axon tracts, is the *corticopontine-cerebellar tract* system. It too begins in the cerebral cortex and descends into the brainstem to reach the pons, where it synapses with a second neuron whose axons sweep up predominantly to the contralateral cerebellar cortex (see Chapter 11). Although this structure is not, strictly speaking, a part of the pyramidal system, its role is to inform the cerebellum of movement intended by the cerebral cortex, so that if the actual movement is not the one intended, the cerebellum can make appropriate adjustments.

PYRAMIDAL SYSTEM AXONS ORIGINATE FROM PARTICULAR REGIONS OF THE CEREBRAL CORTEX

Even though all axons of the pyramidal system originate from neurons in layer V of the cerebral cortex, not all regions of the cerebral cortex give rise to pyramidal system axons. The cerebral cortex, as seen grossly from a lateral view, is anatomically subdivided into four major regions, or lobes: the frontal, parietal, occipital, and temporal lobes (Fig. 9–3). The cerebral cortex is also functionally subdivided. The pyramidal system arises disproportionately from the *motor cortex*, a limited area of the frontal cortex. In humans, the motor cortex is located just rostral to the central sulcus and therefore is called the *precentral gyrus*. Its boundaries are not as well understood in most animals, but the motor cortex is located generally in the region of the cruciate sulcus.

Pyramidal tract axons also arise from three other cortical areas: from an area just rostral to the motor cortex, called the *premotor cortex*; from the *parietal sensory cortex*; and from a *supplementary motor cortex* on the medial surface of the frontal lobe.

These origins of the pyramidal system axons have

end near lower motor neurons on the contralateral side of the spinal cord. The remaining 10% of the axons descend ipsilaterally into the spinal cord, but most of these axons also cross at a segmental level before influencing contralateral lower motor neurons. As the corticospinal axons descend through the medulla oblongata, they pass through a section of the ventral medulla that looks like a pyramid when seen in cross section. This is probably the origin of the term *pyramidal* system. The extrapyramidal system, described later, is so named because as its axons travel through the medulla oblongata, they pass outside these pyramids.

The second pyramidal system tract to leave the cerebral cortex is the *corticobulbar tract* (*bulb* is an archaic term for medulla). These axons follow the same route as the corticospinal tract axons, but they terminate in the brainstem. Hence, they influence brainstem lower motor neurons to muscles of the head, whereas the corticospinal tract influences spinal lower motor neurons.

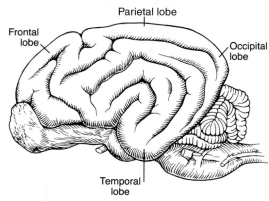

FIGURE 9–3. The cerebral cortex, as seen grossly from the lateral view, is anatomically subdivided into four major regions, or lobes: the frontal, parietal, occipital, and temporal lobes. The cerebral cortex is also functionally divided, and the pyramidal system arises disproportionately from the motor cortex, a limited area of the frontal cortex.

been discovered through anatomic and electrophysiologic techniques and more recently explored by means of special radiographic imaging. Retrograde axonal degeneration can be traced up into the cortex after sectioning of the pyramids of the medulla oblongata. The presence or absence of movement of the contralateral side of the body can be observed also after electrical stimulation of the cerebral cortex. These latter electrical stimulation studies have been best developed in humans, in whom surgical removal of epileptogenic cortical lesions must often be preceded by electrical stimulation studies to ensure that essential areas of the cortex are left intact. Similar studies have been performed with several species of animals.

Phylogenetically, the corticospinal and corticobulbar tracts first appeared in mammals. The higher the mammal phylogenetically, the more sophisticated the motor representation is in the motor cortex. This parallels the increasing ability to carry out skilled, voluntary movement. Hence, in higher mammals, and particularly in primates, the motor cortex can be represented by a distorted somatotopic map of the body. It disproportionately represents muscles of the body responsible for skilled, learned movements. Figure 9–4 depicts the case of the phylogenetically highest mammal, the human, in whom muscles for the hand and mouth are disproportionately represented because these are the muscles needed for grasping and for speech. The map of the motor cortex of the cat is also shown.

The distribution of corticospinal tract axons within the spinal cord is also influenced by phylogeny. In primates and carnivores, corticospinal axons go to both the front and the rear legs, whereas in the horse, most go only to the front legs.

FIGURE 9–4. The map of the motor cortex, noting the origins of axons going to the skeletal muscles of the body, is a disproportionate representation of the body's shape. Note that in the phylogenetically highest mammal, the human *(A)*, muscles of the hand and mouth are disproportionately represented because these muscles are needed for grasping and for speech. The motor cortex of a cat *(B)* is also represented. (*A*, Redrawn from Penfield W, Rasmussen T: The Cerebral Cortex of Man. New York: Macmillan, 1950; used with permission from Berne RM, Levy MN: Physiology, 2nd ed. St. Louis: CV Mosby, 1988. *B*, From Prosser CL: Comparative Animal Physiology, 3rd ed. New York: Wiley, 1988.)

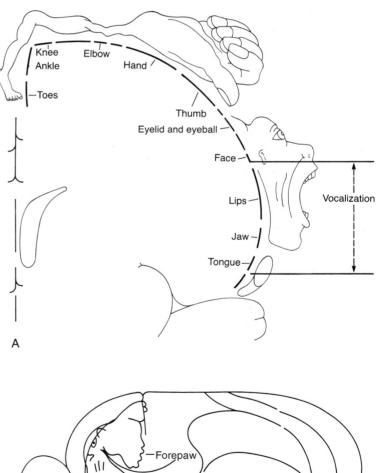

A

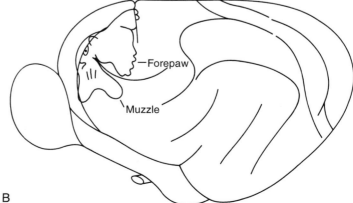

B

THE PYRAMIDAL SYSTEM INITIATES VOLUNTARY, DISCRETE, OFTEN LEARNED MOVEMENTS

The pyramidal system initiates skilled, learned, voluntary movement through its influence on lower motor neurons of the contralateral side of the body. Extrafusal muscle fibers responsible for bringing about such movement tend to be flexor muscles of joints distal to the spine. It is not known how the various areas of the cerebral cortex interact before sending their final action potential commands down the pyramidal tract axons. It seems likely that before the cerebral cortex can send a command to the lower motor neuron, a motor plan of action must be designed. Such a plan would have to include the selection of a sequence of muscular contractions designed to accomplish the desired movement, and it would have to specify how much each muscle must contract. It also seems likely that the premotor cortex and the supplementary motor cortex play important roles in generating such a plan, perhaps in concert with the basal ganglia. The sensory cortex probably also plays an important role in providing spatial information for targeting movement and for some error correction, although the cerebellum and the muscle spindle reflex circuit are probably more important in error correction. This complex interplay of interconnected portions of the cerebral cortex results ultimately in a final set of action potential commands sent down the corticospinal and corticobulbar tract axons to influence the contralateral lower motor neurons. An exact copy of this command of intended movement is sent also to the cerebellum along the corticopontine-cerebellar tract. Here it is compared with the cerebellum's knowledge of what movement is actually occurring so that any appropriate adjustments can be made.

PYRAMIDAL SYSTEM AXONS INFLUENCE BOTH α AND γ LOWER MOTOR NEURONS

The corticospinal tract axons descend the central nervous system to influence lower motor neurons in the contralateral spinal cord; corticobulbar tract axons influence lower motor neurons of the brainstem, usually on the contralateral side. This influence is exerted over both α and γ lower motor neurons (see Chapter 7), usually through short interneurons in the immediate neighborhood of the lower motor neuron. (Some direct, monosynaptic connections to the lower motor neurons are found in primates.)

The simultaneous activation of both α and γ lower motor neurons is known as *coactivation*. These synaptic influences over the α motor neuron allow the pyramidal tract axons to command the intended movement by causing contraction of the appropriate extrafusal muscle fibers. The role of the simultaneous coactivation of the γ motor neuron to the intrafusal muscle fiber, however, is less clear. One likely function of this coactivation is to cause shortening of the intrafusal muscle fiber along with extrafusal muscle fiber. The spindle would shorten along with the whole muscle and therefore would maintain its sensitivity to muscle stretch, regardless of the overall length of the muscle.

An error-correction, or servo-assist, function for coactivation of the γ motor neurons has also been hypothesized, but this concept is not as well accepted by physiologists. In this role, the coactivation of γ motor neurons would lead to additional excitatory postsynaptic potentials (EPSPs) on the α motor neuron, by way of the γ loop, if the initial pyramidal tract stimulation of the α motor neuron failed to cause the intended amount of extrafusal fiber contraction. If the initial stimulation of the α motor neuron motor unit is sufficient, the intended shortening would occur and no servo-assist would be necessary from the γ loop. However, if the initial α stimulation of extrafusal fibers is not sufficient to cause the desired contraction, coactivation of the γ motor neurons would have caused shortening of the intrafusal fibers even though the spindle itself had not shortened. This would lead to more reflex EPSPs onto the α motor neuron by way of the γ loop. In this way, through coactivation, the local, segmental γ loop reflex circuit helps accomplish the intended contraction if the initial α motor neuron stimulation from the pyramidal system is insufficient. This would occur if the load opposing contraction was underestimated by the cerebral cortex. Such coactivation would work much like the power steering in a car, in which a compressor in the motor adds power to the driver's turning of the steering wheel when large resistance is encountered by the tires.

LESIONS IN THE PYRAMIDAL SYSTEM CAUSE CONTRALATERAL WEAKNESS AND LOSS OF PROPRIOCEPTION

The severity of the deficits resulting from lesions of the pyramidal system varies with the evolutionary development of the animal. In primates, such as humans, in whom the pyramidal system is developed extensively, pyramidal tract lesions cause a dense weakness of the contralateral side of the body. Such one-sided weakness is called *hemiparesis* and is most extensive in the hand and facial muscles (e.g., that caused by "stroke" in humans). In most veterinary species, the pyramidal system is not as well developed, and pyramidal system lesions cause much less severe contralateral weakness and almost no alteration of gait. However, pyramidal upper motor neuron lesions in veterinary species do cause important postural response deficits in the contralateral limbs. An example is the *conscious proprioception response*, the ability of an animal to return its paw to a normal, pads-down posture when the paw is turned upside down. This response requires the animal's conscious awareness that the paw is upside down (proprioception) and then requires that the animal be able to respond consciously by returning the paw to its normal posture. This latter motor response, in turn, requires the integrity of the upper motor neurons of the corticospinal tract. When these corticospinal tract neurons are damaged, the animal is slow to return its paw to a normal posture. In addition, toes tend to be dragged on the ground as the leg is drawn forward in normal gait. Noting these conscious proprioception response deficits and other subtle gait changes is important in localizing lesions within the CNS.

▬ THE EXTRAPYRAMIDAL SYSTEM HAS THREE MAJOR TRACTS DESCENDING FROM THE BRAINSTEM TO INFLUENCE SPINAL LOWER MOTOR NEURONS

The pyramidal system has a relatively simple neuroanatomy. Its two tracts begin in the cerebral cortex and end in the spinal cord and brainstem. With the exception of the pyramidal system's corticospinal tract, all other descending upper motor neuron axon tracts that influence spinal lower motor neurons begin in the brainstem. These are all part of the much more complex *extrapyramidal system.*

The extrapyramidal system has three major descending axon tracts that leave the brainstem to influence spinal lower motor neurons. Like most other tracts in the CNS, they are named for the places at which they begin and end. The first is the *reticulospinal tract,* which begins in the reticular activating system in the middle of the medulla oblongata, pons, and mid-brain. It ends on or near a diffuse population of spinal, mostly γ lower motor neurons to more proximal extensor muscles. The second, the *vestibulospinal tract,* begins in the medullary vestibular nuclei and ends on a similarly diffuse population of spinal neurons, although this particular tract may influence more α than γ lower motor neurons. The third, the *tectospinal tract,* begins in the visual tectum and ends on the lower motor neurons of the rostral spinal cord. Each of these extrapyramidal tracts is influenced by other, more rostral parts of the brain.

▬ THE EXTRAPYRAMIDAL SYSTEM MAINTAINS POSTURAL MUSCLE TONE IN PROXIMAL, ANTIGRAVITY EXTENSOR MUSCLES

The responsibility of the extrapyramidal system is to maintain subconscious postural antigravity muscle tone. This muscle tone is found in extensor muscles, whose contraction opposes gravity's pull on the body toward the earth. It is generally found in more proximal muscle groups located near the spinal column. In contrast, the pyramidal system, as mentioned earlier, initiates voluntary movement in more distal, usually flexor muscles. These two systems must work together, because voluntary movement requires postural adjustments. Much of the coordination between these two upper motor neuron systems is performed by the cerebellum. In the paragraphs that follow, the function of the separate, descending extrapyramidal tracts is described to illustrate how the tracts contribute to the general function of antigravity muscle tone.

The *reticulospinal tract* originates in the reticular activating system found in the medial medulla oblongata, pons, and mid-brain. The *reticular activating system,* often called the *reticular formation,* is a complex of small, net-like neurons that anatomically are an extension of the spinal cord into the brainstem. Once thought to be a diffuse and fairly nonspecific system, the reticular formation is now known to contain a number of functionally specific nuclei. One such functionally specific set of neurons consists of those giving rise to the reticulospinal tract. Many neurons of the reticular formation are tonically active, both as the result of stimulation from ascending, sensory axons with branches into the reticular formation and as the result of intrinsic activity of reticular formation neurons themselves.

This tonic activity within the reticular formation gives rise to action potentials departing rostrally into the cerebral cortex to cause general arousal, the absence of which leads to coma, and caudally along the reticulospinal tract to influence particularly γ lower motor neurons of the γ loop (Fig. 9–5). Action potentials on axons of the reticulospinal tract cause EPSPs in γ motor neurons to antigravity extensor muscles. Through the γ loop (see Chapter 7) the extrafusal muscle fibers of these muscles are, in a reflexive manner, made to contract, resulting in postural muscle tone. The reticular activating system is influenced by the more rostral basal ganglia and cerebral cortex, which tends to reduce the EPSP stimulation of the γ loop. Action potentials descending in this system are the major stimulus to antigravity postural muscle tone. Although the relationship among the cerebral cortex, basal ganglia, and the reticular activating system is currently poorly understood, these three struc-

FIGURE 9–5. The reticular activating system stimulates the γ loop, leading to contraction of antigravity extensor muscles. The basal ganglia and cerebral cortex somehow refine the amount of this γ loop stimulation so that movement is appropriate.

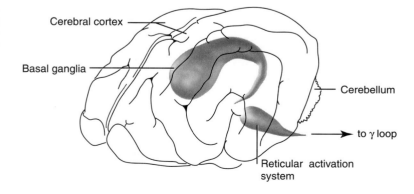

tures somehow collaborate to create the specific amount of antigravity extensor muscle contraction appropriate for normal movement.

Some muscle tone is also contributed by action potentials along the *vestibulospinal tract* axons. These axons arise from the vestibular nuclei in the medulla oblongata and descend to influence some α but mainly γ lower motor neurons to proximal antigravity muscles. Vestibular nuclei neurons are also tonically active as the result of tonic sensory axon input from the inner ear's vestibular system (see Chapter 10). As changes in head position are detected by the vestibular system receptors, the vestibulospinal tract neurons make appropriate adjustments in postural muscle tone to maintain the desired balance.

The functions of these two extrapyramidal system neuron tracts can be better understood by considering the mechanisms of the clinical state called *decerebrate rigidity*. This condition occasionally occurs as the result of severe rostral brain disease. It also results from surgical transection of the brain at the mid-brain level, as discovered by the British neurophysiologist Charles Sherrington. This transection functionally disconnects the EPSP-producing reticulospinal tract from more rostral brain areas that reduced its output. The result is an overactive reticulospinal tract and vestibulospinal tract, causing an excess of EPSPs on γ motor neurons to antigravity muscles. The animal assumes a hobby-horse-like posture, often so rigid that the animal stands in a fixed position. Because this rigidity is the result of overactive γ loop stimulation of the antigravity motor units, if the dorsal roots in one leg of a decerebrate rigid animal are cut, the rigidity is abolished in that leg. Had the overstimulation along the reticulospinal and vestibulospinal tracts led directly to the α extensor motor neuron, cutting the dorsal roots would not have abolished the rigidity. (However, cutting the ventral roots would have abolished such rigidity.) These and other observations of the decerebrate animal yielded the knowledge that postural muscle tone is mediated primarily by the vestibulospinal and reticulospinal tracts, causing a blend of EPSPs and IPSPs on the γ loop and α lower motor neurons to proximal, extensor antigravity muscles.

These mechanisms cause the muscular contraction necessary for antigravity muscle tone, but not the to-and-fro rhythmicity of walking and running. This oscillation in motor neurons is added by interneurons of the spinal cord. It may be these spinal interneurons that are affected by distemper virus, causing the characteristic involuntary, intermittent muscle contractions (chorea) in some dogs with clinical distemper.

The *tectospinal tract*, the third of the extrapyramidal descending tracts, begins in the visual tectum of the mid-brain (superior colliculus) and ends in the cervical spinal cord. It is important in the reflex coordination of the head and eye movements while the animal is watching a moving object.

THE ROLE OF THE BASAL GANGLIA IS POORLY UNDERSTOOD

The *basal ganglia* are a group of nuclei deep within the cerebral hemispheres and have historically been linked to the extrapyramidal system. They include a bilateral set of five large subcortical nuclei: the caudate nucleus, the putamen (known collectively as the striatum), the globus pallidus, the substantia nigra, and the subthalamus. They receive input from the cerebral cortex and project output back to the motor and premotor cortices, among other places. The basal ganglia region is one of the most poorly understood areas of the brain. The basal ganglia appear to play a role in the planning of movement initiated by the pyramidal system and possibly the extrapyramidal system. They may also play a role in coordinating some rhythmic movements, because lesions of the basal ganglia often give rise to rhythmic, tremorous movement disorders.

THE CEREBRAL CORTEX PLAYS A ROLE IN EXTRAPYRAMIDAL SYSTEM FUNCTION

The cerebral and cerebellar cortices influence the extrapyramidal system. Presumably the cerebral cortex adds a sense of purposefulness to posture and locomotion controlled by the extrapyramidal system by choosing, for example, the general direction and speed with which to walk or run. The cerebellum refines movement initiated by the extrapyramidal system on the basis of feedback from several receptor systems of the body.

CLINICAL SYNDROMES RESULTING FROM EXTRAPYRAMIDAL SYSTEM LESIONS MAY INCLUDE EITHER RHYTHMIC OR NONRHYTHMIC MOVEMENT DISORDERS

Focal lesions of the extrapyramidal system (and basal ganglia) cause abnormal, involuntary movements, alterations in muscle tone, and disturbed posture. Such movement disorders are usually categorized as rhythmic and nonrhythmic movement disorders. Rhythmic extrapyramidal disorders include what is known as a *nonintention, or "resting," tremor*. This is a tremor that is worse when the patient is at rest and lessens when the patient intends to move. (A cerebellar tremor gets worse with intended movement and is called an *intention, or "action," tremor*.) Nonintention tremors probably result from a loss of a normal inhibitory pathway. An example of a rhythmic extrapyramidal movement disorder is Parkinson's tremor in humans, and an apparently related condition is star thistle poisoning in horses. In each case, there is a nonintention tremor of muscles of prehension: the hand in humans and the muzzle in horses. In both syndromes, there is a lesion of the substantia nigra, a brainstem structure that projects dopamine-secreting axons to the striatum of the basal ganglia. At least in the case of humans, it appears that the loss of these dopaminergic neurons is important in the mechanism of the disease, because administering dopamine precursor, which crosses the blood-brain barrier, reduces the clinical signs.

An example of a nonrhythmic extrapyramidal movement disorder is the decerebrate rigidity described earlier in this chapter.

CLINICAL CORRELATIONS

Focal lesion of the motor cortex

History You examine an 11-year-old female boxer dog. Her vaccination history is current. She had an adenocarcinoma of the mammary gland removed 6 months before your examination.

The owner states that over the past few days the dog has become progressively weaker in the left front and left rear legs and occasionally stands with the left front paw upside down. On the previous day, the dog suffered a seizure.

Clinical examination On physical examination of the patient you find several routine old-age changes and the results of the mammary surgery. You find also that the dog seems drowsy and is weak on the left front and left rear legs. She has a conscious proprioception response deficit of both the left front and the left rear leg. Radiographic study of the chest reveals metastatic, neoplastic lesions in the lungs.

Comment The conscious proprioception response is tested by turning the animal's paw upside down while gently supporting her weight. A normal dog senses (conscious proprioception) that the paw is upside down and returns it to the normal pads-down posture (motor response). This is called a response, rather than a reflex, because it involves a degree of conscious control. This particular response requires normal function of skin and joint receptors and the peripheral nerve in the tested leg and of the sensory neuron tracts that ascend toward the brain along the ipsilateral (same) side of the spinal cord. They cross to the contralateral (opposite) side of the brain in the brainstem and end in the contralateral cerebral cortex. As the animal becomes consciously aware that the paw is in an unusual position, action potentials are sent back down the corticospinal tract to the lower motor neurons of the muscles of the leg, causing the paw to return to the normal position. With some thought to the wiring diagram of this response, you can imagine that conscious proprioception deficits of the left front and left rear legs could be caused by a lesion of either the left cervical spinal cord or the right motor cortex. The fact that this dog developed seizures (a manifestation of brain disease) at about the same time suggests that this dog's lesion is in the right cerebral cortex. The brain is a common site for metastasis, and the radiographic lung lesions suggest that the mammary tumor has spread to both the lung and the right side of the brain. The lung contains the first capillary bed that a metastatic cancer cell is likely to encounter when it enters the venous system of the mammary gland. Some cells stop here and grow.

Treatment Dogs with metastatic mammary carcinomas are usually not treated except to make them more comfortable.

Bibliography

Guyton AC, Hall JE: Textbook of Medical Physiology, 10th ed. Philadelphia: WB Saunders, 2000, pp 632–664.
Haines DE: Fundamental Neuroscience. New York: Churchill Livingstone, 1997, pp 347–378.
Kandel ER, Schwartz JH, Jessell TM (eds): Principles of Neural Science, 4th ed. New York: McGraw-Hill, 2000, pp 737–781, 816–831, 853–872.

PRACTICE QUESTIONS

1. In order to increase muscle tone (continued contraction of some percentage of muscle fibers) in the body's antigravity muscles, the extrapyramidal system must
   a. increase the IPSPs to γ motor neurons of flexor muscles.
   b. increase the EPSPs to γ motor neurons of extensor muscles.
   c. increase the IPSPs to γ motor neurons of extensor muscles.
   d. increase the EPSPs to γ motor neurons of flexor muscles.
   e. increase the EPSPs to α motor neurons of flexor muscles.

2. Decerebrate rigidity theoretically may be abolished by
   a. removing the cerebellum.
   b. cutting the cervical spinal cord completely in two (complete transection).
   c. removing the cerebral cortex.
   d. cutting the dorsal (posterior) roots.
   e. either b or d.

3. The pyramidal system, in general, initiates what form of movement?
   a. Antigravity movement.
   b. Postural muscle tone.
   c. Skilled, mostly flexor movement.
   d. Tremulous movement.
   e. None of the above.

4. You are presented with a dog with a dense weakness and conscious proprioceptive reflex deficit of his left front and left back legs. A single pathologic site could cause these signs if it were located in
   a. the left side of the cervical spinal cord.
   b. the left cerebral cortex.
   c. the right cerebral cortex.
   d. either a or b.
   e. either a or c.

5. The corticospinal tract simultaneously coactivates both the α and the γ lower motor neurons. If the initial coactivation fails to be sufficient to cause shortening of the whole muscle, the sensory fibers from the muscle spindle of that muscle will have what influence on the motor neurons to the same muscle?
   a. Add EPSPs.
   b. Add IPSPs.
   c. Have no influence.
   d. Add presynaptic inhibition.
   e. Either b or d.

PRACTICE ANSWERS

1. b   2. e   3. c   4. e   5. a

CHAPTER

10

The vestibular system

1 The vestibular system is a bilateral receptor system located in the inner ear

2 Specialized regions of the vestibular system contain receptors

3 The semicircular canals detect rotary acceleration and deceleration of the head

4 The utricle and saccule detect linear acceleration and deceleration and static position of the head in space

5 The vestibular system provides sensory information for reflexes involving spinal motor neurons, the cerebellum, and extraocular muscles of the eye

6 Vestibular reflexes coordinate head and eye movements to maximize visual acuity during movements of the head

In order to coordinate posture and locomotion, the brain needs to know not only what movement it intends to command, but also what movement the body is actually performing. Chapter 7 describes the muscle spindle, an important source of information for the brain about body position and movement. Another important source of information is the vestibular system. This is a bilateral receptor system, located in the inner ear, that informs the brain about the position and motion of the head in space.

The vestibular system is a common site of pathologic lesions. In most veterinary species, lesions of the vestibular system cause a syndrome characterized by head tilt, compulsive rotary movements such as circling or rolling, and nystagmus, which is a spontaneous, oscillating movement of the eyes.

In order to understand how such clinical signs arise and the importance of the vestibular system to the

physiology of movement, its anatomy and function are studied first.

THE VESTIBULAR SYSTEM IS A BILATERAL RECEPTOR SYSTEM LOCATED IN THE INNER EAR

The inner ear, or labyrinth, is made up of two parts: the bony labyrinth and the membranous labyrinth. The *bony labyrinth* is a system of tunnels through the petrous temporal bone of the skull. The bony labyrinth houses both the vestibular system and the receptor for hearing, the *cochlea* (Fig. 10–1) (see Chapter 16). Within the bony labyrinth is the *membranous labyrinth*, so named because it is made up of thin membranes of epithelium. This epithelial membrane is specialized at some locations to become the sensory

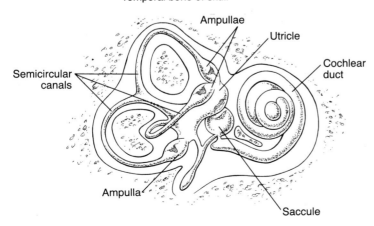

Temporal bone of skull

Ampullae

Utricle

Semicircular canals

Cochlear duct

Ampulla

Saccule

FIGURE 10–1. The bilateral inner ear contains receptor systems for hearing (cochlea) and for sensing the position of the head (vestibular system or labyrinth). The vestibular system on each side of the head contains three semicircular canals, a utricle, and a saccule.

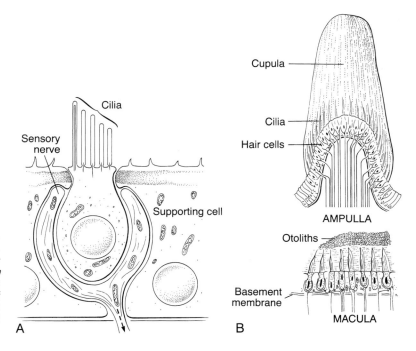

FIGURE 10–2. *A,* Each vestibular structure has a region of epithelial cells that are specialized as receptor cells, or hair cells. *B,* Those in the semicircular canals are clustered in a region called the *ampulla* where all the cilia are glued together by a gelatinous mass called the *cupula.* The hair receptor cells of the utricle and saccule are clustered in the region called the *macula.* Their gelatinous masses contain calcium carbonate crystals called *otoliths.*

receptor cells. The membranous labyrinth is separated from the bony labyrinth by a fluid called *perilymph.* The membranous labyrinth is filled with a fluid called *endolymph.* Each vestibular portion of the labyrinth consists of two major sets of structures: three *semicircular canals,* located at approximately right angles to each other, and a pair of sac-like otolith structures called the *utricle* and *saccule.*

SPECIALIZED REGIONS OF THE VESTIBULAR SYSTEM CONTAIN RECEPTORS

Each structure within the vestibular system has a region of epithelial lining that has become specialized into a set of receptor cells called *hair cells* (Fig. 10–2). Each hair cell has several hair-like cilia projecting into the endolymph and is innervated at its base by a sensory afferent nerve that carries action potentials to the brainstem. The hair-like cilia from all the hair

cells within any one vestibular structure are bound together by a gelatinous mass; displacement of this gelatinous mass causes all the hair cell projections to bend in the same direction. In the utricle and saccule, this gelatinous mass also contains calcium carbonate crystals called *otoliths.* These otoliths are denser than the endolymph and are deflected by gravity.

At rest, sensory nerves innervating vestibular hair cells transmit action potentials spontaneously at about 100 action potentials per second (Fig. 10–3). When the hair cell projections are bent in one direction, the hair cells depolarize and the action potential frequency increases. When the projections are bent in the opposite direction, hair cell membranes hyperpolarize, and the sensory nerve spike frequency decreases. Therefore, displacement of the hair cell projections in either direction can be detected by the brain as either an increase or a decrease from the resting action potential frequency. How the brain uses this information to detect the direction of head movement is described later.

FIGURE 10–3. At rest, sensory nerves innervating vestibular hair cells transmit action potentials spontaneously at a rate of about 100 per second. When hair cell cilia are deflected in one direction, the action potential frequency increases; when they are deflected in the opposite direction, the frequency decreases.

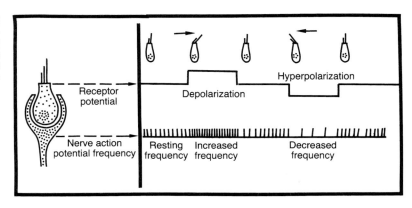

THE SEMICIRCULAR CANALS DETECT ROTARY ACCELERATION AND DECELERATION OF THE HEAD

Three semicircular canals are located within each inner ear (Fig. 10–4). They are positioned at approximately right angles to each other, and both ends of each fluid-filled canal terminate in the utricle. Each semicircular canal has an enlargement, called the *ampulla,* near its junction with the utricle. The ampulla contains the hair cell receptor system, whose hair cells and sensory nerves are attached to its base and whose gelatinous mass (cupula) attaches to the roof of the ampulla (Fig. 10–5).

When the head begins to turn in a rotary direction (acceleration), the semicircular canal rotates with the head, but the endolymph's acceleration lags behind that of the canal owing to inertia. This relative difference in the rate of acceleration of the semicircular canal and its enclosed endolymph causes a displacement of the gelatinous mass in the ampulla and therefore a bending of the hair cells, thus changing the firing rate of their sensory nerves. The opposite happens with deceleration.

Semicircular canals, located on both sides of the head but in approximately the same plane, work as a pair to provide the brain with information about the direction and nature of head movement. For instance,

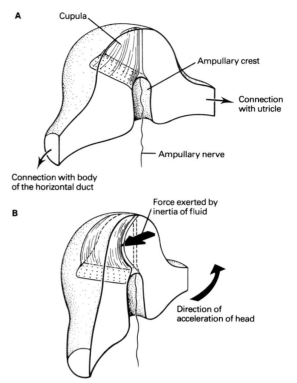

FIGURE 10–5. The ampullae of the semicircular canals contain a hair cell receptor system. *A,* The ampullary crest of the horizontal canal. *B,* Displacement of the cupula by the flow of endolymph caused by head movement. (From Kandel ER, Schwartz JH [eds]: Principles of Neural Science, 2nd ed. New York: Elsevier Science Publishing, 1985.)

a clockwise rotary acceleration of the head would cause bending of the directionally sensitive hair cell projections in one of the semicircular canals on each side of the head. However, the sensory nerve from one side of the head would carry an increased action potential frequency, whereas that of the other side would carry a decreased action potential frequency. The brain has learned to interpret that reciprocal change in sensory action potential frequency as resulting from clockwise or counterclockwise acceleration or deceleration in a given plane of movement. In this way, the bilateral system of six semicircular canals detects the direction of both rotary acceleration and deceleration of the head and alerts the brain for appropriate reflex response.

THE UTRICLE AND SACCULE DETECT LINEAR ACCELERATION AND DECELERATION AND STATIC POSITION OF THE HEAD IN SPACE

In the utricle and saccule, the hair cell receptor region is called the *macula.* Its filamentous projections also extend up into the endolymph and are bound together by a gelatinous mass. As mentioned earlier, in these structures, the gelatinous mass also contains calcium carbonate crystals called *otoliths.* These oto-

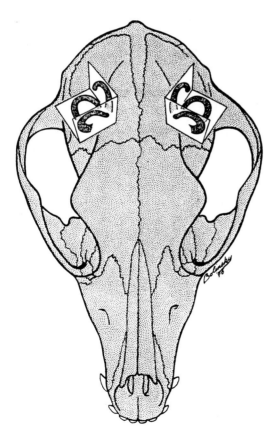

FIGURE 10–4. Three semicircular canals are located on each side of the head and detect rotary acceleration and deceleration of the head.

liths are denser than the endolymph and hence sink toward the earth's center in response to gravity. This gravitational force on the otoliths in the gelatinous mass results in a bending of the hair cells and thus a change in the frequency of action potentials along the sensory nerve fibers. Not all of the hair cell clusters of the utricle and saccule are oriented in the same direction: those of the utricle are oriented in the horizontal plane; those of the saccule, in the vertical plane. The pattern of action potential firing varies, depending on differing head positions as gravity pulls on the otoliths. In this way, the utricle and saccule can inform the brain about the stationary position of the head. Astronauts in low gravitational settings get relatively little information from their utricles and saccules about their stationary head position and must rely more heavily on visual and other sensory cues to detect head position.

▬ THE VESTIBULAR SYSTEM PROVIDES SENSORY INFORMATION FOR REFLEXES INVOLVING SPINAL MOTOR NEURONS, THE CEREBELLUM, AND EXTRAOCULAR MUSCLES OF THE EYE

Action potentials from vestibular receptors arrive in the medulla along axons of the eighth cranial nerve. Nearly all these axons synapse in the vestibular nuclear complex, which is a bilateral group of four distinct nuclei occupying a substantial portion of the medulla beneath the fourth ventricle. From here, second-order neurons project to three important areas of the nervous system. The vestibulospinal tract, part of the extrapyramidal system, receives input from the utricle and saccule and provides excitatory facilitation to γ and some α motor neurons of antigravity muscles (see Chapter 9). Other neurons project to the cerebellum, especially the flocculonodular lobe, where they provide valuable information necessary for the coordination of movement. A third vestibular influence, particularly from the semicircular canals, is over the movements of the eyes.

▬ VESTIBULAR REFLEXES COORDINATE HEAD AND EYE MOVEMENTS TO MAXIMIZE VISUAL ACUITY DURING MOVEMENTS OF THE HEAD

Vestibular reflex control of the extraocular muscles of the eye coordinates eye and head movements. As the head turns, the eyes remain fixed on the field of vision for as long as possible. Imagine that a dog is seated on a piano stool, and you rotated her clockwise to the right. As you rotate her slowly to the right, her eyes would rotate in her head slowly to the left so that the eyes remained fixed on the same field of vision as long as possible. As the eyes reach the limit of their leftward excursion, they swiftly move to the right, in the direction of the head movement, until they fix on a new field of vision. If the head is still

rotating, the cycle is repeated. This allows the animal time to interpret a field of vision despite rotation of the head. This reflex requires normal sensory input from the semicircular canals, the medial longitudinal fasciculus in the brainstem, and the integrity of the motor units in the extraocular muscles. Of course, this reflex can be overwhelmed if head rotation is too fast. Similarly, if the head is tilted to one side, the eyes rotate in the opposite direction, helping to maintain the visual field in the horizontal plane. Voluntary control of the eyes is independent of vestibular reflexes and controlled by the cerebral cortex.

These vestibular movements of the eyes, normal with head movement, appear occasionally under pathologic conditions even when the head is straight and at rest. Unilateral abnormality of one of the vestibular systems results in abnormal, asymmetric action potential frequencies to the brainstem, which cause spontaneous, oscillating movements of the eyes, even when the head is at rest. This condition is known as *nystagmus* and usually has fast and slow directional components because of the normal vestibular reflex control of the eyes. Transient nystagmus can be seen also if a spinning animal or person is suddenly stopped. For a brief period of time, inertia of the endolymph causes it to continue rotating even though the head has stopped. This causes overstimulation of the vestibular eye reflexes, and hence the transient nystagmus. (Humans report dizziness during this time. Try it carefully on a friend; look for postrotatory nystagmus and ask for subjective impressions.)

A persisting head tilt and compulsive circling or rolling often accompany nystagmus in acute vestibular disease in animals, presumably also in association with abnormal, asymmetric action potential inputs from the vestibular systems on either side of the head.

CLINICAL CORRELATIONS

Vestibular syndrome

History A 3-year-old male cocker spaniel is brought to your clinic. The owner states that for the previous 2 days, the dog has held his right ear lower than his left ear. He also tends to walk in circles, clockwise to the right. You have treated this dog previously for an infection of the outer ear.

Clinical Examination On physical examination of the dog, you find that the outer ear infection persists. You also confirm the owner's complaint that the dog persistently tilts his head with the right ear down and circles to the right; you find that he has a horizontal nystagmus. Results of the rest of your physical examination are within normal limits.

Comment Head tilt, circling, and nystagmus constitute a common constellation of clinical signs often called the *vestibular syndrome*. It results from abnormality in the vestibular system, usually in the membranous labyrinth. It is frequently caused by the extension of an infection from the outer and middle ear to the labyrinth of the inner ear. This results in an abnormal balance of action potential frequencies between the normal and abnormal sides of the vestibular system, causing asymmetric stimulation of the ocular and postural reflex mechanisms normally controlled by the vestibular nuclei.

Treatment   When such labyrinthitis is caused by bacterial infection, treatment with appropriate antibiotics is often effective in eliminating the clinical signs by returning the peripheral receptor to its normal function. Spontaneous recovery, without treatment, is common in cats and older dogs.

Bibliography

Guyton AC, Hall JE: Textbook of Medical Physiology, 10th ed. Philadelphia: WB Saunders, 2000, pp 641–646.

Haines DE: Fundamental Neuroscience. New York: Churchill Livingstone, 1997, pp 303–320.

Kandel ER, Schwartz JH, Jessell TM (eds): Principles of Neural Science, 4th ed. New York: McGraw-Hill, 2000, pp 801–815.

PRACTICE QUESTIONS

1. The receptor system detecting rotary acceleration and deceleration of the head is located in the
   a. utricle.
   b. saccule.
   c. semicircular canal.
   d. cochlea.
   e. retina.

2. Astronauts in the low-gravity environment of the moon are most likely to have malfunctions of what sensory system?
   a. Muscle spindle.
   b. Retinal photoreceptor.
   c. Golgi tendon organ.
   d. Utricle and saccule.
   e. Olfaction.

3. The semicircular canals of the vestibular receptor system detect
   a. rotary acceleration of the head.
   b. linear acceleration of the head.
   c. the static position of the head.
   d. whether the visual image is fixed on the retina.
   e. the relative position of the head with respect to the visual horizon.

4. You are presented with a dog with a head tilt, compulsive circling, and nystagmus. The most likely site of this dog's pathologic lesion is the
   a. cerebellar hemisphere.
   b. cerebral cortex.
   c. vestibular system.
   d. cervical spinal cord.
   e. facial (seventh cranial) nerve.

5. Nystagmus, as a clinical sign, is usually a sign of abnormality in the
   a. cerebral cortex.
   b. reticular activating system.
   c. spinal cord.
   d. vestibular system.
   e. oculomotor nerves.

PRACTICE ANSWERS

1. c   2. d   3. a   4. c   5. d

11

The cerebellum

The cerebellum constantly compares the intended movement with the actual movement and makes appropriate adjustments

Cerebellar histology and phylogeny give clues to cerebellar function

1 The vestibulocerebellum helps coordinate balance and eye movements

2 The spinocerebellum helps coordinate muscle tone and movement

3 The cerebrocerebellum helps coordinate the planning of limb movements

The cerebellum plays a role in motor learning

Cerebellar disease causes abnormalities of movement

The preceding chapters, which describe the physiology of posture and locomotion, discuss the function of lower motor neurons, the final common pathway through which the central nervous system can initiate and control movement through the contraction of skeletal muscle. The pyramidal system and the extrapyramidal system are described in those chapters as two of the three major subgroups of upper motor neurons that influence the lower motor neuron. The extrapyramidal system is responsible for involuntary antigravity movement caused largely by contraction of proximal extensor muscles. The pyramidal system is responsible for more skilled, learned, voluntary movements caused by contraction of distal flexor muscles. This chapter also describes the function of the cerebellum, the third upper motor neuron subgroup.

The cerebellum, which is Latin for "little brain," is caudal to the cerebral cortex and dorsal to the brainstem (Fig. 11–1). Although it constitutes only 10% of the total brain, it contains more than half of all the brain's neurons. It has a highly regular, three-layered, cortical histologic appearance, which suggests that all cerebellar regions may perform similar tasks and receive differing afferent inputs from various regions of the nervous system.

The cerebellum is not necessary for sensation or movement. Muscle strength remains largely intact with complete destruction of the cerebellum. But the cerebellum plays a crucial role in the coordination of movement initiated by other parts of the brain, doing so by adjusting the output of the pyramidal and extrapyramidal systems. Lesions of the cerebellum lead to major clinical deficits in the grace with which movement is accomplished.

THE CEREBELLUM CONSTANTLY COMPARES THE INTENDED MOVEMENT WITH THE ACTUAL MOVEMENT AND MAKES APPROPRIATE ADJUSTMENTS

In performing the essential role of choreographer of motor commands, the cerebellum first receives information from the pyramidal and extrapyramidal systems about the movement it has commanded. It also receives information from muscle spindles, the vestibular and visual systems, and other sensory receptors about the movement the body is actually performing. When the intended movement and the actual movement are not the same, the cerebellum's job is to perform the adjustments necessary to make them the same. For example, if the brain intends that a cat

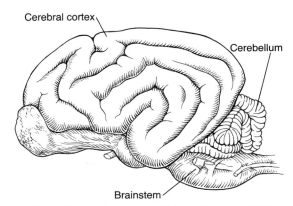

FIGURE 11–1. The cerebellum, which in Latin means "little brain," is caudal to the cerebral hemispheres and dorsal to the brainstem. (Redrawn from Miller ME, Christiansen GC, Evans HE: The Anatomy of the Dog. Philadelphia: WB Saunders, 1964.)

75

move its mouth to a piece of food in a dish but sensory receptors inform the cerebellum that the trajectory of the head will cause the mouth to miss the dish, the cerebellum makes appropriate adjustments in the output of the pyramidal and extrapyramidal systems to correct the head's trajectory.

This chapter describes cerebellar histology and phylogenetic anatomy as clues to cerebellar function. Movement disorders resulting from lesions of the cerebellum are described as further clues to the function of this part of the brain.

CEREBELLAR HISTOLOGY AND PHYLOGENY GIVE CLUES TO CEREBELLAR FUNCTION

The cerebellum occupies most of the posterior cranial fossa. It is composed of an outer layer of gray matter called the *cerebellar cortex*, inner white matter consisting of axons arriving and departing from the cortex, and three pairs of deep cerebellar nuclei within the white matter.

The cortex throughout the cerebellum consists of three layers and only five types of neurons: stellate, basket, Golgi, granule, and Purkinje cells (Fig. 11–2). The outermost layer is the *molecular layer* and consists primarily of granule cell axons, known as *parallel fibers*; dendrites of neurons located in deeper layers; and scattered inhibitory interneurons: the stellate and basket cells. The middle *Purkinje cell layer* consists of the large cell bodies of Purkinje neurons. Axons of the Purkinje neurons go to the deep cerebellar nuclei.

They are the only output neurons of the cerebellar cortex and are all inhibitory, using γ-aminobutyric acid as their transmitter. The innermost *granular cell layer* contains a vast number of small granular cells and occasional Golgi cells.

The two primary groups of input axons to the cerebellum are the mossy fiber and climbing fiber axons. Both are excitatory; they cause excitatory postsynaptic potentials within the cerebellar cortex and, through collateral axons, within the deep cerebellar nuclei. The primary input/output circuit of the cerebellum consists of the climbing and mossy fiber stimulation to the deep cerebellar nuclei, whose output in turn modifies the pyramidal and extrapyramidal systems (Fig. 11–3). However, the output of the deep cerebellar nuclei is itself modified by inhibition from Purkinje cell axons. The Purkinje cell inhibition of deep cerebellar nuclei results from the cerebellar cortex's integration of mossy and climbing fiber inputs with its motor memory. Although the cortical synaptology is understood, just how the cerebellum remembers motor patterns and modifies the output of the deep nuclear neurons is not known. Because the histologic appearance of the cortex is similar throughout the cerebellum, it seems likely that similar modulation processes occur regardless of the cerebellar region. However, inputs from and outputs to different parts of the nervous system would render different motor results. Therefore, it is useful to examine the three major phylogenetically different divisions of cerebellum.

The cerebellum can be divided into three distinct regions from both a functional perspective and a phy-

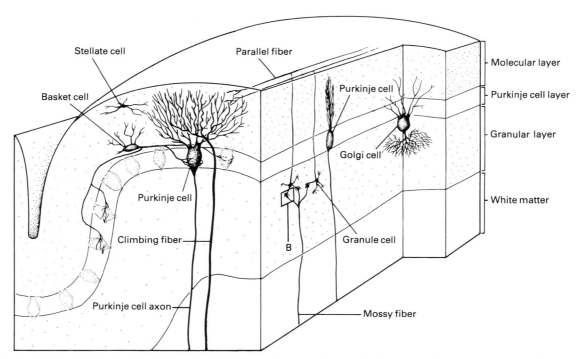

FIGURE 11–2. Five types of neurons are organized into three layers in the cerebellar cortex. A single cerebellar folium is sectioned vertically, in both longitudinal and transverse planes, to illustrate the general organization of the cerebellar cortex. (From Kandel ER, Schwartz JH: Principles of Neural Science, 2nd ed. New York: Elsevier Science Publishing, 1985.)

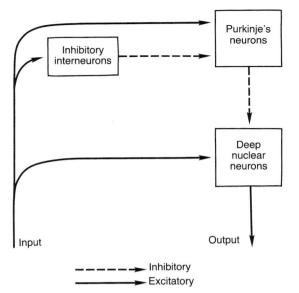

FIGURE 11-3. The input/output organization of the cerebellum involves inhibitory modification of excitatory input.

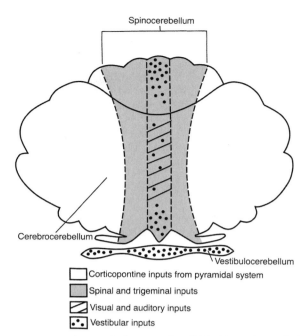

FIGURE 11-5. The cerebellum can be divided into three distinct regions from both a functional perspective and a phylogenetic perspective. These three regions and the area of the nervous system from which sensory axons project are illustrated. (Redrawn from Kandel ER, Schwartz JH: Principles of Neural Science, 2nd ed. New York: Elsevier Science Publishing, 1985.)

logenetic perspective: the *vestibulocerebellum*, the *spinocerebellum,* and the *cerebrocerebellum* (Figs. 11-4 and 11-5).

The vestibulocerebellum helps coordinate balance and eye movements

The vestibulocerebellum occupies the flocculonodular lobe and receives most of its afferent input from the vestibular system and the visual system. Its efferent

output returns to the vestibular nuclei, where it influences balance, controlled by the vestibulospinal tract, and the coordination of head and eye movement. Because this part of the cerebellum was the first to appear in vertebrate evolution, it is sometimes called the *archicerebellum.*

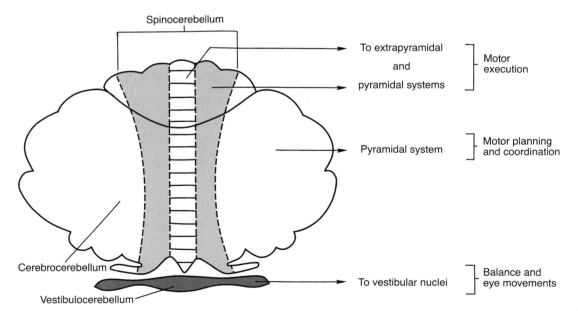

FIGURE 11-4. The cerebellum can be divided into three distinct regions from both a functional perspective and a phylogenetic perspective. These three regions and regions of the brain to which their outputs project are illustrated. (From Kandel ER, Schwartz JH: Principles of Neural Science, 2nd ed. New York: Elsevier Science Publishing, 1985.)

The spinocerebellum helps coordinate muscle tone and movement

The spinocerebellum extends rostrocaudally through the medial portion of the cerebellum. It receives sensory inputs via the spinal cord from muscle and cutaneous receptors. It also receives input from the visual, auditory, and vestibular systems. Its outputs travel, via its deep cerebellar nuclei, to the pyramidal and the extrapyramidal system. Here, when the actual movement being accomplished is not the movement intended by the extrapyramidal system, the spinocerebellum makes the appropriate adjustments. In doing so, it helps control both the execution of movement and muscle tone. Because this portion of the cerebellum appeared next in evolution, it is sometimes called the *paleocerebellum*.

The cerebrocerebellum helps coordinate the planning of limb movements

The cerebrocerebellum occupies the lateral cerebellar hemispheres. They receive input from the motor and sensory cerebral cortices by way of the corticopontine-cerebellar system (see Chapter 9). This area of the cerebellum receives no information from peripheral receptors. Its outputs return to the motor and premotor cerebral cortices by way of the thalamus. The dramatic growth of the cerebrocerebellum and cerebral cortex was the major phylogenetic addition to the brain during primate evolution, and hence it is often called the *neocerebellum*. Presumably this is linked to the primate's ability to coordinate finger movements and the mouth and tongue movements necessary for speech.

It is generally believed that this area of the cerebellum plays an important role in the preparation, or planning, of movement, whereas the spinocerebellum helps coordinate the execution of movement.

THE CEREBELLUM PLAYS A ROLE IN MOTOR LEARNING

There is substantial evidence that the primary cerebellar circuit is the excitatory input of the climbing and mossy fibers on the deep cerebellar nuclei and their output to the extrapyramidal and pyramidal systems. In turn, these deep cerebellar nuclei are modified by the inhibitory Purkinje cell axons from the cerebellar cortex, cells also stimulated by climbing and mossy fiber afferents. This collateral Purkinje cell influence on the deep nuclei can be modified by motor experience. Hence, as a motor skill, such as riding a bicycle, is learned, a person must concentrate on what he or she is doing. But after the skill is learned, presumably in large measure by the cerebellum, the coordination of these motor patterns is taken over by the cerebellum, and the person can concentrate on other things while riding a bike.

CEREBELLAR DISEASE CAUSES ABNORMALITIES OF MOVEMENT

The cerebellum constantly compares the intended movement with the actual movement and makes appropriate adjustments. In cerebellar disease, these appropriate adjustments are not made, resulting in a variety of movement disorders. Affected animals often place their paws far apart (*wide-based gait*) and walk in an uncoordinated manner (*ataxia*), which reflects the inability of the vestibulocerebellum and spinocerebellum to coordinate balance and movement of the axial skeleton. Affected animals also have various degrees of *dysmetria* (inappropriate measure of muscular contraction). In animals, this is often manifested as difficulty in bringing the muzzle to a fixed point in space, such as a food dish, and as exaggerated "goose stepping" walking movements. *Intention tremor* (action tremor), an oscillating movement disorder (tremor) that is worse when the animal is moving, especially near the end of the movement, is also common in cerebellar disease. Unlike the tremors of the extrapyramidal system (see Chapter 9), intention tremors are much less severe when the animal is relaxed and not moving and are worse when a movement is being performed. In animals, intention tremors seem worse in the head and axial (proximal) antigravity muscles. If the vestibular cerebellum is involved, nystagmus may also be seen (see Chapter 10).

This common clinical syndrome resulting from cerebellar disease is one of many examples in which the mechanism of disease can be understood through knowledge of normal physiology.

CLINICAL CORRELATION

Cerebellar hypoplasia

History   An 11-week-old female barn kitten is brought to your clinic for examination. The owner states that this kitten and several others in the litter have been uncoordinated since they began to walk.

Clinical Examination   Physical examination abnormalities are limited to the nervous system. The kitten is bright, alert, and responsive and seems to be of normal size for her age. All cranial nerve and spinal segmental reflexes and intersegmental responses are within normal limits. There is no atrophy. The kitten is uncoordinated (ataxic) when she moves and tends to raise her front paws higher than normal when walking ("goose stepping" hypermetria). She holds her paws far apart when walking. There are coarse, rhythmic movements of her head and proximal antigravity muscles that are absent at rest and severe when she is attempting a precise movement such as getting her head to a food dish (intention tremor). Her complete blood count and serum chemistry results are within normal limits.

Comment   This kitten demonstrates classic signs of cerebellar disease. It is the job of the cerebellum to constantly compare the intended movement with the actual movement and, when these are not the same, make the appropriate adjustments. When the cerebellum cannot do this, movement disorders characterized by wide-based gaits, ataxia, dysmetria, and intention tremor occur. These movement disorders are worse with precise movement and nearly absent at rest.

In this kitten's case, her clinical signs are likely due to cerebellar hypoplasia in which the cerebellum never developed completely in utero. The in utero infection of feline panleukopenia virus results in destruction of the actively dividing granule cells, with an underdevelopment (hypoplasia) of the granular cell layer of the cerebellum. Purkinje cells may also be affected. Barn cats are often not vaccinated for this disease, and often several kittens in a litter are affected.

Treatment   There is no treatment for cerebellar hypoplasia caused by such in utero virus infection. It is not a progressive disease, and if affected kittens are kept in a fairly safe environment, they can have a normal life span.

Bibliography

Guyton AC, Hall JE: Textbook of Medical Physiology, 10th ed. Philadelphia: WB Saunders, 2000, pp 647–656.

Haines DE: Fundamental Neuroscience. New York: Churchill Livingstone, 1997, pp 379–398.

Kandel ER, Schwartz JH, Jessell TM (eds): Principles of Neural Science, 4th ed. New York: McGraw-Hill, 2000, pp 832–852.

PRACTICE QUESTIONS

1. A tremor (abnormal, rhythmic movement) that is worse when the patient is performing a precise movement than when at rest is likely caused by an abnormality of the
   a. cerebral cortex.
   b. extrapyramidal system.
   c. cerebellum.
   d. vestibular system.
   e. lower motor neurons.

2. Which of the following is among the necessary sources of sensory information for the cerebellum?
   a. Muscle spindle
   b. Vestibular system
   c. Visual system
   d. All of the above
   e. None of the above

3. Loss of the cerebellum causes conscious proprioception response deficits.
   a. True
   b. False

4. Loss of the cerebellum causes loss of the muscle stretch reflex.
   a. True
   b. False

5. Cats with congenital malformations of the cerebellum often have ataxia, intention tremor, and wide gait.
   a. True
   b. False

PRACTICE ANSWERS

1. c   2. d   3. b   4. b   5. a

12

The autonomic nervous system and adrenal medulla

1 The autonomic nervous system differs from the somatic motor system in at least two important ways

2 The autonomic nervous system has two major subdivisions

3 The sympathetic nervous system arises from the thoracolumbar spinal cord

4 The parasympathetic nervous system arises from the brainstem and spinal cord

5 Most autonomic neurons secrete either acetylcholine or norepinephrine as a neurotransmitter

6 Acetylcholine and norepinephrine have different postsynaptic receptors

7 There are general differences in sympathetic and parasympathetic function

8 The autonomic nervous system participates in many homeostatic reflexes

9 Preganglionic neurons are influenced by the brain

10 Loss of autonomic neurons results in the hypersensitivity of the target organ to transmitter

The autonomic nervous system is a part of the nervous system that is generally not under conscious control. For this reason, this segment of the nervous system is called *autonomic,* from two Greek words meaning "self-governing" or "independent."

The autonomic nervous system is usually defined as a peripheral motor system innervating smooth muscle, cardiac muscle, and some glandular tissue, although it is subject to reflex and cerebral control. It regulates such subconscious body functions as blood pressure, heart rate, intestinal motility, and the diameter of the eye's pupil.

This system has unique anatomy, synaptic transmission, and effect on its various target organs. It is the site of action of a large number of drugs and is essential for homeostasis. This chapter describes the general anatomy and function of the autonomic nervous system. The autonomic nervous system's specific effect on particular target organs is described in the chapters for each of the body's systems.

THE AUTONOMIC NERVOUS SYSTEM DIFFERS FROM THE SOMATIC MOTOR SYSTEM IN AT LEAST TWO IMPORTANT WAYS

The autonomic nervous system differs from the somatic motor system in its target organ and in the number of neurons in its peripheral circuit. The somatic motor system innervates skeletal muscle, which is the muscle responsible for all movements of the body, as described in Chapters 4 and 5. In contrast, the autonomic nervous system innervates smooth muscle, cardiac muscle, and some glands (Table 12–1). Cardiac muscle is the muscle of the heart (see Chapter 18). Smooth muscle is the muscle in blood vessels, in most of the gastrointestinal tract, in the bladder, and in other hollow visceral structures.

The autonomic nervous system also differs in the number of nerves it has in the peripheral nervous system (Fig. 12–1). The somatic nervous system has one nerve whose cell body is located in the central nervous system (CNS) and whose axon extends, uninterrupted, to the skeletal muscle, where the first peripheral chemical synapse occurs. In contrast, the autonomic nervous system has two peripheral nerves. The first, called a *preganglionic nerve,* also has its cell body in the CNS, but its axon innervates a second neuron in the chain, called the *postganglionic nerve.* Its cell body is in a peripheral structure called a *ganglion.*

TABLE 12–1. Two subdivisions of the motor neurons in the peripheral nervous system

Somatic motor nerves
Skeletal muscle
Autonomic motor nerves
Cardiac muscle
Smooth muscle
Exocrine gland

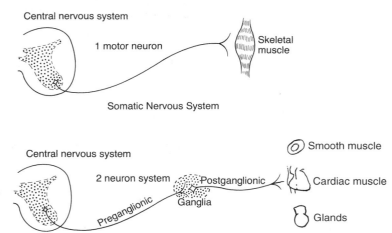

FIGURE 12–1. The autonomic nervous system differs from the somatic nervous system in the number of nerves that it has in the peripheral nervous system. The somatic nervous system has one nerve whose cell body is located in the central nervous system (CNS) and whose axon extends, uninterrupted, to the skeletal muscle, where the first peripheral chemical synapse occurs. In contrast, the autonomic nervous system has two peripheral nerves. The first, called a *preganglionic nerve,* also has its cell body in the CNS, but its axon innervates a second neuron in the chain, called the *postganglionic nerve.* Its cell body is in a peripheral structure called a *ganglion.*

A ganglion is defined as a collection of nerve cell bodies outside the CNS. As another example, remember the dorsal root ganglia along sensory nerves leading to the spinal cord. There are chemically mediated synapses both between the preganglionic and postganglionic neurons and between the postganglionic nerve and its target organ. The autonomic nervous system also differs in the amount of myelin along the peripheral axons—postganglionic neurons are usually unmyelinated—and in a few other, less important ways.

THE AUTONOMIC NERVOUS SYSTEM HAS TWO MAJOR SUBDIVISIONS

The autonomic nervous system is divided into two major subdivisions on the basis of the anatomic origin of their preganglionic neurons and on the basis of their synaptic transmitters at the target organ. These two subdivisions are the *sympathetic nervous system* and the *parasympathetic nervous system.* (Some authors have suggested that the enteric nervous system, found in the gastrointestinal tract, be considered a third subdivision.)

THE SYMPATHETIC NERVOUS SYSTEM ARISES FROM THE THORACOLUMBAR SPINAL CORD

The sympathetic nervous system generally has short preganglionic and long postganglionic axons. Preganglionic axons of the sympathetic nervous system leave the spinal cord by way of the ventral roots of the first thoracic spinal nerve through the third or fourth lumbar spinal nerves (Fig. 12–2). For this reason, the sympathetic nervous system is often called the *thoracolumbar system.* The preganglionic axons pass through a communicating branch to enter the *paraver-*

FIGURE 12–2. The site of origin of preganglionic axons in the central nervous system for both the sympathetic nervous system *(left)* and the parasympathetic nervous system *(right).* Several sites of projection of postganglionic axons are also shown. (From Kandel ER, Schwartz JH: Principles of Neural Science, 2nd ed. New York: Elsevier Science Publishing, 1985, p 219.)

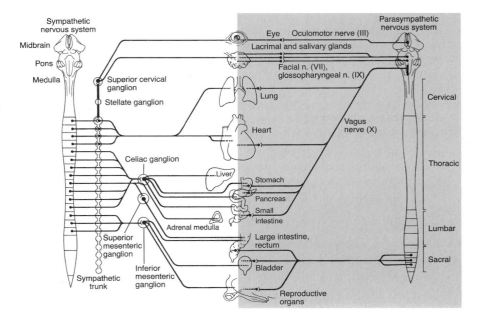

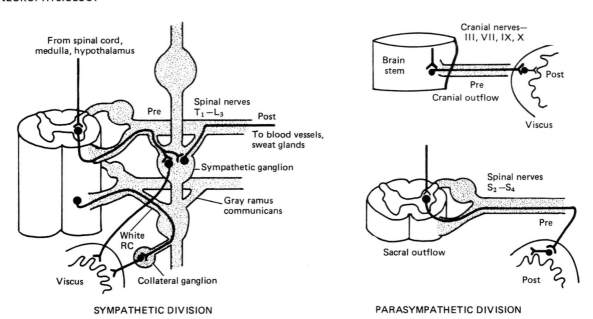

Figure 12–3. The autonomic nervous system. Pre, preganglionic neuron; Post, postganglionic neuron; RC, ramus communicans (communicating branch). (From Ganong WF: Review of Medical Physiology, 13th ed. Norwalk, Conn.: Appleton & Lange, 1987.)

tebral sympathetic ganglion chain, where most synapse with a postganglionic neuron (Fig. 12–3). These postganglionic axons then extend to one of the hollow visceral organs or reenter the spinal nerves to extend to more distal structures. A few preganglionic axons pass through the paravertebral ganglia to synapse with postganglionic neurons in more distal *prevertebral ganglia,* usually named for neighboring blood vessels.

The adrenal medulla is a special variation on this anatomic theme. A few sympathetic preganglionic axons extend all the way to the adrenal medulla, where they synapse with rudimentary postganglionic neurons that make up the adrenal medullary secretory cells. These vestigial postganglionic neurons secrete their transmitter substance directly into the circulating blood. The transmitter substance, acting like a true hormone, is carried by the blood to all tissues of the body.

THE PARASYMPATHETIC NERVOUS SYSTEM ARISES FROM THE BRAINSTEM AND SPINAL CORD

The parasympathetic nervous system generally has long preganglionic and short postganglionic axons. Preganglionic axons of the parasympathetic system leave the CNS by way of cranial nerves III, VII, IX, and X and by way of several sacral spinal nerves. For this reason, it is called the *craniosacral system* (see Fig. 12–2). The long preganglionic axons pass to parasympathetic ganglia in or near the target organ, where they synapse with short postganglionic neurons. (In the gastrointestinal system, postganglionic neurons participate in an extensive enteric neuron network

called the *intrinsic gastrointestinal nervous system.* It is described in Chapter 26.)

MOST AUTONOMIC NEURONS SECRETE EITHER ACETYLCHOLINE OR NOREPINEPHRINE AS A NEUROTRANSMITTER

As described in Chapter 4, acetylcholine is the neurotransmitter at the somatic neuromuscular synapse. Acetylcholine is also the neurotransmitter at all autonomic ganglia (Fig. 12–4), although there is evidence that dopamine-secreting ganglionic interneurons, and some other neurotransmitters, may also play a minor role in sympathetic ganglia. The neurotransmitter secreted by parasympathetic postganglionic neurons is also acetylcholine. Acetylcholine-releasing synapses are often called *cholinergic.* Most anatomically sympathetic postganglionic neurons secrete *norepinephrine.* However, anatomically sympathetic postganglionic neurons traveling to blood vessels of skeletal muscle produce vasodilation and secrete acetylcholine, as do sympathetic, postganglionic nerves to sweat glands in some species. Norepinephrine-releasing synapses are often called *adrenergic.*

In the case of the adrenal medulla, innervating preganglionic axons release acetylcholine, but the vestigial, postganglionic neurons of the adrenal medullary tissue release primarily epinephrine and some norepinephrine into the circulating blood.

It is important that, once released, the neurotransmitter not linger in the synaptic cleft. The neurotransmitter must be either destroyed in the cleft or dissipated so that the postsynaptic membrane can recover its resting potential and be ready for the next synaptic transmission. Because some synapses can transmit

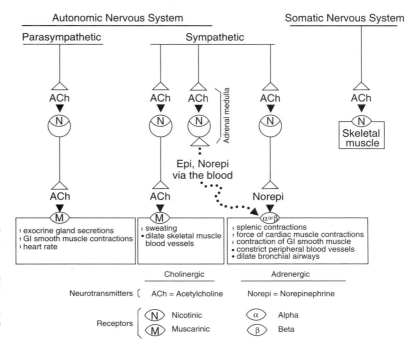

FIGURE 12–4. Classification of autonomic and somatic nerves with regard to their transmitter or mediator released, their postsynaptic receptors, and their general effect on the effector organ. Acetylcholine (ACh), released from the presynaptic membrane, can stimulate either a muscarinic (M) or a nicotinic (N) postsynaptic receptor, depending on the particular location of the synapse. Similarly, norepinephrine (Norepi) can stimulate either α or β receptors, again depending on the location of the synapse. Epi, epinephrine; GI, gastrointestinal.

impulses up to several hundred times per second, neurotransmitter destruction must occur quickly. In the case of acetylcholine, acetylcholinesterase destroys the transmitter in the cleft. In the case of norepinephrine, however, simple diffusion and reuptake by the presynaptic neuron are the most likely ways in which its effect on the postsynaptic membrane is terminated.

ACETYLCHOLINE AND NOREPINEPHRINE HAVE DIFFERENT POSTSYNAPTIC RECEPTORS

The neurotransmitters secreted by the autonomic nervous system all stimulate their target organ by first binding with a postsynaptic receptor. These receptors are proteins in the cell membrane. When the transmitter binds with the postsynaptic receptor, the membrane's permeability to selected ions is changed, and the postsynaptic membrane potential either increases or decreases, with a resulting change in the probability of action potentials in the postsynaptic cell.

Acetylcholine stimulates two different types of receptors (see Fig. 12–4). *Muscarinic* acetylcholine receptors are found on all the target cells stimulated by postganglionic parasympathetic neurons and cholinergic postganglionic neurons of the sympathetic nervous system. *Nicotinic* receptors are found at all synapses between preganglionic and postganglionic neurons and at the somatic neuromuscular junction.

Muscarinic receptors were named because they are stimulated by muscarine, a toadstool poison. Muscarine does not stimulate nicotinic receptors. Nicotine stimulates the nicotinic receptors but not muscarinic receptors. Of course, acetylcholine stimulates both. Different drugs block each receptor. For example, at-

ropine blocks muscarinic receptors, whereas curare blocks nicotinic receptors.

There are two major types of adrenergic receptors, called α and β receptors. The β receptors are further subdivided into β_1 and β_2 receptors, on the basis of the effect of adrenergic blocking and stimulating drugs.

THERE ARE GENERAL DIFFERENCES IN SYMPATHETIC AND PARASYMPATHETIC FUNCTION

Although both the sympathetic and parasympathetic systems are important for homeostasis-maintaining the constancy of the internal environment, there are some important general differences in their function.

In physical and some emotional stress, the sympathetic system discharges as a unit, resulting in widespread stimulation of the body. This causes an increase in heart rate and blood pressure, dilation of the pupil of the eye, an elevation in levels of blood glucose and free fatty acids, and an increased state of arousal. All these widespread effects are useful in responding to an emergency. (Walter Cannon called the sympathetic [noradrenergic] system the "fight or flight" system.) The effect of sympathetic discharge not only is widespread but lasts longer than parasympathetic (cholinergic) discharge because of the prolonged circulation of epinephrine and norepinephrine. Indeed, the adrenal medulla's secretion of epinephrine and norepinephrine into the circulating blood provides prolonged adrenergic stimulation to the entire body, even to some tissues that do not have direct sympathetic postganglionic stimulation.

Although the adrenergic system usually has a wide-

TABLE 12–2. Responses of effector organs to autonomic nerve impulses and circulating catecholamines

Effector organ	Cholinergic impulses: response	Noradrenergic impulses Receptor	Noradrenergic impulses Response
Eye			
Radial muscle of iris		α	Contraction (mydriasis)
Sphincter muscle of iris	Contraction (miosis)	—	—
Ciliary muscle	Contraction for near vision	β	Relaxation for far vision
Heart			
Sinoatrial node	Decrease in heart rate; vagal arrest	β_1	Increase in heart rate
Atria	Decrease in contractility and (usually) increase in conduction velocity	β_1	Increase in contractility and conduction velocity
Atrioventricular (AV) node and conduction system	Decrease in conduction velocity; AV block	β_1	Increase in conduction velocity
Ventricles	—	β_2	Increase in contractility and conduction velocity
Arterioles			
Coronary, skeletal muscle, pulmonary, abdominal visceral, renal	Dilation	α, β_2	Constriction, Dilation
Skin and mucosal, cerebral, salivary gland	—	α	Constriction
Systemic veins	—	α, β_2	Constriction, Dilation
Lung			
Bronchial muscle	Contraction	β_2	Relaxation
Bronchial glands	Stimulation	?	Inhibition (?)
Stomach (monogastric)			
Motility and tone	Increase	α, β_2	Decrease (usually)
Sphincters	Relaxation (usually)	α	Contraction (usually)
Secretion	Stimulation	—	Inhibition (?)
Intestine			
Motility and tone	Increase	α, β_2	Decrease
Sphincters	Relaxation (usually)	α	Contraction (usually)
Secretion	Stimulation	—	Inhibition (?)
Gallbladder and ducts	Contraction		Relaxation
Urinary bladder			
Detrusor	Contraction	β	Relaxation (usually)
Trigone and sphincter	Relaxation	α	Contraction
Ureter			
Motility and tone	Increase (?)	α	Increase (usually)
Reproductive system			
Uterus	Variable*	α, β_2	Variable
Male sex organs	Erection	α	Ejaculation
Skin			
Pilomotor muscles	—	α	Contraction
Sweat glands	Generalized secretion	α	Slight, localized secretion†
Upper abdominal structures			
Spleen capsule	—	α, β_2	Contraction, Relaxation
Adrenal medulla	Secretion of epinephrine and norepinephrine	—	—
Liver	—	α, β	Glycogenolysis
Pancreas			
Acini	Increased secretion	α	Decreased secretion
Islets	Increased insulin and glucagon secretion	α, β_2	Decreased insulin and glucagon secretion; Increased insulin and glucagon secretion
Other glands			
Salivary glands	Profuse, watery secretion	α, β_2	Thick, viscous secretion; Amylase secretion
Lacrimal glands	Secretion	—	—
Juxtaglomerular cells	—	β_1	Increased renin secretion
Pineal gland	—	β	Increased melatonin synthesis and secretion

*Depends on stage of estrous cycle, amount of circulating estrogen and progesterone, pregnancy, and other factors.
†On palms of human hands and in some other locations (adrenergic sweating).
Adapted from Weiner N, Taylor P: Neurohumoral transmission: The autonomic and somatic motor nervous systems. In Gilman AG, Goodman LS, Rall TW, Murad F: Goodman and Gilman's The Pharmacological Basis of Therapeutics, 7th ed. New York: Macmillan, 1985. Copyright 1985, reproduced with permission of The McGraw-Hill Companies.

spread effect, it is also capable of discrete control of particular organs. For example, the dilator smooth muscle in the iris causes enlargement of the pupil in low ambient light without more widespread effects on the body.

In contrast, the parasympathetic (cholinergic) system has more discrete effects on particular organs and is more concerned with the vegetative aspects of daily living. For example, cholinergic stimulation assists digestion and absorption of food by increasing gastric secretion, increasing intestinal motility, and relaxing the pyloric sphincter. For this reason, the parasympathetic nervous system is sometimes called the *anabolic* or *vegetative* nervous system.

Many organs of the body have both sympathetic (adrenergic) and parasympathetic (cholinergic) innervation, each with a reciprocal effect. For example, adrenergic stimulation increases heart rate, whereas cholinergic stimulation decreases heart rate. Adrenergic stimulation enlarges pupillary diameter, whereas cholinergic stimulation causes pupillary constriction.

Table 12–2 gives a more complete listing of the response of various organs to adrenergic and cholinergic stimulation.

THE AUTONOMIC NERVOUS SYSTEM PARTICIPATES IN MANY HOMEOSTATIC REFLEXES

Many of the body's visceral functions are regulated by *autonomic reflexes.* Like reflex arcs in the somatic nervous system (see Chapter 6), autonomic reflex arcs also include a sensory side to the arc, including a visceral receptor; a sensory nerve, often called a *visceral afferent* nerve; and one or more synapses in the CNS. The autonomic nervous system is usually defined as the peripheral motor preganglionic and postganglionic neurons. Visceral afferent neurons are usually not included in this definition but are generally essential parts of the autonomic reflex arc.

Autonomic reflexes are extremely common and are described in detail for each body system in later chapters of this book. A few are described briefly here as examples.

Control of blood pressure. Stretch receptors in the internal carotid artery and the aorta detect systemic blood pressure. As blood pressure rises above normal limits, sympathetic adrenergic vasoconstrictor nerves are inhibited, and blood pressure falls back to within normal limits. (Why this does not happen in hypertensive humans is the subject of much contemporary research.)

Pupillary light reflex. When a flashlight is shone into an animal's eye, light stimulates photoreceptors in the retina (see Chapter 13). Sensory action potentials are then transmitted to the brainstem along the optic nerve, where, through several interneurons, parasympathetic cholinergic neurons stimulate the constrictor smooth muscle of the iris. This causes the pupillary diameter to become smaller.

Gastric secretion of digestive fluids in anticipation of food and emptying of the rectum and bladder in response to filling are but a few of the many other autonomic reflexes that are described in more detail throughout this book.

PREGANGLIONIC NEURONS ARE INFLUENCED BY THE BRAIN

Much as the lower motor neuron of the somatic system is influenced by the upper motor neuron (see Chapter 8), the preganglionic autonomic neuron is also influenced by CNS axons descending from the brainstem, hypothalamus, and even the cerebral cortex. Many brainstem nuclei are known to influence preganglionic neurons in order to control particular visceral functions. Figure 12–5 illustrates several such centers. In turn, each of these brainstem centers can be influenced by the hypothalamus and cerebral cortex, creating a complex system of upper motor neurons within the CNS that helps coordinate autonomic reflexes and directly influences action potential frequency within preganglionic neurons. As more is learned about these central systems controlling the autonomic nervous system, they may be found to play an important role in such conditions as hypertension and various gastrointestinal diseases.

LOSS OF AUTONOMIC NEURONS RESULTS IN THE HYPERSENSITIVITY OF THE TARGET ORGAN TO TRANSMITTER

When the postganglionic neuron to a target organ is lost, the smooth muscle of that organ becomes hypersensitive to any transmitter circulating in the blood. For example, the arterioles of the skin are usually under some adrenergic tone, which results in some vasoconstriction. If the postganglionic adrenergic neuron to the skin is destroyed, vasodilation occurs. However, if norepinephrine is injected into the blood supply to this area of skin, a dramatic (hypersensitive) vasoconstriction occurs. This is thought to

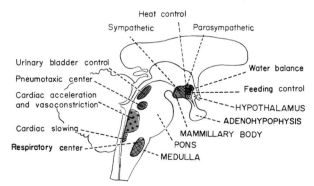

FIGURE 12–5. Autonomic control centers of the brainstem. (From Guyton AC: Textbook of Medical Physiology, 7th ed. Philadelphia: WB Saunders, 1986, p 695.)

be caused, at least in part, by an increase in postsynaptic receptors at the denervated synapse. Why these receptors increase in numbers is not known.

CLINICAL CORRELATIONS

Horner's syndrome

History   A 7-year-old male golden retriever is brought to your clinic for examination. The owner states that during the past 3 weeks, the dog has become progressively weaker in his left front leg and now cannot bear weight on that limb. The owner has also noticed that the dog's left upper eyelid seems to be droopy.

Clinical examination   Physical examination abnormalities are limited to the nervous system. The dog is bright, alert, and responsive. Except for the left front leg, cranial nerve and spinal segmental reflexes and all intersegmental responses are within normal limits. The dog cannot bear weight on the left front leg, and the leg muscles are atrophied. No segmental reflexes (e.g., toe-pinch withdrawal) or intersegmental responses (e.g., conscious proprioception) can be elicited in the left front leg. The left upper eyelid droops lower than the right upper lid, and the left pupil is smaller than the right pupil. The left nictitating membrane (third eyelid) is prolapsed over part of the cornea, and the left eye seems more sunken into the orbit than is the right eye.

Comment   This dog has a lesion of the left brachial plexus, probably a neoplasm. It has caused a lower motor neuron syndrome to the left front leg with atrophy, paralysis, and loss of reflexes. The tumor has damaged the preganglionic neurons of the left sympathetic nervous system as they leave the first two thoracic segments on their way toward the eye. Loss of the sympathetic innervation to the region of the eye causes smallness of the pupil (miosis), drooping of the upper eyelid (ptosis), a sunken appearance in the eye (enophthalmos), and prolapse of the nictitating membrane. This constellation of clinical signs is called *Horner's syndrome*. Sympathetic preganglionic neurons pass through the brachial plexus (where they were damaged in this dog) and ascend in the vagosympathetic trunk to synapse with the postganglionic neurons in the cranial cervical ganglia. The postganglionic cell axons then go to the region of the eye, where they innervate the dilator smooth muscle cells of the iris. When they are paralyzed, the constrictor fibers of the iris are unopposed, and miosis is the result. The sympathetic nervous system also innervates several smooth muscle fibers that lift the upper eyelid and help position the nictitating membrane and the eye within the socket. Because the preganglionic fibers are relatively exposed in the neck, they are commonly damaged. Horner's syndrome can also occur as a result of damage to either the postganglionic neurons or the neurons that descend from the hypothalamus to the rostral thoracic cord to control the preganglionic neurons.

Treatment   Treatment involves removing the cause of sympathetic nerve damage.

Bibliography

Guyton AC, Hall JE: Textbook of Medical Physiology, 10th ed. Philadelphia: WB Saunders, 2000, pp 697–708.

Haines DE: Fundamental Neuroscience. New York: Churchill Livingstone, 1997, pp 417–430.

Kandel ER, Schwartz JH, Jessell TM (eds): Principles of Neural Science, 4th ed. New York: McGraw-Hill, 2000, pp 960–981.

PRACTICE QUESTIONS

1. Choose the *incorrect* statement below:
   a. A ganglion is a collection of nerve cell bodies outside the CNS.
   b. Acetylcholine is the chemical transmitter at the parasympathetic postganglionic–to–target organ synapse.
   c. Sympathetic postganglionic neurons are usually longer than those of the parasympathetic system.
   d. The adrenal medulla secretes mostly norepinephrine and relatively little epinephrine.
   e. Atropine blocks acetylcholine transmission at the parasympathetic postganglionic end organ.

2. The chemical transmitter substance between preganglionic and postganglionic neurons of the sympathetic component of the autonomic nervous system is
   a. norepinephrine.
   b. acetylcholine.
   c. epinephrine.
   d. dopamine.
   e. γ-aminobutyric acid.

3. The neurotransmitter at the sympathetic postganglionic–to–target organ synapse is
   a. norepinephrine.
   b. epinephrine.
   c. acetylcholine.
   d. dopamine.
   e. γ-aminobutyric acid.

4. A drug such as atropine that blocks parasympathetic postganglionic neurons to the eye leads to
   a. an abnormally constricted pupil but normal focusing ability for near vision.
   b. an abnormally dilated pupil but normal focusing ability for near vision.
   c. an abnormally constricted pupil and poor ability to focus on near objects.
   d. an abnormally dilated pupil and poor ability to focus on near objects.
   e. no change in either pupillary diameter or focusing ability.

5. Horner's syndrome is caused by the loss of
   a. sympathetic innervation to the eye.
   b. parasympathetic innervation to the eye.
   c. the acetylcholine transmitter.
   d. acetylcholinesterase.
   e. the smooth muscle of the iris.

PRACTICE ANSWERS

1. d   2. b   3. a   4. d   5. a

The visual system

1 The eye's anatomy is adapted to the eye's role as a visual receptor

2 Through the process of accommodation, the lens changes shape to focus images from various distances onto the retina

3 The vertebrate retina consists of five major cell types

4 The fovea solves a distortion problem found in other areas of the retina

5 Pigment behind the retina either absorbs or reflects light, depending on the animal's habits

6 Photoreception occurs in the rods and cones

7 The electrical response of the photoreceptor to light is transmitted to the ganglion cells by the bipolar cells

8 The electroretinogram records the electrical response of the retina to a flashing light

9 Ganglion cell axons transmit action potentials to the visual cortex by way of the lateral geniculate nucleus

10 The diameter of the pupil is controlled by the autonomic nervous system

11 The retina, optic nerve, and autonomic nerve supply to the pupil can be tested with a flashlight

12 Aqueous humor determines intraocular pressure

The visual system is the sensory modality an animal can least afford to lose. It is also a sensory system commonly involved in clinical disease. Indeed, a whole discipline of veterinary ophthalmology has developed. Hence, an entire chapter is devoted to the visual system.

The eyes are complex sense organs that are basically an extension of the brain. They evolved from primitive light-sensing spots on the surface of invertebrates and in some species have developed many remarkable variations, providing special advantages in various ecologic niches. Each eye has a layer of receptors, a lens system for focusing an image on these receptors, and a system of axons for transmitting action potentials to the brain. This chapter describes how these and other components of the eye work.

▬ THE EYE'S ANATOMY IS ADAPTED TO THE EYE'S ROLE AS A VISUAL RECEPTOR

Figure 13–1 shows the anatomy of the normal eye in the horizontal plane. The white, outer protective layer encasing most of the eyeball is called the *sclera.* It is modified anteriorly into a clear, stratified squamous epithelial layer called the *cornea.* In the posterior two thirds of the eye, the sclera is lined with a vascular and pigmented layer called the *choroid.* Inside the choroid is the retina, the layer containing the photoreceptors.

As light enters the eye, it enters a compartment called the *anterior chamber.* The anterior chamber and the *posterior chamber* are filled with a clear, water-like fluid called *aqueous humor.* Separating the anterior and posterior chambers is a diaphragm of varying size called the *iris.* The iris is a pigmented structure con-

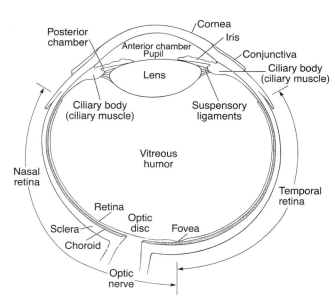

FIGURE 13–1. A schematic diagram of a horizontal section through the right eye as viewed from above. (Redrawn from Walls GL: The Vertebrate Eye and Its Adaptive Radiation. Cranbrook Institute of Science, Bulletin 19, 1942.)

taining dilator and constrictor smooth muscle fibers arranged to vary the diameter of the *pupil*, the hole in the iris through which light passes on its way to the retina. Behind the iris is the *lens.* The lens is suspended in the eye by the *suspensory ligaments,* which attach to the lens and to the *ciliary body,* a muscular structure at the base of the iris. Behind the lens is a chamber filled with a gelatinous fluid called the *vitreous humor.* Behind the vitreous humor is the neural retinal layer. The retina is interrupted at a point where axons of the retina's ganglion cell layer leave the retina on the way to the brain. This point, the *optic disk,* is a recognizable structure when the eye is examined with an ophthalmoscope. The optic disk gives rise to the optic nerve, a cranial nerve so rich in axons that there are more axons in both optic nerves than in all the dorsal roots of the spinal cord.

Also visible through the ophthalmoscope, on the surface of the retina, are the *retinal blood vessels* (Fig. 13–2). These are a network of arteries and veins that enter the retina at the optic disk and provide much of the nutrition to the retina. Vessels of the choroid provide the remaining nutrition to the retina. Examination of retinal vessels often provides valuable clues to abnormalities elsewhere in the cardiovascular system.

Because of pressure generated by the aqueous humor and the inelasticity of the sclera and cornea, the globe of the eye is basically spherical.

The lacrimal gland, located near the lateral canthus of the eye, produces tears in response to parasympathetic nerve stimulation. Tears then flow over the cornea and are drained into the nose by the nasolacrimal duct. A regular flow of tears across the cornea is essential to the health of the cornea.

THROUGH THE PROCESS OF ACCOMMODATION, THE LENS CHANGES SHAPE TO FOCUS IMAGES FROM VARIOUS DISTANCES ONTO THE RETINA

When a camera focuses the images of objects at various distances from the film, the distance between the lens and the film is changed. The eye, however, focuses images by changing the shape of the lens, not by changing the distance between the lens and the retina.

Figure 13–3 shows the primary structures responsible for accommodation. The lens of the eye is made up of an elastic *lens capsule* containing a jelly-like substance. If the eye's lens were taken out of the eye, it would assume a spherical shape because of the elasticity of its capsule, much like a balloon filled with jelly. When suspended in the relaxed eye, however, the elasticity of the suspensory ligaments pulls on the equator of the lens, causing it to flatten in its anterior-posterior dimension. This flattened, less convex lens causes less refraction of light rays and allows the focus onto the retina of objects more than 20 feet away. To focus the image of objects closer to the eye, however, the lens must assume a more spherical, convex shape. This is accomplished by the contraction of the ciliary muscles of the ciliary body. This contraction of the ciliary muscle is much like the contraction of a sphincter and decreases the inner

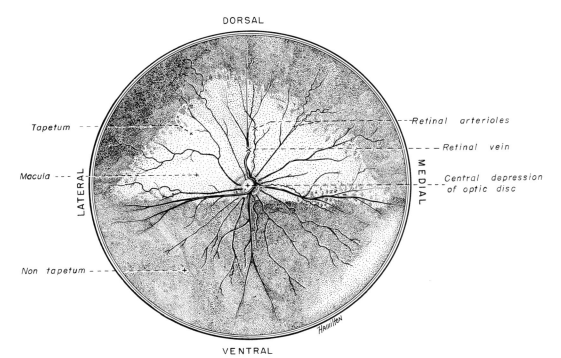

FIGURE 13–2. The ocular fundus of the right eye of a dog as viewed with an ophthalmoscope. (From Evans HE, Christensen GC: Miller's Anatomy of the Dog, 2nd ed. Philadelphia: WB Saunders, 1979.)

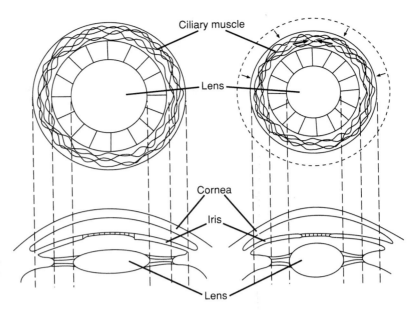

FIGURE 13–3. Primary ocular structures responsible for accommodation. The shape of the lens is shown when the ciliary muscle is relaxed *(left)* and contracted *(right).*

diameter of the ciliary body. In turn, this moves the attachments of the suspensory ligaments to a new position closer to the lens and decreases the pull on the equator of the lens. The result of the inherent elasticity of the lens capsule is a more spherical lens with more light refraction that focuses onto the retina the image of nearer objects. The more the ciliary muscle contracts, the more spherical the lens becomes.

In humans, as the lens ages, it becomes less elastic and tends to become less spherical, even when the ciliary muscles contract. Many people older than 40 years of age need reading glasses to help their less elastic lens focus on objects nearby.

The lens should be clear and free of opacities. However, in *cataracts,* the lens becomes more opaque, causing random refraction of light and blurring vision, often leading eventually to blindness.

THE VERTEBRATE RETINA CONSISTS OF FIVE MAJOR CELL TYPES

Unlike somatic receptors of the skin, the retina is not a peripheral end organ but rather a part of the central nervous system. Skin receptors are derived from conventional ectoderm. The retina is derived from neuroectoderm, a specialized portion of the ectoderm giving rise to the brain. For this reason, the retina is a fairly complex extension of the brain capable of an initial interpretation of the visual image before it is transmitted to the cerebral cortex.

The vertebrate retina consists of five major cell types: photoreceptor cells, bipolar cells, horizontal cells, amacrine cells, and ganglion cells (Fig. 13–4).

There are two types of photoreceptor cells: *rods* and *cones.* Cones are for color vision, whereas rods respond to the entire visual spectrum. Both rods and cones make direct synaptic connection with the interneurons called *bipolar cells,* which connect the receptors with the ganglion cells. Ganglion cell axons

carry action potentials to the brain through the optic nerves.

Modifying the flow of information at the synapses between the photoreceptors, bipolar cells, and ganglion cells are two interneuron cell types: the horizontal cells and the amacrine cells. The *horizontal cells* mediate lateral interactions between the photoreceptors and bipolar cells. The *amacrine cells* mediate lateral interactions between the bipolar cells and the ganglion cells.

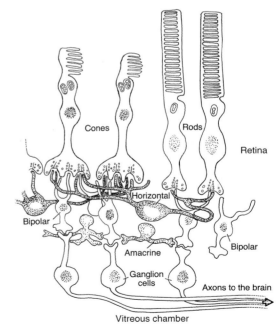

FIGURE 13–4. The vertebrate retina consists of five major cell types: photoreceptor cells (either rods or cones), bipolar cells, horizontal cells, amacrine cells, and ganglion cells. (Redrawn from Kandel ER, Schwartz JH: Principles of Neural Science, 2nd ed. New York: Elsevier Science Publishing, 1985, p 352.)

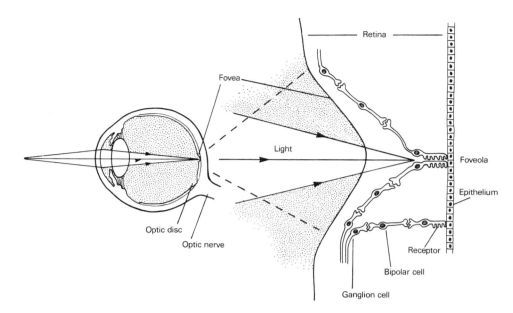

FIGURE 13-5. In most of the retina, light must first pass through overlying layers of nerve cells and their processes before it reaches the photoreceptors. However, in the center of the fovea, an area termed the *foveola*, these proximal neural elements are shifted to the side; therefore, light has a direct pathway to the photoreceptors in this region. An enlarged drawing of the back of the retina is shown on the right. (Reprinted from Kandel ER, Schwartz JH: Principles of Neural Science, 2nd ed. New York: Elsevier Science Publishing, 1985, p 345.)

THE FOVEA SOLVES A DISTORTION PROBLEM FOUND IN OTHER AREAS OF THE RETINA

Throughout most of the retina, light rays travel through ganglion cells, bipolar cells, and occasionally amacrine and horizontal cells before reaching the photoreceptors. Although these inner cell types are unmyelinated and therefore relatively transparent, they still cause some distortion of light rays.

The *fovea* is an area of the retina designed especially to minimize this distortion. It is located at the back of the retina, where light rays would fall from more distant objects (Fig. 13–5). In the center of the fovea, an area called the *foveola*, the inner ganglion and bipolar cells are pushed aside, allowing light rays direct access to the photoreceptors.

Just nasal to the fovea is the *optic disk*. The optic disk is the origin of the optic nerve where ganglion cell axons gather to leave the retina. There are no photoreceptors in the optic disk, so this area is called the *blind spot.*

PIGMENT BEHIND THE RETINA EITHER ABSORBS OR REFLECTS LIGHT, DEPENDING ON THE ANIMAL'S HABITS

In animals that rely heavily on acute, daylight vision, there is a dark pigment in the epithelial layer between the photoreceptors and in the choroid. This pigment absorbs light that has passed by the photoreceptors without stimulating them. If such light were reflected back into the retina, the sharpness of the visual image would be blurred. However, in nocturnal animals, these pigmented layers contain a reflecting pigment and are called the *tapetum.* This allows the retina to make optimal use of what light it gets, but at the expense of visual acuity. Reflection of light off the

tapetum causes the familiar "night shine" from nocturnal animals' eyes.

PHOTORECEPTION OCCURS IN THE RODS AND CONES

The anatomies of the photoreceptors, rods and cones, are similar, but there are some important differences. Both cell types are divided into three parts: a synaptic terminal, an inner segment, and an outer segment (Fig. 13–6). The synaptic terminal synapses with the bipolar cells. The inner segment includes the nucleus, mitochondria, and other cytoplasmic structures. The inner and outer segments are connected by a microtubule-containing cilium. The outer portions are specialized for photoreception. They contain an elaborate array of stacked membranous disks whose membranes contain visual photopigments.

These disks are regularly being formed near the cilium and phagocytized by the pigmented epithelium. Loss of this normal turnover in the outer segment may be important in several retinal diseases. Photopigments are made up of proteins called *opsins* and *retinal*, aldehydes of vitamin A. When light hits the photoreceptor, the photopigment is transformed, leading to a change in the membrane potential of the photoreceptor. Unlike most receptor cell membranes that hypopolarize with stimulation, photoreceptors hyperpolarize when struck by light. In the case of rods, the photopigment is called *rhodopsin*. In the dark eye, many Na^+ channels remain open, allowing leakage of Na^+ ions into the rod, which lowers the electrical membrane potential. When photons of light strike rhodopsin, the retinal is transformed in a way that leads, through a second messenger, to a closing of many Na^+ channels. The result is a hyperpolarization of the receptor cell membrane and a decrease in transmitter released at the synapse with the bipolar cell.

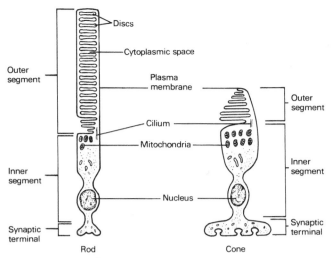

FIGURE 13–6. The two types of photoreceptors, rods and cones, have characteristic structures. Both rod cells and cone cells are differentiated into inner and outer segments connected by a cilium. The inner segments of both cell types contain the nucleus and most of the cell's biosynthetic machinery and are continuous with the synaptic terminals. The outer segments of the membranous disks contain the light-transducing apparatus. The membranous disks in the outer segments of rod cells are separated from the plasma membrane, whereas the disks of cone cells are not. (Adapted from O'Brien DF: The chemistry of vision. Science 218:961–966, 1982. Reprinted from Kandel ER, Schwartz JH: Principles of Neural Science, 2nd ed. New York: Elsevier Science Publishing, 1985.)

Photoreception in cones, although not as well understood, apparently results from a similar breakdown of cone opsin and a hyperpolarization of the cones' electrical membrane potential.

Rods are adapted for night vision. They are highly sensitive to light of all wavelengths, are not selective of the direction from which light comes, and are highly convergent, through bipolar cells, on individual ganglion cells.

Cones, found in many animals, are adapted to acute, daylight color vision. They have a lower sensitivity to light, are directionally sensitive, and in the fovea are linked with almost equal numbers of ganglion cells. According to the *Young-Helmholtz theory*, animals with color vision have inherited at least two—and in higher mammals, three—different types of cones. Each is maximally sensitive to one of three colors: red, green, and blue. Any perceived color can be interpreted as being made up of some proportion of these three colors. People who lack one or more of these cone types as a result of faulty genetic transmission cannot see the colors of a particular spectrum. Such color blindness is linked to the X chromosome.

The extent to which various veterinary species perceive color is the subject of much debate. Some mammals have only rods and are presumably color blind. Most mammals have some cones, but whether this provides them with color vision is debated. On the other hand, some birds, lizards, turtles, frogs, and teleost fish are said to have color vision. Only primates are known to have the classic color vision with which humans are familiar.

THE ELECTRICAL RESPONSE OF THE PHOTORECEPTOR TO LIGHT IS TRANSMITTED TO THE GANGLION CELLS BY THE BIPOLAR CELLS

The hyperpolarizing response of the rods and cones to light influences bipolar cells by a chemically mediated synapse. In turn, the bipolar cell influences action potential frequencies in the ganglion cell axons on their way to the brain. Horizontal cells influence bipolar cells, and amacrine cells influence ganglion cells to make it easier for the brain to detect contrast between brightness and darkness and to distinguish contour. A more detailed description of the synaptic and membrane changes in the chain of transmission within the retina is beyond the scope of this book. To learn more about the many interesting and unusual phenomena occurring in the retina, the reader should refer to the bibliography at the end of this chapter.

THE ELECTRORETINOGRAM RECORDS THE ELECTRICAL RESPONSE OF THE RETINA TO A FLASHING LIGHT

The *electroretinogram* is a clinical electrophysiologic recording from the cornea and skin near the eye. It records the electrical response of the retina to a light flashed into the eye. It has three waves: the A wave, corresponding primarily to the activation of visual pigment and photoreceptors; the B wave, caused primarily by the response of retinal bipolar cells; and a slower C wave, thought to originate in the pigment epithelium.

GANGLION CELL AXONS TRANSMIT ACTION POTENTIALS TO THE VISUAL CORTEX BY WAY OF THE LATERAL GENICULATE NUCLEUS

In order for the image, created in the retina by the visual field, to reach consciousness, the image must be re-created in the visual cerebral cortex. Figure 13–7 shows the visual pathway by which the axons of the ganglion cells project to the lateral geniculate nucleus and by which the lateral geniculate nucleus axons project to the visual cortex. Note that ganglion cell axons from the temporal retina (closest to the ear; see Fig. 13–1) travel along the *optic nerve* to the *optic chiasm* and then project ipsilaterally to the *lateral geniculate nucleus* on the same side of the brain. Ganglion cell axons from the nasal retina (closest to the nose) come to the optic chiasm and cross to the contralateral geniculate nucleus. From there, both lateral geniculate nuclei project to the *visual cortex* in the posterior region of the cerebral cortex by way of the *optic radiations*. Light rays arising in the lateral, or peripheral, field of vision enter the near eye and cross to stimulate photoreceptors and ganglion cells of the nasal retina. Those light rays that can get around the nose to enter the far eye stimulate cells of the temporal

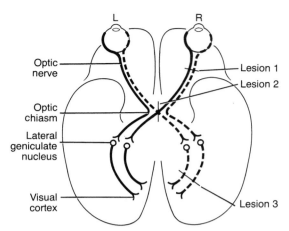

FIGURE 13–7. The visual pathway by which axons of the ganglion cells project to the lateral geniculate nucleus and axons from the lateral geniculate nucleus project to the visual cortex. A lesion in the right optic radiations (lesion 3 on the map) would cause a loss of vision in the left lateral visual field. A lesion at the optic chiasm (lesion 2 on the map) would cause bilateral loss of far lateral, peripheral vision (tunnel vision). A lesion in the right optic nerve (lesion 1 on the map) would cause a loss of vision from the right eye, exactly as if only that eye were closed.

retina. The visual pathway map (see Fig. 13–7) shows that an image arising in the left lateral field of vision would be perceived in the right visual cortex; images arising from the right lateral field of vision would be perceived in the left visual cortex.

THE DIAMETER OF THE PUPIL IS CONTROLLED BY THE AUTONOMIC NERVOUS SYSTEM

The iris of the eye contains two sets of smooth muscle fibers. One set, arranged in a circular pattern around the pupil, causes the pupil to constrict (get smaller) when the fibers contract. These constrictor fibers are innervated by preganglionic parasympathetic nerves found in the oculomotor cranial nerve. Postganglionic neurons begin in the ciliary ganglion, just behind the eye, and secrete acetylcholine as the neurotransmitter to the muscle. The other smooth muscle fibers of the iris are arranged radially from the pupil, like spokes of a wheel. When these radial smooth muscle fibers contract, they cause the pupil to get larger (dilate). These dilator fibers are innervated by the sympathetic nervous system. Sympathetic, preganglionic neurons begin in the first two thoracic segments and course cranially in the vagosympathetic nerve trunk of the neck. Postganglionic axons begin in the cranial cervical ganglion in the anterior neck and course to the region of the eye where they innervate the dilator fibers of the iris, the muscle that helps lift the upper eyelid, and the muscle that helps keep the "third eyelid" in place at the medial canthus of the eye; the sympathetic postganglionic axons also innervate sweat glands and vascular smooth muscle to the face.

THE RETINA, OPTIC NERVE, AND AUTONOMIC NERVE SUPPLY TO THE PUPIL CAN BE TESTED WITH A FLASHLIGHT

When a light is shone into the eye, the pupil of that eye constricts. This action is called the *direct pupillary light reflex.* The light triggers the photoreception mechanism leading to the ganglion cell action potentials transmitted along the optic nerve. Some of the ganglion cell axons go to the pretectal region of the brain that, in turn through interneurons, stimulates the preganglionic parasympathetic neurons of the oculomotor nerve. Through stimulation of the postganglionic neurons, these cause constriction of the pupil by stimulating the constrictor smooth muscle fibers of the iris. A normal direct pupillary light reflex tests the integrity of the retina, the ipsilateral second and third cranial nerves, a limited region of the brainstem, and the iris. This system also crosses the midline in the brainstem, so that when a light is shone into one eye, not only does the pupil on the same side constrict (direct pupillary light reflex) but the contralateral pupil also constricts. This action is called the *indirect pupillary light reflex.* It also requires the integrity of the contralateral oculomotor (third) cranial nerve.

AQUEOUS HUMOR DETERMINES INTRAOCULAR PRESSURE

Aqueous humor is a clear liquid found in the anterior and posterior chambers of the eye. Its rate of production and absorption is sufficiently high to replace the entire chamber's volume several times a day.

Aqueous humor is secreted by the ciliary process, which is a system of finger-like projections on the ciliary body of the posterior chamber. It is thought to be formed by the active transport of sodium, chloride, and, possibly, bicarbonate ions into the posterior chamber. This establishes an osmotic gradient, causing water to flow passively into the posterior chamber.

Aqueous humor flows from the posterior to the anterior chamber through the pupil. Flow is caused by a pressure gradient established by the active process of formation in the posterior chamber.

Aqueous humor is then absorbed into the venous system at the angle between the cornea and the iris. This absorption is driven by a pressure gradient and is assisted, in many species, by a system of trabeculae and canals. If this absorption into the venous system is obstructed, intraocular pressure increases because the production of aqueous humor continues. This pathologic increase in intraocular pressure is called *glaucoma.* As intraocular pressure exceeds intravascular pressure in the blood supply to the retina, blindness results.

CLINICAL CORRELATIONS

Homonymous hemianopia

History You examine a 10-year-old male German shepherd whose owner reports that the dog has recently begun to bump into objects with the left side of his face and has had two seizures. The seizures were characterized by turning of the head to the left and stiffening of the left front leg.

Clinical examination   Physical examination abnormalities are limited to the nervous system. When presented with a maze of unfamiliar objects in the examination room, the dog clearly collides with objects as if he does not see from his left side. He seems somewhat weak in his left front leg. He is otherwise bright, alert, and responsive. His cranial nerve and spinal segmental reflexes are within normal limits, as are his intersegmental, conscious proprioception responses for his right front and right rear legs. However, the conscious proprioception responses for his left front and left rear legs are quite prolonged.

Comment   This dog's history and neurologic examination abnormalities are common in dogs with brain tumors. This dog has a tumor (neoplasm) arising from the meninges over his right posterior cerebral cortex. It is in this posterior (occipital) cortex that the visual image is interpreted from the visual field of the left side (see Fig. 13–7). It is also in the right cerebral cortex that the conscious proprioception response for the left legs is interpreted. His seizures feature turning the head to the left and transient rigidity of the left front leg because the seizure activity arose from the cerebral cortex at the site of the tumor and spread to the right motor cortex but remained limited to the cerebral cortex on the right side. Because the pyramidal system's corticospinal tract controlling the muscles of the left neck and left front leg arise in the right motor cortex (see Chapter 9), seizure activity causes the transient head turning and left leg stiffness.

Treatment   This dog had a meningioma of the right posterior cerebral cortex. Surgical removal was not attempted in this case.

Bibliography

Guyton AC, Hall JE: Textbook of Medical Physiology, 10th ed. Philadelphia: WB Saunders, 2000, pp 566–601.

Haines DE: Fundamental Neuroscience. New York: Churchill Livingstone, 1997, pp 265–284.

Kandel ER, Schwartz JH, Jessell TM (eds): Principles of Neural Science, 4th ed. New York: McGraw-Hill, 2000, pp 492–589.

PRACTICE QUESTIONS

1. A patient whose left pupil diameter is smaller than normal, whose left upper eyelid droops, and whose left eye is sunken into the socket likely has a lesion of which of the following structures?
   a. Left oculomotor nerve.
   b. Left vagosympathetic nerve trunk.
   c. Right oculomotor nerve.
   d. Right vagosympathetic nerve trunk.
   e. Optic chiasm.

2. Your friend, a member of the football team, is trying without much success to explain the cause for the team's recent scoring trend. A variety of implausible explanations are proposed until he mentions that he is progressively losing peripheral vision from the sides of both his visual fields and has frequent headaches. You recommend that he go see a neurologist because he likely has a lesion in
   a. his left optic nerve near the eye.
   b. his right optic nerve near the eye.
   c. his cerebral cortex.
   d. his optic chiasm.
   e. both a and b.

3. You examine a patient's pupillary light reflexes. Shining a light into the left eye produces both a positive direct and a positive indirect pupillary response. However, shining the light into the right eye produces neither a direct nor an indirect pupillary response. This patient's pathologic lesion is located in which of the following structures?
   a. Left optic nerve.
   b. Right optic nerve.
   c. Left oculomotor nerve.
   d. Right oculomotor nerve.
   e. Left optic cortex.

4. You are presented with a dog that is bumping into objects with the left side of his face as if he does not see them. Direct and indirect pupillary light reflexes are normal in both eyes. Where is the most likely location for this dog's pathologic lesion?
   a. Left optic nerve.
   b. Right optic nerve.
   c. Left cerebral cortex.
   d. Right cerebral cortex.
   e. Left oculomotor nerve.

5. You examine a patient whose right pupil is larger than the left pupil. Where in the autonomic innervation of the eyes could the pathologic lesion be located?
   a. Left parasympathetic.
   b. Right parasympathetic.
   c. Left sympathetic.
   d. Right sympathetic.
   e. Either b or c.

PRACTICE ANSWERS

1. b   2. d   3. b   4. d   5. e

14

Cerebrospinal fluid and the blood-brain barrier

1 Cerebrospinal fluid has many functions
2 Most cerebrospinal fluid is formed at the choroid plexus
3 Cerebrospinal fluid flows down a pressure gradient through a predictable anatomic route

4 Cerebrospinal fluid is absorbed into the venous system
5 Hydrocephalus is an increased volume of cerebrospinal fluid in the skull
6 Permeability barriers exist between blood and brain

Cerebrospinal fluid (CSF) is a clear fluid present in the ventricles of the brain, the central canal of the spinal cord, and the subarachnoid space. It has almost no blood cells and little protein. Its rates of formation, flow, and absorption are sufficiently high to cause its replacement several times daily. Sampling its pressure, cell count, and levels of various biochemical constituents is a common diagnostic procedure called a *spinal tap*. Injecting radiopaque dyes into the subarachnoid space is the basis of a common neuroradiographic technique called *myelography*. Obstruction of the flow of CSF is a common cause of hydrocephalus. An understanding of the formation, flow, and absorption of CSF is essential for an understanding of these diagnostic procedures and the pathophysiology of hydrocephalus.

CEREBROSPINAL FLUID HAS MANY FUNCTIONS

One of the most important functions of CSF is to cushion the brain, protecting it against blows to the head. The specific gravities of the brain and CSF are similar. Because of this similarity, the brain floats in the fluid.

Because CSF is in equilibrium with the brain's extracellular fluid, it also helps maintain a constant extracellular environment for the brain's neurons and glial cells.

The CSF may also serve as a conduit for some of the brain's polypeptide hormones and other substances and may help remove harmful metabolites.

MOST CEREBROSPINAL FLUID IS FORMED AT THE CHOROID PLEXUS

The majority of CSF is formed by the *choroid plexuses*. These are small, cauliflower-like growths that stick

out into the CSF of all four ventricles (Fig. 14–1). They consist of tufts of capillaries covered by a thin epithelial layer.

The secretion of CSF, like that of aqueous humor, depends primarily on the active transport of sodium ions into the ventricles. This sets up an osmotic and charge gradient, causing water, chloride, and some other ions to flow passively into the ventricle.

Some CSF is secreted by the ependymal lining elsewhere in the ventricular system. Small amounts also diffuse into the ventricles from the perivascular spaces.

It is important to remember that because the formation of CSF is an active, energy-dependent process, its formation is independent of either CSF pressure or blood pressure. Therefore, if CSF pressure or general intracranial pressure were to rise as a result of an obstruction to flow or a space-occupying mass, for instance, CSF formation would continue.

CEREBROSPINAL FLUID FLOWS DOWN A PRESSURE GRADIENT THROUGH A PREDICTABLE ANATOMIC ROUTE

CSF flows, by bulk, down a pressure gradient from its site of formation at the choroid plexuses through the ventricular system and subarachnoid space into the venous system (see Fig. 14–1). Fluid formed in the *lateral ventricles* passes into the *third ventricle* through the interventricular foramen (foramen of Monro). Here it mixes with fluid formed in the third ventricle. From the third ventricle it passes through the *cerebral aqueduct* (aqueduct of Sylvius) into the *fourth ventricle*. Fluid in the fourth ventricle passes into the *subarachnoid space* through foramina of

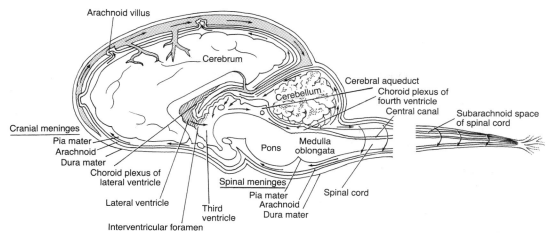

FIGURE 14–1. Sites of origin and routes of flow of cerebrospinal fluid.

Luschka and Magendie. Once in the subarachnoid space, some of the fluid passes down along the spinal cord; most passes up over the convexity of the brain, where it is absorbed into the venous system.

The pressure, cell count, and chemical constituents of CSF can be sampled by placing a styletted spinal needle into the subarachnoid space. Anatomically, the most convenient place to perform this varies with species. In humans, it is usually performed in the lumbar spinal column, because the human cauda equina is located near the first lumbar vertebra and humans have five lumbar vertebrae. This provides a relatively large subarachnoid space in the human midlumbar spinal column from which to sample. However, in most veterinary species, the cauda equina ends near the sixth or seventh lumbar vertebra, leaving only a small subarachnoid space. Instead, most veterinary spinal taps are performed by sampling from the subarachnoid space between the skull

and the first cervical vertebra in anesthetized animals. Here the subarachnoid space is called the *cisterna magna* ("big cistern") and is much deeper than other portions of the subarachnoid space. Spinal taps provide valuable information about such neuropathologic lesions as intracranial space-occupying masses and inflammation.

CEREBROSPINAL FLUID IS ABSORBED INTO THE VENOUS SYSTEM

CSF is absorbed into the venous system. Most of the fluid is absorbed through *arachnoid villi* (Fig. 14–2), which are small, finger-like projections of the arachnoid membrane through the walls of venous sinuses in the dura. How absorption occurs at the arachnoid villi is not clear. It appears to be pressure-dependent, but whether fluid flows into the venous system

FIGURE 14–2. Cerebrospinal fluid is absorbed into the venous system largely through arachnoid villi. (From De Lahunta A [ed]: Veterinary Neuroanatomy and Clinical Neurology, 2nd ed. Philadelphia: WB Saunders, 1983, p 34.)

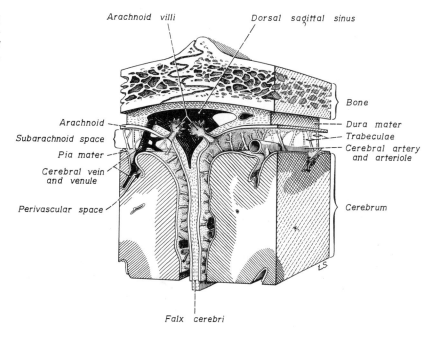

through a membrane (a closed system), through tubules (an open system), or through vacuoles is still a subject of debate.

In normal animals, CSF pressure is regulated primarily by its absorption at the arachnoid villi, because its formation is independent of pressure. CSF pressure is slightly higher than venous pressure, and obstruction of the venous return from the head causes CSF pressure to rise almost immediately. In some pathologic conditions, such as brain tumors or meningitis, CSF pressure can increase dramatically.

HYDROCEPHALUS IS AN INCREASED VOLUME OF CEREBROSPINAL FLUID IN THE SKULL

Hydrocephalus is defined as an increased CSF volume in the skull, usually an increased ventricular volume. In theory, hydrocephalus could be caused by too much fluid production at the choroid plexuses, obstruction to its flow, or impaired absorption at the arachnoid villi. In practice, overproduction seems rare, whereas obstruction to flow seems more common, particularly at such vulnerable sites as the cerebral aqueduct and the exits from the fourth ventricle. Impairment of absorption is also secondary to meningitis or hemorrhage, presumably as a result of cellular debris that obstructs the exit from the arachnoid villi. The pathogenesis of many cases of hydrocephalus is not known. A common form of treatment in humans is to surgically implant a tube that shunts CSF into the atria of the heart or into the peritoneal cavity, thus relieving episodes of increased CSF pressure and preventing further brain damage.

PERMEABILITY BARRIERS EXIST BETWEEN BLOOD AND BRAIN

Many dyes, once injected into the blood, stain other tissues of the body but not the brain. Capillaries in most tissues allow these dyes to escape into the interstitial space, whereas capillaries of the brain do not. In most capillaries (Fig. 14–3), water-soluble compounds leave the capillaries through open clefts between capillary endothelial cells, and exchange is relatively un-

restricted. However, in brain capillaries, passage through intercell clefts is blocked by tight junctions, and exchange of blood solutes is highly selective. Many substances, such as large proteins, toxins, and most drugs, are excluded from the brain, whereas others, such as glucose and many amino acids, penetrate easily by specific, carrier-mediated mechanisms. Cerebral capillaries have a greater number of mitochondria and are surrounded by a layer of glial astrocytic end-feet, although the importance of these end-feet to the blood-brain barrier is controversial.

The blood-brain barrier carefully preserves a stable environment for the neurons and glial cells of the central nervous system. As Claude Bernard pointed out more than a century ago, homeostasis, or constancy of the internal environment, is a precondition for autonomous life. It is not surprising that the brain, the master choreographer of autonomous life, should have a special mechanism for protecting its internal environment from toxins and other outside dangers. Unfortunately for many patients, often it also prevents many antibiotics and other drugs from reaching the brain, particularly drugs with low lipid solubility or drugs bound to plasma proteins.

The blood-brain barrier is apparently not effective in the hypothalamus. This is important because the hypothalamus helps control serum osmolality, glucose levels, and other critical blood parameters and needs to sense the levels of many serum solutes.

CLINICAL CORRELATIONS

Increased intracranial pressure

History You examine a 9-year-old female boxer dog. The owner states that recently the dog has seemed more drowsy than usual and had what you recognize to be a generalized tonic-clonic seizure the preceding night.

Clinical examination Physical examination of the dog reveals a hard, nodular mass of the mammary gland. Other deficits are referable to the nervous system and are characterized by apparent drowsiness and confusion and by a conscious proprioception response deficit of the right front and right rear legs. Lateral radiographs of the chest reveal metastatic, neoplastic lesions in the lungs. The CSF pressure, as measured with a manometer

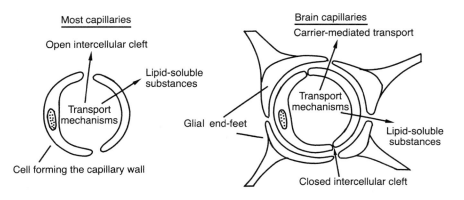

Most capillaries

Open intercellular cleft

Lipid-soluble substances

Transport mechanisms

Cell forming the capillary wall

Brain capillaries
Carrier-mediated transport

Glial end-feet

Transport mechanisms

Lipid-soluble substances

Closed intercellular cleft

FIGURE 14–3. Blood-brain barrier. Unlike most capillaries of the body, cells of brain capillary walls are joined by tight junctions that prevent the passage of material between the cells. All materials leaving brain capillaries must pass through the cells forming the capillary wall.

through a needle placed in the cisterna magna, is 310 mm CSF. (The normal CSF pressure in dogs is less than 180 mm CSF.)

Comment This is a typical case of a dog with a neoplasm of the mammary gland that has spread first to the lungs, which contain the first capillary bed filter encountered by tumor cells as they invade the venous system, and then to the brain. As the tumor mass increases within the fixed encasement of the cranial vault, CSF and other fluid volumes are displaced. Some loss of myelin may compensate temporarily for the expanding intracranial mass, but eventually the expanding tumor, encased in the skull, causes an increase in intracranial pressure, which is reflected in an increased CSF pressure in the cisterna magna. In measuring this pressure, the dog is anesthetized and a styletted spinal needle is placed in the cisterna magna. The stylet is removed, and a rigid glass or plastic tube (manometer) is attached by way of a right-angle, three-way valve. CSF rises up the manometer to a height proportional to intracranial pressure. Its height is measured off the millimeter graduations marked on the tube.

The proprioception response deficits of the right front and right rear legs result from a focal, asymmetric lesion of the left cerebral cortex. The seizure also resulted from this mass. With the mammary mass, metastatic lesions in the lungs, asymmetric neurologic signs, seizures, and elevated CSF pressure, it is reasonable to conclude that this dog has an intracranial neoplasm that probably spread from the mammary gland to the lungs and the brain.

Treatment Extensive treatment in this case would be futile. However, steroids and analgesics may help keep the animal more comfortable.

Bibliography

Guyton AC, Hall JE: Textbook of Medical Physiology, 10th ed. Philadelphia: WB Saunders, 2000, pp 709–717.
Kandel ER, Schwartz JH, Jessell TM (eds): Principles of Neural Science, 4th ed. New York: McGraw-Hill, 2000, pp 1288–1301.

PRACTICE QUESTIONS

1. A drug that would prevent the active transport of Na^+ ions out of cells would lead to
   a. an increased production of both CSF and aqueous humor.
   b. a decreased production of both CSF and aqueous humor.
   c. an increased production of CSF but a decreased production of aqueous humor.
   d. a decreased production of CSF but an increased production of aqueous humor.
   e. no change in the production of either CSF or aqueous humor.

2. You are performing a spinal tap on an anesthetized dog and measuring CSF pressure. While measuring the pressure, you occlude the jugular veins. What would you expect to happen to the CSF pressure?
   a. Pressure would increase.
   b. Pressure would decrease.
   c. No change in pressure would occur.

3. Obstruction of the flow of CSF at the cerebral aqueduct (aqueduct of Sylvius) would lead to dilatation (enlargement) of the
   a. lateral ventricles.
   b. fourth ventricles.
   c. central canal of the spinal cord.
   d. subarachnoid space.
   e. cauda equina.

4. CSF is formed at the
   a. arachnoid villi.
   b. aqueduct of Sylvius.
   c. choroid plexuses.
   d. subarachnoid space.

5. Many dyes injected into the venous system can penetrate most tissues of the body, but not the brain.
   a. True.
   b. False.

PRACTICE ANSWERS

1. b   2. a   3. a   4. c   5. a

15

The electroencephalogram and sensory evoked potentials

1 All areas of the cerebral cortex share common histologic features

2 The electroencephalogram has become a common clinical tool

3 The collective behavior of cortical neurons can be studied noninvasively through the use of macroelectrodes on the scalp

4 Stimulation of sensory tracts can be recorded as evoked potentials

When many excitable cells are present in a living tissue, their electrical behavior can be detected by macroelectrodes placed on the body at a distance from these cells. Several clinically important electrophysiologic diagnostic procedures rely on this concept.

Underlying these procedures is a theory called *volume condition*. This theory describes the spread of ionic currents within the extracellular fluid from a group of nerve or muscle cells to more distant points in the body, such as the skin. These ionic currents can be measured from the skin. Their wave forms are characteristic of the tissues from which they arise. The best known of these electrophysiologic recordings is the electrocardiogram from heart muscle (Chapter 19). The electromyogram from skeletal muscle (Chapter 5) and electroretinogram (Chapter 13) are other examples.

This chapter introduces two additional clinical electrophysiologic tools: the *electroencephalogram* and *sensory evoked potentials*, particularly *brainstem evoked responses*. First, however, it is necessary to understand more about the histology and electrophysiology of the cerebral cortex.

ALL AREAS OF THE CEREBRAL CORTEX SHARE COMMON HISTOLOGIC FEATURES

Different regions of the cerebral cortex have different functions. For example, the motor cortex (Chapter 9) projects to the brainstem and spinal cord to initiate skilled, learned, conscious movement. The occipital cortex processes visual information received from the retina of the eye (see Chapter 13). The temporal cortex processes similar information from the ear (see Chapter 16). However, even though different cortical regions have different functions, their histologic features are basically the same. This suggests that cortical synaptic processing of information is similar in all regions, and the differences between regions are in the origins of their input signals and the destinations of their output signals. In fact, the cerebral cortical cells work collectively in such normal states as sleep and wakefulness and in such disease states as coma and seizures.

The cerebral cortex contains several different cell types, but most belong to two major classes: *pyramidal cells* and *stellate cells* (Fig. 15–1). These cells are arranged in six layers. The pyramidal cells, so called because their cell bodies are shaped like pyramids, have cell bodies located in deeper layers with their dendrites projecting up to the pial surface of the cortex, where they spread out within layer I. Pyramidal cell axons project to other parts of the central nervous system and carry the major output signal of the cerebral cortex. Pyramidal cells are generally excitatory at their axon's synapse. Stellate cells, so named because of their star-like appearance, are interneurons within the cortex and can be either excitatory or inhibitory. Sensory inputs arise from specific nuclei of the lateral thalamus and project to layer IV. Interneurons from other parts of the cortex project to layers I and II.

As with other regions of the brain, the cerebral cortex contains about 10 times more *glial cells* than neurons. Three types of glial cells are present in the cortex: astrocytes, oligodendrocytes, and microglias. They do not develop action potentials and are not thought to play a role in signaling. They probably take up excess potassium ions, neurotransmitter, and toxins from the extracellular space. They may also help stabilize the position of the neurons; hence, the origin of the term *glia* ("glue").

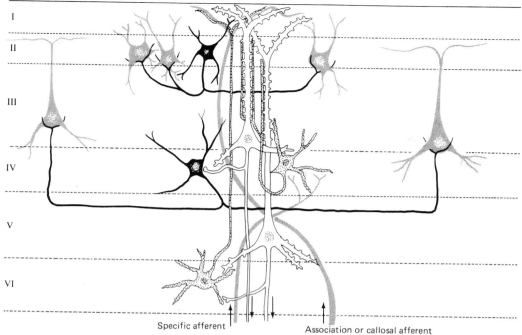

Figure 15–1. The principal neuron types and their interconnections are similar in the various regions of the cerebral cortex. Note that the two large pyramidal cells *(white)* in layers III and V receive multiple synaptic contacts from the star-shaped interneuron (stellate cell, *stippled*) in layer IV. Basket cell *(black)* inhibition is directed to the somata of cortical neurons. Major input to the cortex derives from specific thalamic nuclei (specific afferents) and is directed mostly to layer IV; association and callosal input (association and callosal afferents) are directed largely to more superficial layers. (From Kandel ER, Schwartz JH: Principles of Neural Science, 2nd ed. New York: Elsevier Science Publishing, 1985.)

THE ELECTROENCEPHALOGRAM HAS BECOME A COMMON CLINICAL TOOL

It has been known since the 1930s that a fluctuating electrical voltage reflecting brain activity could be recorded from macroelectrodes on the scalp. Such a recording is known as an *electroencephalogram* (EEG). The frequency of the wave form recorded varies inversely with its amplitude. Both frequency and amplitude change with changes in levels of arousal (Fig. 15–2). An alert animal has a fairly high-frequency, fairly low-amplitude EEG, whereas a more relaxed animal has a slower frequency, higher amplitude EEG. A sleeping animal usually begins sleep exhibiting a slow-wave, high-amplitude EEG. Paradoxically, there are periods of high-frequency, low-amplitude EEG during the sleep cycle. Four frequency ranges have been given names: α (8 to 13 Hz), β (13 to 30 Hz), δ (0.5 to 4 Hz), and υ (4 to 7 Hz).

Since the early 1960s, this technique has been applied clinically. Abnormal EEG activity has been associated empirically with several brain diseases. In human neurology, EEGs have commonly been used to classify the epilepsies, to localize lesions, and more recently to help define brain death. EEGs have not been as widely used in veterinary medicine but still hold promise for veterinary neurology.

Where do these scalp recordings originate and what do they have to do with brain function?

THE COLLECTIVE BEHAVIOR OF CORTICAL NEURONS CAN BE STUDIED NONINVASIVELY THROUGH THE USE OF MACROELECTRODES ON THE SCALP

The scalp EEG records a fluctuating voltage resulting from changes in postsynaptic potentials in thousands of neurons below the electrode. Each change in voltage has a polarity.

By convention, changes in voltage measured by extracellular electrodes such as those on the scalp have a standard direction of pen deflection. When the voltage change is in a positive direction, the deflection is down; when in a negative direction, the deflection is up (Fig. 15–3). The polarity of the voltage change at the scalp depends on the nature and location of the postsynaptic potential change. If an excitatory postsynaptic potential (EPSP) occurs in a deep cortical layer, positive ions (e.g., Na^+) enter the cell there, whereas other positive ions exit the cell nearer to the pial surface (see Fig. 15–3; for simplicity, only one cell is indicated). This results in a positive voltage change at the scalp macroelectrode. If the EPSP occurs at the pial surface (see Fig. 15–3), the voltage recorded from the scalp is negative. The polarity of these changes would be reversed for inhibitory postsynaptic potentials (IPSPs).

Voltage changes recorded from the scalp are the result of the summated extracellular voltage changes caused by the postsynaptic potentials of a large num-

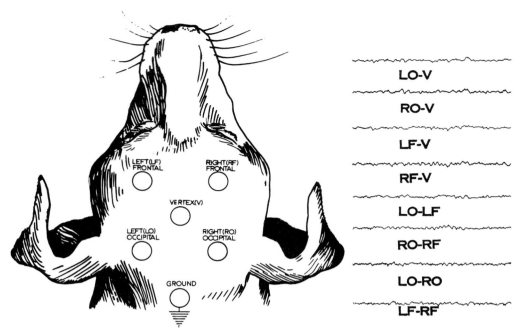

FIGURE 15–2. Points of electrode attachment for recording the electroencephalogram. Recordings obtained from a combination of the lead points are shown. (From Oliver JE, Hoerlein BF, Mayhew IG [eds]: Veterinary Neurology. Philadelphia: WB Saunders, 1987, p 113.)

Illustration continued on opposite page

ber of active cortical neurons, primarily pyramidal cells, because the voltage change from any one neuron is too small to see. Action potentials contribute little to the EEG with scalp electrodes.

The amplitude (height) of voltage fluctuations in the scalp-recorded EEG is a function of how many cortical cells are changing their postsynaptic potentials in the same direction at the same time. Because a high-amplitude voltage change would result from a large number of neurons firing synchronously, a high-amplitude, slow-frequency EEG is said to be a *synchronized EEG.* When neurons are firing more or less at random, a low-amplitude, high-frequency EEG results. This EEG is said to be a *desynchronized EEG.*

The frequency with which EEG voltage changes occur is largely set by medial thalamic nuclei and the reticular activating system through their diffuse connections to the cerebral cortex.

The voltage changes recorded from the scalp result from summated changes in the postsynaptic potentials of large numbers of cerebral cortical neurons. The amplitude and frequency of these changes are influenced by the medial thalamus and the brainstem reticular activating system. However, large areas of the brain and the spinal cord are not reflected in the EEG. There are other clinical electrophysiologic recordings that can help examine the function of these areas.

STIMULATION OF SENSORY TRACTS CAN BE RECORDED AS EVOKED POTENTIALS

Synaptic activity in a sensory pathway can be recorded from the scalp by a computerized technique that averages out the more random background EEG activity and averages in the electrical response to multiple stimulations of a sensory system. Such signals are called *sensory evoked potentials.*

Because scalp macroelectrodes can more easily record the EEG electrical signals generated from the closer cerebral cortical cells, these higher-voltage signals must be eliminated; otherwise, they would mask the sensory evoked potentials. Because the background EEG signals are relatively random, a computer can average them together and functionally erase them from the recording. In addition, the computer averages sensory evoked potential signals recorded simultaneously to multiple stimulations of a sensory pathway. In this way, scalp macroelectrodes can be used to record electrical events generated in brain locations at a great distance from the recording electrode. For this reason, these sensory evoked potentials are often called *far-field potentials.*

One such sensory evoked potential is the *brainstem auditory evoked response* (BSAER). This clinical electrophysiologic procedure records the brainstem electrical events for 10 msec after a click stimulus to the ear (Fig. 15–4). Usually seven waves, thought to be generated by brainstem synaptic relay points in the auditory pathway, are recorded. Recordings longer than 10 msec are sometimes taken. These later waves reflect cortical response to auditory stimulation. BSAER is being used in animals and humans to assess brainstem function in general and auditory function in particular.

Other sensory evoked potentials can be recorded from the visual system, the somatosensory system, and other sensory modalities.

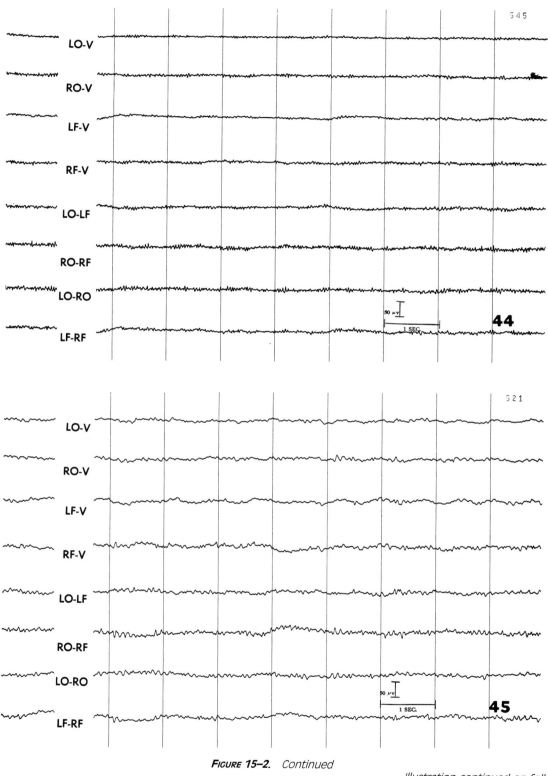

FIGURE 15–2. *Continued*

Illustration continued on following page

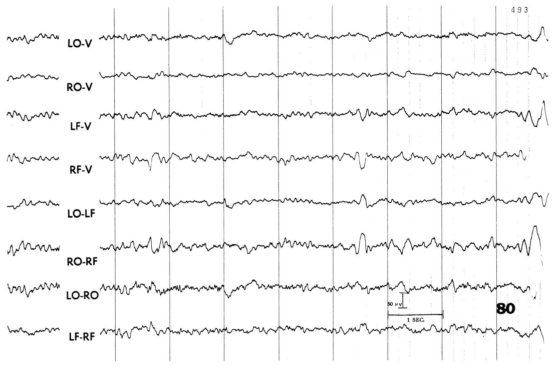

LO-V

RO-V

LF-V

RF-V

LO-LF

RO-RF

LO-RO

LF-RF

493

50 µV

1 SEC.

80

FIGURE 15–2. *Continued*

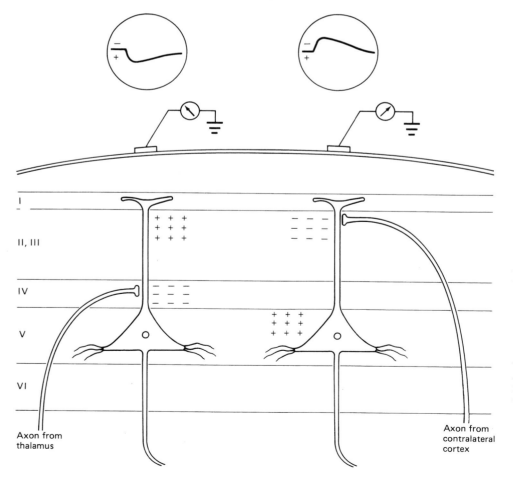

I

II, III

IV

V

VI

+ + +
+ + +
+ + +

− − −
− − −

− − −
− − −

+ + +
+ + +
+ + +

Axon from
thalamus

Axon from
contralateral
cortex

FIGURE 15–3. Scalp recordings and underlying synaptic mechanisms. *Left,* A potential recorded from a scalp electrode after activation of thalamic inputs. The terminals of thalamocortical neurons make excitatory connections on cortical neurons predominantly in layer IV. Thus, the site of inward current flow (sink) is in the superficial cortical layers. Because the recording electrode is located on the scalp, it is closer to the site of outward current flow than to that of inward current flow and, therefore, records a positive potential. By convention, a positive extracellularly recorded potential is, unlike intracellular recordings, a downward deflection. *Right,* A potential recorded from an excitatory input from a callosal neuron in the contralateral cortex. The axons of callosal neurons terminate in the superficial cortical layers. A negative potential (upward deflection) is recorded because the electrode is closer to the site of inward current flow than to that of outward flow. (From Kandel ER, Schwartz JH: Principles of Neural Science, 2nd ed. New York: Elsevier Science Publishing, 1985.)

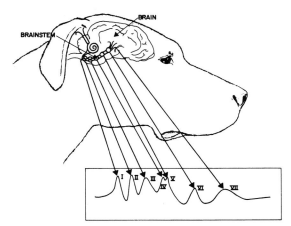

FIGURE 15–4. Brainstem auditory evoked response: idealized diagram of wave forms recorded by signal averaging. Neural elements that are believed to sequentially generate the auditory waves are grouped as follows: wave I reflects the cochlea, spiral ganglia, and cranial nerve VIII; wave II reflects the cochlear nuclei; wave III reflects the nucleus of the trapezoid body; waves IV and V reflect the lateral lemniscus and lemniscal nuclei and caudal colliculus, respectively (these two waves are frequently combined to form one wave); wave VI reflects the medial geniculate body; and wave VII reflects auditory radiations. Positive is upward. (From Oliver JE, Hoerlein BF, Mayhew IG [eds]: Veterinary Neurology. Philadelphia: WB Saunders, 1987, p 173.)

CLINICAL CORRELATIONS

Brain tumor

History You examine a 13-year-old Boston terrier. The owner states that during the past 3 weeks the dog has had seizures of increasing frequency characterized by turning his head to the right, rigidity of the right front and right hind legs, collapsing to the ground, and urination. More recently, he has seemed weak, drowsy, and confused. He tends to walk in circles and seems weak on the right front leg.

Clinical examination Important physical examination deficits are referable to the nervous system. The dog seems weak, drowsy, confused, and unsteady in his gait. He tends to walk in counterclockwise circles. His cranial and spinal segmental reflexes are within normal limits. His conscious proprioception response is abnormal in the right front leg and normal in the other three legs (see Chapter 6). An EEG reveals that the dominant frequency is slower, and the amplitude is higher, over the left parietal cortex than over the rest of the brain. Occasional bursts of electrical spiking activity can also be seen from the area of the left parietal cortex.

Comment This is an old dog, with a recent history of progressive, asymmetric brain disease. The history suggests a focal intracranial lesion, perhaps a brain tumor. A focal lesion is further confirmed by the EEG. Brain tumors within the cerebral hemispheres often cause focal slowing of the EEG frequency with increased amplitude. This is called a *slow-wave focus*. The tumor itself is electrically silent, but its effects on the surrounding cerebral cortex are slowing, and the intermittent bursts of electrical spikes represent seizure activity within the cortex. Between clinical seizures, these spikes can still be seen with the EEG, but they do not spread widely enough within

the cortex to cause a clinical seizure. During a clinical seizure, this abnormal electrical activity spreads more widely to incorporate normal brain, causing the various motor and other events of the seizure. Why such spikes only occasionally spread to incorporate more distant parts of the brain to cause seizures, and why seizures stop, is still unknown.

Treatment Many forms of seizure disorders can be managed successfully by removing the underlying cause, or the frequency of the seizures can be reduced with antiepileptic medication. In this dog's case, the cause is likely a brain tumor, for which there is no reasonable cure. Antiepileptic and steroid medication may improve the quality of the dog's remaining life.

Bibliography

Guyton AC, Hall JE: Textbook of Medical Physiology, 10th ed. Philadelphia: WB Saunders, 2000, pp 689–696.
Kandel ER, Schwartz JH, Jessell TM (eds): Principles of Neural Science, 4th ed. New York: McGraw-Hill, 2000, pp 910–959.

PRACTICE QUESTIONS

1. The EEG is the measurement from the scalp of predominantly what neural event?
   a. Presynaptic inhibition in the cerebral cortex.
   b. Postsynaptic potentials in the cerebral cortex.
   c. Action potentials in the cerebral cortex.
   d. Flow of cerebrospinal fluid in the lateral ventricles.

2. A lesion in which of the following brain structures would have *no* influence over the EEG?
   a. Cerebral cortex.
   b. Medial thalamus.
   c. Internal capsule.
   d. Cerebellum.
   e. Reticular activating system.

3. Which of the following statements is *not* true about the normal EEG?
   a. The EEG should be similar in both cerebral hemispheres.
   b. The EEG should be flat in a dead patient.
   c. Sleep is often characterized by a slow-frequency, high-amplitude EEG.
   d. The left cerebral cortex usually has a much slower frequency than the right cerebral cortex.

4. The BSAER requires the averaging out of the basic EEG before it can be recorded.
   a. True.
   b. False.

5. A brain tumor may cause focal slowing of the EEG from the brain tissue immediately surrounding the tumor.
   a. True.
   b. False.

PRACTICE ANSWERS

1. b   2. d   3. d   4. a   5. a

CHAPTER

16

Hearing

1 Sound waves are alternating phases of condensation and rarefaction (pressure waves) of molecules in the external environment
2 External and middle ears funnel sound waves to the cochlea
3 The cochlea is located in the inner ear

4 The cochlea transduces sound waves to action potentials in the eighth cranial nerve
5 Action potentials from the cochlea are transmitted up through the brainstem to the cerebral cortex
6 Deafness results from an interruption in the hearing process

Our lives are enriched by music and conversation and altered by the sounds of danger. Many mammalian species have a particularly acute sense of hearing. Hearing depends on the remarkable properties of hair cell receptors in the cochlea that transduce sound into action potentials that are then sent to the brain. Fortunately, the auditory system is not often a site of pathologic lesions in veterinary medicine except for occasional congenital defects. Nevertheless, hearing is sufficiently important to warrant a brief discussion of its physiology.

SOUND WAVES ARE ALTERNATING PHASES OF CONDENSATION AND RAREFACTION (PRESSURE WAVES) OF MOLECULES IN THE EXTERNAL ENVIRONMENT

Sound waves are longitudinal vibrations of molecules in the external environment characterized by alternating phases of condensation and rarefaction (increases and decreases in pressure). Sound is the sensation produced when these alternating changes in pressure strike the tympanic membrane. A plot of these changes in pressure on the tympanic membrane per unit time is a series of waves (Fig. 16–1). Such movements in the environment are usually called *sound waves*. In general, the *loudness* of the sound is correlated with the *amplitude* of a sound wave; the *pitch* is correlated with the *frequency* of the waves per unit time. The loudness of a sound is usually quantified according to the *decibel scale,* which expresses the intensity of the sound in comparison with the intensity of a standard sound.

EXTERNAL AND MIDDLE EARS FUNNEL SOUND WAVES TO THE COCHLEA

The external ear and canal funnel sound waves to the *tympanic membrane (eardrum)* (Fig. 16–2). The eardrum

is a membrane between the external and the middle ear. The middle ear is an air-filled cavity in the temporal bone and is connected to the nasopharynx by the auditory (eustachian) tube. Three *auditory bones* (ossicles)—the malleus, incus, and stapes—are connected to each other and are located in the middle ear. They transfer vibrations of the eardrum to the oval window, a membranous separation between the middle and the inner ear. Two small skeletal muscles are also located in the middle ear. Their contraction alters the transfer of vibration between the eardrum and the oval window.

THE COCHLEA IS LOCATED IN THE INNER EAR

The inner ear (labyrinth) contains two receptor systems: the vestibular system, which detects the position of the head (see Chapter 10), and the *cochlea,* a receptor for hearing. The inner ear consists of the *bony labyrinth* and, within the bony labyrinth, the

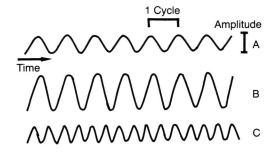

FIGURE 16–1. Characteristics of sound waves. *A,* Record of a pure tone. *B,* Record with a greater amplitude and louder than *A. C,* Record with the same amplitude as in *A* but a greater frequency and with a higher pitch.

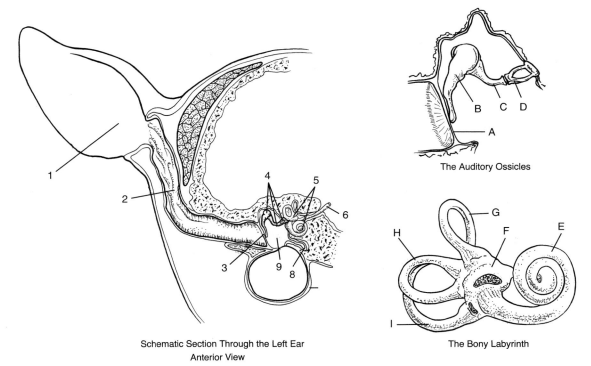

FIGURE 16–2. Schematic sections through the left ear, the auditory ossicles, and the bony labyrinth. 1, pinna; 2, ear canal; 3, tympanic membrane; 4, auditory ossicles; 5, bony labyrinth; 6, eighth cranial nerve; 7, tympanic bulla; 8, auditory (eustachian) tube; 9, middle ear; A, tympanic membrane; B, malleus; C, incus; D, stapes; E, cochlea; F, utricle; G, H, and I, semicircular canals. (From Getty R: Atlas for Applied Veterinary Anatomy, 2nd ed. Ames, Ia.: Iowa State University Press, 1964.)

membranous labyrinth. The bony labyrinth is a series of tunnels within the petrous temporal bone. Inside these tunnels, surrounded by a fluid called *perilymph,* is the membranous labyrinth. The membranous labyrinth follows the contour of the bony labyrinth and contains *endolymph.* This "tunnel within a tunnel" design continues within both the vestibular and the cochlear systems.

The cochlear portion of the labyrinth is a coiled tube. Two membranes, the basilar and Reissner's, divide it into three chambers *(scalae)* throughout its length (Fig. 16–3). The upper and lower scalae contain perilymph and connect with each other at the distal end. The middle scala (scala media) contains endolymph. Along the floor of the scala media, on the basilar membrane, lies the hair cell receptor system called the *organ of Corti,* which transduces sound waves into action potentials.

The organ of Corti contains thousands of hair cell receptors that respond to sound waves and give rise to action potentials in the sensory afferent nerves, which carry action potentials along the eighth cranial nerve to the brainstem's cochlear nucleus.

THE COCHLEA TRANSDUCES SOUND WAVES TO ACTION POTENTIALS IN THE EIGHTH CRANIAL NERVE

Sound waves in the external environment cause vibrations of the tympanic membrane. These vibrations are transmitted through the middle ear by the auditory bones and result in similar vibrations of the oval window. These vibrations produce a series of traveling waves in the perilymph of the scala vestibuli that, in turn, cause vibrations in the basilar membrane. A diagram of this transmission is shown in Figure 16–4. The organ of Corti hair cells along the basilar membrane respond to these traveling waves by generating action potentials along the eighth cranial nerve. Hair cells at differing locations along the basilar membrane are thought to respond to different frequencies of traveling waves (pitch). Loudness is transduced as the intensity with which a given site on the basilar membrane is stimulated.

ACTION POTENTIALS FROM THE COCHLEA ARE TRANSMITTED UP THROUGH THE BRAINSTEM TO THE CEREBRAL CORTEX

Action potentials arising in the cochlea travel along the eighth cranial nerve to the cochlear nuclei in the medulla oblongata. From here, action potentials are transmitted to the ipsilateral and contralateral cerebral cortices by way of various brainstem routings, including the inferior colliculus and the medial geniculate body. Conscious perception of sound and the perception of its location of origin occur in the cerebral cortex.

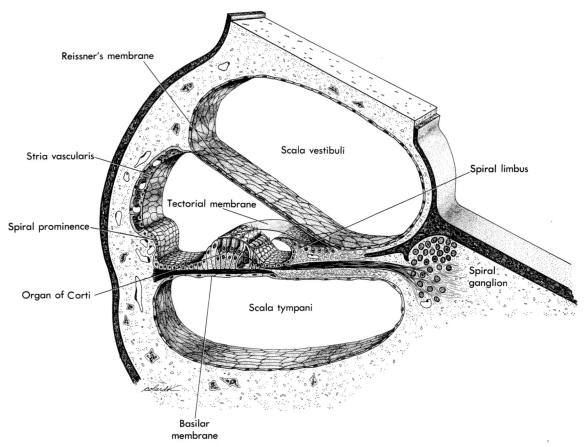

FIGURE 16–3. Schematic representation of a section through one of the turns of the cochlea. (From Bloom W, Fawcett DW: A Textbook of Histology, 10th ed. Philadelphia: WB Saunders, 1975.)

▬ DEAFNESS RESULTS FROM AN INTERRUPTION IN THE HEARING PROCESS

Clinical *deafness* may result from a loss of sound transmission in the external or middle ear, called *conduction deafness,* or from malfunction of the cochlear hair cells or nerve pathways, called *nerve deafness.* In veterinary medicine, deafness in young animals is usually caused by a congenital defect in the cochlea, frequently linked with white coat coloration.

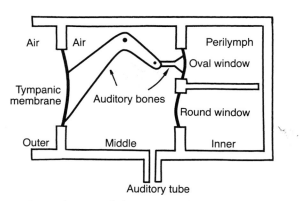

FIGURE 16–4. Diagram of the transmission of vibrations from the outer ear to the inner ear. (Redrawn from Lippold OCJ, Winton FR: Human Physiology, 6th ed. New York: Churchill Livingstone, 1972.)

CLINICAL CORRELATIONS

Congenital deafness

History   An almost completely white male Dalmatian pup is brought to you; the owner reports that the pup does not appear to hear anything.

Clinical examination   Your physical examination reveals an apparently normal, healthy Dalmatian pup except for an apparent deafness. He does not seem to respond to voice commands or loud noises. His vestibular and all other neurologic reflexes are within normal limits. A brainstem auditory evoked response is flat, which suggests that the brain has not received any signal from the cochlea.

Comment   Congenital deafness is fairly common in dogs and other animals with white coat color. It is usually caused by the partial or complete absence of the cochlea and occasionally by the absence of other neural elements of the auditory pathway. This is known as nerve deafness and is usually present at birth (congenital). Why it is linked to white coat coloration is unknown, but the pattern suggests that it is a genetically determined failure, usually bilateral, of the cochlea to develop.

Bibliography

Guyton AC, Hall JE: Textbook of Medical Physiology, 10th ed. Philadelphia: WB Saunders, 2000, pp 602–612.

Haines, DE: Fundamental Neuroscience. New York: Churchill Livingstone, 1997, pp 285–302.

Kandel ER, Schwartz JH, Jessell TM (eds): Principles of Neural Science, 4th ed. New York: McGraw-Hill, 2000, pp 590–624.

PRACTICE QUESTIONS

1. Which of the following cranial nerves transmits sound to the brain?
    a. Cranial nerve II.
    b. Cranial nerve VII.
    c. Cranial nerve VIII.
    d. Cranial nerve X.

2. A fusion of the auditory bones of the middle ear would likely have what effect on hearing?
    a. Improve hearing.
    b. Reduce hearing.
    c. Have no effect on hearing.

3. If the hair cell receptors were missing from the cochlea, what would the animal experience?
    a. Paralysis.
    b. Deafness.
    c. Blindness.
    d. Anesthesia (lack of all sensation).

4. When the frequency of sound waves increases, this is perceived as
    a. increased pitch.
    b. decreased pitch.
    c. increased loudness.
    d. decreased loudness.

PRACTICE ANSWERS

1. c   2. b   3. b   4. a

CARDIOVASCULAR PHYSIOLOGY

Robert B. Stephenson

17

Overview of cardiovascular function

1 Because normal cardiovascular function is essential for life and health, a practical understanding of cardiovascular function and dysfunction is vital to the veterinary clinician

2 Cardiovascular dysfunctions sometimes reflect primary cardiovascular disturbances or diseases, but more often they are secondary consequences of noncardiovascular disturbances or diseases

3 Substances transported by the cardiovascular system include nutrients, waste products, hormones, electrolytes, and water

4 Two modes of transport are used in the cardiovascular system: bulk flow and diffusion

5 Diffusion is very slow, and so every metabolizing cell in the body must be close to a capillary carrying blood by bulk flow

6 The pulmonary and systemic circulations are arranged in series, but the various organs within the systemic circulation are arranged in parallel

7 Cardiac output is the volume of blood pumped each minute by one ventricle

8 The perfusion pressure for the systemic circulation is much greater than the perfusion pressure for the pulmonary circulation

9 Each type of blood vessel has physical properties suited to its particular function

10 Blood is a suspension of cells in liquid (plasma)

11 The cellular component of blood includes red blood cells, white blood cells, and platelets

12 Most of the oxygen in blood is carried in chemical combination with the protein hemoglobin within red blood cells

Because normal cardiovascular function is essential for life and health, a practical understanding of cardiovascular function and dysfunction is vital to the veterinary clinician

Cardiovascular physiology is the study of the function of the heart, the blood vessels, and the blood. The primary function of the cardiovascular system can be summarized in one word: *transport.* The blood stream transports numerous substances that are essential for life and health, including the oxygen and nutrients required by every cell in the body. Blood also carries carbon dioxide and other metabolic waste products away from each cell of the body and delivers them to the lungs, kidneys, or liver, where they are excreted.

To appreciate how cardiovascular transport is essential for life and health, the reader has only to consider what happens if the heart stops completely and circulation ceases: unconsciousness results within about 30 seconds, and irreversible damage to the brain and other sensitive body tissues occurs within a few minutes. Of course, circulation does not have to stop completely in order for significant dysfunc-

tions to occur. For example, the loss of as little as 10% of the normal blood volume can impair exercise performance. In each tissue of the body, normal function depends on the delivery of an adequate amount of blood flow. The higher the rate of metabolism in a tissue, the greater the requirement for blood flow. The condition of inadequate blood flow to any tissue is called *ischemia.* Even transient ischemia leads to dysfunction. Persistent ischemia leads to permanent tissue damage (*infarction*) or cell death (*necrosis*).

Impairment in the transport functions of the cardiovascular system is encountered very frequently in veterinary medicine. Because any cardiovascular impairment inevitably leads to significant dysfunction and loss of health, a practical understanding of cardiovascular function and dysfunction is vital to the veterinary clinician.

Many veterinary students have difficulty understanding cardiovascular physiology. They tend to agree with William Harvey, the father of cardiovascular physiology, whose initial impression was that the motions of the heart and the blood were so complicated that they could be comprehended only by God! Harvey persisted, however, in his careful, deliberate study of cardiovascular function and in 1628 set forth the first proof that the heart propels blood through the blood vessels in a circulatory pattern. Before Harvey's time, it was thought that blood flowed out of the heart into the blood vessels and then returned to the heart by backward flow in the same vessels. In other words, blood was thought to flow in a tidal manner, in much the same way that air flows through a single set of airways: first into the lungs and then back out.

Today it is taken for granted that the cardiovascular system is a *circulatory system,* not a tidal system. However, the circularity of the cardiovascular system is precisely what makes it difficult to understand. It has no clear beginning or ending, and disturbances in one part of the cardiovascular system end up affecting all other parts as well. In recognition of this complexity, Chapters 17 to 25 have been written with the goal of identifying the most basic and important concepts of *normal cardiovascular function* and explaining them in a way that best prepares the reader to understand, diagnose, and treat *cardiovascular dysfunction* (cardiovascular disease).

Cardiovascular dysfunctions sometimes reflect primary cardiovascular disturbances or diseases, but more often they are secondary consequences of noncardiovascular disturbances or diseases

Some of the cardiovascular dysfunctions encountered in veterinary medicine are *primary,* in that the fundamental disturbance or disease process affects the cardiovascular system directly. One example of primary cardiovascular dysfunction is *hemorrhage* (loss of blood from blood vessels). Another is *myocarditis* (literally, "muscle-heart-inflammation"). Myocarditis is caused when a viral or bacterial infection inflames and weakens the heart muscle, impairing the ability of the heart to pump blood.

Cardiovascular dysfunction and disease can be either *congenital* (present at birth) or *acquired* (developing after birth). Myocarditis is an example of an acquired cardiovascular disease, and there are many others. Congenital cardiovascular diseases frequently involve defective heart valves, which either cannot open fully or cannot close completely. Congenital cardiac defects are common in certain breeds of dogs and horses. Although a heart that has a congenital defect or an acquired disease may be able to pump an adequate amount of blood when the animal is at rest, it usually cannot deliver the increased blood flow required by the body during exercise. When a dysfunction in the heart impairs its ability to pump the amount of blood flow normally needed by the body, the condition is called *heart failure.* The patient with heart failure classically exhibits *exercise intolerance.*

Parasites are another common cause of acquired cardiovascular dysfunction. In dogs, for example, adult heartworms *(Dirofilaria immitis)* lodge in the right ventricle and pulmonary artery, where they impede the flow of blood. These worms also release substances into the circulation that disrupt the body's ability to control blood pressure and blood flow. In horses, bloodworms *(Strongylus vulgaris)* lodge in the mesenteric arteries and decrease the blood flow to the intestine. The intestinal ischemia depresses digestive functions (motility, secretion, and absorption), and the horse exhibits signs of gastrointestinal distress *(colic).*

In many other disease states, cardiovascular complications develop even though the cardiovascular system is not the primary target of the disease. These *secondary cardiovascular dysfunctions* often become the most serious and life-threatening aspects of the disease. For example, severe burns or persistent vomiting or diarrhea leads to cardiovascular complications secondary to the substantial losses of water and *electrolytes* (e.g., K^+, Na^+, and Ca^{2+}) from the blood stream. Even if the blood volume is not depleted to dangerously low levels in these conditions, the alteration in electrolyte concentrations can lead to abnormal heart rhythms *(cardiac arrhythmias)* and ineffective pumping of blood by the heart (heart failure). The electrolyte abnormalities in such a patient can be made even worse if incorrect fluid therapy is given. Furthermore, incorrect fluid therapy can lead to an accumulation of excess fluid in the tissues of the body; this accumulation is called *edema.* If the excess fluid gathers in the lung tissue, the condition is called *pulmonary edema.* Pulmonary edema is life-threatening because it slows the flow of oxygen from the pulmonary air sacs *(alveoli)* into the blood stream.

Pulmonary edema is a secondary complication in many disease states. A further example is *shock-lung syndrome,* which results when toxic substances in the body trigger an increase in the permeability of the lung blood vessels. These "leaky" vessels allow water, electrolytes, plasma proteins, and white blood cells to leave the blood stream and accumulate in the lung tissue and airways. The resulting pulmonary edema can lead to death.

Whereas the effects of shock-lung syndrome are most serious in the pulmonary circulation, other kinds of shock depress the cardiovascular system in general. *Hemorrhagic shock* is a generalized cardiovascular failure caused by severe blood loss. *Cardiogenic shock* is a cardiovascular collapse caused by heart failure. *Septic shock* is caused by bacterial infections in the blood stream *(bacteremia). Endotoxic shock* occurs when endotoxins (fragments of bacterial cell walls) enter the blood stream. This often happens when the epithelial cells lining the intestines *(intestinal mucosa)* become damaged. Epithelial damage can result from bacterial infections in the intestines or from ischemia in the intestinal walls (as happens with bloodworms in horses). When the intestinal epithelium breaks down, endotoxins from the intestine enter the blood stream. These endotoxins then cause the body to produce substances that depress the pumping ability of the heart. The resulting heart failure leads to low blood pressure and ischemia in all the vital body organs. Kidney (or renal) failure, respiratory failure, central nervous system depression, and death follow.

Anesthetic overdose is another common clinical problem in which the most serious and life-threatening symptoms are the secondary cardiovascular complications. Most anesthetics depress the central nervous system, and the resulting abnormal neural signals to the heart and the blood vessels can depress cardiac output and lower blood pressure. Some anesthetics, particularly the barbiturates, also depress the pumping ability of the heart directly.

There are many other examples of primary and secondary cardiovascular dysfunction, but the ones just mentioned illustrate the importance and variety of cardiovascular dysfunctions encountered in veterinary medicine. The distinction between primary and secondary cardiovascular dysfunction is sometimes unclear, but this difficulty simply emphasizes how intimately the cardiovascular system is interconnected with all the other body systems and how very dependent all the other systems are on the normal functioning of the cardiovascular system.

The remainder of this chapter mentions the general features of the cardiovascular system. In Chapters 18 to 24, the various elements of the cardiovascular system are considered in detail. Finally, in Chapter 25, cardiovascular function and dysfunction are summarized by descriptions of the overall effects of heart failure, hemorrhage, and exercise.

Substances transported by the cardiovascular system include nutrients, waste products, hormones, electrolytes, and water

The blood transports the metabolic substrates needed by every cell of the body, including oxygen, glucose, amino acids, fatty acids, and various lipids. The blood also carries away from each cell in the body various metabolic waste products, including carbon dioxide, lactic acid, the nitrogenous wastes of protein metabolism, and heat. (Although the heat produced by metabolic processes within cells is not a material waste product, its transport by the cardiovascular system to the body surface is essential, because tissues deep within the body would otherwise become overheated and dysfunctional.)

The cardiovascular system also transports vital chemical messengers: the *hormones.* Hormones are synthesized and released by cells in one organ and are carried by the blood stream to cells in other organs, where they alter organ function. For example, insulin, which is produced by cells of the pancreas, is carried by the blood to cells throughout the body, where it promotes the cellular uptake of glucose. Inadequate insulin production (as happens in diabetes) results in inadequate entry of glucose into cells, whereas glucose concentrations in the blood rise to very high levels. The low intracellular glucose concentration is particularly disruptive to neural function, and the consequences can be serious (diabetic

coma) or lethal. Another hormone, adrenaline (a mixture of epinephrine and norepinephrine), is released into the blood stream by cells in the adrenal medulla during periods of stress. The epinephrine and norepinephrine circulate to various body organs, where they have effects that prepare a threatened animal for fight or flight. These effects include an increase in heart rate and cardiac contractility, a dilation of skeletal muscle blood vessels, an increase in blood pressure, increased glycogenolysis, dilation of the pupils and airways, and piloerection (hair standing on end).

Finally, the blood transports water and electrolytes, including Na^+, K^+, Ca^{2+}, H^+, NCO_3^-, and Cl^- ions. The kidneys are the organs primarily responsible for maintaining normal water and electrolyte composition in the body. The kidneys accomplish this by altering the electrolyte concentrations in blood as it flows through the kidneys. The altered blood then circulates to all other organs in the body, where it affects the water and electrolyte content in the extracellular and intracellular fluids of each tissue.

Two modes of transport are used in the cardiovascular system: bulk flow and diffusion

Blood moves through blood vessels by *bulk flow.* The most important feature of bulk flow is that it is rapid over long distances. For example, blood that is pumped out of the heart travels quickly through the aorta and its various branches, and it reaches distant parts of the body, including the head and limbs, within 10 seconds. Transport requires energy, and the source of energy for bulk flow is a hydrostatic pressure difference; unless the pressure at one end of a blood vessel is higher than the pressure at the other end, flow will not occur. The difference in pressure between two points in a blood vessel is called the *perfusion pressure difference* or, more commonly, simply *perfusion pressure. Perfusion* literally means "flow through," and the perfusion pressure is the pressure difference that causes blood to flow through blood vessels. The muscular pumping action of the heart creates the perfusion pressure differences that provide the driving force for bulk flow of blood through the circulation.

It is important to distinguish between perfusion pressure difference and *transmural pressure difference* (term is commonly shortened to *transmural pressure). Transmural* means "across the wall," and transmural pressure is the difference between the blood pressure inside a blood vessel and the fluid pressure outside the vessel (transmural pressure equals inside pressure minus outside pressure). Transmural pressure is the pressure difference that would cause blood to flow out of a vessel if a hole were poked in the vessel wall. Transmural pressure is also called *distending pressure,* because it corresponds to the magnitude of the net outward "push" on the wall of a blood vessel. To summarize: perfusion pressure is the pressure difference *along the length* of a blood vessel, whereas transmural pressure (distending pressure) is the pressure difference *across the wall* of a blood vessel; perfusion pressure is the driving force for blood flow through the circulation, whereas transmural pressure is the driving force for blood to spill out of a vessel if there is a hole in it.

Diffusion is the second mode of transport in the cardiovascular system. Diffusion is the primary mechanism by which dissolved substances move across the walls of blood vessels, from the blood stream into the interstitial fluid or vice versa. *Interstitial fluid* is the extracellular fluid outside capillaries. It is the fluid that bathes each cell of a tissue. Most of the movement of substances between the blood and the interstitial fluid takes place across the walls of the *capillaries*, the smallest blood vessels. In order for a substance (e.g., oxygen) to move from the blood stream to a tissue cell, it would first have to diffuse across the wall of a capillary and into the tissue interstitial fluid and then diffuse from the interstitial fluid into the tissue cell.

The source of energy for diffusion is a concentration difference. A substance diffuses from the blood stream, across the wall of a capillary, and into the interstitial fluid only if the concentration of the substance is higher in the blood than in the interstitial fluid (and if the capillary wall is permeable to the substance). If the concentration of a substance is higher in the interstitial fluid than in the blood, the substance will diffuse from the interstitial fluid into the capillary blood. It is important to distinguish *diffusion,* in which a substance moves passively from an area of high concentration toward an area of low concentration, from *active transport,* in which substances are forced to move in a direction opposite to their concentration gradient. In general, substances are not transported actively across the walls of capillaries. The movement of substances between the blood stream and the interstitial fluid occurs by passive diffusion.

Diffusion is very slow, and so every metabolizing cell in the body must be close to a capillary carrying blood by bulk flow

To understand more fully how the two types of transport (bulk flow and diffusion) are used in the cardiovascular system, consider the transport of oxygen from the outside air to a neuron in the brain. With each inspiration, fresh air containing oxygen moves (by bulk flow) through the trachea, bronchi, and bronchioles and into the alveolar air sacs (Fig. 17–1A). The wall of each *alveolus* is covered with a meshwork of capillaries (Fig. 17–1B). Blood flowing through these *pulmonary capillaries* passes extremely close to the air in the alveolus (Fig. 17–1C). The blood flowing through the pulmonary capillaries has just returned from the body tissues, where it gave up some of its oxygen. Therefore, the concentration of oxygen in the pulmonary capillary blood is lower than the concen-

tration of oxygen in the alveolar air. This concentration difference causes some oxygen to move, by diffusion, from the alveolar air into the capillary blood.

A large dog has about 300 million alveoli, with a total surface area of about 130 m² (equal to half the surface area of a tennis court). This huge surface area is laced with pulmonary capillaries. Thus, even though only a very tiny amount of oxygen diffuses into each pulmonary capillary, the aggregate uptake of oxygen into the pulmonary blood stream is substantial (typically, 125 mL/minute in a large, resting dog, increasing 10 to 30 times during strenuous exercise). It takes less than 1 second for the blood in a single pulmonary capillary to become oxygenated as it flows past an alveolus. Diffusion can provide such a quick and efficient way for oxygen to move from alveolar air into the blood stream because the distance involved is extremely short; in a normal lung, the distance separating alveolar air from pulmonary blood is less than 1 μm. In summary, both the large surface available for diffusion and the short distance between the alveolar air and the capillary blood promote rapid diffusion.

As it leaves the lungs, each 100 mL of oxygenated blood carries 20 mL of oxygen. About 1% of this oxygen is carried in solution; the other 99% is bound to the protein *hemoglobin* within the *erythrocytes* (red blood cells). The oxygenated blood moves by bulk flow from the lungs to the heart. The heart pumps this oxygenated blood out into the arteries, and it is thereby delivered to all parts of the body, including the brain and skeletal muscles (see Fig. 17–1). Capillaries in the brain bring the oxygenated blood close to each brain neuron (see Fig. 17–1D). Metabolic processes within the neurons consume oxygen, so the oxygen concentration inside neurons is low. Therefore, there exist concentration gradients for the diffusion of oxygen from the capillary blood to the interstitial fluid and from the interstitial fluid into the intracellular fluid of the neurons. The resulting diffusion of oxygen occurs within a few seconds if the capillary is close to the neuron.

Each brain neuron must be within about 100 μm of a capillary carrying blood by bulk flow if diffusion is to deliver oxygen rapidly enough to sustain normal metabolism in the neuron. Diffusional exchange over distances up to 100 μm typically takes only 1 to 5 seconds. If the distance involved were a few millimeters, diffusion would take minutes to occur. Diffusion of oxygen a few centimeters through body fluid would take hours. Therefore, normal life processes require that every metabolizing cell of the body be within about 100 μm of a capillary carrying blood by bulk flow. If this bulk flow is interrupted for any reason, perhaps because of a *thrombus* (blood clot) in the artery that delivers blood to a particular region of a tissue, then that region of tissue becomes *ischemic.* Severe ischemia leads to tissue damage and eventually to tissue death, which is called *necrosis.* An area of tissue damage or death caused by interruption of normal blood flow is called an *infarct.* A cerebral

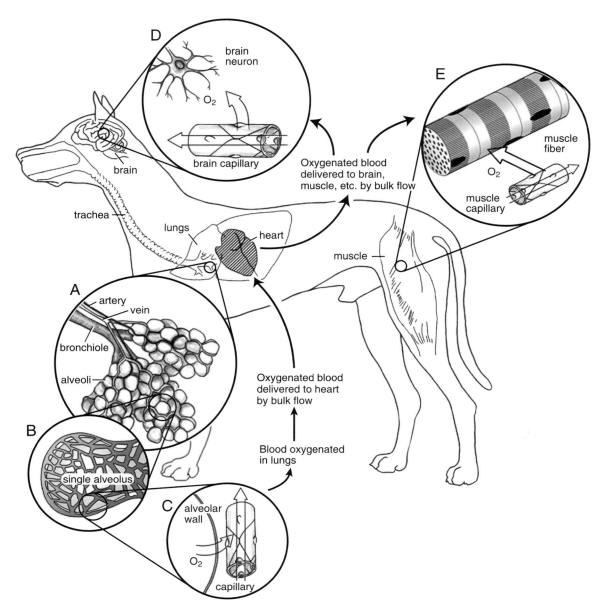

FIGURE 17–1. Oxygen is transported from the atmosphere to cells throughout the body by a combination of bulk flow and diffusion. First, oxygen moves from the atmosphere to the alveolar air sacs of the lungs by bulk flow through the airways. From there it diffuses into the blood that is flowing through pulmonary capillaries *(insets A, B,* and *C).* Bulk flow of blood next carries the oxygen to the heart, from which it is delivered by bulk flow into the capillaries of all the body organs (except the lungs). In the brain *(inset D),* the skeletal muscle *(inset E),* and other tissues, oxygen moves by diffusion from the capillary blood into the interstitial fluid and then into the tissue cells, where it is needed to support oxidative metabolism. Bulk flow is rapid; it can transport oxygen to all parts of the body within a few seconds. Diffusion is slow; it can transport oxygen efficiently only over distances less than 100 μm.

infarction causes the condition commonly known as *stroke.*

Figure 17–1E shows a capillary carrying blood by bulk flow past a skeletal muscle cell (muscle fiber). Oxygen moves by diffusion from the capillary blood into the muscle interstitial fluid and then into the muscle cell, where it is used in the metabolic reactions that provide energy for muscle contraction. The oxygen consumption of a skeletal muscle depends on the severity of its exercise; at a maximum, oxygen consumption may reach levels 40 times greater than the resting level. Because of its tremendous metabolic

capacity, muscle tissue has an especially high density of capillaries. In fact, several capillaries are typically arrayed around each skeletal muscle fiber. This arrangement provides more surface area for diffusional exchange than would be possible with a single capillary and also brings the bulk flow of blood extremely close to all parts of each skeletal muscle cell.

Heart muscle, like skeletal muscle, consumes a large amount of oxygen. Oxygenated blood is carried from the aorta to the heart muscle by a network of branching *coronary arteries.* This blood moves by bulk flow through capillaries that run close to each cardiac muscle cell. If a thrombus interrupts the bulk flow of blood in a coronary artery, the heart muscle cells supplied by that artery become ischemic. Ischemia develops even if the cardiac muscle deprived of blood flow lies within a few millimeters of the left ventricular chamber, which is filled with oxygen-rich blood. Oxygen cannot diffuse rapidly enough from the ventricular chamber to the ischemic cells to sustain their metabolism. Ischemic cardiac muscle loses its ability to contract forcefully, and cardiac arrhythmias may develop. Severe myocardial ischemia causes a *myocardial infarction,* or heart attack.

Coronary artery disease and *cerebral vascular disease* are very commonly encountered in human medicine. These vascular diseases are encountered less frequently in veterinary medicine. In contrast, *cardiac disease* (dysfunction of the heart muscle or valves, as distinguished from disease of the coronary arteries) is more commonly encountered in veterinary medicine than in human medicine. Therefore, in Chapters 18 to 25, more emphasis is placed on cardiac physiology than on vascular physiology. In the remainder of this chapter, the general layout of the circulation is considered, and particular attention is paid to the perfusion pressure differences that drive the bulk flow of blood through the circulation. This chapter then closes with a short description of the properties of blood.

The pulmonary and systemic circulations are arranged in series, but the various organs within the systemic circulation are arranged in parallel

As shown in Figure 17–2, blood is pumped from the left ventricle into the aorta. The aorta divides and subdivides to form many arteries, which deliver fresh, oxygenated blood to each organ of the body, except the lungs. The pattern of arterial branching that delivers blood of the same composition to each organ is called *parallel.* After blood passes through the capillaries within individual organs, it enters veins. Small veins combine to form progressively larger veins, until the entire blood flow is delivered to the right atrium by way of the venae cavae. The blood vessels between the aorta and the venae cavae (including the blood vessels in all organs of the body except the lungs) are collectively called the *systemic circulation.* Blood passes from the right atrium into the right ventricle, which pumps it into the pulmonary artery. The pulmonary artery branches into progressively smaller arteries, which deliver blood to each lung capillary. Blood from lung capillaries is collected in pulmonary veins and brought to the left atrium. Blood then passes back into the left ventricle. The blood vessels of the lungs constitute the *pulmonary circulation.* The pulmonary circulation and the heart are collectively termed the *central circulation.* The pulmonary circulation and the systemic circulation are arranged in *series;* that is, blood must pass through the pulmonary vessels between each passage through the systemic circuit.

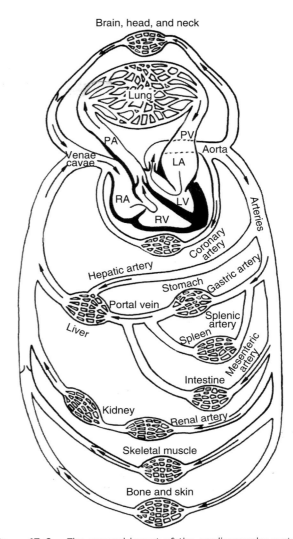

FIGURE 17–2. The general layout of the cardiovascular system, showing that the systemic and pulmonary circulations are arranged in series and that the organs within the systemic circulation are arranged in parallel. LA, left atrium; LV, left ventricle; PA, pulmonary artery; PV, pulmonary vein; RA, right atrium; RV, right ventricle. (Adapted from Milnor WR: Cardiovascular Physiology. New York: Oxford University Press, 1990.)

In one pass through the systemic circulation, blood generally encounters only one capillary bed before being collected in veins and returned to the heart. There are three exceptions to this rule. The first concerns the *splanchnic circulation* (blood supply of the digestive organs). As shown in Figure 17–2, blood that leaves the gastric, splenic, or mesenteric capillaries enters the *portal vein.* The portal vein carries splanchnic venous blood to the liver, where the blood passes through another set of capillaries before it returns to the heart. This arrangement of two systemic capillary beds in series is called a *portal system.* The splanchnic portal system allows nutrients that have been absorbed from the gastrointestinal tract to be delivered directly to the liver. There the nutrients are transformed for storage or allowed to pass into the general circulation. The liver also receives some blood directly from the aorta via the hepatic artery.

The kidneys contain the second example of a portal system. As shown in Figure 17–2, blood enters a kidney via a renal artery and passes through two sets of capillaries (called *glomerular* and *tubular)* before returning to the venous side of the systemic circulation. Large amounts of water, electrolytes, and other solutes are filtered out of the blood as it passes through the glomerular capillaries. Most of this filtered material is subsequently reabsorbed into the blood stream as it flows through the peritubular capillaries. The remainder becomes urine. The kidneys use this *renal portal system* to adjust the amounts of water, electrolytes, and other solutes in the blood.

The third portal system is found in the brain and is important in the control of hormone secretion by the pituitary gland. After traversing capillaries in the hypothalamus, blood enters portal vessels that carry it to the anterior pituitary gland (adenohypophysis) and to another set of capillaries (see Figs. 32–16 and 32–17). As blood traverses the hypothalamic capillaries, it picks up substances that control the release of pituitary hormones. When this blood reaches capillaries in the anterior pituitary gland, these substances diffuse out of the blood stream and into the pituitary interstitial fluid, where they act on pituitary cells to increase or decrease their secretion of specific hormones. This system is called the *hypothalamic-hypophyseal portal system.*

To summarize, the splanchnic, renal, and hypothalamic-hypophyseal portal systems are the only major exceptions to the rule that blood encounters only one capillary bed in a single pass through the systemic circulation.

Cardiac output is the volume of blood pumped each minute by one ventricle

In a resting dog, about 1 minute is typically needed for blood to traverse the entire circulation (from the left ventricle back to the left ventricle). Because the pulmonary and systemic circulations are in series, the volume of blood pumped by the right side of the heart each minute must equal the volume of blood pumped by the left side of the heart each minute. The volume of blood pumped per minute by either the left ventricle or the right ventricle is called *cardiac output.* Among the mammalian species commonly encountered in veterinary medicine, cardiac output at rest is approximately 3 L/minute per square meter of body surface area. A large dog (e.g., German shepherd) typically has a body surface area a little less than 1 m² and a cardiac output at rest of about 2.5 L/minute. Note that the left and right ventricles in such a dog together pump 5.0 L of blood per minute.

In an animal at rest, blood entering the aorta is divided so that approximately 20% of it flows through the splanchnic circulation and 20% to the kidneys. Another 20% goes to the skeletal muscles. The brain receives about 15% of the cardiac output, and the coronary arteries carry about 3% of the cardiac output. The remainder goes to skin and bone.

The perfusion pressure for the systemic circulation is much greater than the perfusion pressure for the pulmonary circulation

When the left ventricle contracts and ejects blood into the aorta, the aorta becomes distended with blood, and aortic pressure rises to a peak value called *systolic pressure* (typically 120 mm Hg). Between ejections, blood continues to flow out of the aorta into the downstream arteries. This outflow of blood from the aorta causes aortic pressure to decrease. The minimal value of aortic pressure, just before the next cardiac ejection, is called *diastolic pressure* (typically 80 mm Hg). The *mean aortic pressure* (average value of the pulsatile pressure in the aorta) is about 98 mm Hg. The mean aortic pressure represents a potential energy for driving blood through the systemic circulation. As blood flows through the systemic blood vessels, this pressure energy is dissipated through friction. The potential energy (blood pressure) remaining by the time the blood reaches the venae cavae is only 3 mm Hg. Therefore, the perfusion pressure for the systemic circuit is 98 − 3 mm Hg, or 95 mm Hg.

The pressures in the pulmonary artery are typically 20 mm Hg (systolic) and 8 mm Hg (diastolic); the typical mean value is 13 mm Hg. Pulmonary venous pressure is typically 5 mm Hg, so the perfusion pressure for blood flow through the lungs is 8 mm Hg (i.e., 13 − 5 mm Hg).

The same volume of blood (the cardiac output) flows each minute through the systemic circulation and through the lungs; however, the perfusion pressure for the systemic circuit is much greater than the perfusion pressure for the lungs. The reason for this difference in perfusion pressure is that the systemic vessels offer more friction against blood flow (have a higher resistance) than do the pulmonary vessels. Therefore, the systemic circulation is referred to as the *high-pressure, high-resistance side of the circulation.* The pulmonary circuit is called the *low-pressure, low-resistance side.*

By convention, blood pressures are always measured with reference to atmospheric pressure. Thus, to say that aortic pressure is 98 mm Hg means that the blood pressure in the aorta is 98 mm Hg higher than the atmospheric pressure outside the body. Also, by convention, blood pressure is measured at heart level. This is why, in human medicine, blood pressure cuffs are typically applied over the brachial artery (in the upper arm); the brachial artery is at the same level as the heart. If blood pressure is measured in an artery or vein at a level different from heart level, an arithmetic correction should be made so that the pressure is reported as if it had been measured at heart level. This correction is necessary, because gravity pulls downward on blood and therefore affects

TABLE 17–1.   **Distribution of blood volume in the cardiovascular system of a normal dog**

Distribution	Percent
Between central and systemic circulations	
Central circulation	25
Systemic vessels	75
Total	100
Within the systemic circulation	
Arteries and arterioles	15
Capillaries	5
Venules and veins	80
Total	100

the actual pressure of blood within vessels. Gravity increases the actual pressure in vessels lying below heart level and decreases the actual pressure in vessels above heart level. The gravitational effect is significant in an animal the size of a dog and substantial in an animal the size of a horse. The correction factor for the effect of gravity is approximately 1 mm Hg for each centimeter above or below heart level.

Each type of blood vessel has physical properties suited to its particular function

In a resting animal, at any one moment, about 25% of the blood volume is in the central circulation and about 75% is in the systemic circulation (Table 17–1). Most of the blood in the systemic circulation is found in the veins. Only 20% of the systemic blood is found in the arteries, arterioles, and capillaries. Therefore, these veins are known as the *blood reservoirs* of the circulation. The arteries are the *high-pressure conduits* for delivery of blood to the capillaries. The arterioles are the "gates" of the systemic circulation; they constrict or dilate to control the blood flow to each capillary bed. Although only a small fraction of the systemic blood is found in capillaries at any one time, it is within these vessels that the important diffusional exchange takes place between the blood stream and the interstitial fluid. The capillaries are the *exchange vessels* of the circulation.

Table 17–2 presents information about the size and number of the various types of vessels in the systemic circulation of a dog. As the aorta branches into progressively smaller vessels, the diameters of the vessels become smaller, but the number of vessels increases. One aorta supplies blood to 45,000 terminal arteries, each of which gives rise to more than 400 arterioles. Each arteriole typically branches into about 80 capillaries. The capillaries are so small in diameter that red blood cells must pass through in single file and must deform somewhat to squeeze through at all. However, because of the sheer number of capillaries, the total cross-sectional area of the capillaries is much greater than the cross-sectional area of the preceding arteries and arterioles. Also, because capillary blood flow is spread out over such a large cross-sectional area, the flow velocity is low. Blood moves rapidly (about 13 cm/second) through the aorta and large arteries. At this speed, blood is delivered from the heart to all parts of the body in less than 10 seconds. The velocity of blood flow decreases as the blood leaves arteries and enters arterioles and capillaries in each tissue. The velocity of blood flow in capillaries is so slow that blood typically takes 1 to 5 seconds to travel the 0.5 mm length of a capillary. During this time, diffusional exchange takes place between the capillary blood and the interstitial fluid. Blood from the capillaries is collected by venules and veins and is carried quite rapidly back to the heart.

Figure 17–3 depicts the branching pattern in the systemic circulation and graphs the velocity of blood flow within the different types of vessels. This figure emphasizes the rapidity of bulk flow through large vessels and the relatively slow flow through the capillaries. Note that the *velocity* of blood flow, not the total flow per minute, is lower in the capillaries. The same *volume* of blood flows each minute through an artery, the capillaries that it feeds, and the veins draining the capillaries.

In addition to having a large cross-sectional area (and therefore slow velocity of blood flow), capillaries have a large surface area. The total surface area of the walls of all the capillaries in the systemic circulation of a large dog is about 20 m^2, which is nearly 30 times greater than the dog's body surface area. The large surface area of capillaries helps promote efficient diffusional exchange between the capillary blood and the interstitial fluid.

TABLE 17–2.   **Geometry of systemic circulation of a 30-kg dog**

Vessel	Number	Inside diameter (mm)	Total cross-sectional area (cm^2)	Length (cm)	Velocity of blood flow (cm/sec)	Mean blood pressure (mm Hg)
Aorta	1	20.0	3.1	40.0	13.0	98
Small arteries	45,000	0.14	6.9	1.5	6.0	90
Arterioles	20,000,000	0.030	140.0	0.2	0.3	60
Capillaries	1,700,000,000	0.008	830.0	0.05	0.05	18
Venules	130,000,000	0.020	420.0	0.1	0.1	12
Small veins	73,000	0.27	42.0	1.5	1.0	6
Venae cavae	2	24.0	9.0	34.0	4.5	3

Adapted from Milnor WR: Cardiovascular Physiology. New York: Oxford University Press, 1990.

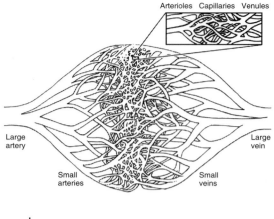

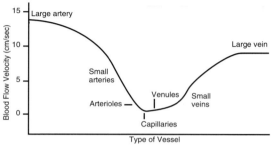

Figure 17–3. As the systemic arteries branch to form small arteries, arterioles, and capillaries *(top)*, the total cross-sectional area of the vessels increases, so the forward velocity of blood flow decreases *(bottom)*. As blood from the capillaries is collected into venules and veins, the total cross-sectional area is reduced, so the velocity of blood flow increases again. Therefore, blood moves quickly from the heart to the microvessels, where it stays for a few seconds before moving rapidly back to the heart.

Blood is a suspension of cells in liquid (plasma)

As shown in Figure 17–4, blood can be separated into its cellular and liquid components by centrifugation. The liquid phase of blood is lighter in weight than are the cells and therefore ends up on the top of the centrifuge tube. This acellular or extracellular liquid in blood is called *plasma*. Water constitutes 93% of the plasma volume. About 5% to 7% of the plasma volume is made up of protein molecules. The presence of proteins gives plasma its typical pale yellow color. The *plasma proteins* are synthesized in the liver and added to the blood stream as it passes through the liver capillaries. Globulin, albumin, and fibrinogen are the primary plasma proteins. Globulin and albumin are important in the immune responses of the body. Fibrinogen is important in the process of blood clotting. If blood is removed from the body and allowed to stand for a few moments, the soluble fibrinogen molecules polymerize to form an insoluble matrix of fibrin. This causes the blood to congeal, or *coagulate*. Coagulation can be prevented by adding an *anticoagulant* to the blood, the most common ones being heparin and citrate. An anticoagulant must be added in preparation for separating blood into its cellular and plasma fractions by centrifugation.

Many important substances, in addition to plasma proteins, are dissolved in plasma. Plasma contains several ions *(electrolytes)* in solution. The dominant cation is Na^+. The predominant anions are Cl^- and HCO_3^-. K^+, Ca^{2+}, H^+, Mg^{2+}, HPO_4^{2-}, $H_2PO_4^-$, and SO_4^{2-} are present in lesser amounts, but their concentrations are critical to normal body function. The body has many mechanisms to regulate the concentrations of all the plasma electrolytes. In general, the plasma electrolytes can diffuse readily across capillary walls; therefore, interstitial fluid and plasma typically have very similar electrolyte concentrations.

Plasma contains small amounts of gases (O_2, CO_2, N_2) in solution. Most (about 99%) of the O_2 in blood is carried in chemical combination with hemoglobin (in the red blood cells). Most of the CO_2 in blood becomes hydrated to form HCO_3^- or combines with hemoglobin or plasma proteins to form carbamino compounds.

The nutrient substances dissolved in plasma include glucose, amino acids, lipids, and some vitamins. The metabolic waste products (in addition to CO_2) include urea, creatinine, uric acid, and bilirubin. Plasma also contains many hormones (e.g., insulin, epinephrine, and thyroxine), which are present in exceedingly tiny, but critically important amounts. Table 17–3 presents a summary of the normal constituents of plasma.

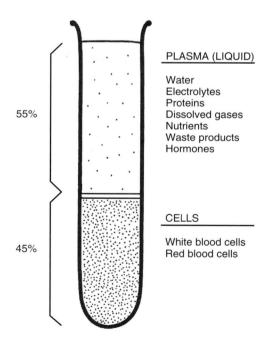

Figure 17–4. Anticoagulated blood can be separated into a liquid component (plasma) and a cellular component (cells) by centrifugation. Plasma is a solution of many important substances in water. The cells are heavier than the plasma, and they settle to the bottom. Most of the cells are red blood cells. The white blood cells are slightly lighter in weight than the red blood cells, and they form a thin "buffy coat" on the top of the red cell layer. The fraction of cells in blood is called the hematocrit. In this example, the hematocrit is 45%.

TABLE 17–3. Some constituents of canine plasma (in addition to water, the main constituent)

Component	Normal range	Units
Plasma proteins (carried in colloidal suspension)		
Globulin (total)	2.7–4.4	g/dL
Albumin	2.3–3.1	g/dL
Fibrinogen	0.15–0.30	g/dL
Electrolytes (dissolved)		
Na^+	140–150	mmol/L
K^+	3.9–5.1	mmol/L
Ca^{2+} (ionized)	1.2–1.5	mmol/L
Mg^{2+} (ionized)	0.5–0.9	mmol/L
Cl^-	110–124	mmol/L
HCO_3^-	20–29	mmol/L
HPO_4^{2-} and $H_2PO_4^-$	1.0–1.4	mmol/L
H^+	36–44	nmol/L*
(H^+ expressed as pH)†	(7.44–7.36)	
Dissolved gases (arterial plasma)		
O_2	0.27–0.30	mL/dL
CO_2	2.2–2.6	mL/dL
Examples of nutrients, waste products, hormones		
Cholesterol	140–280	mg/dL
Glucose	76–120	mg/dL
Triglycerides	40–170	mg/dL
Urea nitrogen	8–28	mg/dL
Creatinine	0.5–1.7	mg/dL
Bile acids (fasting)	0–8	μmol/L
Thyroxine (T_4)	0.019–0.051	μmol/L

*Note that [H^+] is in nmol (nanomolar) units; 10^6 nmol = 1 mmol.
†pH = − log [H^+], where [H^+] is expressed in molar units; pH is dimensionless.
Adapted from Duncan JR, Prasse KW, Mahaffey EA: Veterinary Laboratory Medicine. Ames, Ia.: Iowa State University Press, 1994.

The cellular component of blood includes red blood cells, white blood cells, and platelets

Cells normally constitute 30% to 55% of the blood volume (depending on the species). The fraction of cells in blood is called the *hematocrit* (see Fig. 17–4). The hematocrit is determined by adding an anticoagulant to some blood and then centrifuging it in a tube. The cells are somewhat heavier than plasma and settle to the bottom of the tube during centrifugation. Because centrifugation results in a packing of the blood cells in the bottom of the tube, the hematocrit is sometimes called the *packed cell volume*. Most of the cell component looks red, because most of the blood cells are *erythrocytes (red blood cells)*. The red blood cells get their color from the red-pigmented protein *hemoglobin*.

The *leukocytes,* or *white blood cells,* are slightly lighter in weight than the red blood cells; in a centrifuge tube, they gather in a white "buffy coat" on top of the red blood cells. The buffy coat is normally very thin because there are about 1000 times more red blood cells than white blood cells. Leukocytes are critical in immune and allergic responses of the body. The subtypes of leukocytes include neutrophils, lymphocytes, monocytes, eosinophils, and basophils. A laboratory analysis of the total number and relative distribution of the various white cell subtypes (*differ-*

ential white blood cell count) provides important clues in the diagnosis of disease. Both erythrocytes and leukocytes are made in the bone marrow. They develop, by mitosis and differentiation, from a common line of progenitor cells, the *pluripotent (uncommitted) stem cells.*

The cellular component in a centrifuge tube also contains *platelets (thrombocytes),* which are fragments of the membranes of their precursor cells, the *megakaryocytes.* The megakaryocytes reside in the bone marrow, and they shed platelets into the blood stream. Platelets participate in *hemostasis* (the control of bleeding through coagulation and clotting). In this process, a clumping together of platelets *(platelet aggregation)* begins to create a physical barrier across openings in blood vessels. Then substances released from the platelets, along with fibrinogen and several clotting factors in the plasma, lead to the coagulation of blood and the formation of a stable, fibrin-based blood clot.

Coagulation and clotting involve complex, interconnected sequences of chemical reactions (the *coagulation cascade).* A key step in the coagulation cascade is the formation in the plasma of thrombin, an enzyme that catalyzes the transformation of fibrinogen to fibrin. Several laboratory tests are used to assess the status of an animal's coagulation system. The two most common of these involve determination of the *prothrombin time* (PT) and the *partial thromboplastin time* (PTT).

If blood is allowed to coagulate and then is centrifuged, the fibrin and other plasma clotting factors settle to the bottom along with the red and white blood cells and the platelets. The liquid portion remaining above (essentially plasma without fibrinogen and other clotting factors) is called *serum.* Most of the common clinical blood chemistry analyses are performed on serum. Examples include the determination of concentrations of electrolytes and cholesterol.

If blood is treated with an anticoagulant and then allowed simply to sit in a tube (without centrifugation), the erythrocytes slowly begin to settle. For reasons that are not completely understood, the rate of their settling tends to be increased to above normal in certain disease states and decreased to below normal in others. Therefore the *erythrocyte sedimentation rate* (ESR) is a clinically useful diagnostic measurement. The normal ESR varies substantially between species; for example, it is much more rapid in equine blood than in canine blood.

Blood cell counts are performed by manual or automated scanning of a very small volume (e.g., 1 μL) of anticoagulated whole blood. Table 17–4 presents a summary of normal hematologic values for the dog.

Most of the oxygen in blood is carried in chemical combination with the protein hemoglobin within red blood cells

Of the 20 mL of O_2 normally carried in each 100 mL of oxygenated blood, only 1.5% (0.3 mL) is carried in

TABLE 17–4.   **Canine hematology**

Test	Normal range	Units
Hematocrit	45–57	%
Blood cell counts		
Red blood cells	5000–7900	$\times 10^3/\mu L$
White blood cells	5–14	$\times 10^3/\mu L$
Platelets	210–620	$\times 10^3/\mu L$
Hemoglobin measures		
Blood hemoglobin	12–19	g/dL
MCH	21–26	pg
MCHC	32–36	g/dL

MCH, mean content of hemoglobin per red blood cell; MCHC, mean cell hemoglobin concentration.
Adapted from Duncan JR, Prasse KW, Mahaffey EA: Veterinary Laboratory Medicine. Ames, Ia.: Iowa State University Press, 1994.

dissolved form. The remaining 98.5% is carried in chemical combination with hemoglobin (in the red blood cells). *Oxygenated hemoglobin* (HbO_2) is bright red. When oxygen is released, HbO_2 becomes *reduced hemoglobin* (Hb), which is dark bluish-red. To a degree, the adequacy of oxygenation of an animal's blood can be judged by looking at the color of its nonpigmented epithelial membranes (e.g., gums, nostrils, or inside surfaces of eyelids). Well-oxygenated tissues appear pink. Poorly oxygenated tissues appear bluish *(cyanotic)*, because of the prevalence of reduced hemoglobin.

The ability of blood to carry oxygen is determined by the amount of hemoglobin in the blood and by the chemical characteristics of that hemoglobin. For example, each deciliter of normal dog blood contains about 15 g of hemoglobin. Each gram of Hb can combine with 1.34 mL of oxygen, when fully saturated. Thus, each deciliter of fully oxygenated, normal blood carries 20 mL of oxygen. Several disease states result in the synthesis of chemically abnormal Hb, with a diminished capacity to bind oxygen. In addition to these *hemoglobinopathies*, there are several common toxins, including carbon monoxide and nitrates, that cause life-threatening alterations in the ability of Hb to bind oxygen.

Because hemoglobin is localized inside red blood cells, it is possible to derive several clinically useful relationships among the blood hemoglobin content, red blood cell count, hemoglobin content of each red blood cell, and hematocrit. For example, if a dog has 15 g of hemoglobin per deciliter of blood and a red blood cell count of 6 million cells per microliter of blood, it follows that each red cell (on average) contains 25 pg of hemoglobin:

$$\frac{15 \text{ g of hemoglobin/dL of blood}}{6 \times 10^6 \text{ red blood cells/}\mu L \text{ of blood}}$$

$$= 25 \times 10^{-12} \text{ g of hemoglobin/red blood cell}$$

The value calculated in this way is called the *mean content of hemoglobin per red cell* (MHC). An easier calculation, which serves the same purpose, is to determine how much hemoglobin is contained in each deciliter of packed red blood cells (i.e., what the con-

centration of hemoglobin is in just the red blood cell portion of the blood). For example, if a dog (with 15 g of hemoglobin in each deciliter of blood) has blood that is 50% red cells (i.e., a hematocrit of 50%), then the concentration of hemoglobin in the red cells must be 30 g of hemoglobin per deciliter of packed red cells:

$$\frac{15 \text{ g of hemoglobin/dL of blood}}{0.5 \text{ dL of red blood cells/dL of blood}}$$

$$= 30 \text{ g of hemoglobin/dL of red blood cells}$$

The value calculated in this way is called the *mean cell hemoglobin concentration* (MCHC). For simplicity, the calculation is often summarized as MCHC = [hemoglobin]/hematocrit. (The brackets denote concentration.) An abnormally low value of MCH or MCHC is clinically important, because it points to a deficit in hemoglobin synthesis (i.e., not enough hemoglobin being made to load up each red blood cell). In contrast, an abnormally low value for [hemoglobin] by itself is less helpful. For example, a dog's hemoglobin concentration in the blood could fall below 15 g/dL for several reasons: a deficit in hemoglobin synthesis, a deficit in red blood cell synthesis, or a "watering down" of the blood either by addition of excess plasma fluid or by loss of red blood cells.

Obviously, deviations from a normal hematocrit can have important consequences in terms of the ability of blood to carry oxygen. Hematocrit also affects the *viscosity* of blood, as shown in Figure 17–5. Viscosity is a measure of resistance to flow. For example, honey is more viscous (more resistant to flow) than water. Plasma, by itself, is about 1.5 times more viscous than water because of the presence of plasma protein molecules (albumin, globulin, fibrinogen). The presence of cells in blood has an even bigger effect on viscosity. Blood with a hematocrit of 40% has twice the viscosity of plasma. For hematocrits exceeding

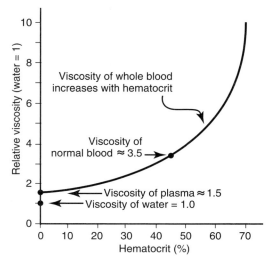

FIGURE 17–5.   Plasma is more viscous than water because of the presence of plasma proteins. Blood is more viscous than plasma because of the presence of blood cells. Blood viscosity increases sharply when the fraction of cells (hematocrit) rises much above 40%.

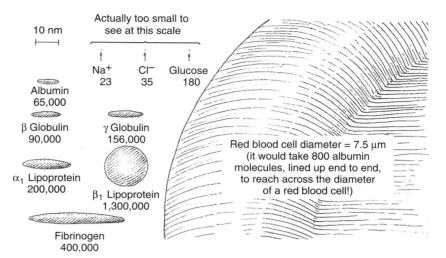

FIGURE 17-6. The relative size and shape of the major constituents of blood. The figure emphasizes that the plasma protein molecules are huge in comparison with the other plasma solutes, such as glucose, Na⁺, and Cl⁻. Furthermore, the blood cells (red and white) are huge in comparison with plasma protein molecules. Numbers under constituents are their molecular weights. The scale (upper left) indicates a length of 10 nm. In comparison, the diameter of the red blood cell is 7.5 μm (7500 nm).

40%, viscosity increases rapidly. An abnormally high hematocrit is called *polycythemia,* which literally means "many cells in the blood." The blood of a patient with polycythemia can carry more than the normal 20 mL of oxygen per dL of blood (provided that the MCHC is normal), and this may be viewed as beneficial. However, the increased viscosity makes it hard for the heart to pump the blood. Therefore, polycythemia creates a heavy workload for the heart and can lead to heart failure if the heart is not healthy.

The opposite problem, in which the hematocrit is too low, is called *anemia.* Anemia literally means "no blood," but it in fact refers to a condition in which there are abnormally few red blood cells in blood. Each deciliter of blood of an anemic patient carries less than the normal 20 mL of oxygen. Therefore, cardiac output must be increased above normal in order to deliver the normal amount of oxygen to the tissues each minute. This need to increase cardiac output also imposes an increased workload on the heart and can lead to the failure of a diseased heart. Thus, hematocrits in the range of 40% to 50% provide the blood with enough hemoglobin to carry an adequate amount of oxygen without putting an undue workload on the heart. For additional information about the transport of oxygen and carbon dioxide in blood, see Chapter 47.

Figure 17–6 provides an idea of the relative sizes and shapes of the major constituents of blood. Red blood cells and white blood cells are many, many times larger than the plasma proteins. In fact, as mentioned earlier, blood cells are so large that they must deform slightly to squeeze through a typical capillary. The plasma proteins, in turn, are much, much larger than the ions and nutrient molecules that are dissolved in plasma.

CLINICAL CORRELATIONS

Colic and endotoxic shock in a horse secondary to *Strongylus* parasitism

History   A 1-year-old Standardbred is brought to your clinic by its new owner because the horse has been rest-less, rolling, kicking at its belly, and pawing the ground. The owner reports that the horse has had a poor appetite for several days and now refuses both hay and grain. The owner says he has wormed the horse recently, but the previous worming history is unknown.

Clinical examination   The horse is underweight and has a dull hair coat. It is obvious that the horse is in pain. Physical examination reveals an abnormally high temperature (103.5°F); fast, labored breathing (40 breaths per minute); and an elevated heart rate (80 beats per minute). All limbs feel cool to the touch. The mucous membranes are abnormally dark, and the capillary refill time is prolonged (both these observations are indicative of sluggish circulation). Abdominal auscultation yields abnormal findings; no abdominal sounds are heard on either the left or the right side. A rectal examination reveals several distended loops of bowel.

You perform abdominocentesis and withdraw some peritoneal fluid. Normally, peritoneal fluid is clear and straw-colored. The fluid from this horse is darker than normal, and it has a turbid appearance. Measurements with a refractometer indicate that the peritoneal fluid contains five times more protein than normal. Microscopic examination of the fluid reveals the presence of four times the normal number of white blood cells, and the cells contain bacteria.

Outcome   You tell the owner that the horse appears to have a badly damaged bowel and that the prognosis is grave. You inform him that surgical treatment is possible, but that expensive postoperative complications are likely, because infection appears to have spread into the peritoneum. After considering the options, the owner decides against surgery. You institute supportive therapy with intravenous fluids and analgesics.

The horse's condition deteriorates over the next 12 hours. The heart rate increases progressively to 100 beats per minute. The mucous membranes show evidence of declining blood flow (darker color and longer capillary refill time). The horse begins to wheeze and becomes lethargic. There are no bowel sounds. Despite the delivery of intravenous fluids, there is no output of urine. With the owner's consent, you euthanize the horse.

Necropsy examination indicates that this horse had thrombi (vascular obstructions) in several major branches of the mesenteric arteries, probably secondary to a severe infestation of bloodworms (*Strongylus vul-*

garis). Several areas of the intestine were necrotic. Gram-negative bacteria were cultured from both the peritoneal fluid and the blood. The lungs were edematous, and fluid was found in the airways and thorax.

Comment In horses, *S. vulgaris* lodges in mesenteric arteries and decreases the blood flow to the intestine. Worming a severely infested horse can precipitate acute intestinal ischemia, because the worms break away from the walls of major arteries and drift into smaller arteries, which they occlude. Also, the dying worms release substances that trigger the formation of blood clots in the mesenteric arteries. Digestive processes become disrupted and may cease entirely. Intestinal ischemia and gaseous distention of the bowel cause severe pain. With persistent ischemia, segments of the bowel become permanently damaged (infarcted). The breakdown of the intestinal epithelium allows bacteria and bacterial products (endotoxins) to enter the peritoneum and the blood. White blood cells move from the blood stream into the peritoneal fluid, where they combat the bacteria by engulfing them (phagocytosis). However, the infection overwhelms the immune system. Bacteria and endotoxins cause the body to produce substances that depress the heart and disrupt the capillary endothelium, especially in the lungs. The combination of heart failure and pulmonary edema leads to respiratory failure and renal failure. The progression of dysfunction becomes irreversible.

Bibliography

Colahan PT, Merritt AM, Moore JN, et al: Equine Medicine and Surgery, 5th ed, vol 1. St. Louis: Mosby–Year Book, 1999, pp 419–420.

Dukes HH, Swenson MJ, Reece WO: Dukes' Physiology of Domestic Animals. Ithaca, N.Y.: Comstock, 1993, pp 1–89.

Duncan JR, Prasse KW, Mahaffey EA: Veterinary Laboratory Medicine: Clinical Pathology, 3rd ed. Ames, Ia.: Iowa State University Press, 1994.

Guyton AC, Hall JE: Textbook of Medical Physiology, 10th ed. Philadelphia: WB Saunders, 2000, pp 96–262.

Hillman RS, Finch CA: Hematologic Pathophysiology, 6th ed. Philadelphia: FA Davis, 1992.

Jain NC: Essentials of Veterinary Hematology. Philadelphia: Lea & Febiger, 1993.

Milnor WR: Cardiovascular Physiology. New York: Oxford University Press, 1990.

Mohrman DE, Heller LJ: Cardiovascular Physiology, 4th ed. New York: McGraw-Hill, 1997.

Patteson MW: Equine Cardiology (Library of Veterinary Practice). Oxford, United Kingdom: Blackwell Scientific, 1996.

Reagan WJ, Sanders TG, Denicola DB: Veterinary Hematology: Atlas of Common Domestic Species. Ames, Ia.: Iowa State University Press, 1998.

Scher AM, Feigl EO: Introduction and physical principles. In Patton HD, Fuchs AF, Hille B, et al (eds): Textbook of Physiology, 21st ed, vol 2. Philadelphia: WB Saunders, 1989, p 771.

Schmidt-Nielsen K: Animal Physiology: Adaptation and Environment. Cambridge, United Kingdom: Cambridge University Press, 1997.

PRACTICE QUESTIONS

1. According to Table 17–2, how long does it take for blood to travel the length of a canine capillary?

   a. 0.05 second.
   b. 0.1 second.
   c. 1 second.
   d. 10 seconds.
   e. 20 seconds.

2. The amount of blood pumped by the left ventricle in 1 minute would equal
   a. the amount of blood that flowed through the coronary circulation (in the same minute).
   b. one half of the cardiac output.
   c. two times the cardiac output.
   d. the amount of blood that flowed through all organs of the systemic circulation except for coronary blood flow.
   e. the amount of blood that flowed through the lungs.

3. A transfusion of plasma would
   a. decrease the hematocrit of the recipient's blood.
   b. increase the viscosity of the recipient's blood.
   c. decrease the mean cell hemoglobin concentration in the recipient's plasma.
   d. increase the number of cells in the recipient's blood.
   e. decrease the concentration of proteins in the recipient's plasma.

4. The walls of most capillaries have pores or clefts in them, which are approximately 4 nm in diameter (4×10^{-9} m). According to Figure 17–6,
   a. a capillary pore is many times larger in diameter than a sodium ion.
   b. an albumin molecule is approximately 2.5 times longer than the diameter of a capillary pore.
   c. the diameter of a red blood cell is many times greater than the diameter of a capillary pore.
   d. a globulin molecule could just about squeeze through a capillary pore if it were lined up exactly right.
   e. All of the above are correct.

5. Which of the following sequences of capillary beds might a red blood cell encounter in a normal circulation?
   a. Lungs, skin, lungs, brain.
   b. Coronary, kidney (glomerular), kidney (tubular), lungs.
   c. Spleen, liver, mesentery, lungs.
   d. Lungs, coronary, stomach, liver.
   e. Brain, lungs, liver, coronary.

PRACTICE ANSWERS

1. c   2. e   3. a   4. e   5. a

CHAPTER

18

Electrical activity of the heart

1 Contraction of cardiac muscle cells is triggered by an electrical action potential

2 The contractile machinery in cardiac muscle is very similar to that in skeletal muscle

3 Cardiac muscle forms a functional syncytium

4 Cardiac contractions are initiated by action potentials that arise spontaneously in specialized pacemaker cells

5 A system of specialized cardiac muscle cells initiates and organizes each heartbeat

6 Cardiac action potentials are very long

7 Membrane calcium channels play a special role in cardiac muscle

8 The long duration of the cardiac action potential guarantees a period of relaxation (and refilling) between heartbeats

9 Atrial cells have shorter action potentials than do ventricular cells

10 Specialized ion channels cause cardiac pacemaker cells to depolarize to threshold and form action potentials

11 Sympathetic and parasympathetic nerves act on cardiac pacemaker cells to increase or decrease the heart rate

12 Cells of the atrioventricular node act as auxiliary pacemakers and also protect the ventricles from beating too fast

13 Sympathetic nerves act on all cardiac cells to cause quicker, more forceful contractions

14 Parasympathetic effects are opposite to those of sympathetic activation but are generally restricted to the sinoatrial node, atrioventricular node, and atria

15 Dysfunction in the specialized conducting system leads to abnormalities in cardiac rhythm (arrhythmias)

16 Atrioventricular node block is a common cause of cardiac arrhythmias

17 Cardiac tachyarrhythmias result either from abnormal action potential formation (ectopic pacemaker) or from abnormal action potential conduction (reentry)

18 Commonly used antiarrhythmic drugs have their effects on the ion channels that are responsible for the cardiac action potential

---

Contraction of cardiac muscle cells is triggered by an electrical action potential

The heart is a muscular pump that propels blood through the blood vessels by alternately relaxing and contracting. As the heart muscle relaxes, the ventricles fill with venous blood. During cardiac contraction, some of this blood is ejected into the arteries. Cardiac contraction takes place in two stages. First, the right and left atria begin to contract. Then, after a delay of 50 to 150 msec, the right and left ventricles begin to contract. Atrial contraction helps to finish filling the ventricles with blood. The delay allows time for this "topping up" of the ventricles. Ventricular contraction ejects blood out of the left ventricle into the aorta and out of the right ventricle into the pulmonary artery. After ventricular ejection, the heart relaxes, and the ventricles begin to refill. The entire contractile sequence is initiated and organized by an electrical signal, an *action potential,* that propagates from muscle cell to muscle cell, through the heart.

This chapter begins with a brief description of how cardiac muscle contracts. Next there is a very detailed description of the action potentials that initiate and organize the heart's contractions. Finally, several common electrical dysfunctions of the heart are discussed.

Throughout much of this chapter, comparisons are made between cardiac and skeletal muscle (Table 18–1). In both cardiac and skeletal muscle, an electrical action potential in each muscle cell is necessary to trigger a contraction. The molecular mechanisms that carry out the contraction are also similar in both types of muscle. However, there are important differences between cardiac and skeletal muscle in the characteristics of the action potentials that initiate contractions.

The contractile machinery in cardiac muscle is very similar to that in skeletal muscle

Cardiac muscle, like skeletal muscle, has a *striated* appearance under the light microscope (Fig. 18–1).

TABLE 18–1. Sequence of events in contraction of skeletal muscle and cardiac muscle

Skeletal muscle	Cardiac muscle
Action potential is generated in somatic motor neuron	Note: Action potentials in autonomic motor neurons are *not* needed to initiate heart beats
Acetylcholine is released	Note: Neurotransmitters are *not* needed to make the heart beat
Nicotinic cholinergic receptors on muscle cell membrane are activated	Note: A completely isolated or denervated heart still beats
Ligand-gated Na^+ channels in muscle membrane open	Pacemaker Na^+ channels spontaneously open (and K^+ channels close) in membranes of pacemaker cells
Muscle membrane depolarizes to threshold level for formation of action potential	Pacemaker cell membranes depolarize to threshold for formation of action potential
Action potential forms in muscle cell but does not enter other cells	Action potential forms in a pacemaker cell and then propagates from cell to cell throughout the whole heart
Note: Skeletal muscle cells do not have slow Ca^{2+} channels	During action potential, extracellular Ca^{2+} (trigger Ca^{2+}) enters cell through "slow" Ca^{2+} channels
Action potential causes Ca^{2+} release from sarcoplasmic reticulum; Ca^{2+} binds to troponin	Entry of extracellular trigger Ca^{2+} causes release of more Ca^{2+} from sarcoplasmic reticulum; Ca^{2+} binds to troponin
Actin's binding sites are made available for actin-myosin cross-bridge formation	Actin's binding sites are made available for actin-myosin cross-bridge formation
Cross-bridge cycling generates contractile force between actin and myosin filaments	Cross-bridge cycling generates contractile force between actin and myosin filaments
Muscle contracts (brief "twitch"); Ca^{2+} is taken up by sarcoplasmic reticulum	Heart contracts (complete "beat" or "systole"; Ca^{2+} is taken up by sarcoplasmic reticulum or pumped back out of cell into extracellular fluid
Muscle relaxes	Heart relaxes

These cross-striations have the same structural basis in cardiac and skeletal muscle. Each striated cardiac *muscle fiber* (muscle cell) is made up of a few hundred myofibrils. Each *myofibril* has a repetitive pattern of light and dark bands. The various bands and lines within a myofibril are given letter designations (A band, I band, Z disk). The alignment of these bands in adjacent myofibrils accounts for the striated appearance of the whole muscle fiber. Each repeating unit of myofibrillar bands is called a *sarcomere*. This name, which means "little muscle," is apt because a single sarcomere constitutes the basic, contractile subunit of the cardiac muscle. By definition, a sarcomere extends from one Z disk to the next, a distance of approximately 0.1 mm, or 100 μm.

Just as in skeletal muscle, each cardiac muscle sarcomere is composed of an array of thick and thin

filaments. The *thin filaments* are attached to the Z disks; they interdigitate with the thick filaments. The thin filaments are composed of *actin* molecules. The *thick filaments* are composed of *myosin* molecules. Each myosin molecule has a flexible end (*myosin head*) that protrudes from the thick filament (for details, see Fig. 1–3). A myosin head can bind reversibly to one of the actin molecules in the nearby thin filament. The binding creates a *cross-bridge* between the thick and thin filaments. In the presence of adenosine triphosphate, cross-bridges undergo a repetitive cycle of flexing, unbinding, unflexing, binding to a different actin molecule, and flexing again (for details, see Fig. 1–4). This cycling of cross-bridges pulls the thin filaments past the thick filaments. As a result, each sarcomere, and therefore the whole muscle cell, gets

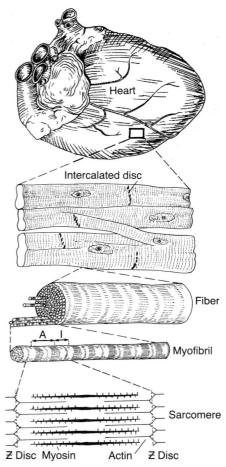

FIGURE 18–1. Under the light microscope, cardiac muscle fibers (cells) are seen to be striated, like skeletal muscle. Electron microscopy reveals that the striations result from an orderly arrangement of actin filaments (thin filaments) and myosin (thick) filaments into muscular subunits called sarcomeres (as shown in bottom drawing). Sarcomeres are the structural and functional subunits of cardiac muscle, just as they are in skeletal muscle. An important difference between cardiac muscle and skeletal muscle is visible under the light microscope: unlike skeletal muscle fibers, cardiac muscle fibers are joined by intercalated disks. Unseen within the intercalated disks are nexi, or gap junctions, which are minute openings that allow action potentials to propagate from cell to cell.

shorter; the muscle cell contracts. (See Chapters 1 and 5 for additional information about filament sliding and sarcomere shortening.)

Cardiac muscle forms a functional syncytium

Although the molecular basis of contraction is the same for cardiac and skeletal muscle, the two muscle types differ in regard to electrical linkages between neighboring cells, and this difference has important consequences. Individual skeletal muscle cells are electrically isolated (insulated) from one another. Action potentials cannot "jump" from one skeletal muscle cell to another. As described in Chapter 4, an action potential is initiated in a skeletal muscle cell by the action of acetylcholine, which is released as a neurotransmitter from a somatic motor neuron. Acetylcholine causes the opening of ligand-gated (see Fig. 1–10) Na$^+$ channels in the skeletal muscle cell membrane, which depolarizes the muscle cell to threshold for the formation of an action potential. Once formed, the action potential propagates along the length of that particular muscle cell and then stops. The muscle action potential causes the cell to contract. Neighboring cells may or may not contract at the same time, depending on whether or not action potentials are initiated in the neighboring cells by their motor neurons.

In contrast, cardiac muscle cells are electrically linked to one another. When an action potential gets started in a single cardiac muscle cell, it propagates along the length of that cell. Then, at specialized points of contact with neighboring cells, ionic currents "jump the gap" and initiate action potentials in the neighboring cells. Because cardiac action potentials propagate from cell to cell through cardiac tissue, neighboring cardiac muscle cells contract in synchrony, as a unit, and then they all relax. In this regard, cardiac muscle tissue behaves as if it were a single cell. Cardiac muscle is therefore said to form a *functional syncytium* (literally, "acts like same cell").

The specialized cellular structures that allow cardiac action potentials to propagate from cell to cell are evident under the light microscope (see Fig. 18–1). Cardiac muscle appears as an array of fibers (individual cardiac muscle cells) that are arranged approximately in parallel but with some branching. Adjacent cells are joined together by dark-appearing structures called *intercalated disks.* Electron microscopy has revealed that within these disks there are tiny openings, tiny channels of cytoplasm, between neighboring cells. These *nexi,* or *gap junctions,* provide points of contact between the intracellular fluid of adjacent cells. When an action potential depolarizes the membrane of the cell on one side of an intercalated disk, positive ions flow through the gap junctions and into the neighboring cell. This local, ionic current depolarizes the neighboring cell to threshold for the formation of an action potential. In effect, an action potential propagates from cell to cell through the nexi, or

gap junctions, that are located within the intercalated disks. Skeletal muscle does not have intercalated disks or nexi (gap junctions).

Cardiac contractions are initiated by action potentials that arise spontaneously in specialized pacemaker cells

Because cardiac muscle tissue forms a functional syncytium, and because a cardiac action potential leads to contraction, any one cardiac muscle cell can initiate a heartbeat. In other words, if a single cardiac muscle cell depolarizes to threshold and forms an action potential, that action potential will propagate from cell to cell, throughout the heart, and cause the whole heart to contract. Most cardiac muscle cells have the property of remaining stable at a resting membrane potential; they never form action potentials by themselves. However, a few specialized cardiac muscle cells have the property of depolarizing spontaneously toward the threshold for the formation of action potentials. When any one of these specialized cells reaches threshold and forms an action potential, a heartbeat results. Cardiac cells that depolarize spontaneously toward threshold are called *pacemaker cells* because they initiate heartbeats and therefore determine the rate, or pace, of the heart.

Although all spontaneously depolarizing cells in the heart are called pacemaker cells, it should be obvious that only one pacemaker cell, the one that reaches threshold first, actually triggers a particular heartbeat. In the normal heart, the pacemaker cells that depolarize most quickly to threshold are located in the *sinoatrial* (SA) *node.* The SA node is in the right atrial wall, at the point where the venae cavae enter the right atrium.

Because it has spontaneously depolarizing pacemaker cells, the heart initiates its own muscle action potentials and contractions. Motor neurons are not necessary for initiating cardiac contractions, whereas they are for initiating skeletal muscle contractions. Motor neurons (sympathetic and parasympathetic) do affect the heart rate, by influencing the rapidity of the pacemaker cells' depolarization to threshold level, but the heart continues to beat even without any sympathetic or parasympathetic influences. Thus, a denervated heart still beats, whereas a denervated skeletal muscle remains relaxed (in fact, paralyzed). The ability of the heart to beat without neural input enables surgically transplanted hearts to function. When a donor's heart is connected to a recipient's circulation during cardiac transplantation, no nerves are attached to the heart. The pacemaker cells in the transplanted heart initiate its action potentials and contractions, just as they do in a normal heart. The only thing missing is control of the heart rate through cardiac sympathetic and parasympathetic nerves.

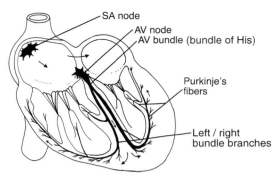

FIGURE 18–2. The specialized conduction system of the heart is responsible for the initiation and organization of cardiac contractions. The system is composed of specialized cardiac muscle fibers, not nerves. AV, atrioventricular; SA, sinoatrial.

A system of specialized cardiac muscle cells initiates and organizes each heartbeat

Each normal heartbeat is initiated by an action potential that arises spontaneously in one of the pacemaker cells in the SA node (Fig. 18–2). Once formed, the action potential propagates rapidly, from cell to cell, across the right and left atria, causing both atria to contract. Next, the action potential works its way, from cell to cell, through a special pathway of cardiac muscle cells that lies between the atria and the ventricles. This pathway consists of the *atrioventricular* (AV) *node* and the first part of the *AV bundle*, also called the *bundle of His*. The AV node and AV bundle provide the only route for the conduction of action potentials from the atria to the ventricles. Elsewhere, the atria and ventricles are separated by a layer of connective tissue. Connective tissue cells neither form nor propagate action potentials. In addition to providing the only conductive pathway between the atria and the ventricles, the AV node and the first part of the AV bundle have the special property of very slow conduction of action potentials. It takes 50 to 150 msec for an atrial action potential to get through the AV node and first part of the AV bundle; that is, it takes 50 to 150 milliseconds for an atrial action potential to propagate into the ventricles. Slow conduction through the *AV junction* creates the delay between atrial and ventricular contractions.

Once past the slowly conducting cells of the AV junction, the cardiac action potential enters a branching network of specialized cardiac cells that have the property of extremely rapid conduction of action potentials from cell to cell. This network begins with the AV bundle, which has slowly conducting cells in its first portion (connected to the AV node) and rapidly conducting cells beyond that. The AV bundle divides to form the rapidly conducting left and right bundle branches. At the ventricular apex, the right and left bundle branches break up into a dispersed network of *Purkinje's fibers*, which carry the action potential rapidly along the inner walls of both ventricles. The Purkinje fibers trigger action potentials in the normal ventricular muscle fibers within the inner walls (*subendocardial layers*) of both ventricles. From there, the action potentials propagate quite rapidly outward, from cell to cell, through the ventricular walls. As the action potential reaches each ventricular muscle fiber, that fiber contracts. The extremely rapid conduction of the cardiac action potential, from cell to cell, through the AV bundle, bundle branches, and Purkinje system results in a nearly synchronous contraction of all the fibers in both ventricles.

The SA and AV nodes, AV bundle, bundle branches, and Purkinje's fibers are collectively called the *specialized conduction system of the heart*. This system is composed of specialized cardiac muscle cells, *not* nerves. These specialized cardiac muscle cells initiate and organize each heartbeat; that is, the particular characteristics of the components in the specialized conduction system cause each heartbeat to follow a specific, patterned sequence. In a normal beat, both atria contract, almost simultaneously. Next, there is a brief pause (caused by slow conduction of the action potential through the AV node). Then the two ventricles contract, almost simultaneously. Finally, the entire heart relaxes and refills.

Figure 18–3 reemphasizes the role of the specialized conduction system in initiating and organizing a normal cardiac contraction. In this "time lapse" illustration, atrial excitation begins at time $t = 0$, when one SA node cell has reached threshold and an action potential is just beginning to propagate out of the SA node and into regular atrial tissue. Within 0.1 second, the action potential has propagated completely across the right and left atria, and a coordinated contraction of both atria is just beginning. As the action potential propagates across the atria, it also depolarizes the first cells in the AV node, beginning at time $t = 0.04$ second. While the atria are in a depolarized (excited) state, the action potential is propagating slowly from cell to cell through the AV node. After traversing the AV node, the action potential reaches the bundle of His and its branches, which carry it rapidly to the ventricular apex. The action potential arrives at the ventricular apex at time $t = 0.17$ second. Note that it takes about 0.13 second (0.17 − 0.04 second) for the action potential to get through the AV node and bundles; that is, 0.13 second represents a typical delay between atrial depolarization and ventricular depolarization. Once the action potential has reached the ventricular apex, Purkinje's fibers propagate it rapidly throughout both ventricles. Ventricular excitation (depolarization) is complete by time $t = 0.22$ second, and both ventricles contract. By this time the atria have repolarized to a resting state and are relaxing. After ventricular excitation and contraction, the whole heart relaxes and remains in a resting state until the next beat is originated by the SA node pacemaker cells.

Cardiac action potentials are very long

As mentioned, there are two major differences between action potentials in skeletal muscle and cardiac

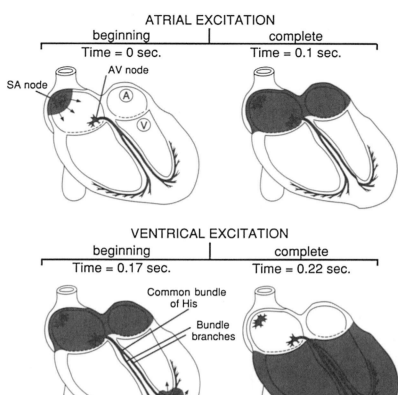

ATRIAL EXCITATION

beginning	complete
Time = 0 sec.	Time = 0.1 sec.

SA node

AV node

A

V

VENTRICAL EXCITATION

beginning	complete
Time = 0.17 sec.	Time = 0.22 sec.

Common bundle
of His

Bundle
branches

Apex

Purkinje fibers

E_m

0

-40

-80

Atrial
cell

Ventricular
cell

0   0.1   0.2   0.3   0.4   0.5

Time (sec)

FIGURE 18–3. The heart is pictured at four instants during the initiation of a normal contraction. *Top left* (time t = 0 seconds), A pacemaker cell in the SA node has just reached threshold, and an action potential has begun to propagate outward across the atria. *Top right* (t = 0.1 second), The action potential has reached all parts of both atria (all atrial cells are at the plateau of their action potentials). *Middle left* (t = 0.17 second), The action potential has passed down the bundle branches and has just reached the ventricular apex. *Middle right* (t = 0.22 second), A short time later, the action potential has just finished propagating outward through the walls of both ventricles (all ventricular cells are at the plateau of their action potentials). *Bottom,* The graph shows the timing of action potentials in a left atrial cell (A, *top left*) and a left ventricular cell (V, *top left*). Their locations make these among the last atrial and ventricular cells to be depolarized as action potentials propagate across the atria and ventricles, respectively. E_m, membrane potential in millivolts.

muscle. First, cardiac muscle cells are electrically connected, whereas skeletal muscle cells are electrically isolated; therefore, action potentials propagate from cell to cell in cardiac muscle but not in skeletal muscle. Second, the heart has pacemaker cells, which form spontaneous action potentials and trigger cardiac contractions; in contrast, skeletal muscle cells only depolarize and form action potentials when "commanded" to do so by motor neurons.

A third important difference between skeletal and cardiac action potentials is their duration (Fig. 18–4). The entire action potential in a skeletal muscle lasts only 1 to 2 msec. A cardiac action potential lasts about 100 times longer (100 to 250 msec). These prolonged action potentials are brought about by prolonged changes in the permeability of the cardiac muscle membrane to Na^+, K^+, and Ca^{2+} ions. Cardiac muscle cell membranes have Na^+ and K^+ channels similar to those found in skeletal muscle, but the timing of their opening and closing is different in cardiac muscle. In

addition, cardiac cell membranes also have special Ca^{2+} channels that are not present in skeletal muscle. The movement of extracellular Ca^{2+} through cardiac Ca^{2+} channels has an especially important role in prolonging the cardiac action potential. The presence of Ca^{2+} channels and the important role of extracellular Ca^{2+} in the action potential is the fourth major difference between cardiac and skeletal muscle.

To understand the special significance of the membrane Ca^{2+} channels in cardiac muscle, it is useful to review the roles of K^+ and Na^+ channels in skeletal muscle and to emphasize some ways in which cardiac K^+ and Na^+ channels are similar to those in skeletal muscle. As explained in Chapter 3, many of the K^+ channels in a neuron or skeletal muscle cell membrane are open when the cell is at rest, and most of the Na^+ channels are closed. As a result, the resting cell is much more permeable to K^+ than to Na^+. The tendency of the positively charged K^+ to leave the cell creates a resting membrane potential (polarization) in

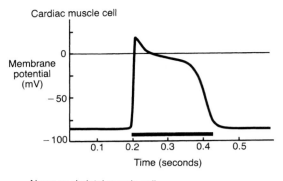

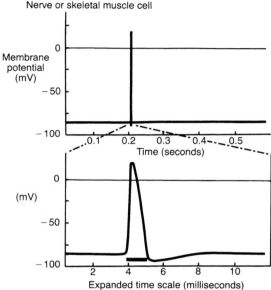

FIGURE 18–4. Action potentials in cardiac muscle cells *(top)* last 100 times longer than action potentials in nerve or skeletal muscle cells *(middle)*. *Bottom,* The nerve or skeletal muscle action potential is shown on a greatly expanded time scale. The prolonged phase of depolarization in cardiac muscle cells is called the *plateau of the action potential.* The dark bars under each action potential indicate the length of the absolute refractory period.

which the inside of the cell membrane is negative in comparison with the outside. The resting membrane potential is typically between −70 and −85 mV (see Fig. 18–4). An action potential is created when something depolarizes the cell (makes it less negative inside). Depolarization to the threshold voltage for opening the voltage-gated Na$^+$ channels allows an influx of extracellular Na$^+$ into the cell. This rapid entry of positive ions causes the cell membrane to become positively charged on its inside surface. This positive membrane potential persists for only a moment, however, because the Na$^+$ channels close very quickly, and the cell rapidly repolarizes to its resting membrane potential. Repolarization is also promoted by the opening of additional K$^+$ channels. In fact, this opening of extra K$^+$ channels may cause nerves and skeletal muscles to become hyperpolarized (even more negative than normal) for a few moments at the end of each action potential (see Fig. 18–4, *bottom).*

In a resting skeletal muscle cell, calcium ions are

stored within the intracellular organelle called the *sarcoplasmic reticulum.* The occurrence of an action potential in the skeletal muscle cell causes Ca^{2+} to be released from the sarcoplasmic reticulum into the free intracellular fluid, which is called the *cytosol.* Some of the cytosolic Ca^{2+} binds to the protein troponin, which is located along the thin (actin) filaments. This binding allows the actin-myosin cross-bridges to begin cycling, which causes muscle contraction. The contraction initiated by a single action potential is very brief, because the cytosolic Ca^{2+} is rapidly pumped back into the sarcoplasmic reticulum by active transport, and the muscle relaxes. Note that the Ca^{2+} responsible for initiating the muscle contraction comes entirely from the intracellular storage site, the sarcoplasmic reticulum. No extracellular Ca^{2+} enters the cell during the action potential, because skeletal muscle cells do not have membrane Ca^{2+} channels. In cardiac muscle, in contrast, membrane Ca^{2+} channels and the entry of extracellular Ca^{2+} into the cells play key roles in both action potentials and contractions.

Membrane calcium channels play a special role in cardiac muscle

Figure 18–5 depicts a cardiac muscle cell action potential and the sequence of changes in K$^+$, Na$^+$, and Ca^{2+} permeability that are responsible for the action potential. As the time line begins (on the left side of each graph), the cardiac cell is at a normal, negative resting membrane potential of about −80 mV. The cardiac membrane potential is negative at rest for the same reason that skeletal muscle cells have negative resting membrane potentials; many K$^+$ channels are open at rest, and most of the Na$^+$ channels are closed. As a result, membrane permeability to K$^+$ is much higher than the membrane permeability to Na$^+$ (see Fig. 18–5, middle two graphs). In resting cardiac cells, the membrane Ca^{2+} channels are closed (see Fig. 18–5, *bottom).* The Ca^{2+} permeability is very low, and extracellular Ca^{2+} ions are prevented from entering the cardiac cells.

Just as in skeletal muscle, a cardiac action potential is created when the cell is depolarized to the threshold voltage for opening the voltage-gated Na$^+$ channels. The rapid influx of extracellular Na$^+$ into the cell causes the cell membrane to become positively charged on its inside surface (phase 0 in Fig. 18–5, *top).* The Na$^+$ channels close again very quickly, and the membrane begins to repolarize (phase 1). However, in cardiac muscle, repolarization is interrupted, and there is a prolonged plateau of depolarization, which lasts about 200 msec (phase 2). The plateau of the cardiac action potential is brought about by two conditions that do not occur in nerves or skeletal muscle fibers: first, some K$^+$ channels close, and so K$^+$ permeability decreases; second, many of the Ca^{2+} channels open, and Ca^{2+} permeability increases. Because the Ca^{2+} concentration is higher in the extracellular fluid than in the intracellular fluid, Ca^{2+} flows

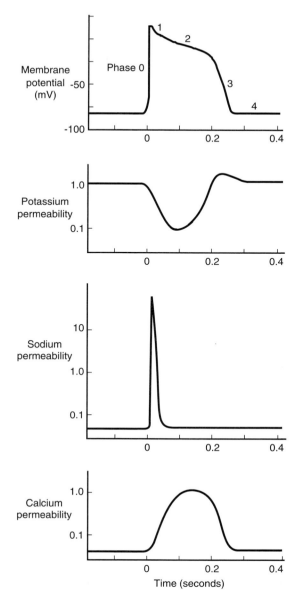

Figure 18–5. The membrane potential of a cardiac muscle cell *(top)* is determined by the relative permeabilities of the cell membrane to K+ *(second from top)*, Na+ *(second from bottom)*, and Ca²⁺ *(bottom)*. At rest (left side of graphs), the cell is much more permeable to K+ than it is to Na+ and Ca²⁺. A cardiac action potential (middle of graphs) is produced by a characteristic sequence of changes in the permeabilities to K+, Na+, and Ca²⁺. The action potential ends when the permeabilities return to their resting state (right side of graphs). Phases 0 to 4 are discussed in the text.

through the open Ca^{2+} channels and into the cytosol. The combination of reducing the exit of K^+ from the cell and allowing the entrance of Ca^{2+} into the cell keeps the cell membrane in a depolarized state. After about 200 msec, the K^+ channels reopen and the Ca^{2+} channels close. K^+ permeability increases and Ca^{2+} permeability decreases. The combination of increasing the exit of K^+ from the cell and shutting off the entrance of Ca^{2+} into the cell causes the cell to repolarize (phase 3) and eventually to reach its stable, negative resting membrane potential (phase 4).

The specialized Ca^{2+} channels in cardiac muscle cell membranes are called *slow Ca^{2+} channels,* because they take much longer to open than do the Na^+ channels, and they stay open much longer. As shown in Figure 18–5, Na^+ permeability increases and then decreases (Na^+ channels open and close) within a few milliseconds. Ca^{2+} permeability, in comparison, is slow to increase (Ca^{2+} channels are slow to open) and Ca^{2+} permeability remains elevated for about 200 msec (Ca^{2+} channels are slow to close). In recognition of their much quicker responses, the Na^+ channels in cardiac muscle are sometimes called *fast Na^+ channels.*

The Ca^{2+} that enters a cardiac cell during an action potential triggers the release of additional Ca^{2+} from the sarcoplasmic reticulum. This process is called *calcium-triggered calcium release.* In less than 0.1 second, the concentration of free Ca^{2+} in the cytosol increases some 100-fold. Just as in skeletal muscle, some of the cytosolic Ca^{2+} binds to the protein troponin. This binding allows the actin-myosin cross-bridges to begin cycling, which causes the cardiac muscle to contract. When the Ca^{2+} channels close, at the conclusion of the action potential, most of the free, cytosolic Ca^{2+} is pumped back into the sarcoplasmic reticulum or pumped back across the cell membrane into the extracellular fluid. Both these processes involve active transport, because the Ca^{2+} is being pumped against its electrochemical gradient. The cytosolic Ca^{2+} concentration is quickly returned to its low, resting level, and the cardiac muscle relaxes. The relationship between an action potential and the resulting contraction in a cardiac muscle cell is depicted in Figure 18–6 *(solid lines).*

The long duration of the cardiac action potential guarantees a period of relaxation (and refilling) between heartbeats

When the Na^+ channels close (at the peak of an action potential), they become *inactivated.* An inactivated Na^+ channel does not reopen, even if the cell membrane potential remains above the threshold that would normally trigger an action potential. As long as the Na^+ channels are inactivated, another action potential cannot occur. The Na^+ channel inactivation ends, and the Na^+ channels become susceptible to reopening, only when the cell membrane potential returns to its resting level. Thus, Na^+ inactivation guarantees that the upstroke of a second action potential cannot occur until the first action potential is completed.

While the Na^+ channels are inactivated, the cell is refractory (resistant) with regard to the formation of an action potential. The time after the beginning of one action potential during which another action potential cannot be initiated is called the *absolute refractory period (refractory period* for short). Because Na^+ inactivation lasts until the membrane potential returns to its resting level, the refractory period lasts about as long as an action potential. Therefore, the

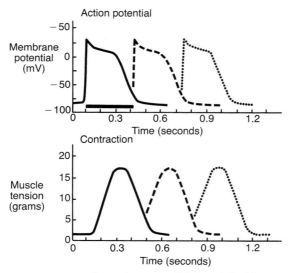

FIGURE 18–6. A cardiac action potential *(top, left side)* causes a cardiac contraction *(bottom, left side)*. Note that the action potential and contraction have similar durations. The heavy *horizontal bar* under the action potential shows the duration of the absolute refractory period. The *dashed lines* in the top graph show the earliest possible occurrence of a second and a third action potential, each occurring right after the absolute refractory period for the preceding action potential; the *dashed lines* in the bottom graph represent the corresponding cardiac contractions. Because of the long refractory period, each contraction is almost over before the earliest possible next contraction can begin. This guarantees a period of cardiac relaxation between contractions.

refractory period in a nerve or skeletal muscle cell lasts about 1 or 2 msec, whereas the refractory period in a cardiac muscle cell lasts 100 to 250 msec (see Fig. 18–4).

The long refractory period in cardiac muscle guarantees a period of relaxation (and cardiac refilling) between cardiac contractions. Figure 18–6 *(top)* depicts the quickest possible succession of three action potentials in a cardiac muscle cell: the second action potential begins immediately after the conclusion of the refractory period for the first action potential. Likewise, the third action potential begins immediately after the conclusion of the refractory period for the second. The bottom graph shows the pattern of muscle contraction that results from the three action potentials. Note that contractile strength reaches a peak late in the plateau phase of each action potential and that the contractile strength decreases (the muscle begins to relax) during the repolarization phase of each action potential. Because the next action potential cannot begin until the first one has ended, the cardiac muscle cell is partially relaxed before it begins to contract again; that is, each action potential produces a cardiac contraction that is distinctly separated from the preceding contraction. Because of its long refractory period, cardiac muscle cannot sustain a continuous contraction. Thus, the heart has a guaranteed period of relaxation (and refilling) between heartbeats.

The pattern of changes in muscle tension depicted in the bottom of Figure 18–6 corresponds closely to the changes in the cytosolic Ca^{2+} concentration. This makes sense, considering that the cytosolic Ca^{2+} concentration determines the degree of activation of troponin, which determines the number of actin binding sites available for forming actin-myosin cross-bridges. Furthermore, the number of cross-bridges formed at any moment determines the strength of muscle contraction at that moment. The fact that contractile tension decreases nearly to its resting level during the repolarization phase of the action potential implies that cytosolic Ca^{2+} concentration is reduced nearly to its resting level by the time the action potential is over. In other words, in the time between closure of the slow Ca^{2+} channels (at the end of the plateau of the action potential) and the return to resting membrane potential, the active transport pumps have moved most of the free, cytosolic Ca^{2+} back into the sarcoplasmic reticulum or out into the extracellular fluid.

In skeletal muscle cells, an action potential lasts only 1 to 2 msec, but the contractile "twitch" resulting from the action potential lasts 50 times longer than that. The action potential in a skeletal muscle cell is so brief that the membrane is repolarized (and the refractory period is over) even before the release of Ca^{2+} from the sarcoplasmic reticulum is finished and many milliseconds before the released Ca^{2+} is pumped back into the sarcoplasmic reticulum. As a result, the cytosolic Ca^{2+} concentration reaches its peak level *after* the action potential is over, and the contractile tension resulting from the action potential also reaches its peak *after* the action potential is over. Because of the very short refractory period in skeletal muscle, several action potentials can occur during the time of a single contractile twitch. Multiple action potentials in quick succession cause the concentration of Ca^{2+} in the cytosol to build to a high level and stay there. The resulting contractile tension is stronger than the tension that results from a single action potential, and it is sustained for a longer time. In effect, the muscle twitches caused by successive action potentials "fuse" together. This phenomenon is called *temporal summation. Fusion* and temporal summation are the mechanisms that permit graded and prolonged tension development in skeletal muscle. In contrast, the long refractory period in cardiac muscle cells prevents the fusion and summation of cardiac contractions. Each contraction of the heart is followed immediately by a relaxation.

Atrial cells have shorter action potentials than do ventricular cells

The preceding description of cardiac ion channels, action potentials, and contractions was based on properties of normal ventricular cells. Atrial cells are basically similar, except that atrial action potentials are shorter than action potentials in ventricular cells. Like ventricular cells, atrial cells have fast Na^+ channels that open briefly at the beginning of an action potential and then become inactivated. Likewise, atrial slow Ca^{2+} channels open during the action potential, and K^+ channels close. The differences between atrial and ventricular cells are that atrial slow Ca^{2+} channels typically stay open a shorter time than do those in ventricular cells, and atrial K^+ channels stay closed for a shorter time. As a result, the plateau of an atrial cell's action potential is shorter and not as "flat" as the plateau of a ventricular cell's action potential (see Fig. 18–3, *bottom*). As a consequence of having a shorter action potential, atrial cells have a shorter refractory period than do ventricular cells. Therefore, the atrial cells are capable of forming more action potentials per minute than are ventricular cells; that is, the atria can "beat" faster than the ventricles. The implications of this difference are discussed later in this chapter.

▄ Specialized ion channels cause cardiac pacemaker cells to depolarize to threshold and form action potentials

As already mentioned, the cardiac pacemaker cells of the SA node spontaneously depolarize to threshold and then form action potentials. The spontaneous depolarization is called a *pacemaker potential,* and it is the distinguishing feature of a pacemaker cell (Fig. 18–7, *top*). The action potentials of cardiac pacemaker cells typically have a rounded appearance; they lack the very rapid (phase 0) depolarization seen in ventricular and atrial cells.

The spontaneous depolarizations and rounded action potentials are consequences of the particular ion channels found in pacemaker cells. Pacemaker cells lack voltage-gated fast Na^+ channels. Instead, these cells have Na^+ channels that close during an action potential and then begin to open again, spontaneously, once an action potential has finished. The spontaneous opening of these *pacemaker Na^+ channels* causes a progressive increase in the cell's Na^+ permeability (see Fig. 18–7). The increase in Na^+ permeability allows Na^+ to enter the cell from the extracellular fluid, which depolarizes the cell toward threshold. K^+ channels also participate in the spontaneous depolarization of pacemaker cells. At the end of one action potential, K^+ permeability in pacemaker cells is quite high, because most K^+ channels are open. Then the K^+ channels begin to close. As K^+ permeability decreases, less K^+ leaves the cells, which makes the cells progressively less negatively charged inside. Ca^{2+} channels also make a small contribution to the pacemaker potential. Late in the pacemaker potential, just before a pacemaker cell reaches threshold, slow Ca^{2+} channels begin to open and Ca^{2+} permeability begins to increase. The resulting entry of Ca^{2+} into the cell speeds its final approach to threshold. Thus, the pacemaker potential is caused by the opening of pacemaker Na^+ channels, the closing of K^+ channels, and (late in the process) the opening of Ca^{2+} channels. These spontaneous changes in Na^+, K^+, and Ca^{2+} channels in pacemaker cells are in contrast to the

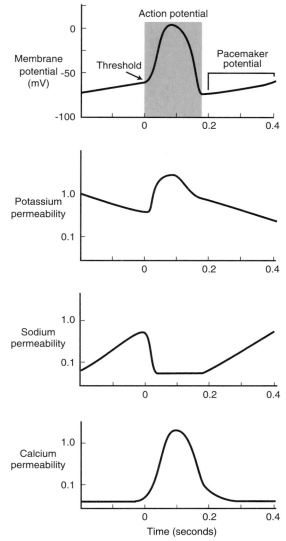

FIGURE 18–7. A pacemaker cell depolarizes spontaneously to threshold and initiates its own action potential *(top).* The spontaneous depolarization (called the *pacemaker potential)* is the result of a spontaneous, progressive decrease in K^+ permeability *(second from top)* and an increase in Na^+ permeability *(second from bottom).* An increase in Ca^{2+} permeability makes a late contribution to the depolarization toward threshold *(bottom).* Once threshold level is reached, an action potential is produced. The action potential is driven primarily by a large, prolonged increase in Ca^{2+} permeability. The absence of fast Na^+ channels in pacemaker cells causes the upstroke of the pacemaker action potential to be much slower than that seen in nonpacemaker cells (compare with Fig. 18–5).

stable status of the ion channels in normal, resting ventricular or atrial cells.

Once threshold is reached in a pacemaker cell, an action potential occurs. The upstroke of the action potential is quite slow, in comparison with the rapid, phase 0 depolarization in a normal ventricular or atrial cell, because there are no fast Na^+ channels in pacemaker cells and therefore no sudden influx of Na^+. The ion primarily responsible for the action potential in a pacemaker cell is Ca^{2+}. Once threshold is reached, many of the cell's slow Ca^{2+} channels

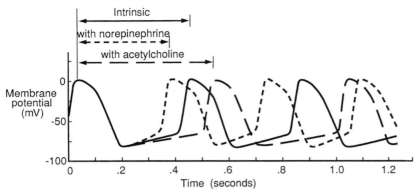

Interval Between Heartbeats

FIGURE 18–8. In the absence of neurohumoral influences, a pacemaker cell of the SA node spontaneously depolarizes to threshold and initiates a series of action potentials *(solid line)*. The interval between action potentials under these conditions determines the intrinsic, or spontaneous, heart rate. Acetylcholine decreases the rate of depolarization and therefore lengthens the interval between action potentials *(long dashes)*. Norepinephrine increases the rate of depolarization and therefore shortens the interval between action potentials *(short dashes)*.

open. The permeability to Ca^{2+} increases, and extracellular Ca^{2+} flows into the cell. The action potentials in pacemaker cells are often called *slow action potentials,* because they lack a rapid, phase 0 depolarization and because they are caused primarily by the opening of slow Ca^{2+} channels. In contrast, normal ventricular or atrial action potentials are called *fast action potentials.* Regardless of whether they are "slow" or "fast," however, all cardiac action potentials have a very long duration in comparison with action potentials in nerve or skeletal muscle cells.

Sympathetic and parasympathetic nerves act on cardiac pacemaker cells to increase or decrease the heart rate

Figure 18–8 shows how the neurotransmitters norepinephrine and acetylcholine affect the pacemaker cells of the heart. Norepinephrine exerts its effect by activating β-*adrenergic receptors* on the pacemaker cells' membranes. Activation of such receptors speeds up the ion channel changes that are responsible for the spontaneous depolarization of pacemaker cells. Because the pacemaker cells reach threshold more quickly in the presence of norepinephrine, there is a shorter interval between heartbeats. Therefore, heart rate is elevated above its intrinsic or spontaneous level.

Acetylcholine has the opposite effect. Acetylcholine slows the spontaneous depolarization of pacemaker cells by activating *muscarinic cholinergic receptors* on the cell membranes. Activation of such receptors causes a slowing of the ion channel changes that are responsible for the pacemaker cell's spontaneous depolarization. Acetylcholine makes it take longer for pacemaker cells to reach threshold. There is a longer time between heartbeats, and so the heart rate is slowed below its intrinsic or spontaneous rate.

Sympathetic neurons release norepinephrine at the SA node cells, and so sympathetic nerve activity increases the heart rate. Parasympathetic neurons release acetylcholine at the SA node cells, and so parasympathetic activity decreases the heart rate. Figure 18–9 illustrates how sympathetic and parasympathetic neurons interact in the control of the heart rate.

In the absence of either norepinephrine or acetylcholine, the heart beats at its intrinsic rate. For a large dog, this rate is typically about 140 beats per minute. However, the heart rate is only about 60 beats per minute during sleep, and about 90 beats per minute when the dog is awake but quiet. Such heart rates (below the intrinsic rate) are achieved by activation of parasympathetic neurons and release of acetylcholine. Accordingly, the graph indicates that parasympathetic activity is very high during sleep. A heart rate of 90 beats per minute is achieved by a somewhat smaller parasympathetic tone. Heart rates above the intrinsic rate occur during exercise or emotional arousal. Such heart rates are achieved by activation of the sympathetic nerves to the heart and release of norepinephrine. Through variation in the level of sympathetic tone, the dog's heart rate is adjusted to meet the demands of each behavioral situation. The highest possible levels of sympathetic activity, and the highest

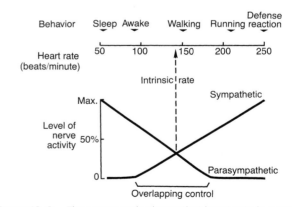

FIGURE 18–9. The upper scale shows that heart rate in a normal large dog ranges from 50 to 250 beats per minute, depending on behavioral state. The graph shows that this wide range of heart rates is brought about by the interactions between parasympathetic nerve activity, which slows the heart below its intrinsic rate, and sympathetic nerve activity, which speeds the heart above its intrinsic rate. Sympathetic and parasympathetic nerves are simultaneously active over a considerable portion of the heart rate range (overlapping control). The heart beats at its intrinsic rate (about 140 beats per minute) either in the absence of any neural influence or when sympathetic and parasympathetic effects are equal and opposite.

possible heart rate, occurs during maximal exercise or a *defense alarm reaction* (fear, fight, or flight response).

Sympathetic and parasympathetic neurons to the heart are sometimes activated simultaneously. When both systems are activated, the resulting heart rate represents the outcome of a sort of tug-of-war between sympathetic action to increase the heart rate and parasympathetic action to decrease the heart rate. Typically, both the sympathetic and parasympathetic systems are partially activated during awake states ranging from quiet rest to moderate exercise (when heart rate is between about 90 and 175 beats per minute). Parasympathetic activity predominates in the lower part of this range, and sympathetic activity predominates in the higher part. When sympathetic activity and parasympathetic activity are equal, their effects cancel, and the heart rate is at its intrinsic, or spontaneous, level. Simultaneous activation of sympathetic and parasympathetic neurons appears to give the nervous system tight control over the heart rate under a wide variety of behavioral conditions.

Cells of the atrioventricular node act as auxiliary pacemakers and also protect the ventricles from beating too fast

Like SA node cells, the cells of the AV node normally exhibit pacemaker activity and slow action potentials. As shown in Figure 18–10, the AV node cells spontaneously depolarize toward threshold, but much more slowly than do the SA node cells. Therefore, under normal circumstances, the SA node cells reach threshold first and initiate an action potential, which then propagates from cell to cell across the atria and into the AV node. As this action potential enters the AV node, it encounters cells that are spontaneously depolarizing toward threshold. The arriving action potential depolarizes these AV node pacemaker cells immediately to threshold, and they form an action potential, which then propagates into the AV bundle and the ventricles. Thus, under normal conditions, each cardiac action potential is triggered by an SA node pacemaker cell, and the pacemaker activity of the AV node cells is irrelevant.

Under certain abnormal conditions, AV node pacemaker function is critical for survival. For example, if the SA node is damaged and does not depolarize to threshold, the AV node pacemaker cells continue to depolarize spontaneously to threshold, and they initiate cardiac action potentials. If not for this *auxiliary pacemaker function* of AV node cells, the heart with a damaged SA node would not beat at all. Because the AV node pacemaker cells depolarize more slowly than normal SA node cells, the heart rate is characteristically very low when the AV node cells are initiating the heartbeats. The heart rate resulting from AV node pacemakers is about 30 to 40 beats per minute in a resting dog, in comparison with a normal rate of 80 to 90 beats per minute when the SA node cells are the pacemakers. Nevertheless, enough heartbeats are

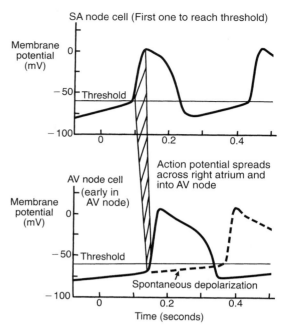

FIGURE 18–10. Both sinoatrial (SA) node cells and atrioventricular (AV) node cells show pacemaker activity (spontaneous depolarization toward threshold). Normally, the SA node cells depolarize more quickly and reach the threshold first *(top)*. The resulting atrial action potential propagates into the AV node (as represented by *hatched band*, which depolarizes the AV node cells to threshold *(bottom graph, solid line)*. However, if the SA node pacemaker cells were nonfunctional or if atrial action potentials were not conducted into the AV node, the AV node cells would eventually depolarize to threshold and initiate action potentials on their own *(bottom graph, dashed line)*. In this way, the AV node cells serve as an auxiliary ventricular pacemaker.

initiated by the AV node to sustain life temporarily if the SA node fails as a pacemaker. Thus, AV node cells are sometimes called the heart's *emergency pacemakers*.

Another important feature of the AV node cells is that they have much longer refractory periods than do normal atrial cells. The long refractory period of AV node cells helps protect the ventricles from being stimulated to contract at rates that are too rapid for efficient pumping. This protective function of the AV node is critical to an animal's survival in cases of atrial flutter or atrial fibrillation, in which atrial action potentials are extremely frequent (as further discussed later in this chapter). The long refractory period of the AV node cells plays an important role, even in a normal heart. Once a normal action potential reaches the ventricles, it is prevented from "circling back" and reactivating the atria by the prolonged refractory state of the AV node cells.

Table 18–2 summarizes the four important electrical characteristics of the AV node that have been discussed. Note that three of these characteristics are influenced by the nervous system. As indicated in the table, sympathetic activity increases the conduction velocity of the AV node cells, shortens their refractory period, and speeds their auxiliary pacemaker activity. Parasympathetic activation has the opposite effects. These sympathetic and parasympathetic effects are

TABLE 18–2. **Electrical characteristics of the atrioventricular (AV) node**

Characteristic (significance)	Sympathetic effect	Parasympathetic effect
Is the only conducting pathway between atria and ventricles (directs atrial action potentials into the rapidly conducting AV bundle and bundle branches)	—	—
Has a slow conduction velocity (creates AV delay)	Increases velocity (shorter AV delay)	Decreases velocity (longer AV delay)
Has a very long refractory period (protective effects: limits maximal rate to which atria can drive ventricles and prevents ventricular action potentials from reexciting atria)	Shortens refractory period (appropriate for high heart rates)	Lengthens refractory period (appropriate for low heart rates)
Spontaneously depolarizes to threshold (acts as auxiliary pacemaker)	Faster depolarization (speeds auxiliary pacemaker)	Slower depolarization (slows auxiliary pacemaker)

appropriate for different heart rates. For example, when sympathetic activity is high and the SA node pacemakers are initiating heartbeats frequently, the whole process of cardiac contraction and relaxation must be sped up. Thus, it is appropriate that sympathetic action also increases the velocity of action potential conduction through the AV node (which shortens AV delay). In addition, sympathetic activation shortens the AV node refractory period, which allows each of the frequent action potentials to be conducted from the atria to the ventricles. Finally, sympathetic activation enhances AV node auxiliary pacemaker activity, which provides the animal with a high enough ventricular rate to cope with some stress, even if the SA node pacemaker has failed. Conversely, when parasympathetic activation causes the SA node pacemakers to decrease the heart rate, all aspects of cardiac contraction and relaxation can proceed at a more leisurely pace. Under these conditions, it is appropriate for AV node conduction velocity to be slowed and the AV node refractory period to be lengthened.

Sympathetic nerves act on all cardiac cells to cause quicker, more forceful contractions

Sympathetic neurons release norepinephrine in all regions of the heart, not just at the SA and AV nodes, and all cardiac muscle cells have β-adrenergic receptors that are activated by norepinephrine. The effects of sympathetic activity (β-receptor activation) on the SA and AV node cells have already been described (see Fig. 18–8 and Table 18–2). In all other atrial and ventricular cells, β-receptor activation leads to higher, shorter action potentials and to stronger, quicker contractions. One reason for these effects is that activation of β receptors increases the number of Ca^{2+} channels that open during the plateau (phase 2) of an action potential, which increases the amount of extracellular Ca^{2+} that enters the cell. Because Ca^{2+} entry is the primary depolarizing influence during the plateau, increased Ca^{2+} entry raises the plateau (makes the membrane potential more positive). A secondary consequence is to shorten the action potential. The

action potential becomes shorter because of a complicated effect of the elevated plateau on the K^+ channels. Recall that K^+ channels close at the beginning of a cardiac action potential and then, after a time, reopen (see Fig. 18–5). Reopening of the K^+ channels helps repolarize the cell to a resting state at the end of the action potential. The length of time before K^+ channels reopen depends on the membrane voltage during the action potential. Specifically, when the plateau is higher (more positive membrane potential) than normal, the K^+ channels reopen sooner. This shortens the action potential and speeds repolarization. Overall, β-receptor activation makes each action potential higher and shorter. An action potential of higher amplitude propagates more quickly along each cell and from cell to cell, leading to faster conduction velocity. The shorter action potential means a shorter refractory period, which facilitates formation of more heartbeats per minute.

Because β-receptor activation increases the entry of extracellular Ca^{2+} into cardiac muscle cells during an action potential, it also increases the strength of the resulting contraction. The increased entry of extracellular "trigger" Ca^{2+} creates a greater stimulus for the release of Ca^{2+} stores from the sarcoplasmic reticulum. Therefore, the cytosolic Ca^{2+} concentration reaches an exceptionally high level during the action potential, which leads to greater-than-normal activation of troponin, more-than-normal binding sites available for actin-myosin cross-bridges, a greater number of active cross-bridges, and therefore a stronger contraction. In addition, the contraction begins more quickly, because of a facilitating effect that β-receptor activation has on the myosin molecules. The contraction is also briefer, because β-receptor activation leads to a speeding up of the pumps that move cytosolic Ca^{2+} back into the sarcoplasmic reticulum and out of the cell into the extracellular fluid. Thus, even though more Ca^{2+} than normal enters the cytosol during an action potential, its removal at the end of the action potential is quicker than normal. Overall, β-receptor activation makes each cardiac contraction stronger and quicker.

In summary, sympathetic nerves act on the SA node pacemaker cells to increase the heart rate, on the AV node cells to increase the conduction velocity and shorten the AV delay, and on all cardiac cells to shorten the refractory period and make each cardiac contraction stronger and quicker. All these changes cause the heart to pump more blood at a higher pressure, which is an animal's normal response during exercise or emotional arousal.

Because sympathetic effects on the heart are all brought about through activation of the β-adrenergic receptors on the cardiac muscle cells, the administration of a drug that activates β receptors (β-*adrenergic agonist*) has the same effects as sympathetic activation. Epinephrine and isoproterenol are two commonly used β-adrenergic agonists. Conversely, the administration of a drug that binds to and blocks β receptors reduces all the effects of sympathetic activation. Propranolol and atenolol are common examples of such β-adrenergic antagonists. Examples of its use are given later.

Parasympathetic effects are opposite to those of sympathetic activation but are generally restricted to the sinoatrial node, atrioventricular node, and atria

Parasympathetic nerves affect the heart by the release of acetylcholine, which activates muscarinic cholinergic receptors on cardiac muscle cells. Qualitatively, all the effects of parasympathetic activation are opposite to those of sympathetic activation, because the effects of activating muscarinic cholinergic receptors are opposite to the effects of activating β-adrenergic receptors. Parasympathetic nerves have very powerful effects on the SA node pacemaker cells (see Fig. 18–8) and on the AV node cells (see Table 18–2). In addition, parasympathetic nerves exert strong, antisympathetic influences on all the atrial cells. However, parasympathetic nerves have relatively weak effects on the ventricular muscle cells. The reason is that very few ventricular cells receive direct parasympathetic innervation. However, all ventricular muscle cells receive direct sympathetic innervation. In summary, the predominant parasympathetic influences on the heart are exerted at the SA node (to decrease the rate), at the AV node (to slow conduction and lengthen the refractory period), and on all supraventricular cells (to lengthen the refractory period and make their contractions weaker and slower).

Parasympathetic neurons do exert a curious, indirect effect on ventricular muscle cells. In the ventricles, parasympathetic neurons release their acetylcholine onto sympathetic neuron terminals. This acetylcholine activates muscarinic cholinergic receptors that are located on the sympathetic neuron terminals. The effect of this activation is to inhibit the release of norepinephrine from the terminals, which weakens the effects of sympathetic activation on ventricular cells.

Parasympathetic effects on the heart can be mimicked by the administration of a muscarinic cholinergic agonist (e.g., muscarine) and blocked by the administration of a muscarinic cholinergic antagonist (e.g., atropine). Some therapeutic applications are mentioned later.

Dysfunction in the specialized conducting system leads to abnormalities in cardiac rhythm (arrhythmias)

Cardiac arrhythmias result either from problems with the formation of action potentials or from problems with the propagation (conduction) of action potentials. One example of a problem with action potential formation has already been mentioned: *sinus arrest*, in which the SA node completely fails to form action potentials. In a patient with sinus arrest, the auxiliary pacemaker function of the AV node keeps the ventricles beating, although at an extremely low rate. Complete cessation of the SA node is the extreme case of the condition called *sick sinus syndrome*. In its more common and less extreme form, sick sinus syndrome is characterized by sluggish depolarization of the SA node pacemaker cells. Patients exhibit an abnormally slow heart rate at rest (*bradycardia*) and an insufficient increase in heart rate during exercise. To be very specific, in sick sinus syndrome, the intrinsic sinus rate is abnormally low.

Even though the problem in sick sinus syndrome is intrinsic to the sinus itself, one treatment strategy is to administer a drug that blocks parasympathetic action on the heart (a cholinergic muscarinic antagonist, such as atropine). The logic behind this treatment is illustrated in Table 18–3. In a normal healthy large dog, the intrinsic rate of the heart is 140 beats per minute. However, the heart rate at rest is about 90 beats per minute, because high parasympathetic tone normally slows the SA node pacemaker to a rate below its intrinsic rate. A drug that blocks parasympathetic effects on the heart would return the heart rate in a normal, resting dog to 140 beats per minute. A dog with a sick sinus has a low intrinsic heart rate, perhaps 80 beats per minute. Parasympathetic tone makes the resting heart rate even lower, approximately 30 beats per minute. A drug that blocks parasympathetic effects restores the heart rate to its intrinsic level, 80 beats per minute. Therefore, a dog with sick sinus syndrome

TABLE 18–3. Treatment of sick sinus syndrome by blocking parasympathetic effects on heart rate with a cholinergic muscarinic antagonist

Heart rate	Normal dog (bpm)	Dog with sick sinus syndrome (bpm)
Intrinsic rate	140	80
Resting rate (with parasympathetic tone)	90	30
Rate after atropine	140	80

bpm, beats per minute.

treated with atropine has a heart rate that closely matches the rate of a normal resting dog.

Another possible therapeutic approach is to increase the heart rate by administering a drug that mimics the action of sympathetic nerves. Specifically, a β-adrenergic agonist (e.g., isoproterenol) could be administered to activate the adrenergic receptors on the SA node cells that are normally activated by norepinephrine. Enough isoproterenol would be given to increase the resting rate from 30 to 80 beats per minute.

If drug treatment of sick sinus syndrome is ineffective, an alternative way to increase the heart rate is through the use of an *artificial cardiac pacemaker.* A cardiac pacemaker periodically applies electric shocks to the heart, and depolarizes cardiac muscle to threshold. Shocks applied to the atria initiate atrial action potentials. If the AV node is functioning normally, these atrial action potentials are conducted to the ventricles, and the ventricles also contract. For temporary or emergency treatment, the pacemaker electrodes can be inserted via the jugular vein and advanced into the right atrial chamber. For long-term treatment, a battery-powered electrical stimulator can be surgically implanted under the patient's skin and attached to electrodes that are either inserted into one of the heart's chambers or attached to the outside surface of the heart.

Atrioventricular node block is a common cause of cardiac arrhythmias

Whereas sick sinus syndrome exemplifies a dysfunction of action potential *formation,* AV node block is a common dysfunction of action potential *conduction.* If damage to the AV node prevents conduction of atrial action potentials into the ventricles, the atria continue to beat at a rate determined by the SA node pacemaker cells. The ventricles also continue to beat, but at a much lower rate. When atrial action potentials are blocked from passing through the AV node, ventricular contractions are initiated by cells low in the AV node that function as auxiliary pacemakers. Recall that the AV node pacemaker cells depolarize more slowly than the SA node pacemaker cells. For example, in a resting dog with AV node block, the ventricles typically beat at 30 to 40 beats per minute. These beats are completely desynchronized with regard to the atrial contractions.

Three degrees of severity of AV node block are recognized. Complete block of the AV node, in which no atrial action potentials are conducted to the ventricles, is called *third-degree AV node block.* If action potentials are conducted sporadically from the atria to the ventricles, so that the AV node transmits some atrial action potentials but not all of them, the condition is called *second-degree AV node block.* In a patient with second-degree block, some atrial contractions are followed by ventricular contractions, and others are not. Strong parasympathetic activity can create or exaggerate second-degree AV node block, because parasympathetic activity increases the refractory period of the AV node cells. For example, in quietly resting horses, parasympathetic activity is often so strong, and AV node refractory period so long, that some atrial beats are not conducted to the ventricles. If the pulse of a relaxed, resting horse is palpated, some "missing" ventricular contractions are likely to be noticed. During exercise, the same horse does not show AV node block, because parasympathetic activity has been reduced and sympathetic activity has been increased. Both these changes shorten the refractory period of the AV node and make it much more certain that every atrial action potential will be conducted to the ventricles.

The mildest degree of AV node block is *first-degree block.* In first-degree block, every atrial action potential is transmitted to the ventricles, but the action potential propagates even more slowly than normal through the AV node. Therefore, the delay between atrial contraction and ventricular contraction is abnormally long. Because the AV node conduction velocity can be slowed by parasympathetic activity and sped by sympathetic activity, the behavioral state of the patient characteristically influences the severity of first-degree block.

AV node block can be caused by toxins, viral or bacterial infections, ischemia, congenital heart defects, or cardiac fibrosis. AV node block is sometimes caused by the inadvertent damage of AV node tissue during a surgical repair of a ventricular septal defect. Second- or third-degree AV node block often involves the electrical phenomenon known as *decremental conduction.* As already mentioned, AV node cells have "slow" action potentials, characterized by a less rapid upstroke, a lower voltage amplitude, and a slower velocity of conduction than the action potentials in regular atrial or ventricular cells. All these differences make conduction of the action potential from cell to cell less reliable in the AV node than in regular atrial or ventricular tissue. When the AV node cells are in an electrically depressed state, an atrial action potential may simply die out within the AV node and not be conducted to the ventricles. This fading and eventual stoppage of a cardiac action potential in a slowly conducting region is called *decremental conduction.*

AV node block must be treated if the resulting ventricular rate is too low to maintain adequate blood flow to the body. Drugs that block parasympathetic actions on the heart (muscarinic cholinergic antagonists such as atropine) might reduce the AV node refractory period and decremental conduction sufficiently to overcome a blocked state. The same effect might be achieved with a drug that mimics the effect of sympathetic nerves by activating β-adrenergic receptors (e.g., isoproterenol) (see Table 18–2). If drug treatment fails to correct AV node block, an artificial pacemaker is needed. In the case of AV node block, the pacemaker needs to be applied to the ventricles. Pacing the atria would not be beneficial, because atrial action potentials would not be conducted to the ventricles.

Cardiac tachyarrhythmias result either from abnormal action potential formation (ectopic pacemaker) or from abnormal action potential conduction (reentry)

Tachyarrhythmias are abnormalities in cardiac rhythm in which the atrial rate, ventricular rate, or both are abnormally high. An isolated, occasional extra atrial or ventricular beat is called a *precontraction* or a *premature beat.* Precontractions often result from an area of abnormal cardiac muscle that acts as a pacemaker by spontaneously depolarizing to threshold before the regular pacemaker does. Certain toxins, electrolyte imbalances, and ischemia can cause such *ectopic pacemaker* activity. Occasional precontractions are common both in animals and in humans, and they usually have no clinical significance. If the precontractions become frequent or continuous, the condition is called *tachycardia,* which means "rapid heart." Tachycardia is a clinically significant sign.

Tachycardia is a heart rate that is more rapid than is appropriate for the behavioral circumstances (e.g., a heart rate of 160 beats per minute in a resting dog). Common causes of tachycardia include cardiac infection, reaction to a drug or toxin, electrolyte imbalances, myocardial ischemia, and myocardial infarction.

The tachycardias are named for the site of the pacemaker at which they originate. If the tachycardia originates from an ectopic pacemaker within the atria, it is called *atrial tachycardia.* Atrial tachycardia is common in some canine breeds, including boxers and wolfhounds. If the tachycardia appears to originate from the SA node pacemaker cells, the condition is called *sinus tachycardia. Junctional tachycardias* originate from ectopic pacemakers within the AV node or first part of the AV bundle. *Supraventricular tachycardia* is a collective term that encompasses sinus tachycardia, atrial tachycardia, and junctional tachycardia. If the ectopic pacemaker causing tachycardia is within the ventricles, the condition is called *ventricular tachycardia.* In this situation, the ventricles beat at a rapid rate, as dictated by the abnormal ventricular pacemaker. In occasional patients, some of the action potentials initiated by an ectopic ventricular pacemaker may be conducted backward through the AV node and cause atrial contractions. More commonly, however, the AV node does not conduct action potentials backward; the atria continue to beat at the rate dictated by the normal SA node pacemaker. In either case, ventricular contractions are not preceded in the normal way by atrial contractions. The major dysfunction associated with ventricular tachycardia is that the ventricles do not relax long enough between contractions for adequate filling, and this problem is exacerbated by the absence of an appropriately timed atrial contraction.

An extremely rapid atrial tachycardia is called *atrial flutter.* Atrial flutter does not lead to ventricular flutter because of the long refractory period of the AV node cells. The AV node conducts some but not all of the atrial depolarizations to the ventricles. In this way, the AV node protects the ventricles from beating at too rapid a rate, even though the atria are in flutter. If atrial contractions become so rapid that they lose synchrony, the condition is called *atrial fibrillation.* Atrial fibrillation is characterized by the continuous, random passage of action potentials through the atria. Fibrillating atria appear to quiver; there is no effective, coordinated contraction, and no blood is pumped. Atrial fibrillation is common in horses and in certain breeds of dogs, including Dobermans. Atrial fibrillation usually does not lead to ventricular fibrillation because of the protective effect of the AV node. With its long refractory period, the AV node does not conduct all of the atrial action potentials to the ventricles. The ventricles continue to contract with a synchronized, effective pumping stroke, at a rate limited by the refractory period of the AV node.

Synchronous ventricular contractions are essential for life. If the synchronization of the ventricular contractions is disrupted and the ventricles begin to fibrillate, ventricular pumping stops. In *ventricular fibrillation,* each tiny region of the ventricular wall contracts and relaxes at random, in response to action potentials that propagate randomly and continuously throughout the ventricles. The condition of ventricular fibrillation is synonymous with *sudden cardiac death.*

Whatever the underlying cause, tachycardia is thought to be triggered either by an ectopic pacemaker or by the phenomenon of reentry. An *ectopic pacemaker* is an area of cardiac muscle (other than the SA node) that depolarizes spontaneously to threshold and initiates a cardiac action potential. *Reentry* occurs when an area of myocardium (other than the AV node) develops the twin properties of slow conduction of action potentials and an ability to conduct action potentials in only one direction. Figure 18–11 illustrates how an area of slow, one-way conduction in the wall of one cardiac chamber can initiate tachycardia. If a normally originating action potential is conducted in only one direction through the abnormal area, and if the conduction is so slow that all the normal tissue is past its refractory period by the time the action potential emerges from the abnormal region, the emerging action potential can trigger another action potential in the normal tissue. If this second action potential then propagates around the cardiac chamber and back into the abnormal region, a self-perpetuating cycle can develop. The action potential once again propagates slowly through the abnormal region, and once again it emerges from the abnormal region after the normal tissue is past its refractory period. The result is another *reentrant action potential* that propagates again through the normal tissue. The pathway taken by a reentrant action potential does not necessarily have to be all the way around the circumference of a cardiac chamber. An ischemic or infarcted area of cardiac muscle can form the nonconducting center around which reentrant action potentials travel. This passage of an action potential around and around a nonconducting center is

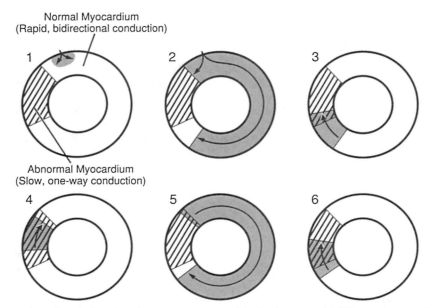

Normal Myocardium
(Rapid, bidirectional conduction)

Abnormal Myocardium
(Slow, one-way conduction)

FIGURE 18–11. A cross section of a cardiac chamber (atrium or ventricle) is shown at six different instants in order to illustrate how reentrant arrhythmias occur. The abnormal region of the myocardium conducts action potentials slowly and only in one direction (upward in this example). *1,* An action potential is just entering this ring of tissue, and only the area shaded gray is depolarized. *2,* The action potential propagates rapidly in both directions through the normal cardiac tissue but is blocked from entering the abnormal myocardium in a counterclockwise direction. *3,* The clockwise-going action potential can enter the abnormal region. *4,* While the action potential propagates slowly through the abnormal region, the normal cardiac tissue repolarizes to a resting state. *5,* The action potential emerges from the abnormal region into normal cardiac tissue and propagates through the normal tissue for a second time. Meanwhile, the abnormal tissue repolarizes to a resting state. *6,* The action potential begins to move slowly through the abnormal region for a second time. States 4, 5, and 6 repeat themselves, so the abnormal region functions as an ectopic pacemaker.

called a *circus movement.* In order for the circus movement of the action potential to be self-regenerating, a portion of the circular, conducting pathway must have the twin properties of slow and one-way conduction. In effect, an area of slow, one-way conduction within a circular conducting pathway (and around a nonconducting center) functions as an ectopic pacemaker. The extra action potentials that are generated can lead to occasional precontractions, continuous tachycardia, or even fibrillation. In any of these cases, the resulting tachyarrhythmia is called a *reentrant arrhythmia.*

In most cases, ventricular fibrillation can be reversed only by electrical *defibrillation.* In this process, a strong electrical current is passed briefly through the heart muscle. This current depolarizes all the cardiac cells simultaneously and holds them in a depolarized state for several milliseconds. It is hoped that when the current is turned off, all the cardiac muscle cells will simultaneously repolarize to a resting membrane potential and that the normal pacemaker of the heart will then have a chance to initiate beats in an organized and synchronized manner once again. Sometimes it works; however, if the cardiac problems that caused ventricular fibrillation to develop in the first place are still present, fibrillation is likely to recur. Usually, defibrillation is performed by placing the stimulating electrodes (the "paddles") on either side of the thorax. The stimulating current passes through, and depolarizes, the skeletal muscles of the thorax as well as the cardiac muscle of the heart. The resulting, involuntary contraction of the skeletal muscles causes the patient to "jump" at the moment of defibrillation.

Commonly used antiarrhythmic drugs have their effects on the ion channels that are responsible for the cardiac action potential

Whereas ventricular fibrillation is generally lethal without electrical defibrillation, other tachycardias can often be treated successfully with *antiarrhythmic drugs.* Because tachyarrhythmias result from extra cardiac action potentials, effective antiarrhythmic drugs must work by counteracting either the formation or the propagation of the extra action potentials.

Local anesthetics (e.g., quinidine or lidocaine) constitute one category of antiarrhythmic drugs. They act by binding to some of the fast Na^+ channels in cardiac muscle cells and preventing them from opening. This counteracts membrane depolarization and action potential formation. In essence, blocking some of the Na^+ channels raises the threshold for action potential formation. This tends to "quiet" ectopic pacemakers and also to stifle reentrant arrhythmias. Incidentally, Na^+ channel blockers, such as lidocaine or procaine (Novocain), are called "local anesthetics" because, when applied to sensory neurons, they prevent the propagation of neural action potentials that would signal pain to the brain. The cardiac, antiarrhythmic effect of local anesthetics is not the result of their blockade of pain pathways.

Another category of antiarrhythmic drugs is the *Ca²⁺ channel blockers*. Examples include verapamil, diltiazem, and nifedipine. These drugs bind to slow Ca^{2+} channels and prevent them from opening, which decreases the entry of Ca^{2+} into cardiac muscle cells during an action potential. Because Ca^{2+} entry is the primary depolarizing influence during the plateau (phase 2) of the cardiac action potential, one major effect of a Ca^{2+} channel blocker is to lower the plateau (make the membrane potential less positive). A secondary consequence is to lengthen the action potential. The action potential is longer because of a complicated effect of the height of the plateau on K^+ channels, which was discussed earlier in connection with sympathetic effects on cardiac action potentials. As mentioned, K^+ channels close at the beginning of a cardiac action potential and then, after a time, reopen (see Fig. 18–5). K^+ channel reopening helps repolarize the cell to a resting state at the end of the action potential. The length of time before K^+ channels reopen depends on the membrane voltage during the action potential. Specifically, when the plateau is lower (less positive membrane potential) than normal, the K^+ channels stay closed for a longer time. This prolongs the action potential and postpones repolarization. Drugs that lengthen the cardiac action potential also lengthen the refractory period, which makes it less likely that early extra action potentials will be formed in ectopic pacemakers or that they will propagate even if they are formed.

The Ca^{2+} channel blockers have especially strong effects on the cells of the SA and AV nodes. As mentioned, these nodal cells do not have fast Na^+ channels; instead, Ca^{2+} entry through slow Ca^{2+} channels is the main event in the slow action potentials of these cells. Not surprisingly, the amplitude of slow action potentials is greatly reduced by Ca^{2+} channel blockers. These action potentials are also lengthened. Low-amplitude, long action potentials propagate very slowly from cell to cell, which decreases the likelihood that early extra action potentials will form or propagate in SA or AV node cells.

Ca^{2+} channel blockers are especially effective in protecting the ventricles from rapid rates in cases of persistent atrial flutter or fibrillation. By increasing the refractoriness and decreasing the conduction velocity of AV node cells, Ca^{2+} channel blockers cause many of the atrial action potentials to dissipate (through decremental conduction) in the AV node and not be conducted to the ventricular bundle branches.

Because Ca^{2+} channel blockers reduce the entry of extracellular Ca^{2+} into cardiac muscle cells during an action potential, they also decrease the strength of the resulting contraction. Less entry of extracellular "trigger" Ca^{2+} means a less powerful stimulus for the release of stored Ca^{2+} from the sarcoplasmic reticulum. Therefore, the cytosolic Ca^{2+} concentration does not increase as much as normal during the action potential, there is less activation of troponin than normal, there are fewer binding sites than normal available for actin-myosin cross-bridges, and therefore there are fewer active cross-bridges. Some clinical

situations in which it is desirable to decrease cardiac contractility are discussed in Chapter 20.

The *cardiac glycosides* (e.g., digitalis) constitute yet another category of antiarrhythmic drugs. Cardiac glycosides act by inhibiting the Na^+, K^+ pump in cell membranes. As mentioned in Chapters 1 and 3, the Na^+,K^+ pump uses energy from adenosine triphosphate to transport Na^+ out of cells and K^+ into cells. The pump also indirectly supplies the energy needed to transport Ca^{2+} back out of cardiac cells after it enters during an action potential. Inhibition of the Na^+,K^+ pump has several important effects on cardiac function. The effects are listed here without much explanation, because the mechanisms are quite complex. First, cardiac cells do not repolarize fully; the resting membrane potential is not as negative as normal. As a consequence, some Na^+ channels remain in an inactivated (closed) state, which makes the cells somewhat refractory with regard to the formation of subsequent action potentials. This tends to quiet ectopic pacemakers. Second, through effects on the central nervous system, there is an increase in the activity of parasympathetic nerves to the heart. This slows the heart rate, quiets atrial ectopic pacemakers, slows conduction through the AV node, and increases the refractory period of AV node cells. The overall effect is to suppress ectopic atrial action potentials and/or to cause extra atrial action potentials to die out in the AV node and not be conducted to the ventricles. A third effect of cardiac glycosides is to allow more Ca^{2+} than normal to accumulate inside cardiac cells. As a consequence, the strength of cardiac contractions is increased. In summary, the cardiac glycosides are antiarrhythmic and also increase cardiac contractility.

β-Adrenergic antagonists (e.g., propranolol) constitute a fourth class of antiarrhythmic drug. β blockers bind to some of the β-adrenergic receptors on cardiac cells and prevent their activation by norepinephrine from sympathetic nerves or by epinephrine from the adrenal medulla. Sympathetic activation tends to promote tachyarrhythmias by increasing heart rate, shortening refractory period, and speeding conduction of action potentials, especially through the AV node. β blockers reduce these effects and therefore reduce the likelihood that extra action potentials will form or propagate. An additional effect of β blockers is to reverse sympathetic activation–induced increases in cardiac contractility.

In summary, of the four types of drugs commonly used to treat tachyarrhythmias, three also have pronounced effects on cardiac contractility. The Ca^{2+} channel blockers and β blockers decrease cardiac contractility, whereas cardiac glycosides increase contractility. Local anesthetics have little effect on contractility. This variety of effects allows a clinician to select the type of antiarrhythmic drug that is best matched to each patient's cardiac contractile state.

Electrical dysfunction of the heart has been discussed in considerable detail in order to illustrate how specific abnormalities in the specialized cardiac conduction system can result in specific and serious arrhythmias. Electrical dysfunction of the heart is encountered often in clinical practice, and its consequences are often serious or even lethal. Because electrical dysfunction is so important, Chapter 19 is devoted to an explanation of the *electrocardiogram*, which is the most commonly used tool for evaluating electrical dysfunction.

CLINICAL CORRELATIONS

Third-degree atrioventricular block

History   A 5-year-old male English bulldog has fainted several times during the past 3 weeks. On each occasion he collapses, is apparently unconscious for a few seconds, and then slowly recovers. These episodes occur most often during exertion. In general, he tends to be less active than normal, but there are no other obvious signs of illness.

Clinical examination   The dog is moderately obese. There are no obvious neurologic deficits. His mucous membranes appear normal; they are pink, and the capillary refilling time is normal (1.5 seconds). Auscultation of the chest reveals a slow, regular heart rate of 45 beats per minute. The femoral pulse rate is also 45 beats per minute and strong. Thoracic radiography reveals a mildly enlarged heart, but the radiograph is otherwise within normal limits.

The electrocardiogram reveals a disparity between the atrial rate (atrial depolarizations occurring regularly, 140 times per minute) and the ventricular rate (ventricular depolarizations occurring regularly, 45 times per minute). There is no consistent time interval between the atrial and ventricular depolarizations.

Comment   Voltage fluctuations are produced at the body surface by atrial and ventricular depolarizations (full explanation in Chapter 19). Electrocardiography detects these voltage fluctuations and produces a graph of voltage as a function of time. The graph is called an *electrocardiogram*. The electrocardiogram of this dog shows a complete dissociation between atrial and ventricular depolarizations, and this provides definitive diagnostic evidence of complete (third-degree) AV node block. The dog's atria are depolarizing 140 times per minute in response to action potentials that are being initiated in the normal manner by pacemaker cells of the SA node. However, the atrial action potentials are not being conducted through the AV node. Ventricular action potentials are being initiated, at the slow rate of 45 per minute, by auxiliary pacemaker cells that are located below the blocked region of the AV node.

The low ventricular rate in this dog allows a longer-than-normal time for ventricular filling between beats. Therefore, the volume of blood ejected with each beat (the stroke volume) is greater than normal. The increased stroke volume causes the femoral pulse to be very strong.

In a normal dog, the heart rate is controlled by sympathetic and parasympathetic nerves acting on the SA node pacemaker cells. These nerves adjust the heart rate so that cardiac output is matched to the metabolic requirements of the body. In a dog with complete AV block, the ventricles do not respond to these autonomi-

cally mediated changes in SA node pacemaker rate. Typically, the rate of ventricular contractions is low at rest and cannot increase much during exercise. Therefore, cardiac output does not increase enough during exertion to meet the increased metabolic needs of exercising skeletal muscle. The inadequate cardiac output results in a decrease in arterial blood pressure during exercise. In this bulldog, the decrease in arterial blood pressure during exertion causes brain blood flow to fall below the level needed to sustain consciousness. As a result, the dog faints.

Treatment   Drug therapy for AV node block involves either blocking the effects of parasympathetic nerves on the AV node (with a muscarinic cholinergic antagonist drug such as atropine) or mimicking the effects of sympathetic activation (with cautious use of a β-adrenergic agonist such as isoproterenol or dopamine). The rationale for these treatments is based on the following physiology: AV node block occurs because atrial action potentials die out in the AV node, a process called *decremental conduction*. The tendency for decremental conduction is increased by parasympathetic activation, because parasympathetic nerves act on AV node cells to increase their refractory period and to decrease the velocity with which action potentials spread from cell to cell. Therefore, blocking parasympathetic effects sometimes (but rather rarely) reverses AV node block. Sympathetic nerves decrease the refractory period of AV node cells and increase their conduction velocity. Therefore, sympathetic activation decreases the tendency for decremental conduction; a sympathomimetic drug (one that mimics the effects of sympathetic activation) has the same effect. In addition, sympathetic nerves act directly on the ventricular auxiliary pacemaker cells to increase their rate. Therefore, even if a sympathomimetic drug does not unblock the AV node, it increases the ventricular rate somewhat.

Many cases of third-degree AV block cannot be managed effectively with drugs, and so an artificial ventricular pacemaker must be installed. Pacemaker electrodes can be inserted into the right ventricle via a systemic vein (e.g., the external jugular vein) with only sedation and local anesthesia.

Bibliography

Berne RM, Levy MN: Cardiovascular Physiology, 7th ed. St. Louis: CV Mosby, 1997.

Dukes HH, Swenson MJ, Reece WO: Dukes' Physiology of Domestic Animals. Ithaca, N.Y.: Comstock, 1993, pp 90–118.

Giles WR: Intracellular electrical activity in the heart. In Patton HD, Fuchs AF, Hille B, et al (eds): Textbook of Physiology—Circulation, Respiration, Body Fluids, Metabolism, and Endocrinology, 21st ed. Philadelphia: WB Saunders, 1989, p 782.

Katz AM: Physiology of the Heart, 3rd ed. Baltimore: Lippincott Williams & Wilkins, 2000.

Lilly, LS: Pathophysiology of Heart Disease (A Collaborative Project of Medical Students and Faculty), 2nd ed. Baltimore: Williams & Wilkins, 1998.

Milnor WR: Cardiovascular Physiology. New York: Oxford University Press, 1990.

Opie LH: The Heart: Physiology, From Cell to Circulation, 3rd ed. Baltimore: Lippincott Williams & Wilkins, 1998.

PRACTICE QUESTIONS

1. An increase in heart rate could result from
   a. an increase in sympathetic nerve activity to the heart.

b. an abnormally rapid decrease in permeability of SA node cells to K^+ during diastole.
c. an abnormally rapid increase in permeability of SA node cells to Na^+ during diastole.
d. a decrease in parasympathetic nerve activity to the heart.
e. all of the above.

2. In which of the following arrhythmias will there be more atrial beats per minute than ventricular beats?
   a. Complete (third-degree) AV block.
   b. Frequent premature ventricular contractions.
   c. Sick sinus syndrome (sinus bradycardia).
   d. First-degree AV block.
   e. Ventricular tachycardia.

3. The normal pathway followed by a cardiac action potential is to begin in the SA node and then propagate
   a. across the atria in the bundle of His.
   b. through the connective tissue layers that separate the atria and ventricles.
   c. across the atria and to the AV node.
   d. from the left atrium to the right atrium.
   e. from the left atrium to the left ventricle and from the right atrium to the right ventricle.

4. Which statement is true?

a. The refractory period of cardiac muscle cells is much shorter than their mechanical contraction.
b. The cardiac action potential propagates from one cardiac cell to another through nexi, or gap junctions.
c. Purkinje's fibers are special nerves that spread the cardiac action potential rapidly through the ventricles.
d. Ventricular muscle cells characteristically depolarize spontaneously to threshold.
e. The permeability of ventricular muscle cells to Ca^{2+} is lower during the plateau of an action potential than it is at rest.

5. Which of the following types of drugs would be the best choice to treat a patient suffering from both a supraventricular tachycardia and an inadequate cardiac contractility?
   a. Local anesthetic (fast Na^+ channel blocker).
   b. Muscarinic cholinergic antagonist.
   c. β-Adrenergic agonist.
   d. Cardiac glycoside (inhibits Na^+, K^+ pump).
   e. Calcium channel blocker.

PRACTICE ANSWERS

1. e   2. a   3. c   4. b   5. d

19

The electrocardiogram

1 An electrocardiogram is simply a graph from a voltmeter that makes plots of voltage as a function of time

2 Atrial depolarization, ventricular depolarization, and ventricular repolarization cause characteristic voltage deflections in the electrocardiogram

3 The electrocardiogram reveals the timing of electrical events in the heart

4 Six standardized electrocardiographic leads are used in veterinary medicine

5 Abnormal voltages in the electrocardiogram are indicative of cardiac structural or electrical abnormalities

6 Electrical dysfunctions in the heart cause abnormal patterns of electrocardiogram waves

---

An electrocardiogram is simply a graph from a voltmeter that makes plots of voltage as a function of time

The *electrocardiogram (ECG)* is the most commonly used clinical tool for diagnosing electrical dysfunctions of the heart. In its most common application, two or more metal electrodes are applied to the skin surface, and the voltages recorded by the electrodes are beamed onto a video screen or drawn onto a paper strip. How the heart produces voltages that are detectable at the body surface is extraordinarily complex. However, elementary physical principles can be used to develop an intuitive model of how the ECG works; this intuitive model is adequate for most clinical applications.

An intuitive understanding of the ECG begins with the concept of an *electrical dipole* in a *conductive medium* (Fig. 19–1). A dipole is a pair of electrical charges (a positive charge and a negative charge) separated by a distance. A common flashlight battery is a good example of a dipole. A battery has a positive end (where excess positive charges are) and a negative end (where excess negative charges are), and the two ends are separated by a distance. If such a dipole is placed within a conductive medium (for example, in a basin of sodium chloride solution), ionic currents flow through the solution. Positive ions in the solution flow toward the negative end of the dipole, and vice versa. The flow of ions creates voltage differences within the salt solution. These voltage differences can be detected by placing the electrodes of a voltmeter at the perimeter of the salt solution. In Figure 19–1, an electrode placed at point A would measure a more positive voltage than an electrode placed at point B. There is a positive voltage at point *A* in comparison with point B; equivalently, there is a positive voltage

difference between point A and point B. Point C and point D are equally near the positive and negative ends of the dipole, so no voltage difference would exist between electrodes placed at points C and D.

In Figure 19–2, the battery in the sodium chloride solution has been replaced with an elongated strip of cardiac muscle. The voltages detected at point A in comparison with point B and at point C in comparison with point D are plotted for five different conditions. In condition 1, all the cells in the strip are at a resting membrane potential. Each cell is charged negatively on its inside and positively on its outside. Because cardiac cells are electrically interconnected via gap junctions, the strip of cardiac muscle behaves electrically as if it were one large cell (a functional syncytium). From the outside, the strip of cells "looks like" one large cell that is symmetrically charged positively around its perimeter. Therefore, no dipole exists; the voltage difference between point A and point B would be zero. The voltage difference between point C and point D would also be zero.

In condition 2, the cells at the left end of the muscle strip have depolarized to threshold level and formed an action potential. The action potential is propagating from cell to cell, through the muscle strip, from left to right. In other words, the cells at the left end of the strip are depolarized and are at the plateau of their action potential, whereas the cells at the right end of the strip are still at a resting membrane potential. Under these conditions, the muscle strip forms an electrical dipole, in which the outside of the cells is charged positively at the right end and negatively at the left end. Therefore, a positive voltage would exist at point A in comparison with point B. Note, however, that the voltage at point C in comparison with point D would still be zero, because neither of these points is closer to the positive end of the dipole.

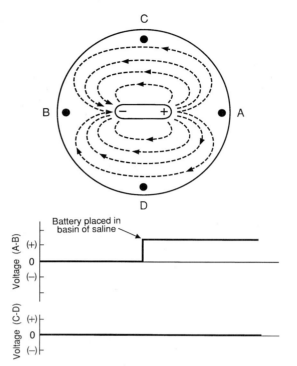

FIGURE 19–1. When an electrical dipole (e.g., a flashlight battery) is placed into a conductive medium (e.g., sodium chloride solution), the flow of ionic currents creates voltage differences within the medium. A simple voltmeter can be used to detect these voltage differences. In this example, point A is positive in comparison with point B (i.e., voltage A-B is positive). No voltage difference exists between point C and point D (i.e., voltage C-D is zero).

In condition 3, the entire muscle strip is depolarized; that is, all the cells are at the plateau of their action potential, with a uniform negative charge outside of each cell. Therefore, no voltage differences exist around the perimeter of the muscle strip, and the recorded voltages (A in comparison with B and C in comparison with D) are zero.

In condition 4, the muscle strip is repolarizing; cells at the left end have returned to a resting state, whereas cells at the right end are still at the plateau of their action potential. Under these conditions, the voltage at point A is negative in comparison with point B, because the outside of the muscle strip is charged negatively at its right end and positively at its left end. The voltage at point C in comparison with point D is still zero.

In condition 5, all the cells in the muscle strip have returned to a resting state (same as condition 1). Again, the voltage at point A in comparison with point B is zero, and the voltage at point C in comparison with point D is zero.

Note that if the repolarization (condition 4) had spread from right to left in the muscle strip (instead of from left to right), the voltage at point A in comparison with point B would have been positive during repolarization. In general, a depolarization spreading from point A toward point B, or a repolarization spreading from point B toward A, creates a positive voltage at A in comparison with B. Conversely, a depolariza-

tion spreading from B toward A, or a repolarization spreading from A toward B, creates a negative voltage at A in comparison with B.

Figure 19–3 takes the development of the ECG one step further by picturing the entire heart (rather than a strip of cardiac muscle) in the basin of saline. The graphs below the drawing show the voltages that would be detected by electrodes at the perimeter of the basin during atrial depolarization.

The plots start at a time between cardiac contractions, when all the cells in the heart are at a resting membrane potential. Every cardiac cell is charged negatively on the inside of its membrane and positively on the outside. Therefore, all around the entire heart, viewed as one big cell, the charge would be positive, and there would be no voltage differences between any of the electrodes.

When the cells in the sinoatrial (SA) node depolarize to threshold level, they initiate an action potential that propagates from cell to cell (spreads) outward from the SA node. As indicated by the arrows in the top diagram of Figure 19–3, the action potential spreads simultaneously downward in the right atrium and also leftward (across the right atrium and into the left atrium). During this spreading atrial depolarization, the right atrial cells near the SA node become negatively charged on their outside, whereas the cells in the left atrium and the cells in the inferior part of the right atrium, which have not yet depolarized, remain positively charged on their outside. Therefore, the depolarizing atria create an electrical

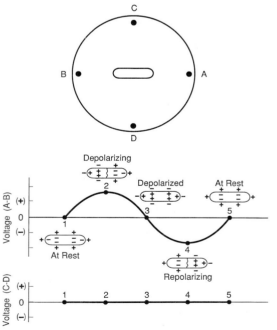

FIGURE 19–2. A strip of cardiac muscle cells in sodium chloride solution produces voltage differences between point A and point B during a phase of spreading depolarization or spreading repolarization, but not when all the cells are in a uniform state of polarization (i.e., not when all the cells are at rest or depolarized). No voltage difference is created between point C and point D. See text for a complete description.

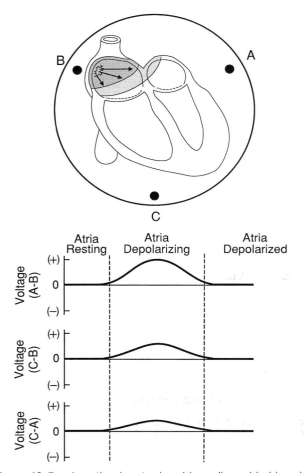

Atria Resting | Atria Depolarizing | Atria Depolarized

Voltage (A-B)

Voltage (C-B)

Voltage (C-A)

FIGURE 19–3. A resting heart, placed in sodium chloride solution, would not create voltage differences among electrodes A, B, and C. However, during depolarization of the atria, a positive voltage would be created at point A in comparison with point B. There would also be positive voltages at point C in comparison with point B and at point C in comparison with point A.

dipole with its positive end angled downward and toward the left atrium. This dipole of atrial depolarization creates a voltage that is positive at point A in comparison with point B. Also, a voltage is created at point C that is positive in comparison with point B. Similarly, there is a positive voltage at point C with regard to point A. These voltage differences are shown in the graphs.

Once the atria are completely depolarized (with every atrial cell at the plateau of its action potential), the voltage differences between all points return to zero.

Atrial depolarization, ventricular depolarization, and ventricular repolarization cause characteristic voltage deflections in the electrocardiogram

In Figure 19–4, the heart is pictured in its normal position in the thorax of a dog. The extracellular fluids of the body contain sodium chloride in solution, so the body can be imagined as a substitute for the basin of saline that was shown in the previous figures. The positions of the left forelimb, right forelimb, and left hind limb in Figure 19–4 correspond with points A, B, and C in Figure 19–3. Figure 19–4A shows that while atrial depolarization is in progress at the beginning of a heart beat, there would be a positive voltage in the left forelimb in comparison with the right forelimb. This is simply a repetition of the idea that was illustrated in Figure 19–3, the left forelimb being equivalent to point A and the right forelimb being equivalent to point B.

The deflection in the ECG trace during atrial depolarization is called the *P wave.* At the end of atrial depolarization (i.e., at the end of the P wave), the ECG voltage returns to zero. At this moment during the actual cardiac cycle, the action potential is propagating from cell to cell through the atrioventricular (AV) node and the first part of the AV bundle. These tissues are so small that their depolarization generally does not create a voltage difference that is detectable at the body surface.

The next voltage differences that are detectable at the body surface are those associated with the depolarization of the ventricles. The first part of ventricular depolarization usually involves a depolarization that spreads from left to right across the interventricular septum, as shown in Figure 19–4B. This first phase of ventricular depolarization usually causes a small voltage difference *(Q wave)* between the left forelimb and the right forelimb; the left forelimb has a slight negative charge in comparison with the right.

The next event in ventricular depolarization usually causes a large, positive voltage *(R wave)* at the left forelimb in comparison with the right, as depicted in Figure 19–4C. To understand why this *R wave* is large and positive, recall that during ventricular depolarization, the left and right bundle branches conduct the spreading action potential to the ventricular apex. From there, Purkinje's fibers carry the action potential rapidly up the inside walls of both ventricles. From there, the depolarization spreads from cell to cell, outward through the walls of both ventricles, as pictured by the small arrows in Figure 19–4C. Each small arrow can be considered a dipole, with its positive end pointing at the outside wall of the ventricle (because the inside surfaces of the ventricles depolarize before the outside surfaces). The net electrical effect of depolarizations spreading outward through the walls of both ventricles is a large electrical dipole pointed diagonally downward (caudad) and toward the dog's left. This *net dipole* points toward the left for two reasons. First, the cardiac axis is tilted toward the left (i.e., the normal orientation of the heart is with the ventricular apex angled toward the left wall of the thorax). Second, the left ventricle is much more massive than the right ventricle, and so the dipoles created by depolarizations spreading outward in the wall of the left ventricle dominate electrically over the dipoles created by depolarizations spreading outward in the wall of the right ventricle. The resulting large, positive R wave is the predominant feature of a normal ECG. Abnormalities in the magnitude or

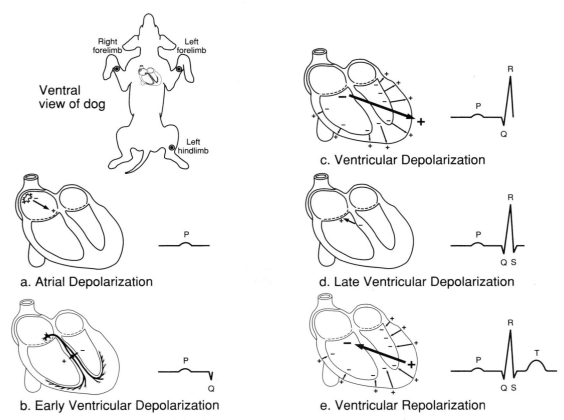

a. Atrial Depolarization

b. Early Ventricular Depolarization

c. Ventricular Depolarization

d. Late Ventricular Depolarization

e. Ventricular Repolarization

FIGURE 19–4. As a normal cardiac action potential is conducted through the atria and ventricles, a characteristic sequence of voltage differences is created between the left forelimb (analogous to point A in Fig. 19–3) and the right forelimb (analogous to point B in Fig. 19–3). See text for a complete description.

polarity of the R wave have great diagnostic significance, as explained later in this chapter.

As the depolarizations finish spreading outward through the walls of both ventricles, the voltage in the left forelimb in comparison with the right forelimb returns to zero and then often becomes slightly negative for a few milliseconds (pictured in Fig. 19–4D). The physical basis of this small, negative S wave is obscure. After the S wave, the voltage in the left forelimb in comparison with the right forelimb returns to zero and stays there for a time, because all the cells throughout both ventricles are uniformly at the plateau of their action potential; no dipole exists.

Altogether, the process of *ventricular depolarization* produces a pattern of voltages in the ECG called the *QRS wave* (or *QRS complex*). The most important feature to understand about the QRS complex is why its predominant component, the R wave, is large and positive.

Figure 19–4E shows the electrical events during repolarization of the ventricles. Whereas the wave of *depolarization* spreads outward through the walls of both ventricles, the wave of *repolarization* is not as predictable. As pictured in Figure 19–4E, the depolarization is spreading inward; that is, the outside surface of the ventricles is the last ventricular tissue to depolarize but the first to repolarize. An inward-going repolarization would create a net dipole with its negative end pointed upward (craniad) and toward

the dog's right, which would create a positive voltage in the left forelimb in comparison with the right forelimb *(T wave)*. In many normal dogs, however, ventricular repolarization proceeds in the same direction as the depolarization (from inside the ventricles to outside). This pattern of repolarization creates a negative voltage in the left forelimb in comparison with the right forelimb; that is, the T wave is negative. Whether positive or negative, T waves are caused by repolarization of the ventricles.

To summarize, the P wave is caused by atrial depolarization, the QRS complex by ventricular depolarization, and the T wave by ventricular repolarization. The pattern of ventricular repolarization varies from dog to dog; the T wave may be positive or negative. No identifiable wave in the normal ECG corresponds to atrial repolarization, because atrial repolarization does not proceed in an orderly enough pattern or direction to create a net electrical dipole.

The electrocardiogram reveals the timing of electrical events in the heart

Because the predominant waves in an ECG correspond to specific electrical events in the heart, the time between these waves can be measured to determine the timing of events in the heart. Figure 19–5 indicates the conventions used to define the important *intervals* and *segments* in the ECG. The *PR*

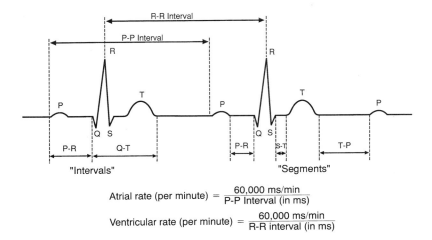

$$\text{Atrial rate (per minute)} = \frac{60,000 \text{ ms/min}}{\text{P-P Interval (in ms)}}$$

$$\text{Ventricular rate (per minute)} = \frac{60,000 \text{ ms/min}}{\text{R-R interval (in ms)}}$$

FIGURE 19–5. The time between various waves of the electrocardiogram corresponds to the timing of specific electrical events in the heart. See text for a complete description. The equations show how the atrial rate and the ventricular rate can be calculated from the PP and RR intervals, respectively. Of course, in a normally functioning heart, atrial rate = ventricular rate = heart rate.

interval corresponds to the time between the start of atrial depolarization and the start of ventricular depolarization. The PR interval is typically about 0.1 second in a resting dog. During this time, the cardiac action potential is conducted slowly through the AV node. The duration of the *QRS complex* corresponds to the time it takes for the ventricles to depolarize, once the cardiac action potential emerges from the AV node and AV bundle. Typically, this is less than 0.1 second. The *QT interval* corresponds to the length of time that the ventricles remain depolarized (i.e., the length of the plateau of the action potential in ventricular tissue). Typically, the QT interval is about 0.2 second. The time between successive P waves *(PP interval)* corresponds to the time between atrial

depolarizations (and hence atrial contractions). The PP interval can be used to calculate the number of atrial contractions per minute (the atrial rate), as illustrated in Figure 19–5. Likewise, the time between successive R waves *(RR interval)* corresponds to the time between ventricular depolarizations (and hence contractions), and so the RR interval can be used to calculate the ventricular rate. Of course, in a normal heart, the atrial rate equals the ventricular rate.

Six standardized electrocardiographic leads are used in veterinary medicine

Figure 19–6 shows actual ECG records obtained from a normal dog. To obtain these recordings, electrodes

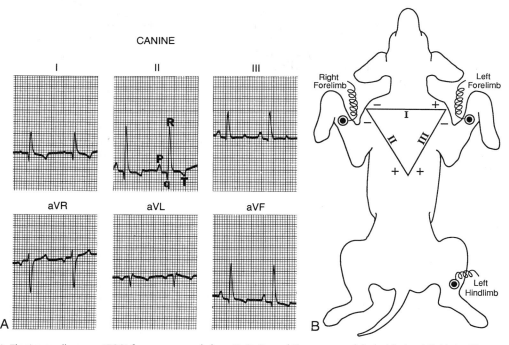

FIGURE 19–6. *A,* Electrocardiogram (ECG) from a normal dog. P, Q, R, and T waves are labeled in lead II. Note: There are no distinct S waves in these ECG records, and the T waves happen to be negative in leads I, II, aV_L, and aV_F. These are not abnormal signs. *B,* Einthoven's triangle depicts the standard conventions for interconnecting the three limb electrodes to obtain lead I, lead II, and lead III ECGs. See text for additional explanation. (From Tilley LP: Essentials of Canine and Feline Electrocardiology: Interpretation and Treatment, 2nd ed. Philadelphia: Lea & Febiger, 1985.)

were placed on the left forelimb, right forelimb, and left hind limb. Electrodes on these limbs are usually envisioned as forming a triangle around the heart (just as electrodes at points A, B, and C form a triangle around the heart in Fig. 19–3). The various ECG traces in Figure 19–6 were obtained by interconnecting these electrodes in standardized combinations that were prescribed by Willem Einthoven, inventor of the ECG. As shown in Figure 19–6B, the voltage in the left forelimb in comparison with the right forelimb is called *lead I*. Note that lead I corresponds to the voltage measurements that were discussed in connection with Figure 19–4. The same pattern of distinct P, R, and T waves is evident in the lead I trace in Figure 19–6, as was seen in Figure 19–4 (although the T wave is negative in Fig. 19–6).

In accordance with Einthoven's convention, the connections for the three standard limb leads are depicted in Figure 19–6 in the form of a triangle (*Einthoven's triangle*). The triangle indicates that to make a *lead I* ECG, the voltage is recorded in the left forelimb (labeled the "+" electrode) in comparison with the right forelimb (called the "−" electrode). Similarly, the diagram indicates that *lead II* is the voltage measured in the left hind limb in comparison with the right forelimb, and *lead III* is defined as the voltage in the left hind limb in comparison with the left forelimb. It is important to remember that the + and − signs on Einthoven's triangle are simply notations about how to hook up the electrodes. They indicate, for example, that lead I is obtained by measuring the voltage in the left forelimb in comparison with the right forelimb (not the other way around). The + and − signs on the triangle do not necessarily correspond to the dipoles that are created in the heart.

As illustrated in Figure 19–6A, the major ECG events (P, R, and T waves) are normally evident no matter whether one is looking at tracings from leads I, II, or III. These standard limb leads simply provide different "angles" for viewing the electrical dipoles created by the heart as it depolarizes and repolarizes. Three additional electrical "views" are provided by the *augmented unipolar limb leads* (aV$_R$, aV$_L$, and aV$_F$). Lead aV$_R$ measures the voltage from the right forelimb electrode in comparison with the average voltage from the other two limb electrodes. Similarly, aV$_L$ and aV$_F$ measure the voltages from the left forelimb and left hind limb electrodes with regard to the average voltage from the other two electrodes.

Leads I, II, and III are used routinely in veterinary electrocardiography. The augmented unipolar limb leads (aV$_L$, aV$_R$, and aV$_F$) are used less commonly. Special additional leads are sometimes recorded by placing ECG electrodes at standardized sites on the thorax. These *precordial (chest) leads* are used more commonly in human medicine than in veterinary medicine. They are helpful in the evaluation of very specific cardiac electrical dysfunctions.

The standardized vertical calibration on an ECG is that two major divisions equal 1 mV. To make it easy to measure time intervals on an ECG, two standard chart speeds, whereby either 5 or 10 major divisions equal 1 second, are used. Five major divisions per second correspond to a paper speed of 25 mm/second. Ten major divisions per second correspond to a paper speed of 50 mm/second.

Abnormal voltages in the electrocardiogram are indicative of cardiac structural or electrical abnormalities

The ECG in Figure 19–7 was obtained from a dog with right ventricular hypertrophy. Note that the sequence of waves in the ECG appears to be normal; that is, each heart beat begins with an upward-going P wave, which is followed by a QRS complex and (in this dog) a positive T wave. The atrial and ventricular rates are equal, at about 100 beats per minute. An abnormality is evident, however, because the predominant polarity of the QRS complex recorded from lead I is negative instead of positive as usual. As mentioned, the QRS complex is caused by ventricular depolarization, and its dominant feature is normally a large, positive R wave. The R wave is normally positive as recorded from lead I, because the cardiac axis is normally angled to the left side of the thorax and because the left ventricular wall is much more massive than the right ventricular wall. Therefore, reversal of this polarity suggests that the cardiac axis has shifted to the right, the mass of the right ventricle

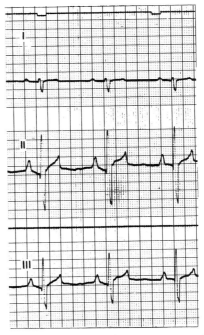

FIGURE 19–7. An ECG from a dog with right ventricular hypertrophy. The paper speed is 50 mm/second; therefore, 10 major grid divisions equal 1 second. (One-second timing marks are visible as small downward deflections at the very top.) Both the PP and RR intervals are 0.6 second, so both atrial and ventricular rates are 100 per minute. The salient abnormalities are (1) predominantly negative QRS complexes recorded from lead I and (2) large-amplitude, bidirectional QRS complexes recorded from leads II and III. (From Ettinger SJ: Textbook of Veterinary Internal Medicine, 3rd ed. Philadelphia: WB Saunders, 1989, p 981.)

has increased, or both. The abnormally high voltages of the QRS complex recorded from leads II and III are also indicative of ventricular hypertrophy. The pronounced negative components in the QRS complexes recorded from leads II and III suggest that during part of ventricular depolarization, the predominant direction of depolarization is away from the left hind limb. This is consistent with a cardiac axis shifted to the right and a massive right ventricle. Right ventricular hypertrophy is a common consequence of cardiac defects that increase either the volume of blood that must be pumped by the right ventricle or the pressure that must be generated within the right ventricle during its contractions. Examples include pulmonic stenosis, patent ductus arteriosus, and ventricular septal defect (these are discussed in Chapter 20).

ECG voltages are also sometimes abnormally low. One common cause of low-voltage ECGs is an accumulation of fluid in the pericardium. This condition is called *cardiac tamponade.* In a sense, the pericardial fluid creates a short circuit for ionic currents, so that less current flows outward toward the body surface. Therefore, voltages smaller than normal are created at the body surface.

An upward or downward shift of the ST segment, in comparison with the rest of the ECG, is often indicative of an area of ischemic or infarcted ventricular muscle. Typically, ischemic or infarcted ventricular muscle cells cannot maintain a normal, negative resting membrane potential; these cells are always more or less depolarized. Therefore, in between ventricular contractions, when normal ventricular cells are at a normal resting membrane potential, a voltage differ-

ence exists between normal and ischemic (or infarcted) ventricular cells. This voltage difference creates an electrical dipole between normal, resting ventricular muscle and ischemic (or infarcted) ventricular muscle. Figure 19–8 *(left)* shows the orientation of the dipole for the case of an ischemic area in the inferior (caudal) part of the ventricles. The dipole creates a negative voltage in lead II during ventricular rest (i.e., during the TP segment). When an action potential enters this ventricle, the normal ventricular tissue becomes depolarized, and a QRS complex is observed. The ischemic area cannot form action potentials; it simply remains depolarized. As a result, during the ST segment, the entire ventricle, normal and ischemic, is depolarized (Fig. 19–8, *right).* During the ST segment, there is no voltage difference (no dipole) between the injured area and the normal area. With no dipole present, the ECG voltage during the ST segment is close to a true zero level. However, the ST segment is elevated in relation to the more negative voltage during the TP segment (ventricular rest). Thus, *ST segment elevation* (which is actually "TP segment depression") is indicative of an ischemic or infarcted area in the inferior (caudal) part of the ventricle. Ischemia or infarction in the anterior (cranial) ventricular area would cause *ST segment depression.*

Making a diagnosis solely on the basis of abnormal ECG voltage is risky. Theoretically, if the structural and electrical properties of a particular heart are known in detail, the appearance of the ECG can be predicted with certainty. However, the reverse situation is not strictly true. Several different cardiac defects may result in similar voltage abnormalities. Thus, a voltage abnormality in an ECG cannot be

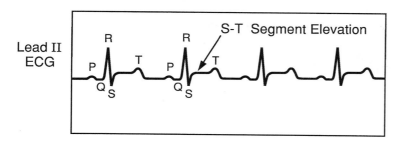

FIGURE 19–8. The voltage recorded during the ST segment is elevated, in comparison with the baseline (TP segment), in this lead II ECG from a dog with an inferior (caudal) ventricular infarction. The drawings show why an ischemic or infarcted area of ventricle creates a net electrical dipole in the resting ventricle (during TP segment) but not in the depolarized ventricle (during ST segment).

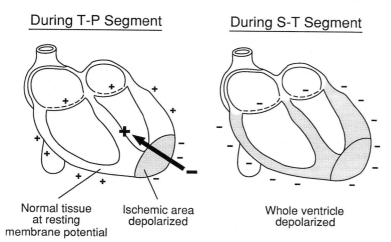

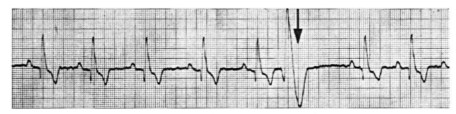

FIGURE 19–9. Lead I ECG of a dog, showing five normal beats followed by one premature ventricular beat. A sixth P wave would be expected at the time marked by the arrow. This P wave is obscured by the large voltages associated with the premature ventricular beat. Also, the refractory period associated with the premature beat prevented the sixth normal ventricular beat from occurring; this creates a long pause (called the *compensatory pause*) between the premature beat and the next regular beat. In this and the remaining ECG examples, paper speed is 50 mm/second (10 major grid divisions equal 1 second). (From Ettinger SJ: Textbook of Veterinary Internal Medicine, 3rd ed. Philadelphia: WB Saunders, 1989.)

ascribed with certainty to a particular cardiac defect. However, in conjunction with other clinical data, ECG abnormalities are often strongly indicative of specific structural or electrical abnormalities in the heart.

Electrical dysfunctions in the heart cause abnormal patterns of electrocardiogram waves

Figure 19–9 is an ECG from a dog with premature ventricular contractions. This lead I strip begins with five normal beats (each QRS complex is preceded by a P wave and followed by a T wave). The P waves are evenly spaced, with a PP interval of 0.5 second (so heart rate is 120 beats per minute). After five normal beats, a large-voltage complex of abnormal shape occurs without a preceding P wave. This is indicative of a premature ventricular depolarization (atrial depolarization could not produce such large voltage deflections). The predominant voltage in the abnormal complex is positive in lead I, indicating that the premature ventricular depolarization spread predominantly from right to left in the ventricles. The abnormal shape and long duration of the complex indicate that the premature depolarization did not spread across the ventricles by way of the rapidly

conducting bundle branches and Purkinje fibers. In other words, the ectopic site that originated the premature depolarization was not within the AV bundle or bundle branches. Instead, the ventricular depolarization must have spread through more slowly conducting pathways. The abnormally large T wave associated with the premature beat further emphasizes the abnormal pattern of spread of the premature action potential across the ventricles.

Had the premature depolarization originated from an ectopic pacemaker within the AV bundle or bundle branches, the pattern of ventricular depolarization and the pattern of ventricular repolarization would have appeared normal; that is, the QRS complex and the T wave of the premature beat would have looked like the other QRS and T waves. They would simply have occurred earlier than expected and would not be preceded by a P wave. Sometimes, premature contractions are initiated by ectopic pacemakers in the atria. In such a case, the QRS complex and T wave would be expected to have a normal size and shape, because normal ventricular pathways would be involved in ventricular depolarization and repolarization.

Figure 19–10 shows additional examples of cardiac electrical dysfunction. The ECG in Figure 19–10*A* was recorded from a resting dog. The R waves are evenly

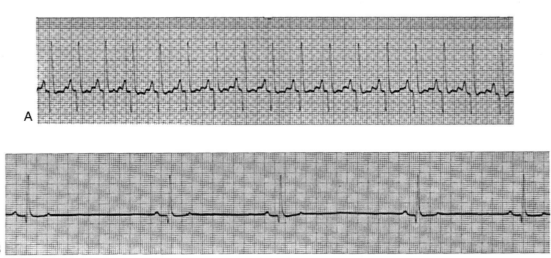

FIGURE 19–10. Sinus tachycardia *(A)* and sinus bradycardia *(B)* are evident in these otherwise normal ECGs from two resting dogs. (From Ettinger SJ: Textbook of Veterinary Internal Medicine, 3rd ed. Philadelphia, WB Saunders, 1989.)

spaced and indicate a ventricular rate of 235 beats per minute. This is fast for a resting dog. However, the pattern of ECG waves appears to be normal; each QRS complex is preceded by a clear, positive P wave and is followed by a positive T wave (which overlaps the next P wave). The most likely diagnosis is *sinus tachycardia* (rapid heart rate initiated by SA node pacemakers). Figure 19–10B shows the opposite extreme. The pattern of ECG waves is normal, but the heart rate is only 55 beats per minute. The diagnosis is *sinus bradycardia* (the SA node is the pacemaker, but its rate is abnormally slow).

The ECG provides an easy way to diagnose AV node block. The ECG in Figure 19–11A looks normal, except that there is an abnormally long PR interval, which is suggestive of abnormally slow conduction of the action potential through the AV node and AV bundle. This would be indicative of *first-degree AV block.* In Figure 19–11B, the P wave spacing indicates an atrial rate of 123 beats per minute. Four of the P waves are followed by faintly visible QRS complexes and large, negative T waves, but the other seven P waves are not followed by QRS complexes. Apparently some, but not all, atrial depolarizations are conducted through the AV node. Therefore, the condition is *second-degree AV block,* which is not life-threatening unless there are so many missed ventricular beats that cardiac output falls to dangerously low levels.

Figure 19–11C shows *third-degree (complete) AV node block* (and, incidentally, ST segment depression). Two large QRS complexes are faintly visible, followed by negative T waves. The RR interval is about 2.9 seconds, indicating that the ventricular rate is only 21 beats per minute. The QRS complexes are not preceded by P waves. Small, evenly spaced, positive P waves are present, indicating a constant atrial rate of 142 beats per minute, but there is no synchronization between the P waves and the QRS complexes. Atrial action potentials are apparently being blocked at the AV node. The ventricles are beating slowly in response to an auxiliary pacemaker in the AV node or in the bundle of His.

Figure 19–12A shows an ECG record of a dog that is drifting in and out of ventricular tachycardia. The first five waves are abnormally shaped ventricular complexes, indicative of an ectopic ventricular pacemaker located outside the normal ventricular conduction system. No P waves are observed. Then there are three normal-appearing P-QRS-T sequences, which suggests that a normal rhythm is being established. However, the ectopic ventricular pacemaker usurps control again, and ventricular tachycardia returns.

Ventricular tachycardia degenerates frequently into ventricular fibrillation. The ECG in Figure 19–12B indicates ventricular fibrillation. The record shows fairly large, irregular voltage fluctuations with no discernible pattern. The atria may or may not be fibrillating; it is possible that regularly occurring P waves

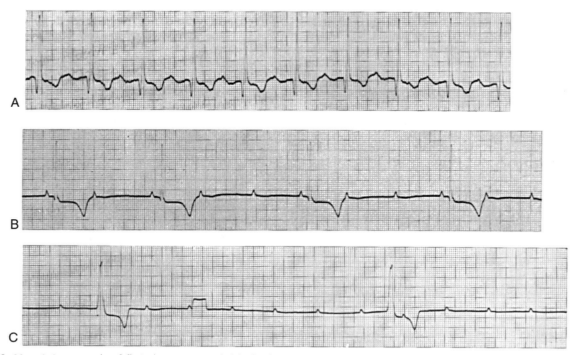

FIGURE 19–11. *A,* An example of first-degree AV node block. The PR interval is 0.2 second (normal for a dog is less than 0.14 second). The heart rate is 120 beats per minute. Each QRS complex is preceded by a positive P wave and followed by a negative T wave. *B,* An example of second-degree AV node block. The small, positive deflections are P waves. The broad, negative deflections are T waves, which follow the faintly visible QRS complexes. Where P waves are followed by QRS complexes, the PR interval is normal. However, only every second or third P wave is followed by a QRS complex; that is, there are two or three atrial beats for every ventricular beat. *C,* An example of third-degree (complete) AV node block. The positive P waves are regularly spaced (two of them are obscured by the two large QRS-T complexes). The QRS-T complexes are not immediately preceded by P waves. ST segment depression is also evident, but this is irrelevant to the diagnosis of AV block. The rectangular deflection one third of the way through the record is a voltage calibration signal. (From Ettinger SJ: Textbook of Veterinary Internal Medicine, 3rd ed. Philadelphia: WB Saunders, 1989.)

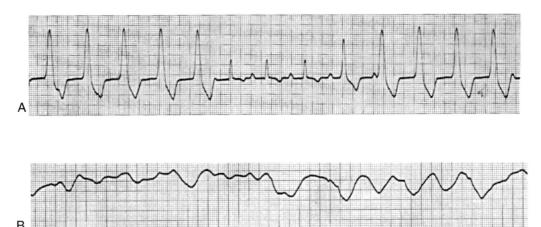

FIGURE 19–12. *A,* An example of ventricular tachycardia, which reverts briefly to a sinus rhythm. The ventricular rate is about 165 beats per minute. This pattern would be typical for a dog with an ectopic ventricular pacemaker functioning at almost the same rate as the SA node pacemaker; some ventricular beats would be initiated by the ectopic pacemaker, and others would be initiated in the normal way through the AV node. *B,* An example of ventricular fibrillation. The random voltage fluctuations generated by the fibrillating ventricles would obscure any P waves that might be present, so it is not possible to determine whether the atria are also fibrillating. (From Ettinger SJ: Textbook of Veterinary Internal Medicine, 3rd ed. Philadelphia: WB Saunders, 1989.)

are present but are obscured by the random electrical activity in the ventricles. However, ventricular fibrillation stops the heart from pumping blood, regardless of whether the atria continue to contract in a synchronized manner.

Atrial fibrillation, like ventricular fibrillation, typically produces random voltage dipoles. However, because the atrial muscle mass is relatively small, the ECG voltages generated by atrial fibrillation are always much smaller than those seen in Figure 19–12*B*. An ECG from an animal with atrial fibrillation would typically show normally shaped QRS and T waves against a background of low-amplitude voltage fluctuations created by the fibrillating atria. In such a case, the AV node is bombarded with very frequent action potentials from the fibrillating atria. Some of these action potentials are conducted to the ventricles, and others are blocked (the long refractory period of the AV node allows it to protect the ventricles from beating too rapidly). Thus, in the case of atrial fibrillation, the QRS-T complexes would typically have normal shape but irregular spacing.

Very sophisticated techniques are widely used in the analysis of ECGs both in human medicine and in many veterinary clinics. The purpose in this chapter is to introduce only enough complexity to illustrate the usefulness of the ECG in the diagnosis of cardiac abnormalities. In addition, this discussion of the ECG is intended to reinforce the student's understanding of electrical dysfunction of the heart, as presented in Chapter 18.

CLINICAL CORRELATIONS

Dilative cardiomyopathy with paroxysmal atrial tachycardia

History   The owner of a 5-year-old male Saint Bernard brings the dog to you because of a distended abdomen, weakness, coughing, and difficulty breathing. The owner believes these signs developed gradually over a period of several weeks; however, there were occasional episodes when the dog suddenly seemed weak and listless.

Clinical examination   Palpation reveals that the dog has muscle wasting and a fluid-filled abdomen *(ascites).* The jugular veins are distended. The arterial pulse is rapid and irregular. There are frequent pulse deficits (missing beats). Thoracic radiography reveals an enlarged heart and an accumulation of fluid near the lung hilus.

You record the dog's ECG for several minutes. The ECG shows that P waves usually occur at a rate of 160 to 170 per minute and that each P wave is followed by a QRS-T complex. However, the ECG also shows frequent episodes when there are 210 to 230 P waves per minute. During these episodes, most P waves are followed by QRS-T complexes, but others are not. As a result, the QRS-T complexes occur irregularly, and there are only about 180 of them per minute.

Echocardiography reveals severe dilation of all four cardiac chambers, particularly the atria. The ventricular contractions are weak.

Comment   The ECG indicates that this dog has atrial tachycardia. The information presented does not establish whether the atrial pacemaker is located in the SA node or somewhere else in the atria. It is likely that one atrial pacemaker area is initiating depolarizations at a rate of 160 to 170 per minute and that another atrial area intermittently preempts the first pacemaker by initiating depolarizations at the more rapid rate of 210 to 230 per minute. When the atrial rate is 160 to 170 per minute, the AV node conducts every atrial action potential to the ventricles, so that the ventricles also contract 160 to 170 times per minute. However, when the atrial rate is 210 to 230 per minute, some of the atrial action potentials arrive at the AV node when the nodal cells are still refractory from the preceding action potential. These atrial action potentials are not conducted into the ventricles. As a result, there are only about 180 ventricular contractions per minute. This is a case in which a second-degree AV-node block, created by the relatively long refractory period of AV-node cells, is beneficial, because it prevents the ventricles from beating too rapidly. The problem with very frequent ventricular contractions is that the time available between contractions becomes too short for adequate ventricular refilling. As ventricular rate increases, the volume of blood pumped with each beat (stroke volume) decreases, and so does cardiac output. At ventricular rates above 180 per minute, cardiac output could fall to such a low level that the dog would collapse.

This dog's primary problem is probably a chronic, progressive weakening of his heart muscle *(cardiomyopathy)*. All the clinical signs, including atrial tachycardia, can be attributed to a primary cardiomyopathy. Dilative cardiomyopathy is common in giant-breed dogs, especially males, and often (as in this case) there is no discernible cause. Even though the cause of the cardiomyopathy could not be determined from the evidence available in this case, the sequence of dysfunctions that resulted from the cardiomyopathy can be inferred with near certainty.

Ventricular weakness (heart failure) caused the cardiac output to fall below normal, especially during exercise. The dog's body attempted to compensate for the heart failure by increasing blood volume, which increased both venous and atrial pressures far above normal. The elevated atrial pressure had the beneficial effect of "supercharging" the ventricles with an extra volume of blood before each contraction, which partially returned the stroke volume toward normal. However, the excessive volume and pressure of blood in the veins caused pulmonary edema (which led to coughing and difficulty breathing) and systemic edema (which led to fluid in the abdomen). Also, distention of the atria made the atrial cells more excitable electrically, which resulted in the formation of ectopic pacemakers and the onset of atrial tachycardia. The tachycardia limited the ventricular refilling time, which brought about a further compromise in cardiac output. A vicious cycle began in which decreased cardiac output caused further venous congestion and atrial distention, which aggravated the arrhythmia, and so forth. The atrial tachycardia is very likely to progress into atrial fibrillation. The prognosis is poor without treatment.

This case of heart failure provides a good preview for the next several chapters, which deal in detail with the physiologic mechanisms of cardiac and vascular control in both normal and heart failure states.

Treatment   A diuretic drug (e.g., furosemide) is administered to promote an increase in urine formation. The goal is to reduce the blood volume and venous and atrial pressures, thereby reducing the signs resulting from congestion and edema. Sometimes the paroxysmal atrial tachycardia resolves after diuretic-induced reductions in atrial size. If it does not, antiarrhythmic drugs (e.g., quinidine or lidocaine, and/or a cardiac glycoside such as digitalis) can be used to try to reduce the electrical excitability of atrial tissue.

Bibliography

Berne RM, Levy MN: Cardiovascular Physiology, 7th ed. St. Louis: CV Mosby, 1997.

Bonagura JD: Diagnosis of Cardiac Arrhythmias. In Ettinger SJ, Feldman EC (eds): Textbook of Veterinary Internal Medicine: Diseases of the Dog and Cat, 5th ed. Philadelphia: WB Saunders, 2000, p 240.

Dukes HH, Swenson MJ, Reece WO: Dukes' Physiology of Domestic Animals. Ithaca, N.Y.: Comstock, 1993, pp 118–144.

Ettinger SJ, Le Bobinnec G, Cote E: Electrocardiography. In Ettinger SJ, Feldman EC (eds): Textbook of Veterinary Internal Medicine: Diseases of the Dog and Cat, 5th ed. Philadelphia: WB Saunders, 2000, p 800.

Katz AM: Physiology of the Heart, 3rd ed. Baltimore: Lippincott Williams & Wilkins, 2000.

Marr C (ed): Cardiology of the Horse. London: WB Saunders, 1999.

Patteson MW: Equine Cardiology (Library of Veterinary Practice). Oxford, United Kingdom: Blackwell Scientific, 1996.

Scher AM: The electrocardiogram. In Patton HD, Fuchs AF, Hille B, et al (eds): Textbook of Physiology—Circulation, Respiration, Body Fluids, Metabolism, and Endocrinology, 21st ed. Philadelphia: WB Saunders, 1989, p 796.

Tilley LP, Burtnick NL: ECG for the Small Animal Practitioner. Teton NewMedia, 1999.

Tilley LP, Goodwin JK (eds): Manual of Canine and Feline Cardiology, 3rd ed. Philadelphia: WB Saunders, 2001.

PRACTICE QUESTIONS

1. In which of the following arrhythmias will the ECG characteristically show the *same number* of P waves and QRS complexes?
   a. Complete (third-degree) AV block.

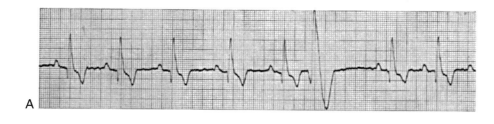

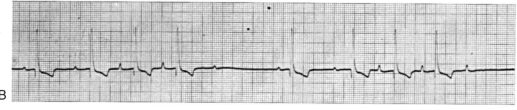

FIGURE 19–13.   Lead I ECG records from two dogs. *A* is the basis for Practice Question 4. *B* is the basis for Practice Question 5. (From Ettinger SJ: Textbook of Veterinary Internal Medicine, 3rd ed. Philadelphia: WB Saunders, 1989.)

b. First-degree AV block.
c. Ventricular tachycardia.
d. Atrial flutter.
e. All of the above.

2. The time required for the conduction of the cardiac action potential through the AV node would be approximately equal to the
   a. RR interval.
   b. PR interval.
   c. ST interval.
   d. PP interval.
   e. QT interval.

3. The T wave in a normal ECG is
   a. always negative.
   b. always positive if the R wave is positive.
   c. also known as the "pacemaker potential."
   d. caused by the delay between atrial and ventricular depolarization.
   e. caused by ventricular repolarization.

4. The ECG in Figure 19–13A indicates
   a. sinus arrhythmia.
   b. right ventricular hypertrophy.
   c. ST segment elevation.
   d. premature ventricular contraction.
   e. atrial fibrillation.

5. The ECG in Figure 19–13B indicates
   a. second-degree AV block.
   b. third-degree AV block.
   c. sinus bradycardia.
   d. ventricular tachycardia.
   e. ST segment elevation.

PRACTICE ANSWERS

1. b   2. b   3. e   4. d   5. a

20

The heart as a pump

1 Each heartbeat is made up of ventricular systole and ventricular diastole

2 Cardiac output equals heart rate multiplied by stroke volume

3 Up to a point, increases in end-diastolic ventricular volume cause increases in stroke volume

4 End-diastolic ventricular volume is determined by ventricular preload, ventricular compliance, and diastolic filling time

5 Increases in ventricular contractility cause decreases in ventricular end-systolic volume

6 Increasing the heart rate does not increase cardiac output substantially unless stroke volume is maintained

7 Murmurs are abnormal heart sounds caused by turbulent flow through cardiac defects

8 Cardiac defects increase the heart's workload because they require one or both ventricles to pump extra blood at an elevated pressure

9 The pathologic consequences of cardiac defects are direct results of the abnormal pressures, volumes, and workloads created in the cardiac chambers

Each heartbeat is made up of ventricular systole and ventricular diastole

The heart is actually two pumps (two ventricles) that work together, side by side. Each ventricular pump works in a cycle, first filling with blood and then emptying. In each *cardiac cycle* (heartbeat), the left ventricle takes in a volume of blood from the pulmonary veins and left atrium and then ejects it into the aorta. The right ventricle takes in a similar volume of blood from the systemic veins and right atrium and ejects it into the pulmonary artery.

The events of a single cardiac cycle are shown in Figure 20–1. A normal electrocardiogram tracing is presented at the top of the figure. Atrial contraction is initiated by atrial depolarization, which is indicated by the P wave. Ventricular contraction is initiated by ventricular depolarization, which is indicated by the QRS complex. The period of ventricular contraction is called *ventricular systole*. Blood is ejected from the ventricles during ventricular systole. Each systole is followed by *ventricular diastole*, during which the ventricles relax and refill with blood before the next ventricular systole.

The ventricles do not empty completely during systole. As shown in the graph of ventricular volume (see Fig. 20–1, *top*), each ventricle of a large dog contains about 60 mL of blood at the end of diastole. This is called *end-diastolic volume*. During systole, about 30 mL of this blood is ejected from each ventricle, but 30 mL remains. This is called *end-systolic*

volume. The volume of blood ejected from one ventricle in one beat is called *stroke volume*, expressed as

$$\text{stroke volume} = \text{end-diastolic volume} - \text{end-systolic volume.}$$

The fraction of end-diastolic volume that is ejected during ventricular systole is called the *ejection fraction*. Thus,

$$\text{ejection fraction} = \frac{\text{stroke volume}}{\text{end-diastolic volume}}.$$

In the example depicted in Figure 20–1, ejection fraction is 50%. Values between 50% and 65% are typical for resting dogs.

As shown in Figure 20–1, left ventricular pressure is low at the beginning of ventricular systole, but the powerful contraction of the ventricular muscle causes the ventricular pressure to increase rapidly. The increase in left ventricular pressure causes a momentary backflow of blood from the left ventricle to the left atrium, which closes the left atrioventricular (AV) valve (the *mitral valve).* Blood is not immediately ejected from the left ventricle into the aorta at the beginning of systole, because the *aortic valve* remains closed until the left ventricular pressure exceeds the aortic pressure. Therefore, ventricular volume remains unchanged during this first phase of systole, which is aptly named *isovolumetric contraction.*

When left ventricular pressure does rise above aortic pressure, the aortic valve is pushed open, and there is a *rapid ejection* of blood into the aorta. Rapid ejection is followed by a phase of *reduced ejection* of blood, as both ventricular pressure and aortic pres-

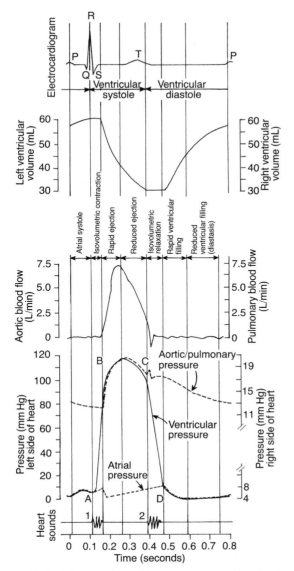

FIGURE 20–1. The events and terminology associated with one cardiac cycle (heartbeat) in a normal dog. The vertical scales on the left side of the graphs are for the left side of the heart. The vertical scales on the right side of the graphs are for the right side of the heart. In the bottom graph, point A is closure of the mitral valve; point B, opening of the aortic valve; point C, closure of the aortic valve; and point D, opening of the mitral valve. See text for details.

sure pass their peak *(systolic)* values and begin to decrease. (During the period of reduced ejection, the ventricular pressure actually falls below the aortic pressure, but ejection continues for a few moments, because the blood flowing out of the ventricle is carried along by the momentum imparted to it during rapid ejection.) As the ventricular pressure continues to decrease, ejection comes to an end. A momentary backflow of blood from the aorta into the left ventricle closes the aortic valve. The closure of the aortic valve demarcates the end of ventricular systole and the beginning of ventricular diastole.

During the first phase of ventricular diastole, the

ventricular muscle relaxes, and left ventricular pressure declines from a value near aortic pressure to a value near left atrial pressure. However, no filling of the ventricle can occur, because the mitral valve remains closed until left ventricular pressure drops below left atrial pressure. This first phase of ventricular diastole is called *isovolumetric relaxation,* because there is neither filling nor emptying of the ventricle.

When left ventricular pressure does fall below left atrial pressure, the mitral valve is pushed open, and ventricular filling commences. First, there is a period of *rapid ventricular filling,* which is followed by a phase of *reduced ventricular filling (diastasis).* Diastasis persists until the sinoatrial node cells initiate an atrial action potential and atrial contraction *(atrial systole).* In a resting dog, as depicted in Figure 20–1, ventricular volume is nearly at its end-diastolic level even before atrial systole. Typically, 80% to 90% of ventricular filling occurs before atrial systole. Atrial systole simply "tops up" the almost-full ventricles. An important clinical consequence of this fact is that dogs can function well at rest even if their atria are in fibrillation and not contracting. During exercise, however, atrial contractions make a relatively greater contribution to ventricular filling, because the rapid heart rate in exercise leaves a shorter time for diastolic filling. Therefore, animals with atrial fibrillation typically exhibit exercise intolerance. Ventricular filling also becomes more dependent on atrial systole in patients with certain valve defects, such as narrowing of the mitral valve *(mitral stenosis).*

At the end of atrial systole, the atria begin to relax. The left atrial pressure drops slightly. Then the ventricles begin to contract, and there is a momentary backflow of blood from the left ventricle to the left atrium. The mitral valve closes, which marks the end of ventricular diastole and the beginning of another left ventricular systole.

By definition, the cardiac cycle is divided into ventricular systole and ventricular diastole. Closure of the mitral valve marks the beginning of ventricular systole. Closure of the aortic valve marks the beginning of ventricular diastole. Atrial systole takes place during ventricular diastole.

The preceding paragraphs discussed pressure changes in the left atrium, left ventricle, and aorta. However, all the events of the cardiac cycle also take place on the right side of the heart. Therefore, all the statements made about the left side of the heart also hold true for the right side of the heart; the right-sided structures corresponding to the aorta, aortic valve, and mitral valve are, respectively, the pulmonary artery, pulmonic valve, and tricuspid valve. The only important difference between the left and right sides of the heart is that the systolic (peak) pressure in the right ventricle and pulmonary artery is only about 20 mm Hg, whereas the systolic pressure on the left side of the heart reaches 120 mm Hg. For this reason, there are different scales on the pressure axes in Figure 20–1 for the left and right sides of the heart.

The timing of the two major heart sounds is also shown in Figure 20–1 *(bottom).* The first heart sound is associated with the closure of the AV valves (the mitral valve on the left side of the heart and the tricuspid valve on the right side of the heart). What makes this sound is not the actual closure of the valves but rather the vibration created in the blood and in the cardiac walls when the valves close. The valve leaflets are very light and could not create much sound by themselves. However, the momentary backflow of blood from the ventricles to the atria at the beginning of ventricular systole causes the AV valves to close quickly. This backflow of blood is brought to a sudden stop against the closing valves, which creates the momentary vibration that is heard as a heart sound.

The second heart sound is associated with closure of the aortic valve on the left side of the heart and the pulmonic valve on the right side of the heart. It is usually briefer, sharper, and higher pitched than the first heart sound. Again, what makes the sound is not the valve leaflets closing but rather the reverberation produced when the momentary backflow of blood into the ventricles is brought to a sudden stop by closure of the valves. The closures of the aortic and pulmonic valves are normally simultaneous. However, under certain circumstances, the two valves close at slightly different times, and the second heart sound is heard as two distinct sounds; this condition is called a *split second heart sound*.

The AV valves close at the beginning of ventricular systole, and the aortic and pulmonic valves close at the end of ventricular systole. Therefore, ventricular systole is sometimes defined as the part of the cardiac cycle between the first heart sound and the second heart sound.

Cardiac output equals heart rate multiplied by stroke volume

All the events diagrammed in Figure 20–1 occur during each heartbeat, and each heartbeat results in the ejection of one stroke volume of blood into the pulmonary artery and aorta. The number of heartbeats per minute is called the *heart rate*. Therefore, the total volume of blood pumped by each ventricle in 1 min-

ute equals stroke volume multiplied by heart rate. Cardiac output can be increased only if heart rate increases, stroke volume increases, or both increase. Therefore, to understand how the body controls cardiac output, one must understand how the body controls heart rate and stroke volume. Figure 20–2 summarizes the factors that affect heart rate and stroke volume. These factors are described in detail in the following three sections.

Up to a point, increases in end-diastolic ventricular volume cause increases in stroke volume

Stroke volume equals end-diastolic volume minus end-systolic volume. Therefore, stroke volume can be increased only by increasing end-diastolic volume (i.e., filling the ventricles more during diastole) or by decreasing end-systolic volume (i.e., emptying the ventricles more completely during systole), or both.

The effect of increasing end-diastolic ventricular volume on stroke volume is plotted in Figure 20–3A. The detailed physiologic mechanisms underlying this relationship are complex. Basically, however, greater ventricular filling during diastole places the ventricular muscle fibers in a more favorable geometry for the ejection of blood during the next systole. Also, stretching the ventricular muscle fibers during diastole causes a greater amount of Ca^{2+} to be released from the sarcoplasmic reticulum during the subsequent systolic contraction, and this enhances the force of contraction. Resting conditions in a normal animal are somewhere around the middle of this *ventricular function curve*. Therefore, increases or decreases from normal ventricular end-diastolic volume result in approximately proportional increases or decreases in stroke volume.

End-diastolic ventricular volume is determined by ventricular preload, ventricular compliance, and diastolic filling time

Ventricular preload is the pressure within a ventricle during diastolic filling. Because ventricular pressure

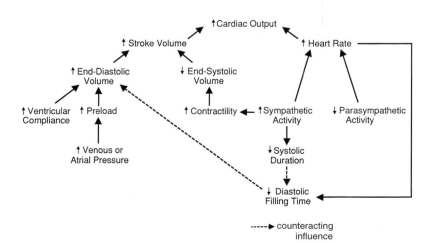

FIGURE 20–2. A summary of the control of cardiac output. The relationships shown here are described in detail in the text.

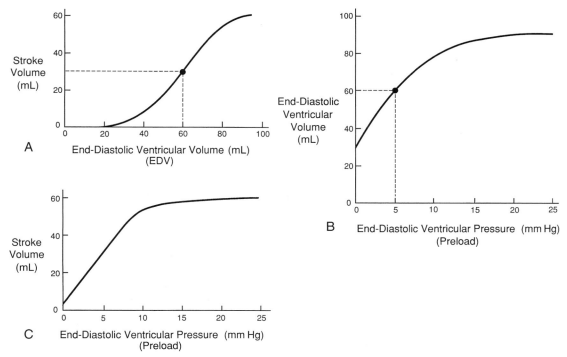

FIGURE 20-3.   *A,* Up to a point, increases in end-diastolic ventricular volume cause increases in stroke volume. The dashed lines indicate the normal values. *B,* Up to a point, increases in end-diastolic ventricular pressure (preload) cause increases in end-diastolic ventricular volume. *C,* The combined relationships of *A* and *B* show that, up to a point, increases in ventricular preload cause increases in stroke volume. In *A* to *C* the numerical data are for the left ventricle of a large dog.

changes throughout filling (see Fig. 20–1), the value of ventricular pressure at the end of diastole is usually accepted as a singular measure of preload. Normal values of preload (ventricular end-diastolic pressure) are about 3 mm Hg for the right ventricle and 5 mm Hg for the left ventricle. In a normal heart, ventricular pressure at the end of diastole is essentially equal to atrial pressure, because the AV valves are open widely up until the end of diastole. Also, because there are no valves between the veins and the atria, the atrial pressure is almost identical to the pressure within the nearby veins. Thus, pulmonary venous pressure, left atrial pressure, and left ventricular end-diastolic pressure are all essentially equivalent measures of left ventricular preload. Similarly, right ventricular end-diastolic pressure, right atrial pressure, and vena caval pressure are all essentially equivalent measures of right ventricular preload. In the clinic, right ventricular preload is measured by introducing a catheter into a peripheral vein (e.g., the jugular vein) and advancing it into the cranial vena cava (precava) or right atrium. Such a catheter is called a *central venous catheter,* and the pressure measured at its tip is called *central venous pressure.* Left ventricular preload is more difficult to measure clinically because there is no easy way to place a catheter tip into the left atrium or pulmonary veins.

Figure 20–3*B* shows that up to a point, increases in preload are associated with increases in end-diastolic ventricular volume. The graph depicts a left ventricle that has a natural volume of 30 mL in a relaxed, nonpressurized state (i.e., when the preload equals 0 mm Hg). Increases in preload distend and fill the

ventricle. A preload of 5 mm Hg brings about the normal left ventricular end-diastolic volume of 60 mL. However, an elastic limit is reached when the ventricular volume approaches 90 mL. Further increases in the preload do not cause much additional ventricular filling.

Increases in ventricular preload cause increases in end-diastolic volume (see Fig. 20–3*B),* and increases in end-diastolic volume cause increases in stroke volume (see Fig. 20–3*A*). Therefore, it follows that increases in preload cause increases in stroke volume. This relationship is shown in Figure 20–3*C*. It is also true that decreases in preload cause decreases in stroke volume. This happens, for example, in response to hemorrhage (detailed in Chapter 25).

The relationships among ventricular preload, end-diastolic volume, and stroke volume were first studied in detail by Ernest Henry Starling. The observation that an increase in preload (or end-diastolic volume) causes stroke volume to increase is called *Starling's law of the heart.* The Starling mechanism plays a critical role in moment-to-moment adjustments of the cardiac stroke volume. For example, if the right ventricle begins to pump an increased stroke volume, the resulting additional pulmonary blood flow causes an increase in the pulmonary venous pressure, which increases left atrial pressure, which in turn increases left ventricular preload, which, furthermore, increases the filling of the left ventricle during diastole. The resulting increase in left ventricular end-diastolic volume leads to a greater stroke volume from the left ventricle. Thus, an increase in right ventricular stroke volume quickly results in a corresponding increase in left ventricular stroke volume. The reverse is also true.

This sequence has a potential for developing into a vicious circle, with runaway increases in stroke volume. Other control mechanisms prevent this from happening, and these are discussed in Chapter 24. The point here is that the Starling mechanism keeps the stroke volumes of the left and right ventricles balanced. If this equality were not maintained (and one ventricle pumped more blood than the other for several minutes), a large part of the body's blood volume would accumulate either in the lungs or in the systemic circulation.

Because of the Starling mechanism's role in controlling the stroke volume, Starling's law of the heart is also referred to as *heterometric autoregulation.* This name implies self-control *(autoregulation)* of cardiac output as a result of different *(hetero)* initial volumes *(metric);* that is, *heterometric* refers to different end-diastolic volumes.

End-diastolic ventricular volume is determined not only by preload but also by *ventricular compliance.* Compliance is a measure of the ease with which the ventricular walls stretch to accommodate incoming blood during diastole. A compliant ventricle is one that yields easily to preload pressure and readily fills with blood during diastole. Compliance is more rigorously defined as the change in volume divided by the change in pressure. Ventricular compliance therefore corresponds to the slope of a ventricular volume-pressure curve like the one shown in Figure 20–3B. This figure shows that a normal ventricle is quite compliant over the range of volumes near the normal end-diastolic ventricular volume. Within this range, small changes in preload result in substantial changes in end-diastolic ventricular volume. However, at preloads higher than about 10 mm Hg, the ventricle becomes less compliant (stiffer). Inelastic connective tissue in the ventricular walls limits further increases in ventricular volume.

Myocardial ischemia, certain cardiac diseases, or mere advancing age can cause the ventricular walls to become stiff and noncompliant even at normal preloads. Figure 20–4 shows a comparison of volume-pressure curves for a normal ventricle and for a noncompliant ventricle. When ventricular compliance decreases, there is a smaller increase in ventricular volume for any given increase in ventricular preload. Another consequence is that larger-than-normal preloads are needed to obtain normal end-diastolic ventricular volumes in a ventricle with decreased compliance. Elevated preloads can lead to edema (detailed in Chapters 22 and 25).

In addition to compliance and preload, the third factor that affects ventricular end-diastolic volume is *diastolic filling time.* Heart rate is the main determinant of diastolic filling time. At normal resting heart rates, there is ample time for ventricular filling during diastole. As mentioned earlier, ventricular filling is nearly complete in a resting dog even before atrial systole occurs. However, as heart rate increases from resting levels, the period available for diastolic filling is reduced more and more. Typically, at heart rates above 150 to 180 beats per minute, insufficient time is available for normal diastolic filling, even though atrial pressure, atrial systolic contraction, and ventricular compliance are normal. This limitation on ventricular filling would dramatically reduce stroke volume when heart rate is high if not for an additional, compensating influence brought about by the sympathetic nervous system, which is discussed later in the chapter.

Increases in ventricular contractility cause decreases in ventricular end-systolic volume

An increase in *ventricular contractility* results in a more complete emptying of the ventricle during systole

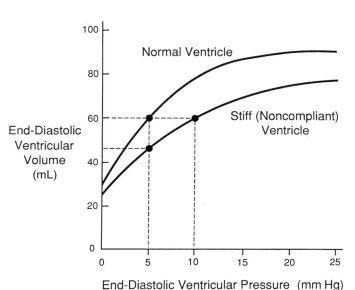

FIGURE 20–4. A stiff, noncompliant ventricle requires a higher filling pressure (preload) in order to reach a normal degree of filling (end-diastolic ventricular volume).

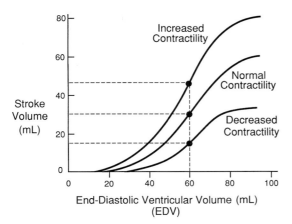

FIGURE 20–5. An increase in cardiac contractility is identifiable graphically as a leftward and upward shift of the ventricular function curve. An increase in contractility means that there will be a larger stroke volume for any given end-diastolic volume. Conversely, a decrease in contractility (rightward and downward shift) means that there will be a smaller stroke volume for any given end-diastolic volume.

and, therefore, a decreased end-systolic volume. Contractility can be defined as the pumping ability of a ventricle. An increase in contractility can bring about an increase in stroke volume without requiring a change in end-diastolic volume. As shown in Figure 20–5, increased contractility results in an increased stroke volume for any given end-diastolic volume. For example, at a normal end-diastolic volume of 60 mL, the end-systolic volume is 30 mL, and so the stroke volume is 30 mL. An increased contractility with no change in end-diastolic volume results in more systolic emptying; if the end-systolic volume is reduced to 15 mL, the stroke volume increases to 45 mL.

Sympathetic nerve activity increases ventricular contractility through the action of the neurotransmitter norepinephrine. Norepinephrine activates β-adrenergic receptors on ventricular muscle cells. As discussed in Chapter 18, activation of β-adrenergic receptors leads to an increased influx of extracellular Ca^{2+} into cardiac cells during an action potential (and to several other effects); the overall result is that cardiac contractions are stronger and quicker. Other β-adrenergic agonist drugs (e.g., epinephrine and isoproterenol) mimic this action of norepinephrine on the heart and likewise increase cardiac contractility. The cardiac glycosides (e.g., digitalis) are another class of drugs that increases cardiac contractility, again by increasing the cytosolic Ca^{2+} concentration during an action potential.

If cardiac contractility becomes depressed, there is less-than-normal ventricular emptying during systole. End-systolic volume increases, and stroke volume decreases. This is shown in Figure 20–5. A decrease in sympathetic activity causes a decrease in cardiac contractility, as do β-adrenergic antagonist drugs, which block the β-adrenergic receptors on cardiac muscle cells. Propranolol and atenolol are the β-adrenergic antagonists used most commonly to decrease

cardiac contractility. These antagonists block the effects of sympathetic nerves on the heart and thereby decrease the concentration of cytosolic Ca^{2+} during a cardiac action potential. Like β-adrenergic antagonists, calcium channel–blocking drugs also decrease cardiac contractility by making less Ca^{2+} available for the activation of the contractile proteins. Barbiturates depress cardiac contractility too, and this must be kept in mind when barbiturates are administered to produce anesthesia or analgesia. A decrease in cardiac contractility causes a decrease in the stroke volume and, therefore, the cardiac output. The blood pressure may fall to dangerously low levels.

A decrease in cardiac contractility is also the hallmark of the general clinical condition called *heart failure*. Although there are many kinds of heart failure, they share one characteristic: a decrease in pumping ability of the ventricle. Heart failure can result from coronary artery disease, cardiac hypoxia, myocarditis, diseases of the cardiac valves, toxins, or electrolyte imbalances.

Although ventricular contractility is usually the predominant factor affecting ventricular end-systolic volume, the effect of arterial blood pressure must also be considered. A substantial increase in arterial blood pressure impairs ventricular ejection, because the left ventricular pressure during systole must exceed aortic pressure before ejection of blood from the ventricle can occur. Arterial pressure is called the *cardiac afterload*. It is the pressure against which the ventricle must pump in order to eject blood. The higher the afterload, the more difficult it is for the ventricle to eject blood. If arterial pressure is excessively high, ventricular ejection is impaired, end-systolic volume increases, and stroke volume decreases. This effect is minor for a normal heart and within the normal range of arterial pressure. However, high afterload can significantly limit stroke volume for a heart that is in failure.

Increasing the heart rate does not increase cardiac output substantially unless stroke volume is maintained

Because cardiac output is equal to stroke volume multiplied by heart rate, cardiac output might be expected to be proportional to heart rate; that is, doubling the heart rate would be expected to double cardiac output (Fig. 20–6, *dashed line*). However, if the heart rate is experimentally increased above its normal level with an electrical pacemaker, cardiac output increases somewhat but not in proportion to the increase in heart rate. As mentioned earlier, when heart rate is increased, diastolic filling time is reduced. The resulting reduction in end-diastolic volume reduces stroke volume, and so cardiac output does not increase in proportion to heart rate (Fig. 20–6, *lower solid line*). In fact, at heart rates of more than 180 to 200 beats per minute, stroke volume falls so much that cardiac output actually decreases with further increases in heart rate. This problem was encountered

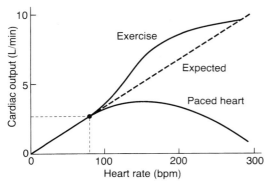

FIGURE 20–6. The *dashed line* shows the expected increase in cardiac output in proportion to increases in heart rate (if stroke volume does not change). However, if the heart is paced to higher and higher rates, the observed increase in cardiac output is less than expected, because stroke volume decreases *(lower solid line)*. In contrast, when a dog increases its own heart rate through sympathetic activation (e.g., during exercise), cardiac output increases even more than expected, because stroke volume increases *(upper solid line)*.

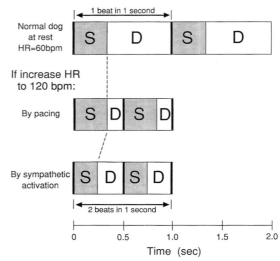

FIGURE 20–7. *Top,* At a heart rate (HR) of 60 beats per minute (bpm), systole takes about one-third second (leaving two thirds of each beat for diastole and filling). *Middle,* If HR is increased to 120 bpm by an artificial pacemaker, the duration of systole remains the same; diastolic duration (filling time) is greatly reduced. *Bottom,* If the same increase in heart rate is brought about by sympathetic activation, systole becomes shorter, which helps to preserve the diastolic filling time.

when early versions of artificial cardiac pacemakers malfunctioned in ways that caused high ventricular rates. Decreases in stroke volume at high heart rates are also encountered in certain cardiac arrhythmias. In *paroxysmal atrial tachycardia,* for example, a rapid heart rate is originated by an ectopic atrial pacemaker. The tachycardia occurs typically in bursts or paroxysms. The rapid heart rate limits diastolic filling so much that cardiac output falls below normal. This causes the blood pressure to fall so low that the patient becomes weak or faints.

Although cardiac pacing does not cause a large increase in cardiac output, increases in heart rate in the course of normal daily activities are accompanied by substantial increases in cardiac output. An example is the increase in cardiac output that normally accompanies exercise. As shown in Figure 20–6 *(upper solid line),* the actual increase in cardiac output during progressively more intense exercise is even greater than would be expected on the basis of the increase in heart rate. The reason that cardiac output increases so much during exercise is that stroke volume also increases. During exercise, increases in heart rate are brought about by increases in sympathetic activity. This sympathetic activation also increases cardiac contractility, so the ventricles empty more completely with each beat. In addition, sympathetic activation shortens the duration of systole, which helps to preserve diastolic filling time. In summary, under sympathetic action, the heart not only contracts more frequently (increased rate) and more forcefully (increased contractility) but also contracts and relaxes more quickly.

Figure 20–7 illustrates how the shortening of systole helps to preserve diastolic filling time. When heart rate is 60 beats per minute, each beat takes 1 second. This 1 second must be composed of one systole and one diastole. Typically, systole lasts about one third of the beat, or one third of a second. If heart rate is increased to 120 beats per minute, each beat lasts only

half a second. If systole remains at one third of a second, there is only one sixth of a second left for diastolic filling. However, if the increase in heart rate occurs because of an increase in sympathetic activity, systole becomes shorter, and this helps preserve the diastolic filling time. Although diastole is shorter under these conditions than at rest, it is longer than it would have been if systole were not shortened. Thus, sympathetic activation is said to help preserve the diastolic filling time. Overall, sympathetic activation (especially when coupled with a decrease in parasympathetic activity) can dramatically increase cardiac output (Table 20–1).

It is useful at this point to review the control of cardiac output, as summarized in Figure 20–2. Cardiac output is determined by stroke volume and heart rate. Stroke volume is determined by end-diastolic volume and end-systolic volume. End-diastolic volume depends on preload, ventricular compliance, and diastolic filling time. End-systolic volume depends on contractility and, to a lesser extent, on arterial pressure or afterload (not shown in the figure). Sympathetic activation increases contractility. Several com-

TABLE 20–1. Typical cardiac changes during vigorous exercise in a large dog

Measurement	Rest	Exercise
Ventricular end-diastolic volume (mL)	60	55
Ventricular end-systolic volume (mL)	30	15
Stroke volume (mL)	30	40
Ejection fraction (%)	50	73
Heart rate (beats/minute)	80	240
Cardiac output (L/min)	2.4	9.6

monly used drugs decrease contractility, and so do several common diseases. Heart rate affects diastolic filling time; the filling time is decreased when heart rate is high. Heart rate is increased by sympathetic activation and parasympathetic withdrawal. Sympathetic activation also shortens systolic duration, which helps to preserve diastolic filling time.

Murmurs are abnormal heart sounds caused by turbulent flow through cardiac defects

Cardiac murmurs are abnormal heart sounds, and they often indicate the presence of cardiac abnormalities. Murmurs can take the form of abnormalities in the first or second heart sound, or they can be additional, abnormal heart sounds. Figure 20–1 indicates that the first heart sound is associated with the closure of the AV valves at the beginning of ventricular systole. The second heart sound is associated with the closure of the aortic and pulmonic valves at the end of ventricular systole. On occasion, normal third and fourth heart sounds are faintly audible with the stethoscope. In comparison, clinically important murmurs are louder. Sometimes murmurs are even louder than the normal first and second heart sounds.

Murmurs are caused by turbulent flow through cardiac defects. The underlying physical principle is that *laminar* or *smooth flow* of blood through the heart or blood vessels is quiet, whereas *turbulent flow* is noisy. An analogy is that a river does not make any sound as it flows smoothly through a broad, relatively flat channel. If the same river enters a channel that is restricted or drops steeply, then a rapid or cataract forms. The flow becomes turbulent, and the turbulent flow makes noise. The same volume of river water passes through the flat area and down the rapids, but the flow is turbulent and noisy only in the area of the rapids. The flow of blood through the heart and blood vessels is normally smooth, and therefore quiet, during all parts of the cardiac cycle, except two. The first moment of turbulent flow occurs at the beginning of ventricular contraction, upon closure of the AV valves. The second moment of turbulent flow normally occurs at the end of ventricular systole, when the aortic and pulmonic valves close. The momentary turbulence and vibration associated with valve closure create the first and second heart sounds.

Table 20–2 lists cardiac valve defects that cause additional instances of turbulent flow and, therefore, murmurs. The table also indicates the timing of the murmurs in relation to the cardiac cycle. *Systolic murmurs* occur during ventricular systole; *diastolic murmurs* occur during ventricular diastole. *Continuous murmurs* occur during both systole and diastole. The timing of each murmur is easy to remember if two basic principles are kept in mind: murmurs are caused by turbulent blood flow, and blood flows in response to pressure differences. In other words, turbulent (noisy) flow through a cardiac defect occurs

TABLE 20–2. Cardiac valve defects and the murmurs they cause

Site of defect	Nature of defect	
	INCOMPETENCE OR INSUFFICIENCY (ALLOWS REGURGITATION)	STENOSIS (NARROW VALVE OPENING, CREATES RESTRICTION)
Atrioventricular valves	Systolic murmur	Diastolic murmur
Aortic or pulmonic valves	Diastolic murmur	Systolic murmur

only if there is a substantial pressure difference from one side of the defect to the other.

Figure 20–8 indicates how these principles can be used to account for systolic murmurs. The numbers in the figure indicate the maximal pressures that normally exist in each cardiac chamber during ventricular systole. Note, for example, that the pressure in the left ventricle is normally much higher than the pressure in the left atrium during ventricular systole. The mitral valve is normally closed during ventricular systole, and so no blood flows backward from the ventricle to the left atrium. However, if the mitral valve fails to close completely during ventricular systole, the large pressure difference between the left ventricle and the left atrium causes a rapid, backward flow of blood through the partially closed valve. This

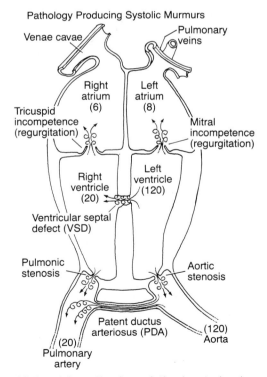

FIGURE 20–8. Schematic view of the heart showing cardiac defects that cause systolic murmurs. The numbers in parentheses indicate normal maximal pressures in millimeters of mercury (mm Hg) during ventricular systole. The *swirled arrows* indicate the sites of turbulent (noisy) flow.

turbulent backflow creates a murmur that is heard during systole. A mitral valve that fails to close completely is said to be *insufficient* or *incompetent.* The backflow across the valve is called *regurgitation.* Mitral regurgitation is present in about 8% of dogs over 5 years of age.

A *ventricular septal defect* (VSD) (hole or cleft in the interventric ular septum) causes a systolic murmur. Blood flows through a VSD from the left ventricle to the right ventricle during ventricular systole, because systolic pressure is much higher in the left ventricle than in the right ventricle. Typically, the flow of blood through a VSD is turbulent, and a systolic murmur is created.

Systolic turbulence is also created if the aortic valve does not open widely enough. Blood ejected from the ventricle accelerates to a high velocity as it squeezes through the restricted aortic opening, and turbulence occurs. A valve that fails to open widely enough is called a *stenotic valve;* the defect of *aortic stenosis* produces a systolic murmur. Likewise, *pulmonic stenosis* causes a systolic murmur. Aortic and pulmonic stenosis are common congenital defects in dogs.

A *patent ductus arteriosus* (PDA) (a persistence after birth of the opening between the aorta and the pulmonary artery; see Chapter 50) produces a murmur during systole, because the pressure in the aorta is much higher than the pressure in the pulmonary artery. Blood flows from the aorta into the pulmonary artery, and turbulence occurs. However, the murmur of a PDA is not restricted to systole, because the aortic pressure remains higher than the pulmonary artery pressure throughout diastole. Therefore, the murmur of PDA is heard in both systole and diastole and is thus a *continuous murmur.* It is also called a *machinery murmur* because it characteristically sounds like the rumble of machinery. PDA is common in dogs, especially females. The murmur of a PDA is characteristically heard best at a specific point on the thorax. The site from which a murmur can be heard best is often indicative of the particular type of defect that causes the murmur.

On occasion, animals exhibit open pathways for blood flow between peripheral arteries and peripheral veins. These openings are called *arteriovenous fistulae.* Arteriovenous fistulae carry flow (and create turbulence) during both systole and diastole and, therefore, create continuous murmurs. The murmur of an arteriovenous fistula is most audible at the body surface close to the point of the fistula.

Figure 20–9 depicts the minimal pressures that normally exist in the various cardiac chambers during ventricular diastole. These pressures form the basis for understanding why certain cardiac defects commonly produce diastolic murmurs. For example, a normal mitral valve opens widely during ventricular diastole, which creates a low-resistance pathway for blood to flow from the left atrium into the left ventricle. However, if the mitral valve fails to open widely (*mitral stenosis),* ventricular filling must occur through a stenotic (restricted) mitral valve. This creates turbulent flow and a diastolic murmur. Mitral stenosis is a common murmur among humans who have developed calcification of the mitral valve as a result of rheumatic heart disease.

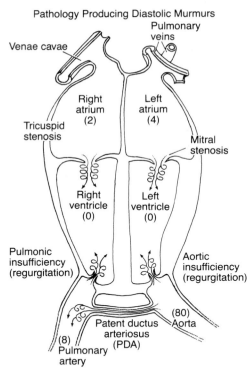

FIGURE 20–9. Cardiac defects that cause diastolic murmurs. The numbers in parentheses indicate normal minimal pressures in millimeters of mercury (mm Hg) during ventricular diastole. The *swirled arrows* indicate the sites of turbulent (noisy) flow.

During diastole, the normal aortic valve is shut tightly, and no blood flows backward from the aorta into the left ventricle. If the aortic valve does not close tightly, blood flows backward (regurgitates) from the aorta to the left ventricle during diastole. Therefore, *aortic regurgitation* produces a diastolic murmur. The defect is called *aortic incompetence* or *aortic insufficiency.* Aortic regurgitation is common in horses but not in dogs. Diastolic murmurs can also be produced by defects on the right side of the heart. Pulmonic regurgitation produces a diastolic murmur, but it is relatively rare. Tricuspid stenosis is uncommon, at least as a congenital defect. However, a heavy infestation of heartworms in the right side of the heart creates a stenosis at the tricuspid valve and a diastolic murmur.

Cardiac murmurs are not harmful in and of themselves. They are clinically important, however, because the defects that cause the murmurs also cause pathologic changes in the body. Cardiac defects typically lead to three different pathologic consequences: (1) abnormally high or low blood flow to one region of the body; (2) abnormally high or low blood pressure in a particular region of the body; and (3) *cardiac hypertrophy* (enlargement of cardiac muscle).

It is not difficult to understand why cardiac defects lead to abnormal blood flows or abnormal blood pressures. For example, in the presence of a ventricular septal defect, the right ventricle receives blood from both the right atrium and the left ventricle, which leads to an abnormally high blood flow through the pulmonary circulation. In the presence of mitral stenosis, blood dams up in the left atrium, which leads to an abnormally high left atrial pressure. It may be more difficult to see why cardiac defects lead to cardiac hypertrophy. The underlying principle is that cardiac defects lead to an increase in the workload of one or both ventricles, and an increase in the workload of cardiac muscle leads to hypertrophy. To develop this concept more fully requires an understanding of cardiac energetics, which is described as follows.

Cardiac defects increase the heart's workload because they require one or both ventricles to pump extra blood at an elevated pressure

Cardiac hypertrophy develops over a period of weeks in response to a persistent increase in the workload of cardiac muscle. Cardiac hypertrophy is analogous to the skeletal muscle hypertrophy that results from a sustained increase in skeletal muscle workload (physical conditioning). To develop this analogy more fully, recall that a skeletal muscle does work by exerting a force while shortening. The mechanical work done by a skeletal muscle is equal to the force developed by the contracting muscle, multiplied by the distance moved during one contraction, multiplied by the number of contractions. Therefore, the mechanical work done by a skeletal muscle can be increased by increasing the forcefulness of contraction, the distance moved, or the number of contractions. In weightlifting conditioning, the emphasis is on performing a few very forceful contractions of skeletal muscle. Weightlifting leads to an increase in the muscle workload and, therefore, muscle hypertrophy. In contrast, conditioning that involves repetitive, low-force contractions of skeletal muscle (such as running or swimming) emphasizes primarily the distance and duration components of skeletal muscle work. "Distance work" also leads to hypertrophy. However, a common observation in skeletal muscle conditioning is that weight work causes more hypertrophy than does distance work.

The function of the heart is to pump blood. The *mechanical (external) work* performed by any pump is equal to the pressure generated by the pump, multiplied by the volume of fluid that is pumped in one pump stroke, multiplied by the number of pump strokes. Therefore, the work done by the left ventricle in one cardiac cycle, called the *stroke work*, is equal to the pressure generated, multiplied by the stroke volume. The work done by the left ventricle in 1 minute is equal to the pressure generated, multiplied by the stroke volume, multiplied by the heart rate. The pressure generated by the left ventricle can normally be approximated by the average pressure in the aorta. Therefore,

the *minute work* done by the left ventricle = average aortic pressure × stroke volume × heart rate.

In accordance with the analogy to skeletal muscle, the average aortic pressure is analogous to the force developed by the contracting skeletal muscle, the stroke volume is analogous to the distance moved during one contraction, and the heart rate is analogous to the number of contractions. Obviously, the external work done by the left ventricle could be increased by increasing the pressure that the left ventricle generates, by increasing the stroke volume, or by increasing the heart rate. A 50% increase in ventricular work can result from a 50% increase in the left ventricular pressure, a 50% increase in the left ventricular stroke volume, or a 50% increase in the heart rate. Any of these changes results, over a period of weeks, in left ventricular hypertrophy. However, a common clinical observation is that an increase in the ventricular pressure causes a much more pronounced hypertrophy than does an increase in the stroke volume or heart rate. This observation is summarized in the clinical aphorism "Pressure work is harder for the heart (and causes more hypertrophy) than volume work." Note the analogy between this observation and the observation that weight work causes more skeletal muscle hypertrophy than does distance work. The basis for this difference is that weight work in skeletal muscle and pressure work in the heart involve the generation of a great deal of *internal, wasted work,* which appears as heat. This greatly increases the *total work* (external work plus internal work) being done by the skeletal or cardiac muscle.

Under normal conditions, about 85% of the metabolic energy consumed by the heart appears as heat, and only 15% appears as external work. A physicist would say that the heart has a thermodynamic efficiency of about 15%. However, the cardiac efficiency depends on the kind of work being done by the ventricles. The heart becomes less efficient when the external work is increased by increasing the pressure. Conversely, the heart becomes more efficient when the external work is increased by an increase in the volume of blood pumped. Thus, an increase in pressure and an increase in volume may cause the same increase in external work, but the increase in pressure causes a much greater increase in the heat produced by the heart than does the increase in volume. It is the total energy consumption of the heart, not just the external work, that is the primary stimulus for ventricular hypertrophy. Again, an increase in pressure work causes greater cardiac hypertrophy than does an increase in volume work.

The dominant role of pressure in determining total ventricular energy consumption is evident from a comparison of the work done by the left and right ventricles. The stroke volume and heart rate are equivalent for the left and right ventricles, but the left ventricle generates about five times more pressure during systole than does the right ventricle. Therefore, the external work done by the left ventricle is approximately five times greater than the external work done by the right ventricle. However, the total metabolic energy consumption of the left ventricle is much more than five times greater than the energy consumption of the right ventricle, because the extra external work performed by the left ventricle is in the form of greater pressure. As a result, almost all of the energy consumed by the heart is consumed by the left ventricle. Therefore, almost all of the coronary blood flow is delivered to the left ventricular muscle, and almost all of the oxygen consumed by the heart is consumed by the left ventricle. Because of the high amount of pressure work done by the left ventricle in comparison with the right ventricle, the left ventricle develops much heavier and thicker muscle walls than does the right ventricle.

A clinical observation from human medicine provides a further illustration of how an increase in the ventricular pressure work leads to ventricular hypertrophy. About 20% of adult humans have hypertension. In most of these patients, cardiac output is normal. Their arterial blood pressure is elevated because of an increased resistance to blood flow in the systemic arterioles. An elevated ventricular pressure is required to force the cardiac output through these constricted systemic arterioles. The increased pressure work done by the left ventricle in hypertensive patients results in a striking left ventricular hypertrophy.

Up to a point, ventricular hypertrophy is an appropriate and beneficial adaptation to an increased workload imposed on the ventricular muscle. However, excessive hypertrophy is deleterious for two reasons. First, enlargement of the ventricular muscle restricts the opening of the aortic or pulmonic valve. A vicious cycle develops. Hypertension leads to increased pressure work for the left ventricle, which leads to left ventricular hypertrophy, which leads to aortic stenosis, which necessitates that the ventricle generate an even greater systolic pressure, which leads to more ventricular hypertrophy, and so on. The second complication of excessive hypertrophy is that the coronary circulation may be unable to provide enough blood flow to meet the increased metabolic demand of the hypertrophic ventricle, particularly during exercise. Inadequate coronary blood flow is especially likely if the coronary vessels have become constricted because of atherosclerosis. A hypertensive patient with coronary artery disease may have adequate blood flow to the hypertrophic ventricle during rest, but the increased need for coronary blood flow in exercise cannot be met. As a result, hypertensive patients with coronary artery disease are at high risk for cardiac ischemia, myocardial infarction, ventricular arrhythmias, and sudden death during periods of exercise. This explains why the all-too-common combination of hypertension and coronary artery disease is such a serious problem in human medicine. Fortunately, coronary artery disease is rare in most animals.

The pathologic consequences of cardiac defects are direct results of the abnormal pressures, volumes, and workloads created in the cardiac chambers

Figure 20–10 summarizes the pathologic consequences associated with some common murmurs.

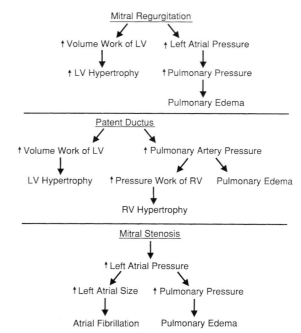

FIGURE 20–10. The pathologic consequences of several common cardiac defects. LV, left ventricle; RV, right ventricle.

First consider mitral regurgitation. With each contraction of the left ventricle, a normal volume of blood is ejected into the aorta, and an additional volume of blood is ejected backward (through the regurgitant valve) into the left atrium. As a result, there is an increase in the volume work performed by the left ventricle. Therefore, mild to moderate left ventricular hypertrophy develops. Also, in a heart with mitral regurgitation, the left atrium becomes distended, and left atrial pressure increases. Blood further backs up, or dams up, in the pulmonary blood vessels, which increases the pressure there. Elevated pressure in the pulmonary blood vessels causes water and electrolytes to be filtered out of the blood stream and into the pulmonary interstitial spaces. The accumulation of water in the lung tissue causes a "waterlogging" or swelling that is called *pulmonary edema.* When left atrial pressures exceed 20 to 25 mm Hg, pulmonary edema becomes so severe that there is a substantial reduction in the ability of the lungs to transfer oxygen into the blood stream. The result is respiratory distress.

The consequences of mitral regurgitation are usually more noticeable during exercise than during rest. One reason is that despite the regurgitation, the left ventricle can usually adapt enough through hypertrophy and an increase in heart rate to maintain a normal cardiac output into the aorta (and therefore into the systemic circulation) at rest. Also, despite some pulmonary edema, the oxygenation of the blood is sufficient to meet the animal's needs during rest. During exercise, however, the output of the left ventricle into the systemic circulation must increase to several times greater than normal if it is to supply adequate blood to exercising skeletal muscle. Also, the delivery of oxygen into the blood must increase to several times greater than normal. Despite the hypertrophy, the left ventricle may not be able to deliver adequate blood flow to the systemic circulation during exercise if mitral regurgitation is serious. Again, if pulmonary edema is serious, the lungs may not be able to deliver enough oxygen into the blood to support the metabolism of the exercising animal.

Consider next the abnormalities associated with aortic stenosis (not shown in Fig. 20–10). In order to eject a normal volume of blood with each beat through a stenotic aortic valve, the left ventricle must develop an abnormally high systolic pressure. This increases the pressure work of the left ventricle, which leads to a marked left ventricular hypertrophy. The hypertrophy has the desirable effect of increasing the contractility of the left ventricular muscle so that it can generate the increased pressure required to maintain normal cardiac output. However, as hypertrophy progresses, the ventricular muscle begins to impinge on the aortic outflow pathway, which further hampers the ability of the ventricle to eject blood. In a sense, the hypertrophic ventricular muscle gets in its own way or becomes muscle-bound. The resulting limitation in aortic outflow is much more likely to be a problem during exercise than at rest. A patient with aortic stenosis may be able to function normally at rest but characteristically exhibits exercise intolerance.

PDA is a defect that typically results in both left and right ventricular hypertrophy (see Fig. 20–10). In a typical patient with a PDA, the left ventricle pumps a nearly normal volume of blood per minute to the systemic circulation and also pumps two to three times that volume of blood per minute through the PDA. As a result, the volume work done by the left ventricle exceeds normal amounts, and this leads to left ventricular hypertrophy. The blood flowing through the PDA enters the pulmonary artery, and so pulmonary arterial pressure exceeds normal levels. This, in turn, increases the pressure work that must be done by the right ventricle. The right ventricle receives a nearly normal volume of blood back from the systemic circulation each minute, and the right ventricle has to generate an elevated systolic pressure in order to eject this blood into the high-pressure pulmonary artery. The increased pressure work for the right ventricle is a powerful stimulus for hypertrophy, and so a pronounced right ventricular hypertrophy develops.

As a patient with PDA grows, exercise intolerance becomes evident. Despite hypertrophy, the left ventricle cannot supply the increased blood flow needed by growing, exercising skeletal muscles in addition to the blood that flows through the PDA. In patients with PDA, pulmonary edema may also develop. The pulmonary artery and the pulmonary blood vessels must carry not only the blood that is pumped by the right ventricle (as in a normal animal) but also the blood that is pumped through the PDA. Therefore, pulmonary blood flow is typically three or four times greater than normal in a patient with a PDA. The resulting increases in pulmonary vascular pressure can lead to pulmonary edema. Surgical repair of a PDA in a young animal leads to a rapid reversal of all these pathologic changes.

An understanding of the preceding examples should make it easy to predict the pathologic consequences of a ventricular septal defect. These consequences include increased volume work of the left ventricle, moderate left ventricular hypertrophy, increased volume and pressure work of the right ventricle, pronounced right ventricular hypertrophy, increased blood flow through the lungs, possible pulmonary edema, and probable exercise intolerance. It should also be clear why pulmonic stenosis leads to increased pressure work for the right ventricle and pronounced right ventricular hypertrophy (see the later Clinical Correlation).

Figure 20–10 also summarizes the pathologic consequences associated with the diastolic murmur of mitral stenosis. The left atrial pressure must exceed normal levels in order to force a normal volume of blood through the stenotic mitral valve and into the left ventricle during each ventricular diastole. The elevated left atrial pressure distends the left atrium. There may be some hypertrophy of the atrial muscle. However, the atrium continues to function mainly as a reservoir to collect and hold blood during ventricular systole rather than as a pumping chamber to force blood into the ventricle during its diastole. One problem is that atrial action potentials tend to become discoordinated in a distended atrium, and atrial fibrillation is a common consequence. Also, the increase in the left atrial pressure causes blood to back up and accumulate in the pulmonary blood vessels, which can cause pulmonary edema. It might be supposed that the backup of blood in the pulmonary vessels would eventually also increase the pressure in the pulmonary artery and thereby increase the pressure work of the right ventricle. In other words, mitral stenosis might be predicted to lead to right ventricular hypertrophy. This prediction is a logical one, but in practice, animals with elevated left atrial pressures usually die from the effects of pulmonary edema before right ventricular pressures have had a chance to become high enough to induce right ventricular hypertrophy. Therefore, mitral stenosis does not generally lead to hypertrophy of either ventricle.

The defect of aortic regurgitation leads to left ventricular hypertrophy. With each systole, the left ventricle has to eject an abnormally large volume of blood into the aorta. Of this, a normal volume of blood goes on into the systemic circuit; the rest is simply regurgitated back from the aorta into the left ventricle during diastole. Thus, the volume work of the left ventricle is increased to above-normal levels, and left ventricular pressures may rise, too. Both these factors stimulate left ventricular hypertrophy. In severe cases of aortic regurgitation, diastolic ventricular pressure becomes elevated (because during diastole the left ventricle receives blood from both the left atrium and the aorta). This leads to an increase in left atrial pressure, and pulmonary edema may develop.

The foregoing consideration of the abnormalities associated with cardiac defects is important for two reasons. First, these defects and their consequences are commonly encountered in the clinic. Second, this discussion illustrates how the symptoms and consequences of disease states can be understood and predicted in a rational way, on the basis of an understanding of basic principles of cardiac physiology.

CLINICAL CORRELATIONS

Pulmonic Stenosis

History A 6-month-old female schnauzer is referred to your clinic because of a heart murmur that was detected during a routine health care visit. The puppy is fairly active but is slightly smaller than her female littermates. She also tires more quickly than her littermates when they play together.

Clinical examination All physical parameters are normal except for a systolic heart murmur that can be heard best over the left third to fourth intercostal space. Femoral pulses are normal, and the jugular veins are not distended. Electrocardiography reveals that the dog is in normal sinus rhythm with a heart rate of 118 beats per minute. The PR interval is normal. However, the major QRS deflection is negative in leads I and aV$_F$. Also, deep S waves are noted in leads II and III, and the QRS complexes are slightly prolonged, as a result of the wide S waves. Thoracic radiographs show right ventricular enlargement; the right border of the cardiac silhouette is more rounded, and closer to the right thoracic wall, than normal.

A catheter is inserted into the jugular vein, and the following pressures are measured as the catheter is advanced through the right side of the heart and into the pulmonary artery: central venous pressure (mean right atrial pressure) is 8 mm Hg; right ventricular systolic pressure is 122 mm Hg; and pulmonary artery systolic pressure is 16 mm Hg.

The jugular catheter is withdrawn until the catheter tip is in the right ventricle. Then additional radiographs are taken while a radiopaque dye is injected through the catheter. These radiographs reveal that the right ventricular outflow tract is narrowed just below the pulmonic valve and that the pulmonic valve does not open widely during ventricular systole.

Comment The young age of this dog and the absence of other signs of illness suggest that the murmur results from a congenital cardiac abnormality. Murmurs are graded on a scale of 1 through 6, 6 being the most severe. This dog's murmur is graded 4. A systolic murmur can result from aortic or pulmonic stenosis, mitral or tricuspid incompetence, or a ventricular septal defect (see Fig. 20–8). On the basis of the location from which this murmur can be heard best, aortic or pulmonic stenosis is the most likely cause. All the additional clinical evidence supports a diagnosis of pulmonic stenosis.

The electrocardiogram indicates that the sinoatrial node is acting as the pacemaker and that the AV node is conducting each atrial action potential into the ventricles. However, the abnormalities observed in the polarity and shape of the QRS complex, when coupled with the radiographic findings, are indicative of right ventricular hypertrophy. Pulmonic stenosis leads to right ventricular hypertrophy, because the right ventricle must generate much higher pressures than normal during systole in or-

der to eject blood through the narrow outflow tract. The right ventricular systolic pressure is 122 mm Hg in this dog; a normal pressure is 20 mm Hg.

Normally, the pulmonic valve opens widely during systole, and the ventricular systolic pressure equals the pulmonary artery systolic pressure. In this dog, there is a difference of 106 mm Hg between right ventricular systolic pressure and the systolic pressure in the pulmonary artery just beyond the pulmonic valve. This difference indicates a severe pulmonic obstruction. The degree of obstruction can be evaluated visually from the radiographs taken during dye injection.

Right ventricular hypertrophy is one of two adaptive responses that help this dog maintain a nearly normal right ventricular stroke volume, despite the pulmonic stenosis. The other adaptive response is that the mean right atrial pressure is higher than normal (8 instead of 3 mm Hg). The right atrial pressure is elevated, because blood backs up or dams up in areas upstream from the stenosis (i.e., in the right ventricle, right atrium, and systemic veins). The elevated atrial pressure is adaptive, because it increases the right ventricular preload, which increases the end-diastolic volume, which (according to Starling's law of the heart) helps keep the right ventricular stroke volume at a normal level, despite the stenosis. The right atrial pressure is not quite high enough in this dog to cause abdominal ascites or systemic edema (detailed in Chapter 22). However, both these signs are sometimes seen in dogs with severe pulmonic stenosis, because excessively elevated right atrial pressure leads to marked increases in capillary hydrostatic pressure (upstream from the right atrium).

The combined effects of right ventricular hypertrophy and elevated right ventricular preload allow this dog's heart to pump a nearly normal stroke volume during rest. However, the pulmonic obstruction limits the increase in the stroke volume that can occur during exercise. The resulting limitation in cardiac output accounts for this dog's lack of stamina during exercise. Over a prolonged period, such a limitation in cardiac output can also stunt growth.

Treatment Theoretically, the best treatment for pulmonic stenosis is to remove the obstruction surgically. A valve dilator can be used, or an artificial conduit can be installed across the stenotic valve. Although seriously affected dogs require interventional treatments such as surgery, dogs with mild to moderate pulmonic stenosis can lead sedentary lives without any treatment.

Some clinicians believe that the adverse effects of pulmonic stenosis can be minimized by the administration of β-adrenergic antagonists (e.g., propranolol) or calcium channel blockers (e.g., verapamil). Although the mechanism and efficacy of these drugs remain unclear, there is speculation that these drugs are beneficial because they limit ventricular contractility, which limits the work of the heart. Because an increase in cardiac work is the stimulus for hypertrophy, a drug that limits the increase in work also limits the hypertrophy. Although moderate hypertrophy can be adaptive (as explained earlier), excessive hypertrophy is detrimental for two reasons. First, the enlarged ventricular muscle can crowd the pulmonic outflow tract, making the stenosis even worse. Second, the coronary circulation may be unable to deliver the increased amounts of blood flow required by the massive ventricular muscle.

Bibliography

Berne RM, Levy MN: Cardiovascular Physiology, 7th ed. St. Louis: CV Mosby, 1997.

de Morais HA: Pathophysiology of heart failure and clinical evaluation of cardiac function. In Ettinger SJ, Feldman EC (eds): Textbook of Veterinary Internal Medicine: Diseases of the Dog and Cat, 5th ed. Philadelphia: WB Saunders, 2000, p 692.

Dukes HH, Swenson MJ, Reece WO: Dukes' Physiology of Domestic Animals. Ithaca, N.Y.: Comstock, 1993, pp 145–183.

Huntsman LL, Feigl EO: Cardiac mechanics. In Patton HD, Fuchs AF, Hille B, et al (eds): Textbook of Physiology, Vol 2. Philadelphia: WB Saunders, 1989, p 820.

Katz AM: Physiology of the Heart, 3rd ed. Baltimore: Lippincott Williams & Wilkins, 2000.

Kvart C, Haggstrom J: Acquired valvular heart disease. In Ettinger SJ, Feldman EC (eds): Textbook of Veterinary Internal Medicine: Diseases of the Dog and Cat, 5th ed. Philadelphia: WB Saunders, 2000, p 787.

Marr C (ed): Cardiology of the Horse. London: WB Saunders, 1999.

Opie LH: The Heart: Physiology, From Cell to Circulation, 3rd ed. Baltimore: Lippincott Williams & Wilkins, 1998.

Patteson MW: Acquired cardiac disease. In Robinson NE (ed): Current Therapy in Equine Medicine 4. Philadelphia: WB Saunders, 1997.

Physick-Sheard PW: Pathophysiology and principles of therapy. In Colahan PT, Merritt AM, Moore JN, et al (eds): Equine Medicine and Surgery, 5th ed., vol 1. St. Louis: Mosby–Year Book, 1999, p 337.

Scher AM: Events of the cardiac cycle: Measurements of pressure, flow, and volume. In Patton HD, Fuchs AF, Hille B, et al (eds): Textbook of Physiology, vol 2. Philadelphia: WB Saunders, 1989, p 834.

Schmidt-Nielsen K: Animal Physiology: Adaptation and Environment. Cambridge, United Kingdom: Cambridge University Press, 1997.

Sisson DD, Thomas WP, Bonagura JD: Congenital Heart Disease. In Ettinger SJ, Feldman EC (eds): Textbook of Veterinary Internal Medicine: Diseases of the Dog and Cat, 5th ed. Philadelphia: WB Saunders, 2000, p 737.

PRACTICE QUESTIONS

1. In the normal cardiac cycle,
   a. ventricular systole and ventricular ejection begin at the same time.
   b. the second heart sound coincides with the beginning of isovolumetric relaxation.
   c. the highest left ventricular pressure is reached just as the aortic valve closes.
   d. aortic pressure is highest at the beginning of ventricular systole.
   e. atrial systole occurs during rapid ventricular ejection.

2. Figure 20–11 shows a plot of the changes in pressure and volume that occur in the left ventricle during one cardiac cycle. Which of the following is true?
   a. Point *D* marks the beginning of isovolumetric relaxation.
   b. Point *B* marks the closure of the aortic valve.
   c. Point *C* marks the opening of the mitral valve.
   d. Point *A* marks the beginning of isovolumetric contraction.
   e. Point *D* marks the beginning of ventricular systole.

3. Which statement is true for a normal heart?
   a. Sympathetic activation causes end-systolic ventricular volume to increase.

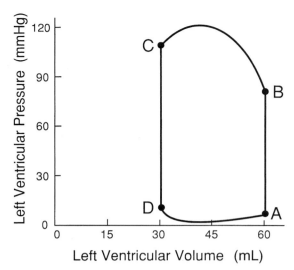

FIGURE 20–11.   The closed loop depicts the changes in left ventricular pressure and volume that occur during one cardiac cycle. Practice Question 2 is based on this graph. The first step in understanding the figure is to determine whether the normal sequence of events proceeds clockwise or counterclockwise around the loop. To make this distinction, recall that the ventricles fill when ventricular pressure is low and empty when ventricular pressure is high. Next, identify the phases of the cardiac cycle that correspond with each limb of the loop. Finally, determine what happens to the mitral and aortic valves at each corner of the loop. Hint: A, B, C, and D in this figure match the similarly labeled events in Figure 20–1, bottom graph.

   b. An increase in ventricular preload causes end-diastolic ventricular volume to decrease.
   c. An increase in ventricular contractility causes systolic duration to increase.
   d. An increase in ventricular contractility causes the external work of the heart to decrease.
   e. Pacing the heart at a high rate causes stroke volume to decrease.

4. Starting at the open circle in Figure 20–12, which point would be reached after the contractility decreased and the preload increased?
   a. Point A.
   b. Point B.

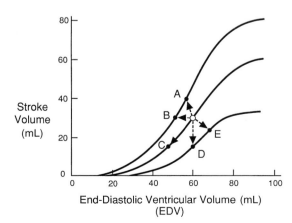

FIGURE 20–12.   Practice Question 4 is based on this graph of three ventricular function curves.

c. Point C.
d. Point D.
e. Point E.

5. You examine a 7-year-old poodle and find evidence of a systolic murmur (no diastolic murmur), pulmonary edema (indicated by rapid, noisy respiration, cough), left ventricular hypertrophy (no right ventricular hypertrophy), and exercise intolerance. The most likely explanation for the symptoms is

a. mitral regurgitation.
b. mitral stenosis.
c. aortic regurgitation.
d. pulmonic stenosis.
e. ventricular septal defect.

PRACTICE ANSWERS

1. b   2. d   3. e   4. e   5. a

21

The systemic and pulmonary circulations

1 Blood pressure represents a potential energy that propels blood through the circulation

2 Vascular resistance is defined as perfusion pressure divided by flow

3 The net resistance of the systemic circulation is called the total peripheral resistance

4 Arterial pressure is determined by the cardiac output and total peripheral resistance

5 The blood flow to each organ is determined by the perfusion pressure and vascular resistance

6 The pulmonary circulation offers much less resistance to blood flow than does the systemic circulation

7 Arterial pressures are measured in terms of systolic, diastolic, and mean levels

8 Pulse pressure increases when the stroke volume increases, heart rate decreases, aortic compliance decreases, or total peripheral resistance increases

---

Blood pressure represents a potential energy that propels blood through the circulation

By definition, the *central circulation* is composed of the right side of the heart, the pulmonary circuit, and the left side of the heart. Blood enters the central circulation from the venae cavae and leaves the central circulation through the aorta. The *systemic circulation* has the aorta as its inlet point and the venae cavae as its outlet. In a normal resting animal, approximately 25% of the blood volume resides in the central circulation and about 75% resides in the systemic circulation. Most of the blood in the systemic vessels is in the systemic veins.

Figure 21–1 shows the normal pressure profile in the systemic circulation. This figure portrays the pressures that would be measured with a miniature pressure gauge inserted into the various vessels that blood encounters in its passage through the systemic circulation. The blood pressure is highest in the aorta (typically, mean aortic pressure is 98 mm Hg) and lowest in the venae cavae (3 mm Hg). It is this pressure difference that forces blood to move (via bulk flow) through the systemic vessels; that is, 98 minus 3 mm Hg is the *perfusion pressure* (difference) that drives systemic blood flow (the concept of perfusion pressure is described in Chapter 17).

Aortic blood pressure can be thought of as the potential energy available to move blood; the decrease in pressure in the sequential segments of the systemic circuit represents the amount of this poten-

tial energy that is "used up" in moving blood through each segment. Pressure energy is used up through *friction,* which is generated as the molecules and cells of blood rub against each other and against the walls of the blood vessels. The energy used up through friction is actually converted to heat, although the increase in the temperature of the blood and blood vessels as a result of friction is very small.

The amount of the blood pressure energy "used up" in each of the sequential segments of the systemic circulation depends on the amount of friction or resistance that the blood encounters. The aorta and large arteries offer very little resistance to blood flow (very little friction), so the blood pressure decreases only a little in these vessels (from 98 to about 95 mm Hg). The greatest pressure decrease (greatest loss of pressure energy through friction) occurs as blood flows through arterioles; that is, the arterioles provide a greater resistance to blood flow than any other segment of the systemic circulation. The capillaries and the venules also offer a substantial resistance to blood flow, but the resistance (and therefore the pressure decrease) is not as great in these vessels as it is in the arterioles. The large veins and the venae cavae are low-resistance vessels, so little pressure energy is expended in driving the blood flow through these vessels.

The pumping of blood by the heart maintains the pressure difference between the aorta and the venae cavae. If the heart stops, blood continues to flow for a few moments from the aorta toward the venae cavae. As this blood leaves the aorta, the aortic walls

169

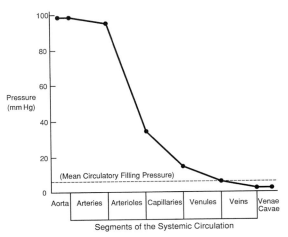

FIGURE 21–1. A graph of the blood pressures (hydrostatic pressures) that typically exist in the systemic circulation of a dog at rest. The actual blood pressure in the aorta and arteries is pulsatile, increasing with each cardiac ejection and falling between ejections. The values plotted here are the average (mean) values of those pulsatile pressures. *Mean circulatory filling pressure (dashed line)* is the pressure that would exist if the heart were stopped (see text for fuller description). All pressures are measured at heart level, with reference to atmospheric pressure (with atmospheric pressure being taken as zero).

become less distended and the blood pressure inside the aorta decreases. As a little extra blood accumulates in the venae cavae, they become more distended than before and the blood pressure inside the venae cavae increases. Soon, there is no pressure difference between the aorta and the venae cavae. Blood flow in the systemic circuit ceases, and the pressure everywhere in the systemic circulation is the same. It has been demonstrated experimentally that this eventual pressure is about 7 mm Hg. This pressure, in a static circulation, is called the *mean circulatory filling pressure.* The mean circulatory filling pressure is above zero, because there is a fullness to the circulation; that is, even if the heart stops, blood still distends the vessels that contain it. The vessel walls, being elastic, recoil ("push back") against this distention. The elastic recoil of the vessel walls accounts for the persistence of pressure in the circulation even if the heart stops. If a transfusion of blood is administered to an animal with the heart stopped, the vessels become more distended and the mean circulating filling pressure rises above 7 mm Hg. Conversely, if blood is removed from an animal with the heart stopped, the pressure everywhere falls to a level below 7 mm Hg.

Consider what happens if the heart is restarted in an animal after the pressure has equalized everywhere at 7 mm Hg. With each heartbeat, the heart takes some blood out of the venae cavae and moves it into the aorta. The volume of blood in the venae cavae decreases, so the venae cavae become less distended and vena caval pressure drops below 7 mm Hg. The volume of blood in the aorta increases, so the aorta becomes more distended and aortic pressure rises above 7 mm Hg. The vena caval pressure drops about 4 mm Hg (from 7 to 3 mm Hg), and the aortic

pressure rises about 91 mm Hg (from 7 to 98 mm Hg). It is important to understand why the pressure decreases only a little in the venae cavae and why it increases so much in the aorta, even though the volume of blood removed from the venae cavae with each heartbeat is the same as the volume of blood added to the aorta. The reason is that the veins are much more compliant than the arteries; that is, one can add or remove blood from veins without changing the venous pressure very much, whereas the addition or removal of blood from arteries changes the arterial pressure a great deal.

A compliant vessel readily distends when pressure or volume is added. It yields to pressure. By definition, *compliance* is the change in the volume within a vessel or a chamber divided by the associated change in pressure. Figure 21–2 shows curves that illustrate the contrast in the relationship between volume and pressure in veins (which have a high compliance) and arteries (which are stiff and have a low compliance). Compliance (Δ volume/Δ pressure) corresponds to the slope on a volume-versus-pressure graph. This graph shows that veins are about 20 times more compliant than are arteries.

The blood volume of the body is not constant but changes with fluid intake (e.g., drinking) and fluid loss (e.g., sweating). The veins are the main site in the circulation that can expand or contract to accommodate changes in blood volume. It is appropriate that veins, the major blood *volume reservoirs* of the body, can accept or give up a large volume of blood without incurring much of a change in pressure. By contrast, the arteries function as *pressure reservoirs.* They are the temporary storage site for the surge of pressure energy created with each cardiac ejection. Arteries must be able to accept a large increase in pressure during cardiac ejection and then hold the pressure high enough to drive blood through the systemic circulation between cardiac ejections. Therefore, it is appropriate that the arteries are tough vessels with low compliance.

Vascular resistance is defined as perfusion pressure divided by flow

Maintenance of a normal blood flow through the systemic tissues requires a high arterial pressure primarily because the arterioles offer such a large resistance to blood flow. In addition to being the site of greatest resistance to blood flow in the systemic circulation, arterioles are the site of adjustable resistance. An increase in arteriolar resistance in a particular organ decreases the amount of blood flow in that organ, and vice versa. The concept of arteriolar resistance and its adjustment is important to an understanding of cardiovascular physiology.

Everyday experience tells us that it is easier to force fluid through a big tube than through a small tube. For example, it is easier to drink a milk shake through a large-diameter straw than through a small-diameter straw. A big tube has a lower resistance to flow (less

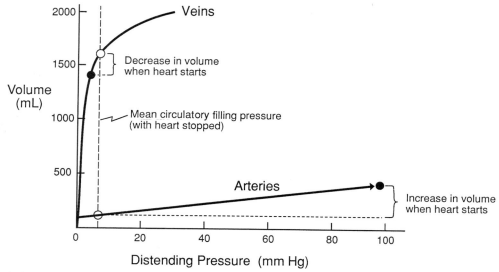

FIGURE 21–2. Typical relationships between the volume (of blood) and the distending pressure for veins and arteries. Veins are more compliant (easier to distend) than arteries, so they hold a greater volume of blood for a given distending pressure. This concept is illustrated for a distending pressure of 7 mm Hg *(vertical dashed line)*, which is a normal value for the mean circulating filling pressure (the pressure in the circulation when the heart is stopped). For a pressure of 7 mm Hg, the veins contain about 1600 mL of blood and the arteries contain only 125 mL *(open circles)*. When the heart is restarted, the venous volume decreases and the arterial volume increases by an identical amount *(filled circles)*. Because the veins are so much more compliant than the arteries, the venous pressure changes very little (decreases from 7 to 3 mm Hg), whereas the arterial pressure increases from 7 to 98 mm Hg.

friction) than a small tube. For a given driving force (perfusion pressure difference), the flow is higher in the tube that has the lower resistance. The perfusion pressure (Δ pressure) is the pressure at the inlet minus the pressure at the outlet. Figure 21–3 presents these concepts in pictorial and graphic form.

The precise definition of resistance is

$$\text{resistance} = \Delta \text{ pressure/flow.}$$

The dashed lines in Figure 21–3 indicate that a pressure difference of 60 mm Hg causes a flow of 1600 mL/min through the large tube. Thus, the resistance of the large tube is 37.5 mm Hg/L/min. The same driving pressure (60 mm Hg) causes a flow of only 100 mL/min through the small tube. The resistance of the small tube is 600 mm Hg/L/min. The resistance of the small tube is 16 times greater than the resistance of the large tube.

In the late 1800s, the French physician J. L. M. Poiseuille demonstrated that the resistance of a tube can be predicted from the following equation:

$$\text{resistance} = 8\eta l/\pi r^4,$$

where l is the length of the tube, r is the radius, η is the viscosity of the liquid, and π has its usual meaning.

This equation is known as *Poiseuille's law*. The equation emphasizes that radius is the primary determinant of the resistance of a tube. The resistance varies inversely with the fourth power of the radius, so that doubling the radius (r) of the tube decreases its resistance by a factor of 16 (2^4). Also, resistance is proportional to the length (l) of the tube. This makes intuitive sense; it is harder to force fluid through a long tube than through a short tube of the same

radius. The final important determinant of resistance is the viscosity (η) of the fluid. The higher the viscosity of the fluid, the higher is the resistance to its flow through a tube. For example, honey is more viscous than water, so a tube would offer a higher resistance to the flow of honey than to the flow of water.

The arterioles are the segment of the systemic circulation that poses the highest resistance to blood flow; there is a larger perfusion pressure (pressure drop) across the arterioles than across any other segment of the systemic circulation. In other words, of the total pressure energy available for systemic blood flow, a larger fraction is expended in forcing blood through the arterioles than through any other segment. It may seem paradoxical that the arterioles are the site of highest resistance when the capillaries are smaller vessels. After all, a smaller tube has a much higher resistance than a bigger tube (as illustrated in Fig. 21–3). The resolution of this paradox is presented in Figure 21–4. It is true that each capillary has a smaller radius and therefore a greater resistance than each arteriole. However, each arteriole in the body distributes blood to many capillaries, and the *net* resistance of all of those capillaries is less than the resistance of the single arteriole that delivers blood to them. It is only because each arteriole delivers blood to so many capillaries that the net resistance of the capillaries is less than the resistance of the arteriole.

Arterioles are the site not only of the highest resistance in the circulation but also of the most variable resistance. Variation in arteriolar resistance is the main factor that determines how much blood flows through each tissue in the body. The length of an arteriole does not change (at least not over the short term), but the radius of an arteriole varies from mo-

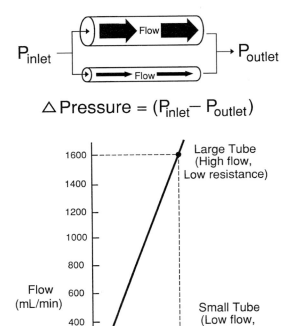

$$\triangle \text{Pressure} = (P_{inlet} - P_{outlet})$$

FIGURE 21–3. The relationship between flow and perfusion pressure (Δ pressure) for two tubes. The perfusion pressure is the pressure at the inlet (P_{inlet}) of the tube minus the pressure at the outlet (P_{outlet}). In this example, the larger tube has twice the radius of the smaller tube. For a given perfusion pressure, the flow through the larger tube is 16 times greater than the flow through the smaller tube. That is, the resistance of the larger tube is one-sixteenth the resistance of the smaller tube.

ment to moment. The walls of arterioles are relatively thick and muscular. Contraction of the arteriolar smooth muscle decreases the radius of arterioles; this *vasoconstriction* substantially increases resistance to blood flow. Relaxation of the smooth muscle increases the radius of the vessels, and this *vasodilation* substantially reduces the resistance to blood flow.

Figure 21–5 illustrates that small changes in the radius of arterioles in an organ bring about large changes in resistance and blood flow. In this example, the arterial pressure is 93 mm Hg and the venous pressure is 3 mm Hg. The brain blood flow is initially 90 mL/min (0.090 L/min). Based on the mathematical definition of resistance, the resistance of the brain blood vessels is calculated to be 1000 mm Hg/L/min. Most of this resistance is provided by the brain arterioles. Consider the consequences of a slight vasodilation, such that the radius of the arterioles increases by 19% (e.g., from a radius of 1.00 to a radius of 1.19). Recall from Poiseuille's law that the resistance varies inversely as the fourth power of the radius. Because 1.19^4 equals 2.00, a 19% increase in radius cuts the resistance in half! Decreasing the brain's resistance by half (to 500 mm Hg/L/min) would double the brain blood flow (to 180 mL/min).

The net resistance of the systemic circulation is called the total peripheral resistance

Like any other resistance, *total peripheral resistance* (TPR) is defined as a pressure difference (perfusion pressure) divided by a flow. In calculation of the resistance of the systemic circulation, the perfusion pressure is the pressure in the aorta minus the pressure in the venae cavae. The flow is the total amount of blood that flows through the systemic circuit, which is equal to the cardiac output:

TPR = (mean aortic pressure − vena caval pressure)/cardiac output.

For a typical dog at rest, the mean aortic pressure is 98 mm Hg, the mean vena caval pressure is 3 mm Hg, and the cardiac output is 2.5 L/min. Under these conditions, TPR is 38 mm Hg/L/min. A TPR of 38 mm Hg/L/min means that it takes a driving pressure of 38 mm Hg to force 1 L/min of blood through the systemic circuit.

Because the pressure in the venae cavae is usually close to zero, it is sometimes ignored in the calculation of TPR. The resultant simplified equation states that TPR is approximately equal to the aortic pressure divided by the cardiac output. Usually, this equation is rearranged to form the statement that the mean aortic blood pressure (BP) is approximately equal to the cardiac output (CO) multiplied by TPR:

$$BP \approx CO \times TPR.$$

This equation expresses one of the central concepts in cardiovascular physiology; it points out that the mean aortic blood pressure is determined by two, and only two, factors. Thus, if the aortic pressure is increased, it must be because the cardiac output increased, the

Resistance of arteriole is less than resistance of capillary

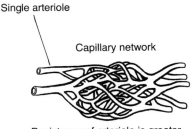

FIGURE 21–4. The resistance of a single arteriole is less than the resistance of a single capillary, because arterioles are larger in diameter. However, each arteriole supplies blood to a whole network of capillaries, and the resistance of an arteriole is greater than the resistance of the capillary network that it supplies with blood.

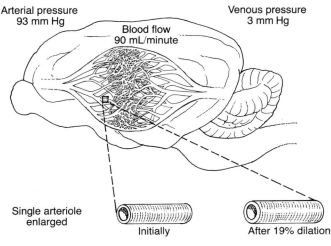

Initially,

$$\text{Resistance} = \frac{\Delta \text{Pressure}}{\text{Blood Flow}} = \frac{(93-3)\text{ mm Hg}}{90\text{ mL/minute}} = 1000\text{ mm Hg/L/minute}$$

After dilation of arterioles, resistance = 500 mm Hg/L/minute

$$\text{Blood Flow} = \frac{\Delta \text{Pressure}}{\text{Resistance}} = \frac{(93-3)\text{ mm Hg}}{500\text{ mm Hg/L/minute}} = 180\text{ mL/minute}$$

FIGURE 21–5. An example to illustrate how a small arteriolar dilation could substantially increase blood flow to the brain (see text for further discussion).

TPR increased, or both. There are no other possibilities.

Arterial pressure is determined by the cardiac output and total peripheral resistance

Three examples illustrate the application of the concept that the mean aortic blood pressure is determined by the cardiac output and TPR. First, in the most common form of human essential hypertension, the cardiac output is normal. The blood pressure is elevated because of excessively constricted systemic arterioles, which increase TPR above normal. What remains unclear about human essential hypertension is why the arterioles are constricted and why the body does not compensate for the elevated TPR by lowering the cardiac output below normal (which would keep the arterial pressure close to normal). High blood pressure is a serious health problem in human medicine, because patients with uncontrolled hypertension often develop cardiac hypertrophy and they are at high risk for cardiac arrhythmias, myocardial infarction, renal failure, and stroke. Naturally occurring hypertension is rare in veterinary species, although several techniques have been developed to induce hypertension in laboratory animals for research purposes.

Severe hemorrhage or dehydration is another condition in which the arterial pressure becomes abnormal, and it provides several distinct contrasts to chronic hypertension. For one thing, hemorrhage and dehydration are commonly encountered in veterinary medicine. Next, the arterial pressure is reduced in these conditions, not elevated. The cause of the abnor-

mal pressure is an abnormal cardiac output. Hemorrhage or dehydration characteristically reduces the cardiac preload, which reduces the stroke volume and cardiac output, and this leads to the decrease in arterial pressure. TPR is actually increased above normal, because compensating reflexes (discussed later) constrict the arterioles in the kidneys, splanchnic circulation, and resting skeletal muscle. Vasoconstriction in these organs minimizes the fall in arterial pressure and diverts the available cardiac output to the brain, heart, and any exercising skeletal muscle.

The response to vigorous exercise provides a third application of the concept that the mean aortic blood pressure is determined by the cardiac output and TPR. Like hemorrhage, exercise causes the cardiac output and TPR to change in opposite directions. However, in exercise, the cardiac output is elevated and TPR is decreased. TPR decreases because the arterioles in the working skeletal muscle dilate to increase the skeletal muscle blood flow. During vigorous exercise, TPR decreases to about one fourth of its resting value. The cardiac output increases about fourfold. The result is that the aortic pressure is negligibly changed. Figure 21–6 depicts the cardiovascular adjustments to vigorous exercise.

The blood flow to each organ is determined by the perfusion pressure and the vascular resistance

If the equation that defines resistance is solved for flow, the result is

$$\text{flow} = \Delta \text{ pressure} / \text{resistance}.$$

As applied to the blood flow through any organ, this equation points out that the blood flow is determined

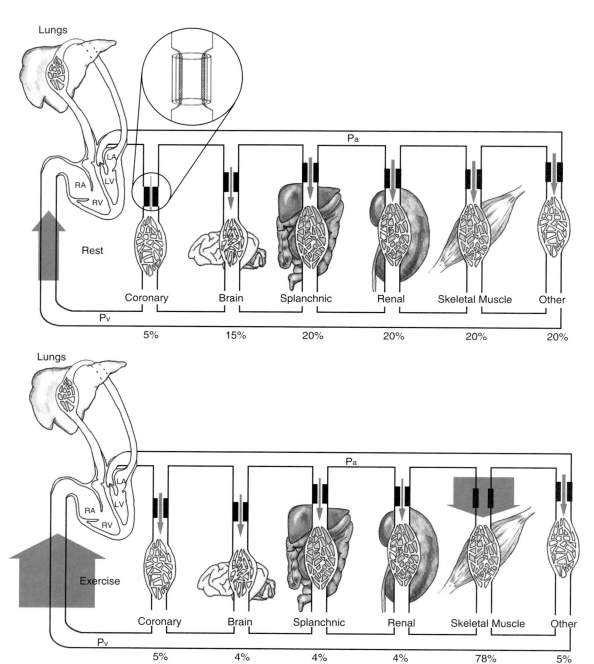

FIGURE 21–6. Cardiac output and its distribution compared during rest *(top)* and vigorous exercise *(bottom)* in a typical large dog. The width of the shaded arrows denotes the amount of blood flow. The flow of blood into the right side of the heart (which, of course, is equal to the cardiac output) is represented by the very wide arrows on the left. The cardiac output is 2.5 L/min at rest and increases to 10.0 L/min during exercise (fourfold increase). The entire cardiac output passes through the lungs and then is pumped by the left ventricle (LV) into the systemic arterial system *(horizontal tube across top)*. The systemic arteries deliver blood to each of the systemic vascular beds, which are grouped here into coronary, brain, splanchnic, renal, skeletal muscle, and other. In each systemic organ, blood must pass through high-resistance arterioles *(heavy bars)* before reaching the capillaries. The arterioles act as adjustable cuffs or constrictors (see magnified view, *top*). The proportion of the total cardiac output that goes to the different organs is indicated by the percentages across the bottom. Because each organ is exposed to the same arterial pressure (P_a) and venous pressure (P_v), the proportion of cardiac output that each organ receives is determined by their relative resistances. Resistance is determined mainly by the arteriolar diameter, which is drawn to scale in this figure. During vigorous exercise, skeletal muscle arterioles dilate maximally, and the blood flow to the exercising muscles increases 16-fold (from 0.5 L/min at rest to 7.8 L/min). Coronary arterioles also dilate, and the coronary blood flow increases about fourfold, which meets the increased demand by the heart muscle for oxygen. Vasoconstriction causes a small decrease in blood flow to the splanchnic and renal circulations. Blood flow to the brain is basically unchanged. Of course, the percentage of total cardiac output received by the brain decreases. RV, right ventricle; LA, left atrium; RA, right atrium.

by the perfusion pressure (arterial pressure minus venous pressure) and by the resistance of the blood vessels of the organ. There are no other factors. All of the organs of the systemic circulation are exposed to the same perfusion pressure. Therefore, the differences in blood flow to the various organs result solely from their different vascular resistances. As explained earlier, the vascular resistance of an organ is determined mainly by the diameter of its arterioles. Thus, arteriolar vasodilation and vasoconstriction are the mechanisms that increase or decrease the blood flow in one organ relative to another organ.

This point is illustrated pictorially in Figure 21–6. In a typical dog at rest, the arteriolar resistances are similar (diameters are the same) in the splanchnic, renal, and skeletal vascular beds. Therefore, each of these beds receives about the same blood flow (shown by arrows of an equal width in the figure). During exercise, the skeletal muscle arterioles nearly double in diameter, which decreases their resistance to blood flow by a factor of almost 16. Therefore, the skeletal muscle blood flow increases almost 16-fold (from 0.5 to 7.8 L/min). By contrast, the arterioles in the splanchnic and renal circulations constrict slightly during exercise, which causes splanchnic and renal resistance to increase by about 20%. Therefore, the splanchnic and renal blood flows decrease by about 20% (from 0.5 to 0.4 L/min). Also during exercise, coronary arterioles dilate, so the coronary blood flow increases; brain arterioles remain the same, so the brain blood flow is unchanged.

This discussion of blood flow during exercise assumes that the heart can meet the demands of exercise. A normal dog with a healthy heart can increase its cardiac output during exercise to meet the increased blood flow needs of the skeletal and cardiac muscle. As a result, the arterial pressure and the perfusion pressure are very similar during rest and exercise. By contrast, a dog with heart failure cannot increase the cardiac output much above its resting level. Therefore, the arterial pressure (and perfusion pressure) declines during exercise, and none of the organs receive the blood flow that they require. That is why animals with heart failure exhibit weakness, fatigue, and exercise intolerance. (Additional complications of heart failure are discussed in Chapter 25.) The point for now is that the equation that relates blood flow, perfusion pressure, and vascular resistance is fundamental and inescapable; this relationship is profoundly important to an understanding of cardiovascular function and dysfunction.

The pulmonary circulation offers much less resistance to blood flow than does the systemic circulation

Like any other resistance, pulmonary resistance is calculated as a pressure difference (perfusion pressure) divided by a flow. The perfusion pressure that forces blood through the pulmonary circuit is the pressure in the pulmonary artery minus the pressure in the pulmonary veins. The flow that traverses the pulmonary circuit is equal to the cardiac output:

$$\text{pulmonary vascular resistance} = (\text{pulmonary artery pressure} - \text{pulmonary venous pressure})/\text{cardiac output}.$$

For a typical dog at rest, the mean pulmonary arterial pressure is 13 mm Hg, the mean pulmonary venous pressure is 5 mm Hg, and the cardiac output is 2.5 L/min. Thus, pulmonary resistance is 3.2 mm Hg/L/min. Note that this is only about one twelfth of the resistance of the systemic circulation.

During exercise, pulmonary blood vessels dilate and pulmonary resistance decreases. An increase in cardiac output is the cause of the pulmonary vasodilation. Cardiac output may increase to five times its resting value during vigorous exercise. Therefore, the pulmonary blood flow also is five times higher than normal. This raises the pulmonary artery pressure. Pulmonary blood vessels are compliant, and the increase in pulmonary arterial pressure distends the pulmonary vessels. Because resistance is inversely proportional to the fourth power of the vessel radius (Poiseuille's law, as mentioned earlier), a small increase in the radius of the pulmonary vessels greatly decreases their resistance.

The distention of pulmonary blood vessels during exercise is advantageous because it lowers the pulmonary resistance, which allows the pulmonary flow to increase greatly without necessitating a large increase in the pulmonary arterial pressure. However, in other circumstances, the distention of pulmonary vessels can lead to adverse consequences. An example is the effect of gravity on pulmonary blood flow. Gravity pulls downward on the blood within lung blood vessels, which increases the distending pressure in vessels low in the lungs compared with vessels that are higher (Fig. 21–7). The distended vessels have a lower resistance to blood flow, so more of the pulmonary blood flow traverses the lower (*dependent*) regions of a lung than the higher regions. Gravity also affects the airways of the lungs. For reasons explained later (see Chapter 45), the effect of gravity on the airways causes more air to be delivered to the dependent regions of the lungs than to the higher regions. However, gravity has a greater effect on blood flow than on air delivery, so there is a tendency for blood flow to be excessive (relative to air delivery) in the dependent region of a lung. Any such imbalance in the lungs between air delivery and blood flow is called a *ventilation-perfusion mismatch*. This inherent problem is most severe in large animals, in which the large size of the lungs leads to substantial gravitational effects.

Hypoxic vasoconstriction is an important mechanism that helps offset ventilation-perfusion mismatches in the lungs regardless of whether these mismatches result from gravitational effects or from any other cause. The pulmonary blood vessels are sensitive to the local concentration of oxygen (measured as oxygen partial pressure [P_{O_2}]). A low P_{O_2} (*hypoxia*) causes pulmonary vessels to constrict. Hypoxic vasoconstriction takes place in any region of the lung where

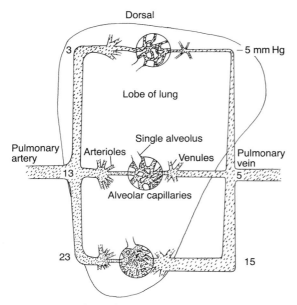

FIGURE 21–7. Gravity pulls downward on the blood within the lungs, which increases the pressure within blood vessels low in the lungs (see values in the figure). The pressure outside the blood vessels (intrapleural pressure) is not affected much by gravity (because air is so much lighter than blood). Therefore, the low-lying blood vessels become distended, which decreases their resistance to blood flow. As a result, more blood flows through the lower parts of the lungs than through the upper parts.

ventilation (the delivery of fresh air and oxygen) is reduced relative to blood flow. The vasoconstriction increases the resistance of blood vessels in that lung region and thereby reduces blood flow (perfusion). In this way, hypoxic vasoconstriction brings about a better match between ventilation and perfusion.

Like many compensatory mechanisms, hypoxic vasoconstriction can have undesirable consequences. For example, consider what happens if ventilation becomes depressed throughout both lungs. This occurs acutely during an allergic constriction of the airways (*asthma*) or chronically as the result of long-term pulmonary disease that obstructs the airways (*chronic obstructive pulmonary disease*, which is common in horses). The depressed ventilation causes hypoxia throughout the lungs. The hypoxia causes pulmonary vasoconstriction, which increases pulmonary vascular resistance. The increased resistance necessitates a substantial increase in pulmonary arterial pressure to maintain pulmonary blood flow. The condition of elevated pulmonary arterial pressure is called *pulmonary hypertension*. Pulmonary hypertension greatly increases the workload of the right ventricle. In extreme cases, it leads to right ventricular failure.

Arterial pressures are measured in terms of systolic, diastolic, and mean levels

The pressures in the aorta and pulmonary artery are not constant but rather are pulsatile, as shown in

Figure 21–8 (femoral artery pressure, also shown in Figure 21–8, is discussed later). With each cardiac ejection, the aorta and pulmonary artery become distended with blood, which causes the aortic and pulmonary artery pressures to increase to peak values, called *systolic pressures*. Between cardiac ejections (i.e., during ventricular diastole), blood continues to flow out of the aorta and pulmonary artery into the systemic and pulmonary circulations, respectively. As the volume of blood in these large arteries decreases, the arteries become less distended, so arterial pressure decreases. Pressure continues to decrease until the next cardiac ejection begins. The minimal pressure reached before each new ejection is called the *diastolic pressure*. Figure 21–8 provides typical values for systolic and diastolic pressures.

The amplitude of the pressure pulsations in an artery is called the *pulse pressure*; specifically,

aortic pulse pressure = (aortic systolic pressure −
aortic diastolic pressure)

and

pulmonary artery pulse pressure = (pulmonary
artery systolic pressure − pulmonary artery
diastolic pressure).

Typical values for pulse pressure are also given in Figure 21-8. Note how much lower the systolic, diastolic, and pulse pressures are in the pulmonary artery than in the aorta. These differences illustrate why the pulmonary circulation is called the "low-pressure circulation" and the systemic circulation is called the "high-pressure circulation."

It is important to distinguish among systolic pressure, diastolic pressure, and pulse pressure and to distinguish all of them from *mean pressure*. Mean aor-

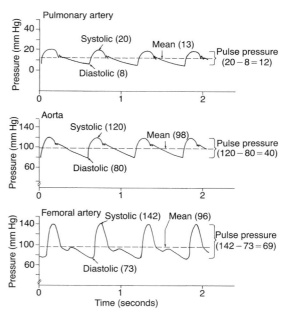

FIGURE 21–8. Blood pressure in the large arteries is pulsatile. The pressure patterns typical of the pulmonary artery, aorta, and femoral artery of the dog are shown.

tic pressure is the average pressure in the aorta over the course of one or more complete cardiac cycles. Likewise, mean pulmonary artery pressure is the average pressure in that vessel. Obviously, the mean pressure in an artery is somewhere between the systolic (maximal) and diastolic (minimal) pressure levels. However, because the pressure patterns in arteries are asymmetric, the mean pressure is not necessarily midway between the systolic and diastolic pressures.

A popular rule is that mean pressure is about one third of the way up from diastolic toward systolic pressure; that is,

$$\begin{array}{c}\text{mean} \\ \text{arterial} \\ \text{pressure}\end{array} \approx \left(\begin{array}{c}\text{diastolic} \\ \text{pressure}\end{array} + \frac{1}{3}\text{ pulse pressure}\right).$$

Figure 21–8 reveals that this is *not* a valid approximation for the determination of mean pressure in the aorta. However, the approximation is a good one for pressures measured in the femoral artery or in most other major arteries distal to the aorta. The reason that the rule applies in the distal arteries but not in the aorta is that the pattern of the arterial pressure pulsations changes as the pulses move out away from the heart. The pressure pulses become narrower and more sharply peaked. This pronounced asymmetry of the pressure pulses causes the mean level in distal arteries to be closer to the diastolic pressure than to the systolic pressure (see Fig. 21–8).

For complex reasons, the pulse pressure typically *increases* as blood flows from the aorta into the distal arteries. However, the mean pressure *decreases* in accordance with the principle of the conservation of energy. Mean arterial pressure is a measure of the potential energy in the blood stream, and this potential energy is used up (converted into heat by friction) as blood flows from the aorta through the systemic circulation. As stated earlier, most of the resistance to blood flow is found in the arterioles and capillaries. Therefore, the largest decrements in *mean pressure* occur in these segments of the systemic circulation (see Fig. 21–1). The aorta and large arteries offer only a small resistance to blood flow; mean arterial pressure decreases only 1 to 3 mm Hg between the aorta and the femoral artery (see Fig. 21–8).

Mean pressures are the pressures that must be used in calculation of vascular resistance from the following equation:

$$\text{resistance} = \text{perfusion pressure}/\text{blood flow}.$$

In the calculation of TPR, the perfusion pressure is *mean* aortic pressure minus *mean* vena caval (or right atrial) pressure. In the calculation of pulmonary resistance, the perfusion pressure is *mean* pulmonary arterial pressure minus *mean* pulmonary vein (or left atrial) pressure.

Unfortunately, the only way to measure mean vascular pressures is by inserting a needle or catheter into the vessel of interest. The first direct measurement of mean arterial blood pressure was carried out by Stephen Hales, an English clergyman. In about 1730, Hales inserted a tube (catheter) into the femoral

artery of a conscious horse and found that blood rose in the tube to a height of more than 8 feet. An 8-foot column of blood represents a pressure of more than 180 mm Hg, almost twice the mean arterial pressure expected in a normal resting animal. The high pressure undoubtedly reflected the physical and emotional distress of the horse, which was restrained upside down during the episode. Nowadays, arterial catheterization (with anesthetic agent to reduce pain) is routine in human medicine (e.g., in cardiac catheterization laboratories) and is becoming more common in veterinary medicine. However, the lesson that physical or emotional distress can dramatically increase blood pressure is as relevant today as it was in Hales' time.

In human medicine, systolic and diastolic arterial pressures can be measured quite accurately with a blood pressure cuff and stethoscope. Blood pressure cuffs are less commonly used on veterinary species, but the pulse is commonly palpated by placing the fingertips over a major artery, such as the femoral artery. Palpation of an artery allows the clinician to sense the pulse pressure on the basis of the magnitude of the pulsations felt in the artery. A low pulse pressure is referred to as a "thready," or weak, pulse. A high pulse pressure may be called a "bounding," or strong, pulse.

Pulse pressure increases when the stroke volume increases, heart rate decreases, aortic compliance decreases, or total peripheral resistance increases

Because the arterial pulse is so frequently palpated in patients, it is important for the veterinary clinician to understand the factors that commonly influence pulse pressure. First, an increase in stroke volume tends to increase pulse pressure. Because cardiac ejections create the arterial pulsations in the first place, it is not surprising that larger ejections create bigger pulsations. Figure 21–9A depicts this effect and shows that an increase in stroke volume also increases mean arterial pressure. Mean pressure increases, because an increased stroke volume increases cardiac output.

A second factor that tends to increase pulse pressure is a decrease in heart rate. Between cardiac ejections, blood continues to run out of the aorta and through the systemic circulation, and aortic pressure decreases. It falls to a minimal (diastolic) level before being boosted again by the next cardiac ejection. When heart rate decreases, there is a longer time between beats (ejections) and therefore a longer time for blood to run out of the aorta and into the systemic circulation. The blood pressure in the aorta falls to a lower level before the next cardiac ejection, and pulse pressure is increased (see Fig. 21–9B). A decrease in heart rate decreases the mean arterial pressure, because a decreased heart rate results in a decreased cardiac output.

Figure 21–9C shows the effect of a simultaneous

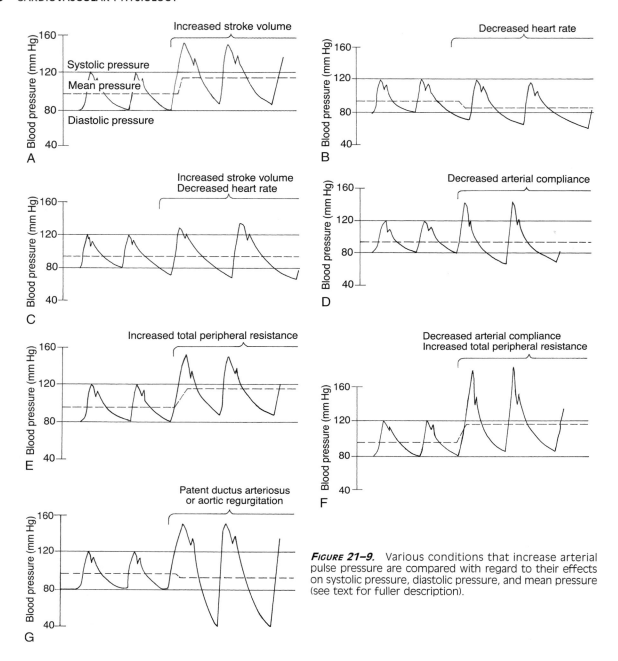

FIGURE 21–9. Various conditions that increase arterial pulse pressure are compared with regard to their effects on systolic pressure, diastolic pressure, and mean pressure (see text for fuller description).

increase in stroke volume and decrease in heart rate. In this example, cardiac output, which is stroke volume multiplied by heart rate, remains unchanged. Therefore, mean arterial pressure remains unchanged. However, pulse pressure is markedly increased as a result of the combined effects of an increase in stroke volume and a decrease in heart rate. Aerobic conditioning in humans, and in some animals, leads to increased stroke volume and decreased heart rate at rest. Therefore, in a well-trained athlete, mean arterial pressure is typically normal but pulse pressure is greater than normal. Palpation of the arteries of an athlete at rest reveals a strong, slow pulse.

A decrease in arterial compliance (stiffening of the arteries) is a third factor that tends to increase pulse pressure (see Fig. 21–9D). With each ventricular sys-

tole, the heart ejects blood into the aorta and large arteries, which distends these vessels. The stiffer the walls of the large arteries, the greater is the increase in pressure required to distend them. Arterial stiffening also decreases diastolic arterial pressure. This effect is harder to grasp intuitively but should not be surprising. Just as aortic pressure rises to higher than normal levels when the heart ejects blood into a stiff aorta, so also does aortic pressure fall to lower than normal levels when blood runs out of the stiff aorta between cardiac ejections. The higher systolic pressure and lower diastolic pressure are simply two direct consequences of the same phenomenon: decreased arterial compliance. The major arteries tend to become stiffer as a result of the normal aging process, and this accounts for the increase in pulse pressure that is typical in older humans and some animals.

In general, neither cardiac output nor TPR is affected by arterial stiffening. A healthy ventricle is able to generate the higher systolic pressures needed to eject blood into a stiff arterial system, although ventricular hypertrophy is sometimes triggered. TPR is not usually affected, because the arterioles remain normal. Even though the arteries are stiff, they retain their large diameters and therefore low resistance. *Mean* arterial pressure, the product of cardiac output and TPR, is generally unchanged by arterial stiffening.

Arteriolar vasoconstriction is a fourth factor that commonly increases pulse pressure (see Fig. 21–9E). In actuality, vasoconstriction does not affect pulse pressure directly but acts through a stiffening of the arteries. The mechanism is as follows: (1) vasoconstriction leads to an increase in total peripheral resistance, (2) blood backs up or accumulates in the large arteries, (3) mean arterial pressure increases, (4) the arteries become more distended than normal, and (5) distention forces the arteries toward their elastic limit, so they become stiffer than arteries under normal pressurization (Fig. 21–10). This stiffening of the arteries causes pulse pressure to increase.

Many human patients develop both stiffening of arteries (as a consequence of aging) and essential hypertension (caused by increased TPR). This combination produces dramatic increases in pulse pressure (see Figure 21–9F). An older person with severe hypertension might have a pulse pressure of 110 mm Hg (200 mm Hg systolic minus 90 mm Hg diastolic). Arterial hypertension and arterial stiffening are both less common in veterinary species.

In summary, pulse pressure tends to be increased by increased stroke volume, decreased heart rate, decreased arterial compliance, or vasoconstriction.

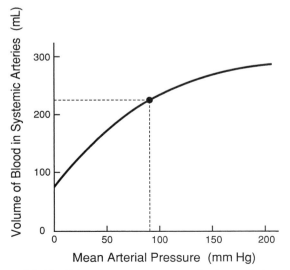

FIGURE 21–10. This volume-pressure graph shows that normal systemic arteries become stiffer (less compliant) when they are distended by an above-normal arterial pressure. (Recall that compliance is equal to the slope of a volume-pressure curve.)

Some of the cardiac defects that produce murmurs also cause characteristic changes in a pulse pressure. For example, a patient with patent ductus arteriosus has a large left ventricular stroke volume, which elevates aortic systolic pressure. Aortic diastolic pressure is much lower than normal because between cardiac ejections, blood runs out of the aorta by two pathways: into the systemic circuit and through the open ductus. Pulse pressure is dramatically increased. Aortic regurgitation causes a similar, characteristic increase in pulse pressure (see Fig. 21–9G). During diastole, blood leaves the aorta via two pathways: forward into the systemic circuit and backward (through the incompetent valve) into the left ventricle. Stroke volume is elevated because with each systole, the left ventricle ejects both the blood that has returned to it via the normal pathway and the regurgitant blood.

CLINICAL CORRELATIONS

Canine heartworm disease with pulmonary embolism

History You examine a 6-year-old male beagle that has been used as a hunting companion by his owner for several years. The owner reports that the dog tires more easily than usual and has developed a cough that is worse when exercising. You had treated this dog for a laceration when he was 3 years old, and your records indicate that the dog was otherwise in excellent health at that time. The owner acknowledges that the dog has not been given any immunizations or heartworm prophylactic medication for the past 2 years.

Clinical examination On physical examination of the dog, you note the cough reported by the owner and an apparent, modest accumulation of fluid in the abdominal cavity (ascites). You also note a systolic murmur that is heard the loudest over the left third and fourth intercostal spaces. The chest radiograph and electrocardiogram show evidence of right ventricular enlargement. In addition, the pulmonary vessels are more prominent than normal on the radiograph, and they are tortuous. You obtain a blood sample for centrifugation and use a pipette to apply a bit of the buffy coat onto a glass slide for microscopic examination. You see microfilaria of the type shed by adult canine heartworms *(Dirofilaria immitis)*. You diagnose canine heartworm parasitism.

Comment Mosquitoes transfer the microfilaria from the blood stream of an infected dog to the blood stream of a noninfected dog. The microfilaria develop into adult worms, which grow to a length of 10 to 20 cm while clinging to the walls of the pulmonary artery and its major branches. Heartworm infestation typically causes pulmonary arterial vessels to become enlarged and tortuous (twisted). In heavily infested dogs, adult worms also reside in the right ventricle and right ventricular outflow tract, where they cause pulmonic stenosis. The resulting turbulence during right ventricular ejection accounts for the murmur heard in this dog. The pulmonic stenosis and the increased pulmonary resistance created by the worms also lead to right ventricular hypertrophy, exercise intolerance, and ascites (review the Clinical Correlation in Chapter 20 for an explanation of why these complications develop). An additional problem is that the adult worms release substances into the circulation that disrupt some of the normal mechanisms of the body that adjust arteriolar diameter, control blood flow, and regulate arterial pressure. Heavily infested dogs become very ill.

Treatment   You advise the owner that the dog should be treated with an arsenic-containing medication that kills adult worms over a period of several days. You also warn the owner that the treatment of severely infested dogs is risky. Dead adult worms break away from the right ventricle and pulmonary artery and lodge in smaller pulmonary vessels. These vascular occlusions *(pulmonary emboli)* restrict pulmonary blood flow and reduce cardiac output. Therefore, it is necessary to keep the dog in a quiet, unstressed state for 8 to 10 days after beginning treatment. In addition to restricting pulmonary blood flow, the emboli are likely to cause inflammation and blood clots in the lungs. Pulmonary edema is expected. Pulmonary blood vessels may break down, allowing blood to enter the airways of the lungs. Respiratory failure is possible. Anti-inflammatory drugs are sometimes administered to reduce these complications.

With the owner's consent, you keep the dog at your clinic for 2 days (to allow him to become accustomed to the surroundings) and then begin treatment. During the next week, the dog becomes even more lethargic than before and begins to cough up blood. The dog has a low-grade fever (102° to 103°F), and his ascites becomes worse. However, his systolic murmur begins to fade. After 1 week, all the clinical signs have improved markedly. The dog is sent home for a prolonged period of recuperation. The long-term prognosis is good.

Bibliography

Berne RM, Levy MN: Cardiovascular Physiology, 7th ed. St. Louis: Mosby, 1997.

Butler J: The circulation of the lung. In Patton HD, Fuchs AF, Hille B, et al (eds): Textbook of Physiology, vol 2. Philadelphia: WB Saunders, 1989, p 961.

Dillon R: Dirofilariasis in dogs and cats. In Ettinger SJ, Feldman EC (eds): Textbook of Veterinary Internal Medicine: Diseases of the Dog and Cat, 5th ed. Philadelphia: WB Saunders, 2000, p 937.

Feigl EO: The arterial system. In Patton HD, Fuchs AF, Hille B, et al (eds): Textbook of Physiology, vol 2. Philadelphia: WB Saunders, 1989, p 849.

Milnor WR: Cardiovascular Physiology. New York: Oxford University Press, 1990.

Mohrman DE, Heller LJ: Cardiovascular Physiology, 4th ed. New York: McGraw-Hill, 1997.

PRACTICE QUESTIONS

1. If aortic compliance is decreased while heart rate, cardiac output, and TPR remain unchanged,
   a. pulse pressure will be unchanged.
   b. pulse pressure will increase.
   c. pulse pressure will decrease.
   d. one cannot know the effect on pulse pressure because stroke volume may have changed.
   e. one cannot know the effects on pulse pressure because mean aortic pressure may have changed.

2. Mean aortic pressure increases if
   a. stroke volume increases from 30 to 40 mL and heart rate decreases from 100 to 60 beats per minute.
   b. arterial compliance decreases.
   c. heart rate decreases.
   d. arterioles throughout the body dilate.
   e. TPR increases.

3. The following measurements are made on a dog: heart rate, 80 beats per minute; stroke volume, 30 mL; mean aortic pressure, 96 mm Hg; mean pulmonary artery pressure, 30 mm Hg; left atrial pressure, 5 mm Hg; and right atrial pressure, 12 mm Hg. TPR (taking into account both arterial and atrial pressures) is exactly
   a. 10.42 mm Hg/L/min.
   b. 12.50 mm Hg/L/min.
   c. 35.00 mm Hg/L/min.
   d. 37.92 mm Hg/L/min.
   e. 40.00 mm Hg/L/min.

4. A change from breathing normal air (21% O_2 and 0% CO_2) to breathing a gas mixture of 10% O_2 and 5% CO_2 causes pulmonary blood vessels to _____ and pulmonary resistance to _____.
   a. constrict; increase.
   b. constrict; decrease.
   c. dilate; increase.
   d. dilate; decrease.
   e. remain unchanged; remain unchanged.

5. Which of the following would cause the biggest decrease in coronary blood flow?
   a. Coronary arterioles constrict to half their normal diameter.
   b. Coronary arteries develop atherosclerosis, and lipid plaques plug up half of their normal cross-sectional area.
   c. Mean aortic pressure decreases to half its normal level.
   d. The resistance to coronary blood flow doubles.
   e. The resistance to coronary blood flow decreases to one-fourth its normal value.

PRACTICE ANSWERS

1. b   2. e   3. c   4. a   5. a

22

Capillaries and fluid exchange

1 Capillaries, the smallest blood vessels, are the sites for the exchange of water and solutes between the blood stream and the interstitial fluid

2 Lipid-soluble substances diffuse readily through capillary walls, whereas lipid-insoluble substances must pass through capillary pores

3 Fick's law of diffusion is a simple, mathematical accounting of the physical factors that affect the rate of diffusion

4 Water moves across capillary walls through both diffusion (osmosis) and bulk flow

5 The Starling equation quantifies the interaction of oncotic and hydrostatic forces acting on water

6 Several common physiologic changes alter the normal balance of Starling's forces and increase the filtration of water out of capillaries

7 Edema is a clinically noticeable excess of interstitial fluid

Capillaries, the smallest blood vessels, are the sites for the exchange of water and solutes between the blood stream and the interstitial fluid

Because of their small size, the capillaries are sometimes called the *microcirculation.* They are also called the *exchange vessels,* because the exchange of water and solutes between the blood stream and the interstitial fluid takes place across the walls of the capillaries. Each type of blood vessel in the body is structurally suited for its primary function, and the walls of the capillaries are especially well adapted for their exchange function.

Figure 22–1 shows the contrasting features of the walls of the various types of blood vessels. The distinguishing feature of the walls of the aorta and large arteries is the presence of a large amount of elastic material along with the smooth muscle. These vessels are called the *elastic vessels;* elasticity is necessary because the aorta and large arteries must distend with each pulsatile ejection of blood from the heart.

The arterial walls are also strong and quite stiff (low compliance). There is no contradiction in saying that the arteries are elastic and have low compliance. *Elasticity* denotes distensibility and an ability to return to the original shape after the distending force or pressure is removed. *Compliance* is a measure of how much force or pressure is required to achieve distention. The arteries are elastic, but a high pressure (systolic pressure) is required to distend them.

Small arteries, and particularly arterioles, have relatively thick walls with less elastic tissue and a predominance of smooth muscle, so they are called the *muscular vessels.* The muscle enables these vessels to constrict or dilate, which varies their resistance to blood flow. The muscular vessels vary the total peripheral resistance and direct blood flow toward or away from particular organs or particular regions within an organ.

Capillaries are the smallest vessels, being about 8 μm in diameter and about 0.5 mm long. Capillaries are so small that red blood cells (7.5 μm in diameter) must squeeze through in single file. Capillary walls consist of a single layer of endothelial cells. The small diameter of the capillaries and the thinness of their walls permit the blood within capillaries to pass close to the interstitial fluid outside the capillaries.

Venules and veins are larger than capillaries, and they have thicker walls. Venules and veins have both elastic tissue and smooth muscle in their walls. However, the walls of veins are not as thick or as muscular as the walls of arteries or arterioles. The primary role of veins is to serve as *reservoir vessels.* Veins are very compliant. In addition, it is normal for many veins in the body to be in a state of partial collapse. Therefore, substantial changes in venous blood volume can occur without much change in venous pressure.

Capillaries form a network (see Fig. 17–3). In most tissues, the capillary network is so dense that each cell of the tissue is within 100 μm of a capillary. However, not all of the capillaries of a tissue carry blood at all times. In most tissues, the arterioles alternate between constriction and dilation, so blood flow is periodically reduced or even stopped in most capillaries. Also, in some tissues (e.g., intestinal circulation), tiny cuffs of smooth muscle encircle capillaries at the points where they branch off from arterioles. Contraction of these *precapillary sphincters* can reduce or stop the flow of blood in individual capillaries. When the metabolic rate of a tissue increases (and therefore its need for blood flow increases), the arteri-

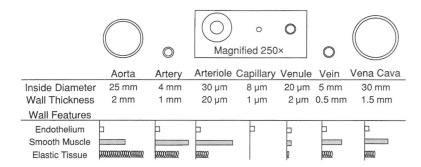

FIGURE 22–1. Each type of blood vessel in the systemic circulation is specifically suited to its particular function by its size, wall thickness, and wall composition. In this drawing, each type of vessel is shown in cross section. The drawings are to scale (the arteriole, capillary, and venule are magnified 250 times to make them visible). Also shown are the relative proportions of the three most important types of tissue found in blood vessel walls.

	Aorta	Artery	Arteriole	Capillary	Venule	Vein	Vena Cava
Inside Diameter	25 mm	4 mm	30 μm	8 μm	20 μm	5 mm	30 mm
Wall Thickness	2 mm	1 mm	20 μm	1 μm	2 μm	0.5 mm	1.5 mm

Wall Features

Endothelium
Smooth Muscle
Elastic Tissue

oles and precapillary sphincters still constrict periodically, but they spend more time in the dilated (relaxed) state. This increases the fraction of capillaries in which blood is flowing at any one time. At maximal metabolic rate (e.g., maximal exercise in a skeletal muscle), blood flows through all of the capillaries all the time. Sending blood flow to all of the capillaries simultaneously not only increases the total blood flow through a tissue but also minimizes the distance between each cell of the tissue and the nearest capillary carrying blood by bulk flow. Both these effects speed up diffusional exchange between the capillary blood and the tissue cells.

Lipid-soluble substances diffuse readily through capillary walls, whereas lipid-insoluble substances must pass through capillary pores

The rate of diffusional exchange between capillary blood and the surrounding interstitial fluid depends both on the features of the capillary wall and on the properties of the substance being exchanged. In most tissues, there are *water-filled pores*, or *clefts*, between the endothelial cells that form capillary walls (Fig. 22–2). These pores provide channels through which water and water-soluble (lipid-insoluble) substances can move from the capillary lumen to the interstitial space, or vice versa. Plasma electrolytes, glucose, and amino acids are among the lipid-insoluble substances that must pass through these water-filled channels. By contrast, lipid-soluble substances in blood, such as dissolved oxygen and carbon dioxide, fatty acids, ethanol, and some hormones, can diffuse through the endothelial cells that form the capillary wall. In the process of diffusion through an endothelial cell, a lipid-soluble substance passes through the cell membranes on both sides of the cell and through the cell cytoplasm. For a lipid-soluble substance, this process takes only a fraction of a second. In fact, the diffusional exchange of lipid-soluble substances is much more rapid than that of lipid-insoluble substances, because the lipid-insoluble substances are restricted to passage through the capillary pores, which constitute only about 1% of the total wall surface area of a typical capillary.

The characteristics of the capillary pores vary from tissue to tissue. Two extremes are found in the liver

and the brain. The capillary pores, or clefts, in the liver are so large that even plasma proteins like albumin and globulin can pass through them. This is an appropriate feature for the liver capillaries, because the plasma proteins are produced in the liver. The large clefts permit the newly synthesized protein molecules to enter the blood stream. The large pores in liver capillaries are also appropriate for the role of the liver in detoxification. Some toxins that become bound to plasma proteins are removed from the blood stream by the liver and chemically changed into less toxic substances. Because of their large pores, capillaries in the liver are called *fenestrated capillaries* ("capillaries with windows") (see Fig. 22–2, *bottom*).

The brain capillaries represent the other extreme in pore size. The pores of brain capillaries are so small that only water and electrolyte molecules can pass through them; not even glucose and amino acid molecules can pass through these tiny pores. The tight

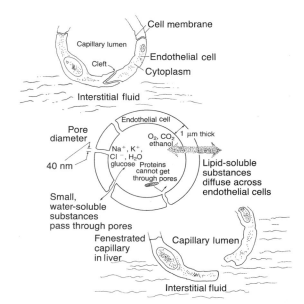

FIGURE 22–2. Capillaries in cross section. Most capillaries have pores, or clefts, between endothelial cells *(top)*. Water and lipid-insoluble compounds move between the capillary plasma and the interstitial fluid through these water-filled channels *(center)*. Lipid-soluble substances diffuse right through the capillary endothelial cells. The size of the capillary pores varies greatly from tissue to tissue, with the largest capillary pores being found in the liver *(bottom)*.

barrier provided between the blood stream and the brain tissue by the small pores is called the *blood-brain barrier* (see Chapter 14). One function of the blood-brain barrier is to protect brain neurons from exposure to toxic substances. Glucose is moved across the brain capillary endothelial cells by means of specialized protein carrier molecules that are embedded in the cell membranes of the endothelial cells. The energy to drive this *facilitated diffusion* comes from the glucose concentration difference between the blood and the brain interstitial fluid. Brain neurons require glucose to carry out their normal metabolism.

Fick's law of diffusion is a simple mathematical accounting of the physical factors that affect the rate of diffusion

Most of the factors that affect the rate of diffusional exchange between capillary blood and interstitial fluid have been mentioned. These factors include the distance to a capillary that is carrying blood by bulk flow, the size of the capillary pores, and the properties of the diffusing substance (i.e., lipid soluble versus lipid insoluble). The German physiologist Adoph Fick incorporated all of these factors into an equation: *Fick's law of diffusion.* Figure 22–3 shows how Fick's law applies to the diffusional exchange between capillary fluid and interstitial fluid. The rate of diffusion of any substance S depends, first, on the *concentration difference* between the substance in the capillary fluid and the substance in the interstitial fluid. Diffusion is driven by this concentration difference. Diffusion always proceeds from the area of higher concentration toward the area of lower concentration. Next, the rate of diffusion is determined by the *area available for diffusion.* For lipid-soluble substances, this area is equivalent to the total surface area of the capillaries. For lipid-insoluble substances, this area is much smaller, being equal to the area of the capillary pores or clefts.

The term Δx in the equation represents the *distance* over which diffusion must occur. The distance Δx equals the distance from a tissue cell to the nearest capillary that is carrying blood by bulk flow. The greater the distance from the tissue cells to the capillaries, the slower the rate of diffusional exchange of substances between that cell and the capillary blood. Therefore, Δx appears in the denominator in the equation.

The term D in the equation is a *diffusion coefficient.* The value of D increases with temperature, because diffusion is dependent on the random brownian motion of particles in solution, and the velocity of that motion increases with temperature. D is different for different substances. For example, D for carbon dioxide is about 20 times greater than D for oxygen. As a result, carbon dioxide diffuses much more rapidly than does oxygen for a given concentration difference, area, and diffusion distance. This difference is inconsequential under normal physiologic conditions. However, in certain disease states, the area available for diffusion decreases and the diffusion distance increases. Under these conditions, the delivery of oxygen to the metabolizing cells of a tissue generally becomes inadequate before the removal of carbon dioxide from the cells becomes inadequate. In other words, physiologic diffusion limitations generally cause bodily tissues to exhibit *hypoxia* (low oxygen levels) before they exhibit *hypercapnia* (elevated carbon dioxide levels).

Several of the factors that affect the rate of diffusion are physiologically adjustable. For example, in skeletal muscle at rest, the arterioles cycle between open and closed, and even when open, their diameter is small. At any one moment, blood flows through only about one fourth of the skeletal muscle capillaries. Blood sits still in the remainder of them. Nevertheless, this low and "part-time" blood flow through capillaries is adequate to deliver oxygen and nutrients to the resting skeletal muscle cells and to remove the small amounts of carbon dioxide and other waste products being produced by those cells. During exercise, however, the metabolic rate of the muscle cells increases by severalfold. To supply the needed blood flow, the

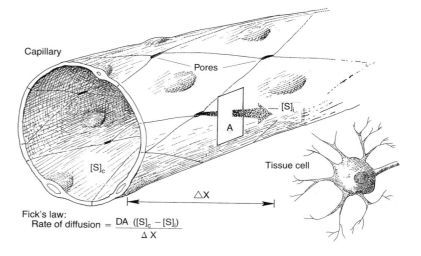

FIGURE 22–3. According to Fick's Law, the factors that affect the rate of diffusion of a substance S from the capillary plasma to the interstitial fluid next to a tissue cell are $[S]_c - [S]_i$, the concentration difference between the capillary plasma and interstitial fluid. A, the area available for diffusion; Δx, the distance involved; D, the diffusion coefficient.

Capillary

Pores

$[S]_i$

A

Tissue cell

$[S]_c$

$\triangle X$

Fick's law:
$$\text{Rate of diffusion} = \frac{DA\,([S]_c - [S]_i)}{\Delta X}$$

skeletal muscle arterioles dilate, and increasingly more of them remain open on a "full-time" basis as the level of exercise increases. Capillary blood flow likewise increases and becomes more continuous.

These changes act in three ways to speed the delivery of oxygen and metabolic substrates to the exercising muscle cells and to facilitate the removal of carbon dioxide and other metabolic waste products. First, when more capillaries carry blood, the area available for diffusion (A in Fick's diffusion equation) is increased. Second, because more capillaries carry blood, the distance between each exercising skeletal muscle cell and the nearest open capillary (Δx in the diffusion equation) is decreased. Third, the driving force for diffusion of oxygen (the oxygen concentration difference between the capillary blood and the interstitial fluid) is increased. The concentration difference is increased, first, because the greater blood flow brings more oxygenated blood into the tissue, which increases the concentration of oxygen in capillary blood. Second, the rapid utilization of oxygen by the exercising skeletal muscle cells decreases the concentration of oxygen within the skeletal muscle cells and in the surrounding interstitial fluid.

The same factors that increase the rate of oxygen diffusion during exercise increase the rate of delivery of glucose and other nutrients. Furthermore, the same factors act to increase the rate at which carbon dioxide and other metabolic products are removed from the tissue cells and into the blood stream. In the case of carbon dioxide and other metabolic products, the concentration is highest in the cells and lowest in the capillary plasma, so diffusional movement is from the cells toward the blood stream.

Water moves across capillary walls through both diffusion (osmosis) and bulk flow

The exchange of water between the capillary plasma and the interstitial fluid merits special consideration for two reasons. First, the forces that govern water movement are more complicated than the forces that affect solute movement. Second, the important clinical sign *edema* results from the accumulation of an excessive amount of water in the interstitial space.

As the preceding discussion emphasized, solutes such as oxygen, carbon dioxide, glucose, electrolytes, and fatty acids move between the capillary plasma and the interstitial fluid by diffusion. Water also moves by diffusion; the diffusional movement of water is called *osmosis*. The physical prerequisites for osmosis are (1) the presence of a *semipermeable membrane* (a membrane that is permeable to water but not to specific solutes) and (2) a difference in the total concentration of *impermeable solutes* on the two sides of the membrane.

The capillary wall constitutes a semipermeable membrane. Water readily passes through the capillary pores; however, in most organs the capillary walls are impermeable to the plasma proteins. (The molecules of albumin, globulin, and the other plasma proteins are just slightly too large to pass through the pores in most capillaries.) Normally, there are different concentrations of these impermeable proteins on the two sides of capillary walls. The normal concentration of plasma proteins is 7 g/dL within the capillary plasma and only 0.2 g/dL in the interstitial fluid. The higher protein concentration within the capillaries creates a tendency for water molecules to move through osmosis from the interstitial fluid into the capillary blood plasma. (Remember, when water moves through osmosis, it moves toward the side of the membrane with the higher concentration of impermeable solute.)

The tendency for water to move through diffusion is quantified by *osmotic pressure* (for details, review Chapter 1). The normal osmotic pressure created by the proteins in the plasma is 25 mm Hg; that is, the osmotic effect of the plasma proteins is equivalent to a pressure of 25 mm Hg driving water into the capillaries. The osmotic pressure created by the plasma proteins is also called *plasma oncotic pressure* or *colloid osmotic pressure*. (The term *colloid* is used because the plasma proteins are not in a true solution but rather in a colloidal suspension.)

Recall that a low concentration of plasma proteins is normally found in the interstitial fluid. The oncotic pressure created in the interstitial fluid by these proteins is normally only about 1 mm Hg. On balance, the osmotic effect of the capillary fluid is much greater than the osmotic effect of the interstitial fluid, so water would move through osmosis from the interstitial fluid into the capillaries. The movement of water in this direction is called *reabsorption*. The movement of water in the opposite direction, from the capillary plasma into the interstitial fluid, is called *filtration*.

The *net oncotic pressure difference* favors reabsorption. Net oncotic pressure difference is calculated by subtracting the oncotic pressure of interstitial fluid from the oncotic pressure of capillary blood (e.g., 25 mm Hg − 1 mm Hg = 24 mm Hg).

In addition to being affected by diffusional (osmotic) forces, water responds to hydrostatic pressure differences across the capillary wall. Hydrostatic pressure differences between the capillary plasma and the interstitial fluid cause water to move through bulk flow through the capillary pores. The hydrostatic pressure within the capillaries (capillary blood pressure) is higher at the arteriolar end of capillaries than at the venous end (see Fig. 21–1). However, a pressure of 18 mm Hg is taken as a representative average. Interstitial fluid hydrostatic pressure is normally about −7 mm Hg. (The negative sign simply means that interstitial fluid pressure is *less*, but only slightly less, than atmospheric pressure.) The negative interstitial fluid pressure (−7 mm Hg) together with the positive capillary hydrostatic pressure (18 mm Hg) creates a hydrostatic pressure difference of 25 mm Hg across the wall of a typical capillary. This hydrostatic pressure difference tends to force water out of the capillaries and into the interstitial spaces; that is, the *net hydrostatic pressure difference* favors filtration.

The net hydrostatic pressure difference (which favors filtration) nearly balances the net oncotic pressure difference (which favors reabsorption). However, the balance is rarely perfect. Usually, the hydrostatic pressure difference slightly exceeds the oncotic pressure difference, so there is a small, net filtration of water out of the capillaries. This water would simply accumulate in the interstitial spaces and cause swelling there were it not for the lymph vessels, which collect excess interstitial fluid and return it to the blood stream via the subclavian veins (Fig. 22–4).

The hydrostatic pressures in the capillaries and in the interstitial fluid are, by convention, always measured relative to atmospheric pressure. Thus, to say that interstitial pressure is normally negative does not imply that a vacuum exists but only that the interstitial pressure is slightly below atmospheric pressure. If the interstitial spaces of the body were always pressurized more than atmospheric pressure, then all parts of the body would bulge outward. The subatmospheric interstitial fluid pressure probably accounts for the fact that the skin normally stays snug against the underlying tissue and that some body surfaces normally have a concave shape (e.g., the axillary space or the orbits of the eyes).

The Starling equation quantifies the interaction of oncotic and hydrostatic forces acting on water

The following equation expresses mathematically the interaction between osmotic pressures and hydrostatic pressures in determination of the net force (net pressure) acting on water. Nominal values for each pressure are also listed:

$$\text{net pressure} = (P_c - P_i) - (\pi_c - \pi_i),$$

where P_c is capillary hydrostatic pressure, P_i is interstitial fluid hydrostatic pressure, π_c is capillary plasma oncotic pressure, and π_i is interstitial fluid oncotic pressure.

Nominal values for systemic capillaries are as follows: P_c of 18 mm Hg; P_i, -7 mm Hg; π_c, 25 mm Hg; and π_i, 1 mm Hg. The solution of the equation with nominal values is therefore

$$\begin{aligned}\text{net pressure} &= (18\,\text{mm Hg} - -7\,\text{mm Hg}) \\ &\quad - (25\,\text{mm Hg} - 1\,\text{mm Hg}) \\ &= +1\,\text{mm Hg}.\end{aligned}$$

A positive net pressure favors filtration (a negative net pressure would indicate that reabsorption is favored). The small magnitude of the net pressure (1 mm Hg) indicates that the hydrostatic and osmotic forces that affect water are nearly in balance (i.e., there is only a slight tendency for filtration). The quantitative analysis of how oncotic and hydrostatic pressures affect water movement across capillary walls was first derived by Ernest Henry Starling (the same scientist for whom Starling's law of the heart is named). Therefore, the oncotic and hydrostatic pressures that act on water are often called *Starling forces*. Furthermore, the tendency for the net oncotic effect to be closely balanced by the net hydrostatic effect is often referred to as *the balance of Starling forces*. Star-

ling realized that the actual rate of water movement across capillary walls is affected both by the magnitude of the imbalance between hydrostatic and oncotic forces and by the permeability of the capillary wall to water. These ideas are expressed in the following equation, which indicates that the movement of water is equal to the permeability of the capillary wall (given as the filtration coefficient K_f) multiplied by the net difference between the hydrostatic and oncotic pressures:

$$\begin{array}{l}\text{transcapillary} \\ \text{water flux}\end{array} = K_f\,[(P_c - P_i) - (\pi_c - \pi_i)].$$

Examination of this equation reveals that the tendency for the filtration of water out of capillaries can be enhanced by (1) increasing the hydrostatic difference between capillary blood and interstitial fluid, (2) decreasing the osmotic tendency for water to be reabsorbed, or (3) increasing the permeability of the capillary to water (i.e., increasing the filtration coefficient).

Several common physiologic changes alter the normal balance of Starling forces and increase the filtration of water out of capillaries

An increase in capillary hydrostatic pressure (P_c) favors the greater filtration of water. Capillary hydrostatic pressure can be increased by an increase in arterial blood pressure or by a decrease in arteriolar resistance. An increase in arterial pressure causes more pressure to be transmitted down through the arterioles and into the capillaries. Likewise, a decrease in arteriolar resistance (e.g., a dilation of the arterioles) allows a greater portion of the arterial pressure to be transmitted into the capillaries. Capillary hydrostatic pressure can also be increased by a "backing up" ("damming up") of venous blood. For example, an increase in central venous pressure causes blood to accumulate in the capillaries and raises capillary pressure. An obstruction to venous outflow (e.g., too tight a dressing on a limb) also causes blood to back up in the capillaries, which increases capillary hydrostatic pressure.

Although several factors commonly affect capillary hydrostatic pressure, the only important determinant of interstitial fluid hydrostatic pressure is the volume of fluid present in the interstitial space. An accumulation of interstitial fluid increases interstitial hydrostatic pressure. Removal of interstitial fluid decreases the pressure. As stated earlier, interstitial fluid hydrostatic pressure is usually slightly subatmospheric (e.g., -7 mm Hg). When interstitial fluid hydrostatic pressure rises above atmospheric pressure, the accumulation of interstitial fluid becomes clinically noticeable as a swelling, or *edema*.

The net oncotic pressure depends on the concentrations of proteins in the capillary plasma and in the interstitial fluid. The normal protein concentration in plasma is 7 g/dL, which results in a plasma oncotic pressure of 25 mm Hg. Any alteration in the concen-

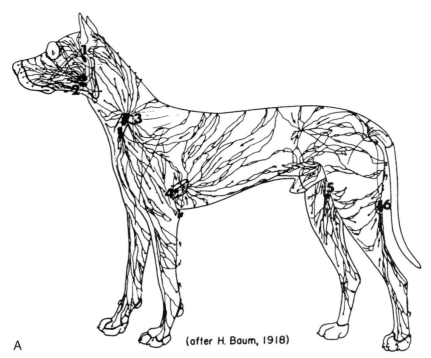

A

(after H. Baum, 1918)

FIGURE 22–4. Anatomic *(A)* and schematic *(B)* overviews of the lymphatic system. The lymphatic vessels collect excess interstitial fluid from tissues throughout the body (including the lungs) and carry it to the subclavian veins, where the lymph reenters the blood stream. Lymph moves through lymph vessels via bulk flow. The driving force for this flow is interstitial fluid hydrostatic pressure minus subclavian vein pressure. Lymph flow is also promoted by the massaging action exerted on lymph vessels by contraction and relaxation of skeletal muscles. The lymph vessels contain one-way valves, which prevent the backflow of lymph. Thus, the massaging action of skeletal muscles propels lymph in one direction only: toward the subclavian vein. In addition, some lymph vessels have smooth muscle in their walls, and the alternating contraction and relaxation of this smooth muscle also propels lymph flow toward the subclavian veins. The numbers in *A* identify the major lymph nodes. *(A* from Getty R: Sisson and Grossman's The Anatomy of the Domestic Animal, vol 2. Philadelphia: WB Saunders, 1975, p 1653.)

tration of proteins in the capillary plasma alters the plasma oncotic pressure.

Similarly, changes in the interstitial protein concentration alter interstitial fluid oncotic pressure. Under normal circumstances, protein molecules are slightly too large to pass through the capillary pores or clefts. The main route for the delivery of plasma proteins into the interstitial fluid is through the process of *pinocytosis*. Pinocytosis involves the invagination of the capillary endothelial cell membrane to form an intracellular vesicle that contains plasma, including plasma proteins. This is also called *endocytosis*. Next, these vesicles cross the capillary endothelial cell from the side facing the blood stream to the side facing the interstitial fluid. Then, the vesicles containing plasma fuse with the outer membrane of the capillary endothelial cells; the vesicles discharge their contents into the interstitial space. This is called *exocytosis*. An increase in pinocytotic activity increases the delivery of plasma proteins into the interstitial space and increases interstitial fluid oncotic pressure. In addition, abnormal circumstances (e.g., tissue inflammation) can cause the capillary pores to open wide enough that plasma proteins can pass through.

Plasma proteins are removed from the interstitial space through lymph flow. The lymphatic vessels carry the interstitial fluid, including any plasma pro-

teins that are contained in it, to the thorax, where the fluid enters the subclavian veins.

The role of lymphatic flow in prevention of the accumulation of excessive interstitial fluid is especially important in the lungs. Lung capillaries are more permeable to plasma proteins than are most capillaries in the systemic circulation. As a result, the oncotic pressure of interstitial fluid in the lungs is normally about 18 mm Hg. Capillary hydrostatic pressure in the lungs is generally about 12 mm Hg. (This value is lower than the capillary hydrostatic pressure for systemic capillaries, because pulmonary arterial pressure is so much lower than systemic arterial pressure.) Interstitial hydrostatic pressure in the lungs is generally about −5 mm Hg (the same as intrapleural pressure). Summation of these Starling forces for lung capillaries yields the following:

$$\begin{aligned} \text{net pressure} &= (P_c - P_i) - (\pi_c - \pi_i) \\ &= (12 \text{ mm Hg} - -5 \text{ mm Hg}) \\ &\quad - (25 \text{ mm Hg} - 18 \text{ mm Hg})] \\ &= +10 \text{ mm Hg} \end{aligned}$$

A net pressure of +10 mm Hg indicates that there is a substantial driving force for filtration of fluid out of the capillaries and into the lung interstitial spaces. The lung interstitial spaces would fill rapidly with water, and pulmonary edema would develop, were it

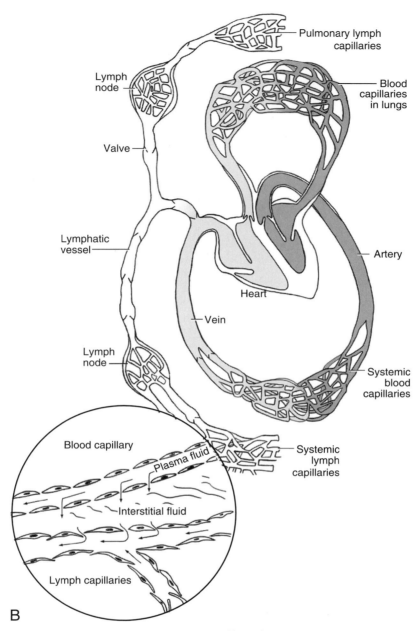

Pulmonary lymph
capillaries

Lymph
node

Blood
capillaries
in lungs

Valve

Lymphatic
vessel

Artery

Heart

Vein

Lymph
node

Systemic
blood
capillaries

Blood capillary

Plasma fluid

Interstitial fluid

Systemic
lymph
capillaries

Lymph capillaries

B

FIGURE 22–4 Continued.

not for the well-developed system of lymph vessels in the lungs. These vessels continuously remove interstitial fluid and prevent its excessive accumulation.

Edema is a clinically noticeable excess of interstitial fluid

Edema is a common clinical problem. Edema results either from excessive filtration of fluid out of capillaries or from depressed lymphatic function. One common cause is increased venous pressure. Increased venous pressure can result from the application of a too-tight dressing on the extremity of an animal. The resulting constriction of the veins impedes the out-

flow of venous blood from the limb. Blood backs up in the limb veins, which increases venous pressure. Blood then backs up in the capillaries and increases capillary hydrostatic pressure. As shown in Figure 22–5, the increase in capillary hydrostatic pressure leads to an excessive filtration of capillary fluid into the interstitial space. When this accumulation of fluids becomes clinically noticeable, the patient is said to exhibit edema.

Three factors (safety factors) limit the degree of edema. All three safety factors depend on the fact that an increased interstitial fluid volume leads to an increase in interstitial fluid hydrostatic pressure. The first safety factor is that the increased interstitial fluid pressure acts directly to oppose or limit filtration.

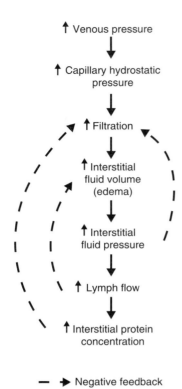

Figure 22–5. An increase in venous pressure leads to an increase in interstitial fluid volume (edema). The *dashed lines* indicate the effects of the three safety factors against edema. First, an increase in interstitial fluid hydrostatic pressure reduces the rate of filtration back toward normal. Second, an increase in lymph flow reduces interstitial fluid volume back toward normal. Third, a decrease in interstitial fluid protein concentration reduces the rate of filtration back toward normal.

Interstitial fluid pressure does not have to rise above capillary hydrostatic pressure to limit edema. Any increase in interstitial fluid pressure (e.g., from a normal value of −7 to +2 mm Hg) helps to change the net balance of the Starling forces in the direction of reducing excessive filtration.

The second safety factor against edema is that increased interstitial fluid pressure promotes lymph flow. Lymph flow removes edema fluid from the tissue and therefore helps to limit the degree of edema.

The third safety factor is an indirect consequence of increased lymph flow. Recall that interstitial fluid normally has a small amount of plasma protein present in it, usually as the result of pinocytosis. This protein exerts a small but significant oncotic pressure that favors filtration. As lymph carries away interstitial fluid under these circumstances, the proteins originally present in the interstitial fluid are carried away by the lymph, and fluid relatively free of proteins is being added to the interstitial space by the increased filtration. Therefore, the interstitial protein concentration and interstitial fluid oncotic pressures decrease, and this helps reduce filtration.

To summarize, venous obstruction causes capillary hydrostatic pressure to increase, which increases filtration. Edema develops. Then, three safety factors

come into play to limit the degree of edema. A steady-state degree of edema is eventually reached, wherein interstitial fluid is removed by lymph vessels as fast as it is filtered.

Another common clinical situation that leads to an increased venous pressure (and therefore edema) is heart failure. If the right ventricle fails (i.e., if the right ventricular contractility decreases), blood backs up or pools in the right atrium and the venae cavae. This increase in venous and atrial pressures is beneficial in one respect: it increases preload, which helps promote diastolic filling of the failing ventricle. An increased diastolic ventricular volume helps restore the stroke volume of the failing right ventricle back toward its normal level (recall Starling's law of the heart). Although the increased venous pressure is beneficial in terms of restoring the stroke volume toward normal, the increased venous pressure often leads to excessive capillary filtration and edema in the systemic organs. *Systemic edema* therefore is a common complication of right-sided heart failure. The edema is often most noticeable in the dependent regions of the body, such as the lower extremities, particularly if the patient remains standing for a long time. Systemic edema also is commonly noted in the abdomen. When edema develops in the abdominal organs, excess interstitial fluid tends to ooze out and accumulate in the peritoneal space. Excessive fluid in the peritoneum is called *ascites*. Marked ascites is common in patients with right-sided heart failure.

Failure of the left ventricle leads to increased left atrial pressure and increased pulmonary venous pressure. The result is an increase in capillary filtration in the lungs, which leads to an increase in the amount of interstitial fluid in the lung tissue, or *pulmonary edema*. In extreme cases, some of the excess interstitial fluid oozes into the alveolar and bronchial air spaces of the lungs, so that frank fluid is found in the airways. Such a patient typically coughs up a frothy fluid.

A decreased plasma protein concentration is another common cause of edema (Fig. 22–6). One common cause of decreased plasma protein concentration is a decrease in the rate of plasma protein production by the liver. This occurs in malnutrition and leads to the clinical syndrome of *kwashiorkor*. Victims of kwashiorkor typically look emaciated, except that the abdomen is grossly distended by ascites (edema fluid in the peritoneum). Another cause of abnormally low plasma protein concentration is an increase in the rate of loss of proteins from the body. Protein loss occurs in kidney disease. For example, in *nephrotic syndrome*, the kidney glomerular capillaries become permeable to plasma proteins. Plasma proteins leave the blood stream and enter the urinary tubules (nephrons) of the kidney. A chronic loss of proteins in the urine reduces the plasma protein concentration. Hence, the presence of substantial amounts of plasma protein in the urine is an alarming clinical sign.

Severe burns are another common cause of the loss of plasma proteins from the body. The capillaries of

Edema Caused by Hypoproteinemia

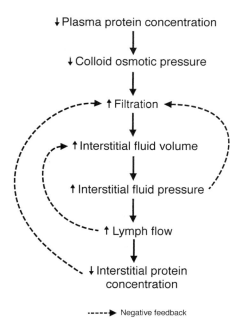

----→ Negative feedback

FIGURE 22-6. A decrease in plasma protein concentration leads to edema, but three safety factors limit the degree of the edema, just as shown in Figure 22-5.

burned skin become permeable to both fluid and proteins. Substantial amounts of plasma can leave the body through these damaged capillaries. The presence of plasma proteins in the fluid weeping from a burn site accounts for the typical yellow color of that fluid. If the water and electrolytes lost through burns are replaced through the intravenous administration of saline or lactated Ringer's solution or through the ingestion of salt and water and if the plasma proteins are not replaced, the plasma protein concentration decreases.

Whether a decrease in plasma protein concentration results from decreased production or increased loss, it leads to a decrease in plasma colloid osmotic pressure. This alters the balance of the Starling forces in a direction that favors excessive filtration of fluid from the capillaries (see Fig. 22-6). Interstitial fluid accumulates and edema is noticed. However, the same three safety factors that limited edema in the case of increased venous pressure (see Fig. 22-5) also operate in the case of decreased plasma protein concentration. The degree of edema is limited by (1) an increased interstitial fluid pressure, (2) an increased lymph flow, and (3) a decreased interstitial protein concentration.

Another cause of edema is lymphatic obstruction. Clinically, this situation is called *lymphedema.* Inflammatory diseases and cancers that produce obstruction of the lymphatic vessels cause lymphedema. Also, in certain parasitic diseases, microfilaria lodge in the lymph nodes and obstruct lymph flow. Filarial parasites cause the pronounced edema seen in cases of *elephantiasis.* Lymphedema also occurs as a second-

ary consequence of surgical procedures that damage lymph nodes. A common example of this in human medicine is the edema of the arm that follows radical mastectomy. The removal of axillary lymph nodes during radical mastectomy creates scar tissue that impairs lymphatic drainage from the arm.

Figure 22-7 traces the causes of edema after lymphatic obstruction and shows why lymphedema is clinically so troublesome. Lymphatic obstruction decreases lymph flow. Interstitial fluid accumulates instead of being removed, and edema results. The accumulation of edema fluid raises interstitial fluid pressure, which acts as a safety factor to limit the excess capillary filtration. However, the second and third safety factors that were discussed earlier are absent in the case of lymphedema, because these safety factors depend on an increase in lymph flow. In lymphedema, a decreased lymph flow is the causative problem, so there cannot be an increased lymph flow (second safety factor) to compensate for the edema. An additional complicating factor with lymphatic obstruction is that interstitial proteins accumulate instead of being carried away by the lymph. Therefore, the third safety factor that protects against edema (decreased interstitial fluid oncotic pressure) is also compromised in lymphedema.

Another cause of edema is physical injury or allergic reactions to antigen challenges. Physical trauma, like a scratch or a cut on the skin, results in a localized bump or swelling. A similar swelling is observed when the skin reacts to an irritating agent or antigen challenge. An allergic swelling can also occur in bronchial tissue during an asthmatic reaction. The edema of asthma can be life threatening, because it limits air

Edema Caused by Lymphatic Obstruction

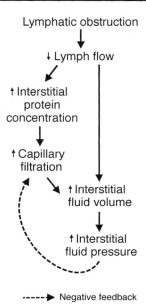

----→ Negative feedback

FIGURE 22-7. Lymphatic obstruction leads to edema. Lymphedema is clinically troublesome because only one of the normal three safety factors is operative to limit the degree of edema.

flow to the lungs. As shown in Figure 22–8, an injury or antigen challenge leads to the release of the chemical *histamine* from mast cells in the affected tissue. Histamine has two effects that cause edema. First, histamine increases the permeability of capillaries to proteins. As proteins leave the blood stream and accumulate in the interstitial space of the damaged tissue, they increase the interstitial fluid oncotic pressure, which promotes filtration of fluid. Second, histamine promotes filtration by relaxing arteriolar smooth muscle. The arterioles dilate, and the resulting decrease in arteriolar resistance allows more of the arterial blood pressure to impinge on the capillaries. This leads to an increase in the capillary hydrostatic pressure, which promotes filtration. Although histamine promotes excess filtration and edema through two mechanisms, all three safety factors that protect against edema are intact and act to limit the degree of edema.

Other situations also cause edema, but the examples discussed here cover some of the most common causes of clinical edema and reinforce an understanding of the interplay of the osmotic and hydrostatic forces that act on water to govern its filtration out of capillaries or reabsorption into capillaries.

CLINICAL CORRELATIONS

Acute protein-losing enteropathy in a horse

History   You are called to a home a few miles from your clinic by parents who are concerned about their daughter's 4-year-old quarter horse. They report that the horse is listless and has had diarrhea for 2 days.

Clinical examination   You arrive at the client's home to find that the horse is stabled in a small barn with no access to pasture. Poor-quality grass hay is stacked in the barn. On physical examination, you find the horse to be somewhat emaciated, with dry mucous membranes, a foul-smelling diarrhea, and a fast heart rate (tachycardia). When you pinch up a section of the horse's skin, it falls back to the normal position slowly, which indicates dehydration.

You take a blood sample and then begin an intravenous administration of polyionic fluid (lactated Ringer's solution). You tell the clients that you will return later. Analysis of the blood sample indicates a hematocrit of 55% (the normal range for the horse is 35% to 45%) and a plasma protein concentration of 4.5 g/dL (the normal range is 5.9 to 7.8 g/dL). You become concerned that the administration of fluids, without replacement of plasma proteins, will exaggerate the horse's hypoproteinemia, so you arrange to obtain plasma from a donor horse, and you return to examine the sick horse. You find the horse is still listless. Edema is now evident along the ventral abdomen and in the limbs.

Comment   Acute enteropathy (intestinal disorder) often causes diarrhea. The loss of water and solutes leads to dehydration. Before treatment, blood volume and interstitial fluid volume are both reduced. The hematocrit (fraction of cells in blood) is typically elevated, because fluid is removed from the blood stream but blood cells are not. In some forms of enteropathy (called protein-losing enteropathy), the capillaries in the intestine become leaky to plasma proteins. Albumin, in particular, moves from the blood stream into the intestinal lumen and is eliminated in the feces.

This horse has a severe shortage of plasma proteins. The shortage of plasma proteins probably resulted from a combination of poor nutrition (which depresses the production of plasma proteins by the liver) and the protein-losing enteropathy. The deficit of plasma proteins in this horse is even more severe than might be suspected on the basis of the plasma protein concentration of 4.5 g/dL, because this value is the net result of two opposing processes. The loss of protein in the diarrhea lowers the plasma protein concentration, but the dehydration raises the plasma protein concentration.

The administration of intravenous fluids added water and electrolytes to the circulating blood volume, but the plasma proteins remaining in the blood stream were further diluted. As a result, plasma oncotic pressure decreased even further, and this led to excess filtration of water out of capillaries and into the interstitial space. The result was edema, especially in the dependent regions of the body (ventral abdomen and legs). Restora-

Edema Caused by Injury or Allergic Reaction

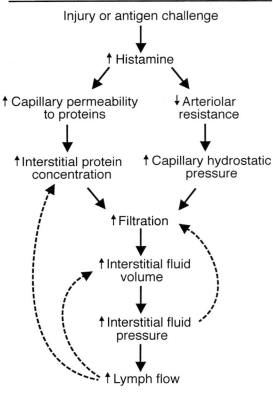

FIGURE 22–8. Histamine mediates the changes that lead to edema in the case of a physical injury or antigen challenge. The normal three safety factors against edema are intact and help to limit the degree of edema. Treatment with an antihistamine (a drug that blocks histamine receptors on arterioles and capillaries) also helps to reduce edema in these cases.

tion of a normal plasma protein concentration would reverse the edema.

Treatment The enteropathy in cases such as this one is often self-limiting. Therefore, the aim of treatment should be to remedy the dehydration, the electrolyte loss, and the plasma protein deficit. Intravenous administration of both polyionic fluids and plasma is usually effective. Better nutrition, regular worming, and improved stable management would be important steps for long-term health.

Bibliography

Berne RM, Levy MN: Cardiovascular Physiology, 7th ed. St. Louis: Mosby, 1997.

Bolton GR, Ettinger SJ: Peripheral edema. In Ettinger SJ (ed): Textbook of Veterinary Internal Medicine. Philadelphia: WB Saunders, 1989, p 41.

Cunningham SL: The physiology of body fluids. In Patton HD, Fuchs AF, Hille B, et al (eds): Textbook of Physiology, vol 2. Philadelphia: WB Saunders, 1989, p 1098.

Guyton AC, Hall JE: Textbook of Medical Physiology, 10th ed. Philadelphia: WB Saunders, 2000, pp 162–174, 444–451.

Milnor WR: Cardiovascular Physiology. New York: Oxford University Press, 1990.

Renkin EM: Microcirculation and exchange. In Patton HD, Fuchs AF, Hille B, et al (eds): Textbook of Physiology, vol 2. Philadelphia: WB Saunders, 1989, p 860.

Taylor FGR: Differential diagnosis of dependent edema. In Robinson NE (ed): Current Therapy in Equine Medicine 4. Philadelphia: WB Saunders, 1997, p 269.

Ware WA, Bonagura JD: Pulmonary edema. In Fox RR (ed): Canine and Feline Cardiology. New York: Churchill Livingstone, 1988, p 205.

PRACTICE QUESTIONS

1. Which of the following will *not* cause pulmonary edema?
   a. An increase in pulmonary capillary permeability to protein.
   b. A blockage of pulmonary lymph vessels.
   c. An increase in left atrial pressure.
   d. A constriction of pulmonary arterioles.
   e. Left-sided heart failure.

2. A patient with a form of protein-losing kidney disease has a plasma colloid osmotic pressure of 10 mm Hg. The patient has edema but is not getting any worse. Blood pressure and heart rate are normal.

Which of the following is probably preventing further edema?
   a. Increased interstitial fluid hydrostatic pressure.
   b. Increased capillary hydrostatic pressure.
   c. Decreased lymph flow.
   d. Increased plasma sodium ion concentration.
   e. Increased interstitial fluid oncotic pressure.

3. The following parameters were measured in the microcirculation of a skeletal muscle: P_c (capillary hydrostatic pressure), 34 mm Hg; P_i (interstitial fluid hydrostatic pressure), 10 mm Hg; π_c (capillary plasma oncotic pressure), 24 mm Hg; and π_i (interstitial fluid oncotic pressure), 1 mm Hg. Which of the following is true?
   a. These conditions would favor filtration.
   b. These conditions would favor reabsorption.
   c. These conditions would favor neither filtration nor reabsorption.
   d. It is not clear what these conditions favor because the concentration of plasma protein is not specified.

4. During a 30-minute hemorrhage, the mean arterial pressure of a horse decreases from 90 to 75 mm Hg. The heart rate increases from 40 to 90 beats per minute. The skin becomes cold. After the hemorrhage, you take a blood sample and measure the hematocrit, which is 28%. It is most likely that
   a. capillary hydrostatic pressure is increased.
   b. interstitial fluid volume is decreased.
   c. interstitial fluid pressure is increased.
   d. capillary colloid osmotic pressure is increased.
   e. arteriolar resistance has decreased.

5. The rate of diffusion of glucose molecules from capillary blood to interstitial fluid is most directly affected by
   a. the voltage difference between capillary blood and interstitial fluid.
   b. the interstitial fluid hydrostatic pressure.
   c. the size and number of capillary pores.
   d. the amount of oxygen in the blood.
   e. the hematocrit.

PRACTICE ANSWERS

1. d   2. a   3. a   4. b   5. c

23

Local control of blood flow

1 Vascular resistance is affected by intrinsic and extrinsic control mechanisms

2 Metabolic control of blood flow is a local mechanism that matches the blood flow of a tissue to its metabolic rate

3 Autoregulation is a relative constancy of blood flow in an organ despite changes in perfusion pressure

4 Regardless of the status of arterioles, mechanical compression can reduce blood flow to a tissue

▬ Vascular resistance is affected by intrinsic and extrinsic control mechanisms

As described in Chapter 21, the blood flow through any organ or tissue is determined by the perfusion pressure (arterial pressure minus venous pressure) and by the resistance of the blood vessels of the organ and no other factors:

blood flow = perfusion pressure/vascular resistance

All of the organs of the systemic circulation are exposed to the same perfusion pressure. The differences in blood flow to the various organs result solely from their different vascular resistances. The vascular resistance of an organ is determined mainly by the diameter of its arterioles. Thus, arteriolar vasodilation and vasoconstriction are the mechanisms that increase or decrease the blood flow in one organ relative to another organ.

In general, the factors that affect arteriolar resistance can be divided into intrinsic and extrinsic factors. *Extrinsic control mechanisms* act from outside a tissue, through nerves or hormones, to alter arteriolar resistance. *Intrinsic control* is exerted by local mechanisms within a tissue. For example, as described in Chapter 22, histamine is released from mast cells of tissues in response to injury or during allergic reactions. Histamine acts locally on the arteriolar smooth muscle to relax it. Dilation of the arterioles decreases arteriolar resistance and therefore increases the blood flow to the tissue. Histamine is an example of a *paracrine*: a substance released from one type of cell in a tissue that acts on another cell type in the same tissue to alter its function. A second example of intrinsic control is the arteriolar dilation and increased blood flow during exercise in skeletal muscle. This example illustrates the general phenomenon of *metabolic control* of blood flow: tissues tend to increase their blood flow whenever their metabolic rate increases.

Although the arterioles in all tissues are affected by both intrinsic and extrinsic mechanisms, intrinsic mechanisms predominate over extrinsic mechanisms in the control of arterioles in the coronary circulation, brain, and working skeletal muscle. By contrast, extrinsic mechanisms predominate over intrinsic mechanisms in the control of blood flow to the kidneys, splanchnic organs, and resting skeletal muscle. Skin is an example of a tissue in which both intrinsic and extrinsic control mechanisms have strong influences. In general, local (intrinsic) control dominates extrinsic control in the so-called *critical tissues*: those that must have sufficient blood flow to meet their metabolic needs on a second-by-second basis for an animal to survive. Extrinsic control dominates intrinsic control in tissues that can withstand temporary reductions in blood flow (and metabolism) to make extra blood available for the critical tissues.

▬ Metabolic control of blood flow is a local mechanism that matches the blood flow of a tissue to its metabolic rate

Metabolic control of blood flow is the most important local control mechanism. For example, metabolic control accounts for the huge increase in blood flow through a skeletal muscle as it goes from rest to maximal exercise. The functional significance of metabolic control of blood flow is that it matches the blood flow in a tissue to the metabolic rate of the tissue. An increase in tissue blood flow in response to increased metabolic rate is called *active hyperemia* (*hyper* means "elevated," *emia* refers to blood, and the word *active* implies an increased metabolic rate).

Metabolic control of blood flow works by means of chemical changes in the tissue. When the metabolic rate of a tissue increases, its consumption of oxygen increases and there is an increased rate of production

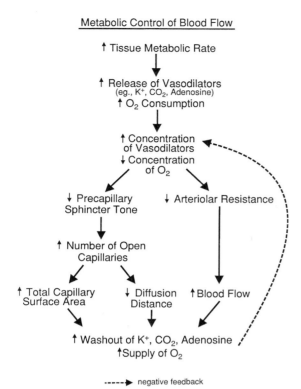

Metabolic Control of Blood Flow

FIGURE 23–1. Metabolic control of blood flow is a local (intrinsic) mechanism that acts within a tissue to match blood flow to the metabolic rate. As a tissue becomes more active metabolically, the metabolic control mechanism increases blood flow and thereby regulates the concentration of oxygen and metabolic products in the tissue.

of metabolic products, including carbon dioxide, adenosine, and lactic acid. Also, some K^+ moves from the intracellular fluid to the interstitial fluid. Therefore, as the metabolism of a tissue increases, the interstitial concentration of oxygen decreases and the interstitial concentrations of metabolic products and K^+ increase. All of these changes have the same effect on arteriolar smooth muscle: they relax it. The arterioles dilate and vascular resistance decreases. More blood flows through the tissue. Low levels of oxygen and high concentrations of metabolic products and K^+ also cause relaxation of the precapillary sphincters (in the tissues that have them), which opens more of the capillaries in the tissue to blood flow. As explained in Chapter 22, the opening of more capillaries decreases the diffusion distance between fresh, oxygenated blood and the metabolizing cells of the tissue. Opening more capillaries also increases the total capillary surface area for diffusional exchange. The net result of the increased blood flow, the decreased diffusion distance, and the increased total capillary surface area is a more rapid delivery of oxygen and other metabolic substrates to the tissue and a more rapid removal of metabolic waste products from the tissue.

Metabolic control of blood flow involves negative feedback. The accumulation of metabolic products and the lack of oxygen initiate vasodilation and increase blood flow, which removes the accumulating

metabolic products and delivers additional oxygen. A new balance is reached when the increased blood flow closely matches the increased metabolic needs of the tissue. The major features of metabolic control of blood flow are summarized in Figure 23–1.

Reactive hyperemia is a temporary increase above normal in the flow of blood to a tissue after a period when blood flow was restricted. In this case, the hyperemia (increased flow) is a response (reaction) to a period of inadequate blood flow. Mechanical compression of blood vessels is one cause of inadequate blood flow. It is easy to demonstrate reactive hyperemia in nonpigmented epithelial tissue after mechanical compression: press a finger against nonpigmented skin hard enough to occlude the blood flow; maintain the pressure for about 1 minute, and then release. The previously compressed area of skin looks darker (redder) for a short time. The red color results from reactive hyperemia; blood flow becomes greater than normal when the compression is released.

The same metabolic control mechanisms that account for active hyperemia also explain reactive hyperemia. During the period of restricted blood flow, metabolism continues in the compressed area, so metabolic products accumulate, and the local concentration of oxygen decreases. These metabolic effects cause dilation of the arterioles and a decrease in arteriolar resistance. When the mechanical obstruction to flow is removed, blood flow increases above normal until the "oxygen debt" is repaid and the excess metabolic products have been removed from the compressed tissue. Active and reactive hyperemia are compared in Figure 23–2.

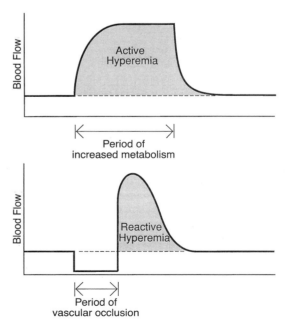

FIGURE 23–2. Both active and reactive hyperemia involve increases above normal in blood flow, and both are brought about by the same mechanisms for the local, metabolic control of blood flow.

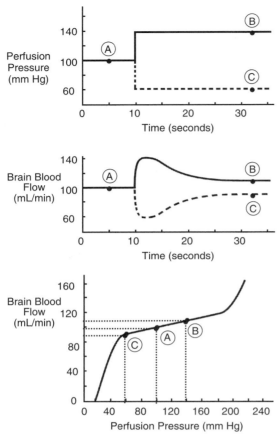

FIGURE 23–3. The experiment summarized here demonstrates autoregulation of brain blood flow. Perfusion pressure was artificially set to various levels *(top)*, and the resulting steady-state values of blood flow were measured *(middle)*. Then, the steady-state values of brain blood flow were plotted against the perfusion pressure *(bottom)*. Circled points A, B, and C are discussed in the text.

▬ Autoregulation is a relative constancy of blood flow in an organ despite changes in perfusion pressure

Metabolic control mechanisms also appear to account for the phenomenon known as *blood flow autoregulation*. Autoregulation is evident in denervated organs and organs in which local control of blood flow is predominant over neural and humoral control (e.g., in coronary circulation, brain, and working skeletal muscle).

Figure 23–3 summarizes an experiment that demonstrates autoregulation in the brain. Initially, the perfusion pressure (arterial pressure minus venous pressure) in this animal is 100 mm Hg, and the blood flow to the brain is 100 mL/min (point A). When perfusion pressure is increased suddenly to 140 mm Hg, brain blood flow rises initially to 140 mL/min but returns toward its initial level over the next 20 to 30 seconds. Eventually, blood flow reaches a stable level of about 110 mL/min (point B). The dashed lines in the top and middle graphs show what happens if the perfusion pressure is decreased suddenly from 100 to 60 mm Hg. Brain blood flow decreases initially

to 60 mL/min but returns toward its initial level over the next 20 to 30 seconds. Eventually, blood flow reaches a stable level of about 90 mL/min (point C). These stable responses are plotted in the bottom graph. The remainder of the bottom graph is obtained in a similar way; that is, perfusion pressure is set artificially to various levels, ranging from 40 to 220 mm Hg, and the resulting steady-state levels of blood flow are plotted.

Over a considerable range of perfusion pressure (from about 60 to 190 mm Hg), there is relatively little change in blood flow to the brain; that is, brain blood flow is autoregulated. The range of perfusion pressures over which flow remains relatively constant is called the *autoregulatory range.* Autoregulation fails at very high and very low perfusion pressures. Extremely high pressures result in marked increases in blood flow, and extremely low pressures result in marked decreases in blood flow. Nevertheless, over a considerable range of perfusion pressure, autoregulation keeps brain blood flow relatively constant.

Figure 23–4 shows how the metabolic control mech-

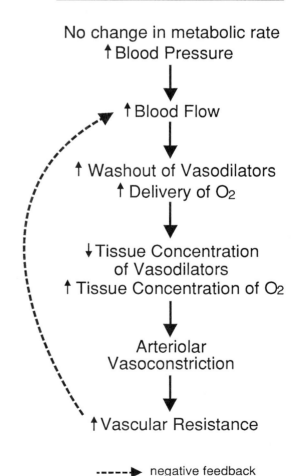

FIGURE 23–4. The same metabolic mechanism that is responsible for active hyperemia and reactive hyperemia can also account for autoregulation.

anisms previously described can account for the phenomenon of autoregulation. If the metabolic rate of an organ does not change but perfusion pressure is increased above normal, the increased pressure forces additional blood flow through the organ. The additional blood flow accelerates the removal of metabolic products from the interstitial fluid and increases the rate of oxygen delivery to the interstitial fluid. Therefore, the concentration of vasodilating metabolic products in the interstitial fluid decreases and the concentration of oxygen in the interstitial fluid increases. These changes cause the arterioles of the tissue to constrict, which increases the resistance to blood flow above normal and decreases blood flow back toward its initial level, despite the continuation of the elevated perfusion pressure.

To summarize, metabolic control mechanisms can account for active hyperemia (the increase in blood flow in an organ in response to an increased metabolic rate, in the absence of any blood pressure change). The same metabolic mechanisms can also account for reactive hyperemia (the increase in blood flow above normal in an organ after a period of flow restriction). In addition, the same metabolic mechanisms can account for autoregulation (the relative constancy of blood flow in an organ when there has been no change in metabolic rate but blood pressure has either increased or decreased). There are other mechanisms that contribute to autoregulation, and the student may encounter discussions of these under the terms *myogenic hypothesis* and *tissue pressure hypothesis*. However, metabolic control is the most likely explanation for autoregulation of blood flow in the critical tissues of a body (brain, coronary vessels, and exercising skeletal muscle).

Regardless of the status of arterioles, mechanical compression can reduce blood flow to a tissue

Mechanical compression can reduce blood flow in a tissue by literally squeezing down on all of its blood vessels. The example of mechanical compression of the epithelial blood vessels has been mentioned as a way to trigger a readily visible reactive hyperemia. Long-term mechanical pressure on the skin must be avoided, however, because a prolonged period of subnormal blood flow (ischemia) leads to irreversible tissue damage and cell death (infarction). Pressure sores are an unfortunate and common example. Three other specific instances of mechanical compression are also mentioned because of their clinical importance.

Figure 23–5 is a diagram of the effect of mechanical compression on coronary blood flow. The top tracing shows the changes in arterial (aortic) blood pressure during one whole cardiac cycle and the beginning of a second one. The periods of ventricular systole and ventricular diastole are labeled at the bottom of the figure. One would expect that left coronary blood flow would be highest during ventricular systole (when the aortic pressure is highest) and lowest dur-

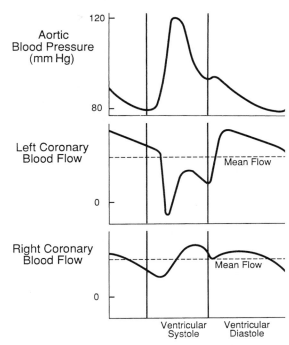

FIGURE 23–5. Left coronary blood flow is greatly reduced during ventricular systole by mechanical compression of left ventricular blood vessels. Right coronary flow is less affected by mechanical compression.

ing diastole (when the aortic pressure is lowest). However, the tracings of left coronary blood flow indicate that blood flow is actually depressed during systole and much higher during diastole. Flow even reverses (blood flows backward, in a negative direction) for a brief period near the beginning of systole. The fact that coronary blood flow is much lower during systole, even though the perfusion pressure is higher, implies that coronary resistance must be substantially higher during systole than during diastole.

Coronary resistance is high during systole because the contracting ventricular muscle squeezes down on the coronary blood vessels, which increases their resistance to blood flow. The coronary vessels are not constricted in this way during diastole because the ventricular muscle is relaxed. Therefore, coronary vascular resistance decreases dramatically (and blood flow increases) during diastole. The bottom tracing in Figure 23–5 indicates that mechanical compression does not have much influence on right coronary blood flow; that is, the magnitude of right coronary blood flow closely follows the changes in arterial pressure (being highest during systole and lowest during diastole). Right coronary flow is not restricted by mechanical compression during systole because the right ventricle contracts with much less force than the left ventricle. The right ventricle does not develop sufficient compressive force to constrict its own blood vessels.

Most of the blood that is needed to support left ventricular metabolism must be delivered during ventricular diastole, when the vessels are not compressed.

This fact has great clinical significance. In a resting animal with a low heart rate, there is adequate time during diastole for the coronary vessels to supply the amount of blood needed by the ventricular tissue. During exercise, both heart rate and cardiac contractility increase, which greatly increases the metabolic rate of the ventricular muscle cells. To support the increased metabolic rate, the ventricular tissue needs much more blood flow than normal. However, the duration of diastole is reduced during exercise, so there is less time available for blood flow delivery. Nevertheless, normal, healthy coronary vessels have a sufficiently low resistance during diastole to supply the needed blood flow, even during maximal exercise. The situation is different, however, in animals with coronary artery disease. In animals whose coronary vessels are narrowed because of atherosclerosis, there cannot be sufficient blood flow during diastole to supply the needs of the vigorously working ventricular muscles. Therefore, ventricular ischemia develops during exercise in patients with coronary artery disease. The ischemic areas of the ventricle fail to contract normally. Ischemia can also cause arrhythmias or even ventricular fibrillation (sudden death). Coronary artery disease is more common in humans than in veterinary species, so this scenario is actually more likely to occur in the veterinarian than in the veterinarian's patients.

Mechanical compression caused by muscle contraction can also restrict blood flow through skeletal muscles. The blood vessels within skeletal muscles become compressed during strenuous, sustained contractions of the muscle. The compression reduces blood flow and can create ischemia. Ischemic muscles cannot contract with normal vigor. Ischemia also activates sensory nerve endings in the muscle, which causes pain. Activation of these muscle ischemia re-

ceptors also triggers a reflex increase in arterial pressure. The high arterial pressure is advantageous, because it partially overcomes the effects of mechanical compression on blood flow. In other words, a high arterial pressure helps to force blood flow through the skeletal muscle blood vessels, despite the compressive effects of the muscle contraction. The high arterial pressure of ischemic exercise is risky, however, for patients with coronary artery disease, because high arterial pressure causes a tremendous increase in the cardiac workload. This is why patients with coronary artery disease are cautioned against types of exercise that involve strenuous, sustained muscle contractions, such as weightlifting.

Mechanical compression has very important effects on the pulmonary circulation. Pulmonary arterial pressure is much lower than systemic arterial pressure, so mechanical compression can easily reduce pulmonary blood flow. Figure 23–6 is a diagram of an example of mechanical interference with pulmonary blood flow, showing a pulmonary blood vessel passing between two alveoli. Figure 23–6A depicts normal conditions, in which the pulmonary vessels are not compressed. The arterial pressure is 13 mm Hg, and the venous pressure is 5 mm Hg. The pressure in the alveolar air spaces is near zero (i.e., near atmospheric pressure). Alveolar pressures typically vary between −1 mm Hg (during inspiration) and +1 mm Hg (during expiration).

Figure 23–6B depicts a situation in which abnormally high alveolar pressure compresses pulmonary blood vessels. This could happen during the administration of a general anesthetic agent if a patient has a tracheal tube inserted into the airway and the tracheal tube is attached to a source of elevated pressure. The elevated pressure could be generated by a mechanical respirator or by an anesthetist when he or she

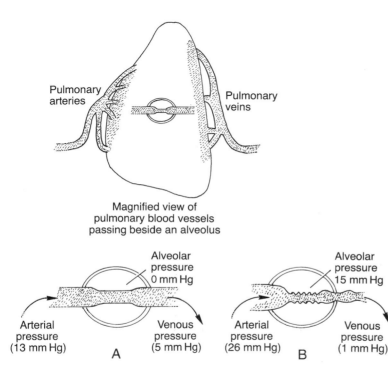

Pulmonary arteries

Pulmonary veins

Magnified view of
pulmonary blood vessels
passing beside an alveolus

Alveolar
pressure
0 mm Hg

Arterial
pressure
(13 mm Hg)   A   Venous
pressure
(5 mm Hg)

Alveolar
pressure
15 mm Hg

Arterial
pressure
(26 mm Hg)   B   Venous
pressure
(1 mm Hg)

FIGURE 23–6. Pulmonary vessels are susceptible to mechanical compression. Normally, pulmonary arterial and venous pressures are both higher than alveolar pressure, so pulmonary vessels stay open *(A)*. However, if alveolar pressure increases to 15 mm Hg *(B)*, the pulmonary blood vessels are compressed. The resulting increase in pulmonary vascular resistance causes pulmonary blood flow to decrease, arterial pressure to increase, and venous pressure to decrease.

squeezes the bag on an anesthesia machine that is attached to the tracheal tube. In either case, the pressures generated in the tracheal tube are transmitted to the alveoli. An increase in alveolar pressure increases the external compressing pressures applied around the pulmonary blood vessels.

Alveolar pressures in excess of 10 to 15 mm Hg compress pulmonary blood vessels sufficiently to raise the resistance to blood flow through the lungs, so pulmonary blood flow decreases. Two things happen as a result. First, less blood reaches the left atrium and left ventricle, which causes left ventricular stroke volume and aortic blood pressure to decrease. Second, blood ejected by the right ventricle dams up in the pulmonary arteries. This causes pulmonary arterial pressure to increase. An elevated pulmonary arterial pressure helps force blood through the compressed vessels. However, the increased pulmonary artery pressure also places an increased workload on the right ventricle. If the alveolar pressure is not excessively high, the right ventricle generates sufficient pulmonary arterial pressure to restore pulmonary blood flow to near normal. However, with extremely high alveolar pressures, the right ventricle is unable to raise pulmonary arterial pressure high enough to sustain flow. Under these conditions, pulmonary blood flow and, consequently, systemic blood flow fall substantially below normal and systemic hypotension and ischemia develop in the patient. The consequences can be fatal. The veterinary clinician must be mindful of the risks of high airway pressures whenever a patient is intubated and attached to a mechanical respiratory device.

CLINICAL CORRELATIONS

Patent ductus arteriosus

History   A 3-month-old female Welsh corgi is brought to your clinic by its owner, who has noticed a "rumbling noise" in the dog's chest. The dog is smaller than her littermates and a little less playful. The dog coughs occasionally, but the cough does not produce fluid.

Clinical examination   The dog appears to be in good health except for an occasional cough. The mucous membranes are pink, and the capillary refill time is normal (1.5 seconds). However, when you place your hand on the anterior left chest, you feel an abnormal vibration *(thrill)* with each heartbeat. With a stethoscope, you can auscultate a cardiac murmur that is loudest during systole but continues throughout both systole and diastole. The murmur is heard most loudly at the ventral third intercostal space on the left side. Expiratory sounds are slightly louder than normal. The pulse rate is 152 beats per minute, which you consider to be above normal for a dog of this size and age.

The electrocardiogram indicates that the dog has sinus tachycardia; the atrial and ventricular rates are both 152 beats per minute. The R waves are abnormally large in leads II and III (2.5 and 3.5 mV, respectively). The QRS complex in lead I shows a large negative deflection followed immediately by an equally large positive deflection.

Thoracic radiographs show a generalized enlargement of the heart. The initial portion of the pulmonary artery is also substantially larger than normal, and the pulmonary blood vessels appear generally to be more prominent than normal.

Comment   A murmur in a young, otherwise healthy dog is most likely the result of a congenital cardiac abnormality. A continuous murmur can occur only if there is a defect that causes turbulent flow throughout both diastole and systole. Because flow can occur only when there is a pressure gradient, the defect in this dog must be located where a substantial pressure gradient is present during both systole and diastole. No single intracardiac defect meets this criterion; that is, a stenotic or regurgitant valve produces either a systolic murmur or a diastolic murmur, but not both. A valve that is both stenotic and regurgitant produces two murmurs: one in systole and one in diastole. However, in such a case, there are moments during the cardiac cycle when no pressure gradient exists across the valve, so there are moments of silence between the systolic murmur and the diastolic murmur. (Admittedly, if the heart rate is high, these moments of silence are difficult to detect, and the two murmurs can be mistaken for a continuous murmur, particularly in the case of combined aortic stenosis and regurgitation.)

The most common cardiac defect that causes turbulent flow throughout both systole and diastole is a patent ductus arteriosus (PDA). This vessel is normal in the fetus but should close shortly after birth. The flow through a PDA is continuous, because aortic pressure is higher than pulmonary artery pressure throughout the cardiac cycle. The resulting murmur is usually heard best in the left third intercostal space. All of the other clinical signs in this dog are also consistent with the diagnosis of PDA. The prominence of the pulmonary vessels on the radiographs indicates that pressure and flow are abnormally high in the pulmonary artery and its branches. In a dog with a PDA, a large volume of blood flows from the aorta into the pulmonary artery, and this increases both pulmonary arterial pressure and pulmonary flow.

The radiographs and electrocardiograms indicate that this dog has both right and left ventricular hypertrophy. The large R waves in leads II and III indicate left ventricular hypertrophy, and the large negative deflection during the QRS complex in lead I suggests that the right ventricle is hypertrophic, too. The left ventricle becomes hypertrophic in a dog with PDA because it is called on to pump three to five times the normal cardiac output. (It pumps a near-normal volume to the organs of the systemic circulation and two to four times that much through the PDA.) The flow through the PDA is large, because the PDA offers little resistance to flow. The demand on the left ventricle to pump so much blood (increased volume work) leads to left ventricular hypertrophy. The volume of blood pumped by the right ventricle is nearly normal; it only has to pump the blood that returns through the venae cavae from the systemic organs. However, the right ventricle has to develop higher systolic pressures than normal to eject this blood into the pulmonary artery, because pulmonary artery pressure is higher than normal, as explained earlier. This increase in pressure work often leads to right ventricular hypertrophy.

Because the PDA carries so much blood away from the aorta, dogs with PDA tend to have an abnormally low aortic pressure. Diastolic pressure is particularly reduced because of the rapid outflow of blood from the aorta during ventricular diastole. Therefore, PDA is typically associated with low mean aortic pressure but elevated pulse pressure (review Fig. 21–9C).

Two mechanisms work together to keep blood flow to the systemic organs nearly normal despite the fact that a large fraction of cardiac output is "lost" through the PDA. First, reflex mechanisms (which are discussed in detail in Chapter 24) increase sympathetic activity to the heart, which increases heart rate and contractility above normal. These sympathetic effects keep left ventricular output (and aortic pressure) sufficiently high to supply blood to the systemic organs, in spite of the PDA. Second, metabolic control mechanisms cause the systemic organs to vasodilate, which keeps their blood flow nearly normal despite the subnormal aortic pressure.

The compensatory mechanisms just described allow most dogs with a PDA to maintain a nearly normal blood flow to the systemic organs at rest. Many months may pass before the dog's owner notices limitations in the dog's activity or growth. In some cases, however, the heart cannot increase its output sufficiently to supply the systemic blood flow needed by the muscles during exercise, and a puppy with a PDA appears less playful and energetic than its normal littermates. Also, if the heart is unable to supply the blood flow needed by metabolically active tissues, the owner may notice some stunting of growth. In any case, a dog with a widely open ductus has a poor long-term prognosis, unless treated.

Treatment   You show the dog's owner a diagram of the fetal circulation and explain that the ductus arteriosus normally closes and seals itself within 1 to 6 weeks after birth but that the ductus fails to close spontaneously in about 1 of every 700 newborns (the condition is four times more common in female pups than in male pups). Treatment involves closure of the ductus, either by ligation during open-chest surgery or by insertion of a specially designed plug during a cardiac catheterization procedure. Most dogs treated before the age of 6 months go on to lead completely normal lives. However, you advise the owner that PDA is hereditary and that this puppy should probably not be used for breeding.

The owner elects to have the dog treated surgically, and the surgery is successful. The murmur and cough disappear immediately. Within 1 week, the dog is noticeably more energetic than before. By the time she is 6 months old, the dog has "grown into" her enlarged heart, and all physical findings are within normal limits.

Bibliography

Berne RM, Levy MN: Cardiovascular Physiology, 7th ed. St. Louis: Mosby, 1997.

Guyton AC, Hall JE: Textbook of Medical Physiology, 10th ed. Philadelphia: WB Saunders, 2000, pp 175–183.

Kittleson MD, Kienle RD: Small Animal Cardiovascular Medicine. St. Louis: Mosby–Year Book, 1998.

Milnor WR: Cardiovascular Physiology. New York: Oxford University Press, 1990.

Mohrman DE, Heller LJ: Cardiovascular Physiology, 4th ed. New York: McGraw-Hill, 1997.

Sisson DD, Thomas WP, Bonagura JD: Congenital heart disease. In Ettinger SJ, Feldman EC (eds): Textbook of Veterinary Internal Medicine: Diseases of the Dog and Cat, 5th ed. Philadelphia: WB Saunders, 2000, p 737.

PRACTICE QUESTIONS

1. The increase in coronary blood flow during exercise is
   a. called Starling's law of the heart.
   b. caused by sympathetic activation of α-adrenergic receptors.
   c. caused by compression of the coronary blood vessels during systole.
   d. closely matched to the metabolic requirements of the heart.
   e. called reactive hyperemia.

2. A dog with an arterial blood pressure of 120/80 mm Hg has a cerebral blood flow of 100 mL/min. When blood pressure is increased to 130/100 mm Hg, the cerebral blood flow increases to 105 mL/min. This is an example of
   a. active hyperemia.
   b. autoregulation.
   c. reactive hyperemia.
   d. the blood-brain barrier.
   e. hypoxic vasoconstriction.

3. Local, metabolic control of blood flow through skeletal muscle
   a. characteristically dominates over neurohumoral control.
   b. characteristically is subservient to neurohumoral control.
   c. can either dominate or be subservient to neurohumoral control, depending on whether the muscle is exercising or resting.
   d. depends primarily on changes in the resistance of the arteries of the muscle.
   e. involves the release of histamine from mast cells within the skeletal muscle.

4. In response to an increase in perfusion pressure, the arterioles of an autoregulating organ _____ and the vascular resistance of the organ _____.
   a. constrict; increases.
   b. constrict; decreases.
   c. dilate; increases.
   d. dilate; decreases.

5. When a young dog with a PDA begins to exercise,
   a. arterioles in the exercising skeletal muscle constrict.
   b. oxygen concentration in the skeletal muscle interstitial fluid decreases.
   c. left ventricular output decreases.
   d. right ventricular output decreases.
   e. mean arterial pressure increases to very high levels.

PRACTICE ANSWERS

1. d   2. b   3. c   4. a   5. b

24

Neural and hormonal control of blood pressure and blood volume

1 Neurohumoral mechanisms regulate blood pressure and blood volume to ensure adequate blood flow for all body organs

2 The autonomic nervous system affects the cardiovascular system through the release of epinephrine, norepinephrine, and acetylcholine

3 The arterial baroreceptor reflex regulates arterial blood pressure

4 The atrial volume receptor reflex regulates blood volume and helps to stabilize blood pressure

5 The cardiovascular state of conscious subjects is determined by an ongoing and ever-changing mixture of reflex effects and psychogenic responses

Neurohumoral mechanisms regulate blood pressure and blood volume to ensure adequate blood flow for all body organs

The influences of the nervous system and hormones on the cardiovascular system are referred to collectively as the *neurohumoral* mechanisms of cardiovascular control. The neurohumoral mechanisms are also called *extrinsic control mechanisms,* because they act on organs from the outside. As described in Chapter 23, the mechanisms of cardiovascular control that act locally, within individual tissues, are referred to as *intrinsic control mechanisms.* The local, or intrinsic, mechanisms predominate over extrinsic mechanisms in the control of blood flow to the "critical" organs, which include the heart (i.e., coronary circulation), brain, and working skeletal muscle. In contrast, neurohumoral, or extrinsic, control mechanisms predominate over the intrinsic mechanisms in the control of blood flow to the "noncritical" organs, which include the kidneys, the splanchnic organs, and resting skeletal muscle.

Neurohumoral mechanisms also control the heart rate and cardiac contractility. This allows cardiac output to be adjusted to provide adequate blood flow for all the systemic organs, or at least for the critical organs. An important distinction is that cardiac muscle is under neurohumoral control, whereas the coronary blood vessels are primarily under local control. When neurohumoral mechanisms increase the heart rate and cardiac contractility, the cardiac metabolic rate also increases. The increased metabolic rate triggers local metabolic control mechanisms to dilate coronary arterioles, which increases coronary blood flow.

To appreciate the importance of neurohumoral control mechanisms, consider what would happen in their absence. For example, consider what would happen during exercise if all of the body organs simply relied on local control mechanisms to adjust their blood flows. At the onset of exercise, metabolic control mechanisms would cause vasodilation in the exercising skeletal muscles. Vascular resistance would decrease in the exercising muscles, and the blood flow through the muscles would increase. However, the decrease in resistance in skeletal muscles would also lower the total peripheral resistance (TPR). As a consequence, arterial blood pressure would decrease. This would decrease the perfusion pressure for all of the systemic organs, and blood flow would therefore decrease below normal levels in the brain, kidneys, splanchnic organs, and so forth.

The decreased blood flow in these organs would trigger autoregulatory responses, and these organs would vasodilate. However, the vasodilation would lower the TPR even further, which would reduce arterial pressure even more. This in turn would limit the increase in skeletal muscle blood flow. The end result would be increased blood flow in the exercising muscle and decreased blood flow elsewhere, but none of the organs (including skeletal muscle) would be receiving sufficient blood flow to meet their metabolic needs. Arterial pressure would be dangerously low, and the animal would exhibit profound exercise intolerance.

Neurohumoral control mechanisms allow an animal to avoid these complications. First, cardiac output is increased sufficiently to meet the increased need for blood flow in the exercising muscle (and in the coronary circulation, too), while keeping all of the other organs supplied with a normal blood flow. If cardiac output cannot be increased sufficiently to meet all of these needs, the control mechanisms take the additional step of temporarily reducing blood flow in the noncritical organs and making this extra flow available to the critical organs.

How do the neurohumoral control systems "know" whether cardiac output is sufficiently high to meet the needs of all of the organs and whether to initiate vasoconstriction in the noncritical organs? An indirect "strategy" is used: cardiac output is sufficiently increased to keep arterial pressure at a normal level. As long as arterial pressure can be maintained, then local metabolic control mechanisms can successfully match blood flow to metabolic need in each individual organ. If cardiac output cannot be sufficiently increased to keep arterial pressure from falling, vasoconstriction of the noncritical organs is initiated. Thus, neurohumoral control mechanisms may deprive noncritical organs of an ideal level of blood flow if more flow is needed by the critical organs than can be supplied by the heart.

There are many important neurohumoral control mechanisms, but four are emphasized in the following presentation. Two of them are cardiovascular reflexes. The arterial baroreceptor reflex works to keep arterial pressure at its "set-point" through the continual adjustment of cardiac output and vascular resistance (in the noncritical organs). The atrial volume receptor reflex works in conjunction with the arterial baroreceptor reflex to regulate arterial pressure by adjusting cardiac preload. The other two neurohumoral mechanisms described in this chapter are the defense-alarm reaction and vasovagal syncope (the "playing dead" reaction). These two are examples of psychogenic influences on the cardiovascular system.

The autonomic nervous system affects the cardiovascular system through the release of epinephrine, norepinephrine, and acetylcholine

The autonomic nervous system is the "neural" arm of neurohumoral control. Sympathetic and parasympathetic neurons influence the cardiovascular system through the release of the neurotransmitters norepinephrine and acetylcholine. In addition, sympathetic nerves affect the cardiovascular system through the release of epinephrine and norepinephrine from the adrenal medulla. The adrenal secretions enter the blood stream as hormones and circulate throughout the body. Chapter 12 contains additional, basic information about the autonomic nervous system.

Whether acting as neurotransmitters or as hormones, epinephrine, norepinephrine, and acetylcholine exert their cardiovascular effects by activating membrane receptors on the cardiac muscle cells or on the endothelial cells or the smooth muscle cells of blood vessels. Epinephrine and norepinephrine activate *adrenergic* (named after *adrenal) receptors.* There are two major subtypes: α-*adrenergic receptors* and β-*adrenergic receptors.* Each of these is subdivided again into α_1, α_2, β_1, and β_2, and the four have important cardiovascular roles.

Acetylcholine activates *cholinergic receptors.* There are two major subtypes: *muscarinic cholinergic receptors* and *nicotinic cholinergic receptors.* The main cardiovascular effects of acetylcholine are mediated through muscarinic cholinergic receptors. Of five known types of muscarinic receptors, the M_2 and M_3 muscarinic receptors are those with the greatest cardiovascular importance.

Table 24–1 summarizes the main cardiovascular consequences of the activation of adrenergic and cholinergic receptors. α-Adrenergic receptors (both α_1 and α_2) are located on the cell membranes of the smooth muscle cells of the arterioles in all organs of the body as well as on the smooth muscle cells of the abdominal veins. The α-adrenergic receptors on arterioles and abdominal veins are innervated by postganglionic sympathetic neurons. Activation of the α-adrenergic receptors leads to constriction of the arterioles or the veins.

Arteriolar *vasoconstriction* increases the resistance and decreases the blood flow through an organ. If one or more major body organs are vasoconstricted, the TPR increases. TPR (along with cardiac output) determines arterial blood pressure, so widespread α-adrenergic vasoconstriction in the body leads to an increase in arterial blood pressure. The increase in arterial pressure increases blood flow to the nonvasoconstricted organs. In this way, the sympathetic nervous system can use vasoconstriction in some organs to direct blood flow to other, nonvasoconstricted organs.

The major role of veins is to act as reservoirs for blood. *Venoconstriction* displaces venous blood toward the central circulation, which increases central venous pressure, ventricular preload, and stroke volume. Venoconstriction in the abdominal organs is particularly important in the control of central blood volume and, therefore, central venous pressure. Venoconstriction causes only a small increase in the resistance to blood flow through an organ, because the veins, whether constricted or dilated, offer much less resistance to blood flow than do the arterioles.

Sympathetic control of the heart is exerted through the β_1-adrenergic receptors, which are found on every cardiac muscle cell. The β receptors are activated by norepinephrine or epinephrine. Details of the effects of activation of the cardiac β receptors are given in Chapters 18 and 20. In brief, the pacemaker rate increases, the cell-to-cell conduction velocity increases, and the refractory period decreases. In addition, the contractions are quicker and stronger (contractility is increased). The overall effect is increased heart rate and stroke volume.

β_2-Adrenergic receptors are found on the arterioles, particularly in the coronary circulation and in skeletal muscles. The activation of arteriolar β_2-adrenergic receptors causes relaxation of the vascular smooth muscle and dilation of the arterioles. However, these β_2-adrenergic receptors are not innervated by the

TABLE 24–1.   Receptors involved in autonomic control of the cardiovascular system

Receptor type	Location	Usual activator	Effect of activation	Function
α_1- and α_2-adrenergic	Arterioles (all organs)	Norepinephrine from sympathetic neurons; circulating epinephrine and norepinephrine	Vasoconstriction	Decreases blood flow to organs; increases total peripheral resistance (major effect)
	Veins (abdominal organs)	Norepinephrine from sympathetic neurons; circulating epinephrine and norepinephrine	Venoconstriction	Displaces venous blood toward heart
β-Adrenergic β_1	Heart (all cardiac muscle cells)	Norepinephrine from sympathetic neurons; circulating epinephrine and norepinephrine	Increased pacemaker rate; faster speed of conduction; decreased refractory period; quicker, stronger contractions	Increases heart rate, stroke volume, and cardiac output (major effects)
β_2	Arterioles (coronary and skeletal muscle)	Circulating epinephrine and norepinephrine	Vasodilation	Increases coronary blood flow; increases skeletal muscle blood flow
Muscarinic cholinergic M_2	Heart (all cardiac muscle cells, but sparse direct innervation of ventricular muscle cells)	Acetylcholine from parasympathetic neurons	Opposite of β_1	Decreases heart rate and cardiac output (major effect)
	Sympathetic nerve endings at ventricular muscle cells	Acetylcholine from parasympathetic neurons	Inhibition of norepinephrine release from sympathetic neurons	Decreases magnitude of sympathetic effects on ventricular muscle cells
M_3	Arterioles (coronary)	Acetylcholine from parasympathetic neurons	Vasodilation (via nitric oxide)	Increases coronary blood flow (minor effect)
	Arterioles (genitals)	Acetylcholine from parasympathetic neurons	Vasodilation (via nitric oxide)	Causes engorgement and erection
	Arterioles (skeletal muscle)	Acetylcholine from specialized sympathetic neurons	Vasodilation (via nitric oxide)	Increases muscle blood flow (in anticipation of exercise)
	Arterioles (most other organs)	Normal activator unknown	Vasodilation (via nitric oxide)	Function unknown

sympathetic nervous system, so they are not activated directly by sympathetic nerves. Instead, they respond to circulating epinephrine and norepinephrine, which are released by the adrenal medulla. The adrenal medulla releases epinephrine and norepinephrine in situations that involve trauma, fear, or anxiety. Dilation of arterioles in the coronary circulation and in skeletal muscles is appropriate in such "fear, fight, or flight" situations, because the dilation results in an anticipatory increase in blood flow to the heart and skeletal muscle. Note that β_2-adrenergic vasodilation can overpower α-adrenergic vasoconstriction in the coronary circulation and in skeletal muscles.

Cholinergic muscarinic receptors of the M_2 type are located in the cell membranes of cardiac muscle cells. The natural stimulus for the cardiac M_2 receptors is acetylcholine, released from postganglionic parasympathetic neurons. Cells of the sinoatrial and atrioven-

tricular nodes are densely innervated by postganglionic parasympathetic neurons. Atrial cells also receive strong parasympathetic innervation. In the sinoatrial node, atria, and atrioventricular node, the activation of M_2 receptors has effects basically opposite to those of the activation of β_1-adrenergic receptors. Parasympathetic activation powerfully slows the pacemaker rate, decreases the cell-to-cell conduction velocity, and increases the refractory period. By contrast, few ventricular muscle cells receive direct parasympathetic innervation. Therefore, parasympathetic activation has very minor, direct effects on cardiac contractility. Still, parasympathetic activation can profoundly decrease cardiac output by decreasing the heart rate. In addition, parasympathetic neurons do exert an interesting, indirect effect on ventricular muscle cells. Some parasympathetic neurons release their acetylcholine onto sympathetic neuron terminals, rather than directly onto ventricular muscle cells. This acetylcholine activates muscarinic cholinergic receptors on the sympathetic neuron terminals, which inhibits the release of norepinephrine from the terminals and in turn weakens the effects of sympathetic activity on ventricular cells.

Cholinergic muscarinic receptors of the M_3 type are found on the endothelial cells and on the smooth muscle cells of most arteries and arterioles. Activation of M_3 receptors on smooth muscle cells causes them to contract (and the blood vessels to constrict). However, this *vasoconstrictor* effect is usually overridden by the *vasodilatory* effect of activating the M_3 receptors on the vascular endothelial cells. In this strange arrangement, activation of M_3 receptors on endothelial cells causes the synthesis of *nitric oxide,* which then diffuses out of the endothelial cells and into the nearby smooth muscle cells, where it acts as a vasodilator. The vasodilatory effect of stimulating the M_3 receptors on endothelial cells is stronger than the vasoconstrictor effect of stimulating the M_3 receptors on smooth muscle cells.

The M_3 receptors on vascular endothelial cells are innervated in only three tissues. In the coronary circulation, parasympathetic neurons innervate vascular M_3 receptors and bring about vasodilation. This vasodilatory effect is minor, however, and the function of this innervation is unclear. In the external genital organs, parasympathetic neurons lead to vasodilation, which results in engorgement and erection. The third tissue in which vascular M_3 receptors are innervated is skeletal muscle. In some species (e.g., cats and dogs) but not in others (e.g., primates), the M_3 receptors of skeletal muscle blood vessels are innervated by special postganglionic sympathetic neurons that release acetylcholine (rather than norepinephrine) as a neurotransmitter. These *sympathetic-cholinergic neurons* appear to be activated specifically in anticipation of muscular exercise and during the "fear, fight, or flight" (defense-alarm) reaction. The resulting vasodilation increases blood flow through the skeletal muscle just before and during the initiation of exercise. Primates do not have sympathetic cholinergic vasodilatory nerves. However, primates can bring about an anticipatory vasodilation of skeletal muscle arterioles in another way (via activation of β-adrenergic receptors by circulating epinephrine and norepinephrine, which are released from the adrenal medulla), as mentioned earlier.

To summarize, although arteries and arterioles throughout the body dilate when exposed to acetylcholine, only the arterioles of the heart, external genitalia, and (in some species) skeletal muscle are innervated by acetylcholine-releasing autonomic neurons. The functional significance of the M_3 receptors on arterioles in other organs is unclear, because no neurons (either sympathetic or parasympathetic) appear to innervate them.

Of all of the autonomic influences on the cardiovascular system just mentioned, three stand out as most important. The first is α_1- and α_2-adrenergic vasoconstriction in the arterioles of all body organs, which is brought about by the sympathetic nervous system. The second is β_1-adrenergic excitation of cardiac muscle, which is brought about by the sympathetic nervous system and results in an increased heart rate and stroke volume. The third is the decrease in heart rate brought about by activation of cardiac M_2 receptors.

The arterial baroreceptor reflex regulates arterial blood pressure

Arterial blood pressure is monitored by pressure-sensitive nerve endings known as *baroreceptors*. The baroreceptors send afferent impulses to the central nervous system, which reflexly alters cardiac output and vascular resistance (in noncritical organs) to keep blood pressure at a set-point. The reflex is called the *arterial baroreceptor reflex.*

The arterial baroreceptors are specialized nerve endings that are embedded in the walls of the carotid arteries and aortic arch (Fig. 24–1). The baroreceptors are concentrated at the origin of each internal carotid artery in enlarged parts of the arteries called the *carotid sinuses.* Similar nerve endings are found in the

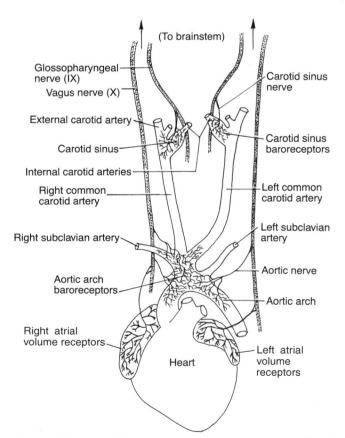

FIGURE 24–1. Arterial baroreceptors are located in the walls of the carotid sinuses and in the walls of the aortic arch and its major branches. The atrial volume receptors are located in the walls of the right and left atria. See text for a description of the neural pathways followed by the baroreceptor and volume receptor afferents.

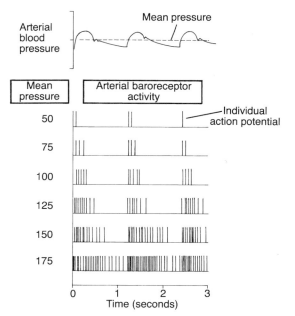

FIGURE 24–2. Each arterial pressure pulse causes action potentials to be generated in baroreceptor afferent neurons. The number of action potentials generated per heartbeat increases dramatically with increases in mean arterial pressure.

wall of the aortic arch, especially at the origin of its major branches. These nerve endings are sensitive to stretch *(distention)* of the arterial wall. In effect, they sense arterial pressure, because blood pressure is the natural force that distends these arteries. Therefore, these nerve endings are called *baroreceptors* (literally, "pressure sensors"), even though the actual physical factor being sensed is not pressure but rather stretch or distortion.

With every systolic ejection from the heart, blood distends the aorta and arteries, including the carotid sinuses, and the baroreceptors initiate neural impulses (action potentials). The frequency of impulses is proportional to the arterial blood pressure. The afferent neurons from the aortic arch baroreceptors run in the vagus nerves. In some species, the aortic baroreceptor afferents form a distinct bundle within

the vagal nerve sheath, called the *aortic depressor nerve.* The stretch receptors in the carotid sinuses have their afferents in the carotid sinus nerves (Hering's nerves), which join into the glossopharyngeal (ninth cranial) nerves. By way of these afferent neurons, the brain receives beat-by-beat information about the level of arterial blood pressure.

Figure 24–2 depicts the effect of different arterial blood pressures on the sensory afferent nerve activity of arterial baroreceptors. The tracing on the top shows the pulsatile arterial pressure on three successive heartbeats. The mean level of arterial pressure is indicated by the dashed line. Below the tracing is the typical pattern of action potentials that is seen in a baroreceptor afferent neuron when the mean arterial pressure is lower than normal, in this case 50 mm Hg. Note that there are only one or two action potentials with each heartbeat. These action potentials occur during the rapid upstroke of the pressure wave, because the baroreceptors are sensitive to the rate of change of pressure as well as to mean pressure. If the mean arterial pressure is at a higher level, perhaps 75 mm Hg, more action potentials are formed during each heartbeat, but the action potentials still tend to occur during the rapid pressure increase at the beginning of the cardiac ejection. The higher the mean arterial pressure, the more action potentials are formed in each heartbeat. Thus, the arterial baroreceptors signal increases in pressure by increasing their action potential frequency. Because the baroreceptors are active when arterial pressure is normal (mean pressure near 100 mm Hg), they can also signal a decrease in arterial pressure by decreasing their action potential frequency.

The reflex consequences of a decrease in afferent baroreceptor activity are summarized in Figure 24–3. The brain responds to a decrease in the afferent activity from the baroreceptors by increasing sympathetic activity. In the heart, sympathetic activation results in increased stroke volume and heart rate, which increases cardiac output. The increase in cardiac output helps to restore blood pressure toward normal. The sympathetically driven increase in heart rate is augmented by a simultaneous reduction in parasympa-

FIGURE 24–3. The arterial baroreceptor reflex responds to decreases in blood pressure *(top left)* by increasing cardiac output (CO), total peripheral resistance (TPR), or both *(far right)*. These reflex effects offset the initial fall in blood pressure *(dashed line)*. SA, sinoatrial.

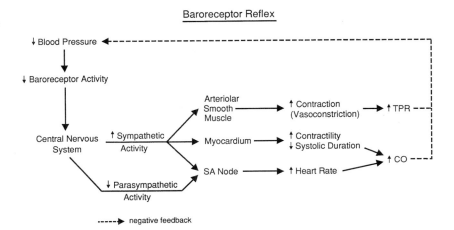

thetic activity to the sinoatrial node. Thus, the baroreceptor reflex uses reciprocal changes in sympathetic and parasympathetic activity to control heart rate. Sympathetic activity is also increased to the arterioles of all organs but particularly to the arterioles of non-critical organs (kidney, splanchnic organs, and resting skeletal muscle). Sympathetic activation causes vasoconstriction of these arterioles, which increases the resistance to blood flow through these organs and therefore increases TPR. The increase in peripheral resistance helps to restore arterial blood pressure back toward its normal level and directs blood flow to the critical organs.

To correctly understand the function of the baroreceptor reflex, it is important to recognize that the reflex does not *reverse* disturbances in blood pressure but only minimizes them. Also, it is important to distinguish between cause and effect when thinking about the baroreflex. For example, what *causes* blood pressure to decrease *below normal* is a decrease *below normal* in cardiac output, TPR, or both. *There is no other way to lower blood pressure.* When TPR falls below normal and *causes* blood pressure to decrease below normal, the *compensatory response* of the baroreceptor reflex is (1) to increase cardiac output above normal through increased sympathetic (and decreased parasympathetic) activation of the heart and (2) to minimize the decrease in peripheral resistance by initiating a sympathetic vasoconstriction in the noncritical organs. After compensation by the baroreceptor reflex, cardiac output is *above* normal. Peripheral resistance is still *below* normal but not as far below normal as in the uncompensated state. Blood pressure is still *below* normal but not as far below normal as in the uncompensated state.

All of the reflex responses just illustrated for a decrease in arterial blood pressure occur in reverse in response to an increase in arterial blood pressure above its normal level. Hence, the baroreceptor reflex acts to combat either decreases or increases in blood pressure.

As a regulator of arterial blood pressure, the baroreflex is both powerful and rapid. It can initiate compensations for changes in blood pressure within 1 second. A hemorrhage that would decrease blood pressure by 40 to 50 mm Hg if there were no baroreflex decreases blood pressure by only 10 to 15 mm Hg with intact baroreflexes. The baroreflex also acts to maintain blood pressure close to normal during changes in posture or activity. In a dog without baroreflexes, changes in posture are accompanied by large, uncontrolled variations in blood pressure, as shown in Figure 24–4. By minimizing fluctuations in blood pressure, the baroreflex functions to ensure an adequate blood flow to the critical organs.

Although the baroreceptor reflex is essential for the moment-to-moment stability of blood pressure, it does not appear to be the major mechanism responsible for setting the long-term level of arterial blood pressure, because baroreceptors adapt slowly or *reset* to the prevailing level of arterial pressure. In other

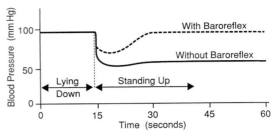

FIGURE 24–4. The baroreflex is essential for normal, moment-to-moment stability of blood pressure. Dogs in which baroreflexes are eliminated exhibit much larger swings in blood pressure in response to postural changes than do dogs with intact baroreflexes.

words, the baroreceptors come to accept whatever the prevailing blood pressure is as if it were the normal pressure. Baroreceptor resetting causes the baroreflex to "lose track of" normal blood pressure. For example, in an animal or a human who has been hypertensive for a few days or weeks, the baroreflex functions to regulate blood pressure at the elevated level rather than to restore blood pressure toward its normal level. Also, the baroreflex can become reset in a downward direction during a period of sustained hypotension. For example, in chronic heart failure, in which arterial pressure may be below normal for a period of days or weeks, the baroreflex appears to regulate blood pressure at a depressed level rather than to push it back toward its normal level. In summary, the baroreflex responds quickly and powerfully to counteract sudden changes in blood pressure, but it has little influence on the long-term level of blood pressure over a period of days or weeks.

The atrial volume receptor reflex regulates blood volume and helps to stabilize blood pressure

The *atrial volume receptor reflex* is initiated by specialized sensory nerve endings that are located in the walls of the left and right atria (see Fig. 24–1). These nerve endings are activated by stretch, but they are called *volume receptors*, because it is the volume of blood in each atrium that determines how much the atrial wall is stretched. For example, a decrease in the total blood volume of an animal (e.g., a hemorrhage) results in a decrease in the amount of blood in the major veins and in the atria. When atrial volume decreases, atrial pressure decreases, and so does the stretch on the atrial walls. This decreases the frequency of action potentials generated in atrial stretch receptors. Conversely, increases in blood volume result in increased atrial stretch and an increased frequency of action potentials generated by the atrial stretch receptors. Therefore, these atrial stretch receptors are sensitive detectors of atrial blood volume and, indirectly, of total blood volume.

Figure 24–5 summarizes the reflex effects of a

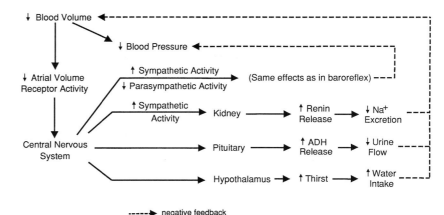

FIGURE 24–5. The atrial volume receptor reflex responds to a decrease in blood volume by decreasing sodium and water loss in the urine and by increasing oral water intake. The reflex also helps support blood pressure by increasing cardiac output and total peripheral resistance (similar to baroreflex). ADH, antidiuretic hormone.

change in the activity of the atrial volume receptors. If blood volume decreases, the result is a decrease in the afferent activity from the atrial volume receptors. The central nervous system responds reflexly to this decreased afferent activity by increasing sympathetic efferent activity to the heart and systemic arterioles and decreasing parasympathetic efferent activity to the heart.

Note that the atrial volume receptor reflex and the baroreceptor reflex exert synergistic effects; that is, a decrease in blood volume leads via the atrial volume receptor reflex to an increase in cardiac contractility, a decrease in systolic duration, and an increase in heart rate and to arteriolar vasoconstriction in the noncritical organs. All of these changes help combat the decrease in arterial blood pressure that would otherwise result from a decreased blood volume. In effect, the atrial volume receptor reflex augments the effectiveness of the baroreceptor reflex as a regulator of blood pressure.

The volume receptor reflex also acts in three additional ways to help restore lost blood volume (see Fig. 24–5). First, the reflex acts through the hypothalamus to increase the sensation of thirst. If water is available, the animal drinks. This provides the fluid necessary to increase blood volume back toward normal. Second, the atrial volume receptor reflex acts via the hypothalamus and pituitary gland to increase the release of *antidiuretic hormone* (ADH). ADH is synthesized in the hypothalamus, but it is transported to the posterior pituitary gland for storage and release. ADH acts on the kidneys to decrease urine production. ADH is also called *arginine vasopressin* (AVP). The third effect of the atrial volume receptor reflex on blood volume is to increase the release of the hormone *renin* from the kidneys. Renin acts to increase the production of the hormone *angiotensin II*, which acts to increase production of the hormone *aldosterone,* which acts to decrease the amount of sodium excreted by the kidneys; that is, activation of the *renin-angiotensin-aldosterone system* causes the body to conserve available sodium.

The combination of decreased sodium excretion (by the actions of renin) and decreased urine flow (by the actions of ADH) results in the conservation of body fluid. The conservation of body fluid, combined with an increased water intake, eventually restores blood volume back toward normal.

Although not diagrammed in Figure 24–3, the arterial baroreceptor reflex also responds to decreases in arterial pressure by increasing thirst, ADH release, and renin release. An increase in arterial pressure above normal initiates the opposite effects. Thus, the arterial baroreceptor reflex and the atrial volume receptor reflex are synergistic partners in the interrelated tasks of regulating arterial pressure and blood volume.

The cardiovascular state of conscious subjects is determined by an ongoing and ever-changing mixture of reflex effects and psychogenic responses

The baroreceptor reflex and the atrial volume receptor reflex are just two of several important cardiovascular reflexes. They are primarily responsible for the regulation of blood pressure and blood volume, and they illustrate several properties common to all cardiovascular reflexes. First, these reflexes originate from changes detected by peripheral sensory receptors. Second, the reflexes occur at a subconscious level, through neural pathways that primarily involve cardiovascular centers in the brainstem and midbrain. Third, cardiovascular reflexes persist in unconscious and anesthetized subjects, although the strength and character of the reflexes are altered by anesthesia. Finally, the reflexes use sympathetic and parasympathetic neurons as well as hormonal and behavioral responses to bring about cardiovascular changes.

In conscious subjects, neurohumoral control of the cardiovascular system involves both cardiovascular reflexes and psychogenic effects. Psychogenic responses originate from conscious perceptions or emotional reactions. They are eliminated by unconsciousness or general anesthesia. They involve neural pathways of the midbrain and forebrain, including the limbic system and cerebral cortex. Psychogenic responses are often triggered by sensory stimuli. For example, the sights, sounds, and smells of a veterinary clinic may trigger perceptions and emotions that cause increases in heart rate and blood pressure in both animal patients and their human companions. Psychogenic responses can also occur without any obvious sensory triggers. For example, anxiety about a future event can increase heart rate and blood pressure, at least in humans. Cardiovascular reflexes and psychogenic reactions use the same sympathetic and parasympathetic neurons and some of the same hormonal responses to bring about cardiovascular changes.

Two important psychogenic responses are the defense-alarm reaction and vasovagal syncope (the "playing dead reaction"). The *defense-alarm reaction (fear, fight, or flight response)* is an emotional response to a threatening situation, physical injury, or trauma. This reaction involves increased sympathetic activity and decreased parasympathetic activity. The sympathetic activation may be sufficiently strong to cause the release of epinephrine and norepinephrine from the adrenal medulla. The cardiovascular responses during a defense-alarm reaction include an increased heart rate, increased stroke volume, vasoconstriction in noncritical organs (kidneys, splanchnic organs, resting skeletal muscle) and skin, vasodilation in coronary vessels and in working skeletal muscle, and increased blood pressure. The cardiovascular responses during the defense reaction are also enhanced by other circulating hormones, including ADH, angiotensin II, and corticotropin (formerly called adrenocorticotropic hormone [ACTH]). The elevated blood pressure helps to ensure adequate blood flow for the critical organs (exercising skeletal muscles, heart, and brain).

During a defense-alarm reaction, the baroreceptor reflex is reset by the central nervous system so that it regulates blood pressure at an elevated level rather than acting to oppose the increased pressure. This is analogous to resetting the cruise control on a car so that it regulates speed at an elevated level rather than acting to oppose an increased speed. Thus, it is more accurate to say that the baroreceptor reflex regulates blood pressure at a variable set-point (set by the central nervous system) than to say that the baroreflex regulates arterial pressure at any single "normal" pressure.

It is important to recognize that the defense-alarm reaction is simply the extreme form of a continuum of states of emotional arousal. Sleep is at the opposite end of this cardiovascular and emotional continuum. In quiet rest or sleep, sympathetic activity is minimal and parasympathetic activity is maximal. During a full-blown defense-alarm reaction, sympathetic activity is maximal and parasympathetic activity is minimal. Between these extremes lie all of the levels of emotional arousal experienced by animals and humans from moment to moment during ordinary and extraordinary daily activities. Cardiovascular variables, such as heart rate and blood pressure, are sensitive to these changes in emotional state (Fig. 24–6). For example, a large dog may normally have a heart rate of 80 beats per minute while resting at home; it would be entirely normal for the same dog to have a heart rate of 130 beats per minute while "resting" in a clinic, if the dog is frightened in that setting. Another important point for the clinician to remember is that emotional responses are subjective. Situations that severely agitate one animal may cause only a mild alerting response in another animal. The clinician must evaluate heart rate, blood pressure, and other cardiovascular signs with respect to the patient's emotional state.

Vasovagal syncope is another psychogenic response that may be encountered in veterinary practice. This response is also called the "playing dead reaction" or "playing 'possum." In response to certain threatening or emotional situations, some humans and animals experience a psychogenic decrease in blood pressure and may faint. In many ways, this response is the opposite of the defense-alarm reaction. As shown in Figure 24–7, vasovagal syncope involves a decrease in sympathetic activity and an increase in parasympathetic activity. These neural changes bring about a vasodilation in the noncritical organs and a decrease in TPR. Heart rate and cardiac output also decrease, so there is a large drop in arterial blood pressure. The expected compensatory reflex responses do not take place. If blood pressure falls so low that there is inadequate cerebral blood flow, then *syncope* (fainting) results. The term *vasovagal syncope* denotes *vaso*dilation, *vagal* (parasympathetic) activation, and *syncope* (fainting). It is not clear why some animals respond to a threatening situation with a defense-alarm reaction, whereas others exhibit vasovagal syncope. Also unclear is the survival value of "playing dead," although this response seems to have served opossums well over several million years.

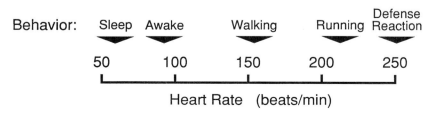

FIGURE 24–6. The defense-alarm reaction is simply the extreme on a continuum of emotional and physical arousal. The cardiovascular system (e.g., heart rate) responds sensitively to every change along this arousal scale.

Vasovagal Syncope

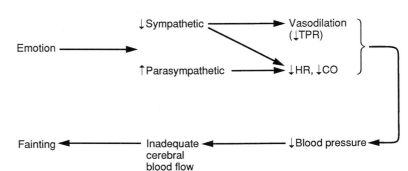

FIGURE 24–7. Vasovagal syncope ("playing dead reaction") is an emotional response that involves decreases in sympathetic activity and increases in parasympathetic activity. CO, cardiac output; HR, heart rate; TPR, total peripheral resistance.

CLINICAL CORRELATIONS

Intraoperative hemorrhage

History Four hours after abdominal surgery for a splenic sarcoma, a 30-kg, 9-year-old Labrador retriever is severely lethargic and recumbent. An abnormally large amount of hemorrhage occurred during the surgical removal of the spleen, because the dog had a hereditary blood-clotting defect (von Willebrand's disease).

Clinical examination The dog's gums are pale, and his capillary refilling time is abnormally prolonged (3 seconds). His extremities are cool to the touch. The femoral pulse is rapid and weak. An electrocardiogram indicates sinus tachycardia at a rate of 185 beats per minute. The hematocrit (packed cell volume) is 38%, and the plasma protein concentration is 5.6 g/dL; both these values are below normal. A jugular catheter is inserted, and central venous pressure is measured and found to be −1 mm Hg (normal is from 0 to +3 mm Hg). Despite the intravenous administration of 600 mL of lactated Ringer's solution during surgery, the dog has not produced any urine.

Through abdominocentesis, 100 mL of bloody fluid is removed from the dog's abdomen.

Comment This case illustrates the clinical signs that are typical of hemorrhage. Most of the blood in a dog is in the systemic veins, so most of the blood missing after hemorrhage is missing from the veins. The result is an abnormally low central venous pressure, as observed in this dog. The decreased central venous pressure causes a decreased ventricular preload and a decreased ventricular end-diastolic volume. This leads to decreases in stroke volume (Starling's law of the heart), cardiac output, and arterial blood pressure. Inadequate cardiac output and blood pressure lead to behavioral depression.

Neurohumoral compensations for the hemorrhage are initiated by the atrial volume receptor reflex and the arterial baroreceptor reflex. Heart rate is increased by the combination of increased sympathetic activation and decreased parasympathetic activation. The combination of high heart rate and low stroke volume accounts for the rapid but weak (low pulse pressure) femoral pulse. Sympathetic activity also causes vasoconstriction in the mucous membranes, resting skeletal muscle, splanchnic organs, and kidneys. The reduced blood flow in these tissues accounts for the pale gums, the slow refilling of capillaries, the cool limbs, and the lack of production of urine by the kidneys. Urine formation by the kidneys is

also being depressed by the combined hormonal effects of ADH and the renin-angiotensin-aldosterone system.

Hemorrhage per se does not reduce either the hematocrit or the plasma protein concentration, because whole blood is being lost. However, two factors caused the hematocrit and plasma protein concentration to decrease in this dog. First, the fluid administered intravenously during surgery (lactated Ringer's) contained neither red blood cells nor plasma proteins, so the cells and proteins remaining in the blood stream were diluted by the addition of the fluid. Second, the hemorrhage reduced not only venous and arterial pressures but also capillary hydrostatic pressure, and this changed the balance of hydrostatic and oncotic forces ("Starling forces") across the capillary walls in favor of reabsorption. The interstitial fluid that was reabsorbed into the blood stream contained no red blood cells and almost no plasma proteins. This caused a further dilution of the cells and proteins in the blood.

Treatment Therapy for this case involves measures to stop ongoing blood loss and to restore the lost blood volume. In this dog, the hemorrhage is predominantly seepage from small intra-abdominal vessels as a result of the coagulation defect. Transfusions of fresh blood or plasma, or concentrated preparations of clotting proteins, would promote clotting, limit subsequent hemorrhage, and expand the intravascular fluid volume. Additional crystalloid solutions (such as lactated Ringer's) also can be infused into this dog, because the hematocrit and plasma protein concentration are not dangerously low. If crystalloid solutions are administered, the hematocrit and plasma protein concentration should be monitored closely to avoid the hypoxia that results from too much dilution of the red blood cells or the edema that results from too much dilution of the plasma proteins.

Bibliography

Berne RM, Levy MN: Cardiovascular Physiology, 7th ed. St. Louis: CV Mosby, 1997.

Dukes HH, Swenson MJ, Reece WO (eds): Dukes' Physiology of Domestic Animals. Ithaca, N.Y.: Comstock, 1993, pp 184–226.

Guyton AC, Hall JE: Textbook of Medical Physiology, 10th ed. Philadelphia: WB Saunders, 2000, pp 96–262.

Milnor WR: Cardiovascular Physiology. New York: Oxford University Press, 1990.

Mohrman DE, Heller LJ: Cardiovascular Physiology, 4th ed. New York: McGraw-Hill, 1997.

Shepherd JT, Vatner SF: Nervous Control of the Heart. Amsterdam: Harwood, 1996.

Sisson DD, Thomas WP, Bonagura JD: Congenital heart disease. In

Ettinger SJ, Feldman EC (eds): Textbook of Veterinary Internal Medicine: Diseases of the Dog and Cat, 5th ed. Philadelphia: WB Saunders, 2000, p 737.
Scher AM: Cardiovascular control. In Patton HD, Fuchs AF, Hille B, et al (eds): Textbook of Physiology. Philadelphia: WB Saunders, 1989, p 972.

PRACTICE QUESTIONS

1. The dilation of arterioles that occurs during steady-state exercise in active skeletal muscles could be eliminated by
 a. pharmacologic blockade of all sympathetic and parasympathetic nerves.
 b. complete surgical removal of sympathetic innervation of the skeletal muscles.
 c. administration of a muscarinic cholinergic–blocking agent.
 d. administration of a β-adrenergic receptor–blocking agent.
 e. none of the above.

2. A drug is injected intravenously into a dog and causes a transient increase in mean arterial pressure and a transient decrease in heart rate. The baroreceptor nerves are cut; the drug is reinjected and now causes a greater increase in blood pressure but no change in heart rate. Which choice is most likely to explain the results caused by the first injection of the drug?
 a. It caused activation of muscarinic cholinergic (M_3) receptors of arterioles.
 b. It caused a reflex slowing of the heart.
 c. It caused activation of $β_1$-adrenergic receptors of the pacemaker cells of the atrium.
 d. It blocked α-adrenergic receptors of peripheral arterioles.
 e. It decreased the activity of arterial baroreceptors.

3. A dog has had a hemorrhage. The heart rate is increased above normal, and the skin is cold. The mucous membranes are pale. In this situation (compared with normal)
 a. the baroreceptor nerves are firing at a higher rate.
 b. the sympathetic nerves to the heart are firing at a decreased rate.
 c. the sympathetic nerves to the blood vessels of the skin and mucous membranes are firing at an increased rate.
 d. the parasympathetic fibers to the blood vessels are firing at an increased rate.
 e. the release of renin by the kidney is decreased.

4. Vasovagal syncope
 a. involves decreased blood pressure and heart rate.
 b. involves increased sympathetic activity.
 c. involves a decrease in cardiac parasympathetic activity.
 d. repares an animal for fight or flight.
 e. involves constriction of splanchnic arterioles.

5. Blood (250 mL) is taken from a vein of a dog. Mean arterial pressure does not decrease measurably. Nevertheless, it is likely that
 a. stimulation of atrial stretch receptors has decreased.
 b. stroke volume has increased.
 c. stimulation of aortic arch baroreceptors has increased.
 d. TPR has decreased.
 e. secretion of ADH by the pituitary has decreased.

PRACTICE ANSWERS

1. e   2. b   3. c   4. a   5. a

CHAPTER

25

Integrated cardiovascular responses

1 Heart failure is compensated for by both Starling's mechanism and the arterial baroreflex

2 Serious complications secondary to heart failure include exercise intolerance, edema, salt and water retention, uremia, kidney failure, septic shock, and decompensation

3 The immediate cardiovascular effects of hemorrhage are minimized by compensations initiated by the atrial volume receptor reflex and the arterial baroreceptor reflex

4 The blood volume lost in hemorrhage is restored through a combination of capillary fluid shifts and hormonal and behavioral responses

5 The initiation of exercise involves an interplay of local and neural changes to increase cardiac output and to deliver increased flow to exercising muscle

In the preceding chapters, the various elements of cardiovascular function and control were described. However, an understanding of these individual elements is not sufficient to provide a basis for the diagnosis and treatment of cardiovascular dysfunction. The veterinary clinician must understand the interaction of these elements in both normal and abnormal situations. Therefore, in this chapter, three fundamentally important, integrated cardiovascular responses are described (1) the response to heart failure, (2) the response to hemorrhage, and (3) the response to exercise. In addition to elucidating important, integrated responses, this discussion provides a review and summary of key concepts of cardiovascular physiology.

Heart failure is compensated for by both Starling's mechanism and the arterial baroreflex

There are many kinds and causes of *heart failure*. Some clinicians use the term very broadly to refer to any condition in which a problem in the heart limits its ability to deliver a normal cardiac output to the body tissues. Such conditions would include various valve defects, arrhythmias, and even heartworm infestation. A more restrictive definition, and one favored by physiologists, is that *heart failure* is any condition in which a depressed *cardiac contractility* limits the ability of the heart to deliver a normal cardiac output. The broad definition of heart failure encompasses virtually any problem with the heart as a pump; a com-

mon synonym is *pump failure*. The more restrictive definition (which is used in this chapter) equates heart failure with *myocardial failure*, a depressed contractility of the heart muscle itself.

A depressed cardiac contractility can result from coronary artery disease, cardiac hypoxia, myocarditis, toxins, drug effects, or electrolyte imbalances. If the decrease in contractility affects both sides of the heart, the condition is called *bilateral heart failure.* In other circumstances, failure may be restricted primarily to either the left ventricle or to the right ventricle and so is called *left-sided heart failure* or *right-sided heart failure.*

Ventricular function curves provide a helpful way to envision the consequences of heart failure and the compensations for heart failure. In Figure 25–1, the curve labeled *normal* indicates the relationship between stroke volume and preload for a normal ventricle (for a review, see Fig. 20–3C). The curve labeled *initially severe failure* shows that a ventricle in failure has a depressed contractility (i.e., a smaller stroke volume for any given preload). If a normal heart suddenly goes into severe failure, stroke volume decreases from its normal value (shown by point 1) to the low value (shown by point 2). For purposes of illustration, imagine that these curves define the function of the left ventricle and that the left ventricle is the one that fails. A decrease in left ventricular stroke volume causes a decrease in left ventricular output, which results in a decrease in mean arterial blood pressure. If there is inadequate compensation for this fall in blood pressure, severe exercise intolerance is certain, inadequate perfusion of the critical organs is likely, and death is probable. However, several

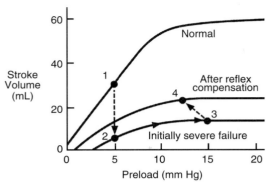

FIGURE 25–1. Ventricular function curves depicting the consequences and compensations for heart failure in terms of changes in preload and stroke volume. Details are given in the text.

mechanisms act to compensate for heart failure and to minimize its adverse effects.

One compensation for heart failure is *Starling's mechanism.* If the left ventricle suddenly decreases its stroke volume, blood backs up (dams up or accumulates) in the left atrium and pulmonary veins, because the right ventricle, at least for a few heartbeats, maintains a higher stroke volume than does the failing left ventricle. Some of the excess blood pumped by the right ventricle accumulates in the left atrium, so left atrial pressure increases. The increase in left atrial pressure creates an increase in left ventricular preload, which leads to an increase in left ventricular end-diastolic volume and (by Starling's mechanism) an increase in stroke volume. In other words, instead of remaining at the point on the graph labeled 2, the function of the left ventricle moves to the right along the curve of initially severe failure, to point 3, with a higher preload and a somewhat higher stroke volume. This sequence of events, whereby an increase in preload helps offset the fall in stroke volume, is also diagrammed in Figure 25–2 (top left loop). Note that this compensation does not return stroke volume to its normal value but does bring it to a level somewhat higher than that before the compensation.

Another compensatory mechanism for heart failure involves the arterial baroreflex. Because stroke volume remains below normal, even after compensation by the Starling mechanism, left ventricular output also remains below normal, and so does arterial blood pressure. Therefore, baroreceptor activity is below normal. The central nervous system responds reflexly by increasing sympathetic efferent activity to the heart and blood vessels and by decreasing parasympathetic activity to the heart.

The sympathetic effect on the heart increases ventricular contractility. Contractility is not restored to normal but is brought to a higher level than existed in the absence of reflex compensation. Graphically, the effect of the baroreflex is to move the failing ventricle to a function curve that is intermediate between the normal curve and the curve of initially severe failure (see point 4 in Fig. 25–1). Note that the

increase in contractility also brings stroke volume back toward (but does not reach) its normal level.

Sympathetic actions on the heart increase heart rate above normal and decrease the systolic duration; these changes also help to restore cardiac output back toward normal despite the persistently depressed stroke volume. Finally, sympathetic activation causes vasoconstriction in the noncritical organs, which increases total peripheral resistance (TPR) above normal. This also helps to return blood pressure toward its normal level.

The net effect of the compensations by way of Starling's mechanism and the baroreflex is that blood pressure can be maintained near its normal level, at least when the animal is at rest, despite a severe ventricular failure. These reflex effects are summarized in Figure 25–2. Note that after compensation by the Starling mechanism and the baroreflex, contractility, stroke volume, cardiac output, and blood pressure remain at least somewhat below normal; preload, sympathetic activity, heart rate, and TPR are above normal.

Serious complications secondary to heart failure include exercise intolerance, edema, salt and water retention, uremia, kidney failure, septic shock, and decompensation

Even though Starling's mechanism and the baroreflex can compensate to a remarkable degree for severe heart failure, important, secondary complications often develop. These complications make heart failure a serious clinical problem, even in cases where arterial

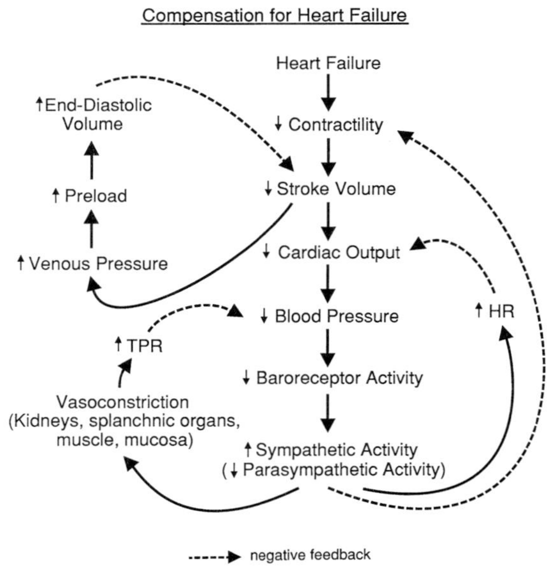

FIGURE 25–2. The consequences and compensations for heart failure. The changes described here include those presented graphically in Figure 25–1. Details are given in the text. HR, heart rate; TPR, total peripheral resistance.

Integrated cardiovascular responses **211**

pressure is maintained near normal levels in the resting animal.

The first complication secondary to heart failure is *exercise intolerance.* In a normal animal, the ability of the heart to increase cardiac output during exercise depends on sympathetically ediated increases in stroke volume and heart rate. However, in a patient with heart failure, the ability of sympathetic activation to increase cardiac output is nearly exhausted simply to restore cardiac output toward normal in the resting state. Therefore, the patient's attempt to exercise is not accompanied by an effective, further increase in sympathetic activity; the failing heart cannot provide the increased cardiac output required to meet the blood flow requirements of exercising skeletal muscle. Metabolic vasodilation in the exercising muscle, in the absence of an adequate increase in cardiac output, results in a large decrease in arterial

pressure and inadequate blood flow to all organs, including the exercising muscle. The patient exhibits lethargy and weakness; even mild exercise leads quickly to exhaustion.

Edema is the second serious complication secondary to heart failure. As noted, blood backs up or dams up in the veins and the atrium behind a failing ventricle. In the case of left ventricular failure, left atrial pressure increases, and so does pressure in the pulmonary veins and pulmonary capillaries. The increase in pulmonary capillary hydrostatic pressure leads to an increase in the filtration of capillary fluid into the interstitial spaces of the lungs. As fluid accumulates in the interstitial space, *pulmonary edema* develops. These events are summarized in Figure 25–3 (*top left*). Excess interstitial fluid in the lungs slows the transfer of oxygen from the lung alveoli into the lung capillaries and can result in systemic hypoxia. In extreme cases,

FIGURE 25–3. Heart failure leads to exercise intolerance. Several additional life-threatening complications secondary to heart failure are diagrammed here; these include edema, salt and water retention, uremia, kidney failure, and septic shock. See text for details and for a discussion of an additional complication, *decompensation.*

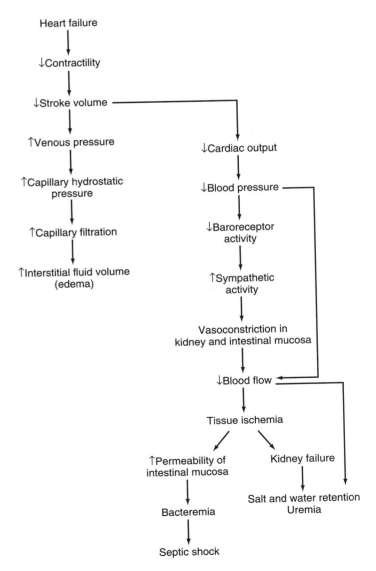

pulmonary edema results in the actual accumulation of fluid in the intrapleural space (*pleural effusion*) or in the alveolar air spaces, and this causes a further reduction in lung function. The resulting systemic hypoxia can lead to death. In a case of right ventricular failure, the increase in venous pressure occurs in the systemic circulation. Therefore, the resulting edema occurs in the systemic organs, particularly in dependent extremities and in the abdomen.

Whether the edema is in the lungs or in the systemic circulation, its degree is limited by the three safety factors previously discussed (see Fig. 22–5). These safety factors would probably keep the edema of heart failure well controlled were it not for an additional factor that exaggerates the elevation of venous pressure in heart failure. As long as arterial pressure remains subnormal in a patient with heart failure, the baroreceptor reflex works to raise blood volume above normal. The volume-increasing mechanisms activated by the arterial baroreflex include increasing thirst (which raises fluid intake), increasing the release of antidiuretic hormone (ADH) from the pituitary (which decreases fluid loss in the urine), and activating the renin-angiotensin-aldosterone system (which decreases Na^+ loss in the urine). These effects of the baroreflex were mentioned briefly in Chapter 24, and the mechanisms of action of ADH and the renin-angiotensin-aldosterone system are covered in more detail in Chapters 40 and 42.

The point for now is that the patient with severe heart failure experiences substantial and persistent increases in blood volume. The excess blood accumulates particularly in the veins and capillaries upstream from the failing ventricle and often leads to an increase in capillary filtration that overwhelms the normal safety factors against edema. In fact, one of the main goals in the clinical treatment of heart failure is to counteract the buildup of excessive blood and interstitial fluid volume. Diuretic drugs are the main therapies used for this purpose (see a further discussion in Chapter 42).

Arteriolar vasoconstriction leads to the additional complications of uremia, kidney failure, and septic shock in severe heart failure. When the baroreceptor reflex responds to an abnormally low arterial pressure in heart failure, it brings about arteriolar vasoconstriction, primarily in the kidneys, splanchnic organs, and resting skeletal muscle (the "noncritical organs"). In severe failure, the skin and mucous membranes may also be vasoconstricted. Vasoconstriction in these organs helps compensate for heart failure by permitting the available cardiac output to be routed to the critical organs (brain, heart, and working skeletal muscle). However, persistent vasoconstriction leads to several adverse effects.

Vasoconstricted kidneys cannot form urine in a normal manner and therefore do not rid the body of the excess volume of blood and interstitial fluid that accumulates in heart failure. Vasoconstricted kidneys also allow nitrogenous and acidic waste products to accumulate in the body. The condition is called *uremia*, which literally means "urine in the blood." To make matters worse, after a prolonged period of intense vasoconstriction, the kidney tissue becomes irreversibly damaged. At that stage, uremia, acidosis, and salt and water retention may persist even if clinical treatment is successful in restoring cardiac output and blood pressure to normal. In fact, *renal failure* often is the terminal event in chronic heart failure.

Intense and prolonged vasoconstriction in the splanchnic circulation can also have lethal consequences. The mucosa of the gastrointestinal tract is very susceptible to ischemic damage. Normally, the intestinal mucosa creates a barrier between the intestinal lumen and the blood stream. Prolonged intestinal vasoconstriction damages the mucosa, with the consequence that bacteria and bacterial toxins pass into the blood stream or the peritoneum. The resulting bacteremia or peritonitis can lead to septic shock and death. The causes and consequences of renal and splanchnic ischemia are summarized in Figure 25–3 (*bottom right*).

Cardiac decompensation is an additional (and frequently terminal) complication secondary to heart failure. The basic concept of decompensation is that when heart failure reaches a certain degree of severity, the compensations by the body for heart failure end up making the heart failure worse. Vicious "decompensating" cycles develop and lead to death within a few hours unless there is vigorous medical intervention.

The specific mechanisms of the decompensating cycles are very complex, but two examples illustrate the concept. As explained, in the case of left ventricular failure, the damming up of blood in the left atrium is compensatory because it increases left ventricular preload, which helps boost stroke volume toward normal. However, the increased left ventricular preload can lead to the secondary complication of pulmonary edema. If it is severe, pulmonary edema interferes with the oxygenation of blood. One tissue that depends critically on an adequate supply of oxygen is cardiac muscle; hypoxia depresses the contractility of cardiac muscle. Thus, a vicious cycle can develop, in which severely depressed ventricular contractility leads to severe pulmonary edema, which leads to inadequate oxygenation of blood, which leads to hypoxia of the left ventricular muscle, which further depresses ventricular contractility.

For a second example of a decompensatory vicious cycle, consider again the effects of the baroreflex on the kidneys. Renal vasoconstriction is compensatory for heart failure in that it helps increase TPR, which helps raise arterial pressure back toward normal, which helps keep perfusion pressure high enough to deliver adequate blood flow to the critical organs. However, intense and prolonged renal vasoconstriction leads to the secondary complications of reduced excretion of acidic and nitrogenous metabolic waste products. Accumulation of these waste products in the blood (uremia) causes their accumulation in various body tissues, including the heart. The accumulation of acidic and nitrogenous waste products in cardiac muscle tissue depresses cardiac contractility.

Thus, another vicious cycle can develop, in which severe ventricular failure leads to intense and prolonged renal vasoconstriction, which leads to uremia, which causes metabolic waste products to accumulate in cardiac muscle, which further depresses ventricular contractility.

Other decompensatory cycles develop in cases of severe heart failure, but these examples illustrate the basic concept and show why decompensation is such a serious development.

In summary, in addition to exercise intolerance, the life-threatening complications secondary to heart failure include edema, salt and water retention, uremia, kidney failure, septic shock, and decompensation. Careful clinical diagnosis and prompt treatment of heart failure are imperative, even in cases in which compensatory mechanisms have maintained blood pressure near its normal level.

In the evaluation of the severity of heart failure and the extent of compensation, it is clinically useful to group the signs of heart failure into two categories. The first category is referred to as *backward heart failure*. The signs of backward heart failure include the changes in the circulation *upstream* from the failing ventricle: namely, increased atrial pressure, increased venous pressure, excessive capillary filtration, edema, and the functional changes secondary to edema (e.g., respiratory failure). The category *forward heart failure* refers to the consequences of heart failure *downstream* from the failing ventricle and include decreased cardiac output, decreased arterial blood pressure, and the consequences of excessive vasoconstriction in the systemic organs, especially the kidneys and intestines.

The immediate cardiovascular effects of hemorrhage are minimized by compensations initiated by the atrial volume receptor reflex and the arterial baroreceptor reflex

The cardiovascular responses to hemorrhage are summarized in Figures 25–4 and 25–5. The curve labeled *Normal* in Figure 25–4 shows that the maintenance of a normal stroke volume is dependent on the maintenance of a normal level of ventricular preload. When hemorrhage occurs, blood is lost from the whole cardiovascular system, and particularly from the veins, which are the blood reservoirs of the body. Hemorrhage decreases central venous volume, central venous pressure, and atrial pressure. The decrease in atrial pressure decreases ventricular preload and end-diastolic ventricular volume. In the absence of any compensations, the stroke volume decreases from point 1 in Figure 25–4 to point 2. Note that the normal ventricular function curve is rather steep to the left of the normal operating point (point 1). Therefore, a 40% hemorrhage results in approximately 40% reductions in central venous pressure, left atrial pressure, ventricular preload, and stroke volume. In the absence of compensations, cardiac output and mean arterial pressure would also decrease by 40%. The mean arte-

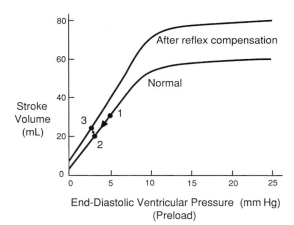

FIGURE 25–4. The direct effect of hemorrhage is to decrease ventricular preload, which decreases stroke volume (transition from point 1 to point 2). Stroke volume is restored *toward normal* by a reflex increase in sympathetic activity, which increases ventricular contractility *above normal* (transition from point 2 to point 3).

rial pressure would then be inadequate to sustain normal function in the critical organs, and the animal would die. However, with intact compensatory mechanisms, a normal animal can withstand a 40% hemorrhage without death and have only an approximately 10% decrease in mean arterial pressure.

The immediate compensations for hemorrhage are initiated by the arterial baroreflex and atrial volume receptor reflex. Hemorrhage decreases mean arterial pressure, which decreases the activity of arterial baroreceptors. The baroreflex response is to increase sympathetic activity and to decrease parasympathetic activity. The increased sympathetic activity acts on the

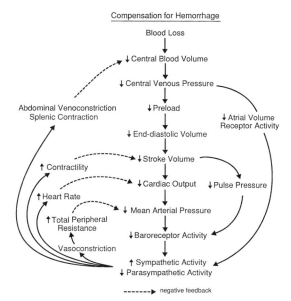

FIGURE 25–5. Summary of the consequences of hemorrhage and of the immediate compensations brought about by the arterial baroreflex and by the atrial volume receptor reflex. The changes described here include those presented in Figure 25–4.

heart to increase cardiac contractility. This helps restore stroke volume back toward normal, despite a persistent, subnormal preload and end-diastolic volume. The effect of this sympathetic compensation is diagrammed in Figure 25–4 as point 3. Note that the stroke volume is not returned to normal; after compensation for a 40% hemorrhage, the stroke volume may remain 25% below normal. However, the stroke volume is closer to normal than it was before compensation.

Additional compensations help restore blood pressure closer to normal. First, heart rate increases above normal, which brings cardiac output back to within about 20% of its normal level, despite the persistent low stroke volume. In addition, sympathetic vasoconstriction in the noncritical organs raises TPR above normal, resulting in a mean arterial pressure that remains within approximately 10% of its normal level, despite a persistent 20% drop in cardiac output. The reader may wish to review the compensations described thus far by locating them on Figure 25–5.

The perceptive reader may wonder why baroreflex compensatory actions continue if mean arterial pressure is returned most of the way toward normal. Compensatory baroreflex responses are sustained because baroreceptors are responsive to changes in pulse pressure as well as to changes in mean arterial pressure, and pulse pressure remains low. There are two reasons for the subnormal pulse pressure: (1) the persistent decrease in stroke volume and (2) the increase in heart rate above normal. Thus, even if the mean arterial pressure were returned completely to normal after a hemorrhage, arterial baroreceptor action potential frequency would remain below normal because of the persistent subnormal pulse pressure.

The atrial volume receptor reflex also contributes to the sustained increase in sympathetic activity after hemorrhage. As shown in Figure 25–5, hemorrhage leads to a persistent decrease in central venous pressure and atrial pressure. Therefore, the activity of the atrial volume receptors is decreased below normal. The central nervous system responds to this decreased afferent activity from atrial volume receptors by elevating sympathetic efferent activity and by decreasing cardiac parasympathetic efferent activity. Thus, the atrial volume receptor reflex and the arterial baroreflex work synergistically to compensate for hemorrhage.

In extreme hemorrhage, the reflex increases in sympathetic activity affect not only the heart and resistance vessels but also the veins. The abdominal veins, in particular, are constricted when sympathetic activation is intense. Sympathetic venoconstriction displaces blood from the abdominal veins and moves it toward the central circulation, which helps to increase central venous pressure, atrial pressure, and preload back toward normal (see Fig. 25–5). In addition, a substantial volume of blood can be moved from the spleen into the central circulation in species that have large spleens, such as dogs and horses. Sympathetic activation constricts both the blood vessels within the spleen and the muscular capsule around the spleen.

The blood that is sequestered in the spleen is expelled into the abdominal veins, and then it moves toward the heart. In the dog and the horse, splenic contraction can mobilize a volume of blood equal to 10% of the total blood volume. An additional, adaptive feature of the blood sequestered in the spleen is that it has a higher-than-normal hematocrit. The mobilization of these sequestered red blood cells helps to offset the fall in hematocrit that is a normal consequence of interstitial fluid reabsorption after hemorrhage (see later).

The arterial baroreceptor reflex and the atrial volume receptor reflex act within a few seconds to restore blood pressure toward its normal level after a hemorrhage. Other compensations come into play in the minutes and hours after hemorrhage to restore the lost fluid volume.

The blood volume lost in hemorrhage is restored through a combination of capillary fluid shifts and hormonal and behavioral responses

Hemorrhage causes both venous and arterial pressures to fall below normal, so capillary hydrostatic pressure also falls below normal throughout the body. This alters the balance of hydrostatic and oncotic pressures acting on water in a direction that favors reabsorption of interstitial fluid back into the capillaries (Fig. 25–6). The volume of interstitial fluid that can be reabsorbed by this process in 1 hour is approximately 10% of the volume lost in the hemorrhage.

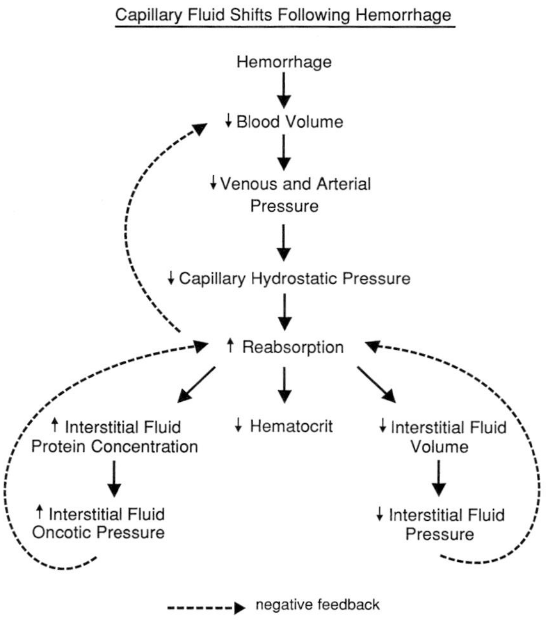

Capillary Fluid Shifts Following Hemorrhage

FIGURE 25–6. During the first 3 to 4 hours after a hemorrhage, interstitial fluid is reabsorbed into the blood stream, which helps compensate for the lost blood volume. A complication is that the hematocrit decreases. Reabsorption is limited by decreases in interstitial fluid hydrostatic pressure and by increases in interstitial fluid oncotic pressure.

However, the rate of reabsorption of interstitial fluid becomes limited after 3 to 4 hours, because as interstitial fluid is reabsorbed, there is a decrease in interstitial fluid hydrostatic pressure (it becomes even more negative than normal), and this opposes further reabsorption. Also, as interstitial fluid is reabsorbed, the interstitial fluid protein concentration increases, because proteins in the interstitial fluid are not reabsorbed. The resulting increase in interstitial fluid oncotic pressure also opposes further reabsorption. Despite these limits, the reabsorption of interstitial fluid is an important compensation for hemorrhage in the first few hours.

A complication that results from the reabsorption of interstitial fluid after hemorrhage is that the reabsorbed fluid contains no plasma proteins or blood cells. Therefore, the proteins and cells that are in the blood stream are diluted as interstitial fluid is reabsorbed. The concentration of plasma proteins in blood decreases, as does the hematocrit. This is why a decreasing hematocrit over a period of a few hours in an otherwise normal patient is presumptive evidence that a hemorrhage has occurred recently or is continuing to occur. In the absence of an obvious hemorrhage, such a patient should be examined for evidence of internal bleeding.

The restoration of blood volume after hemorrhage also involves hormonal and behavioral responses (Fig. 25–7). As mentioned, hemorrhage leads to a decrease in the action potential frequency of both the arterial baroreceptors and the atrial volume receptors. In addition to immediate sympathetic and parasympathetic responses (already described, and depicted in Fig. 25–5), the arterial baroreflex and the atrial

volume receptor reflex trigger important hormonal effects. The increase in sympathetic activity (coupled with a decrease in arterial pressure) acts on the kidneys to increase their release of the hormone renin. As mentioned in Chapter 24, renin works through the additional hormones angiotensin and aldosterone to decrease sodium excretion by the kidneys. Also, there is increased ADH secretion from the pituitary gland. ADH circulates to the kidneys, where it reduces urine formation. Through the combined actions of renal vasoconstriction, the renin-angiotensin-aldosterone system, and ADH, both sodium excretion and water excretion are decreased. Note that these actions *conserve* the available blood volume after hemorrhage, but they do not *restore* it to normal. The actual restoration of blood volume after hemorrhage requires increased fluid intake. The baroreceptor reflex and the atrial volume receptor reflex act through the hypothalamus to increase the sensation of thirst. If water is available, there is an increase in fluid intake until the lost blood volume is restored to normal. This may take 1 to 2 days.

The final compensations for hemorrhage involve the restoration of the lost plasma proteins and blood cells. The plasma proteins are synthesized by the liver, and the blood cells are produced by the bone marrow. The time required may be several days for the plasma proteins and a few weeks for the blood cells.

The preceding discussion focused on the effects of severe hemorrhage. All of the same compensations occur to a milder degree after mild hemorrhage. For example, when a human donates blood, 0.5 L (about 10% of the blood volume) is removed. All of the compensations just described are evident after this 10% hemorrhage.

In humans and in some large animals, the transition from a supine to a standing posture elicits many of the same cardiovascular responses as hemorrhage. The reason for this can be understood if one considers the effect of gravity on the blood contained within the blood vessels of the body. In a standing subject, gravity increases the distending pressure in the dependent vessels (those below heart level), particularly in the leg vessels. The gravitational effect does not result in much accumulation of blood in the arteries and arterioles, because these vessels are not easily distensible (they have low compliance). However, the gravitational effect results in a significant distention of the dependent veins, because of their much greater compliance. The extra blood in the dependent veins is blood that would otherwise be returned to the central circulation. Therefore, in an upright subject, there is a decrease in central blood volume and central venous pressure, just as there would be after hemorrhage. Thus, upright posture causes decreased cardiac filling, decreased stroke volume, decreased cardiac output, and so on. In a normal human, the assumption of an upright posture is equivalent to a 10% hemorrhage. All of the compensations for hemorrhage that have been described also occur in response to upright posture. The gravitational effect of standing is negligible in small animals. In large animals,

Fluid Volume Replacement Following Hemorrhage

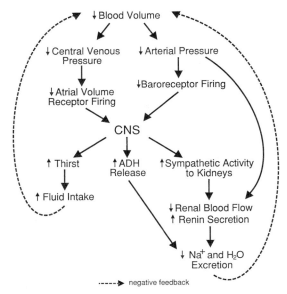

FIGURE 25–7. The behavioral and humoral responses after hemorrhage include increased fluid intake and retention of body fluid and electrolytes. ADH, antidiuretic hormone; CNS, central nervous system.

such as cattle and horses, the pooling of blood in leg veins is minimized by the relatively small size of veins in the extremities.

The initiation of exercise involves an interplay of local and neural changes to increase cardiac output and to deliver increased flow to exercising muscle

Local metabolic control mechanisms dilate skeletal muscle arterioles during exercise. As discussed in Chapter 23, when skeletal muscle begins to exercise, metabolic products accumulate in the muscle tissue, and the local oxygen concentration decreases. The metabolic products and hypoxia both cause dilation of the arterioles within the exercising muscle. This vasodilation is a local response, not dependent on nerves or hormones. This metabolic control mechanism results in an increased blood flow to the exercising muscle. The increased blood flow delivers more oxygen and removes some of the accumulated metabolic vasodilating products. In this way, muscle blood flow is matched to metabolic rate (Fig. 25–8, *top right*).

Metabolic control of blood flow in exercising muscle can succeed only if arterial blood pressure is maintained at a level sufficient to provide the needed additional blood flow. This necessitates a substantial increase in cardiac output and, in extreme exercise, vasoconstriction in the noncritical organs, to make more blood flow available for the critical organs. These adjustments are brought about by three neural mechanisms: central command, the exercise reflex, and the arterial baroreflex.

Central command is a psychogenic effect. In preparation for exercise (and continuing during exercise), the central nervous system increases sympathetic activity to the heart and blood vessels and decreases parasympathetic activity to the heart. The sympathetic and parasympathetic changes are graded, depending on the intensity of the exercise. In effect, central command represents the "best guess" by the brain as to the levels of sympathetic and parasympathetic activity that will be needed during the exercise to match cardiac output to the needs of the systemic organs.

The *exercise reflex* is the second mechanism that helps set the level of sympathetic and parasympathetic activity during exercise. The exercise reflex is initiated by specialized nerve endings within muscles and joints. An increase in muscular work and in the movement of the body joints causes an increased frequency of action potentials in these muscle and joint receptors. The increased afferent activity results reflexly in an increased sympathetic and decreased parasympathetic efferent drive. Although the mechanism for excitation of the muscle and joint receptors is not completely understood, it is clear that the activation of these receptors is necessary to keep blood pressure from falling during exercise.

The arterial baroreceptor reflex is the third major

controller of sympathetic and parasympathetic activity during exercise. The baroreflex serves to fine-tune autonomic drive to the heart and arterioles to keep arterial pressure at its set-point. If central command and the exercise reflex do not set sympathetic activity to a sufficiently high level during a particular bout of exercise, arterial pressure falls below normal. The arterial baroreceptors detect this low pressure, and the baroreflex responds by increasing sympathetic activity. Conversely, if central command and the exercise reflex set sympathetic activity too high in a particular case, arterial pressure rises above normal. The response of the baroreflex is to decrease sympathetic activity.

In effect, central command and the exercise reflex initiate the autonomic adjustments for exercise, and the arterial baroreflex performs the fine-tuning to keep arterial pressure near its set-point (see Fig. 25–8).

Two additional, non-neural mechanisms also help

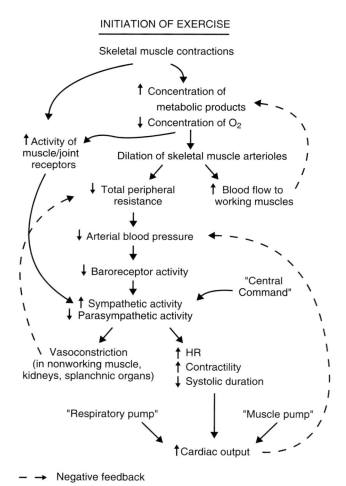

INITIATION OF EXERCISE

FIGURE 25–8. The cardiovascular responses to exercise involve a complex interplay of local metabolic control mechanisms: central command, reflexes, and the blood-pumping effects of muscle contraction and respiration. The overall result is increased blood flow in exercising muscle, decreased blood flow in the noncritical organs, decreased total peripheral resistance, increased cardiac output, and maintenance of arterial blood pressure.

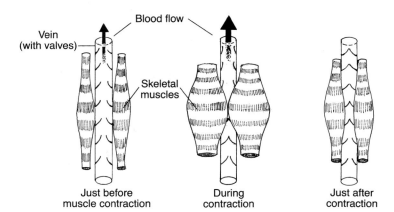

FIGURE 25–9. During dynamic exercise, the rhythmic contractions of the skeletal muscles squeeze venous blood out of the muscles and back toward the central circulation. This so-called muscle pump helps increase central venous pressure in an exercising animal.

to increase the cardiac output during exercise. The first of these is the *muscle pump* (Fig. 25–9). When skeletal muscles contract, they tend to squeeze down on the blood vessels contained within them. One effect of this, as already mentioned, is the tendency for a muscle to restrict its blood flow during a sustained contraction. However, if the contractions are rhythmic, each contraction causes blood to be expelled out of the muscle veins and hence toward the central circulation. There is minimal backflow of blood from the central circulation into the veins during muscular relaxation, because the veins have one-way valves within them. Thus, the pumping action of muscle, which massages the veins, displaces venous blood toward the central circulation and increases central venous pressure. In this way, the muscle pump increases ventricular preload above the level that would otherwise exist.

The second non-neural mechanism that helps to increase cardiac output during exercise is the *respiratory pump.* Vigorous exercise involves an increase in the rate and the depth of respiration. With each inspiration, a subatmospheric pressure is generated within the thorax. This negative pressure "pulls" outward on the airways of the lungs to expand them. It also pulls outward on the central veins and the heart and distends them. In this way, the negative intrathoracic pressure during inspiration helps draw blood from the abdominal veins into the central veins and the atria. In addition, the diaphragm muscle moves caudally during inspiration and compresses the abdominal organs. This increases intra-abdominal pressure and squeezes blood out of the abdominal veins and back toward the central veins. This respiratory pumping action helps to increase venous return, central venous volume, and ventricular preload during exercise. The combined effect of sympathetic and parasympathetic responses, the muscle pump, and the respiratory pump is that cardiac output can increase to four to six times its resting level during vigorous exercise.

Note that the success of the mechanisms that increase cardiac output during exercise depends on an ability of the heart to respond normally both to increased sympathetic drive and to increases in preload.

As mentioned earlier, during heart failure, the autonomic mechanisms available to increase cardiac contractility and heart rate are invoked simply to maintain a normal cardiac output in the resting stage. Therefore, the autonomic nervous system in a patient with heart failure has a limited ability to bring about further increases in cardiac output during the initiation of exercise. For this reason, patients with heart failure typically exhibit exercise intolerance.

Maximal exercise ability in normal humans and animals appears to be limited by cardiac output; that is, the respiratory system can oxygenate as much blood as the heart can deliver to the lungs, and skeletal muscle can take up and metabolize as much oxygen as the heart can deliver to it. However, when cardiac output has reached a maximal level, oxygen transport from the lungs to the skeletal muscle also is maximized. This sets the upper limit to the level of exercise that can be sustained.

CLINICAL CORRELATIONS

Exercise intolerance secondary to congestive heart failure

History An 8-year-old female Great Dane has been diagnosed previously with idiopathic dilative cardiomyopathy. Severe, generalized cardiac enlargement is evident on thoracic radiographs. The dog is losing weight and is unable to complete daily walks with her owners.

Clinical examination Femoral pulses are weak but regular at 140 beats per minute. The mucous membranes are pale, and the capillary refilling time is prolonged. Respiration is rapid at 45 breaths per minute. The abdomen is distended, and the abdominal organs are difficult to palpate. The electrocardiogram shows sinus tachycardia with broad, high-voltage QRS complexes. Thoracic radiography reveals a greatly enlarged heart and moderate pulmonary edema.

Additional diagnostic tests are conducted to help assess the degree of complications secondary to the heart failure. The percentage saturation of hemoglobin in arterial blood is 78% (normal 95% to 100%), the difference in oxygen content between arterial and venous blood is 8.5 mL of O_2 per deciliter of blood (normal 4 to 6 mL), the serum creatinine concentration is 3 mg/dL (normal is less than 1 mg/dL), urine specific gravity is 1.036 (high normal), and central venous pressure is 14 mm Hg (normal 0 to 3 mm Hg).

When persuaded to exercise, the dog appears to become tired after walking less than one block. Her legs begin to tremble, and then she collapses. Her pulse rate is 180 beats per minute, and her mucous membranes are dark and cyanotic (blue).

Comment Chronic heart failure secondary to cardiomyopathy is common in large dogs older than 4 years. Often, the cardiomyopathy is idiopathic (of unknown cause). The case presented here is fairly typical of advanced heart failure. All of the clinical findings are either direct consequences of the heart failure or consequences of attempts by the body to compensate for the heart failure (see Figs. 25–1 to 25–3). In brief, ventricular failure (decreased contractility) leads to decreased stroke volume, cardiac output, and blood pressure.

Compensations for the heart failure involve reflex decreases in parasympathetic activity, increases in sympathetic activity, and increases in the release of ADH and renin. Heart rate is increased, which helps raise cardiac output back toward normal. Pulse pressure, judged by palpation of the femoral pulse, is reduced (because heart rate is high and stroke volume is low). The mucosa, splanchnic organs, kidneys, and resting skeletal muscle are vasoconstricted, which helps support arterial pressure and reserves the available cardiac output for the heart and brain. The vasoconstriction is evident in the pale color and slow refilling of the mucous membranes. Renal vasoconstriction reduces the rate of urine formation. Urinary loss of salt and water is further reduced by the actions of ADH and renin. The urine that is formed has a high solute concentration (high specific gravity). Metabolic products (e.g., creatinine) that are normally eliminated by the kidneys accumulate in the blood. Salt and water retention increases blood volume above normal.

Most of the excess blood volume is in the veins, so venous and atrial pressures are above normal. The elevated atrial pressure (preload) increases ventricular end-diastolic volume above normal, which helps the failing heart to pump a larger stroke volume than it otherwise would. However, the excessive volume and pressure of blood in the veins also cause systemic edema (distended abdomen) and pulmonary edema (visible on the radiograph). Pulmonary edema impairs the ability of the lungs to oxygenate blood. Therefore, the hemoglobin saturation and the oxygen content of arterial blood are both below normal in this dog. The tissues of the body respond to the low rate of oxygen delivery by unloading as much oxygen as they can from the blood as it flows through the tissue. This makes the arteriovenous difference in oxygen content greater than normal. The general inadequacy of cardiovascular transport leads to metabolic stresses on the tissues of the dog, and weight loss occurs.

Despite many compensatory mechanisms, this dog is unable to deliver a normal amount of well-oxygenated blood to the body tissues, even at rest. When the dog tries to exercise, cardiac output increases little. Therefore, when exercise-induced vasodilation occurs in the exercising muscles and TPR decreases, blood pressure falls dramatically. There is a further decrease in blood flow in the tissues of the systemic circulation that were already vasoconstricted (e.g., the mucous membranes),

and these tissues become hypoxic and cyanotic. Inadequate blood flow in the exercising skeletal muscles leads to hypoxia and acidosis, and the dog collapses.

Treatment The ideal treatment strategy for this dog is to improve the contractile performance of the myocardium. Theoretically, β-adrenergic agonists or cardiac glycosides could be administered to increase cardiac contractility. However, currently available drugs are either ineffective or only mildly effective in dogs with severe, chronic heart failure. Therefore, treatment should emphasize symptomatic therapy, with the goals of controlling pulmonary congestion and improving cardiac output. Diuretics or venodilators reduce venous pressures and are usually effective in controlling signs of congestion. They must be used cautiously, however, because they create the risk of lowering preload and therefore exacerbating the low cardiac output. Arteriolar vasodilators can augment the output of a failing heart by reducing the afterload (arterial pressure) against which the heart must eject blood. An appropriate initial treatment for this dog includes a diuretic (furosemide) and a cardiac glycoside (digitalis). If digitalis fails to improve cardiac contractility in this advanced case of cardiomyopathy, an arteriolar vasodilator (hydralazine) or a mixed vasodilator-venodilator (enalapril) can be added to the furosemide regimen. Despite therapy, the prognosis for a dog with severe chronic heart failure is poor.

Bibliography

Berne RM, Levy MN: Cardiovascular Physiology, 7th ed. St. Louis: CV Mosby, 1997.

de Morais HA: Pathophysiology of heart failure and clinical evaluation of cardiac function. In Ettinger SJ, Feldman EC (eds): Textbook of Veterinary Internal Medicine: Diseases of the Dog and Cat, 5th ed. Philadelphia: WB Saunders, 2000, p 692.

Dukes HH, Swenson MJ, Reece WO (eds): Dukes' Physiology of Domestic Animals. Ithaca, N.Y.: Comstock, 1993, pp 244–262.

King AS: The Cardiorespiratory System: Integration of Normal and Pathological Structure and Function. London: Blackwell Scientific, 1999.

Kittleson MD: Therapy of heart failure. In Ettinger SJ, Feldman EC (eds): Textbook of Veterinary Internal Medicine: Diseases of the Dog and Cat, 5th ed. Philadelphia: WB Saunders, 2000, p 713.

Kittleson MD, Kienle RD: Small Animal Cardiovascular Medicine. St. Louis: Mosby–Year Book, 1998.

Lilly LS: Pathophysiology of Heart Disease (A Collaborative Project of Medical Students and Faculty), 2nd ed. Baltimore: Williams & Wilkins, 1998.

Marr C (ed): Cardiology of the Horse. London: WB Saunders, 1999.

Opie LH: The Heart: Physiology, From Cell to Circulation, 3rd ed. Baltimore: Lippincott Williams & Wilkins, 1998.

Patteson MW: Equine Cardiology (Library of Veterinary Practice). Oxford, United Kingdom: Blackwell Scientific, 1996.

Rowell LB: Human Cardiovascular Control. New York: Oxford University Press, 1993.

PRACTICE QUESTIONS

1. During experimental trials on a new artificial aortic valve, a dog is anesthetized and placed on cardiac bypass for 1 hour (i.e., a heart-lung machine is substituted for the dog's own heart and lungs). After successful installation of the artificial valve, the dog is taken off bypass, and the normal circulation is restored. Ten minutes later, the dog's central venous pressure is 20 mm Hg, mean arterial pressure is 90

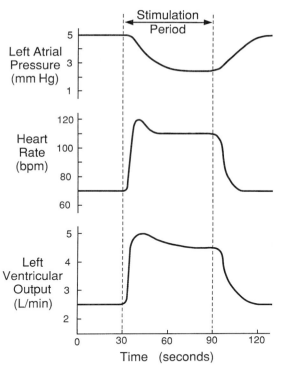

FIGURE 25–10. The cardiovascular data for Practice Question 2.

mm Hg, and heart rate is 130 beats per minute. The cardiac output is not measured, but the surgeon suspects that it is too low and that therefore the patient's tissues are not being adequately supplied with blood. Which of the following measures would be best to improve the patient's condition?

a. Transfusion with 500 mL of whole blood.

b. Administration of isoproterenol (a selective β-adrenergic agonist).

c. Increasing the heart rate by electrical pacing.

d. Administration of norepinephrine (a nonselective α/β-adrenergic agonist).

e. Administration of a β-adrenergic antagonist, such as propranolol.

2. One of the nerves leading to a dog's heart is stimulated for 1 minute while left atrial pressure, heart rate, and left ventricular output are measured (Fig. 25–10). During this stimulation,

a. venous return to the left atrium transiently exceeds left ventricular output.

b. the increase in left ventricular output at the beginning of stimulation can be explained by Starling's law of the heart.

c. stroke volume is lower after 15 seconds of stimulation than before stimulation.

d. the effects of stimulation are the same as those caused by sympathetic activation.

e. the progressive decline in left ventricular output during the stimulation is probably caused by a progressive increase in ventricular end-diastolic volume.

3. One hour after a severe hemorrhage, a dog's arterial pulse pressure, mean pressure, and hematocrit are all below normal. Which of the following statements is true?

a. The diminished pulse pressure reflects decreased aortic compliance.

b. The diminished mean pressure probably results from decreased TPR.

c. The diminished hematocrit probably results from reabsorption of interstitial fluid into the blood stream.

d. Under these conditions, the action potential frequency of the arterial baroreceptors is greater than normal.

e. Under these conditions, sympathetic activity is probably less than normal.

4. When a sheep is held in a vertical, head-up position, arterial pressure decreases because

a. the baroreceptor reflex causes an increase in TPR.

b. valves in the leg veins promote the return of blood to the heart.

c. the respiratory pump promotes movement of abdominal venous blood into the thorax.

d. central blood volume is increased.

e. right atrial pressure is decreased.

5. During exercise in a normal animal

a. TPR is decreased.

b. cardiac output is increased.

c. stroke volume is increased.

d. blood pressure is nearly normal.

e. all of the above are true.

PRACTICE ANSWERS

1. b   2. d   3. c   4. e   5. e

GASTROINTESTINAL PHYSIOLOGY AND METABOLISM

Thomas Herdt

26

Regulation of gastrointestinal function

1   An independent, intrinsic enteric nervous system lies within the wall of the gut

2   The enteric nervous system contains receptors, sensory neurons, interneurons, and motor neurons

3   The gut also receives extrinsic innervation from the autonomic nervous system

4   The gastrointestinal system has an intrinsic endocrine system

5   Regulatory peptides may originate from neurons, as well as from endocrine cells

6   The immune system participates in regulation of gastrointestinal activity

7   Regulatory peptides exert a trophic effect on gastrointestinal epithelial cells

The gastrointestinal (GI) system is regulated at two levels. One level of control is applied by the central nervous and endocrine systems and is exerted in a manner similar to that for other organ systems. The second level of control is unique to the GI system and is exerted by intrinsic nervous and endocrine components located within the gut. This *intrinsic* level of control allows the gut to autonomously regulate its functions based on local conditions, such as the amount and type of food contained in the lumen. Control of the gut by the central nervous system is mainly secondary; the central nervous system applies an influence on the intrinsic systems (nervous and endocrine), which then directly regulate gut function (Fig. 26–1).

An independent, intrinsic enteric nervous system lies within the wall of the gut

The intrinsic enteric nervous system is extensive and highly sophisticated, containing about as many neurons as the spinal cord. The enteric nervous system consists of cell bodies and their associated neurons, all of which lie within the gut wall. Anatomic characteristics of the GI wall are illustrated in Figure 26–2, which depicts the small intestine for an example. Within the gut wall, cell bodies of the enteric nervous system are arranged into two systems of ganglia: the *myenteric* (Auerbach) plexus and the *submucosal* (Meissner) plexus. (See Chapter 12 for a more general discussion of ganglia.) The myenteric plexus consists of ganglia located between the circular and longitudi-

nal muscle layers. The submucosal plexus has its ganglia in the submucosal layer. Axons from the cell bodies project in rich networks near the ganglia. A thick net of neurons runs in the plane between the circular and longitudinal muscle layers, connecting the ganglia of the myenteric plexus. Individual neurons leave the neuronal network to innervate structures within the gut wall and to intercommunicate between the myenteric and submucosal plexuses (Fig. 26–3). Interneuronal connections within the myenteric plexus are very extensive and traverse long segments of gut, whereas there are limited interneurons within the submucosal plexus. The greater intricacy of the myenteric plexus has earned it the name "little brain" within the gut.

The enteric nervous system contains receptors, sensory neurons, interneurons, and motor neurons

The plexuses of the enteric nervous system contain sensory (afferent) neurons, interneurons, and motor (efferent) neurons. Sensory input comes from *mechanoreceptors* within the muscular layers and *chemoreceptors* within the mucosa. Mechanoreceptors monitor distention of the gut wall, whereas chemoreceptors in the mucosa monitor chemical conditions in the gut lumen (Fig. 26–4).

Enteric motor nerves supply vascular muscle, gut muscle, and glands within the gut wall. Motor innervation of gut smooth muscle is less intimate than that found in skeletal muscle; there is no direct synaptic-type junction between enteric nerve endings and

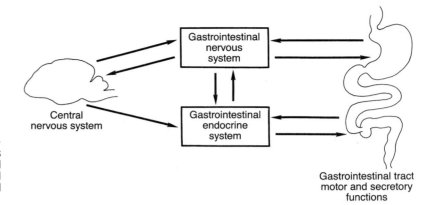

FIGURE 26–1. Gut function is under direct regulation by the intrinsic gastrointestinal (GI) nervous system and the GI endocrine system. Most central nervous system influence on the gut is mediated through indirect effects on the GI endocrine and intrinsic nervous systems.

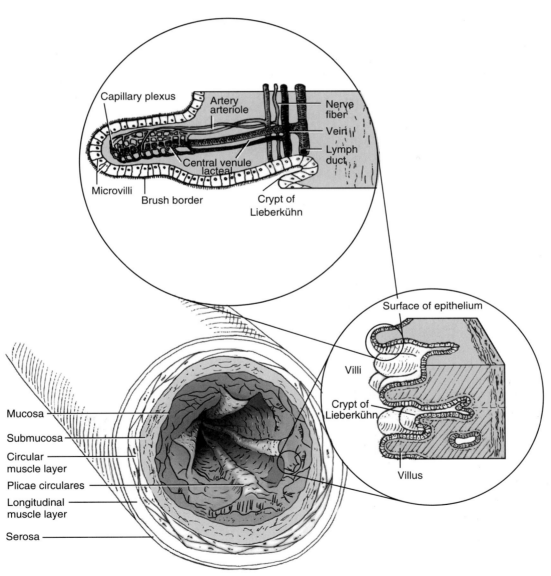

FIGURE 26–2. Schematic of the cross-sectional anatomy of the gut wall.

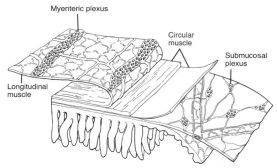

FIGURE 26–3. Schematic of the organization of the gastrointestinal intrinsic nervous system. Note the arborizations of nerve fibers that run between the individual ganglia of the myenteric and the submucosal plexus. (Adapted from Furness JB, Costa M: Types of nerves in the enteric nervous system. Neuroscience 5:1, 1980. Copyright 1980, with permission from Elsevier Science Ltd.)

smooth muscle fibers. Rather, axons end in arborizations that contain many vesicular structures called *varicosities* (see Fig. 26–4). The varicosities contain *neuroregulatory transmitter* substances that are secreted by the nerves in response to action potentials and affect the activities of nearby muscle or glandular cells. There are two general types of efferent neurons: stimulatory and inhibitory. Many of the stimulatory, or excitatory, neurons are cholinergic, having *acetylcholine* as their neuroregulatory transmitter substance. Other stimulatory neurons have peptide transmitters known as *substance P* or *substance K* as neuroregulatory transmitters. Inhibitory enteric neurons contain one of several neuroregulatory transmitters, most of which are peptides. There are a wide variety of these inhibitory neuroregulatory transmitters, including such peptide examples as *vasoactive intestinal peptide* and *somatostatin,* as well as such nonpeptide regulators as *nitric oxide* and *adenosine triphosphate.*

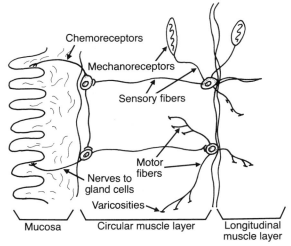

FIGURE 26–4. The arrangement of nerve fibers and receptors within the intrinsic gastrointestinal nervous system. Varicosities release neuroregulatory substances in the vicinity of muscle fibers.

The gut also receives extrinsic innervation from the autonomic nervous system

The parasympathetic and sympathetic nervous systems form the link between the enteric nervous system and the central nervous system. Most of the GI tract receives parasympathetic innervation by way of the vagus nerve, except the terminal portions of the colon, which receive parasympathetic innervation from the sacral cord by way of the pelvic nerve (Fig. 26–5). By classical description, the parasympathetic nervous system is composed of preganglionic and postganglionic fibers (see the discussion of preganglionic and postganglionic autonomic fibers in Chapter 12). However, this division of parasympathetic fiber types is not clearly defined for the gut. This lack of clarity occurs because extrinsic preganglionic fibers of the parasympathetic system become integrated with fibers of the enteric nervous system. Parasympathetic, preganglionic fibers reach the gut and synapse on cell bodies of the enteric system, so in that way the enteric ganglia of the gut serve as peripheral autonomic ganglia of the parasympathetic system. However, the enteric nervous system must be perceived as being much more than postganglionic parasympathetic neurons. Unlike typical postganglionic parasympathetic neurons, the enteric neurons receive input from sources other than preganglionic parasympathetic fibers. These include afferent neurons and interneurons of the enteric system. Thus, the classical description of the organization of the parasympathetic nervous system does not strictly apply to the gut (Fig. 26–6). *Acetylcholine* is the neurotransmitter agent between the preganglionic parasympathetic fibers and the enteric neurons.

In contrast to the extrinsic parasympathetic fibers, extrinsic sympathetic fibers that enter the gut are primarily postganglionic. Postganglionic sympathetic fibers arise from cells in the prevertebral ganglia (see Chapter 12 for a discussion of prevertebral ganglia) and follow the splanchnic nerves and vascular arteries into the gut wall (see Fig. 26–5). Some sympathetic fibers synapse on neurons of the enteric system, whereas others exert a direct effect on GI muscles and glands. The sympathetic fibers that exert a direct effect do so in a manner similar to that of the enteric nerve fibers (i.e., by the release of neuroregulatory substances in the vicinity of their target cells). The neuroregulatory substance of the postganglionic sympathetic cells is *norepinephrine.*

The gastrointestinal system has an intrinsic endocrine system

The GI system has an extensive number and variety of endocrine cells. Endocrine cells are usually grouped together into glands, but the GI endocrine cells are distributed diffusely throughout the gut epithelium. Typically, the GI endocrine cells are columnar with a broad base and a narrow apex (Fig. 26–7).

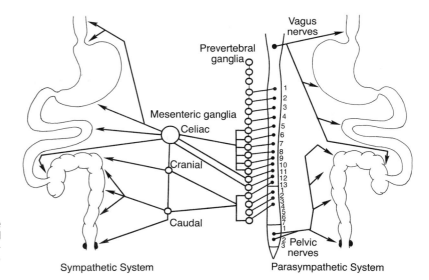

FIGURE 26–5. The distribution of autonomic nerve fibers to the gut. The spinal cord is represented in the center, with the sympathetic system extended to the left and the parasympathetic system to the right.

They are positioned individually among the other mucosal cells in both the secretory and the absorptive areas of the mucosa. The narrow apex of the endocrine cells is exposed to the lumen of the gut, allowing them to "sample" or "taste" the luminal contents. The base of these cells contains *secretory granules,* which are storage forms of hormones. This anatomic arrangement provides a mechanism for the cells to sense changes in luminal contents and to respond by releasing hormones into the submucosal area, where they may be absorbed into the blood stream. The hormones are not secreted into the lumen of the gut. There are many types of endocrine cells within the gut epithelium, all of which are morphologically similar. However, despite their similar appearance, there are many distinct populations of cells that produce a wide variety of hormones and hormone-like substances.

Hormonal products of the GI endocrine cells are released into the submucosa. From there they may be picked up by the blood vascular system and transported out of the gut to distant sites, or they may simply diffuse through the extracellular fluid to have effects on local target cells. When transported by the blood to distant sites, the products of the GI endocrine cells are functioning as classical hormones. By strict definition, a hormone is a substance that is transported through the blood from its site of production to a distant site of effect. When functioning as hormones (i.e., by transport through the blood), the products of the GI endocrine cells are said to be *endocrines,* or to have *endocrine activity.* In contrast, when these molecules elicit their effects by means of local diffusion, their activity is referred to as *paracrine.* Therefore, the distinction between endocrine and paracrine activity is based on whether the active molecule reaches its target cell by transport through the blood stream or by local diffusion. One additional

FIGURE 26–6. The interface between the autonomic and gastrointestinal intrinsic nervous systems. Note that parasympathetic fibers reaching the intrinsic system are preganglionic, whereas sympathetic fibers are postganglionic.

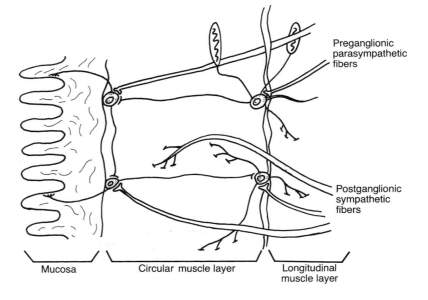

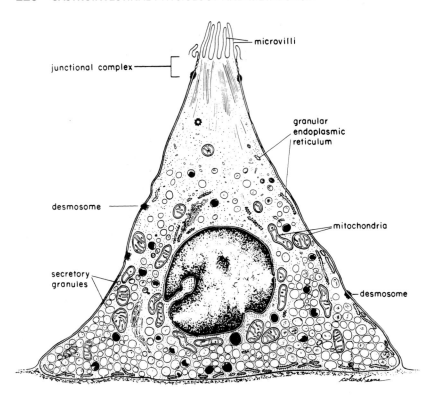

Figure 26–7. Schematic illustration of a gastrointestinal endocrine cell. All of the gastrointestinal endocrine cells have a similar structure, but each cell produces only one type of hormone. Note the narrow apex that is exposed to the intestinal luminal contents and the broad base for storage of secretory granules. (From Johnson LR, Christensen J, Jacobsen ED, et al [eds]: Physiology of the Gastrointestinal Tract, vol. 1, 2nd ed. New York: Raven Press, 1987.)

definition is necessary to complete the discussion of the types of actions of the products of GI endocrine cells. The term *autocrine* is used to describe the action of a molecule when it is released into the extracellular environment but feeds back on its cell of origin. In the case of autocrine activity, the target cell and the cell producing the active molecule are the same. There are many different active molecules produced by the various GI endocrine cells; some have endocrine activity, whereas others have paracrine or autocrine activity, and many probably function in all three ways. All of the GI endocrine cell products—endocrine, paracrine, and autocrine—are peptides and can be referred to collectively as *regulatory peptides.*

Each type of endocrine cell has a characteristic distribution within the GI tract. *Gastrin-producing cells,* for example, are found primarily in the distal portion of the stomach, and few are found elsewhere in the gut. *Cholecystokinin-producing cells* are found in the small intestine, especially in the proximal region. Thus, although endocrine cells are distributed throughout the GI tract, the production of individual hormones may be confined to specific areas. This is not always the case, however, as in the instance of *enteroglucagon-producing cells,* which are distributed along the entire length of the gut. The sites of production and actions of the major GI regulatory peptides are listed in Table 26–1. A more extensive list of peptides and their modes of activity is in Table 26–2.

The GI regulatory peptides influence various gut functions and in many instances form part of the regulatory feedback loops. An example is the feedback loop that involves gastrin and gastric acid. After a meal, gastrin-producing cells, which are located in

the stomach, secrete gastrin. Gastrin stimulates gastric acid production and lowers the stomach pH. The gastrin-producing cells monitor the pH of the distal stomach, and when the pH is reduced to a critical point, gastrin secretion is inhibited, removing the stimulus for the production of more gastric acid and stabilizing the stomach pH. Thus, the pH of the stomach is regulated closely by the actions of the gastrin-producing endocrine cells. Other specific examples of GI regulatory peptide effects are discussed in subsequent chapters in the context of the actions they regulate (Fig. 26–8).

Regulatory peptides may originate from neurons, as well as from endocrine cells

All products of GI endocrine cells are regulatory peptides, but not all regulatory peptides of the GI system originate from endocrine cells. Most of the neuroregulatory transmitter substances produced by the noncholinergic neurons of the intrinsic nervous system are also peptides and have mechanisms of action much like those of the endocrine and paracrine substances. These substances of neuronal origin are also grouped in the category of regulatory peptides and sometimes are referred to specifically as *neurocrines.* Several regulatory peptides appear to be produced by both neurons and endocrine cells. Thus, some GI regulatory peptides have endocrine, paracrine, autocrine, and neurocrine modes of activity. Regardless of the mode of activity, all regulatory peptides elicit their effects after binding to specific receptors on the

TABLE 26–1. **Major gastrointestinal hormones**

Hormone	Site of Production	Action	Release Stimulus
Gastrin	Distal stomach	*Primary:* Stimulates acid secretion from stomach glands. *Secondary:* Stimulates gastric motility, growth of stomach epithelium	Protein in stomach; high gastric pH; vagal stimulation
Secretin	Duodenum	*Primary:* Stimulates bicarbonate secretion from pancreas. *Secondary:* Stimulates biliary bicarbonate secretion	Acid in duodenum
Cholecystokinin (CCK)	Duodenum to ileum, with highest concentration in duodenum	*Primary:* Stimulates enzyme secretion from pancreas. *Secondary:* Inhibits gastric emptying	Proteins and fats in small intestine
Gastric inhibitory polypeptide (GIP)	Duodenum and upper jejunum	*Primary:* Inhibits gastric motility and secretory activity. *Secondary:* Stimulates insulin secretion provided sufficient glucose is present; may be most important action in many species	Carbohydrate and fat in small intestine
Motilin	Duodenum and jejunum	*Primary:* Probably regulates motility pattern of the gut in period between meals. *Secondary:* May regulate tone of lower esophageal sphincter	Acetylcholine

surface of their target cells. Once these receptors are occupied, responses by the cells are elicited. The general mode of action of peptide hormones and other regulatory peptides is described in detail in Chapter 32.

A list of known or suspected regulatory peptides of gut origin is given in Table 26–2. Although the list is extensive, it is probably incomplete, because new regulatory peptides continue to be discovered. Some peptides, such as substance P and bombesin, have strange, nondescriptive names that reflect historical incidents in their discovery. Others, such as vasoactive intestinal peptide and gastric inhibitory peptide, have names that describe their first-discovered action but do not describe what is now believed to be their primary action. Gastrointestinal regulatory peptide function is an area of active research and rapidly expanding knowledge. The *clinical* use of GI hormones and their analogues, as well as specific agents that block their activity, is just beginning to occur in human and veterinary medicine. As GI regulatory peptide physiology becomes better understood, these substances will probably become an important part of the treatment of GI disease.

The immune system participates in regulation of gastrointestinal activity

Like the intrinsic nervous and endocrine systems, the gut has a somewhat autonomous immune system.

Although the role of this system in disease resistance and inflammation has long been appreciated, only recently has its role in the regulation of physiologic GI functions been realized. From a physiologic point of view, it is important to realize that the intestinal mucosa is richly populated with immune cells, including lymphocytes and phagocytes. Because of the variety of materials that animals eat, these cells are exposed to a wide range of antigens. In response to an antigen to which the animal has been specifically sensitized, lymphocytes secrete regulatory transmitters known as *cytokines*. The cytokines are well known to elicit inflammatory responses, but it is now known that they can also elicit physiologic responses in the gut by influencing the intrinsic nervous and endocrine systems.

An example of the interaction of the GI immune system with the other regulatory systems might involve the response to a noxious antigen, perhaps a bacterial toxin, to which the gut had been sensitized. In response to such an antigen, lymphocytes would be stimulated to release cytokines that in turn could stimulate the intrinsic nervous and endocrine systems to increase the glandular secretion and motility of the gut. This response would have the effect of diluting the antigen with secretions and washing it away by the action of increased gut motility. Such action would remove the antigen from the gut and protect the animal. The extensive nature, structure, and func-

TABLE 26–2. Peptides of the gastrointestinal tract with their likely role as endocrine, neurocrine, or paracrine substances

Endocrine Peptides	Neurocrine Peptides	Paracrine Peptides
Somatostatin*	Somatostatin*	Somatostatin*
Cholecystokinin (CCK)	CCK	Peptide YY
Gastrin	Gastrin-releasing peptide	
Secretin	Opioids	
Insulin	Substance P	
Glucagon	Vasoactive intestinal peptide (VIP)	
Enteroglucagon	Neuropeptide Y	
Pancreatic polypeptide	Neurotensin	
Neurotensin	Peptide HM	
Motilin	Pancreastatin	
Glucose-dependent insulinotropic peptide (GIP)	Galanin	
	Motilin	
Peptide YY	Peptide YY	
Urogastrone		

*Some peptides may serve multiple functions. Adapted from Brand SJ, Schmidt WE: Gastrointestinal hormones. In Yamada T (ed): Textbook of Gastroenterology, 2nd ed. Philadelphia: Lippincott Williams & Wilkins, 1995, p 39.

tion of the GI immune system are outside the realm of this textbook. For further information on this topic, students are referred to textbooks of immunology.

Regulatory peptides exert a trophic effect on gastrointestinal epithelial cells

In addition to regulating cell functions, several GI regulatory peptides exert *trophic*, or growth-regulating, effects on epithelial cells of the GI system. For example, gastrin promotes growth of the gastric mucosa, and enteroglucagon and cholecystokinin pro-mote growth of the intestinal mucosa. This is one mechanism by which the gut can adapt to increased digestive requirements; that is, as appetite and food intake increase, GI regulatory peptide production is stimulated and the gut mucosa hypertrophies to meet the increased functional demand.

An important example that illustrates this trophic effect is found in animals exposed to a cold environment. In these cold-adapted animals, it has been observed that appetite increases in response to their need for additional dietary energy with which to maintain body temperature. In addition to an increase in appetite, the length of the intestinal villi increases. This is an important response that allows the animal to digest and absorb the increased amount of nutrients consumed. The hypertrophy of the intestinal villi probably occurs in response to high and sustained blood and tissue fluid concentrations of such regulatory peptides as cholecystokinin and enteroglucagon. Secretion of these peptides is in turn stimulated by the increased concentration and frequency of nutrients present in the gut. In this manner, increased food consumption leads to an adaptive response of the GI epithelium.

Bibliography

Buchan AM: Nutrient tasting and signaling mechanisms in the gut III. Endocrine cell recognition of luminal nutrients. Am J Physiol 277:G1103–G1107, 1999.

Collins SM: The immunomodulation of enteric neuromuscular function: Implications for motility and inflammatory disorders. Gastroenterology 111:1683–1699, 1996.

Furness JB, Bornstein JC, WAA Kunze, N Clerc: The enteric nervous system and its extrinsic connections. In Yamada T, Alpers DH, Kaine L (eds): Textbook of Gastroenterology, vol. 1, 3rd ed. Philadelphia: Lippincott Williams & Wilkins, 1999, pp 11–35.

Furness JB, Clerc N: Responses of afferent neurons to the contents of the digestive tract, and their relation to endocrine and immune responses. Prog Brain Res 122:159–172, 2000.

Johnson LR, Alpers DH, Christensen J, et al (eds): Physiology of the Gastrointestinal Tract, vol. 1, 3rd ed. New York: Raven Press, 1994.

Johnson LR: Regulation: Peptides of the gastrointestinal tract. In Johnson LR (ed): Gastrointestinal Physiology, 6th ed. St. Louis: CV Mosby, 2001, pp 1–14.

Johnson LR: Regulation: Nerves and smooth muscle. In Johnson LR (ed): Gastrointestinal Physiology, 6th ed. St. Louis: CV Mosby, 2001, pp 17–26.

Kunze WA, Furness JB: The enteric nervous system and regulation of intestinal motility. Annu Rev Physiol 61:117–142, 1999.

Miller LJ: Gastrointestinal Hormones and Receptors. In Yamada T, Alpers DH, Kaine L (eds): Textbook of Gastroenterology, vol. 1, 3rd ed. Philadelphia: Lippincott Williams & Wilkins, 1999, pp 35–66.

Qian B, Danielsson A: Vagal regulation of the gastrointestinal neuroendocrine system. Scand J Gastroenterol 31:529–540, 1996.

Stevens CE, Hume ID: Comparative Physiology of the Vertebrate Digestive System, 2nd ed. Cambridge, United Kingdom: Cambridge University Press, 1996, pp 268–286.

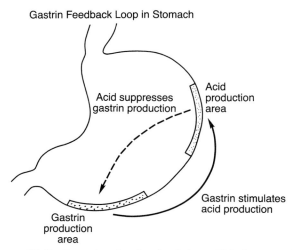

FIGURE 26–8. Example of a feedback loop. This is a negative feedback loop in that acid production, which is stimulated by gastrin, suppresses gastrin secretion.

PRACTICE QUESTIONS

1. Which statement is the most accurate anatomic description of the intrinsic nervous system of the gut?
   a. Intrinsic neuronal fibers and their cell bodies are diffusely spread throughout the length and thickness of the stomach and intestine.

b. Intrinsic neuronal fibers traverse the length of the stomach and intestine in discrete nerve bundles.
c. Intrinsic neuronal cell bodies are aggregated in a discrete "gut brain" that is positioned near the pylorus.
d. Intrinsic neuronal cell bodies lie in discrete planes within the thickness of the gut wall and are diffusely distributed throughout its length.
e. Intrinsic neuronal fibers exist only in the longitudinal muscle layer of the stomach and intestine.

2. Which statement is true with regard to the parasympathetic fibers that innervate the cells of the intrinsic nervous system?
a. The fibers exit the central nervous system from lumbar segments of the spinal cord.
b. The fibers have vasoactive intestinal peptide as a neurotransmitter.
c. The fibers are inhibitory.
d. The fibers are preganglionic.
e. There are no parasympathetic fibers that innervate cells of the intrinsic nervous system.

3. Which statement is true with regard to the GI endocrine cells?
a. Secretory activity is influenced by the luminal contents of the gut.

b. Hormones are secreted directly into the gut lumen and affect the activity of glands "downstream" from the point of secretion.
c. Endocrine cells are aggregated into discrete bundles known as intestinal glands.
d. The secretory products of the GI endocrine cells are steroid hormones.
e. Each GI endocrine cell can produce many different kinds of hormones, depending on the stimulus applied to it.

4. It is important for clinicians to understand GI endocrinology because
a. GI hormones are involved in abnormal, as well as normal, gut activity.
b. some tumors can produce copious and unrestricted amounts of GI hormones.
c. GI hormones and their analogues and antagonists will probably become important agents of therapy in GI disease.
d. All of the above.

PRACTICE ANSWERS

1. d   2. d   3. a   4. d

27

Movements of the gastrointestinal tract

1   Slow waves of electrical depolarization are a unique feature of gut smooth muscle

2   When spreading slow waves reach primed smooth muscle cells, action potentials and contraction result

3   Coordinated motility enables the lips, tongue, mouth, and pharynx to grasp food and propel it down the gastrointestinal tract

4   Motility of the esophagus propels food from the pharynx to the stomach

5   The function of the stomach is to process food into a fluid consistency and release it into the intestine at a controlled rate

6   The proximal stomach stores food awaiting further gastric processing in the distal stomach

7   The distal stomach grinds and sifts food entering the small intestine

8   Control of gastric motility differs in the proximal and distal stomach

9   The rate of gastric emptying must match the small intestine's rate of digestion and absorption

10   Between meals, the stomach is cleared of indigestible material

11   Vomiting is a complex reflex coordinated from the brainstem

12   Motility of the small intestine has a digestive and interdigestive phase

13   The ileocecal sphincter prevents movement of colon contents back into the ileum

14   Motility of the colon causes mixing, retropulsion, and propulsion of ingesta

15   In the carnivore colon, absorption and storage occur

16   Despite anatomic differences in herbivore colons, similar motility patterns are found

17   The anal sphincter has two layers with separate innervation

18   The rectosphincteric reflex is important in defecation

19   Major differences between avian and mammalian digestive systems include, in birds, both the lack of teeth and the separation of gastric functions into distinct anatomic regions

The walls of the gastrointestinal (GI) tract, at all levels, are muscular and capable of movement. Movements of the GI muscles have direct actions on ingesta in the gut lumen. GI movements have several functions: (1) to propel ingesta from one location to the next; (2) to retain ingesta at a given site for digestion, absorption, or storage; (3) to physically break up food material and mix it with digestive secretions; and (4) to circulate ingesta so that all portions come into contact with absorptive surfaces. The dynamics of fluid movement in the gut are not as well understood as in other organ systems, particularly the cardiovascular system. The heart and great vessels behave in a manner similar to that of most mechanical pumping systems: there is a central pump that pushes fluid through a conduit of relatively fixed diameter. Because of this configuration, the cardiovascular system more or less conforms to physical laws that are well established and studied reasonably easily; sophisticated quantitative analyses of cardiovascular function can be made clinically. In contrast to the situation in the heart, the fluid pump and the conduit are the same organ in the gut. This makes study of the fluid dynamics of the gut extremely complex. At this time, the mathematically defined physical laws of fluid dynamics, as applied to the gut, are of little clinical usefulness. Therefore, the physiology of GI motility is usually applied clinically on a qualitative, rather than quantitative, basis.

Movement of the gut wall is referred to as *motility*, and motility may be of a propulsive, retentive, or mixing nature. The time it takes material to travel from one portion of the gut to another is referred to as the *transit time*. An increase in propulsive motility decreases the transit time, whereas an increase in retentive motility increases the transit time. Selectively increasing retentive motility and reducing propulsive motility are important aspects of diarrhea therapy.

Slow waves of electrical depolarization are a unique feature of gut smooth muscle

In both the longitudinal and circular layers, GI smooth muscle cells are arranged in a network of interconnected, indistinct bundles, so that each muscle layer is a continuous, interlocking sheet of muscle cells. The individual muscle cells are connected to each other by *gap junctions,* also called *nexuses.* These junctions create an electrical connection between the cells and allow changes in membrane potential to be transferred from cell to cell. The arrangement permits the gut musculature to function as a *syncytium* (i.e., a multinucleate mass of protoplasm produced by the merging of cells) that allows waves of electrical activity to spread over the muscle layers, in much the same way as the transmission of electrical activity in heart muscle.

The first level of control of GI motility lies in the intrinsic electrical properties of the smooth muscle mass. Smooth muscle cells of the gut, like other excitable cells, maintain an electrical potential difference across their cell membranes, the inner surface being electrically negative in comparison with the outer surface. The events responsible for cellular membrane potentials are similar in most cells and involve selective transport of ions into or out of the cell. These mechanisms are described in Chapter 3.

The membrane potentials of GI smooth muscle cells, in contrast to those of many other types of excitable cells, fluctuate rhythmically. In the resting state, the baseline membrane potential is usually −70 to −60 mV (Fig. 27–1). But the membrane potential

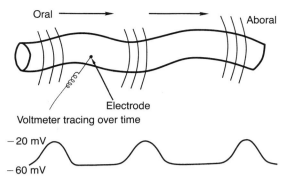

FIGURE 27–2. The partial membrane depolarizations of GI smooth muscle cells occur in a coordinated manner, creating waves of depolarization that sweep over large segments of muscle. Electrodes placed on or near the surface of the muscle record changes in potential as waves of depolarization pass toward or away from them. Coordinated changes in membrane potential among cells are necessary for these waves to be measured, because random changes among cells would cancel each other out, and no changes would be recorded by electrodes placed extracellularly.

depolarizes or hyperpolarizes from this baseline level by as much as 20 to 30 mV (see Fig. 27–1). Thus, under resting conditions, the depolarization is only partial, and the membrane potential never reaches 0 mV. Because the cells are connected electrically, the variation in membrane potential is spread, or propagated, over large areas of muscle. In the intestine, the spontaneous, rhythmic changes in membrane potential occur most rapidly in the duodenum. Because of this, changes in membrane potential are propagated aborally (away from the mouth) along the length of the small intestine (Fig. 27–2). These aborally moving waves of partial depolarization are called *slow waves* or *basic electrical rhythm,* and they are similar to an excitatory postsynaptic potential in nerve cell membranes (see Chapter 3). In the dog, slow waves occur about 20 times per minute in the small intestine. In the stomach and colon, they are considerably less frequent, occurring about five times per minute. However, the slow waves are present throughout the smooth muscle portions of the GI tract. The frequency of slow waves varies among the domestic species, but their presence does not.

The origin of the slow waves appears to be the *interstitial cells of Cajal.* These are specialized cells that lie at the junctions between the submucosa and circular muscle and between the longitudinal and circular muscle. These cells extend the length of the gut and act as pacemakers. Electrical activity in these cells is spontaneous. The interstitial cells of Cajal are connected to the smooth muscle cells by tight junctions, allowing the spontaneous electrical activity of the cells of Cajal to be transmitted to the smooth muscle mass.

The slow waves are an intrinsic property of the GI smooth muscle and associated cells of Cajal. Whereas the amplitude and, to a lesser extent, the frequency of the slow waves can be modulated by the nervous or endocrine systems, the presence of the slow waves

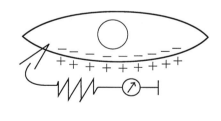

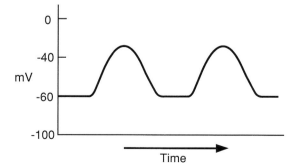

FIGURE 27–1. Spontaneous changes in the membrane polarity of gastrointestinal (GI) smooth muscle cells. The upper illustration represents a single cell with a voltmeter measuring the transmembrane electrical potential. The graph illustrates spontaneous changes in electrical potential (in millivolts) that would be measured across the cell membrane.

is dependent only on the cells of Cajal. The link between slow waves and muscle contractions, however, is under control of nervous and endocrine factors.

When spreading slow waves reach primed smooth muscle cells, action potentials and contraction result

Slow waves have an important relationship with muscle contractions, but they are not the direct stimuli for contractions. Slow waves are constantly passing over GI smooth muscle, whether it is actively contracting or not. GI smooth muscle cells, like other muscle cells, contract in association with action, or spike, potentials. These potentials are characterized by complete depolarization of the membrane for a short period of time. (A more complete discussion of action potentials can be found in Chapter 3.) Action potentials in the GI smooth muscle occur only at the crest of slow waves. Thus, muscle contractions can occur at no higher a frequency than the frequency of the slow waves. This can be seen in the activity of muscle in the stomach of the dog. Slow waves in the canine stomach occur about five times per minute. The crest of each slow wave may or may not be accompanied by action potentials. Therefore, during a given minute, the muscle in a localized area may not contract at all or may contract up to five times. If the passing slow waves generate no action potentials, the muscle does not contract at all. If there are action potentials associated with one slow wave, the muscle contracts once. Action potentials on two slow waves result in two contractions and so on up to a maximum of five contractions per minute, but no more than five, because there are no more slow waves.

The function of the slow waves appears to be to synchronize the contractions of the GI muscle mass. In order for the muscle to function efficiently, all or many of the muscle cells in one layer of a segment of gut must contract simultaneously. This can best be visualized by considering the circular muscle layer. The contents of the circle cannot be "squeezed" effectively unless all the muscles of the circumference contract simultaneously; it would have little effect on luminal pressure if one portion of the circle contracted while another portion relaxed. The nervous system cannot direct an individual circle of GI smooth muscle fibers to contract simultaneously in a manner similar to that of nervous control of skeletal muscle contraction. This is because there is no direct connection between the nervous system and the musculature, such as exists in the neuromuscular end-plates of skeletal muscle.

The combined effects of the enteric nervous system and the slow waves achieve control of smooth muscle contraction, without the presence of direct nerve-muscle connections. To achieve this control, the enteric nervous system releases neuroregulatory substances from nerve endings near muscle cells. The neuroregulatory substances sensitize the cells to make them more likely to generate an action potential and contract in the presence of a slow wave. When a slow wave passes over a sensitized group of cells, the entire group contracts. Thus, the nervous system "primes" the smooth muscle for contraction, whereas the slow waves signal the simultaneous contraction of a group of primed muscle fibers (Fig. 27–3).

Whether action potentials, and an associated muscle contraction, will occur as a given slow wave passes over an area of gut muscle is dependent on the height of the slow-wave crest. If the crest reaches a threshold value, a characteristic action potential, with short-term membrane depolarization and muscle contraction, occurs. The enteric nervous system regulates

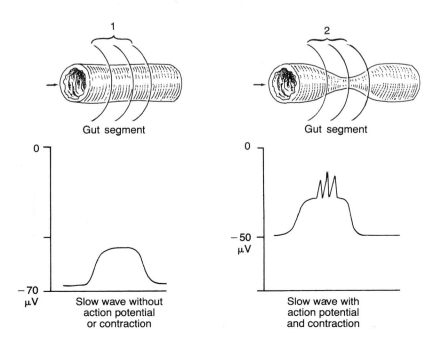

Gut segment

Gut segment

0

0

−50
µV

−70
µV

Slow wave without
action potential
or contraction

Slow wave with
action potential
and contraction

Figure 27–3. No muscle contraction occurs in the absence of action potentials (1). Muscle contracts when the crest of the slow waves reaches a critical point of depolarization, allowing action potentials to occur (2). The probability of action potentials occurring during the passage of a slow wave over a segment of gut muscle is influenced by the degree of baseline depolarization. Norepinephrine lowers the baseline (increases its absolute value), whereas acetylcholine raises the baseline (decreases its absolute value).

the likelihood of action potential occurrence by altering the baseline membrane potential and amplitude of the slow waves (see Fig. 27–3). Motor nerves that are stimulatory to the gut muscle raise the baseline and amplitude of the slow waves, whereas inhibitory nerves lower them (i.e., create more negative values). Parasympathetic stimulation (through cholinergic nerves of the enteric nervous system) tends to raise the slow-wave baseline and stimulate muscular activity in the gut, whereas sympathetic stimulation has the opposite effect.

The overall motility pattern of the gut is achieved by local variations in the activity of the enteric nervous system, in concert with the endocrine and autonomic nervous systems. Some areas of muscle may be "primed" for contraction, whereas others are not. Slow waves passing over primed areas incite action potentials and hence contractions; in unprimed areas the slow waves pass by, without stimulating muscle activity (see Fig. 27–3).

This discussion of control of GI muscle activity applies most directly to the small intestine. The general principles also apply to both the stomach and the colon, but the system appears to be more intricate in those areas than in the small intestine.

Coordinated motility enables the lips, tongue, mouth, and pharynx to grasp food and propel it down the gastrointestinal tract

Before digestion can begin, food must be directed into the GI tract. To ingest food, quadruped animals must first grasp it with the lips, teeth, or tongue. This involves highly coordinated activity of small, voluntary skeletal muscles. The muscles of the face, lips, and tongue appear to be among the most delicately controlled voluntary muscles of most domestic animals. The exact method of food prehension varies greatly among different species. For example, horses use their lips extensively, whereas cattle often use their tongues for grasping food. In all domestic animals, however, prehension is a highly coordinated process involving direct control by the central nervous system. Problems of prehension may develop because of abnormalities in the teeth, jaws, muscles of the tongue and face, cranial nerves, or central nervous system. The facial cranial nerve, the glossopharyngeal cranial nerve, and the motor branch of the trigeminal cranial nerve control the muscles of prehension.

Mastication, or chewing, involves the actions of the jaws, tongue, and cheeks and is the first act of digestion. It serves not only to break food particles down to a size that will pass into the esophagus but also to moisten and lubricate food by thoroughly mixing it with saliva. Abnormalities of the teeth are a common cause of digestive disturbances in animals.

Deglutition, or swallowing, involves voluntary and involuntary stages and occurs after food has been well masticated. In the voluntary phase of swallowing, food is molded into a bolus by the tongue

and then pushed back into the pharynx. When food enters the pharynx, sensory nerve endings detect its presence and initiate the involuntary portion of the swallow reflex.

The involuntary actions of the swallow reflex occur primarily within the pharynx and esophagus. The pharynx is the common opening of both the respiratory and digestive tracts. The major physiologic function of the pharynx is to ensure that air, and only air, enters the respiratory tract and that food and water, and only food and water, enter the digestive tract. The involuntary portion of the swallow reflex is the action that directs food into the digestive system and away from the upper airway. This reflex involves the following series of highly coordinated actions (Fig. 27–4). Breathing stops momentarily. The soft palate is elevated, closing the pharyngeal opening of the nasopharynx and preventing food from entering the internal openings of the nostrils. The tongue is pressed against the hard palate, closing off the oral opening of the pharynx. The hyoid bone and larynx are pulled forward; this action pulls the glottis under the epiglottis, blocking the laryngeal opening. Concurrently, the arytenoid cartilages constrict, further closing the opening of the larynx and preventing the movement of food into the respiratory system. When all openings to the pharynx are closed, a wave of muscular constriction passes over the walls of the organ, pushing the bolus of food toward the opening of the esophagus. As the food reaches the esophagus,

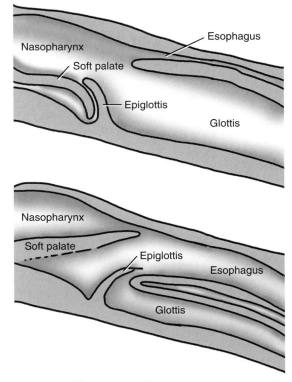

Figure 27–4. Midline cross-sectional schematic showing the position of the structures of the larynx and pharynx during breathing *(top)* and swallowing *(bottom)*.

the upper esophageal sphincter relaxes to accept the material.

The complex reactions of deglutition are controlled by lower motor neurons located in various centers of the brainstem. Efferent nerve fibers from these centers travel in the facial, vagus, hypoglossal, and glosso-pharyngeal cranial nerves as well as the motor branch of the trigeminal nerve. Clinically, problems with pre-hension, mastication, and deglutition frequently are related to neurologic lesions, either peripherally in the cranial nerves or centrally in the brainstem.

Motility of the esophagus propels food from the pharynx to the stomach

The esophagus, like other tubular portions of the gut, contains an outer longitudinal and inner circular layer of muscle. The esophagus is unique with regard to other areas of the gut, however, in that much of its muscular wall is composed of striated skeletal muscle fibers. In most domestic animals, the entire length of esophageal musculature is striated. In horses, pri-mates, and cats, however, a portion of the distal esophagus is smooth muscle. The striated muscle por-tions of esophagus are under control of somatic (not parasympathetic) motor neurons in the vagus nerve, whereas the smooth muscle portions are under direct control of the enteric nervous system and indirect control of the autonomic nervous system. A myenteric plexus exists throughout the entire length of the esophagus. In the area of striated muscle, the myen-teric plexus probably serves a sensory function and acts to coordinate the movements of the striated mus-cle portion with the esophageal smooth muscle seg-ments and stomach.

In terms of motor activity, the esophagus may be thought of as consisting of an upper sphincter, body, and lower sphincter. The upper esophageal sphincter is called the *cricopharyngeal muscle*. This muscle and the upper end of the esophagus are attached to the cricoid cartilage of the larynx. When deglutition is not taking place, the muscle compresses the end of the esophagus against the cartilage of the larynx, tightly closing the upper esophageal opening. During deglutition, the cricopharyngeal muscle relaxes and the larynx is pulled forward. The ventral portion of the upper end of the esophagus is attached to the larynx; the dorsal portion, to the cervical spine. Be-cause of these attachments, the forward motion of the larynx tends to passively pull open the upper esophageal orifice (see Fig. 27–4).

The body of the esophagus serves as a relatively simple conduit, rapidly transferring food from the pharynx to the stomach. Food is propelled through the esophagus by propulsive movements known as *peristalsis*. Peristalsis consists of a moving ring of con-striction in the wall of a tubular organ. In the esopha-gus, these rings start at the cranial end and progress toward the stomach. The rings reduce or obliterate the esophageal lumen, thus pushing the bolus of food ahead of them in much the same manner as a person

would push material out of a soft rubber tube by stripping it with the fingers. In addition to the con-striction of the circular muscles, there may be some contraction of longitudinal muscles just ahead, or ab-oral, to the ring of circular muscle contraction. This longitudinal muscle activity would increase the size of the esophageal lumen to accommodate the advanc-ing food bolus (Fig. 27–5). Peristalsis is a universal type of GI propulsive motility that exists at all levels of the gut.

During deglutition, the upper esophageal sphincter relaxes as the pharynx constricts; food is pushed into the upper portion of the esophageal body, and a wave of peristalsis propels the material toward the stomach. As the food bolus reaches the distal end of the esoph-agus, the lower sphincter relaxes and the ingested matter enters the stomach. If the esophagus is not cleared of food material by the primary wave of peri-stalsis, secondary peristaltic waves are generated. One or more secondary waves are almost always adequate for pushing material into the stomach and clearing the esophagus. If food or foreign bodies become lodged in the esophagus, secondary waves of peristal-sis may lead eventually to muscle spasms that con-strict tightly around the lodged material. These spasms frequently interfere with attempts to remove the obstructing object.

When deglutition is not taking place, the body of the esophagus is relaxed, but the upper and lower sphincters remain constantly constricted. The con-striction of these sphincters is important because of the differences in external pressure applied to the esophagus at different points along its length. During the inspiratory phase of breathing, the portion of the esophagus within the thorax is subjected to less-than-atmospheric pressure. If the two esophageal sphinc-ters were not tightly closed, inspiration would cause aspiration of air from the pharynx and reflux of in-gesta from the stomach into the body of the esopha-gus, in the same manner as inspiration draws air into

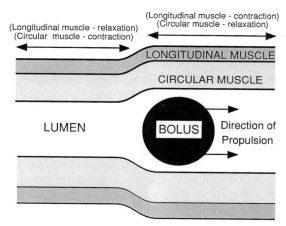

FIGURE 27–5. Peristalsis consists of a moving ring of luminal constriction preceded by an area of luminal distention. The area of constriction is created by contractions of the circular muscle, whereas the dilation is created by contractions of the longitudi-nal muscle. The net action is to propel a bolus of ingesta.

the lung. Stomach contents would be drawn into the esophagus, because inspiratory pressures in the thorax are lower than intra-abdominal pressure. It is particularly important that the lower esophageal sphincter remain closed during inspiration, because the mucosa of the esophagus is not equipped to resist the caustic actions of gastric contents; thus, movement of stomach contents into the esophagus would cause damage to the esophageal mucosa.

In many species, the action of the lower esophageal sphincter is aided by the anatomic nature of the attachment of the esophagus and stomach. The esophagus enters the stomach obliquely, allowing distention of the stomach to block the esophageal opening in a valve-like manner. During deglutition, the longitudinal muscle of the esophagus contracts, shortening the esophagus and opening the valve at the junction with the stomach. This anatomic arrangement, along with the lower esophageal sphincter, is particularly well developed in the horse, making reflux of stomach material into the esophagus extremely rare in this species. In many instances in which the intragastric pressure of the horse is pathologically raised, the stomach ruptures before vomiting or esophageal reflux takes place.

The function of the stomach is to process food into a fluid consistency and release it into the intestine at a controlled rate

Among animals there is tremendous diversity in the anatomy and motility patterns of the stomach. The following discussion applies best to the animals with the simplest stomachs, such as the dog and cat, but is probably also a reasonable description of the activity of the somewhat more complex stomachs of the pig, horse, and rat. The complex motility patterns of the ruminant stomach are discussed in Chapter 30.

The function of the stomach is to serve food to the small intestine. There are two important aspects of this function: rate of delivery and consistency of material. The stomach serves as both a storage vat to control the rate of delivery of food to the small intestine and as a grinder and sieve that reduces the size of food particles and releases them only when they are broken down to a consistency compatible with small-intestinal digestion.

The stomach is divided into two physiologic regions, each of which has a different impact on gastric function. The proximal region, at the esophageal end of the stomach, serves a storage function, retaining food as it awaits eventual entry into the small intestine. The distal region serves a grinding and sieving function, breaking solid pieces of food down into particles small enough for small-intestinal digestion.

The proximal stomach stores food awaiting further gastric processing in the distal stomach

The major muscular activity in the proximal region of the stomach is of a weak, continuous-contraction nature. These *tonic* contractions tend to shape the gastric wall to its contents and provide gentle propulsion of material into the distal stomach. The major muscular reflex of the proximal stomach is *adaptive relaxation* (Fig. 27–6). This reflex is characterized by relaxation of the muscles as food enters the stomach. Because of this relaxation, the stomach can dilate to accept large quantities of food without an increase in intraluminal pressure. Thus, the proximal stomach serves as a food storage area. A consequence of the rather passive muscular activity of the proximal stomach is that little mixing occurs there. In fact, food boluses tend to become layered in the stomach in the order in which they are swallowed. As the stomach empties, tension on the wall of the proximal stomach increases slightly, pushing food distally in the stomach, where it can be processed for transport into the duodenum.

The distal stomach grinds and sifts food entering the small intestine

The muscular activity of the distal stomach and pylorus (sphincter-like junction between stomach and duodenum) is completely different from that of the proximal stomach. In the distal stomach, known as the

FIGURE 27–6. Adaptive relaxation refers to the stretching of the stomach wall that occurs as the organ fills during eating. This stretching occurs as a result of muscle relaxation and is accompanied by little or no change in intraluminal pressure.

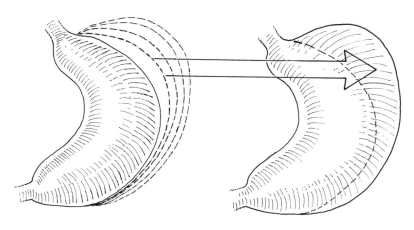

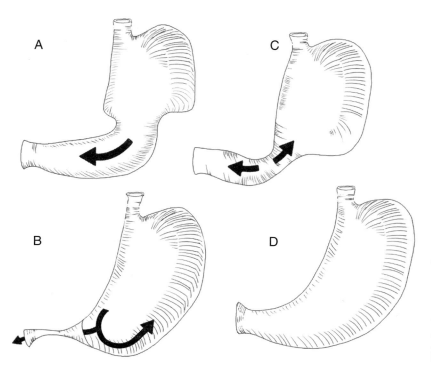

FIGURE 27–7. The grinding and churning activity of the distal stomach. *A,* A wave of peristalsis begins at the junction of the proximal and distal areas of the stomach and moves toward the pylorus. *B,* As the peristaltic wave approaches the pylorus, the pylorus constricts, causing some of the ingesta to be crushed within the peristaltic ring and propelled back toward the proximal stomach. *C,* As the peristaltic wave reaches the pylorus, some finely ground and liquefied material passes through into the duodenum, but the majority of material has been propelled back into the stomach. *D,* Between contractions, no gross movement of gastric contents occurs. (From Johnson LR [ed]: Gastrointestinal Physiology. St. Louis: CV Mosby, 1985.)

antrum, there is intense slow-wave activity, and muscular contractions are frequently present. Strong waves of peristalsis begin at about the middle of the stomach and migrate, with the slow waves, toward the pylorus. As the waves of peristalsis near the pylorus, the pylorus constricts, blocking the gastric exit of all but the smallest particles (Fig. 27–7). Particles leaving the stomach during the digestive phase of activity are less than 2 mm in diameter. Particles too large to pass the pylorus are crushed and ejected back into the antrum by the passing wave of peristalsis. Thus, the peristaltic actions of the distal stomach walls serve not only to propel food but also, and perhaps of more importance, to grind and mix it.

Control of gastric motility differs in the proximal and distal stomach

The motility of the stomach, like that of other smooth muscle portions of the gut, is under both nervous and endocrine control. Fibers of the vagus nerve synapse on nerve cell bodies of the extensive gastric myenteric plexus and exert a high degree of control over gastric motility. The effects of vagal stimulation on the proximal and distal regions of the stomach are opposite; in the proximal stomach, vagal activity suppresses muscular contractions and leads to adaptive relaxation, whereas in the distal stomach, vagal stimulation causes intense peristaltic activity. Vagal stimulation of distal antral motility is mediated by acetylcholine, but vagal inhibition of proximal stomach motility is not. The identity of the inhibitory mediator is not well established, but it may be vasoactive intestinal peptide.

Vagal action on the stomach is stimulated by events occurring within the central nervous system, as well as within the stomach and intestine. The anticipation of food consumption causes vagal stimulation of the stomach and thus primes the stomach to receive a meal. Reactions of the GI tract that originate in the central nervous system in response to anticipated food intake are often referred to as the *cephalic phase* of digestion. Reactions to the cephalic phase of digestion are then augmented as food enters the stomach. In response to food in the stomach, vagal activity increases as sensory receptors in the stomach create a positive feedback loop.

The exact role of hormones in regulation of gastric motility is not completely established. Gastrin, which is secreted from cells in the gastric antrum, appears to enhance gastric motility. Cholecystokinin, secretin, and gastric inhibitory peptide appear to suppress gastric motility, at least in the dog. The roles of the various GI hormones are difficult to determine from available information, because many of the experimental results reported have been in response to administration of GI hormones at amounts far greater than those normally occurring.

The rate of gastric emptying must match the small intestine's rate of digestion and absorption

The rate at which food leaves the stomach must match the rate at which it can be digested and absorbed by the small intestine. Because some types of foods can be digested and absorbed more rapidly than others, the rate at which the stomach empties has to be regulated by the contents of the small intestine. Thus, there are reflexes that regulate gastric emptying and allow the stomach to serve as a storage site. The afferent receptors of these reflexes are in the duodenum and are activated by low pH, high osmolality, and the presence of fat. It appears that there are separate sensory receptors for each of these stimuli, but those receptors have not been identified anatomically.

Many reflexes occur within the GI system. Their names usually reflect the site of origin of the afferent stimulus and the site of the efferent response. Thus, reflex control of gastric emptying by the duodenum is referred to as the *enterogastric reflex*. *Entero-* is a prefix referring to the intestine.

The arc of the enterogastric reflex probably involves the central nervous system and the enteric nervous system, as well as the endocrine system (Fig. 27–8). The extrinsic reflex pathway appears to involve afferent fibers of the vagus, which receive stimuli in the duodenum. These stimuli are integrated in the brainstem, and the response is mediated by vagal efferent fibers to the stomach. The enteric reflex arc involves receptors in the duodenum and nerve fiber connections in the enteric nervous system that directly affect gastric emptying.

A contribution of the GI endocrine system to the enterogastric reflex has long been suspected, but the exact hormones responsible for the reflex are not known. It is suspected that cholecystokinin and secretin may be important. Both hormones are secreted by cells in the duodenum; cholecystokinin is secreted in response to fat, and secretin, in response to low pH;

both appear to have suppression of gastric emptying as secondary effects. Gastric inhibitory peptide is a hormone produced in the duodenum in response to the presence of carbohydrate. In the dog, gastric inhibitory peptide may function as an inhibitor of gastric emptying, although stimulation of insulin secretion is probably its major action.

Enterogastric reflexes control gastric emptying by regulating stomach motility. The manner in which motility affects gastric emptying of solids is different from that for liquids. The rate at which solids are expelled from the stomach is regulated by the rate at which they are broken down into particles small enough to pass through the pylorus. This, in turn, is controlled by the motility of the antrum, or distal stomach; the greater the motility of the antrum, the faster material is broken down. Thus, antrum motility regulates the rate of release of solid material from the stomach. Liquid material leaves the stomach more quickly than solid matter, and the release of liquid may be less dependent on antral motility than on the motility of the proximal stomach.

There is little mixing activity in the proximal stomach. Because of this, liquids and solids tend to separate, the liquids moving to the outside and the solids to the center of the mass of food in the proximal stomach. Increased tension in the wall of the stomach body forces liquid into the antrum. Liquid may leave the antrum quickly, dependent on the activity of the pylorus. On the other hand, increased tension in the stomach body has little effect on the transport of solid material, because such material cannot leave the gastric body until sufficient space has been made available in the antrum. Thus, motility of the stomach body appears primarily responsible for the liquid-emptying rate, whereas motility of the antrum is most responsible for the solid-emptying rate. The effect of the pylorus itself on gastric emptying is not as great as might be expected; removal of the pylorus results in a slight increase in the liquid-emptying rate and little increase in the rate of emptying of solid material. It appears that the distal portion of the antrum can account for much of the sieving action usually attributed to the pylorus. The rate of emptying of an isotonic liquid from the stomach is exponential and dependent on the initial volume of the liquid meal. Under usual circumstances, a liquid meal in the canine stomach has a half-life of about 18 minutes and is essentially gone by 1 hour after ingestion. Solid material is emptied more slowly, and its rate is dependent on its fat content. Low-fat meat meals are usually gone from the stomach in 3 to 4 hours after ingestion.

Between meals, the stomach is cleared of indigestible material

It is obvious that ingested material often cannot be reduced to particles less than 2 mm in diameter. During the digestive phase of gastric motility, such material does not leave the stomach. To clear the stomach of indigestible debris, a particular type of motility

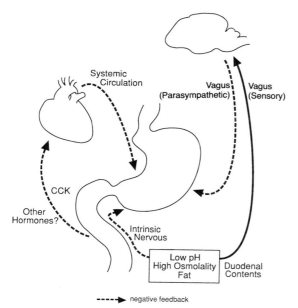

FIGURE 27–8. Inhibitory arcs of the enterogastric reflex. Low pH, high osmolality, and the presence of fat in the duodenum stimulate vagal, enteric neuronal, and hormonal reflexes that inhibit stomach emptying. After the duodenal pH and osmolality have moderated and some of the fat has been absorbed, the inhibitory influences on the stomach are removed. CCK, cholecystokinin.

occurs between meals. This motility pattern is called the *interdigestive motility complex*. In association with this complex, the pylorus relaxes as strong waves of peristalsis sweep over the antrum, forcing less digestible material into the duodenum. This type of motility appears to have a "housekeeping" function in clearing the stomach of indigestible material.

The peristaltic waves of the interdigestive motility complex occur at approximately 1-hour intervals during the periods when the stomach is relatively empty of digestible material. Eating disrupts the complex and causes the resumption of the digestive motility pattern. Herbivores, which eat nearly constantly, have a slightly different pattern; the interdigestive motility complex occurs at approximately hourly intervals, even with digestible food present in the stomach.

Vomiting is a complex reflex coordinated from the brainstem

Vomiting is a complex reflex activity whose integration, or coordination, is centered in the brainstem. The act of vomiting involves many striated muscle groups and structures outside the GI tract. Vomiting is associated with the following actions:

1. Relaxation of the muscles of the stomach and lower esophageal sphincter and closing of the pylorus.
2. Contraction of the abdominal musculature, creating an increase in intra-abdominal pressure.
3. Expansion of the chest cavity while the glottis remains closed; this action lowers intrathoracic pressure.
4. Opening of the upper esophageal sphincter.

The efferent limb of this reflex arc involves motor fibers in many different peripheral nerves.

Afferent stimulation of the vomiting reflex comes from a large number of receptors. Of particular importance are mechanoreceptors in the pharynx and tension receptors and chemoreceptors in the gastric and duodenal mucosa. Stimulation of these receptors sends signals to the *vomit center* in the brainstem. Thus, noxious tactile or chemical stimulation of the GI mucosa can result in vomiting that clears, or attempts to clear, the offending stimulus from the GI tract. Direct irritation of GI structures is not, however, the only stimulus for vomiting. The vomit center receives afferent input from a variety of organs; thus, vomiting is not always an indication of a primary GI problem.

An important structure outside the GI tract that supplies afferent input in the vomit center is the *chemoreceptor trigger zone*. This is an area of the brainstem that lies in contact with the third ventricle. The chemoreceptor trigger zone is sensitive to the presence of some drugs and toxins in the blood. When stimulated, the chemoreceptor trigger zone sends signals to the vomit center and induces vomiting. Some of the products of inflammation stimulate the chemoreceptor trigger zone. Thus, inflammatory disease,

even outside the GI tract, can sometimes lead to vomiting. The semicircular canals of the inner ear are other important structures that supply afferent input to the vomit center. Constant stimulation of the semicircular canals may induce vomiting, as occurs in motion sickness. Other sites in the body may stimulate the vomit center also; thus, vomiting is a rather nonspecific sign of disease.

Motility of the small intestine has a digestive and interdigestive phase

Motility of the small intestine occurs in two distinct phases: one during the digestive period after food intake, and another during the interdigestive period when little food is present in the gut. In the digestive phase there are two primary motility patterns: propulsive and nonpropulsive. The nonpropulsive pattern is referred to as *segmentation*. Segmentation results from localized contractions of circular muscle. Portions of small intestine, usually 3 to 4 cm long, contract tightly, dividing the gut into segments of constricted and dilated lumen. Within a few seconds, the constricted portions relax and new areas constrict (Fig. 27–9). This action tends to "milk" gut contents back and forth within the small intestine, mixing them with digestive juices and circulating them over the absorptive mucosal surfaces. This type of motility does not contribute much to the net aboral propulsion of ingesta. In fact, segmentation tends to slow down the aboral movement of material because of closure of the intestinal lumen in the constricted segments. Propulsive activity during the digestive phase consists of peristaltic contractions that migrate down the gut in phase with the slow waves. Digestive phase peristaltic contractions, in contrast to interdigestive phase peristalsis, pass over short segments of intestine and then die out. Thus, ingesta is pushed down the gut for a short distance and then subjected to additional segmentation contractions and mixing activity.

The interdigestive phase of small intestinal motility is characterized by waves of powerful peristaltic contractions that sweep over a large length of small intestine, sometimes traversing the entire organ. These waves are referred to as the *migrating motility complex* (MMC) or, alternatively, the *migrating myoelectric complex*. The MMC begins in the duodenum as groups of

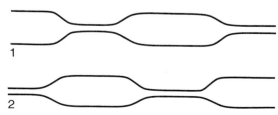

FIGURE 27–9. Segmentation in the small intestine. Areas of circular muscle constriction close the lumen and divide the gut into dilated segments containing ingesta. At periodic intervals the areas of constriction and dilation alternate, exerting a mixing and circulating action on the ingesta.

slow waves that stimulate intense action potential and muscular contraction activity. The complex migrates down the intestine at the rate of the slow waves. Some of the MMCs die out before reaching the ileum, but some travel the entire length of the small intestine.

The MMC probably has a housekeeping function and serves to push undigested material out of the small intestine. The MMC may also be important in controlling the bacterial population in the upper gut. Normally the duodenum harbors a relatively small population of bacteria, and the population increases distally into the ileum, which has a moderately large number of bacterial organisms. The colon is heavily colonized by numerous species of bacteria. It is important for digestive function that this relative distribution of bacteria be maintained within the gut. The MMC may help to impede the migration of bacteria from the ileum to the duodenum.

The ileocecal sphincter prevents movement of colon contents back into the ileum

The *ileocecal sphincter* is at the junction of the small and large bowel and prevents the retrograde movement of colon contents into the ileum. It consists of a well-developed ring of circular muscle that remains constricted at most times. In addition to the muscular sphincter, in many species there is a flap of mucosa that acts as a one-way valve, further blocking movement of colon contents into the ileum. During periods of peristaltic activity in the ileum, the sphincter relaxes, allowing movement of material into the colon. When colonic pressure increases, the ileocecal sphincter constricts more tightly.

Motility of the colon causes mixing, retropulsion, and propulsion of ingesta

The colon acts in (1) absorption of water and electrolytes, (2) storage of feces, and (3) fermentation of organic matter that escapes digestion and absorption in the small intestine. The relative importance of these functions varies with the species, and tremendous differences in colon size and shape exist among animals. The major determinant of colon size is the importance of colonic fermentation to the energy needs of the animal. Some species, such as the horse and rabbit, make extensive use of fermentation products for nutritional needs and have large and complex colons. (The ruminant's fermentation chamber is in the stomach.) Other species, such as the dog and cat, do not rely on fermentation products and have relatively simple colons. Differences in colonic anatomy among four species with different needs for fermentative digestion are illustrated in Figure 27–10.

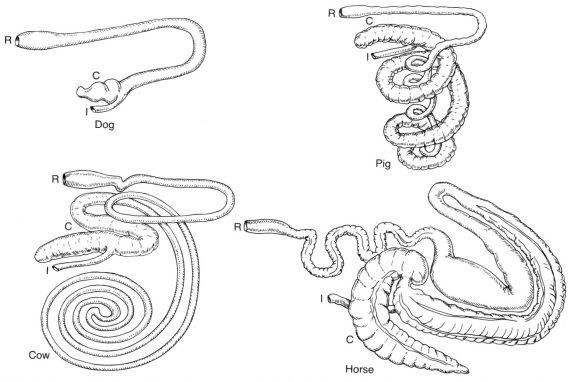

Figure 27–10. Variations of colon anatomy of four mammals. Animals with simple colons, such as the dog, are not dependent on colonic fermentation to supply energy needs. Horses, which have tremendous colonic development, rely on colonic fermentation for a large portion of their energy needs. In animals such as pigs and cattle, the importance of colonic fermentation to digestive needs is intermediate between the those of the horse and dog, and this intermediate position is noted in their colon development. C, cecum; I, ileum; R, rectum.

Considerable similarity appears to exist in colon motility patterns among animals, in spite of the anatomic diversity. Mixing activity is prominent in the colons of all species, because mixing and circulating is important to both absorptive and fermentative functions. Mixing is achieved by segmentation contractions along with other types of motility. In many species, such as the horse and pig, colonic segmentation is pronounced and in some areas results in the formation of sacculations known as *haustra*, which are visible even after death.

A particular characteristic of colonic motility is retropulsion, or *antiperistalsis*. This is a type of peristaltic contraction that migrates orally, the opposite of normal peristaltic movement. This type of motility appears to result from colonic slow-wave activity that is somewhat more complex than that of the small intestine. The site of slow-wave origin in the colon, in contrast to that in the small intestine, is determined by the enteric nervous system. Under resting conditions in the colon, slow waves originate from "pacemakers" in one or more central sites. The pacemakers are not anatomic structures; rather, they are areas defined by activities of the enteric nervous system. Thus, the pacemakers are not always the same areas but can disappear and form in different locations in response to the need for different motility patterns. Antiperistaltic contractions occur in the segments in which slow waves migrate in an oral direction. Antiperistaltic contractions are retropulsive and impede the movement of ingesta, causing intense mixing activity and forcing material to accumulate in the proximal portions of the colon. Retropulsion appears to be particularly strong near the pacemakers, and the pacemakers therefore represent sites of high resistance to the flow of colonic ingesta.

Because of continued inflow of material from the ileum into the colon, some ingesta escapes the retropulsive, antiperistaltic motility and moves into areas of propulsive, peristaltic activity and proceeds along the colon. In addition, there are periods of intense propulsive activity that involve the entire colon. These are called *mass movements* and frequently involve the distal translocation of the entire colonic content.

In the carnivore colon, absorption and storage occur

The colon of the dog and cat is a relatively simple organ consisting of a short cecum, an ascending part, a transverse part, and a descending part. During the resting phase, there is a colonic pacemaker at about the junction of the transverse and descending colons (Fig. 27–11). This gives rise to antiperistaltic activity in the proximal colon, with resultant accumulation of ingesta in the cecum and ascending colon areas. Moderate peristaltic activity usually occurs in the descending colon, whereas the distal colon and rectum are usually constricted and empty.

Material entering the carnivore colon is of a fluid

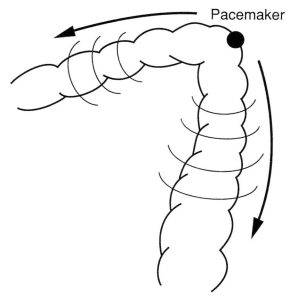

FIGURE 27–11. A pacemaker is present at the junction of the transverse and descending parts of the colon of the cat and probably in other mammals with similar colonic anatomy. Slow waves and peristaltic activity emanate in both directions from the pacemaker. Retrograde, or reverse, peristalsis in the proximal portions of the colon causes ingesta to be retained there, promoting the storage and absorptive functions of the colon.

consistency. It is thoroughly mixed in the ascending and transverse colons, and much of the water and many of the electrolytes are absorbed. By the time it reaches the descending colon, it is semisolid and becoming feces-like.

Despite anatomic differences in herbivore colons, similar motility patterns are found

The functions of the herbivore colon are discussed more extensively in Chapter 30. Here it is important to point out the between-species comparisons in colon motility. In spite of the extreme between-species differences in colon anatomy, there are numerous similarities in colon motility.

The equine hindgut is complex and highly developed (see Fig. 27–10). The cecum is large and formed into a haustrum, and it is unique among those of most species because there is a distinct, sphincter-like orifice joining it to the colon. The colon is divided into a large and a small portion, and the large colon is folded on itself so that there are three distinct flexures. The longitudinal muscles of the cecum and most areas of the colon are not evenly dispersed around the circumference of the gut. Instead, they form discrete bands, or *teniae*, that course along the longitudinal axis of the gut. The teniae divide the haustra longitudinally, giving the equine cecum and large colon a sacculated appearance.

Motility in the equine cecum consists of active segmentation and mixing, along with occasional mass movements that appear to transfer large amounts of ingesta to the colon. Motility in the colon consists of segmentation, antiperistalsis, and peristalsis. A colonic pacemaker appears to exist at the pelvic flexure and creates an area of high resistance to flow that results in prolonged retention of material in the ventral portions of the large colon. Little is known about regulation of motility in the equine small colon. The characteristic ball-shaped form of equine feces probably represents intense segmentation-type motility in the small colon, where the feces are formed. The motility and function of the equine colon are discussed in more detail in Chapter 30.

In ruminants and swine, the hindgut consists of a cecum of intermediate complexity, a spiral colon, and a straight colon. In comparison with other species, less is known about the hindgut motility of animals with spiral colons. It seems that there is an area of high flow resistance at the flexure, or central point, of the spiral colon. This may represent a pacemaker and result in generation of antiperistaltic motility in the centripetal portion of the colon.

The anal sphincter has two layers with separate innervation

The anal opening is constricted by two sphincters: an internal sphincter of smooth muscle, which is a direct extension of the circular muscle layer of the rectum; and an external sphincter of striated muscle. The internal anal sphincter remains tonically contracted most of the time and is responsible at most times for anal continence. The internal sphincter receives parasympathetic innervation from the sacral spinal segments through the pelvic nerve and sympathetic innervation from the lumbar spinal segments through the hypogastric nerve. In most species, sympathetic stimulation results in constriction of the sphincter, and parasympathetic stimulation results in relaxation.

The external sphincter maintains some degree of tonic contraction, but the consistent tone of the anus is primarily regulated by the internal sphincter. The external sphincter is innervated by general somatic efferent fibers that have cell bodies in the cranial sacral spinal segments and course in the pudendal nerve.

The rectosphincteric reflex is important in defecation

The entry of feces into the rectum is accompanied by the reflex relaxation of the internal anal sphincter, followed by peristaltic contractions of the rectum. This is known as the *rectosphincteric* reflex and is an important part of the act of defecation (Fig. 27–12). The reflex normally results in defecation, but in trained animals its effects can be blocked by voluntary constriction of the external anal sphincter. When defecation is voluntarily prevented, the rectum soon relaxes to accommodate the fecal bolus, and the inter-

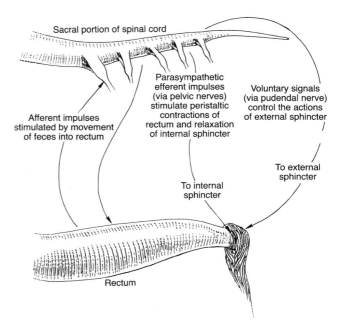

FIGURE 27–12. Arcs of the rectosphincteric reflex. The reflex is initiated by the movement of feces into the rectum and results in peristaltic movements of the rectal wall and relaxation of the internal anal sphincter. Fecal passage is the normal effect of the reflex, but voluntary constriction of the external anal sphincter can prevent the passage of feces and eventually override the reflex, apparently enabling trained animals to suppress the urge to defecate.

nal anal sphincter regains its tone. In humans, and presumably in dogs and cats, relaxation of the rectum and constriction of the internal sphincter is associated with fading of the urge to defecate, until another bolus of feces enters the rectum.

Uninhibited animals respond to the presence of feces in the rectum with a number of voluntary actions associated with defecation. In carnivores, the diaphragm and abdominal muscles contract to increase intra-abdominal pressure, and striated muscles of the anal canal relax as the animal assumes the defecation posture. These acts are important for complete evacuation of the rectum.

Major differences between avian and mammalian digestive systems include, in birds, both the lack of teeth and the separation of gastric functions into distinct anatomic regions

There are important anatomic differences between the digestive systems of birds and mammals. These differences affect motility functions more than other aspects of digestion, such as secretion, digestion, and absorption. Therefore, the digestive tract of birds is covered in this chapter as a separate topic. In other chapters of this section, aspects of avian digestion are integrated into the general discussion.

The general anatomy of the avian digestive system is illustrated in Figure 27–13. The pharynx of birds is

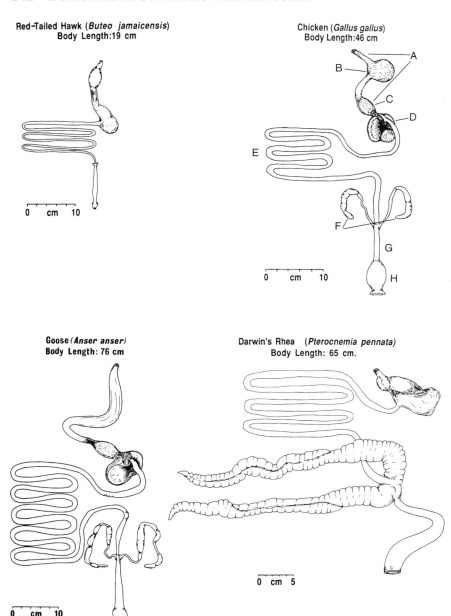

Red-Tailed Hawk (*Buteo jamaicensis*)
Body Length:19 cm

Chicken (*Gallus gallus*)
Body Length:46 cm

Goose *(Anser anser)*
Body Length: 76 cm

Darwin's Rhea   (*Pterocnemia pennata*)
Body Length: 65 cm.

FIGURE 27–13. Comparative anatomy of the digestive tracts of four avian species. Note the variation in crop and cecal development. The carnivorous red-tailed hawk has a small crop and rudimentary ceca. The chicken has a well-developed crop, and the rhea has tremendous cecal development. A, esophagus; B, crop; C, proventriculus; D, gizzard or ventriculus; E, small intestine; F, ceca; G, rectum; H, cloaca. (From Stevens CD: Comparative Physiology of the Vertebrate Digestive System. Cambridge, United Kingdom: Cambridge University Press, 1988, p 37.)

simpler than that in mammals with no soft palate. There are no teeth, although in carnivorous species, the beak is modified for tearing of food into pieces small enough to swallow. The esophagus has a large diameter, so as to accommodate unmasticated food. There is an outpouching of the esophagus known as the *crop.* The extent of development of the crop varies widely among avian species. The glandular portion of the stomach is the *proventriculus,* which is separated by an isthmus, known as the *ventriculus* or *gizzard,* from the muscular stomach. The small intestine varies greatly in length among species but is generally rather short in comparison with that of mammals of similar size. The ceca are usually paired and vary tremendously in development among avian species. In some carnivorous species, such as the hawk, the ceca are rudimentary, whereas in some of the nonflying herbivores such as the ostrich, cecal

development is extensive (see Fig. 27–13). The colon and rectum are very simple; the rectum ends in the *cloaca,* which is a common passageway for digestive, urinary, and reproductive discharges.

The crop performs a storage function. In some species the crop is little more than a pouch in the esophagus, whereas in others, such as the chicken, there is a distinct sphincter-like opening between the esophagus and crop. In general, ingesta do not begin to accumulate in the crop until the gizzard is full. The crop is richly populated with mucus-secreting cells, but no digestive glands are present. However, there are digestive glandular secretions that originate from the salivary glands and proventriculus. In many species, it appears that ingesta and secretions pass in a retrograde manner up the esophagus from the gizzard and proventriculus to the crop. The motility of the crop is under regulation of vagal in pulses. Crop motility and rate of emptying are coordinated so as to release ingesta at a rate matching the emptying rate of the proventriculus and gizzard. In some avian species, the crop also functions as a storage place for food being transported to the young. In this case, food is swallowed into the crop and later regurgitated as feed for offspring.

The proventriculus is a low-volume organ with a glandular epithelium resembling that of the stomach of mammals (see Chapter 28). Motility functions of the proventriculus are to propel ingesta and digestive secretions into the gizzard for mixing and grinding. The gizzard is a very muscular organ that grinds and liquefies ingesta. In addition, particle size discrimination occurs in the gizzard; small particles are passed into the duodenum, whereas large particles are retained for further comminution or are ejected back into the proventriculus for further addition of digestive secretions. In carnivorous birds, concretions of bone, hair, feathers, and other indigestible material accumulate in the gizzard and are occasionally regurgitated in an action known as *egestion*. In grain-eating birds, small stones or gravel are swallowed and retained in the gizzard to aid in the comminution of ingesta. This material is referred to as *grit*, and its presence increases digestive efficiency, although it is not essential. The mucosa of the gizzard is covered by a tough coating known as *koilin*. This coating is composed of glandular secretions and desquamated cells. It protects the mucosa from the physical grinding actions of the gizzard.

The motility and function of the various stomach areas of birds are easily comparable with gastric motility and function in mammals. The crop and proventriculus function in much the same manner as the fundus and body of the mammalian stomach, with storage and secretory functions. The gizzard functions in much the same way as the antrum of the mammalian stomach, with grinding and particle-size discrimination functions. The major functional differences between birds and mammals include the physical separation of the stomach compartments in birds and the very advanced grinding function of the gizzard.

The motility patterns of the avian small intestine appear to be generally similar to those in mammals. The motility of the hindgut similarly shares some of the same characteristics of other animals. Reverse peristalsis is a dominant characteristic of the colon and rectum. This moves ingesta into the ceca. Urinary excretions arriving at the cloaca become incorporated with ingesta and move in a retrograde manner into the ceca, thus facilitating reabsorption of the remaining water and electrolytes from urine. Cecal motility is characterized primarily by mixing and reverse peristalsis, with occasional mass movements resulting in the evacuation of the ceca. These mass movements are followed by defecation.

CLINICAL CORRELATIONS

Equine rabies

History Owners report that their horse has not "been itself" for the past few days. Today the animal is ex-tremely lethargic and stands with forelegs wide apart and head held low. The nostrils are soiled, and the owners report that water and feed come out of the nostrils when the animal attempts to eat or drink.

Clinical examination From the history and presenting signs, you recognize that the horse may have paralysis of muscles of the pharynx and larynx. Because these lesions are commonly associated with rabies in horses, you don a pair of plastic gloves and sleeves and proceed with your examination. To assess the function of the swallow reflex, you attempt to pass a stomach tube. You observe that the swallow reflex appears to be diminished, but that with some persistence the tube can be passed. This indicates that there is no physical obstruction in the pharynx or esophagus and that the problem is of a functional nature. These findings support, but do not confirm, a diagnosis of rabies.

Comment Rabies in herbivorous animals may take a number of forms. One of the most common signs in cattle and horses is paralysis of the pharynx and larynx as a result of viral lesions in the brainstem nuclei supplying the appropriate cranial nerves. If rabies is suspected, no one should come into direct contact with the excretions of the animal, especially saliva.

Treatment In this case, treatment should consist of oral fluid and electrolyte therapy administered through an indwelling stomach tube. If there is no response to this conservative therapy, and if the animal's condition appears to deteriorate, euthanasia is necessary, and the animal's head should be submitted for evaluation for a positive diagnosis of rabies.

Bibliography

Biancani P, Harnett KM, Behar J: Esophageal motor function. In Yamada T, Alpers DH, Laine W, et al (eds): Textbook of Gastroenterology, 3rd ed. Philadelphia: Lippincott Williams & Wilkins, 1999, pp 158–173.

Duke GE: Alimentary canal: Anatomy, regulation of feeding and motility. In Sturkie PD (ed): Avian Physiology. New York: Springer-Verlag, 1986, pp 269–288.

Hagger R, Finlayson C, Jeffrey I, et al: Role of the interstitial cells of Cajal in the control of gut motility. Br J Surg 84:445–450, 1997.

Hasler WL: Motility of the small intestine and colon. In Yamada T, Alpers DH, Laine W, et al (eds): Textbook of Gastroenterology, 3rd ed. Philadelphia: Lippincott Williams & Wilkins, 1999, pp 188–215.

Hasler WL: The physiology of gastric motility and gastric emptying. In Yamada T, Alpers DH, Laine W, et al (eds): Textbook of Gastroenterology, 3rd ed. Philadelphia: Lippincott Williams & Wilkins, 1999, pp 188–215.

Horowitz B, Ward SM, Sanders KM: Cellular and molecular basis for electrical rhythmicity in gastrointestinal muscles. Annu Rev Physiol 61:19–43, 1999.

Johnson LR, Alpers DH, Christensen J, et al (eds): Physiology of the Gastrointestinal Tract, 3rd ed. New York: Raven Press, 1994, pp 771–1024.

Kerlin P, Zinsmeister A, Phillips S: Relationship of motility to flow of contents in the human small intestine. Gastroenterology 82:701–706, 1982.

Makhlouf GM: Smooth muscle of the gut. In Yamada T, Alpers DH, Laine W, et al (eds): Textbook of Gastroenterology, 3rd ed. Philadelphia: Lippincott Williams & Wilkins, 1999, pp 82–105.

Merrit AM: Normal equine gastroduodenal secretion and motility. Equine Vet J Suppl 29: 7–13, 1999.

Rasmussen OO, Christiansen J: Physiology and pathophysiology of anal function. Scand J Gastroenterol Suppl 216:169–174, 1996.

Stevens CE, Hume ID: Comparative Physiology of the Vertebrate Digestive System, 2nd ed. Cambridge, United Kingdom: Cambridge University Press, 1996, pp 94–150.

Weisbrodt NW: Gastric emptying. In Johnson LR (ed): Gastrointestinal Physiology, 6th ed. St. Louis: CV Mosby, 2001, pp 37–46.

Weisbrodt NW: Motility of the small intestine. In Johnson LR (ed): Gastrointestinal Physiology, 6th ed. St. Louis: CV Mosby, 2001, pp 47–55.

Weisbrodt NW: Regulation: Nerves and smooth muscle. In Johnson LR (ed): Gastrointestinal Physiology, 6th ed. St. Louis: CV Mosby, 2001, pp 17–26.

Weisbrodt NW: Swallowing. In Johnson LR (ed): Gastrointestinal Physiology, 6th ed. St. Louis: CV Mosby, 2001, pp 28–35.

Weisbrodt NW: Motility of the large intestine. In Johnson LR (ed): Gastrointestinal Physiology, 6th ed. St. Louis: CV Mosby, 2001, pp 57–64.

PRACTICE QUESTIONS

1. A unique feature of GI smooth muscle cells is that
   a. their resting transcellular electrical potential has the positive pole on the outside surface of the cell membrane.
   b. action potentials, or spikes of membrane depolarization, are not associated with muscle contractions.
   c. muscle contractions are stimulated by partial depolarization of the membrane.
   d. there are spontaneous, rhythmic undulations in the electrical potential across the cell membrane.
   e. contraction of the muscles is never influenced by nervous activity.

2. The term *slow waves* as applied to the gut refers to
   a. slowly moving fronts of electrical activity that are propagated down the enteric nervous system.
   b. slowly moving fronts of electrical activity that result from coordinated changes in cell membrane potential occurring throughout the smooth muscle of the intestinal wall.
   c. slowly moving fronts of ingesta that proceed down the intestine in response to peristaltic movement.
   d. slowly moving fronts of action potentials that are constantly passing over the gut smooth muscle.
   e. slowly moving fronts of peristaltic contractions that pass uniformly over the entire small intestine during the digestive period.

3. An animal is presented to you with aspiration pneumonia (the result of food material entering the lower respiratory tract). Which of the following lesions would be a likely cause?
   a. Loss of myenteric plexus function in the pharynx and upper esophagus.
   b. Loss of slow-wave activity in the pharynx and upper esophagus.
   c. A lesion in the brainstem.
   d. A lesion in the trachea.
   e. None of the above.

4. The term *cephalic phase* is used in reference to a number of activities occurring in the GI tract. In general, the term means
   a. the early phases of digestion, when food is nearest the head.
   b. any actions stimulated directly by the presence of food in the stomach.
   c. any actions stimulated directly by the presence of food in the mouth.
   d. digestive events stimulated by the presence of food in the GI tract, but requiring reflexes integrated in the central nervous system.
   e. digestive events that occur before the ingestion of food and in response to central nervous system stimulation that is brought on by the anticipation of eating.

5. Conditions in the duodenum, such as low pH or high fat concentration, can in a reflexive manner inhibit gastric emptying. Which reflex arc is involved in this inhibition?
   a. Parasympathetic nervous system.
   b. GI enteric nervous system.
   c. GI endocrine system.
   d. All of the above.

PRACTICE ANSWERS

1. d   2. b   3. c   4. e   5. d

28

Secretions of the digestive tract

The salivary glands
1 Saliva moistens, lubricates, and partially digests food
2 Salivary secretions originate in the gland acini and are modified in the collecting ducts
3 Salivary glands are regulated by the parasympathetic nervous system
4 Ruminant saliva is a bicarbonate-phosphate buffer secreted in large quantities

Gastric secretion
1 Depending on the species, there may be two general types of gastric mucosa: glandular and non-glandular
2 The gastric mucosa contains many different cell types
3 The gastric glands secrete hydrochloric acid
4 Pepsin is secreted by gastric chief cells in an inactive form and subsequently activated in the gut lumen
5 The parietal cells are stimulated to secrete by the action of acetylcholine, gastrin, and histamine

The pancreas
1 Pancreatic exocrine secretions are indispensable for the digestion of the complex nutrients: proteins, starches, and triglycerides
2 Acinar cells secrete enzymes, whereas centroacinar cells and duct cells secrete a sodium bicarbonate solution
3 Pancreatic cells have cell surface receptors stimulated by acetylcholine, cholecystokinin, and secretin

Bile secretion
1 The liver is an acinar gland with small acinar lumina known as canaliculi
2 Bile contains phospholipids and cholesterol maintained in aqueous solution by the detergent action of bile acids
3 The gallbladder stores and concentrates bile during the periods between feeding
4 Bile secretion is initiated by the presence of food in the duodenum and stimulated by the return of bile acids to the liver

Digestion and absorption can take place only in the aqueous milieu of digestive secretions. Synthesis and secretion of these fluids is a well-controlled process, regulated by endocrine as well as neural events.

THE SALIVARY GLANDS

Saliva moistens, lubricates, and partially digests food

As food is chewed, it is mixed with salivary secretions that allow it to be molded into a well-lubricated bolus that facilitates swallowing. In addition, saliva may have antibacterial, digestive, and evaporative cooling functions, depending on the species.

The antibacterial activity of saliva is due to antibodies and lysozyme. *Lysozyme* is an enzyme that has antibacterial properties. It may appear that the antibacterial properties of saliva are inefficient, because the mouth normally contains a large, thriving population of bacteria. However, saliva aids in keeping this population in check, and animals with impaired salivary function are prone to infectious diseases of the oral cavity.

In omnivorous animals, such as rats and pigs, saliva contains a starch-digesting enzyme known as *salivary amylase*. This enzyme is usually absent from the saliva of carnivorous animals, such as dogs and cats. The saliva of some species also contains a fat-digesting enzyme known as *lingual lipase*. This enzyme is frequently present in young animals, such as calves, while they are on a milk diet; the enzyme disappears as they mature.

Salivary enzymes probably have their major digestive effect in the proximal stomach, because food is not retained in the mouth long enough to permit extensive digestion. The lack of mixing activity in the proximal stomach may be essential in the starch-digesting function of saliva. This is because the amylase enzyme is functional at neutral to slightly basic pH, which characterizes saliva. The low pH of the distal stomach probably inactivates the enzyme; therefore, it may be important that food entering the stomach not be mixed with gastric secretions. Some birds have salivary amylase that is active in the environment of the crop.

The evaporative cooling function of saliva is covered in Chapter 52.

Salivary secretions originate in the gland acini and are modified in the collecting ducts

Saliva is initially secreted into the lumen of the *acini,* or end-pieces, of the salivary glands. The glandular cells lining the acini secrete water, electrolytes, enzymes, and mucus. As the newly formed saliva progresses through the collecting ducts, its composition is modified. The duct epithelium reabsorbs electrolytes, especially sodium and chloride, in a manner similar to that in the proximal tubules of the kidneys (Fig. 28–1). The final product, saliva, is hypotonic and has a sodium concentration substantially less than that of extracellular fluid. The extent to which the acinar secretion is modified in the collecting ducts is dependent on the rate of saliva production. At high rates of salivary flow, there is little modification, which results in higher tonicity and electrolyte concentration, in comparison to low rates of flow.

Most mammals have at least three pairs of salivary glands: the *parotid* glands, which lie just under the ear and behind the vertical ramus of the mandible; the *mandibular* glands, which are in the intramandibular space; and the *lingual* glands, which lie in the base of the tongue. Each of these glands drains into a main duct that has a single opening into the mouth. In addition to these major glands, there are minor glands in the tongue and buccal mucosa. These are small, indistinct glands that often have numerous secretory ducts emptying into the mouth. The concentration of mucus is different in the secretions of the various salivary glands. The parotid gland secretes watery, or *serous,* saliva, whereas many of the minor glands se-

crete highly mucous saliva. Other glands secrete a mixed type of saliva containing both mucous and serous material. Avian salivary glands secrete a copious amount of mucus in order to lubricate unmasticated food for swallowing.

Salivary glands are regulated by the parasympathetic nervous system

Autonomic, parasympathetic nerve fibers of the facial and glossopharyngeal nerves end on the secretory cells of the salivary gland acini and stimulate the cells by way of cholinergic receptors. All phases of salivary activity are stimulated by this mechanism, including electrolyte, water, and enzyme secretion. The anticipation of eating can initiate a parasympathetic response that results in salivary secretion. In Pavlov's famous experiment, parasympathetic stimulation of the salivary gland was evoked in dogs by the sound of a ringing bell. The dogs had been trained to anticipate eating after hearing the bell. This well-known experiment was one of the first demonstrations that the central nervous system could regulate digestive functions. Chewing and stimulation of taste buds, in addition to the anticipation of eating, are afferent stimuli for salivation.

Salivary secretory cells also contain β-adrenergic receptors that are activated by sympathetic nerve stimulation or circulating catecholamines. This form of stimulation probably has little to do with normal digestive activity but is related to the salivation and drooling that is seen in carnivores preparing to attack. Among digestive glands, the salivary glands are unique because there is no endocrine regulatory component.

Ruminant saliva is a bicarbonate-phosphate buffer secreted in large quantities

The normal composition of ruminant parotid saliva is quite different from the saliva of monogastric animals. Bovine and canine saliva are compared in Figure 28–2. Ruminant saliva is isotonic and, in comparison with blood serum, has high concentrations of bicarbonate and phosphate and a high pH. This well-buffered solution is necessary for neutralizing acids formed by fermentation in the rumen, and ruminants secrete it in enormous quantities. An adult cow may secrete 100 to 200 L of saliva per day. This volume is approximately equivalent to the extracellular fluid volume of most adult cattle. It is obvious that much of the water and electrolytes secreted in saliva must be reabsorbed rapidly and recirculated through the total body water, or the cow would die of dehydration. In abnormal circumstances, such as blockage of the esophagus, in which the flow of saliva is diverted from the gastrointestinal tract, cattle quickly become dehydrated and acidotic.

In general, the salivary glands of domestic animals

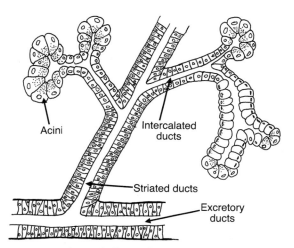

FIGURE 28–1. Schematic illustration of the salivary gland. Saliva is initially secreted by the acinar cells and is then modified as it passes through the intercalated, or collecting, ducts. Modification of acinar secretions by duct epithelia is a physiologic phenomenon common among several types of glands, including the pancreas.

Acini

Intercalated ducts

Striated ducts

Excretory ducts

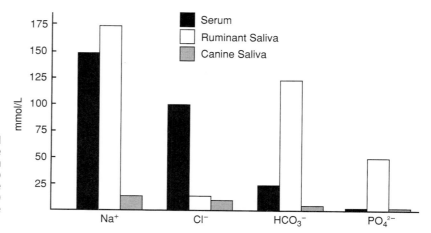

FIGURE 28–2. Electrolyte composition of blood serum and of canine and ruminant saliva. Note that the electrolyte concentration of canine saliva is much lower than that of serum, in contrast to the concentration in ruminant saliva. Also note the high concentrations of bicarbonate (HCO_3^-) and phosphate (PO_4^{2-}) in ruminant saliva; these ions give ruminant saliva its alkalizing quality.

are seldom involved in disease processes and infrequently require veterinary attention.

GASTRIC SECRETION

Depending on the species, there may be two general types of gastric mucosa: glandular and nonglandular

Most domestic animals have only glandular mucosa, but horses and rats have an area in the proximal portion of their stomachs that is covered by nonglandular, stratified squamous epithelium. This area is visibly different from the glandular area, to which it adjoins with a sharp line of demarcation. The function of the nonglandular area of gastric mucosa is not known with certainty. The nonglandular area may serve as a place where a small amount of fermentative (rumen-like) digestion could occur. Because there is little mixing activity in the proximal stomach, food in the nonglandular area would be protected from the secretions of the gastric glands. These acid secretions kill bacteria and thus would prevent fermentation.

The glandular area of the stomach is divided into three regions: *cardiac mucosa, parietal mucosa,* and *pyloric mucosa.* These areas contain glands of similar structure but with different types of secretions, as described later. In most species, the cardiac mucosa forms a narrow band around the gastric opening of the esophagus. In the pig, however, the cardiac mucosa covers a substantial portion of the proximal stomach.

The gastric mucosa contains many different cell types

The glandular mucosa of the stomach has frequent invaginations, or pores, known as *gastric pits.* The size of the pits is such that the pores leading into them can be seen with a hand-held magnifying glass. At the base of each pit is a narrowing, or isthmus, that continues into the opening of one or more gastric glands (Fig. 28–3).

The major surface areas of the stomach, as well as the lining of the pits, are covered with *surface mucous cells.* These cells produce thick, tenacious mucus that is a special characteristic of the stomach lining. The mucous cells and their associated secretion are important for protecting the stomach epithelium from the acid conditions and grinding activity present in the lumen. When the mucous cells are injured, stomach ulcers result.

Each region of the mucosa contains glands with characteristic cell types. Within the parietal area, the glands contain *parietal* cells. These cells are clustered in the neck, or proximal area, of the gland. It is their function to secrete hydrochloric acid (HCl). Distributed among the parietal cells in the neck of the gland is another type of cell, the *mucous neck cells.* These mucous cells secrete thin mucus, less viscous than that of the surface mucous cells. The mucous neck cells, in addition to their secretory function, appear to be the progenitor cells for the gastric mucosa. They are the only cells of the stomach lining that are capable of division. As they divide, they migrate either down into the glands or up into the pits and onto the surface epithelium. As they migrate, they differentiate into any of the several types of mature cells of the gastric surface and glands. In the base of the gastric glands is yet a third type of cell, the *chief* cells. These secrete *pepsinogen,* precursor to the digestive enzyme *pepsin.*

The glands of the cardiac and pyloric mucosal regions resemble those of the parietal area in structure but contain different cell types. The cardiac glands secrete only mucus. Their mucus is alkaline and probably serves to protect the adjacent esophageal mucosa from the acid secretions of the stomach. The pyloric glands have no parietal cells but contain the gastrin-producing G cells. According to most reports, pyloric glands do secrete pepsinogen.

The gastric glands secrete hydrochloric acid

When the gastric glands are stimulated maximally, the HCl solution secreted into the lumen is isotonic

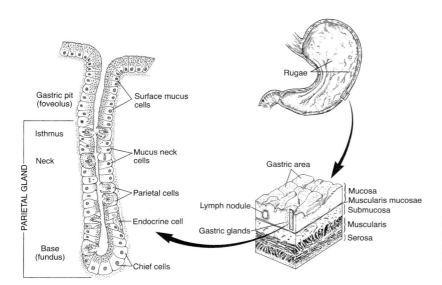

FIGURE 28–3. Anatomic illustration of glands of the stomach body. Other portions of the glandular stomach mucosa have similar structures but may differ somewhat in the cell types present in the glands. The gland openings are large enough to be seen with a hand-held magnifying glass.

and has a pH of less than 1. Both the hydrogen and chloride ions are secreted by the parietal cells but apparently by different cellular mechanisms. Hydrogen ion is secreted through an H^+,K^+-ATPase (adenosine triphosphatase) pump located on the luminal surface of the cell. This enzyme exchanges hydrogen ions for potassium ions, pumping one potassium ion into the cell for each hydrogen ion secreted into the lumen. In the exchange process, one molecule of adenosine triphosphate (ATP) is hydrolyzed to adenosine diphosphate (ADP), representing an expenditure of energy. The potassium cations that accumulate within the cells are released back into the lumen in combination with chloride anions. This allows the recycling of potassium ions as they are pumped back into the cells in exchange for hydrogen, resulting in the net secretion of hydrogen and chloride, with little net movement of potassium.

Hydrogen ions for secretion come from the dissociation of intracellular carbonic acid (H_2CO_3), leaving a bicarbonate ion (HCO_3^-) in the cell for each hydrogen ion secreted into the lumen (Fig. 28–4). Carbonic acid originates from water and carbon dioxide through the

action of *carbonic anhydrase*, an enzyme found in high concentration in the gastric mucosa.

As hydrogen cations are secreted, bicarbonate anions accumulate in the cell. To counterbalance this accumulation, bicarbonate anions are exchanged for chloride anions at the cell's nonluminal surface. In this manner, additional chloride is made available to the cell for secretion into the glandular lumen, and bicarbonate is secreted into the blood. During periods of intense secretion by the gastric glands, large amounts of bicarbonate are released into the blood. This alkalization of the blood is known as the "alkaline tide" and is associated with digestion. Normally, the alkaline tide is reversed when bicarbonate in the blood is consumed indirectly during the neutralization of gastric secretions as they enter the intestine (see the section on pancreatic secretions). Thus, on a total-body basis, gastric acid production results in only small and transient changes in blood pH; however, in disease states in which the secretions of the stomach are prevented from entering the intestine or are lost from the body because of vomiting, the pH of the blood can rise to dangerously high values.

Pepsin is secreted by gastric chief cells in an inactive form and subsequently activated in the gut lumen

Pepsin is usually referred to as a single compound, but it is actually a family of protein-digesting enzymes that are secreted from the gastric glands. They are formed in the chief cells as inactive proenzymes called *pepsinogens*. Pepsinogens are stored in the chief cells as granules until secreted into the lumen of the gastric glands. After secretion, pepsinogens are exposed to the acid contents of the stomach; this results in cleavage of a small portion of the protein molecule, which results in activation of the enzymes.

Digestive enzymes that are synthesized and stored

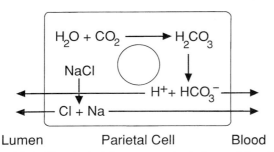

FIGURE 28–4. The electrolyte movements during gastric acid secretion. The production of hydrogen and bicarbonate ions from water and carbon dioxide is stimulated by the action of the enzyme carbonic anhydrase, the activity of which is high in gastric mucosa.

as inactive proenzymes and activated in the lumen of the gut are known by the general name of *zymogens*. The general pattern of zymogen formation and activation is necessary because the active enzymes could digest and destroy the cells that synthesize them.

The parietal cells are stimulated to secrete by the action of acetylcholine, gastrin, and histamine

Gastric acid secretion is stimulated by the anticipation of eating and the presence of undigested food in the stomach. When an animal anticipates eating, parasympathetic vagal impulses stimulate cells of the enteric nervous system, which in turn release acetylcholine into the vicinity of G cells and parietal cells. These secretory cells have acetylcholine receptors on their surfaces and respond by secreting gastrin and HCl, respectively. Gastrin circulates in the blood stream and eventually finds its way to the parietal cells, which have gastrin receptors, in addition to acetylcholine receptors, on their surfaces. The combined actions of gastrin and acetylcholine on the parietal cells result in high rates of HCl flow. The response of the stomach to anticipatory stimuli originating in the brain is referred to as the *cephalic phase* of gastric secretion.

Food entering the stomach initiates the second phase, or "gastric phase," of gastric secretion. Distention of the stomach by food stimulates stretch receptors of the enteric nervous system; the system responds by direct nervous (acetylcholine) stimulation of the G and parietal cells. In addition, food acts as a buffer, raising the stomach pH. This removes the inhibiting effect of acid on G cell secretion, further stimulating the production of gastrin, which leads to even greater enhancement of acid production by the parietal cells.

Histamine plays a role as an amplifying substance in gastric acid secretion. Parietal cells have surface receptors for gastrin, acetylcholine, and histamine. They are stimulated maximally when all three receptors are occupied. Histamine is secreted by *mast cells* and *enterochromaffin-like cells* in the parietal mucosa and acts on parietal cells in a paracrine manner. The histamine-secreting cells are stimulated to secrete by gastrin and acetylcholine. Thus, the effects of gastrin and acetylcholine on gastric acid secretion are amplified through their stimulation of histamine secretion.

As gastric secretion and digestion proceed, the pH of the stomach decreases. When the stomach pH falls to about 2, gastrin secretion is depressed, and at a pH of 1, gastrin secretion is completely abolished; thus, the gastrin stimulus to the parietal cells is removed, and acid secretion is reduced (see Fig. 26–8).

In addition to the gastrin-mediated negative feedback on acid secretion in the stomach, there is also an intestinal negative feedback mechanism. As acid contents from the stomach flow into the duodenum and the duodenal pH is reduced, gastric acid production is suppressed. The exact mechanism by which duodenal acidification exerts negative feedback on the parietal cells is not known with certainty. The hormone *secretin*, produced in the duodenum, may be involved, as well as neuronal reflexes acting through the enteric nervous system. The secretion of pepsinogen appears to be under the same regulatory influences as the secretion of HCl. However, regulation of pepsin secretion has been subjected to much less research than has the regulation of HCl secretion.

THE PANCREAS

Pancreatic exocrine secretions are indispensable for the digestion of the complex nutrients: proteins, starches, and triglycerides

The pancreas is composed of two functionally separate types of glandular tissue. A small but important portion of the pancreatic tissue is arranged into discrete islets within the parenchyma of the gland. These cells are collectively called the *endocrine pancreas*, because they secrete hormones into the blood stream. The endocrine pancreas is discussed in Chapter 33. The large majority of the pancreatic tissue is involved with the elaboration of digestive secretions. This portion is known as the *exocrine pancreas*, because its secretions are delivered into the intestinal lumen. The exocrine pancreas is the subject of this section.

Acinar cells secrete enzymes, whereas centroacinar cells and duct cells secrete a sodium bicarbonate solution

The exocrine pancreas is a typical acinar gland in which the end-pieces, or acini, are connected by an arborizing system of ducts, so that the gland conceptually resembles a bunch of grapes. In general structure it resembles the salivary gland, as illustrated in Figure 28–1. The cells of the acini contain a generous portion of rough endoplasmic reticulum, upon which large amounts of secretory proteins, the digestive enzymes, are synthesized. Each pancreatic acinar cell can produce all of the more than 10 different enzymes secreted by the pancreas. The major digestive enzymes of the pancreas are listed in Table 29–1. The functions of these enzymes are further discussed in Chapter 29. Protein-digesting enzymes, which are potentially harmful to the pancreatic cells, are synthesized as zymogens in a manner completely analogous to that of pepsinogen synthesis in the gastric glands. After synthesis, the enzymes and proenzymes are stored in vesicles, or *zymogen granules*, near the cellular apex. When the cells are stimulated, the zymogen granules fuse with the plasma membrane and release their contents into the lumen of the gland and eventually into the duodenal lumen, where they are converted to the activated form of the enzyme.

Specialized cells near the junction of the acini and ducts are called *centroacinar cells*. These cells, and the lining cells of the ducts, produce a watery secretion rich in sodium bicarbonate. Within the cells, carbonic acid (H_2CO_3) for the generation of bicarbonate ion (HCO_3^-) is produced by the action of carbonic anhydrase on H_2O and CO_2. The H_2CO_3 dissociates to form H^+ and HCO_3^-. Hydrogen ion is pumped from the cell in exchange for Na^+, allowing the accumulation of HCO_3^- within the cell. As HCO_3^- accumulates in the cell, it flows down its concentration gradient into the lumen of the pancreatic duct. In general, the ion transport activities of the pancreatic duct cells are opposite in direction to those of the parietal cells, as illustrated in Figure 28–4.

The ducts of the pancreatic lobules coalesce in an arborizing pattern to form either one or two main pancreatic ducts, depending on the species. The pancreatic duct or ducts may empty directly into the duodenum or, as in sheep, into the common bile duct. In the latter case, the pancreatic secretions enter the intestinal lumen along with bile.

Pancreatic cells have cell surface receptors stimulated by acetylcholine, cholecystokinin, and secretin

When binding sites on the surfaces of pancreatic acinar or duct cells are occupied, the cells are stimulated to secrete. Each type of cell, acinar and duct cells, appears to have receptors for the neurotransmitter acetylcholine as well as the gastrointestinal hormones cholecystokinin (CCK) and secretin. Acetylcholine, released from nerve endings near the cells, stimulates secretion, as do CCK and secretin arriving in the blood. CCK is the primary hormonal stimulus for acinar cells, whereas secretin is the primary hormonal stimulus for duct cells. It appears, however, that maximal stimulation of the cells occurs when all receptors are occupied. Thus, acinar cells secrete most actively in the presence of all three ligands: acetylcholine, CCK, and secretin. In this manner, secretin is said to potentiate, or increase, the action of CCK on acinar cells, and CCK potentiates the action of secretin on duct cells.

Nerve fibers ending in the vicinity of pancreatic acinar glands originate from cell bodies in the enteric nervous system. These neurons are stimulated to release acetylcholine by impulses arriving from other neurons of the enteric system, or by parasympathetic fibers arriving by way of the vagus nerve. Vagal stimulation of pancreatic secretion may arise as the result of several stimuli. The sight and smell of food induce centrally integrated vagal responses leading to pancreatic secretion; as mentioned, this is referred to as the *cephalic phase* of pancreatic secretion. Distention of the stomach causes a vagovagal reflex stimulating pancreatic secretion, and this is called the *gastric phase* of pancreatic secretion. The effects of the cephalic and gastric phases of pancreatic secretion are to "ready" the intestine for the imminent arrival of food by prior stimulation of pancreatic secretions.

The third phase, or *intestinal phase,* of pancreatic

secretion is the most intense and involves endocrine as well as neuronal stimuli. This phase commences as food material from the stomach enters the duodenum. This leads to distention of the duodenum, which appears to produce enteric nerve impulses, resulting in acetylcholine stimulation of pancreatic secretory cells. This stimulation reinforces and enhances the vagally mediated neuronal stimulation of the cephalic and gastric phases. The endocrine portion of the intestinal phase of pancreatic secretion occurs in response to the chemical stimulation that results from the presence of gastric contents in the duodenum. Peptides in the duodenal lumen, arising from the digestion of food protein, stimulate CCK production from endocrine cells in the duodenum. Fats in gastric ingesta also stimulate CCK secretion, whereas the low pH of material entering the duodenum from the stomach stimulates the secretion of secretin.

This stimulatory pattern is logical and results in a coordinated pattern of digestion. Proteins (peptides) and fats stimulate, through CCK, the secretion of protein- and fat-digesting enzymes. These enzymes function best in an alkaline environment, and so the acid secretions of the stomach must be neutralized. Acid conditions in the duodenum stimulate pancreatic bicarbonate secretion through secretin, leading to alkalization of the ingesta. As food is digested and absorbed and acid is neutralized, the stimuli for pancreatic secretion are removed and the amount of secretion diminishes to low, basal rates.

BILE SECRETION

One of the functions of the liver is that of a secretory gland of the digestive system. Its secretion, bile, has an important role in fat digestion.

The liver is an acinar gland with small acinar lumina known as canaliculi

The liver is composed of "plates," or one-cell-thick layers of hepatocytes that are bathed on either side by blood from the hepatic sinusoids. Between each row of cells is a small space created by cavitations in the plasma membranes of two apposing cells. The portions of the plasma membranes lining the spaces are isolated from the remainder of the plasma membrane by tight junctions, which seal off the spaces from the surrounding extracellular environment. Within the plates of cells, these spaces join to form channels, or *canaliculi,* that connect to the bile ductules. Bile is secreted from the hepatocytes into the canaliculi, from which it flows into the bile duct system. From a functional standpoint, the canaliculi may be perceived as acini lined by hepatocytes and emptying into the biliary duct system, as schematically illustrated in Figure 28–5. The bile duct epithelium is metabolically active and capable of altering the composition of canalicular bile by adding additional water and electrolytes, especially bicarbonate.

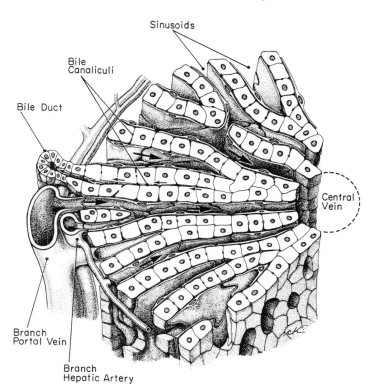

Figure 28–5. Hepatic microanatomy is complex and can be visualized in several ways. Note the relationship of the bile canaliculi to the bile ducts; the biliary system may be imagined as an acinar gland with the bile canaliculi forming a long, narrow acinus. (Modified from Ham AW: Textbook of Histology, 5th ed. Philadelphia: JB Lippincott, 1965.)

Bile contains phospholipids and cholesterol maintained in aqueous solution by the detergent action of bile acids

Hepatocytes form bile acids from cholesterol. The chemical changes necessary to convert cholesterol to cholic acid, a representative bile acid, are shown in Figure 28–6. Cholesterol is almost totally insoluble in water, but the chemical changes involved in the conversion of cholesterol to bile acids result in a molecule with a water-soluble (*hydrophilic,* or "water-loving") side and a lipid-soluble (*hydrophobic,* or "water-hating") side. This combination hydrophobic-hydrophilic attribute is the characteristic property of a detergent. Because of this dual solubility, detergents can render lipids soluble in water. The function of the bile acids is to emulsify dietary lipids and to solubilize the products of fat digestion.

Bile acids are produced in the smooth endoplasmic reticulum of the hepatocytes. As they are secreted from the cells into the lumen of the canaliculi, bile acids "dissolve away" some of the cell membrane components: phospholipids and cholesterol. These constituents—phospholipids, cholesterol, and bile acids—are the major functional components of bile and are important for the digestion and absorption of fats. The mechanism by which bile aids in fat digestion is discussed in Chapter 29.

Bile acids are secreted into the canaliculi as their sodium salts. The presence of bile acid salts and sodium in the canaliculi draws water, by osmosis, from the cells into bile. The electrolyte composition of canalicular bile usually resembles that of plasma but

may be somewhat lower in chloride. As bile flows through the bile ducts, water and electrolytes are added. Bicarbonate may be secreted by the duct cells, so that the bicarbonate concentration of bile is often higher than that in blood serum.

In addition to bile acids, phospholipids, and choles-

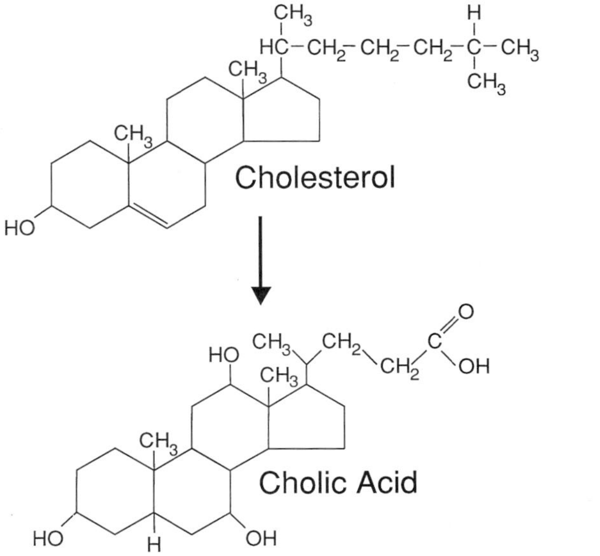

Figure 28–6. The conversion of cholesterol to cholic acid, a representative bile acid. Note the presence of two additional hydroxyl groups on the ring structure of cholic acid, in comparison with cholesterol. These hydroxyl groups enhance the water solubility and detergent action of the bile acid molecule. Other bile acids differ from cholic acid in the number and position of hydroxyl groups.

terol, bile contains other lipid-soluble organic substances. Of these, the *bile pigments* are present in the highest concentration. Bile pigments are breakdown products of heme porphyrin, a portion of the hemoglobin molecule. The principal bile pigment is *bilirubin,* which is produced during the normal process of red blood cell turnover. Bilirubin gives bile its characteristic green color. In the lumen of the gut, bilirubin is converted by bacterial action to other compounds. These secondary compounds are responsible for the characteristic brown color of the feces of nonherbivorous animals. Bile pigments serve no useful digestive function: the body simply uses bile, and ultimately feces, as a route for the excretion of these waste products.

The liver serves as an excretory organ for many lipid-soluble substances in addition to bilirubin. The detergent action of the bile acids makes the liver an ideal excretory organ, in comparison with the kidney, for these types of compounds. Substances metabolized and secreted by the liver include many important drugs and toxins. This is important clinically, because the actions of these agents can be potentiated by impaired liver function.

The gallbladder stores and concentrates bile during the periods between feeding

When there is little or no food in the intestinal lumen, the *sphincter of Oddi,* at the union of the common bile duct and duodenum, is closed, and bile cannot enter the intestine and is diverted into the gallbladder. The gallbladder epithelium absorbs sodium, chloride, and bicarbonate from bile; water is absorbed passively. Thus, in the gallbladder the organic constituents of bile are concentrated, whereas the volume of bile is reduced. In species that have no gallbladder, such as horses and rats, the sphincter of Oddi is apparently nonfunctional, and bile is secreted into the intestine during all phases of the digestive cycle.

Bile secretion is initiated by the presence of food in the duodenum and stimulated by the return of bile acids to the liver

When food, especially fat-containing food, reaches the duodenum, the gastrointestinal endocrine cells are stimulated to secrete CCK. CCK causes relaxation of the sphincter of Oddi and contraction of the gallbladder, forcing stored bile into the intestine. Bile acids aid in the digestion and absorption of fats in the jejunum (see Chapter 29) but are not absorbed themselves until they reach the ileum. After absorption in the ileum, the bile acids travel in the portal blood to the liver. In the liver, bile acids are almost completely absorbed from the portal blood. As a result, almost no bile acids reach the posterior vena cava, and they are consequently found only in low concentrations in

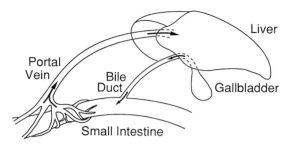

FIGURE 28–7. Bile acids and other molecules circulate in an enterohepatic cycle. Phases of the cycle include the portal vein, biliary system, and intestinal lumen.

the systemic circulation. The flow of bile acids from liver to intestine to portal blood to liver and back to intestine is known as *enterohepatic circulation* (Fig. 28–7).

Bile acids arriving at the liver, by way of the portal circulation, stimulate bile synthesis. Thus, a positive feedback system is initiated when the gallbladder contracts: the absorption of gallbladder bile from the intestine stimulates additional bile synthesis by the hepatocytes. Rapid bile synthesis continues as long as the sphincter of Oddi is open and the gallbladder is contracted. When fats are digested, CCK secretion ceases, the sphincter of Oddi closes, and bile is diverted to the gallbladder. Because bile acids are no longer reaching the intestine, they are no longer being absorbed, and thus the stimulus for bile secretion is reduced and bile flow slows down.

In addition to the effect of CCK on bile secretion, secretin influences secretion from the bile duct epithelium. Secretin stimulates water and bicarbonate secretion from the bile ducts in a manner similar to that of its effects on the duct cells of the pancreas. Thus, bile may participate in the neutralization of stomach acids.

Bibliography

Boyer JL: Bile secretion—Models, mechanisms, and malfunctions. A perspective on the development of modern cellular and molecular concepts of bile secretion and cholestasis. J Gastroenterol 31:475–481, 1996.

Del Valle J, Todisco A: Gastric secretion. In Yamada T, Alpers DH, Laine W, et al (eds): Textbook of Gastroenterology, 3rd ed. Philadelphia: Lippincott Williams & Wilkins, pp 278–319, 1999.

Johnson LR: Gastric secretion. In Johnson LR (ed): Gastrointestinal Physiology, 6th ed. St. Louis: CV Mosby, 2001, pp 75–94.

Johnson LR: Pancreatic secretion. In Johnson LR (ed): Gastrointestinal Physiology, 6th ed. St. Louis: CV Mosby, 2001, pp 95–106.

Johnson LR: Salivary secretion. In Johnson LR (ed): Gastrointestinal Physiology, 6th ed. St. Louis: CV Mosby, 2001, pp 65–74.

Johnson LR, Alpers DH, Christensen J, et al (eds): Physiology of the Gastrointestinal Tract, 3rd ed. New York: Raven Press, 1994, pp 1025–1576.

Moseley RH: Bile secretion. In Yamada T, Alpers DH, Laine W, et al (eds): Textbook of Gastroenterology, 3rd ed. Philadelphia: Lippincott Williams & Wilkins, 1999, pp 380–403.

Nauntofte B, Jensen, JL: Salivary secretion. In Yamada T, Alpers DH, Laine W, et al (eds): Textbook of Gastroenterology, 3rd ed. Philadelphia: Lippincott Williams & Wilkins, 1999, pp 263–277.

Owyang C, Williams JA: Pancreatic secretion. In Yamada T, Alpers DH, Laine W, et al (eds): Textbook of Gastroenterology, 3rd ed. Philadelphia: Lippincott Williams & Wilkins, 1999, pp 355–379.

Parsons ME: Control of gastric secretion. Proc Nutr Soc 55:251–258, 1996.
Prinz C, Zanner R, Gerhard M, et al: The mechanism of histamine secretion from gastric enterochromaffin-like cells. Am J Physiol 277:C845–C855, 1999.
Stevens CE, Hume ID: Comparative Physiology of the Vertebrate Digestive System, 2nd ed. Cambridge, United Kingdom: Cambridge University Press, 1995, pp 229–266.
Weisbrodt NW: Bile production, secretion, and storage. In Johnson LR (ed): Gastrointestinal Physiology, 6th ed. St. Louis: CV Mosby, 2001, pp 107–118.

PRACTICE QUESTIONS

1. In monogastric animals, saliva produced during periods of rapid secretion has a higher electrolyte concentration than saliva produced during periods of slow salivary secretion. From your understanding of salivary gland physiology, which appears to be the most likely explanation?
a. During periods of slow salivary secretion, the acinar cells are inactive and low-electrolyte saliva is secreted by the duct cells.
b. Parasympathetic stimulation of the acinar cells results in the elaboration of a more electrolyte-rich saliva.
c. Gastrin stimulation increases the electrolyte concentration of saliva.
d. During rapid secretion, fluid produced by the acinar cells is exposed to the actions of the duct cells for a shorter period of time than during slow rates of secretion.
e. Different cell types within the acinus are responsible for salivary production, depending on the type of stimulus.

2. Some nutritionists are experimenting with a drug that increases salivary secretion in cattle. What effect do you think this would have on rumen pH?
a. Increase rumen pH.
b. Decrease rumen pH.
c. Have no effect on rumen pH.

3. Inhibition of the enzyme carbonic anhydrase is likely to have what effect on gastric pH?
a. Decrease gastric pH.
b. Increase gastric pH.
c. Have no effect on gastric pH.

4. Which of the following is *not* a potential stimulus for gastric acid secretion?
a. Norepinephrine secretion resulting from stimulation of sympathetic nerves.
b. Vagal nerve activity resulting from the sight of food.
c. The presence of undigested protein in the pyloric antrum.
d. Acetylcholine release stimulated by gastric stretch receptors acting on nerves of the enteric system.
e. Histamine release from cells in the gastric mucosa.

5. Which of the following is *not* a natural ligand for receptors in the pancreas?
a. CCK.
b. Acetylcholine.
c. Gastrin.
d. Secretin.

PRACTICE ANSWERS

1. d   2. a   3. b   4. a   5. c

29

Digestion and absorption: the nonfermentative processes

1 Digestion and absorption are separate, but related, processes

2 The small intestinal mucosa has a large surface area and epithelial cells with "leaky" junctions between them

3 At the intestinal surface, there is a microenvironment made up of glycocalyx, mucus, and an unstirred water layer

Digestion

1 Breaking down food particle size by physical action is an important part of the digestive process

2 Chemical digestion results in the reduction of complex nutrients into simpler molecules

3 Luminal-phase carbohydrate digestion results in the production of short-chain polysaccharides

4 Luminal-phase digestion of carbohydrates applies only to starches, because sugars are all digested in the membranous phase

5 Proteins are digested by a variety of luminal-phase enzymes

6 Membranous-phase digestive enzymes are a structural part of the intestinal surface membrane

7 Membranous-phase digestion occurs within the microenvironment of the unstirred water layer, intestinal mucus, and glycocalyx

8 A specific membranous-phase enzyme exists for the digestion of each type of polysaccharide

9 Complete digestion of peptides to free amino acids takes place both on the enterocyte surface and within the cells

Intestinal absorption

1 Specialized nutrient transport systems exist in the apical and basolateral membranes

2 Secondary and tertiary active transport utilize the transcellular sodium ion electrochemical gradient as their source of energy

3 Passive transport occurs either through ion channels in cell membranes or directly through the tight junctions

4 The products of membranous-phase digestion are absorbed by sodium co-transport

Absorption of water and electrolytes

1 There are at least three distinct mechanisms of sodium absorption

2 There are three major mechanisms of chloride absorption

3 Bicarbonate ion is secreted by several digestive glands and must be recovered from the gut if body acid-base balance is to be maintained

4 Potassium is absorbed primarily by passive diffusion through the paracellular route

5 The major mechanisms of electrolyte absorption are selectively distributed along the gut

6 All intestinal water absorption is passive, occurring because of the absorption of osmotically active solutes

Intestinal secretion of water and electrolytes

1 Passive increases in luminal osmotic pressure occur during hydrolytic digestion and result in water secretion

2 Active secretion of electrolytes from the crypt epithelium leads to intestinal water secretion

Gastrointestinal blood flow

1 Water and solute movement between the lateral spaces and villous capillaries is subject to the same forces that govern water and solute movement between the extracellular and vascular fluids in other tissues

2 Absorbed nutrients enter the capillaries by diffusion from the lateral spaces

3 A countercurrent, osmotic-multiplier system may increase the osmolality of blood at the tips of the villi, further promoting absorption of water into the blood

4 Disturbances in the venous drainage from the intestine can markedly affect the mechanisms of capillary absorption in the villi

Digestion and absorption of fats

1 Detergent action as well as enzymatic action is necessary for the digestion and absorption of lipids

2 Lipids are absorbed through the apical membrane by carrier proteins and simple diffusion

3 Bile acids are reabsorbed from the ileum by a sodium co-transport system

4 Absorbed lipids are packaged into chylomicrons before leaving the enterocytes

Growth and development of the intestinal epithelium

1 The length of intestinal villi is determined by the relative rates of cell loss at the tips and cell replenishment at the base

Digestion in the neonate

1 During the first few hours of life, proteins are not digested but are absorbed intact

2 The major intestinal disaccharidase switches from lactase to maltase with maturity

Pathophysiology of diarrhea

Diarrhea occurs when there is a mismatch between secretion and absorption

Digestion and absorption are separate, but related, processes

Digestion is the process of breaking down complex nutrients into simple molecules. In contrast, *absorption* is the process of transporting those simple molecules across the intestinal epithelium (Fig. 29–1). The two processes are the result of different biochemical events occurring within the gut. Both processes are necessary for the assimilation of nutrients into the body; absorption cannot occur if food is not digested, and the process of digestion is fruitless if the digested nutrients cannot be absorbed.

Disturbances of nutrient assimilation are common in veterinary medicine and may be caused by a variety of diseases, some of which affect digestion, and others absorption. The overt signs of failure of nutrient assimilation are often similar, but the biochemical lesions and specific therapies associated with maldigestive disease can be quite different from those associated with malabsorptive disease. Therefore, diagnosing the cause of failure of nutrient assimilation is a frequent challenge faced by veterinary clinicians,

a challenge that requires a thorough understanding of the physiology of nutrient digestion and absorption. In this chapter, the structural characteristics of the small intestinal epithelium that are of particular importance to the digestive and absorptive processes are reviewed first.

The small intestinal mucosa has a large surface area and epithelial cells with "leaky" junctions between them

Contact between the small intestinal mucosa and the luminal contents is facilitated by an extensive intestinal surface area. Three levels of surface convolutions serve to expand the surface area of the small intestine (see Fig. 26–2). First, large folds of mucosa known as *plicae circulares* add to the intestinal surface area of some animals but are not present in all species. Second, the mucosal surface is covered with finger-like epithelial projections known as *villi*. These structures are present in all species and increase the intestinal surface area by some 10- to 14-fold compared with a flat surface of equal size. Last, the villi themselves are covered with a brush-like surface membrane known as the *brush border*. The brush border is composed of submicroscopic *microvilli* that further enlarge the surface area (Fig. 29–2). At the base of the villi are gland-like structures known as *crypts of Lieberkühn* (Fig. 29–3). The villi and crypts are covered with a continuous layer of cellular epithelium.

The epithelial cells covering the villi and crypts are called *enterocytes*. Each enterocyte has two distinctly different types of cell membranes (Fig. 29–4). The cell surface facing the lumen is called the *apex* and is covered by the *apical membrane*. The apical membrane contains the microvilli. Under the light microscope, the microvilli give the cell surface a brush-like appearance, leading to the name *brush border*, which is synonymous with the apical membrane. Covering the apical membrane, and encasing the microvilli, is a jelly-like layer of glycoprotein known as the *glycocalyx*. Important digestive enzymes and other proteins are attached to the microvilli and project into the glycocalyx. Under the intense magnification of the electron microscope, these enzyme molecules, as well as other proteins, give the glycocalyx a fuzzy appearance (see Fig. 29–2). The apical membrane is a complex and unusual cellular membrane with a high protein content.

The remaining portion of the enterocyte plasma

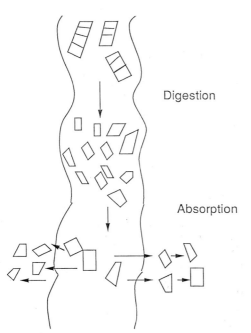

Digestion

Absorption

FIGURE 29–1. *Digestion* is the process of reducing macromolecules to their constituent monomers. *Absorption* is the transport of the resultant monomers across the intestinal epithelium into the blood stream.

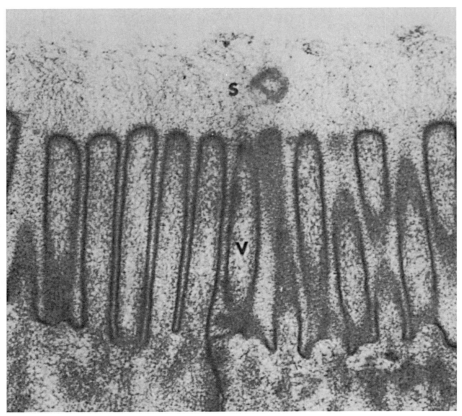

FIGURE 29–2. Electron micrograph of the microvilli of the intestinal brush border. The brush border is composed of the apical membranes of enterocytes. Note the indistinct array of molecular material (S) that radiates away from the microvilli (V); membranous-phase digestion occurs within this array of molecular material, which includes the membrane-bound digestive enzymes. (From Johnson LR, Christensen J, Jacobsen ED, et al [eds]: Physiology of the Gastrointestinal Tract, 2nd ed. New York, Raven Press, 1987, p 1215.)

membrane, that part not facing the gut lumen, is called the *basolateral membrane,* referring to the base and sides of the cell. This membrane is not especially unusual and indeed has many similarities to cell

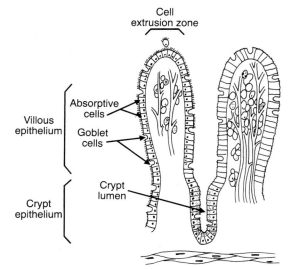

FIGURE 29–3. A layer one cell thick, the intestinal epithelium is continuous over the villi and the crypts of Lieberkühn.

membranes of other tissues. Although the basolateral membrane is not in direct contact with ingesta in the gut lumen, it serves an important role in intestinal absorption; nutrients that are absorbed into the enterocytes through the apical membrane must exit the cell through the basolateral membrane before gaining access to the blood stream.

The attachments between adjacent enterocytes are called *tight junctions.* These connections serve a special function in the process of digestion and absorption. The tight junctions form a narrow band of attachment between adjacent enterocytes. The band is near the apical end of the cells and divides the apical membrane from the basolateral membrane. The junctions may be called "tight," but from a molecular standpoint, they are rather loose. This is especially true in the duodenum and jejunum, where the tight junctions are loose enough to allow the free passage of water and small electrolytes. However, organic molecules do not penetrate the tight junctions.

The narrow band of tight junctions leaves the majority of the basolateral membrane unattached to its neighboring membrane on the adjacent enterocyte. This arrangement creates a potential space between enterocytes. This area between the lateral surfaces of the enterocytes is called the *lateral space*. The lateral spaces are normally distended and filled with extra-

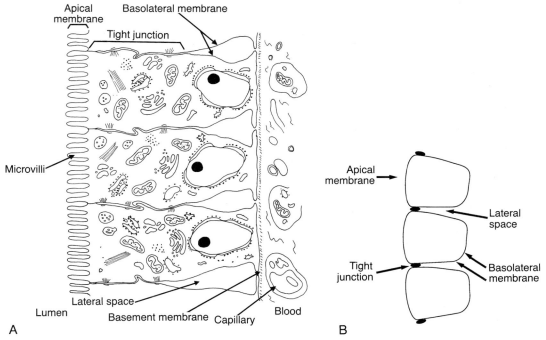

FIGURE 29–4.   Understanding the anatomic relationships of the enterocytes, tight junctions, apical membrane, basolateral membrane, and lateral spaces is critical to an understanding of the physiology of intestinal absorption. *A,* An anatomic illustration of the intestinal epithelium. *B,* A stylized sketch of the epithelium, including a capillary containing formed elements of blood. It is important to understand the relationship between part *A* and part *B* of this diagram.

cellular fluid. At the end of the lateral spaces nearest the apical membrane, the extracellular fluid is separated from the fluid of the intestinal lumen only by the tight junctions. At the opposite end of the lateral spaces, the fluid is separated from the blood by only the basement membrane of the intestinal capillaries. Both the tight junctions and the capillary endothelium are permeable barriers that allow the free passage of water and small molecules. Thus, there is relatively free flow of water and most electrolytes between the fluid in the lumen of the intestine, the extracellular fluid in the lateral spaces, and the blood.

At the intestinal surface, there is a microenvironment made up of glycocalyx, mucus, and an unstirred water layer

Liberally interspersed among the enterocytes are *goblet cells,* which secrete a rich layer of mucus that covers the mucosa. At the brush border surface, the mucus blends into the glycocalyx, the two layers forming a viscous coating that tends to trap molecules near the apical membrane. In addition to the mucus and glycocalyx layers, there is an area near the intestinal surface known as the *unstirred water layer.* With respect to the unstirred water layer, the intestine can be likened to a large stream or river; that is, the water in the center flows relatively rapidly, whereas the water near the edge or bank is quiet and flows slowly. Because of the same fluid-friction phenomenon that causes the water on the banks of rivers to be less

turbulent and to flow at a slower rate than water in center stream, the water very near the intestinal surface is quiet and flows at a much slower rate than water in the central part of the lumen. The unstirred water layer, mucus, and glycocalyx form an important diffusion barrier through which nutrients must pass before entering the enterocytes.

DIGESTION

Breaking down food particle size by physical action is an important part of the digestive process

The overall process of digestion is the physical and chemical breaking down of food particles and molecules into subunits suitable for absorption. Physical reduction of food particle size is important, not only because it allows food to flow through the relatively narrow digestive tube but also because it enlarges the surface area of the food particles, thus increasing the area exposed to the actions of digestive enzymes. Physical reduction of food particle size begins with mastication (chewing) but is completed by the grinding action of the distal stomach. In the distal stomach, the physical action of grinding is aided by the chemical actions of pepsin and hydrochloric acid. The chemical actions of these stomach secretions break down connective tissue and thus aid in breaking apart food particles, especially foods of animal origin. The reduction of food particle size by physical means is essentially complete when food leaves the stomach, as described in Chapter 27 in the discussion of motility of the distal stomach.

Chemical digestion results in the reduction of complex nutrients into simpler molecules

Chemical digestion of each major nutrient is accomplished by the process hydrolysis. As its name implies, *hydrolysis* is the splitting of a chemical bond by the insertion of a water molecule. Glycosidic linkages in carbohydrates, peptide bonds in proteins, ester bonds in fats, and phosphodiester bonds in nucleic acids are all cleaved by hydrolysis during digestion. Hydrolytic splitting of these various chemical bonds is illustrated in Figure 29–5.

Hydrolysis in the digestive tract is catalyzed by the action of enzymes. There are two general classes of digestive enzymes: those that act within the lumen of the gut, and those that act at the membrane surface of the epithelium. Enzymes acting within the lumen originate from the major gastrointestinal (GI) glands, including the salivary gland, gastric glands, and especially the pancreas. The secretions of these glands become thoroughly mixed with ingesta and exert their actions throughout the lumen of their associated gut segments; thus, the actions they catalyze are referred to as the *luminal phase* of digestion. In general, luminal-phase digestion results in the incomplete hydrolysis of nutrients, resulting in the formation of short-chain polymers from the original macromolecules (Fig. 29–6).

The hydrolytic process is completed by enzymes that are chemically bound to the surface epithelium of the small intestine. These enzymes break the short-chain polymers resulting from luminal-phase digestion into monomers that can be absorbed across the epithelium. This final phase, which occurs at the epi-

thelial membrane surface, is referred to as the *membranous phase* of digestion. Membranous-phase digestion is followed closely by absorption.

Luminal-phase carbohydrate digestion results in the production of short-chain polysaccharides

Carbohydrates are nutrients containing carbon, hydrogen, and oxygen atoms arranged as long chains of repeating simple-sugar molecules. Dietary carbohydrates originate primarily from plants. There are three general types of plant carbohydrates: fibers, sugars, and starches. Fibers, the structural parts of plants, form an important energy source for herbivorous animals; however, plant fibers are not subject to hydrolytic digestion by mammalian enzymes and, therefore, cannot be digested directly by animals. Digestion of plant fibers is discussed along with fermentative digestion in Chapter 30.

Sugars are energy-transport molecules in plants. Sugars, or *saccharides*, may be *simple* (made up of a single molecular unit, monosaccharides) or *complex* (made up of two or more repeating saccharide subunits, polysaccharides). *Glucose, galactose,* and *fructose* are the most important simple sugars in animal diets. These monosaccharides are present, preformed in small quantities, in normal diets; however, most monosaccharides absorbed from the gut arise from the enzymatic hydrolysis of more complex carbohydrates. Complex sugars are referred to as disaccharides, trisaccharides, and oligosaccharides, depending on the number of repeating simple-sugar subunits. Oligosaccharides contain several monomer units, usually between 3 and 10. Important complex sugars in animal diets are *lactose*, or milk sugar, and *sucrose*, or table sugar. Lactose is a disaccharide composed of glucose and galactose, whereas sucrose is a disaccharide com-

A Hydrolysis of glycosidic bond

B Hydrolysis of peptide bond

C Hydrolysis of two ester bonds in a triglyceride molecule

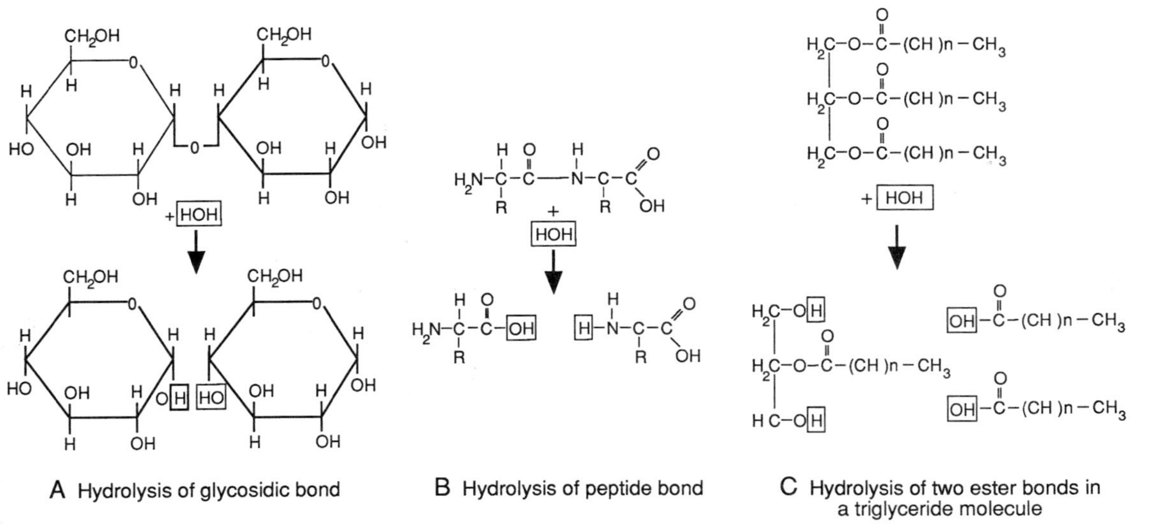

FIGURE 29–5. The major polymeric molecules forming food nutrients can be split into their constituent monomers by the insertion of a water molecule. This process, referred to as *hydrolysis*, is the major action of the digestive enzymes.

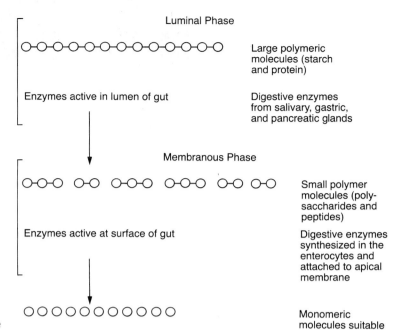

FIGURE 29–6. Luminal-phase and membranous-phase oligosaccharides.

posed of glucose and fructose. Other important complex sugars are *maltose, isomaltose,* and *maltotriose*; these three sugars are composed of two or three repeating glucose units (Fig. 29–7). They are seldom present preformed in the diet but rather are formed in the gut as intermediate products of starch digestion.

Starch is an energy-storage carbohydrate of plants that forms the major energy-yielding nutrient in the diets of many omnivorous animals, such as pigs, rats,

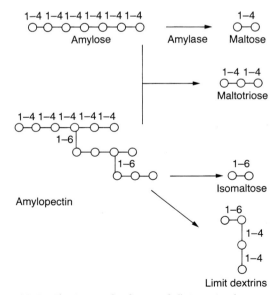

FIGURE 29–7. The two major forms of dietary starch are amylose and amylopectin. Amylose is composed of repeating glucose units joined by α[1–4] linkages. Amylopectin is a similar molecule, except that it has branch points formed by α[1–6] linkages. Because of the different linkage points, various polysaccharides result from luminal-phase digestion, as illustrated.

and primates. There are two chemical forms of starch, known as *amylose* and *amylopectin*. They are both long-chain glucose polymers, but amylose is a straight-chain molecule containing glucose monomers linked by α[1–4] glycosidic linkages. Amylopectin also contains glucose chains joined by α[1–4] glycosidic linkages, but the amylopectin chains are branched, having an α[1–6] linkage at each branch point (see Fig. 29–7). Although the chemical structure of starch is limited to these two molecular types, the physical structure and encapsulation of starches vary among plant sources. This variation results in the unique characteristics of starches from different sources, such as wheat, corn, and barley.

Luminal-phase digestion of carbohydrates applies only to starches, because sugars are all digested in the membranous phase

The enzyme involved in luminal starch digestion is α-amylase, which is actually a mixture of several similar molecules. This enzyme arises from the pancreas in all species and, in addition, from the salivary glands of some species (see Chapter 28). The α[1–4] linkages of either amylose or amylopectin are attacked by α-amylase. Characteristic of luminal-phase digestion, α-amylase does not break off, or cleave, single glucose units from the ends of the chain. Rather, the starch chains are broken in their midsections, resulting in the production of polysaccharides of intermediate chain length, known as *dextrins*. These chains continue to be attacked until disaccharide (maltose) and trisaccharide (maltotriose) units are formed.

This digestive process proceeds for amylopectin in

the same way as it does for amylose, except that the α[1–6] linkages at the chain branch points of amylopectin are not hydrolyzed. Because these branch points are not hydrolyzed, branch-chain oligosaccharides, known as *limit dextrins*, as well as an α[1–6]-linked disaccharide, known as *isomaltose*, are formed (see Fig. 29–7). The end result of luminal-phase carbohydrate digestion is the creation of many disaccharides, trisaccharides, and oligosaccharides from large starch molecules. These complex sugars are not hydrolyzed further in the luminal phase.

Proteins are digested by a variety of luminal-phase enzymes

Proteins are a source of amino acids, essential components of all animal diets. Dietary proteins come from both plant and animal sources. The general pattern of protein digestion is similar to that of carbohydrate digestion, in that large molecular proteins are broken down into small peptide chains by luminal digestion. Subsequent digestion of the peptide chains to individual amino acids occurs to a large extent by membranous-phase digestion, although, unlike in carbohydrate digestion, a portion of free monomers, that is, amino acids, is released in the luminal phase.

A major difference between protein digestion and carbohydrate digestion is in the number of different enzyme types involved. The relatively larger number of enzymes involved in protein digestion could be expected if one considers that starch molecules are made up of only one kind of monomer, glucose. Therefore, only bonds between glucose molecules have to be broken. On the other hand, proteins are made up of infinite combinations of up to 20 individual types of amino acids; the various proteolytic enzymes are necessary for digestion because they differ in their efficiency in cleaving peptide bonds between specific kinds of amino acids.

The major luminal-phase proteolytic enzymes are listed in Table 29–1. Most proteolytic enzymes are *endopeptidases*, meaning that they break proteins at internal points along the amino acid chains, resulting in the production of short-chain peptides from complex proteins. Endopeptidases produce essentially no free amino acids. Two *exopeptidases*, which release individual amino acids from ends of peptide chains, are secreted also from the pancreas and are active in luminal-phase digestion.

The proteolytic enzymes are secreted from the stomach glands or pancreas in the form of inactive *zymogens* (see Chapter 28 for a discussion of zymogens), which are activated in the stomach or intestinal lumen, respectively. These enzymes must be secreted in an inactive form, because otherwise the active enzymes would digest the cells in which they are synthesized. Activation of the zymogens occurs in the gut lumen. The stomach enzymes pepsinogen and chymosinogen are activated by hydrochloric acid (HCl) in the stomach. Pepsinogen is also activated by pepsin in an autocatalytic feedback loop. Trypsinogen from the pancreas is activated by *enterokinase*, an enzyme elaborated by the duodenal mucosal cells. The active enzyme, trypsin, then serves as an autocatalytic agent to activate additional trypsinogen as well as the other pancreatic protein-digesting enzymes. The cascade of intraluminal zymogen activation is illustrated in Figure 29–8.

Luminal-phase protein digestion begins in the stomach. Gastric digestion of protein is facilitated not only by the stomach enzymes but also by HCl, which has hydrolytic properties of its own. The acid environment of the stomach is suited to the action of pepsin, which has its optimal activity at pH 1 to 3. Gastric hydrolysis of protein is probably important to the physical as well as chemical digestion of protein, because most connective tissue of animal origin is protein; digestion of connective tissue aids in breaking food down into particles small enough to pass the pylorus. Although stomach action is important in initiating protein digestion, it is not essential; animals without stomachs can digest proteins, provided they have a functional pancreas and are fed small, frequent meals of soft, moist food. Luminal-phase digestion of proteins is completed in the small intestine by the action of pancreatic enzymes.

Membranous-phase digestive enzymes are a structural part of the intestinal surface membrane

Membranous-phase digestion, like its luminal counterpart, occurs because of the hydrolytic action of enzymes. The difference between the two phases is that membranous-phase enzymes are chemically bound to the surface membrane of the intestine; thus, the enzyme substrates must be in contact with the

TABLE 29–1. **Luminal-phase enzymes of protein digestion**

Enzyme	Action	Source	Precursor	Activator
Pepsin	Endopeptidase	Gastric glands	Pepsinogen	Hydrochloric acid, pepsin
Chymosin (rennin)	Endopeptidase	Gastric glands	Chymosinogen	?
Trypsin	Endopeptidase	Pancreas	Trypsinogen	Enterokinase, trypsin
Chymotrypsin	Endopeptidase	Pancreas	Chymotrypsinogen	Trypsin
Elastase	Endopeptidase	Pancreas	Proelastase	Trypsin
Carboxypeptidase A	Exopeptidase	Pancreas	Procarboxypeptidase A	Trypsin
Carboxypeptidase B	Exopeptidase	Pancreas	Procarboxypeptidase B	Trypsin

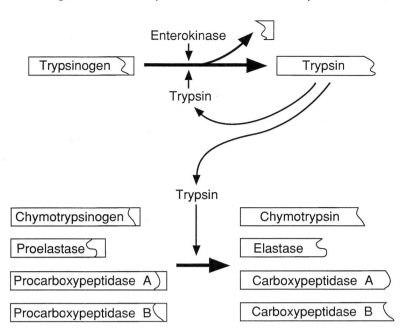

FIGURE 29–8. The activation of pancreatic zymogens. Note that trypsinogen is activated by trypsin as well as by the duodenal enzyme enterokinase. The autocatalytic action of trypsin on trypsinogen forms a positive feedback loop that ensures the rapid and complete activation of trypsinogen in the gut. Trypsin then activates the other zymogens.

epithelium before hydrolysis can occur. These membrane-bound digestive enzymes are synthesized within the enterocytes and are subsequently transported to the luminal surface of the apical membrane. They remain attached to the surface by a short anchor segment while the large, catalytic portion of the enzyme molecule projects away from the surface, toward the gut lumen.

Membranous-phase digestion occurs within the microenvironment of the unstirred water layer, intestinal mucus, and glycocalyx

As previously described, the unstirred water layer, mucus, and glycocalyx form a diffuse zone separating the mucosal surface from the lumen of the intestine. The membranous-phase digestive enzymes project from the apical membrane into this surface layer. The quiet surface layer forms a microenvironment in which membranous-phase digestion occurs. Peptides and polysaccharides in the intestinal lumen must diffuse into the surface layer before membranous-phase digestion can take place. Furthermore, most of the products of membranous-phase digestion never diffuse away from the surface environment back into the lumen of the intestine; instead, they are absorbed, soon after formation, into the underlying epithelial cells. This arrangement is efficient, because it ensures that the final products of carbohydrate and protein digestion are formed near their site of absorption, avoiding the need for long diffusion distances (Fig. 29–9).

A specific membranous-phase enzyme exists for the digestion of each type of polysaccharide

The membranous-phase enzymes of carbohydrate digestion have as their substrates dietary complex carbohydrate, such as sucrose and lactose, as well as the polysaccharide products of luminal-phase starch digestion, including maltose and isomaltose. The specific membranous-phase enzymes are named ac-

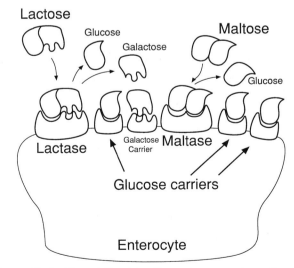

FIGURE 29–9. The relationship of membranous-phase digestion to absorption. The enzymes responsible for digestion and the carrier molecules responsible for absorption are both part of the apical membrane. The products of digestion are thus formed in the immediate vicinity of the carrier proteins, avoiding long diffusion distances. Specific enzymes and carrier molecules are present for the various substrates, as illustrated.

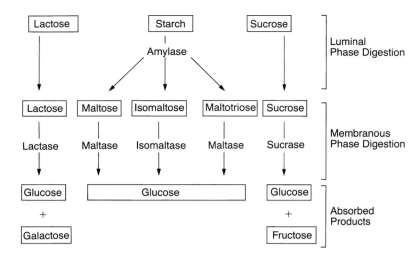

FIGURE 29-10. Luminal-phase and membranous-phase digestion of carbohydrate. Note that specific enzymes exist for each polysaccharide and that a limited number of monomers are formed eventually from a relatively large number of starches and polysaccharides.

cording to their substrates and include *maltase, isomaltase, sucrase,* and *lactase.* The sole product of maltose and isomaltose digestion is glucose, whereas in addition to glucose, fructose and galactose are produced from the digestion of sucrose and lactose, respectively. All polysaccharides are digested to monosaccharides before absorption (Fig. 29–10).

Complete digestion of peptides to free amino acids takes place both on the enterocyte surface and within the cells

Membranous-phase digestion of peptides is, in some respects, similar to that of carbohydrates; peptide-digesting enzymes, or *peptidases,* are present on the enterocyte surface membrane and extend into the glycocalyx. These enzymes hydrolyze the peptide products of luminal-phase protein digestion, yielding free amino acids. Some of the longer-chain peptides are incompletely digested, yielding dipeptides and tripeptides. A large portion of dietary amino acids is absorbed directly in the form of dipeptides and tripeptides. This mode of absorption contrasts with that of carbohydrates, in which only monomeric, simple sugars may pass the apical membrane. Dipeptides and tripeptides that are absorbed intact are subsequently hydrolyzed by the action of intracellular peptidases, which results in the formation of free amino acids that are then available for passage into the blood. Thus, the final digestion of peptides to free amino acids may occur at either of two sites: on the surface membrane of the enterocyte, or within the cell. In either case, the final product of protein digestion is free amino acid (Fig. 29–11).

INTESTINAL ABSORPTION

Absorption refers to the movement of the products of digestion across the intestinal mucosa and into the vascular system for distribution. To better understand the physiologically eloquent and clinically important

processes of intestinal absorption, the reader might need to review several of the earlier chapters of this book: the processes of diffusion across membranes (Chapter 1), the difference in composition of intracellular and extracellular fluid (Chapter 1), the electrical polarity across cell membranes (Chapters 1 and 3), the function of the Na^+,K^+ adenosine triphosphatase (ATPase) pump, and the function of selective ion channels (Chapters 1 and 3).

In considering intestinal absorption, one must keep in mind that molecules move across membrane barriers in response to chemical and electrical gradients.

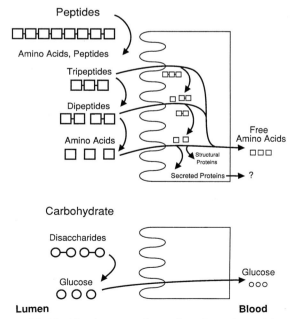

FIGURE 29-11. Membranous-phase digestion of peptides and carbohydrates. Note that tripeptides and dipeptides may be hydrolyzed to their constituent amino acids either on the apical membrane or within the enterocyte. In carbohydrate digestion, however, all disaccharide hydrolysis occurs at the apical membrane. Regardless of the site at which the final hydrolysis of peptides occurs, the product absorbed into the blood is free amino acid (see Fig. 29–16).

When molecules can freely penetrate a membrane, their movement across it is completely determined by the laws of diffusion and differences in chemical and electrical gradients: molecules flow to areas of lower concentration and charged particles move to areas of opposite charge. However, charged ions and most organic nutrient molecules do not freely penetrate the GI epithelium. Therefore, they do not move in accordance with the laws of diffusion unless there is some mechanism to facilitate their transport across membranes.

Specialized nutrient transport systems exist in the apical and basolateral membranes

Specialized *transport mechanisms* exist for the movement of molecules across membranes in the intestinal epithelium. These mechanisms are interactions of events involving specific proteins that lie embedded in the matrix of the cell membranes of the epithelial cells. These proteins provide the *transport pathway* for the passage of ions and organic molecules across the plasma membranes of cells. As we shall discuss, there are a large number of transport pathways. In general, the different pathways are polarized within the enterocytes, meaning that specific transport pathways exist on either the apical or the basolateral membrane, but not both. The transport pathway proteins chemically interact with specific organic nutrients and inorganic ions to effect their transport across the membrane. The transport mechanisms can be classified as active transport, secondary active transport, tertiary active transport, and passive transport.

Active transport involves the direct consumption of metabolic energy. During active transport, energy stored as ATP is expended to move ions or molecules across membranes against an electrical or chemical gradient. In the large and small intestine, the active transport pathway of greatest importance is the Na^+,K^+-ATPase pump. This protein pathway lies on the basolateral membrane and uses energy from the hydrolysis of one molecule of ATP to drive three ions of sodium out of the cell, in exchange for the entry of two potassium ions into the cell. This important transport pathway exists in a wide variety of cells, in addition to enterocytes. The Na^+,K^+-ATPase pump is the mechanism by which (1) the interior of cells is kept electrically negative with respect to the extracellular fluid and (2) the concentration of sodium is kept very low in the intracellular fluid. The Na^+,K^+-ATPase pump is covered in greater detail in Chapter 1.

Secondary and tertiary active transport utilize the transcellular sodium ion electrochemical gradient as their source of energy

Just as a large stone resting atop a hill represents potential energy, so does the electrochemical gradient of sodium ions across the enterocyte membrane. Gravity imparts potential energy to the stone, whereas diffusion forces impart potential energy to sodium ions outside cells. Transport mechanisms that harness the potential energy of the sodium gradient are referred to as *secondary active transport*. Various transport pathway proteins exist for secondary active transport.

One type is referred to as a *co-transport* protein or *symport*. The characteristic of a co-transport protein is that it has binding sites for one or more sodium ions as well as an additional binding site for some other specific molecule. For example, the glucose co-transport protein has one binding site for glucose and two for sodium ions. Co-transport proteins exist in the apical membrane of enterocytes. When the binding sites are unoccupied, they face the intestinal lumen. When all binding sites are occupied, a change in molecular configuration results such that the binding sites, with their ligand molecules, flip to the interior of the cell. When this happens, the sodium ions along with the co-transported molecule are released into the intracellular fluid. Thus, there is transport of sodium and another molecule, such as glucose, across the apical membrane. When the ligand molecules are released, the protein is reconfigured so that the binding sites are again on the extracellular surface of the apical membrane, ready to transport additional molecules (Fig. 29–12).

This process proceeds only as long as there is an electrochemical gradient for the sodium ion. When this gradient is large, as is normally the case, it can provide the energy to "pull" the co-transported molecule, such as glucose, from an area of lower concen-

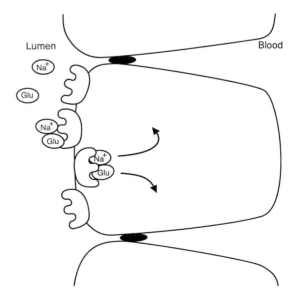

FIGURE 29–12. During co-transport, sodium moves down its electrochemical gradient. The favorable gradient for sodium movement is maintained by the continuous action of the Na^+,K^+-ATPase pump. During absorption, the glucose concentration difference appears to become unfavorable for transport, but absorption continues because of the sodium gradient (see Fig. 29–14).

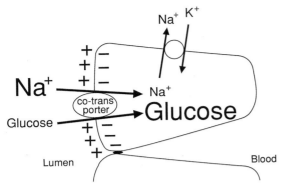

FIGURE 29–13. During co-transport, glucose is transported against an unfavorable concentration gradient. This diagram illustrates that the large sodium concentration difference across the apical membrane provides energy to transport glucose against its concentration gradient.

tration to one of higher concentration, as illustrated in Figures 29–13 and 29–14. Although the movement of a molecule against its concentration gradient represents expenditure of energy, there is no direct expenditure of metabolic energy by the sodium co-transport process. The energy expenditure is indirect and results from the direct expenditure of energy by the Na$^+$,K$^+$-ATPase pump in creating and maintaining the sodium electrochemical gradient. Many organic nutrients, including glucose, amino acids, several vitamins, and bile acids, are absorbed by this sodium co-transport process.

In addition to sodium co-transport, there are other

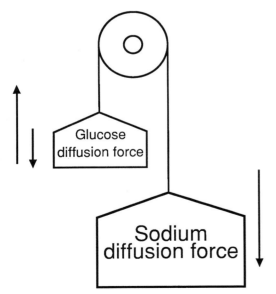

FIGURE 29–14. Sodium-glucose co-transport. Transport is mediated by a protein in the apical membrane. The protein has ligand sites for sodium ion and glucose; when both sites are occupied, the protein alters its configuration so that the sodium and glucose are released on the inner face of the apical membrane. The protein, then free of its ligands, reverses its orientation, ready to transport another sodium-glucose pair.

types of secondary active transport pathways. These pathway proteins are known as *exchangers* or *antiports*. Exchangers are usually involved with ion transport and are similar to co-transport proteins in that they have binding sites for selected ions. The difference between exchangers and co-transport proteins is that in exchangers, the binding sites for the two different ligands are on opposite sides of the plasma membrane. For example, an important exchanger is the Na$^+$/H$^+$ exchanger in the apical membrane. The protein has a binding site for Na$^+$ and another for H$^+$. When the sites are unoccupied, the Na$^+$ site faces the intestinal lumen and the H$^+$ site faces the interior of the enterocyte. When both sites are occupied, the protein flips, transporting H$^+$ out of and Na$^+$ into the cell, thus explaining the name *exchanger*, as H$^+$ is exchanged for Na$^+$. As with co-transport, the force driving the exchange is the Na$^+$ electrochemical gradient across the cell membrane.

There is one additional form of active transport, referred to as *tertiary active transport*. Tertiary transport occurs via transport pathway proteins and is driven by electrochemical gradients that are established by secondary active transport. The best example of tertiary active transport is the Cl$^-$/HCO$_3^-$ exchanger. This mechanism occurs in response to gradients established by the Na$^+$/H$^+$ exchanger, a secondary active transport mechanism. The Cl$^-$/HCO$_3^-$ exchanger is discussed in more detail later, in the section on absorption. In essence, the term *tertiary* is used because the Na$^+$,K$^+$-ATPase system (primary) establishes the gradient that drives the Na$^+$/H$^+$ exchanger (secondary), which then establishes the gradient that drives the Cl$^-$/HCO$_3^-$ exchanger (tertiary).

Passive transport occurs either through ion channels in cell membranes or directly through the tight junctions

Ion channels, which are protein constituents of cell plasma membranes, are the transport pathways of passive diffusion into cells. Ions move through the channels in a completely passive manner, responding only to electrochemical gradients. No metabolic energy is directly required to effect ion movement. The only regulatory influence the cell can exert over this form of transport is in opening or closing of the channels. For a more detailed description of ion channels, see Chapter 1.

A second form of passive molecular movement through the intestinal epithelium is via the tight junctions. As previously mentioned, the tight junctions are not so tight, especially in the duodenum and upper jejunum. In these areas, the tight junctions are freely permeable to water and small, inorganic ions. Thus, water and ions move across the tight junctions in response to osmotic pressure and electrochemical gradients. Movement of materials through the tight junctions is called *paracellular* (around the cells) *ab-*

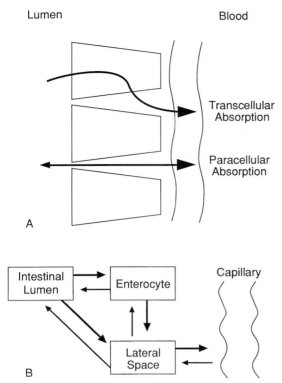

Lumen   Blood

Transcellular
Absorption

Paracellular
Absorption

A

Intestinal
Lumen   Enterocyte   Capillary

Lateral
Space

B

FIGURE 29–15. Transcellular and paracellular absorption. *A,* Substances move from the intestinal lumen to the capillary by either transcellular (through the enterocyte) or paracellular (through the tight junction) absorption. *B,* The intestinal lumen, enterocytes, and lateral spaces form three separate pools that may contain nutrients in different concentrations. Note that nutrients move into the capillaries from the lateral spaces and that reverse transport (from the capillary to the intestinal lumen) is possible for some substances.

sorption, in contrast to absorption through the apical membrane, which is called *transcellular* (through the cells) *absorption.* Transcellular absorption and paracellular absorption work in a complementary manner to produce an efficient absorptive process (Fig. 29–15).

The products of membranous-phase digestion are absorbed by sodium co-transport

Sodium co-transport proteins for glucose and galactose are located in the apical membrane, in proximity to the membranous-phase digestive enzymes. As these saccharide monomers are produced by the action of membranous-phase enzymes on polysaccharides, they move very short distances to binding sites on co-transport proteins. When both the glucose-binding (or galactose-binding) and sodium-binding sites on these proteins are occupied, absorption occurs as described previously.

In the initial phases of digestion of a starch-containing meal, the glucose concentration at the apical membrane is very high because there is ample substrate. Sodium is also readily available as a result of its presence in the various gastrointestinal secretions.

At this time, movement of both sodium and glucose into the enterocytes is down a concentration gradient. As digestion and absorption proceed, the glucose concentration at the apical membrane diminishes. Thus, toward the end of the digestive and absorptive process, the concentration of glucose at the luminal surface of the enterocyte apical membrane becomes small. At this point, the concentration of glucose within the enterocyte can be higher than in the intestinal lumen, thus creating an unfavorable concentration gradient for glucose absorption. However, the transcellular sodium concentration gradient is maintained, driving the continued absorption of glucose (see Fig. 29–14). The process of glucose absorption by this mechanism is very efficient, and little free glucose escapes the absorptive process.

To complete the process of carbohydrate absorption, the glucose must move through the basolateral membrane, into the lateral spaces, and on into the capillaries. Movement of glucose through the basolateral membrane occurs by *facilitated diffusion,* in which there is a transport pathway protein but the direction of transport is driven only by the concentration gradient. As sodium co-transport from the gut lumen raises the intracellular glucose concentration of the enterocytes, glucose diffuses from the cells into the lateral spaces. From the lateral spaces, it diffuses through the capillary basement membrane into the blood.

Absorption of the products of membranous-phase protein digestion occurs in a manner similar to that of carbohydrates. Sodium co-transport systems exist for free amino acids and might also exist for dipeptides and tripeptides. At least three co-transport proteins are necessary for absorption of free amino acids. The mechanism of transport for dipeptides and tripeptides might also involve sodium co-transport, but this issue is not established with certainty (Fig. 29–16).

ABSORPTION OF WATER AND ELECTROLYTES

Conservation of the body's supply of water and electrolytes, primarily sodium, potassium, chloride, and bicarbonate, is a high priority for sustaining life. The gut plays a major role in this conservation, not only because it is the portal of entry for replenishment of the nutrients but also because water and electrolytes in GI secretions must be efficiently reclaimed to maintain body composition. The most immediate clinical ramifications of GI disease usually involve the loss of water and electrolytes. Here, the absorption of the major ions and electrolytes is discussed sequentially.

There are at least three distinct mechanisms of sodium absorption

The first pathway of sodium absorption is via sodium co-transport proteins, as previously discussed. This secondary active transport pathway is not only the mechanism for glucose and amino acid absorption

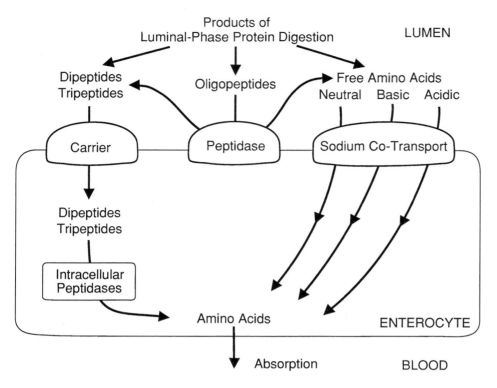

Products of
Luminal-Phase Protein Digestion

LUMEN

FIGURE 29–16. At least three different sodium co-transport proteins exist for the transport of amino acids: those for neutral, basic, and acidic amino acids. A sodium co-transport process might be involved in the absorption of dipeptides and tripeptides, but this possibility is not well established.

(Fig. 29–17a) but also a major means of sodium absorption.

The second sodium absorption mechanism is via the Na^+/H^+ exchanger (Fig. 29–17b), which was mentioned previously as an example of an ion exchanger, or antiport. Via this mechanism, intracellular H^+ is exchanged for luminal Na^+ across the apical membrane. The H^+ for this exchange is formed by the action of carbonic anhydrase, which generates HCO_3^- as well as H^+. As H^+ is exchanged for Na^+, HCO_3^- concentrations build up in the cell. The resulting transcellular HCO_3^- gradient drives the action of the Cl^-/HCO_3^- exchanger, which results in the exchange of intracellular HCO_3^- for luminal Cl^-. Because of the close connection between Na^+ and Cl^- absorption by these pathways, this transport mechanism is often called *coupled sodium chloride transport*, as illustrated in Figure 29–17b. One must appreciate, however, that it is only the intracellular balance of H^+ and HCO_3^- that couples the two exchange pathways. There are instances in which the intracellular pH is such that Na^+/H^+ exchange occurs without Cl^-/HCO_3^- exchange, and vice versa.

Coupled sodium chloride absorption is usually most active in the ileum and colon, where the sodium concentration in the gut is usually relatively low compared with that in the duodenum and jejunum. As usual, sodium entering the enterocytes is transported across the basolateral membrane to the lateral spaces via the action of the Na^+,K^+-ATPase pump. Chloride, however, remains in the enterocyte until its concentration is high enough to promote the diffusion of chloride through special channels in the basolateral membranes. The rate of absorption of sodium and chloride by the coupled mechanism appears to depend on the permeability of the chloride channels; when the

permeability is high, chloride passes rapidly out of the enterocyte, allowing continued chloride absorption. Conversely, when chloride channels are relatively closed, the intracellular chloride concentration

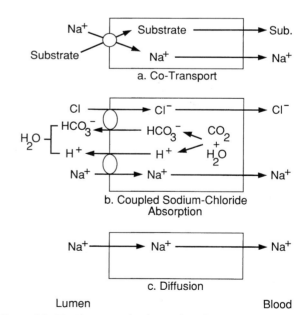

FIGURE 29–17. Three mechanisms of sodium absorption. *a,* Sodium co-transport with organic molecules is a major means of sodium uptake during active digestion and absorption. *b,* Chloride-coupled sodium absorption is also an important means of sodium absorption and requires the action of carbonic anhydrase and the existence on the apical membrane of bicarbonate-chloride and sodium-hydrogen exchange mechanisms. *c,* Simple diffusion of sodium across the apical membrane may occur because of the large favorable concentration gradient, but it is a relatively minor means of sodium absorption.

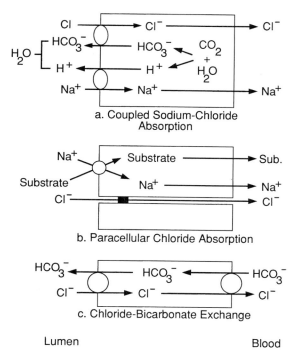

a. Coupled Sodium-Chloride
Absorption

b. Paracellular Chloride Absorption

c. Chloride-Bicarbonate Exchange

Lumen   Blood

Figure 29–18. Three mechanisms of chloride absorption. *a,* Chloride-coupled sodium absorption is directly related to sodium uptake. *b,* Paracellular chloride absorption is indirectly related to sodium absorption that occurs during co-transport. *c,* Chloride-bicarbonate exchange occurs especially in areas where bicarbonate secretion into the intestinal lumen is important.

rises, diminishing chloride absorption by the creation of an unfavorable concentration gradient.

The third mechanism of sodium absorption is via simple diffusion through ion channels in the apical membrane (Fig. 29–17c). The large electrochemical gradient that can exist for sodium across the enterocyte apical membrane allows direct, uncoupled movement of sodium across the membrane when the ion channels are open. Although some sodium absorption probably occurs by this mechanism, its overall importance in body sodium homeostasis is probably not large.

There are three major mechanisms of chloride absorption

One mechanism of chloride absorption is coupled sodium chloride absorption, as discussed previously in relation to sodium (Fig. 29–18a). Another mechanism is paracellular chloride absorption, which occurs in association with sodium co-transport of glucose and amino acids (Fig. 29–18b). Paracellular chloride transport occurs because of an electrical gradient. Sodium co-transport leads to the net movement of positive electrical charges (sodium ions) across the apical membrane, because neither glucose nor most amino acids are charged molecules. As the sodium cations are transferred to the lateral spaces, the spaces develop a positive polarity with respect to the gut lumen. Chloride from the gut lumen passes directly

into the lateral spaces through the tight junctions, because the tight junctions are readily permeable to small anions. This provides a major mechanism for the absorption of chloride ion while maintaining electrical neutrality, although a small electrical potential is maintained across the gut surface, the lumen being negative with respect to the lateral spaces.

The last mechanism of chloride absorption is by direct exchange for bicarbonate (Fig. 29–18c) without coupled sodium absorption. With this mechanism, there is a net movement of bicarbonate into the gut lumen, resulting in an increase in luminal pH.

Bicarbonate ion is secreted by several digestive glands and must be recovered from the gut if body acid-base balance is to be maintained

Much bicarbonate is in essence "absorbed" by the neutralization of HCl from the stomach. Sodium bicarbonate entering the intestine reacts with HCl to form water, carbon dioxide, and sodium chloride, effectively resulting in the absorption of bicarbonate and hydrogen ions. (See Chapter 28 for an explanation of the counterbalancing effects of gastric acid secretion and pancreatic bicarbonate secretion.) However, considerable bicarbonate remains in the intestine after the neutralization of stomach acid. This remaining bicarbonate is reabsorbed, primarily in the ileum and colon via an ion-exchange mechanism.

Bicarbonate anions in the gut are electrically balanced, primarily with sodium cations, and reabsorbed essentially as sodium bicarbonate. In the absorptive process, hydrogen and bicarbonate ions are first generated within the enterocytes from water and carbon dioxide. Hydrogen ion is then exchanged for sodium ion across the apical membrane. Within the cell, sodium ion is electrically balanced by the remaining bicarbonate ion, whereas the bicarbonate ion remaining in the gut lumen is neutralized by the secreted hydrogen ion (Fig. 29–19). The result is that sodium is transferred through the membrane. However, luminal bicarbonate is converted to water and carbon dioxide in the gut lumen, whereas bicarbonate anion is regenerated intracellularly. The net effect is the absorption of sodium bicarbonate. This mecha-

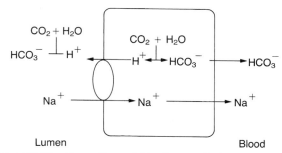

Figure 29–19. Absorption of bicarbonate is facilitated by sodium-hydrogen exchange at the apical membrane. The bicarbonate ion is regenerated by the action of carbonic anhydrase.

nism is essentially one half of chloride-coupled sodium absorption, except that the bicarbonate ion remains within the enterocyte rather than being exchanged for chloride.

Potassium is absorbed primarily by passive diffusion through the paracellular route

Potassium, although a highly important ion in the body, is present in abundance in most animal diets, unlike sodium, which is present in nutritionally inadequate amounts in most natural animal feeds. Therefore, frequently the concentration of potassium in the material entering the intestinal lumen is relatively high compared with that of sodium. In addition, dietary potassium is concentrated in the gut lumen because of the absorption of other nutrients, electrolytes, and water, unaccompanied by active potassium absorption. Thus, the potassium concentration within the gut lumen increases as digestion and absorption of other osmotically active molecules proceed.

As potassium reaches relatively high concentrations in the intestinal lumen, a concentration gradient favorable for the diffusion of potassium across the intestinal epithelium is created. Furthermore, the concentration gradient is enhanced by the normally low concentration of potassium in the lateral spaces. The primary mechanism of potassium absorption is paracellular passive diffusion, which occurs in response to this concentration gradient (Fig. 29–20). A clinical ramification of this absorptive mechanism is that potassium absorption is directly coupled to water absorption. In diarrhea conditions, in which net absorption of water is impaired, potassium absorption is impaired also, because potassium in the gut lumen is diluted so that a concentration gradient favorable for passive diffusion of potassium never develops. In addition to passive diffusion, it appears that an H^+,K^+-ATPase exists in the distal colon. This transport pathway may be important for recovering the last remaining potassium from the colonic ingesta of animals with diets low in potassium.

The major mechanisms of electrolyte absorption are selectively distributed along the gut

The activity of the assorted electrolyte absorption mechanisms discussed earlier varies along the length

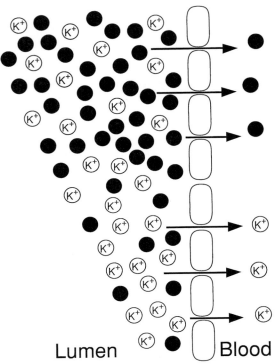

Lumen **Blood**

FIGURE 29–20. Potassium is absorbed by simple diffusion through the paracellular route. Water absorption in the upper intestine results in an increase in the potassium concentration in the lower intestine, creating a favorable diffusion gradient for potassium. Note that the removal of water (*solid black circles*) in the upper part results in a relative increase in the number of potassium ions in the lower part.

of the gut. The distribution of activity is listed in Table 29–2.

All intestinal water absorption is passive, occurring because of the absorption of osmotically active solutes

Water moves through the intestinal mucosa by either the paracellular or the transcellular route, but always by osmosis. The general discussion of osmosis is in Chapter 1 and should be reviewed by those who do not have a clear understanding of the process. The intestinal mucosa is freely permeable to water, allowing it to move in whatever direction is dictated by changes in osmotic pressure. As electrolytes and other soluble nutrients are actively absorbed, water

TABLE 29–2. Distributions of electrolyte absorptive mechanisms throughout the gut

Mechanism			Duodenum	Jejunum	Ileum	Colon
Sodium co-transport	+ + + + +	+ + + +			+	−
Chloride coupled sodium absorption	+		+		+ +	+ + +
Chloride-bicarbonate exchange	−		−		+ +	+ + +
Bicarbonate absorption		−		−	−/+	+ + +
Potassium absorption	−		−		+	+ + +

is drawn along passively from lumen to intestinal capillaries. Water may move also into the intestinal lumen at times when the intraluminal osmotic pressure is high, as discussed later.

INTESTINAL SECRETION OF WATER AND ELECTROLYTES

In addition to the water and electrolytes that are secreted into the intestine by the pancreas, liver, and other glandular organs, a considerable portion of GI water and electrolyte secretion occurs directly from the intestinal surface. All water secretion is osmotic, but the osmotic gradient driving water secretion may occur in response to either passive or active processes.

Passive increases in luminal osmotic pressure occur during hydrolytic digestion and result in water secretion

Food entering the intestine may be hyperosmotic because of its composition, such as salty foods and foods with high sugar content. Alternatively, food may become hyperosmotic after digestion. Digestion of foods creates many osmotically active molecules from one giant precursor molecule; thus, the osmotic activity of ingesta is increased initially by digestion. When starchy meals, for example, first enter the duodenum, intraluminal digestion creates thousands of osmotically active disaccharide and trisaccharide molecules from single starch molecules. These osmotically active saccharide molecules draw water from the lateral spaces into the intestinal lumen. Water in the lateral spaces is quickly replaced by water from the intestinal capillaries, so that water is essentially drawn into the intestine from the vascular system. As digestion proceeds, the saccharide molecules are absorbed, thus reducing the number of particles and lowering the osmotic pressure of the intestinal lumen. As solute molecules are absorbed, water follows them osmotically back through the epithelium and, hence, into the blood vascular system. *The cardinal rule of water movement in the intestine is that water moves in whatever direction necessary to keep ingesta iso-osmotic,* entering the gut when ingesta is hyperosmotic and leaving the gut when ingesta is hypo-osmotic. This fact has important clinical implications in the pathophysiology of diarrhea, as discussed later.

Active secretion of electrolytes from the crypt epithelium leads to intestinal water secretion

In contrast to the absorptive function of the villous cells, the crypt cells have a secretory function. This secretory function appears to use a chloride transport mechanism. The mechanism seems to be similar to coupled sodium chloride transport, as occurs in the villous enterocytes, except that the direction of transport is reversed. In the crypt cells, the coupled sodium chloride transport mechanism is on the basolateral membrane, in contrast to its position on the apical membrane of the villous cells. The effect of this arrangement is to pump sodium and chloride into the crypt enterocytes from the lateral spaces. As these ions are transported into the enterocytes, sodium is quickly pumped out by the Na^+,K^+-ATPase pump. In contrast, chloride is trapped within the cells, reaching relatively high intracellular concentrations. Under appropriate stimuli, chloride channels in the apical membranes of the crypt cells are opened, and the pent-up chloride from within the cells flows down its concentration gradient into the lumen of the crypt. (Ion channels and their regulation in cellular membranes are discussed in Chapter 1). Movement of the chloride anion into the lumen of the crypts creates an electrical attraction for sodium cations, which move into the luminal fluid from the lateral spaces through the paracellular route. Water follows sodium and chloride osmotically; thus, chloride, sodium, and water are secreted from the crypt epithelium (Fig. 29–21).

The triggering mechanism that activates water secretion from the crypts is the opening of the chloride gates in the crypt enterocyte apical membrane. Much study has been devoted to determining the factors controlling the opening of the chloride gates in crypt cells. One important factor in regulating chloride gates appears to be the activity of the adenylate cyclase enzyme and the intracellular concentration of cyclic adenosine 3′,5′-monophosphate (cyclic AMP, or cAMP). (The role of adenyl cyclase and cAMP in cellular regulation is discussed in Chapter 1). As cAMP concentrations rise, chloride gates open, and

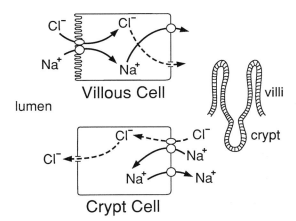

FIGURE 29–21. Water and electrolyte secretion in the crypts is affected by the secretion of chloride from the apical membrane of crypt enterocytes. Sodium moves into the lumen by the paracellular route and electrically balances chloride secretion. Water follows osmotically, the net effect being secretion of a sodium chloride solution into the crypt lumen. In the crypts, the coupled sodium chloride absorption mechanism appears to exist on the basolateral membrane, with chloride gates present on the apical membrane. The opening of the chloride gates on the crypt cell apical membranes initiates crypt secretion. The membrane position of the coupled sodium chloride transport process reverses itself, moving from the basolateral membrane to the apical membrane as the cells mature and move up the villi.

secretion of water and electrolytes is stimulated. The physiologic, or normal, activators of adenyl cyclase on crypt cells are not known for sure. Vasoactive intestinal peptide originating from effector neurons of the mucosal plexus is probably one very important normal regulator of cAMP and chloride gates in crypt apical membranes. Of perhaps greater medical significance than the normal regulation of this process is the existence of pathologic, or abnormal, activators of crypt cell adenyl cyclase; these are discussed later, in the section on the pathophysiology of diarrhea.

The physiologic function of water and electrolyte secretion by the crypts is not completely understood. It can be speculated that such secretion may have a function in maintaining the concentration of sodium and water near the villous surface during sodium co-transport–stimulated absorption. It may be that at certain times during digestion, the amount of sodium near the absorptive surface of the villi becomes insufficient to promote the maximal absorption of glucose and amino acids by sodium co-transport. If this is the case, crypt secretion could provide a mechanism to supply additional sodium for villous absorption. According to this hypothesis, water, sodium, and chloride would circulate from the crypt to the villi and back during the process of glucose and amino acid absorption by sodium co-transport.

GASTROINTESTINAL BLOOD FLOW

Water and solute movement between the lateral spaces and villous capillaries is subject to the same forces that govern water and solute movement between the extracellular and vascular fluids in other tissues

Water and all other nutrients, whether they are absorbed through the transcellular or paracellular routes, enter the extracellular fluid of the lateral spaces before entering the vascular system. Therefore, the movement of extracellular fluid components into capillaries is of particular importance to intestinal absorption. The physical laws determining the distribution of water between the intravascular and extravascular fluid are the same in the villi as in other tissues. These Starling laws (which can be reviewed in Chapters 1 and 22) simply state that the movement of water is determined by the algebraic sum of osmotic and hydrostatic (created by water pressure) forces.

Absorbed nutrients enter the capillaries by diffusion from the lateral spaces

The collective action of the various intestinal absorptive mechanisms concentrates solutes (nutrients) in the lateral spaces. When the concentrations of individual solutes in the lateral spaces exceed their concen-

trations in blood, a gradient favoring the diffusion of nutrients from lateral spaces into the capillaries is established. The movement of solutes by diffusion into the capillaries creates an osmotic force that draws water into the capillaries (water follows solute). In addition, the oncotic force (the osmotic force exerted by plasma proteins; see Chapters 1 and 22) also tends to draw water into the capillary lumen. Moreover, hydrostatic pressure in the lateral spaces may force water directly into the capillaries. Lateral-space hydrostatic pressure can be created by the osmotic effect of absorbed solutes. As these solutes attract water from the intestinal lumen, the lateral spaces become distended, developing a small amount of hydrostatic pressure. There are two exits for the relief of this pressure: the tight junctions and the capillary endothelium, with the endothelium presenting the route of least resistance to water flow. Thus, water under slight pressure within the lateral spaces tends to flow into the capillaries rather than into the intestinal lumen (Fig. 29–22).

A countercurrent, osmotic-multiplier system may increase the osmolality of blood at the tips of the villi, further promoting absorption of water into the blood

The villous vascular system consists of an arteriole rising up the central portion of the villi and dividing

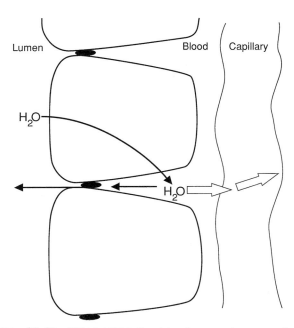

FIGURE 29–22. Water enters the lateral spaces because of osmotic effects created by absorbed solutes, thus creating a hydrostatic pressure head in the lateral spaces. Under pressure, the lateral-space solution can exit through the tight junctions or through the basement membrane of the capillaries. Under normal conditions, the route of least resistance is into the capillaries, resulting in little movement of water from the lateral space into the intestinal lumen.

at the tip into many capillaries, which course down the outer portion of the villous stroma between the mucosa and artery. This arrangement provides for direct countercurrent flow of blood; that is, blood coming down the venules passes close to blood flowing in the opposite direction up the arteriole. Because blood in the venules contains absorbed nutrients, its osmolarity could be expected to be slightly higher than that of blood entering the villi in the arteriole. This slight difference in osmolarity can be multiplied and perpetuated by the countercurrent flow characteristics of the arterial and venous blood supplies. These conditions create a potential for the creation of an osmotic gradient along the villi; some researchers calculate osmolalities near the tips of the villi to be as high as 600 mosm, approximately twice that of blood entering the base of the villi. (The characteristics of a countercurrent osmotic multiplier are further explained in Chapter 42 in reference to the renal loop of Henle.) The existence of the villous countercurrent osmotic multiplier is still somewhat controversial, and its presence may depend on the species in question. The effect of this osmotic-multiplier system would be to accentuate all the osmotic forces that result in the movement of water from lumen to lateral spaces and from lateral spaces to capillaries.

Disturbances in the venous drainage from the intestine can markedly affect the mechanisms of capillary absorption in the villi

With the exception of blood from the terminal colon and rectum, all venous blood from the GI tract is collected into the hepatic portal vein and passes through the liver before entering the vena cava and returning to the heart (Fig. 29–23). Because of this system, the nutrient-rich blood leaving the intestine may be modified by the liver. The liver can thus regulate the nutrient concentration of blood reaching general body tissues, keeping it relatively constant. This particular vascular arrangement of the GI system results in the passage of blood through two capillary beds, one in the gut wall and one in the liver, before its return to the heart. In most tissues, arterial hydrostatic pressure forces blood through the capillary beds. In the liver, however, this is not the case, because most of the arterial hydrostatic pressure has been dissipated during flow of blood through the intestinal capillaries. Two circumstances tend to overcome this problem and allow hepatic blood flow to occur:

1. The capillaries (referred to as *sinusoids*) of the liver are comparatively large and thus offer little resistance to flow; therefore, they can function in a low-pressure system.
2. The venous outflow of the liver goes directly into the thoracic vena cava.

The bellows-like action of the thorax transmits a negative pressure to the thoracic vena cava, which tends to aspirate blood from the hepatic veins and abdominal vena cava. Under normal circumstances, these conditions allow blood to flow readily from the intestine through the liver. However, small changes in circulatory function can have a large impact on GI blood flow. If the pumping capacity of the heart becomes reduced, it cannot remove returning venous blood quickly. Accumulation of blood and an increase in pressure in the thoracic vena cava result. This increase in pressure interferes with the flow of blood out of the liver, which in turn reduces blood flow out of the intestine. This sequence of events makes the GI system particularly susceptible to right-sided heart failure, in which the heart's pumping action is compromised.

Diffuse liver disease, in addition to right-sided heart failure, can also interfere with GI blood flow. In this condition, the resistance to blood flow through the liver is increased because of pressure on the sinusoids. Small rises in hepatic flow resistance can have large effects on intestinal blood flow, because the pressure gradient across the hepatic portal vein is normally small. When the flow of blood out of the intestine is impaired, hydrostatic pressure in the capillaries of the villi is increased; the higher pressure tends to offset the osmotic and hydrostatic forces promoting water absorption, and thus, water absorption is impaired.

DIGESTION AND ABSORPTION OF FATS

Detergent action as well as enzymatic action is necessary for the digestion and absorption of lipids

Lipids, or fats, present a special digestive problem to the animal because they do not dissolve in water, the major medium in which most body processes,

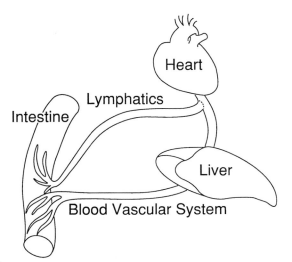

FIGURE 29–23. All blood exiting the gut flows through the liver before returning to the heart. Lymphatic drainage from the gut bypasses the liver, entering the blood stream through the thoracic duct.

including digestion, occur. Detergent action is necessary to emulsify or dissolve lipids, so that they may be subjected to the actions of water-soluble hydrolytic enzymes in the gut. The problem of solubility makes the mechanics of digestion and absorption of lipids somewhat different from that of proteins and carbohydrates. For that reason, lipid assimilation is discussed here in a separate section.

Lipids make up a large portion of the diets of carnivores, whereas they usually form a minor portion of the natural diets of adult herbivores. Nonetheless, it appears that herbivorous species have the capacity to digest and absorb lipids in quantities considerably higher than found in their natural diets, and frequently, supplemental lipids are added to the diets of performance horses and high-producing dairy cows. The neonates of all mammalian species have a high capacity for lipid digestion and absorption, because milk has a high fat content.

The primary dietary lipid is *triglyceride*, which may originate from either plant or animal sources. Other important dietary lipids are *cholesterol* and *cholesterol ester* from animal sources, waxes from plant sources, and *phospholipids* from both plant and animal sources. The structures of these dietary lipids are illustrated in Figure 29–24. In addition, the lipid-soluble vitamins A, D, E, and K are absorbed along with the other dietary lipids.

Lipid assimilation can be divided into four phases: (1) emulsification, (2) hydrolysis, (3) micelle formation, and (4) absorption. *Emulsification* is the process of reducing lipid droplets to a size that forms stable suspensions in water or water-based solutions. In the gut, the emulsification phase begins in the stomach as the lipids are warmed to body temperature and subjected to the intense mixing, agitating, and sieving actions of the distal stomach. This distal-stomach activity tends to break lipid globules up into droplets that pass into the small intestine. In the small intestine, emulsification is completed by the detergent action of bile acids and phospholipids. (See Chapter 28 for a discussion of bile formation and secretion.) These bile products reduce the surface tension of the lipids and allow the droplets to become even further divided and reduced in size (Fig. 29–25).

While in the bile-coated, or emulsified droplet, stage, the lipids are subject to the actions of hydrolytic enzymes. *Hydrolysis* of triglyceride, the major dietary lipid component, occurs because of the combined action of the pancreatic enzymes *lipase* and *co-lipase*. Lipase is an enzyme secreted, in its active form, from the pancreas. However, lipase cannot directly attack the emulsified lipid droplets in the gut because it cannot penetrate the coat of bile products surrounding the droplets. The function of co-lipase, a relatively short peptide, is to "clear a path" through the bile products, giving lipase access to the underlying triglycerides. Lipase cleaves the fatty acids off each end of the triglyceride molecule but does not attack the central fatty acid, resulting in the formation of two *free*, or *nonesterified, fatty acids* and a *monoglycer-*

ide from each molecule of triglyceride hydrolyzed (Fig. 29–26).

Other lipid-digesting pancreatic enzymes are *cholesterol esterase* and *phospholipase*. The products of these enzymes are nonesterified fatty acids, cholesterol, and lysophospholipids.

The products of hydrolytic lipid digestion (fatty acids, monoglycerides, and so forth) combine with bile acids and phospholipids to form *micelles*, small water-soluble aggregations of bile acids and lipids. Micelles are considerably smaller than the emulsified fat droplets from which they are derived (see Fig. 29–25). The soluble micelles allow the lipids to diffuse through the gut lumen into the unstirred water layer and into close contact with the absorptive surface of the apical membrane (Figs. 29–26 and 29–27).

Lipids are absorbed through the apical membrane by carrier proteins and simple diffusion

The process of lipid absorption into the enterocytes is incompletely understood. As the micelles come close to the surface of the enterocytes, the various lipid components diffuse the short distance through the glycocalyx to the apical membrane by means of special *fatty acid–binding proteins* (not shown in Fig. 29–27). Fatty acids in the micelles appear to be taken up and transported across the apical membrane by special fatty acid–binding proteins in the apical membrane. Other micellar components appear to simply diffuse into the apical membrane; they include such lipids as monoglycerides, cholesterol, and vitamin A. The apical membrane, like other cellular membranes, is composed primarily of phospholipids (see Chapter 1 for a description of cellular membranes). The highly hydrophobic products of lipid digestion are soluble in the phospholipid matrix of the membrane and thus may diffuse freely through the apical membrane and into the cell. Lipid absorption from micelles is illustrated in Figure 29–27.

Bile acids are reabsorbed from the ileum by a sodium co-transport system

All components of the micelle diffuse into the enterocytes except the bile acids. Bile acids remain in the lumen of the gut, being separated from the other micellar elements as absorption proceeds. By the time bile acids reach the ileum, they are in a relatively free state, devoid of other lipids. Localized in the ileum is a specific bile-acid transport system. This system operates by sodium co-transport and results in the nearly complete reabsorption of bile acids. After absorption, bile acids are transported directly back to the liver by the portal vasculature. The liver efficiently extracts bile acids from the portal blood, so normally, the concentration of bile acids in the nonportal blood (systemic circulation) is small. The bile acids extracted by the liver are recycled into the bile. This recycling

LIPIDS WITH POLAR GROUPS

chemical structure   schematic illustration

$$H_2C - O - \overset{\overset{\displaystyle O}{\|}}{C} - (CH_2)_n - CH_3$$
$$H_2C - O - \overset{\overset{\displaystyle O}{\|}}{C} - (CH_2)n - CH_3$$
$$H_2C - O - \overset{}{\underset{\overset{\displaystyle |}{OH}}{P}} - O - X$$

Phospholipid

$$H_2C - O - \overset{\overset{\displaystyle O}{\|}}{C} - (CH_2)_n - CH_3$$
$$HC - OH$$
$$H_2C - O - \overset{}{\underset{\overset{\displaystyle |}{OH}}{P}} - O - X$$

Lysophospholipid

$$HCOH$$
$$H_2C - O - \overset{\overset{\displaystyle O}{\|}}{C} - (CH_2)_n - CH_3$$
$$HCOH$$
$$H$$

Monoglyceride

$$CH_3$$
$$HC - CH_2 - CH_2 - CH_2 - \overset{\overset{\displaystyle H}{|}}{C} - CH_3$$
$$CH_3 \qquad\qquad CH_3$$

Cholesterol

$$HO$$

$$HO \quad CH_3 \quad CH_2 \quad \overset{\overset{\displaystyle O}{\|}}{C}$$
$$CH_3 \quad\quad CH_2 \quad OH$$
$$CH_3$$
$$HO \quad H \quad OH$$

Bile Acid
(cholic acid)

$$\overset{\overset{\displaystyle O}{\|}}{\underset{HO}{C}} - (CH_2)_n - CH_3$$

Nonesterified Fatty Acid

LIPIDS WITHOUT POLAR GROUPS

chemical structure   schematic illustration

$$H_2C - O - \overset{\overset{\displaystyle O}{\|}}{C} - (CH_2)n - CH_3$$
$$HCC - O - \overset{\overset{\displaystyle O}{\|}}{C} - (CH_2)n - CH_3$$
$$H_2C - O - \overset{\overset{\displaystyle O}{\|}}{C} - (CH_2)n - CH_3$$

Triglyceride

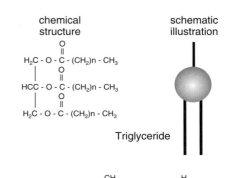

$$CH_3 \qquad\qquad H$$
$$HC - CH_2 - CH_2 - CH_2 - \overset{\overset{\displaystyle |}{}}{C} - CH_3$$
$$CH_3 \qquad\qquad CH_3$$
$$CH_3$$
$$\overset{\overset{\displaystyle O}{\|}}{O - C}$$
$$(CH_2)n$$
$$CH_3$$

Cholesterol Ester

FIGURE 29–24. Chemical structures and their schematic representations for lipid molecules involved in fat digestion and absorption. n, number of carbon atoms in fatty acid chains; X, phospholipid head group, most commonly choline.

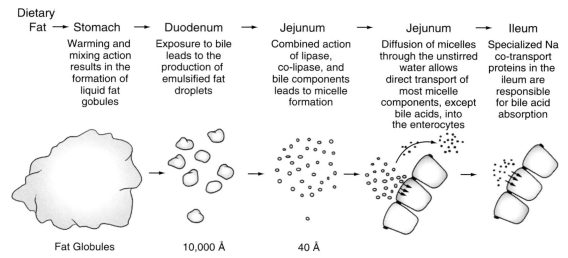

FIGURE 29–25. The sites and reactions involved in fat digestion and absorption.

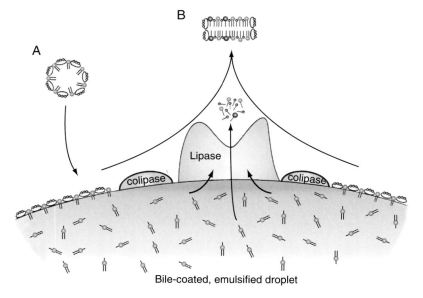

FIGURE 29–26. A portion of the surface of a bile-coated, emulsified fat droplet. Bile components reach the surface of the droplet through micelles *(A)* coming from the gallbladder. Co-lipase clears bile constituents from an area of the surface of the droplet, allowing the attachment of lipase. Lipase catalyzes the formation of fatty acids and monoglycerides from triglycerides. The surface components and products of lipase action combine to form micelles *(B)* containing fatty acids and monoglycerides as well as bile constituents.

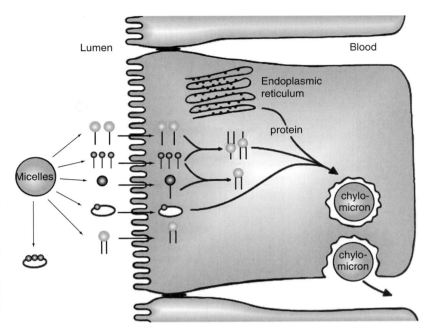

FIGURE 29–27. Lipid absorption from micelles with subsequent formation of chylomicrons. As micelles come into close proximity with the apical membrane, lipid constituents, except bile acids, are transported through the membrane into the cell. Once in the enterocyte, triglycerides are re-formed from fatty acids and monoglycerides. Triglycerides are then packaged into the core of chylomicrons for transport out of the cell. The chylomicron surface is coated with phospholipids, cholesterol, and proteins.

process occurs repeatedly, so the entire mass of bile acids within the body is circulated through the intestine several times per day.

Absorbed lipids are packaged into chylomicrons before leaving the enterocytes

After passing the apical membrane, the absorbed lipids are quickly picked up by carrier molecules and transported intracellularly to the endoplasmic reticulum. Once on the smooth endoplasmic reticulum, the major lipids are re-esterified to form triglyceride and phospholipids. The re-esterified lipids are then packaged with cholesterol, minor dietary lipids, and proteins from the rough endoplasmic reticulum into structures known as *chylomicrons*. Chylomicrons are spherical structures with a core of triglyceride and cholesterol ester and a surface of phospholipid and cholesterol. The phospholipid and cholesterol are arranged with their *hydrophobic* (water-repelling) ends facing the core lipids and their *hydrophilic* (water-attracting) ends facing the surface of the chylomicron particle (Fig. 29–28). This arrangement of surface lipid makes the chylomicron water-soluble. A small number of special protein molecules are also present on the chylomicron surface. These proteins help to stabilize the surface and to direct the metabolism of the particle.

After their formation, chylomicrons are expelled from the basolateral membrane into the lateral spaces. Unlike most other nutrients entering the lateral spaces, chylomicrons are too large to pass through the basement membrane of the intestinal capillaries. Thus, chylomicrons cannot be absorbed through the intestinal blood system. Rather, they travel through the intestinal lymphatics, which eventually form a

major abdominal lymph duct that passes through the diaphragm and into the *thoracic duct*. The major lymph-collecting vessel of the body, the thoracic duct empties into the vena cava. Through this means, chylomicrons eventually reach the blood vascular system. During absorption of a fatty meal, the character of intestinal lymph changes from water-clear to milky white because of the presence of chylomicrons. After a fatty meal, this milky white color can even be seen

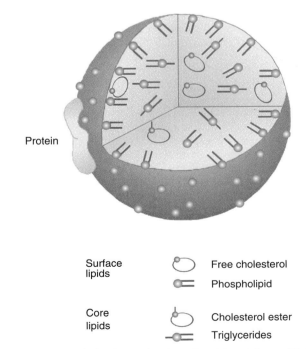

Surface lipids		Free cholesterol
Core lipids		Phospholipid
		Cholesterol ester
		Triglycerides

FIGURE 29–28. Chylomicron structure. Special proteins and lipids with polar groups form the surface coat, whereas nonpolar lipids form the core of the particle.

in blood plasma. In normal animals this white color in blood plasma, known as *lipemia,* is transient, disappearing within 1 to 2 hours after digestion of the meal. The metabolic fate of the chylomicrons is discussed in Chapter 31.

GROWTH AND DEVELOPMENT OF THE INTESTINAL EPITHELIUM

The length of intestinal villi is determined by the relative rates of cell loss at the tips and cell replenishment at the base

Replication of enterocytes occurs in the crypts. Crypt enterocytes are highly mitotic and regenerate rapidly. In fact, the intestinal crypt cells are among the most rapidly regenerating cells of the body, representing the single greatest need for protein synthesis in non-growing animals. As crypt cells multiply, they migrate onto the base of the villi, pushing other villous cells ahead of them, so that there is a continuous progression of cells migrating up the villi. As the cells migrate they mature, changing from relatively undifferentiated cells in the crypts to highly specialized absorptive cells on the villi. As the cells reach the tips of the villi, they are lost because of age and exposure to gut contents. The length of the villi is determined by the rate at which cells are lost at the tips of the villi and the rate at which they are replaced by cells from the crypts. The time taken for an enterocyte to migrate from its site of origin in the crypt to the tip of a villus varies with species and physiologic state; on average, however, the turnover time of enterocytes is 4 to 7 days.

The rate of cell replication in the crypts appears to be stimulated by several of the GI hormones. When appetite and feed intake increase, there is an overall increase in the secretion of GI hormones. This in turn leads to a rise in crypt cell proliferation, resulting in longer villi. Appetite and feed intake may increase because of conditions of greater energy need, such as lactation, exercise, and cold environmental temperatures. The greater villi length provides a greater digestive and absorptive capacity to match the need created by higher feed intake. Thus, the functional capacity of the intestine is adjusted to match the nutrient needs of the animal.

DIGESTION IN THE NEONATE

During the first few hours of life, proteins are not digested but are absorbed intact

In general, a major function of digestion is to break down proteins by hydrolysis. Under most circumstances, this process is a benefit to the animal, not only from a nutritional and digestive standpoint but also from a toxicologic and allergic standpoint; poten-

tially toxic or allergenic proteins are broken down before they are absorbed into the body. In the special case of some neonates, however, there is a need to absorb proteins intact. In most livestock species, including horses, cattle, sheep, and swine, essentially no antibodies are passed from the mother to fetus through the placenta, in contrast to some other animals such as primates. Thus, young livestock are born without the immunologic protection of their mother's antibodies. In these species, antibodies from the mother must be acquired through ingestion of colostrum, the special mammary secretion present at the time of birth. At birth in these animals, the digestive tract is altered from the adult state so that the antibody proteins are absorbed intact rather than after digestion.

There are three primary alterations:

1. Acid secretion from the stomach is delayed for several days after birth.
2. A similar delay appears in the development of pancreatic function, and thus, acid and trypsin digestion of proteins are avoided.
3. A specialized intestinal epithelium develops that is capable of engulfing soluble proteins in the intestinal lumen and discharging them into the lateral spaces.

The fetal epithelium has the same villous structure as the mature epithelium, but the villi are covered with special enterocytes capable of protein absorption. Immediately after birth, this special epithelium starts to disappear, and it is essentially gone after 24 hours. The loss of the protein-absorptive function in the neonate is referred to as *gut closure.*

The major intestinal disaccharidase switches from lactase to maltase with maturity

Lactose from milk is the major carbohydrate in the diets of neonatal and young mammals; thus, all mammals are born with high intestinal lactase activity. In contrast, maltase activity, necessary for digesting the products of luminal starch digestion, is weak or absent for several weeks after birth. As the animals progress toward weaning, lactase activity wanes and maltase activity increases, allowing the animals to shift from lactose to starch as a carbohydrate source. In many species of adult animals, lactase activity is practically nonexistent.

PATHOPHYSIOLOGY OF DIARRHEA

Diarrhea refers to an increase in the frequency of defecation or in the volume of feces. This discussion is mainly concerned with the volume of feces. Fecal volume rises in diarrhea primarily because of an increase in water content. The amount of water passed in feces is the algebraic sum of GI water input and water absorption. As discussed earlier, water in the gut results from ingested water, water secreted by

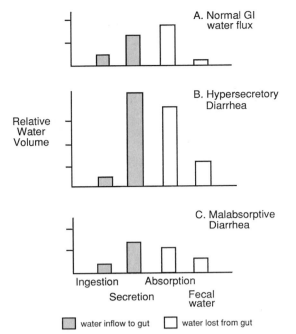

FIGURE 29–29. Pathophysiology of diarrhea. The *bars* represent the relative amounts of water entering or leaving the gut. Fecal volume is the sum of the water ingested and the water secreted minus the water absorbed. Therefore, fecal volume depends not on the amount of water entering the gut but, rather, on the balance between water influx and efflux.

glands of the GI system, and water secreted or lost directly through the mucosal epithelium. Under most circumstances, the amount of water secreted into the gut greatly exceeds the amount ingested. Normally, the amount absorbed is just slightly less than the sum of the amounts secreted and ingested, leaving a small remainder for passage in the feces (Fig. 29–29A).

Diarrhea occurs when there is a mismatch between secretion and absorption

The amount of water in the feces is the result of the balance between secretion and absorption. *Malabsorptive diarrhea* occurs when absorption is inadequate

to recover a sufficient portion of secreted water, as illustrated in Figure 29–29C. Malabsorptive diarrhea usually occurs because of the loss of GI epithelium. In most instances, such losses occur because of viral, bacterial, or protozoal infections. Viral infections often cause particularly severe destruction of villous epithelium. These infections result in the loss of enterocytes from the villi. As pointed out previously, villous length is determined by the relative rates of cell loss and cell replacement (Fig. 29–30).

Intestinal infections result in decreased villous length, because the rate of cell loss is higher than the rate of cell replacement. Short villi cause impaired absorption for two reasons: (1) there is an absolute loss of absorptive intestinal surface area and (2) the cells that are lost are the mature cells from the upper regions of the villi. It is these mature cells that possess the enzymes of membranous-phase digestion and the transport proteins for sodium co-transport; loss of these cells results in impairment of digestion and absorption of nutrients. Because nutrient absorption is necessary for the osmotic absorption of water, water absorption is diminished when nutrient absorption is impaired.

Secretory diarrhea occurs when the rate of intestinal secretion increases and overwhelms the absorptive capacity. Most cases of hypersecretory diarrhea result from inappropriate secretion from the small intestinal crypts. This occurs when the normal secretory mechanism of the crypt epithelium (as discussed earlier) is abnormally stimulated. Toxins, known as *enterotoxins*, are produced by some types of pathogenic bacteria. These toxins bind to enterocytes and stimulate adenyl cyclase activity and the production of cAMP within the cells, resulting in opening of the chloride gates and the secretion of water and electrolytes from crypt epithelium. If the stimulation is mild, the gut may respond with an increase in absorption, and diarrhea does not result. However, when the secretion exceeds the capacity of the gut to increase absorption, as illustrated in Figure 29–29B, diarrhea results. Hypersecretory diarrhea has devastating effects on the water, electrolyte, and acid-base status of animals, especially neonates. Hypersecretory diarrhea due to enterotoxin-producing *Escherichia coli* is an extremely common disease of neonatal calves and pigs that causes large

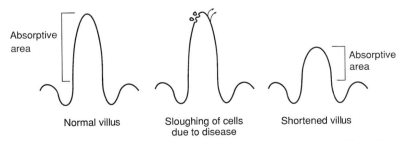

FIGURE 29–30. Shortening of villi because of increased cell loss. Many infectious diseases result in an increased rate of cell sloughing from the villi. As cells are lost, the villus shrinks to fill in the gap in the epithelial coat. If villous height is to be maintained in the presence of rapid loss of enterocytes, the rate of recruitment of new cells, generated in the crypts, must be raised. Therefore, when the rate of cell loss exceeds the capacity for cell replacement, shortened villi with reduced absorptive surfaces and relatively immature enterocytes appear.

economic losses in the cattle and swine industries due to death and treatment costs.

CLINICAL CORRELATIONS

Calf diarrhea with dehydration and acidosis

History You are asked to examine a 2-day-old calf. The owner reports that the calf appeared normal the night before, but this morning she is recumbent and will not rise. In addition, she shows no interest in suckling a bottle.

Clinical and laboratory examination The calf's body temperature is subnormal. The mouth is dry, and the eyes are sunken into the orbits. The ears, tail, and distal legs are cool to the touch. The tail and perineum of the calf are wet. As you remove your thermometer, the calf passes a stream of liquid feces. The feces are nearly clear and slightly yellow; they have the consistency of water. Simple laboratory tests indicate that the packed cell volume is 50% (normal, 30% to 35%), and the serum total-solids concentration is 7.5% (normal, 5.5% to 6.5%).

Comment The calf has diarrhea, and the physical examination and laboratory findings indicate a state of advanced dehydration. Loss of body fluid volume is so severe that the calf appears to be in or near a state of hypovolemic shock. Although you cannot be absolutely sure from the information you collect while examining the calf at the farm, the severity of dehydration, the rapidity of onset, and the age of the calf all suggest a hypersecretory diarrhea due to enterotoxigenic *E. coli* bacteria. Animals with such clinical signs are usually severely acidotic, although blood pH is seldom measured in field cases. Diarrhea, acidosis, and dehydration occur because toxins produced by the bacteria stimulate opening of chloride gates in the apical membranes of crypt cells, stimulating copious secretion of water and electrolytes, including bicarbonate. The sodium co-transport system on the villi is unaffected by the bacterial toxin, but the simultaneous presence of glucose and sodium in the lumen is necessary to promote co-transport, which can offset some of the fluid and electrolyte losses caused by hypersecretion from the intestinal crypts.

Treatment Vascular volume expansion and correction of acidosis are primary concerns in such cases. A calf such as this should receive 2 L of alkalizing fluids by rapid intravenous administration. An additional 2 L or more should be given intravenously over the next 24 hours. Frequently, the response of calves to such treatment is remarkable, and calves that appear almost dead can often be saved by vigorous fluid therapy. After the initial replacement of lost fluids by intravenous therapy, further dehydration due to ongoing fluid losses can be prevented by oral administration of glucose- and sodium-containing fluids.

Juvenile pancreatic atrophy

History You are presented with a thin, 3-year-old German shepherd. The owners report that the dog appeared normal up until 6 months ago. At that time they noticed that he started losing weight and began to develop the disgusting habit of eating his own feces. Re-

cently, the weight loss has become more severe, even though he has had a good appetite and seems normal otherwise. Lately, the owners have noted that the dog seems to pass a large amount of feces, and the fecal material is soft and gray with a clay-like consistency.

Clinical and laboratory examination Physical examination reveals an extremely thin dog with a dull, uneven hair coat. Other physical findings are unremarkable, and the dog seems bright and friendly. You hospitalize the animal for further testing and note that he readily eats two cans of commercial dog food per day. Laboratory analysis of feces collected over a 24-hour period reveals that the dog is passing 25 g of fat in the feces per day (normal is less than 5 g, assuming a normal type of diet).

Comment This degree of fat malabsorption is characteristic of pancreatic exocrine insufficiency. Because there is insufficient pancreatic lipase, fats cannot be hydrolyzed to fatty acids for absorption; thus, they pass unabsorbed through the gut. Several other laboratory tests are available for assessing pancreatic exocrine function. Other tests have as their basis such activities as the examination of blood for the presence of orally administered markers that require pancreatic enzymes for digestion and absorption and the direct examination of feces for the presence of pancreatic enzymes or undigested nutrients.

Treatment Feeding highly digestible diets mixed with commercially prepared pancreatic enzymes is commonly successful in promoting adequate nutrient absorption in animals with juvenile pancreatic atrophy. Digestion may not be completely normal but is sufficient for the dog to attain a normal body weight. Treatment must be continued for life. You may wonder how orally administered pancreatic enzymes can survive intact through the proteolytic environment of the stomach. Undoubtedly, a portion of them are destroyed, but enough appear to make it through the stomach to be effective.

Bibliography

Argenzio RA, Whipp SC: Pathophysiology of diarrhea. In Anderson NV (ed): Veterinary Gastroenterology. Philadelphia: Lea & Febiger, 1980, pp 220–232.

Davidson NO: Intestinal lipid absorption. In Yamada T, Alpers DH, Laine L, et al (eds): Textbook of Gastroenterology, 3rd ed. Philadelphia: JB Lippincott, 1999, pp 428–455.

Ganapathy V, Leibach FH: Protein digestion and assimilation. In Yamada T, Alpers DH, Laine L, et al (eds): Textbook of Gastroenterology, 3rd ed. Philadelphia: JB Lippincott, 1999, pp 456–467.

Hall EJ: Clinical laboratory evaluation of small intestinal function. Vet Clin North Am Small Anim Pract 29:441–469, 1999.

Johnson LR: Digestion and absorption. In Johnson LR (ed): Gastrointestinal Physiology, 6th ed. St. Louis: Mosby, 2001, pp 119–140.

Johnson LR: Fluid and electrolyte absorption. In Johnson LR (ed): Gastrointestinal Physiology, 6th ed. St. Louis: Mosby, 2001, pp 37–46.

Johnson LR, Alpers DH, Christensen J, et al (eds): Physiology of the Gastrointestinal Tract, 3rd ed. New York: Raven Press, 1994, pp 1577–2183.

Montrose MH, Keely SJ, Barrett KE: Electrolyte secretion and absorption: Small intestine and colon. In Yamada T, Alpers DH, Laine L, et al (eds): Textbook of Gastroenterology, 3rd ed. Philadelphia: JB Lippincott, 1999, pp 320–354.

Nagy B, Fekete PZ: Enterotoxigenic *Escherichia coli* (ETEC) in farm animals. Vet Res 30:259–284, 1999.

Naylor JM: Oral electrolyte therapy. Vet Clin North Am Food Anim Pract 15:487–504, 1999.

Stevens CE, Hume ID: Comparative physiology of the vertebrate digestive system Argenzio RA: Comparative physiology of the gastrointestinal system. In Anderson NV (ed): Veterinary Gastroenterology. Philadelphia: Lea & Febiger, 1980, pp 172–198.

Traber PG: Carbohydrate assimilation. In Yamada T, Alpers DH, Laine L, et al (eds): Textbook of Gastroenterology, 3rd ed. Philadelphia: JB Lippincott, 1999, pp 404–427.

PRACTICE QUESTIONS

1. Finding triglycerides and starch in the feces of a thin dog with a normal feed intake would suggest
    a. malabsorption.
    b. maldigestion.

2. Which statement about the tight junctions is false?
    a. Tight junctions encircle the enterocyte near its apical end.
    b. Tight junctions form the dividing line between the apical membrane and the basolateral membrane.
    c. Tight junctions are impermeable to water.
    d. Tight junctions separate the lateral space from the intestinal lumen.
    e. Tight junctions are the only points that attach enterocytes together.

3. Which of the following molecules is consumed during the process of hydrolytic digestion?
    a. Glucose.
    b. Alanine.
    c. Dipeptides.
    d. Fatty acids.
    e. Water.

4. A drug that blocks the activity of the Na^+,K^+-ATPase pump could be expected to have what effect on sodium-glucose co-transport?
    a. Increased sodium-glucose co-transport.
    b. Decreased sodium-glucose co-transport.
    c. No effect on sodium-glucose co-transport.

5. During sodium absorption by glucose co-transport,
    a. chloride is absorbed by the paracellular route.
    b. chloride absorption is not affected.
    c. chloride is absorbed in exchange for bicarbonate.
    d. chloride absorption is coupled with potassium absorption.
    e. chloride is absorbed in exchange for hydrogen ion.

6. Before entering the intestinal capillaries, all nutrients pass through the
    a. apical membrane.
    b. tight junction.
    c. lateral space.
    d. basolateral membrane.
    e. enterocyte cytoplasm.

PRACTICE ANSWERS

1. b   2. c   3. e   4. b   5. a   6. c

Digestion: the fermentative processes

1 Fermentation is the metabolic action of bacteria

2 The sites of fermentative digestion must be conducive to microbial growth

The microbial ecosystem of fermentative digestion

1 The microbes responsible for fermentative digestion include bacteria, fungi, and protozoa

2 Cooperation and interplay among the many species of microbes give rise to a complex ecosystem in the forestomach and hindgut

Substrates and products of fermentative digestion

1 Plant cell walls are important substrates for fermentative digestion and significant nutrient sources for many species

2 Nutrients other than cell walls are also subject to fermentative digestion

3 Anaerobic conditions in the rumen result in metabolic activities leading to the production of volatile fatty acids

4 Volatile fatty acids are important energy substrates for the host animal

5 Fermentative digestion of protein results in the deamination of a large portion of amino acids

6 When protein and energy availability in the forestomach are well matched, there is rapid microbial growth and efficient protein utilization

7 Microbial protein can be synthesized in the rumen from nonprotein nitrogen sources

Reticulorumen motility and maintenance of the rumen environment

1 The physiologic functions of the reticulorumen maintain an environment favorable to fermentation patterns that are beneficial to the host

2 Rumen fermentation is maintained by selectively retaining actively fermenting material while allowing unfermentable residue to pass on to the abomasum

3 Gravity and reticulorumen motility combine to create the selective flow of particulate matter out of the rumen

4 Functional specific gravity determines the rate at which particulate matter (solids) moves through the zones of the reticulorumen

5 Digestibility and physical characteristics of feed have important influences on both the rate of particle passage from the rumen and the rate of feed intake

6 Rumination, or cud chewing, has an important effect on the reduction of particle size and the movement of solid material through the rumen

7 Water moves through the rumen at a much faster rate than particulate matter

8 Rumen dilution rate has important influences on fermentation and microbial cell yield

Control of reticulorumen motility

1 Reticulorumen motility is controlled by the central nervous system and affected by intraluminal conditions

Omasal function

1 Passage of material from the reticulum to the omasum occurs during reticular contraction

Volatile fatty acid absorption

1 Volatile fatty acids, representing 60% to 80% of the energy needs of the animal, are absorbed directly from the forestomach epithelium

Rumen development and esophageal groove function

1 Tremendous changes in forestomach size and function occur with dietary changes in early life

2 The esophageal groove diverts the flow of ingested milk past the forestomach and into the abomasum

Function of the equine large hindgut

1 The equine hindgut has a tremendous capacity for fermentation

2 The types of substrate and fermentation patterns are essentially identical for forestomach and hindgut fermentation

3 The motility functions of the cecum and colon retain material for fermentation and separate particles by size

4 The rate of fermentation and volatile fatty-acid production in the equine colon is similar to that in the rumen

5 There are tremendous variations in hindgut anatomy and function among the many species of veterinary interest

Fermentation is the metabolic action of bacteria

In fermentative digestion, molecular substrates are broken down by the action of bacteria and other microorganisms. Enzymatic hydrolysis of large molecules is an essential part of fermentative digestion, just as it is for glandular digestion. The major difference between the two processes is that the enzymes of fermentative digestion are microbial in origin, rather than coming from the host animal. Other major differences between fermentative and glandular digestion are the rates of reactions and the extent of alteration of the substrate molecules. In general, fermentative digestion is much slower than glandular digestion, and the substrates are altered to a much greater degree.

The sites of fermentative digestion must be conducive to microbial growth

Fermentative digestion occurs in specialized compartments that are positioned either before or after the stomach and small intestine. Fermentative compartments positioned before the stomach are called *forestomachs* and are most highly developed in the ruminants and cameloids. There are tremendous species variations in the size and development of the forestomach fermentation compartments; many species have distinct forestomachs that are less developed than those of ruminants. In some species, including the horse, pig, and rat, there is no anatomically distinct forestomach; however, there is a nonglandular portion of the proximal stomach in which some fermentative digestion may occur.

Fermentation compartments positioned distal to the small intestine are the cecum and colon, often collectively called the *hindgut*. As with the forestomachs, there are tremendous anatomic differences in the hindguts of various species. This variation can be so great as to make it appear that the cecum and colon are functionally different organs in different species; however, when the variations are evaluated critically, important similarities can be seen in hindgut function among species.

The forestomach and hindgut can support fermentative digestion, because their pH, moisture, ionic strength, and oxidation-reduction conditions are maintained in a range compatible for the growth of suitable microbes. In addition, the flow of ingesta through these areas is comparatively slow, allowing microbes time to maintain their population size. The importance of these factors can be illustrated through comparison of the forestomach and colon to the stomach and small intestine. In the stomach, bacterial numbers are kept low by the acid pH, whereas in the small intestine, bacterial numbers are kept in check by the constant flushing action of ingesta and secretions. In contrast, the pH in the forestomach and large colon is close to neutral, and the flow rate is comparatively slow.

In general, the fermentative patterns of the hindgut appear to be similar to those of the forestomach, although forestomach fermentation, especially that of the rumen, appears to be the better studied of the two. The following discussion concerns rumen digestion specifically, but comments on hindgut digestion are included. A specific discussion of digestion in the equine cecum and colon can be found at the end of the chapter.

THE MICROBIAL ECOSYSTEM OF FERMENTATIVE DIGESTION

The microbes responsible for fermentative digestion include bacteria, fungi, and protozoa

The bacterial population associated with fermentative digestion is vast, with at least 28 different functionally important species occurring in the rumen. Some of the major species found in the rumen are listed, with their preferred substrates, in Table 30–1. Total bacterial numbers in the forestomach or hindgut normally range from 10^{10} to 10^{11} cells per gram of ingesta. Most of these bacteria are strict anaerobes that cannot survive in the presence of oxygen, although facultative organisms are also present. In the rumen, fungi are present, and research suggests that they may play an important role in the digestion of plant cell walls.

There is also a large population of protozoa in the rumen as well as in the cecum and colon. Protozoal numbers average about 10^5 to 10^6 cells per gram of rumen contents. Although this number is considerably smaller than the number of bacteria, the relatively larger size of the individual protozoa, compared with bacteria, results in a total rumen protozoal cell mass approximately equal to the bacterial cell mass, under most dietary conditions. Most of the rumen protozoa are ciliated and belong to the genus *Isotricha* or *Entodinium*, although flagellate species are also present, especially in young ruminants. Like the other organisms of the rumen, the protozoa are anaerobic.

The digestive abilities, or capacities, of protozoa and bacteria are similar; thus, either type of organism can perform most of the fermentative functions of the rumen. Protozoa ingest large numbers of bacteria and hold rumen bacterial numbers in check. However, none of the actions of protozoa appears essential to rumen function, because ruminants can survive well without protozoa. Thus, the role of protozoa in the total ecologic picture of the rumen is uncertain. One potentially important function of protozoa may involve their ability to slow down the digestion of rapidly fermentable substrates, such as starch and some proteins. Protozoa are capable of ingesting particles of starch and protein and storing them in their bodies, protected from bacterial action. The starch and protein remain engulfed until digested by the

TABLE 30-1. Grouping of rumen bacterial species according to the type of substrates that are fermented

Major cellulolytic species
Bacteroides succinogenes
Ruminococcus flavefaciens
Ruminococcus albus
Butyrivibrio fibrisolvens

Major hemicellulolytic species
Butyrivibrio fibrisolvens
Bacteroides ruminicola
Ruminococcus species

Major pectinolytic species
Butyrivibrio fibrisolvens
Bacteroides ruminicola
Lachnospira multiparus
Succinivibrio dextrinosolvens
Treponema bryantii
Streptococcus bovis

Major amylolytic species
Bacteroides amylophilus
Streptococcus bovis
Succinimonas amylolytica
Bacteroides ruminicola

Major ureolytic species
Succinivibrio dextrinosolvens
Selenomonas species
Bacteroides ruminicola
Ruminococcus bromii
Butyrivibrio species
Treponema species

Major methane-producing species
Methanobrevibacter ruminantium
Methanobacterium formicicum
Methanomicrobium mobile

Major sugar-utilizing species
Treponema bryantii
Lactobacillus vitulinus
Lactobacillus ruminis

Major acid-utilizing species
Megasphaera elsdenii
Selenomonas ruminantium

Major proteolytic species
Bacteroides amylophilus
Bacteroides ruminicola
Butyrivibrio fibrisolvens
Streptococcus bovis

Major ammonia-producing species
Bacteroides ruminicola
Megasphaera elsdenii
Selenomonas ruminantium

Major lipid-utilizing species
Anaerovibrio lipolytica
Butyrivibrio fibrisolvens
Treponema bryantii
Eubacterium species
Fusocillus species
Micrococcus species

From Church DC (ed): The Ruminant Animal. Digestive Physiology and Nutrition. Englewood Cliffs, NJ: Prentice-Hall, 1988, p. 126.

protozoa, or until the protozoa die or are swept from the rumen into the lower digestive tract. Thus, protozoa may have the effect of delaying, or prolonging, the digestion of these substrates. Especially in the case of starch, this protozoal effect may be beneficial to the host through modulation or delay of the digestion of rapidly fermentable substrate.

Cooperation and interplay among the many species of microbes give rise to a complex ecosystem in the forestomach and hindgut

The digestive process in the rumen or colon involves the interplay among the many species of bacteria and other microbes. The ecosystem of fermentative digestion is extremely complex, with the waste products of one microbial species serving as substrate for another. For example, *Ruminococcus albus* and *Bacteroides ruminicola* appear to exist synergistically. *R. albus* digests cellulose (is *cellulolytic*) but cannot digest protein. *B. ruminicola,* on the other hand, can digest protein but cannot digest cellulose. When the microbes are grown together, cellulose digestion by *R. albus* provides hexoses for the energy needs of *B. ruminicola,* and protein digestion by *B. ruminicola* provides ammonia and branch-chain fatty acids for the growth needs of *R. albus.*

In addition to substrate needs, growth factor needs are also supplied synergistically within the rumen ecosystem. As an example, B vitamins are necessary for the growth of several rumen microbes, and yet these nutrients are generally not necessary in ruminant diets. The synergistic effect of B vitamins results from cross-feeding between species of those microbes that produce various B vitamins and those microbes that require them.

In spite of tremendous ecologic complexity, however, the entire pattern of fermentation may be viewed as a holistic process, without consideration of the roles and interactions of individual microbial species. Fermentative digestion is examined here in that light, with the actions of the entire rumen biomass considered as an overall digestive process, irrespective of the specific needs and actions of individual microbial species.

SUBSTRATES AND PRODUCTS OF FERMENTATIVE DIGESTION

Plant cell walls are important substrates for fermentative digestion and significant nutrient sources for many species

Forages, or the foliage of plants, are both the major feedstuff of large herbivores and an important substrate for fermentative digestion. Some appreciation of the physical and chemical nature of plants is important to an understanding of the fermentative digestion of forages. This understanding may be aided by a brief comparison of plant and animal tissue structure.

At the cellular level, a major difference between plants and animals is the existence of a *cell wall* in plants. The cell wall is a complex of various carbohydrate molecules. The structural parts of plants, the leaves and stems, contain a large portion of cell-wall material. This material gives the plants their rigid framework and protects them from weather and other elements during growth. The cell-wall structure of plants can be roughly compared to the connective tissue structure of animals. Long, fiber-like molecules of *cellulose* have a strength-giving role similar to that of collagen, whereas *hemicellulose, pectin,* and *lignin* cement the cellulose together, much as hyaluronic acid and chondroitin sulfate do in animal connective tissue. With the exception of lignin, all these cell-wall molecules are carbohydrate.

Cellulose is composed of nonbranching chains of glucose monomers joined by $\beta[1–4]$ glycosidic linkages, in contrast to the $\alpha[1–4]$ linkages in starch. Pectin and hemicellulose are chemically more heterogeneous than cellulose, being composed of various proportions of several sugars and sugar acids. None of the cell-wall materials is subject to hydrolytic digestion by mammalian glandular digestive enzymes. However, cellulose, hemicellulose, and pectin are subject to the hydrolytic action of a complex of microbial enzymes known as *cellulase.* This enzyme system releases monosaccharides and oligosaccharides from the complex carbohydrates of cell walls, but the released saccharides are not directly available for absorption by the animal. Rather, they are further metabolized by the microbes, as discussed later.

Lignin, a heterogeneous group of phenolic chemicals, is resistant to the action of either mammalian or microbial enzymes, and only a small portion of lignin is digested by either process. Lignin is important, not only because it is indigestible itself but also because it tends to encase the cell-wall carbohydrates, reducing their digestibility by protecting them from the action of bacterial cellulase. The lignin concentration of plants increases with age and ambient temperature; thus, young, cool-season plants are more digestible than mature plants grown in hot weather.

Nutrients other than cell walls are also subject to fermentative digestion

The fermentative digestion of plant cell-wall material and its importance to herbivore digestion are well known. It must not be forgotten, however, that essentially all protein and carbohydrate nutrients that can provide substrate for energy and growth in mammals can also support the similar needs of microbes. Therefore, nearly all dietary protein and carbohydrate are potentially subject to fermentative digestion. This fact is especially important in ruminants, in which food is exposed to fermentative digestion in the forestomach before its arrival at sites of glandular digestion. This temporal arrangement leads to the fermentative digestion of many nutrients that would otherwise have been available to the animal through glandular digestion. Thus, forestomach fermentative digestion, which provides for the efficient use of plant cell walls, can potentially lead to the inefficient use of other nutrients because of microbial alteration.

Anaerobic conditions in the rumen result in metabolic activities leading to the production of volatile fatty acids

When carbohydrate material enters the rumen or colon, it is attacked by hydrolytic microbial enzymes. In the case of insoluble carbohydrates, attack requires the physical attachment of bacteria to the surface of the plant particle, the enzymes themselves being part of the surface coating of the bacteria. Enzymatic action liberates glucose, other monosaccharides, and short-chain polysaccharides into the fluid phase, outside the microbial cell bodies. Although free in solution, these products of microbial enzyme action do not become immediately available to the host animal; rather, they are quickly subjected to further metabolism by the microbial mass. Glucose and other sugars are absorbed into the cell bodies of the microbes.

Once within the microbial cells, glucose enters the glycolytic, or Embden-Meyerhof, pathway. This is the same glycolytic pathway that exists in mammalian cells, and as in mammalian tissues, catabolism of glucose through this pathway yields two molecules of pyruvate for each molecule of glucose. In the process, two molecules of oxidized nicotinamide adenine dinucleotide (NAD) are reduced to NAD hydrogen (NADH), and two molecules of adenosine triphosphate (ATP) are formed from adenosine diphosphate (ADP). The potential energy represented by the ATP formed in this reaction is not directly available to the host animal but is the major source of energy for maintenance and growth of microbes.

If fermentative digestion were to occur under aerobic conditions, which it does not, the pyruvate produced by the glycolytic process would enter the citric acid (Krebs) cycle and would be metabolized to carbon dioxide and water, as occurs under the aerobic conditions in mammalian cells. Furthermore, in an aerobic system, the NADH produced would be oxidized in the cytochrome oxidase system with additional production of ATP and the regeneration of NAD. But fermentative digestion is not an aerobic system; on the contrary, it proceeds in a reductive, highly anaerobic environment. Therefore, a different mechanism must be provided for the oxidation of NADH and other reduced cofactors, such as flavin adenine dinucleotide hydrogen ($FADH_2$). If such a mechanism were not available, all the oxidized cofactors present would soon be reduced, and metabolism would come to a halt. Because no atmospheric oxygen is available, some other compound must serve as an electron sink for the oxidation of enzyme cofactors.

In fermentative digestion, pyruvate can act as an electron sink, being further reduced to provide for regeneration of NAD and the general removal of excess electrons, with an additional yield of ATP. Also, carbon dioxide can be reduced to methane, accepting electrons for the regeneration of NAD and flavin adenine dinucleotide (FAD). The metabolic pathways of these reactions are illustrated in Figure 30–1. These pathways lead to the major end products of the fermentative digestion of carbohydrate, the *volatile fatty*

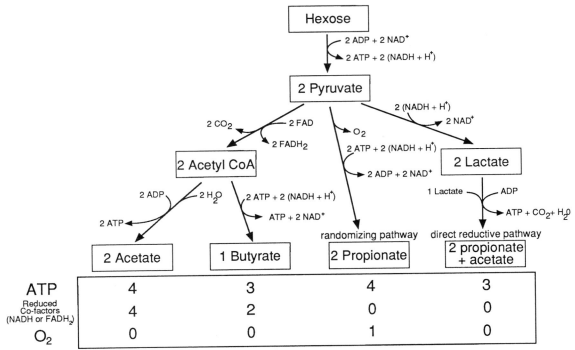

FIGURE 30–1. Pathways of volatile fatty acid (VFA) production by the rumen or colonic biomass. The production of methane is necessary for the production of oxidized cofactors in the pathways leading to acetate and butyrate production, but not in the pathways leading to propionate production. The production of oxygen by the randomizing pathway results in the net production of oxidized cofactors.

acids (VFAs). The primary VFAs are *acetic acid, propionic acid,* and *butyric acid*; the VFAs are often referred to as their dissociated ions: acetate, propionate, and butyrate, respectively. Other quantitatively minor but metabolically important VFAs are valeric acid, isovaleric acid, isobutyric acid, and 2-methylbutyric acid. The chemical structures of the VFAs are shown in Figure 30–2.

From Figure 30–1, it can be seen that production of propionic acid from pyruvate results in the efficient regeneration of NAD with no net production of NADH. In fact, production of available oxygen by the *randomizing branch* of the propionic acid pathway leads to oxidation of excess NADH originating from the acetic or butyric acid pathways, as illustrated (see Fig. 30–1). The production of acetic acid leads to the efficient generation of ATP but, in contrast to the production of propionic acid, does not result in the regeneration of NAD from NADH. In the acetic acid pathway, excess NADH is produced. In this case, NAD is regenerated by the formation of free hydro-

gen, which is subsequently used to reduce carbon dioxide to methane and water (Fig. 30–1, *lower portion*).

Thus, there is a direct relationship between acetic acid production and methane production; as the amount of pyruvate entering the acetic acid pathway increases, there must be a concomitant rise in methane production. Likewise, there is a reciprocal relationship between methane production and propionic acid production; as pyruvate is diverted to propionic acid production, there is less need for methane synthesis. These relationships are illustrated in the stoichiometric equations of Table 30–2. These reactions do not, however, fully describe the flow of hydrogen, or reducing substances, in rumen or colonic metabolism. The chemical reactions of fermentation are extremely complex and interdependent, and NADH can donate its electrons to reactions other than those described in Table 30–2, such as the synthesis of microbial protein and the saturation of unsaturated fatty acids.

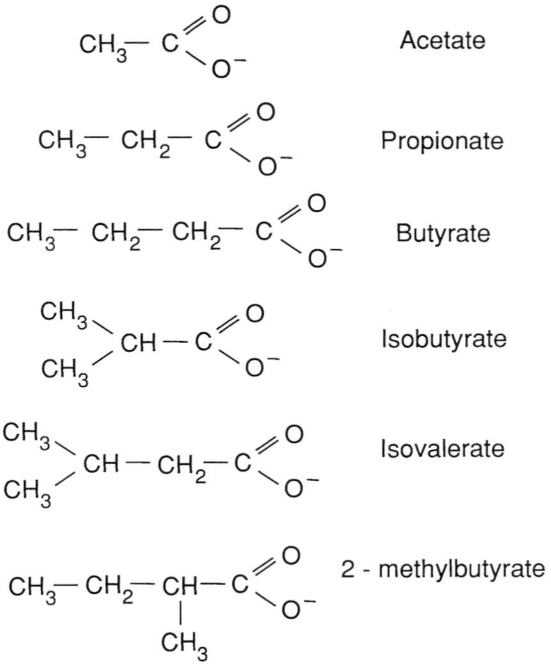

FIGURE 30–2. Chemical structures of the major volatile fatty acids produced by fermentative digestion.

In the rumen, methane production is facilitated by methanogenic bacteria, such as *Methanobacterium ruminantium*. This fragile bacterium is sensitive to changing conditions in the rumen. When conditions are unfavorable for the survival of *M. ruminantium*, methane production is reduced, shifting the metabolic pathways toward propionic acid production. Some conditions that suppress methanogenic species are high levels of feed intake, use of finely ground or

TABLE 30–2. Theoretical stoichiometric carbon-hydrogen balance equations describing conversion of glucose in the rumen

Case 1

glucose → 2 acetate + 2 CO_2 + 8 H
glucose → butyrate + 2 CO_2 + 4 H
glucose + 4 H → 2 propionate + 2 H_2O
CO_2 + 8 H → CH_4 + H_2O

Net*
  3 glucose → 2 acetate + butyrate + 2 propionate + 3 CO_2 + CH_4 + 2 H_2O

Case 2

3 glucose → 6 butyrate + 2 CO_2 + 24 H
glucose → butyrate + 2 CO_2 + 4 H
glucose + 4 H → 2 propionate + 2 H_2O
3 CO_2 + 24 H → 3 CH_4 + 6 H_2O

Net*
  5 glucose → 6 acetate + butyrate + 2 propionate + 5 CO_2 + 3 CH_4 + 6 H_2O

From Van Soest PJ: Nutritional Ecology of the Ruminant. Ithaca, NY: Cornell University Press, 1982.
*Note that in case 1, the acetate-to-propionate ratio is 1:1 and the methane-to-glucose ratio is 1:3, whereas in case 2, the acetate-to-propionate ratio is 3:1 and the methane-to-glucose ratio is 3:5.

pelleted feeds, and high-grain or high-starch diets. Under these circumstances, the rate of methane production is reduced, resulting in a lower rate of acetic acid production with a concomitant increase in the propionic acid production rate.

The proportional rates at which acetic acid, propionic acid, and butyric acid are produced are reflected in their relative concentrations in the rumen fluid. The relative concentrations of the VFAs have important nutritional and metabolic consequences, and although seldom measured for medical purposes, VFA concentrations are frequently reported in research literature. Typically, the ruminal acetic-to-propionic-to-butyric acid concentration ratio in ruminants ranges from 70:20:10 for animals eating high-forage diets to 60:30:10 for animals eating high-grain diets. It must be appreciated that these values represent relative proportions and not absolute amounts. The total amount of VFA produced with a high-starch diet is usually much higher than that produced with a high-fiber diet, such that total acetic acid production may be higher with a high-starch diet than with a high-fiber diet, even though the acetic acid production relative to the other VFAs may be reduced. This principle is illustrated in Figure 30–3.

Volatile fatty acids are important energy substrates for the host animal

One can appreciate the elegance and beauty of the symbiotic relationship represented by fermentative digestion by considering the metabolism of VFAs. These molecules are the end products, indeed, the waste products, of anaerobic microbial metabolism, just as carbon dioxide is the waste product of aerobic metabolism. If the VFAs were allowed to accumulate, they would suppress or alter the fermentative process by lowering the pH of the gut or forestomach. However, the host animal maintains conditions for fermentation both by buffering pH changes and by removing VFAs from the gut by absorption. The benefit derived by the host is from the chemical energy that is contained in the VFAs. These bacterial "waste products" represent spent compounds within the framework of the anaerobic fermentation system, but they still contain considerable energy that can be derived from aerobic metabolism. In ruminants and other large herbivores, the VFAs are the major energy fuels, to a large extent serving the role played by glucose in omnivorous monogastric animals. The metabolic fates of the VFAs are discussed further in Chapter 31.

Fermentative digestion of protein results in the deamination of a large portion of amino acids

To this point, the discussion of fermentative digestion has centered primarily on carbohydrates, but as previously mentioned, other energy-yielding substrates are subject to microbial attack as well. Proteins are particularly vulnerable, because they are composed

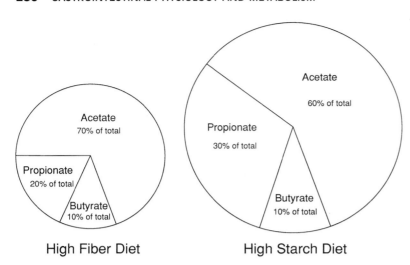

FIGURE 30–3. VFA production on high-fiber and high-starch diets. Although the percentage of acetate is lower on the high-starch diet, the total amount of acetate produced is greater on the high-starch diet. In contrast, propionate increases in both amount and proportion on the high-starch diet.

of carbon compounds that can be further reduced to provide energy for anaerobic microbes. As proteins enter fermentative areas of the gut, they are attacked by extracellular microbial proteases. The majority of these enzymes are "trypsin-like" endopeptidases that form short-chain peptides as end products. These peptides are formed extracellularly and are absorbed into the microbial cell bodies, much as glucose is formed from carbohydrate and then absorbed. Within the microbial cells, the peptides either can be used for the formation of microbial protein or can be further degraded for the production of energy through the VFA pathways (Fig. 30–4).

To enter the VFA pathways, the individual amino acids are first deaminated to yield ammonia and a carbon skeleton. The carbon structures of many of the amino acids can fit directly into various steps of the VFA pathways, leading to the production of the three major VFAs. The three branch-chain amino acids (BCAAs) are exceptions, however, and lead to the production of branch-chain VFAs by the following reactions:

$$valine + 2\,H_2O \rightarrow isobutyrate + NH_3 + CO_2$$

$$leucine + 2\,H_2O \rightarrow isovalerate + NH_3 + CO_2$$

$$isoleucine + 2\,H_2O \rightarrow 2\text{-methylbutyrate} + NH_3 + CO_2$$

These branch-chain VFAs are important growth factors for several species of bacteria, as described later.

Although many species of rumen microbes appear capable of using preformed amino acids, which they derive from absorbed peptides, for the synthesis of

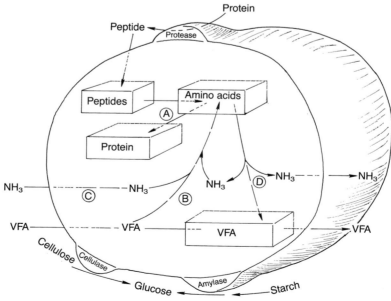

FIGURE 30–4. Protein metabolism by rumen microbes. Protease enzymes on the microbe surfaces generate peptides that are then taken up by many types of organisms. Absorbed peptides contribute to an intracellular pool of amino acids from which microbial proteins are synthesized (A). Another source of amino acids is from intracellular synthesis (B), using ammonia and VFA. Many microbes appear capable of deriving their amino acids from either extracellular peptides or intracellular synthesis; however, several types of bacteria seem incapable of using peptides for an amino acid source and are thus dependent on an extracellular source of ammonia (C) for amino acid synthesis. Amino acids not used for protein synthesis can be metabolized to VFA and ammonia (D).

protein, several species cannot do so. These species must synthesize amino acids from ammonia and the various carbon metabolites of the VFA pathways. For synthesis of the BCAAs, however, the branch-chain VFAs are required. Among the microbial species that require ammonia and branch-chain fatty acids are some of the important cellulose-digesting bacteria.

When protein and energy availability in the forestomach are well matched, there is rapid microbial growth and efficient protein utilization

Because a large part of preformed dietary protein is fermented in the rumen, ruminant animals depend, to a large extent, on microbial protein to meet their own protein needs. Microbial protein reaches the abomasum and small intestine when microbes are washed out of the rumen and into the lower tract. Digestive efficiency is optimized in ruminants when the growth rate of the microbial mass is maximal and so results in maximal delivery of microbial protein to the host animal. These conditions are best met by rapidly growing populations of microbes. The microbial growth rate depends on the supply of nutrients and the rate at which microbes are washed from the rumen. Here we consider the effect of nutrient supply on microbial growth rate; factors affecting the rate of microbial removal are discussed later in the chapter.

The overall reaction in the rumen may be greatly simplified, for the purposes of this discussion, to Equation 1:

$$\text{glucose + peptide =} \quad (1)$$
$$\text{microbes + VFA + NH}_3 \text{ + CH}_4 \text{ + CO}_2$$

where glucose and peptide represent ruminally available carbohydrate and protein, respectively. In this context, *available* means available to the microbes for fermentation. Carbohydrate or protein that is not susceptible, or accessible, to microbial attack is classified as *unavailable* and is not included in Equation 1. Glucose was chosen to represent carbohydrate, and peptide to represent protein, because all carbohydrates must be broken down to simple sugars, and proteins to peptides, before becoming available to bacteria. The term *peptide* in this equation could be replaced by other forms of nitrogen, but for now, the discussion is confined to peptide as a nitrogen source. Peptide is the only nitrogen-containing substrate on the left in the equation, but there are two nitrogen-containing products on the right: microbes (as protein) and NH_3. Both substrates, glucose and peptide, contain carbon, oxygen, and hydrogen and thus can contribute to the formation of microbial carbon, VFA, CH_4, and CO_2.

Equation 1 always balances, but the distribution of products varies according to the relative concentrations of substrates, as illustrated in Figure 30–5. For microbial cells to be produced, both energy and nitrogen are required. Energy can come from either glucose or peptide, but nitrogen must come from peptide. When glucose and peptide availability are appropriately matched (Fig. 30–5A), energy for cellular growth comes primarily from glucose, with pep-

tides directed toward microbial protein synthesis. Under these conditions, the products of Equation 1 favor microbial cells with little ammonia production. Glucose fermentation with accompanying VFA production must be high to meet the large energy demands necessary to support the rapid growth of the microbial mass. Ammonia production is low, because most peptide nitrogen is being incorporated into microbial protein.

When the availability of glucose is high relative to peptide (Fig. 30–5B), there is ample energy but insufficient nitrogen to support adequate protein synthesis, and thus, microbial replication is not maximal. In this case, microbial energy utilization becomes inefficient as energy is used for the maintenance of nondividing cells, rather than for the energy-requiring synthetic processes of growing cells. The maintenance energy needs of the microbes still drive some fermentation of glucose with moderate VFA production, but production of both microbial cells and ammonia is limited because of lack of nitrogen.

When peptide availability exceeds glucose availability (Fig. 30–5C), there is ample nitrogen to support growth, but growth is limited owing to insufficient energy supplies. These conditions force the microbes to use peptides to meet energy needs instead of to synthesize proteins. Microbial growth rate is low, and VFA production is moderate, because fermentation is driven only by the maintenance energy needs of the microbes. Much of the VFA production comes from the carbon portions of the peptides, whereas the amine groups are shunted to ammonia production; thus, the products of equation 1 favor ammonia.

The relationship between available glucose (carbohydrate) and peptide (or nitrogen) has a tremendous effect on the production of microbial cells and, thus, a profound impact on the nutrition of the host. This relationship, as illustrated in Figure 30–5, is quantified by expressing microbial growth in terms of grams of microbial dry matter produced per mole of energy-producing substrate used. This value, referred to as *microbial yield*, is usually designated by a capital Y subscripted with the abbreviation of the energy substrate to which it is referenced. A convenient but somewhat theoretic substrate with which to reference microbial cell yield is ATP. Microbial yield is then written as $Y_{ATP} = x$, where x is the number of grams of microbial dry matter produced per mole of ATP used. The value of Y_{ATP} varies between about 10 and 20 g of microbes per mol of ATP. Nitrogen availability, from either peptide or nonprotein sources, has an important affect on the Y_{ATP} value. When microbial growth is limited by *low* nitrogen availability, a large portion of available ATP is used for maintenance rather than cell growth; thus, the number of cells produced per ATP is small, and the Y_{ATP} value is low.

Microbial protein can be synthesized in the rumen from nonprotein nitrogen sources

If there is sufficient available carbohydrate, most rumen microbes, even those capable of utilizing pre-

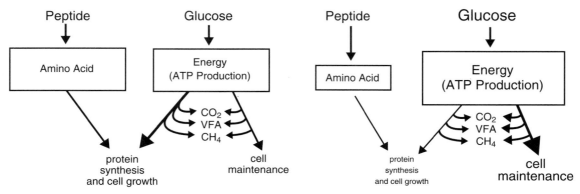

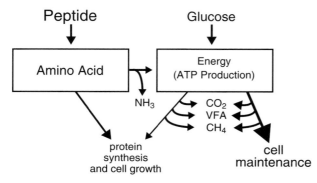

FIGURE 30–5. The efficiency with which dietary energy is used for protein synthesis in the rumen depends on the balance between energy and nitrogen sources. The proportion of energy used for protein synthesis and cell maintenance (as indicated by the size of the *arrows*) changes in relation to the balance of peptide (nitrogen) and glucose supplies.

formed peptides, can synthesize protein from ammonia (see Fig. 30–4). Thus, protein can be produced in the rumen from such nonprotein sources as ammonia, nitrates, and urea. From a nutritional and economic point of view, this capability has been exploited by the inclusion of inexpensive nonprotein nitrogen sources in place of expensive protein in ruminant diets, allowing the microbes to synthesize protein for the amino acid needs of the host. This process also can be exploited physiologically by the recycling of endogenous urea.

Urea, the nitrogenous waste product of protein catabolism, is formed in the liver. In ruminant animals, hepatic urea production is from two sources: (1) nitrogen arising from the deamination of endogenous amino acids and (2) nitrogen absorbed as ammonia from the rumen (Fig. 30–6). Ammonia absorption from the rumen is proportional to the ruminal ammonia production rate, which is subject to the influences of ruminal carbohydrate and protein availability, as discussed earlier. Ammonia, which is toxic at moderate concentrations, is absorbed from the rumen and delivered to the liver through the hepatic-portal blood vascular system. The liver extracts ammonia from the portal blood efficiently; thus, little of the potentially toxic ammonia reaches the systemic circulation.

In monogastric animals, urea is excreted from the body nearly exclusively by the kidneys. In ruminants,

however, urea also may be excreted into the rumen (see Fig. 30–6). Such excretion can occur by direct absorption of urea into the rumen from the blood or by excretion of urea into saliva. In either case, the urea reaches the rumen, where it is quickly transformed to ammonia, and enters the general pool of rumen nitrogen from which microbial proteins are synthesized.

The direction of nonprotein nitrogen flow, either into the rumen as urea or out of the rumen as ammonia, depends on rumen ammonia concentrations. During times of high nitrogen availability in the rumen, relative to carbohydrate availability, this system results in high blood urea concentrations and the extensive loss of precious nitrogen through urinary excretion, making ruminants nutritionally inefficient under these dietary conditions. However, during times of high carbohydrate availability relative to nitrogen availability, the major flow of urea nitrogen is from the blood into the rumen. Under these circumstances, in which ruminal ammonia concentrations are low, most of the blood urea is from endogenous protein catabolism. A portion of this urea, which in monogastric animals would be unavailable for protein synthesis, is excreted into the rumen, where it can be resynthesized into protein that will contribute eventually to the amino acid needs of the host. Thus, under conditions of low dietary protein, ruminants are efficient conservers of nitrogen.

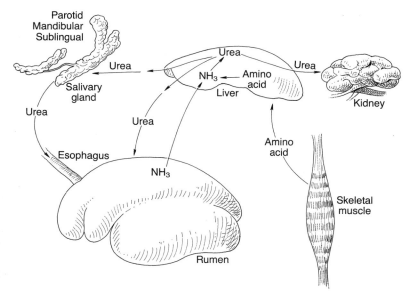

FIGURE 30–6. Interorgan nitrogen cycling in ruminants. The diagram shows the effects of rumen ammonia concentration on the formation and utilization of urea. When rumen ammonia concentrations are high, the net movement of nonprotein nitrogen is toward the liver, resulting in high urea production rates and poor nitrogen conservation. When rumen ammonia concentrations are low, the net movement of nonprotein nitrogen is from liver to rumen, resulting in protein production from endogenous urea.

RETICULORUMEN MOTILITY AND MAINTENANCE OF THE RUMEN ENVIRONMENT

The physiologic functions of the reticulorumen maintain an environment favorable to fermentation patterns that are beneficial to the host

The host animal has no direct control over the metabolism of the microbes in its gut. Yet there are important physiologic factors that influence the gastrointestinal fermentation process. In order for the host to ensure that the proper type of fermentation patterns occur, it must maintain within the rumen (or colon) conditions that promote the growth and favorable metabolic patterns of the most beneficial bacteria and other microbes. The following requirements must be met by the host for proper fermentation to occur:

1. Substrate for fermentation must be supplied.
2. Temperature must be maintained at or near 37°C.
3. Ionic strength (osmolality) of the rumen fluid must be kept within an optimal range (near 300 mosm).
4. A negative oxidation-reduction potential must be maintained (-250 to -450 mV).
5. Indigestible waste (solid material) must be removed.
6. The rate of removal of microbes must be compatible with the regeneration times of the most favorable microbes.
7. Acid products of anaerobic fermentation (VFAs) must be buffered or removed.

The first of these requisites, delivery of substrate, requires only eating; others—temperature and ionic strength—are met by the same homeostatic mechanisms that maintain these physiologic conditions within the host body in general. Maintenance of an appropriate oxidation-reduction potential requires only that oxygen be kept away from the fermentation site. The remaining requisites for fermentation, however, have required the development of special physiologic functions associated with the forestomach (or hindgut). These specialized functions include the motility patterns characteristic of the reticulorumen, the direct absorption of VFA, and the production of tremendous amounts of saliva.

Rumen fermentation is maintained by selectively retaining actively fermenting material while allowing unfermentable residue to pass on to the abomasum

The walls of the reticulorumen are muscular, possess an extensive intrinsic nervous system, and are capable of highly complex and coordinated motility patterns. The selective ruminal retention of fermenting material and the release of unfermentable residue are accomplished by these motility patterns. An understanding of reticulorumen anatomy is necessary for comprehension of the effects of reticulorumen motility patterns. Figure 30–7 illustrates the division of the reticulorumen into compartments, or *sacs*. These divisions are created by muscular pillars that project into the lumen of the organ. It should be appreciated that the reticular fold and rumen pillars, in addition to the walls themselves, are motile. During reticulorumen contractions, the pillars elevate and relax alternately, either accentuating or reducing the divisions within the lumen of the reticulorumen. Students who are accustomed to studying the reticulorumens of embalmed specimens may find it difficult to visualize the extent of rumen movement. At times during contractions, the excursions of the walls and pillars are so great that the total shape of the reticulorumen

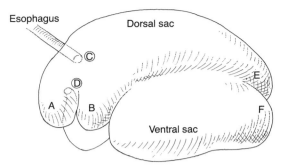

FIGURE 30–7. Rumen anatomy. A, reticulum; B, cranial sac; C, cardia; D, reticulo-omasal orifice; E, caudal-dorsal blind sac; F, caudal-ventral blind sac.

is distorted; sacs and compartments become nearly obliterated, and pillars elevate to the extent that compartmental divisions become nearly complete. When the magnitude of these contractions is recognized, it is not difficult to appreciate the tremendous effect that reticulorumen motility has on the flow of rumen ingesta.

Two patterns of reticulorumen motility are generally described: *primary* or *mixing contractions*, and *secondary* or *eructation contractions*. Primary contractions start with a double, or biphasic, contraction of the reticulum. In the first phase of this reticular contraction, the organ is reduced to about half its relaxed size, whereas the second contraction is strong, nearly obliterating the lumen of the reticulum. The next action of the primary contraction pattern is a caudal-moving peristaltic contraction of the dorsal sac. Upon completion of the dorsal sac contraction, there is a similar caudal-moving contraction of the ventral sac, followed by a cranial-moving contraction of the dorsal sac. The primary contraction pattern is completed by a cranial-moving contraction of the ventral sac (Fig. 30–8). The primary contraction pattern serves to mix ingesta and to aid in the separation of large and small particles. Secondary contractions, when they occur, follow immediately after the primary contractions.

The secondary contractions consist of a cranial-moving wave that starts in the caudal-dorsal blind sac and continues over the dorsal sac (see Fig. 30–8). The function of the secondary contraction is to force gas toward the cranial portion of the rumen. As the secondary contraction moves gas toward the cardia, the cranial sac relaxes and the cranial pillar elevates, allowing liquid ingesta to move away from the cardia so that gas can enter the esophagus and be eructated. Secondary contractions are important, because large amounts of gas, primarily CO_2 and CH_4, are formed during fermentation, and they must be removed rapidly to prevent distention of the rumen.

In general, reticulorumen contractions occur with a frequency of 1 to 3 per minute; contractions occur most frequently during eating and disappear entirely during deep sleep. The rate and strength of contractions depend on the character of the diet: coarse, fibrous feeds stimulate the most frequent and strongest contractions. Secondary contractions usually occur in association with half of the primary contractions, although this relationship is variable and depends on the rate of gas formation. Reticulorumen contractions have an important influence on the flow of fluid and particulate matter through the rumen.

Gravity and reticulorumen motility combine to create the selective flow of particulate matter out of the rumen

Rumen ingesta are stratified and segregated by the effects of gravity and reticulorumen motility. In cattle receiving forage diets, there are distinct zones or phases of rumen ingesta. In the dorsal rumen there is a gas cap, or zone, created by the fermentation gases. Below this is a *solid zone* composed of intertwined particles of fermenting forage. The solid zone is sometimes referred to as the *rumen mat* because of the braided or woven nature of its particles. The solid zone is kept afloat by buoyancy created by air trapped in the feed particles and also by small bubbles of fermentation gases that form around bacteria that adhere to the plant material as fermentation takes place. At the bottom of the rumen there is a *liquid zone* with a water-like consistency. The area between the solid and liquid zones is the *slurry zone*. The

FIGURE 30–8. Contraction sequence in the reticulorumen. These drawings were derived by taking tracings directly from radiographs. The open regions represent the rumen gas cap, whereas the stippled region represents ingesta. The heavy lines indicate portions of the wall that are actively contracting. Drawings 1 through 16 represent the sequence of events in a primary contraction in a normally fed sheep. Drawings 17 through 21 represent the sequence of events in a secondary or eructation contraction. The individual drawings represent the following events: *1,* Resting stage. *2,* Initiation of sequence with elevation of reticuloruminal fold. *3,* End of first phase of reticular contraction. *4,* End of second phase of reticular contraction; note dilation of cranial sac. *5 to 7,* Contraction of cranial sac followed by contraction of cranial pillar and dorsal sac. *8,* Contraction of caudal-dorsal blind sac and caudal pillar, causing cranial displacement of gas cap toward reticulum, under cranial pillar, and into caudal-ventral blind sac. *9,* Contraction of longitudinal pillar and cranial ventral rumen; in anorectic sheep, the sequence frequently ceases at this point, and the occurrence of the remaining steps in the sequence varies according to the degree of filling of the reticulorumen. *10 to 12,* Wave of contraction migrating caudally onto the caudal-ventral blind sac, associated with a ventral displacement of the caudal pillar. *13,* Contraction of the pole of the caudal-ventral blind sac displacing gas cap around the caudal pillar. *14 to 16,* Cranial migration of contraction if no secondary contraction sequence occurs. *17,* When a secondary contraction follows a primary, the terminal contraction of the caudal-ventral blind sac may be maintained over a prolonged period or may be repeated simultaneously with a second contraction of the caudal pillar. *18,* Contraction of caudal pillar and dorsal blind sac start to push gas cap cranially; contraction starts to move cranially across caudal-ventral blind sac. *19,* Contraction has moved rapidly across dorsal rumen, and cranial pillar has moved for the second time; eructation, if it occurs, occurs at this point. *20 to 21,* Contraction migrates cranially onto ventral rumen, causing contraction of ventral coronary pillars and second ventral displacement of the caudal pillar; cycle terminates with a contraction of the cranial ventral rumen. (From Ruckebusch Y, Thivend P: Digestive Physiology and Metabolism in Ruminants. Westport, Conn.: AVI Publishing, 1980, p 40.)

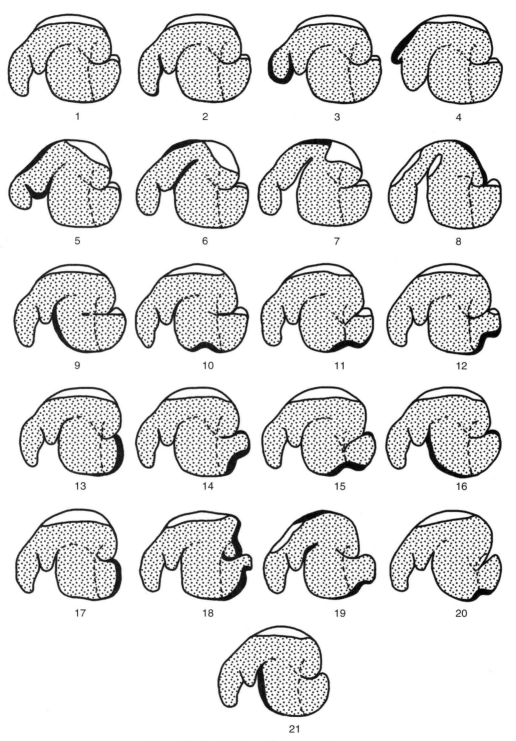

1

2

3

4

5

6

7

8

9

10

11

12

13

14

15

16

17

18

19

20

21

FIGURE 30–8 *See legend on opposite page*

slurry zone has indistinct boundaries and forms a continuum of consistency from the liquid to the solid zones. These four major zones are created primarily by the effect of gravity; two additional functional zones are created by the motility patterns. These are the *ejection zone* and the *zone of potential escape*, which constitute the dorsal and ventral areas, respectively, of the reticulum and cranial sac (Fig. 30–9).

Functional specific gravity determines the rate at which particulate matter (solids) moves through the zones of the reticulorumen

As forage is consumed by ruminants, the particles are only partially comminuted by the initial mastication and thus arrive at the reticulum as a tangled, masticated bolus of fairly long forage pieces. The bolus has a functional specific gravity of less than 1 because of air that is trapped both within and between the feed particles. (The term *functional* is applied to specific gravity in this context to indicate that the effects of trapped air are taken into consideration.) Because of the low specific gravity, the bolus floats in the ejection zone until a reticulum contraction occurs, when the pressure exerted by the reticular contraction washes, or ejects, the bolus from the reticulum into the solid zone of the dorsal sac.

In the dorsal sac, bacteria adhere to the forage particles, and fermentation begins. As fermentation proceeds, small bubbles of fermentation gases form and help keep the functional specific gravity of the particles low. Motility in the dorsal sac mixes ingesta in the solid zone in a counterclockwise (when viewed from the left side of the animal) circle Fig. 30–10). As the ingesta are mixed, the particles begin to break up because of fermentative destruction of structural carbohydrates in the plants. As fermentation pro-

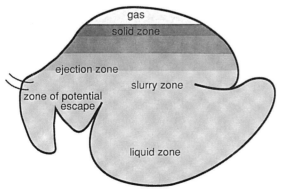

FIGURE 30–9. The rumen is stratified into indistinct zones, varying in consistency of ingesta. The dorsal solid zone contains relatively undigested forage material and continues imperceptibly into the slurry and liquid zones. The ejection zone, near the cardia, is the area that receives newly swallowed feed; contractions of the reticulum eject feed material from this area into the solid zone. As material becomes digested, it sinks into the liquid zone, eventually returning from the liquid zone to the cranial sac and reticulum. Once in the reticulum and cranial sac, material is in a zone of potential escape, from which it may enter the reticulo-omasal orifice.

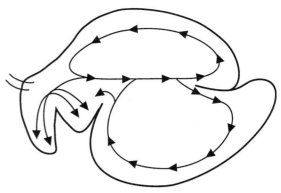

FIGURE 30–10. Patterns of movement of rumen ingesta. Rumen motility results in more or less circular patterns of ingesta movement. (From Ruckebusch Y, Thivend P: Digestive Physiology and Metabolism in Ruminants. Westport, Conn.: AVI Publishing, 1980, p 40.)

ceeds, particle size is reduced, entrapped air escapes, and there is a lower rate of fermentation gas formation. Because of these events, the functional specific gravity of the feed particles increases.

As functional specific gravity rises, particles tend to sink and separate into a slurry zone between the solid and liquid zones of the rumen, where further fermentation and size reduction occur. In the ventral sac, the motility pattern creates a clockwise movement of ingesta (see Fig. 30–10). As the flowing ingesta move against the cranial pillar of the rumen, material that still has a relatively low functional specific gravity tends to remain in suspension in the slurry zone and is retained in the circulating mass within the ventral sac. Material that has become relatively dense tends to fall over the cranial pillar and into the cranial sac, thus into the zone of potential escape. During contractions of the cranial sac, dense material can move into the reticulum, from which it can exit the rumen through the reticulo-omasal orifice.

One can appreciate the effectiveness of the particle separation system in the rumen by considering particle sizes at different points in the digestive process. Long forage material is reduced by initial mastication to particles of 1 to 2 cm or shorter. Most of the material in the dorsal rumen is of similar particle size. Particle size diminishes in the more ventral portions of the rumen. Most particles that move through the reticulo-omasal orifice are 2 to 3 mm long. The selection of small particles for passage into the omasum occurs even though the reticulo-omasal orifice, when dilated for food passage, is probably about 2 cm in diameter, indicating that size discrimination is not based on sieving action at the orifice.

Digestibility and physical characteristics of feed have important influences on both the rate of particle passage from the rumen and the rate of feed intake

As indicated by the earlier discussion, feed does not leave the rumen until it is broken down into small particles. Microbial action and remastication (as discussed later) are primarily responsible for particle size reduction in the rumen, and the rate of breakdown of fiber is chiefly a function of its digestibility. Poorly digestible fiber takes longer to be broken down sufficiently to enter the zone of potential escape compared with fiber of greater digestibility. This means that poorly digestible fiber remains in the rumen longer than fiber of greater digestibility. Because there are fixed limits to the volume of the rumen, the rate of feed intake cannot exceed the rate of ingesta outflow; therefore, intake of poorly digestible feeds is always less than intake of highly digestible feeds.

Feed preparation can influence this relationship. Chopping, or grinding, of poorly digestible forages increases their rate of passage from the rumen, because less particle size reduction is necessary before pieces can pass into the omasum. Chopping or grinding usually increases the amount of material that an animal can eat, because the rumen throughput is increased. Often, however, digestibility is decreased by chopping or grinding of forages, because the duration of exposure to microbial action is reduced as a result of rapid passage of feed through the rumen. Thus, physical form (length) and digestibility each has an effect on rate of passage from the rumen and also on feed intake. In general, forage material of relatively high digestibility has a rumen half-life of approximately 30 hours, whereas poorly digestible material has a half-life of up to 50 hours.

Rumination, or cud chewing, has an important effect on particle size reduction and the movement of solid material through the rumen

Rumination is the act of remasticating rumen ingesta. The initial act of rumination is regurgitation, which occurs just before the initiation of a primary rumen contraction. When regurgitation occurs, there is an extra contraction of the reticulum, which takes place just before the regular biphasic reticular contraction that initiates the primary cycle. Simultaneous with the extra reticular contraction, the cardia relaxes, and there is an inspiratory excursion of the ribs with the glottis closed. The latter action creates a negative pressure within the thorax, favoring the movement of food into the esophagus. When food enters the esophagus, a reverse peristaltic wave propels the material cranially into the mouth. As soon as the food bolus reaches the mouth, excess water is expressed by action of the tongue; the water is swallowed, and remastication of the material begins. The duration of remastication depends on the character of the diet, with coarse material appearing to require more time for remastication than finely ground or highly digestible feeds.

Regurgitated material for remastication comes from the dorsal portion of the reticulum, in which particle size and functional specific gravity are characteristic of the slurry zone. Thus, the ingesta selected for rumination are not the coarsest material in the rumen but, rather, are material that has already been through the digestive actions of the solid zone. This appears to be an efficient system in which some of the structural material of the plant is softened by soaking and removed or weakened by microbial action in the solid zone. The partially fermented material then reaches the slurry zone and is subjected to remastication, causing further comminution and exposing additional fermentable substrate that may not have been directly exposed to previous microbial action.

Rumination may also aid the particle separation process: as the regurgitated bolus reaches the mouth, it is squeezed by the tongue and cheeks before mastication begins. Water and small particles are expressed from the bolus by this squeezing action and are swallowed before mastication of the remaining bolus. Thus, this squeezing or expressing action tends to separate small particles from large particles. The small particles, when reswallowed, tend to sink into the zone of potential escape, whereas the larger particles, when swallowed after remastication, are ejected back into the slurry zone.

Rumination occurs during times when the animal is not actively eating, usually during times of rest, but not during deep sleep. The time spent ruminating depends on the type of diet and appears to range from almost none for high-grain diets to a maximum of about 10 hours per day for high-forage diets. The feed intake level also influences the amount of rumination time, with high intakes stimulating greater rumination.

Water moves through the rumen at a much faster rate than particulate matter

The flow of water has important effects on rumen dynamics. In order for small particles and soluble material to exit the rumen, liquid from the liquid zone of the ventral sac, cranial sac, and reticulum must constantly be moving through the reticulo-omasal orifice. This means that water must be constantly flowing through the mass of solid material. In effect, the reticulorumen functions like a giant strainer, holding the fermenting mass of particulate matter while water flows through it and washes small particles and soluble material away. Therefore, the transit rate of water must be considerably greater than the transit rate of particulate matter through the rumen. The relative differences in the rates of movement of solid-phase and liquid-phase material through the rumen can be appreciated from their respective rumen half-lives: 30 to 50 hours for particulate matter and about 15 to 20 hours for liquid.

The rate of liquid flow through the rumen is often measured as the dilution rate, which is expressed as the percentage of total liquid that leaves the rumen in an hour. The term *dilution rate* comes from the way liquid turnover is measured; some soluble marker substance is mixed into the rumen, and its concentration is measured as soon as it is thoroughly dispersed into the liquid phase. Then, samples are taken over time, and the rate at which the marker substance becomes diluted is measured. The rate of dilution depends on the rate at which water that contains marker leaves the rumen and is replaced with new, unmarked water; thus, the dilution rate is an indirect measure of the rate of water flow through the rumen. Normal dilution rate values vary with diet and feed intake and are usually in the range of 5% to 30% per hour. One other point should be appreciated from the concept of dilution rate: water leaves the rumen only as it is replaced from some other source.

Nearly all water that enters the rumen does so through the esophagus, from salivary flow, drinking, or succulent feeds. Thus, the dilution rate depends on rates of salivation and drinking. The salivation rate is influenced by the chewing time and feed type; feeds such as long-stemmed dry roughages, which require relatively high rates of mastication, stimulate high rates of both salivary flow and dilution. Salivation occurs during rumination as well as during initial mastication; therefore, those feeds that stimulate high rumination rates, such as forages, also stimulate high dilution rates. Conversely, feeds that do not stimulate extensive rumination, like concentrates, result in relatively low dilution rates. The rate of drinking is influenced by (1) the rate of feed intake and (2) the salt, or electrolyte, content of the diet. Thus, high rates of intake or diets with high electrolyte contents stimulate high dilution rates.

Little water enters the rumen by way of the mucosa. The mucosa of the forestomachs is stratified squamous epithelium and is aglandular; thus, there is no direct fluid secretion. Some water can enter the rumen through osmosis, but under normal conditions, the amount appears to be little. Normal rumen osmolality is about 280 mosm/kg, compared with a normal of approximately 300 mosm/kg in blood and extracellular fluid. Thus, the usual osmotic flow of water is out of the rumen. After consumption of relatively digestible feeds, rumen osmolality increases briefly because of VFA production; however, it appears that osmolalities in excess of 340 mosm/kg are necessary for water to flow osmotically into the rumen. Under normal conditions, osmolalities this high are not sustained for long, and thus, there is usually little osmotic flow of water into the rumen.

Rumen dilution rate has important influences on fermentation and microbial cell yield

Small particles, including microbes, leave the rumen with the liquid phase. Therefore, high dilution rates result in rapid removal of microbes and reductions in microbial cell concentrations. Because high microbe concentrations suppress microbial cell division, the growth of microbes is stimulated by high dilution rates. High growth rates are nutritionally desirable, because a larger portion of the energy available to the microbes is used for growth instead of for maintenance, as occurs in older, relatively stable microbial populations. Thus, high dilution rates usually increase Y_{ATP} values, provided that adequate protein is available to support cell growth.

In addition to its effect on Y_{ATP}, the dilution rate may affect the microbial makeup of the rumen biomass and also may have some influence on the fermentation pattern. The rate of microbial washout increases with the dilution rate. At high dilution rates, microbial species with slow growth rates diminish in population size, because their replication rate is not great enough to match the rate at which they are removed. Thus, selection pressure favors species with faster growth rates during times of high rumen dilution rates. Exceptions to this pattern occur, because some microbes are able to attach themselves to the particulate matter in the solid and slurry zones. Such microbes then exit the rumen according to the kinetics of particle size reduction rather than dilution rate. In general, the changes occurring in the rumen microbial population with high dilution rates appear to favor acetic acid production and to increase the acetic acid/propionic acid ratio.

CONTROL OF RETICULORUMEN MOTILITY

Reticulorumen motility is controlled by the central nervous system and affected by intraluminal conditions

In the dorsal vagal nucleus of the brainstem, there is a motility control center for the regulation of reticulo-ruminal motility. This center sends action potentials along afferent fibers to the forestomach by way of the vagus nerve. There is an extensive intrinsic nervous system within the reticulorumen, but vagal innervation is necessary for coordination of normal motility patterns. When the vagal nerves are destroyed, motility of the rumen musculature ceases initially but returns within several days; however, the motility that develops after vagotomy is erratic, uncoordinated, and incapable of supporting the normal flow of ingesta through the reticulorumen. Vagotomized ruminants do not survive.

The dorsal vagal nucleus receives afferent stimuli that affect the control of forestomach motility. Important afferent signals come from the lumen of the reticulorumen and monitor distention, ingesta consistency, pH, VFA concentration, and ionic strength. Rumen volume, or distention, appears to be monitored by stretch receptors in the walls and, especially, in the pillars. Moderate distention increases rumen motility and rumination. Increased motility and rumination have the effect of raising the rate at which particles are broken down, leading to a higher passage rate. Thus, rumen throughput is enhanced when increased intake expands rumen volume. Severe distention, as occurs pathologically in bloat, causes cessation of rumen motility.

The consistency of ingesta also has an important influence on rumen motility. Consistency is determined largely by diet type. When the diet consists of succulent plants, grain, or finely chopped forage, there is little material in the solid zone, or rumen mat, and the slurry zone is fluid. This type of fluid ingesta offers little resistance to the movement of the rumen pillars; thus, the rumen musculature has to apply relatively little force to mix and circulate the rumen contents. Tension receptors in the reticuloruminal muscle appear to monitor the force necessary to move the pillars through the ingesta. Highly fluid rumen ingesta are associated with low muscle tension and have a negative influence on reticulorumen motility. At the other dietary extreme, when animals are eating dry, long-stem hay, the rumen contents are solid and create a large and highly interwoven rumen mat. Resistance to movement of the pillars through the solid mass of ingesta is high and leads to stimulation of tension receptors, resulting in a positive feedback on motility. The motility rate is directly related to the rate of particle breakdown; this arrangement appears to be a self-regulatory mechanism that increases the rate of particle comminution when animals consume diets with large particle size.

Chemoreceptors appear to exist in the walls of the rumen and reticulum. These receptors monitor pH, VFA concentration, and ionic strength (or osmolality). The pH of the reticulorumen is normally slightly acid, reflecting the acidity of the VFAs, but extreme acid conditions are undesirable. Increasing VFA concentrations or decreasing pH results in a suppression of rumen motility. The normal rumen pH is in the range of 5.5 to 6.8, depending on the type of diet. When the rumen pH falls much below 5.0, motility is severely depressed. This response appears to be protective, because fermentation tends to be enhanced by motility-induced mixing; thus, suppression of motility slows down fermentation, allowing VFA absorption to catch up with VFA production.

Osmolality may influence rumen motility also, although motility appears less sensitive to osmotic changes than it does to pH changes. Normal osmolality in the rumen is about 280 mosm, but the osmolality increases during active fermentation. Osmotically active solutes in the rumen include organic acids as well as salivary and dietary electrolytes. As organic acid formation increases during fermentation, osmolality increases also, tending to reduce motility. The rumen epithelium creates a relatively impermeable barrier to water, so that wide swings in rumen osmolality can occur without large shifts in water between the rumen and the vascular compartment. At abnormally high osmolalities, however, water can be drawn into the rumen.

OMASAL FUNCTION

Passage of material from the reticulum to the omasum occurs during reticular contraction

The omasum is composed of a body and a canal. The body is filled with multiple muscular folds, or *leaves*, that project from the greater curvature into the lumen. The canal, which is located on the lesser curvature, connects the reticulum to the abomasum. Ingesta move into the omasum during reticular contractions. The omasal orifice usually remains open, but dilates especially during the second phase of the reticular contraction, during which ingesta flows rapidly into the omasal canal. After the reticular contraction, the omasal orifice closes briefly as the canal contracts, forcing newly arrived ingesta up into the leaves. Intermittently, the body and leaves of the omasum contract, forcing the material from the body of the organ into the canal and on into the abomasum.

Proper functioning of the omasum and reticulum appears to be particularly important to the passage of ingesta out of the rumen. Occasionally, traumatic injury due to ingested foreign bodies causes severe adhesions of the reticulum and omasum to the body wall. In addition, damage to vagal fibers entering the organs may occur. In such cases, motility of the rumen proper may continue normally, but the ability to move food out of the forestomachs and into the abomasum is severely impaired. The rumen becomes greatly distended with finely comminuted feed, and the entire rumen becomes a slurry zone. In spite of the distended rumen, there is little movement of ingesta into the abomasum, and the animals eventually suffer severe inanition. This condition is variably known as *omasal transport failure* and vagal indigestion; usually, little can be done to correct it.

The structure of the omasum, with its many leaves and large mucosal surface area, suggests that it has an absorptive function, but the exact nature of this function is still incompletely understood. One important possibility is that it exists to remove residual VFAs and bicarbonate from ingesta before material is transported to the abomasum. VFAs appear to cause unfavorable reactions in the abomasum, so it is important that the major portion of them be removed before abomasal entry. Also, it appears desirable to absorb, before abomasal entry, any bicarbonate remaining in the ingesta. Bicarbonate remaining in ingesta and entering the abomasum would only neutralize abomasal hydrochloric acid, making the abomasal glands work harder to maintain appropriate abomasal pH.

VOLATILE FATTY ACID ABSORPTION

Volatile fatty acids, representing 60% to 80% of the energy needs of the animal, are absorbed directly from the forestomach epithelium

VFAs are bacterial waste products and, if allowed to accumulate, will suppress fermentation. Furthermore, the VFAs are tremendously important energy substrates for the host, supplying 60% to 80% of the dietary energy to ruminants with most types of diets. Therefore, it is important, from the standpoint of both digestion and host metabolism, that an efficient and high-capacity mechanism for VFA absorption be present. The forestomach epithelium supplies such a system, absorbing nearly all the VFAs, with only small amounts escaping to the lower digestive tract. In addition, the absorptive process helps maintain rumen pH by removing acid from the forestomach ingesta and contributing bicarbonate in the process.

The epithelium responsible for this tremendous absorption is structurally much different from other absorptive epithelia of the gastrointestinal system. However, there is an interesting nature to the rumen epithelium that may impart to it functional characteristics similar to those of the absorptive epithelium of the small intestine and colon. The forestomach surface is of the stratified squamous type and, like the stratified squamous epithelium of the skin and other surfaces, consists of several layers of cells of varying maturity. The deepest layer is the *stratum basale,* from which cells divide and migrate into the *stratum spinosum.* Cells of the stratum spinosum begin the process of keratinization and continue into the *stratum granulosum,* which is covered by the outermost and most keratinized layer, the *stratum corneum.* Although the forestomach epithelium is seemingly completely different from the columnar epithelium of the small intestine, an interesting similarity between forestomach and intestinal epithelia is noted when the cellular attachments and intercellular spaces of the forestomach are examined (Fig. 30–11).

The cells of the stratum granulosum are tightly joined by junctions that may functionally resemble

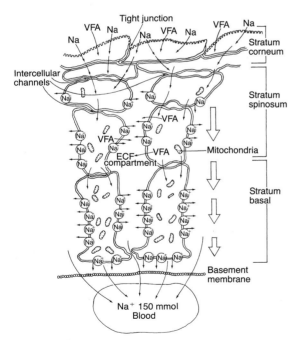

FIGURE 30–11. The stratified squamous epithelium of the rumen, although anatomically much different, shares functional similarities with the columnar epithelium of the intestine. Note the tight junctions of the cells of the stratum corneum and the lateral space–like compartment between adjacent cells of the stratum spinosum and stratum basale. Although the cells of the stratum spinosum are metabolically inactive, the intercellular channels allow the metabolic actions of the stratum basale to be reflected in the more superficial layers. VFA, volatile fatty acid; Na, sodium; ECF, extracellular fluid. (Modified from Steven DH, Marshall AB: Organization of the rumen epithelium. In Phillipson AT [ed]: Physiology of Digestion and Metabolism in the Ruminant. Newcastle upon Tyne, U.K.: Oriel Press, 1970, p 98.)

the tight junctions of the enterocytes (see Chapter 29 for a description of enterocyte tight junctions). Deeper in the epithelium, the cells of the stratum spinosum and stratum basale are separated by intercellular spaces that increase in size as the basement membrane is approached. These intercellular spaces are reminiscent of the lateral spaces of columnar absorptive epithelia. If these observations are combined with the existence of the intercellular bridges that characterize the forestomach epithelium, an interesting analogy to columnar absorptive epithelia can be constructed. VFAs, electrolytes, and water apparently are initially absorbed through the stratum corneum and passed cell to cell by way of intercellular bridges to the cells of the stratum spinosum and stratum basale, from which the absorbed substances are passed into the intercellular spaces before entering the capillaries.

This arrangement of the forestomach epithelium is very similar to the three-compartment characteristics of the columnar absorptive epithelia, with solutes passing from lumen to cell to lateral spaces. Although the keratinized cells of the stratum corneum do not appear to retain adequate metabolic machinery (mitochondria and so forth) to maintain appropriate gradients for diffusion, the cells of the stratum spinosum and stratum basale do seem to be metabolically active. Because of the intercellular bridges, absorbed solute can be transferred directly from the outer keratinized cells to the deeper, more metabolically active cells. Thus, the metabolic activity deep in the epithelium appears to maintain conditions for absorption at the epithelial surface.

The molecular mechanism of VFA absorption is incompletely understood but seems to involve local alterations in pH near the absorptive surface. Differences in pH can have an important influence on VFA absorption because of shifts in the dissociation state of the VFA molecules. The pKa of the VFA is approximately 4.8, well below the normal pH of the rumen; thus, most of the VFAs exist in the rumen in the dissociated, or ionic, form. However, sodium-hydrogen ion exchange by the epithelial cells may decrease the local pH at the absorptive surface. Such a drop in pH would lead to a shift in the VFA from the ionic to the free-acid state. Cell membranes are permeable to VFA free acids, and absorption proceeds because of the concentration gradient between the lumen and cells. The high CO_2 tension in the rumen, due to the production of fermentation gases, may also enhance the conversion of VFA to the free-acid state. As shown in Figure 30–12, when one VFA molecule is absorbed, one molecule of bicarbonate is generated in the lumen; thus, VFA absorption helps buffer rumen pH both by generating base and by removing acid.

All the VFAs appear to be absorbed by the same mechanism, but they are handled differently within the epithelial cells. Some acetate seems to be completely oxidized within the cells, with the remainder absorbed unchanged. Most propionate is absorbed, but a small portion is converted to lactate by the epithelial cells. Butyrate is modified extensively, and essentially all molecules are changed to β-hydroxybutyrate before absorption. β-Hydroxybutyrate is an im-

LUMEN CELL BLOOD

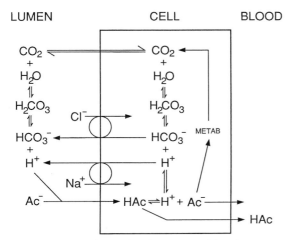

FIGURE 30–12. VFA absorption is promoted by the conversion of VFA anions (Ac⁻) to free acids (HAc) in the microenvironment near the epithelial surface. This diagram illustrates two proposed means, one intracellular and one extracellular, by which hydrogen ions could be locally generated to effect the formation of VFA free acids; both mechanisms could exist simultaneously. (From Stevens CE, Argenzio RA, Roberts MC: Comparative physiology of mammalian colon and suggestions for animal models of human disorders. Clin Gastroenterol 15:763, 1986.)

portant metabolite that is known as a *ketone body.* Ketone bodies are metabolites that frequently have special medical significance and are discussed in greater detail in Chapter 31. It is important to point out here that in ruminants, the rumen itself is a significant source of ketone bodies. In monogastric animals, however, ketone bodies arise exclusively from the partial oxidation of long-chain fatty acids.

The rumen epithelium is arranged in *papillae,* finger-like projections that increase the absorptive surface area. Although they serve the same area-expanding function as the villi of the small intestine, papillae are much larger and easily visible to the unaided eye. The size and shape of the papillae are quite dynamic and responsive to changes in diet. Papillary growth is stimulated by VFAs, especially butyrate and propionate. Diets with high digestibility result in high rumen VFA concentrations, which stimulate the growth of long papillae. In contrast, animals receiving little feed or diets of low digestibility have short rumen papillae. It is important to adapt ruminants gradually when changing them from diets of low digestibility to those of high digestibility. Part of the reason for this may be to allow time for sufficient adjustment of papillary size, so that VFA absorption will match VFA production.

RUMEN DEVELOPMENT AND ESOPHAGEAL GROOVE FUNCTION

Tremendous changes in forestomach size and function occur with dietary changes in early life

At birth, the forestomach is about equal in size to the abomasum in both lambs and calves, a stark contrast

to the normal adult proportions, in which the forestomach accounts for more than 90% of the total stomach volume. Enlargement of the forestomach occurs rapidly after birth, but the rate depends on diet type. When young ruminants are given access to solid feeds soon after birth, the forestomach development rate is maximal.

In cattle, the period of forestomach development is arbitrarily divided into the nonruminant period, from birth to 3 weeks, and the transitional period, from 3 to 8 weeks. Approximate adult distribution of stomach proportions is achieved usually by 8 weeks, if the calves have access to solid feeds. Calves can be seen eating grain and forage as early as 2 weeks of age and are frequently seen to ruminate by 3 weeks, indicating considerable forestomach development by this time. Withholding solid feed dramatically reduces the rate of rumen development. In calves that are given diets of only milk or milk substitute ("replacer"), forestomach development remains rudimentary for 14 to 15 weeks or longer.

Development of forestomach epithelium parallels the general development of the organ. At birth, the epithelium is thin, with small or nonexistent papillae. Exposure of the epithelium to VFAs appears to stimulate papillary development and general organ development as well. Highly digestible feeds, such as concentrates, result in the greatest VFA production and fastest epithelial development. Some dietary forage may aid in muscular development of the forestomachs, but calves and lambs in the transitional period should receive most of their solid feed as grain, because their energy needs are high compared with their ability to ferment forages.

The forestomach is sterile at birth but is quickly colonized by environmental bacteria, mostly facultative organisms. As bacterial fermentation proceeds in the anaerobic confines of the forestomach, the electromotive force, becomes low, as the typical reductive environment of the rumen is created by bacterial action. This environment creates conditions necessary for the growth and establishment of the strict anaerobes. The development of forestomach bacterial flora occurs independently of any special inoculation process, and indeed, it is impossible to prevent it from occurring except by raising calves under gnotobiotic conditions. Protozoal inoculation, in contrast to bacterial inoculation, seems to require some exposure to other cattle: calves raised in complete isolation do not develop protozoal fauna. It appears that aerosol spread of protozoa can occur, because no direct physical contact among cattle is necessary to establish a protozoal fauna.

The esophageal groove diverts the flow of ingested milk past the forestomach and into the abomasum

For proper rumen development in the suckling animal, it is important for milk to be diverted away from the developing rumen. This is accomplished by the actions of the *reticular groove* (also called the *esophageal groove*). This structure is a gutter-like invagination traversing the wall of the reticulum from the cardia to the reticulo-omasal orifice. When stimulated, muscles of the groove contract, causing it to shorten and twist. The twisting action causes the lips of the groove to close together, forming a nearly complete tube from the cardia to the omasal canal. Milk entering the cardia when the groove is contracted is directed into the omasum, with 10% or less entering the rumen. Milk quickly traverses the omasum and enters the abomasum. Reticular groove closure is a reflex action, with efferent impulses arriving from the brainstem through the vagus nerve. Afferent stimuli arise centrally and from the pharynx. Anticipation of suckling invokes central stimulation of reticular groove closure, which may be considered a cephalic phase. Fluid, especially sodium-containing fluid in the pharynx, stimulates afferent fibers that reinforce the cephalic phase of groove closure. The posture of the calf or lamb when suckling does not appear to have a large influence on reticular groove function, but rapid drinking from an open pail, in contrast to suckling from a nipple, frequently results in inefficient groove function and spillage of milk into the rumen. Milk in the rumen results in the formation of improper fermentation patterns.

The reticular groove has its primary function in suckling animals, and the activity of the groove reflex appears to diminish after weaning and with advancing age. However, the groove reflex is stimulated by antidiuretic hormone (see Chapter 42), indicating that it may have some physiologic function in adult life. Antidiuretic hormone is secreted by the posterior pituitary in response to dehydration or increases in plasma osmolality. Antidiuretic hormone is associated with thirst, and because it stimulates the reticular groove, a large portion of the water drunk by water-deprived animals may bypass the rumen. This may be a functional mechanism to ensure that water arrives quickly at the site of most rapid absorption, the small intestine.

FUNCTION OF THE EQUINE LARGE HINDGUT

The equine hindgut has a tremendous capacity for fermentation

A general function of the cecum and colon, as mentioned in Chapter 29, is to recover fluid and electrolytes from ingesta leaving the ileum. In many herbivorous species, this function has been expanded to include fermentative digestion. Absorptive and fermentation functions complement each other in the colons of nonruminant herbivores. This arrangement leads to an elegantly interactive system of fermentation and absorption; however, it also results in an interdependence between the two processes, meaning that disturbances in fermentation can result in important abnormalities in absorption, and vice versa.

The types of substrate and fermentation patterns are essentially identical for forestomach and hindgut fermentation

Structural and nonstructural carbohydrates as well as proteins form the major substrates for hindgut fermentation. However, the passage of material through the stomach and small intestine before its arrival at the cecum and colon may have some important effects on fermentative digestion. First, hindgut fermentation may be aided by prior gastric action. The effects of soaking and acid exposure on plant particles in the stomach may increase their susceptibility to microbial attack and, thus, raise their rate of digestion in the hindgut. Second, some of the readily available carbohydrate, particularly sugars and starches, may be digested and absorbed before the other material arrives in the cecum. Most evidence indicates, however, that glandular digestion of carbohydrate in the horse is not extremely efficient and that substantial amounts of starch and sugars reach the cecum. Further, cell-wall carbohydrate appears to interfere with the digestion or absorption of nonstructural carbohydrate, so that diets high in cell-wall content result in relatively little starch digestion and absorption in the equine small intestine. Even with a high-grain diet, up to 29% of dietary starch may reach the cecum and colon.

Protein as well as carbohydrate is absorbed in the small intestine, potentially leading to a deficiency of nitrogen for colonic microbes. However, there is extensive urea recycling into the colon and cecum similar to that occurring in the rumen (see Fig. 30–6). Thus, urea plus protein escaping small intestinal digestion supplies the nitrogen needs of the microbes. In contrast to ruminants, horses do not have an efficient means of recovering the microbial protein synthesized in the hindgut, and most of it passes out in the feces. Some experiments have shown a small amount of amino acid absorption from the equine cecum or colon, but the amount does not compare with microbial protein availability in the ruminant.

The motility functions of the cecum and colon retain material for fermentation and separate particles by size

The functions of the equine hindgut in maintaining fermentation are similar to those of the rumen: favorable conditions must be maintained to support optimal fermentation. As in the rumen, these conditions are (1) substrate supply, (2) control of pH and osmolality, (3) anaerobiosis, (4) retention of fermenting material, and (5) continual removal of waste products and the residue of spent fermentation substrate. Separation of fermenting material from residue appears to be accomplished by selective retention of particles according to size, just as in the rumen; however, the means by which the cecum and colon accomplish size separation and discriminate passage are quite different from those of the forestomach. Anatomic characteristics and motility patterns in the cecum and colon are responsible for selective retention of long particles, allowing sufficient exposure for microbial digestion to occur. In general, the fermentative digestive process in the horse is not as efficient as that in the ruminant, and digestible energy values for forages are usually lower for horses than for cattle.

Before the motility of the equine cecum and colon is discussed, a brief review of the anatomy of the equine hindgut is important. A diagram of the equine digestive system, separated from its mesenteric attachments and laid out in a linear fashion, is shown in Figure 30–13. The hindgut commences with the cecum, which is separated from the large colon by a well-defined orifice. The large colon is folded on itself three times, forming four major anatomic divisions: the *right* and *left ventral* and the *left* and *right dorsal colon* segments. Ingesta enter the right ventral colon and course to the left ventral colon, from which the material enters the left dorsal portion through the *pelvic flexure*. From the left dorsal colon, material moves to the right dorsal colon before entering the small colon. A description of the arrangement of the large colon in the abdomen can be found in textbooks of anatomy. For the purposes of physiologic study, the reader should note in Figure 30–13 the tremendous size and volume of the cecum and colon compared with the small intestine. The differences in diameter that occur throughout the colon should also

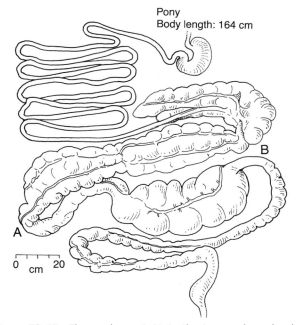

FIGURE 30–13. The equine gut. Note the tremendous development of the colon, compared with the small intestine. Note also the relative areas of constriction at the junctions of the ventral and dorsal colons (A) and the large and small colons (B). (From Stevens CE: Comparative physiology of the digestive system. In Swenson MJ [ed]: Dukes' Physiology of Domestic Animals, 9th ed. Ithaca, NY: Cornell University Press, 1977. Used by permission of the publisher, Cornell University Press.)

be noted, particularly the reductions in diameter that occur at the pelvic flexure and at the junction of the large and small colons. The sac-like evaginations that occur in the wall of the cecum and most segments of the colon are called *haustra*. Functionally, the equine hindgut can be divided into four sections: cecum, ventral colon, dorsal colon, and small colon.

Ingesta reach the cecum after a relatively short time in the stomach and small intestine. A large portion of soluble ingesta usually reaches the cecum by 2 hours after ingestion, whereas solids take somewhat longer, depending on particle size and consistency. The material in the cecum and throughout the large colon has a high water content and a slurry-like consistency.

The majority of cecal motility is of a mixing nature, with frequent low-amplitude contractions that transport ingesta from haustrum to haustrum and back in a mixing pattern. The mixing action of the cecum maintains the cecal contents in a homogeneous state. About once every 3 to 4 minutes, there is a strong contraction of cecal muscles in a mass-movement type of action (see Chapter 27 for a description of *mass movement*) in which the *body* and *apex* of the organ shorten and constrict, lifting ingesta into the *base*. Constriction of the base forces material through the *cecocolic* orifice and into the right ventral colon. The motility pattern functionally separates the cecum from the ventral colon with no apparent mixing of contents between the two hindgut segments. Thus, there is no retrograde flow of material from the colon to the cecum, so the composition of ingesta in these two organs usually differs somewhat.

Three types of motility patterns exist in the right and left ventral colon: haustral segmentation, propulsive peristalsis, and retropulsive peristalsis. Segmentation serves a mixing function that aids in promoting fermentation and bringing VFAs in contact with the mucosa for absorption. Mixing occurs throughout the ventral colon, and the right and left segments may be regarded as one functional unit with homogeneous ingesta. Propulsive activity, or aboral peristalsis, in the ventral colon originates near the cecum and appears to occur as a continuation of the cecal mass movements. Peristaltic activity in the proximal ventral colon propels ingesta distally into the left ventral colon. In the left ventral colon, retropulsive or antiperistaltic movements are encountered, which resist the flow of ingesta and result in the retention of material in the ventral colon, allowing time for microbial digestion and preventing the washout of microbes. In addition, the retropulsive actions of the left ventral colon aid in creating differential flow rates of liquid and particulate matter through the colon. The antiperistaltic motility appears to originate from a pacemaker in the *pelvic flexure*, the area of restricted diameter where the left ventral and dorsal colons meet.

The motility of the ventral colon can be roughly compared with that of the stomach, with the pelvic flexure and distal left ventral colon acting as the pylorus and antrum, respectively. The pumping action of cecal mass movements, combined with the propulsive action of the proximal ventral colon, continually moves ingesta toward the pelvic flexure. In the distal ventral colon, however, antiperistaltic activity and the narrow diameter of the pelvic flexure retard the movement of material, causing it to be retained in the ventral colon. The squeezing action of the pelvic flexure mimics the action of the pylorus in selectively retaining relatively large particulate matter while allowing liquid and small particles to pass. As particle size is reduced by fermentative action and the mixing activity of the colon, particles eventually become small enough to flow with the fluid phase and leave the colon. The action of the pelvic flexure is not as efficient as that of the pylorus, and some large particles do escape the ventral colon. In addition, there are periods during which propulsive movements occur in the left ventral colon and pelvic flexure. These factors allow the movement of particulate matter into the left dorsal colon.

The actions of the dorsal colon appear to mimic those of the ventral colon. Impedance to ingesta flow

is created by the size restriction at the junction of the right dorsal colon and small colon. In addition, there may be retropulsive motility originating in the area of the distal right dorsal colon, near the junction with the small colon. These actions tend to impede the movement of ingesta through the dorsal colon, subjecting the material to another round of fermentative digestion, as occurred in the ventral colon. The delay in the flow of ingesta created by the combined actions of the ventral and dorsal colons results in significant retention of material, with most particulate matter taking from 24 to 96 hours to pass the large colon. The efficiency of the large colon in retaining and separating ingesta of different particle sizes can be understood from Figure 30–14.

Understanding the motility of the equine colon is important, because problems of colon impaction in horses are common. Impactions usually occur near or within the pelvic flexure, probably because the pelvic flexure is a site of flow restriction and differential flow of solid and liquid material. It is easy to imagine

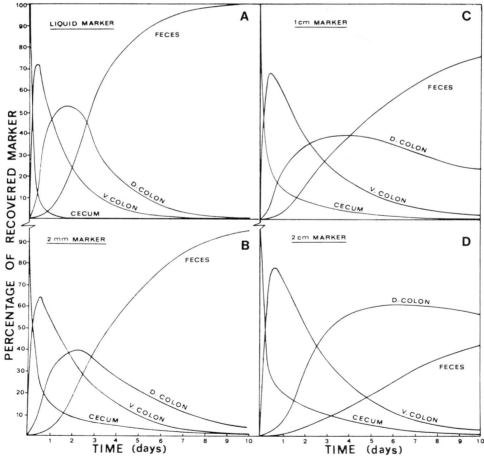

FIGURE 30–14. Retention of liquid and particles of various sizes in the compartments of the equine large intestine. Marker liquid *(A)* and marked particles of various sizes *(B,* 2 mm; *C,* 1 cm; *D,* 2 cm) were placed in the cecum of ponies, and the distribution of marked materials among colon segments was measured at 2-hour intervals. The lines of the graph were mathematically fitted to the data. Each line indicates the percentage of marker in a given segment at any time. Note in graph *A* that at 7 days after infusion, nearly all of the liquid marker had been recovered in the feces, with little or none remaining in the intestinal segments. Increasing particle size has a relatively small effect on the movement of particles out of the cecum. In contrast, as particle size increases, there is significant retention of material in the colon and slow passage to the feces. D, dorsal; V, ventral. (From Argenzio RA, Lowe JE, Pickard DW, et al: Digesta passage and water exchange in the equine large intestine. Am J Physiol 226:1035–1042, 1974.)

how the normal motility pattern could allow solid material to accumulate in this area and cause obstructions.

The general understanding of small colon motility is limited, but it appears to consist primarily of segmentation and propulsion. The characteristic fecal balls of horses are formed by segmentation within the small colon.

The rate of fermentation and volatile fatty acid production in the equine colon is similar to that in the rumen

In the equine colon, efficient means of buffering and VFA absorption must be present. Salivary buffering, as occurs in ruminants, cannot aid in buffering the colon, because of the changes in ingesta pH that occur during transit through the stomach and small intestine. In the horse, large quantities of fluid, rich in bicarbonate and phosphate buffers, are secreted by the ileum and transferred to the cecum, thus mimicking the actions of the salivary glands in ruminants. In addition, because of the glandular nature of the colonic mucosa, there is more direct addition of bicarbonate and other electrolytes to the lumen fluid in the cecum and colon than in the rumen.

Large fluxes of water traverse the cecal and colonic mucosa during the course of digestion. When horses are meal-fed, feed starts to enter the cecum about 2 hours after eating, and VFA production rapidly commences. As ingesta are transported from the cecum, VFA production continues in the large colon. During the period of active VFA production, large quantities of water enter the hindgut from the blood through the mucosa. Although this water flux may be a response to increased osmolality created by the generation of osmotically active VFA molecules, it is more likely a response to direct fluid secretion from the crypts of the colonic epithelium (see Chapter 28 for a description of colonic epithelium). Secretion of sodium-, bicarbonate-, and chloride-containing fluid from the colonic mucosa appears to occur in response to high concentrations of VFA in the lumen. This secretory response, in combination with the ileal secretions, is responsible for buffering of the lumen contents. Figure 30–15 illustrates the magnitude of water fluxes that occur during hindgut digestion in the pony. Note that there is considerable inward and outward movement of water across the mucosa in each of the major fermentation compartments, ventral and dorsal colons, and cecum. Inward (into the lumen) water movement results from mucosal secretion, whereas outward water movement occurs in association with absorption of VFA.

The molecular mechanisms of VFA absorption in the equine colon appear to be identical to those in the rumen (see Fig. 30–12). Note in Figure 30–12 that sodium absorption accompanies VFA absorption and that bicarbonate is generated in the lumen. The absorption of VFA and sodium leads to osmotic absorption of water, probably through the transcellular path-

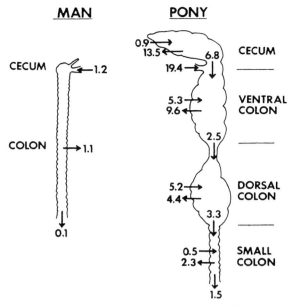

FIGURE 30–15. Net movement of water through the large intestine of a 70-kg man and a 160-kg pony. Values are in liters per day. Note the relatively large amount of fluid delivered to the pony's colon from the ileum (19.4 L/day), compared with humans. Also note the inward and outward movement of fluid in the various compartments of the pony's large intestine. (From Argenzio RA, Lowe JE, Pickard DW, Stevens CE: Digesta passage and water exchange in the equine large intestine. Am J Physiol 226:1035–1042, 1974.)

way. The dynamics of water and electrolyte absorption in the gut may be reviewed in Chapter 29.

The function of the small colon is to recover water, electrolytes, and VFAs that were not absorbed in the large colon. There appears to be little VFA production in the small colon, but considerable absorption of water, sodium, and phosphate occurs there.

The large water and electrolyte fluxes that occur in the colon make horses vulnerable to colonic diseases. Colonic disease in the horse has consequences in terms of fluid and electrolyte loss that are more characteristic of small intestinal disease in many other animals.

There are tremendous variations in hindgut anatomy and function among the many species of veterinary interest

All the variations in hindgut anatomy and function among the species cannot be discussed here, but it should be remembered that in addition to Equidae, rabbits, rats, guinea pigs, swine, and some large birds depend on hindgut fermentation for a significant portion of their energy needs. It must also be appreciated that ruminants have a reasonably extensive hindgut and that fermentative digestion occurs there, even after material has been through the rumen.

The basic scientific understanding of colonic function in general is not as advanced as that of small intestinal function. This dichotomy probably exists because in humans, problems of the small intestine occur as more important and life-threatening diseases than do problems of the colon. However, interest in colonic physiology and pathophysiology has increased among basic scientists and physicians. Veterinary physiologists have long been interested in colonic function and have become leaders in the exploration of this area.

CLINICAL CORRELATIONS

Grain engorgement toxemia

History In mid-January, a cattle feeder has asked you to examine a feedlot full of 400-kg steers. The steers have been on free-choice grain from a self-feeder for several weeks. Three days ago, a blizzard prevented the caretaker from delivering feed to the feeders, and they were empty for 36 hours. Yesterday, the feeders were filled, and all the steers ate ravenously. Today, 2 of the 40 steers are dead, and many appear lethargic and uncoordinated and have diarrhea.

Clinical and laboratory examination Two steers are isolated for physical examination. They are lethargic and have to be coaxed to move. Their heart rates are all above 100 bpm (normal, <80 bpm), and their body temperatures are less than 101.0°F (normal, 101.5 to 103.0°F). Their rumens appear distended, and there is no evidence of rumen motility. The eyes are sunken in the orbits, and the oral mucosa is dry and sticky, indicating clinical dehydration. Necropsy examination of a dead steer reveals a greatly distended rumen filled with grain and fluid. A pH-paper test indicates that the rumen fluid pH of the dead animal is below 4.5, but above 3 (normal, 5.5 to 7.0).

Comment Ruminants may be fed large amounts of grain if they are accustomed to it and receive it on a regular and frequent basis. In this case, even though the steers had been accustomed to a high-grain diet, the lack of grain for more than a day followed by a large grain intake set up conditions for grain engorgement toxemia.

In grain engorgement, there is an abundant supply of starch, leading to the rapid growth and proliferation of rumen streptococci. These bacteria produce VFA rapidly, causing the rumen pH to diminish. As the rumen pH becomes lower, conditions become unfavorable for the growth and survival of cellulose-fermenting organisms and favorable for the growth of lactic acid–producing bacteria. This leads to the accumulation of lactic acid, a stronger acid than the VFAs. Thus, rumen pH becomes even lower, killing many of the normal microflora. Some of the lactic acid is absorbed, leading to a reduced blood pH and a life-threatening situation. Moreover, the large ruminal concentration of lactic acid and VFA results in a high osmotic pressure, drawing water out of the vascular fluid compartment and into the rumen. This leads to systemic hypovolemia, which may proceed to hypovolemic shock.

Treatment This is a grave situation, and it is likely that the farmer will lose additional steers. Treatment is aimed at expanding the intravascular fluid volume, correcting the systemic acidosis, and reestablishing a normal ru-

men environment. Severely affected steers should be evaluated to determine whether their prognosis is good enough to warrant the expense of therapy: if not, euthanasia should be employed. Initial treatment should consist of rapid intravenous administration of large quantities of alkalizing fluid. After the correction of fluid and acid-base disturbances, ideally the rumen should be emptied, either by intubation with a large-bore stomach tube or by rumenotomy. In some cases, oral administration of an antifermentation agent, such as oil of turpentine, mineral oil, or an antibiotic, along with an alkalizing agent, is an acceptable alternative to emptying the rumen. After the rumen environment is brought back to normal, it may be helpful to re-inoculate the rumen with material taken from the rumen of a normal animal.

Impaction colic

History You are presented with a 20-year-old gelding that has been showing signs of abdominal discomfort (colic) for 16 hours. When left alone in his stall, the horse lies down, frequently preferring to lie on his back. There is little fresh manure in the stall. When taken out of the stall, the gelding leads normally but then lies down and rolls whenever he is released from the lead rope.

Clinical and laboratory examination The heart rate is slightly elevated, at 60 bpm; respiratory rate and temperature are normal. The hydration state, as well as the color and perfusion of the mucous membranes, is normal. Simple laboratory evaluation reveals the packed cell volume to be 41% (normal, 35% to 45%) and the plasma total solids to be 7.8 g/dL (normal, 6.5 to 8.0 g/dL). Borborygmi (intestinal sounds) are softer and less frequent than normal, especially on the left side. Examination by rectal palpation reveals the pelvic flexure to be firm with a dough-like consistency; normally, the contents of the pelvic flexure have a fluid consistency. When you examine the teeth, you find that the molar surfaces are irregular, and one of the molars has a crack extending from the table surface to below the gum line.

Comment The pelvic flexure is a site of flow restriction and particle size separation. As water moves through the pelvic flexure, large forage particles accumulate and are retained for further fermentation and mixing in the ventral colon. A horse with poor teeth may not chew its forage adequately; as a result, many large particles may be swallowed. These particles tend to accumulate in the pelvic flexure and may cause an impaction and obstruction, as occurred in this case.

Treatment Treatment involves the oral administration of softening agents, such as mineral oil. Drugs such as dioctyl sodium sulfosuccinate, which stimulate water secretion from the intestinal mucosa, are also beneficial. Prevention in this case involves correction of the dental problems so that forage is more thoroughly chewed. Feeding pelleted feeds may also be beneficial.

Bibliography

Argenzio RA: Functions of the equine large intestine and their interrelationship in disease. Cornell Vet 65:303–330, 1975.
Engelhardt W von, Leonhard-Marek S, Breves G, Giesecke D (eds): Ruminant Physiology: Digestion, Metabolism, Growth and Reproduction. Albany, Germany: Delmar Publishers, 1995.

Forbes JM (ed): Quantitative Aspects of Ruminant Digestion and Metabolism. Wallingford, U.K.: CAB International, 1993.

Church DC: The Ruminant Animal: Digestive Physiology and Nutrition. Prospect Heights, Ill.: Waveland Press, 1993.

Hungate RE: The Rumen and Its Microbes. New York: Academic Press, 1966.

McDonald W, Warner ACI (eds): Digestion and Metabolism in the Ruminant. Armidale, Australia: University of New England Publishing, 1975.

Phillipson AT (ed): Physiology of Digestion and Metabolism in the Ruminant. Newcastle upon Tyne, U.K.: Oriel Press, 1970.

Ryckebusch Y, Thivend P: Digestive Physiology and Metabolism in Ruminants. Westport, Conn.: AVI Publishing, 1980.

Stevens CE, Hume ID: Comparative Physiology of the Vertebrate Digestive System, 2nd ed. Cambridge, U.K.: Cambridge University Press, 1995, pp 188–266.

Van Soest PJ: Nutritional Ecology of the Ruminant, 2nd ed. Ithaca, N.Y.: Comstock Publishing, 1994.

PRACTICE QUESTIONS

1. In which of the following respects is fermentative digestion different from glandular digestion?
a. Enzymes are not involved in fermentative digestion.
b. Chemical bonds are not split by hydrolysis in fermentative digestion.
c. Only carbohydrates are digested by fermentative digestion.
d. Substrates are more extensively altered in fermentative digestion than in glandular digestion.
e. Proteins are digested to amino acids by fermentative digestion and to dipeptides by glandular digestion.

2. In a comparison of hindgut fermentation and forestomach fermentation, which of the following statements is true?
a. The microbial populations are considerably different, but the products of digestion are the same.
b. The microbial populations are the same, but the products of digestion are considerably different.
c. Both the microbial populations and the digestion products are similar.
d. Structural carbohydrates of plants are not digested by hindgut fermentation.

e. A nitrogen source is not required by the microbes of the hindgut.

3. The three VFAs—acetate, propionate, and butyrate—are
a. net-reaction products of the fermentative action of the entire rumen biomass.
b. the individual products of cellulose, starch, and hemicellulose digestion, respectively.
c. the individual products of bacterial, protozoal, and fungal digestion, respectively.
d. volatile products that leave the rumen with the gas phase during eructation.
e. intermediate metabolites that are passed between microbial species.

4. Matching protein and energy availability in the rumen is an important nutritional goal in feeding ruminants. Which of the following completions of this statement concerning protein and energy availability in the rumen is false? Diets well matched in available protein and energy result in
a. the most efficient use of energy for microbial growth.
b. maximal delivery of protein to the host.
c. minimal breakdown of protein in the rumen.
d. loss of a minimal amount of dietary amino acids due to formation of excess ammonia.
e. optimal rumen ammonia concentrations.

5. Which of the following statements is true of both methane and propionate?
a. They are waste products of anaerobic fermentation but contain potential energy that is recoverable by the host.
b. They are highly oxidized molecules.
c. They are eructed from the rumen.
d. Their formation results in the generation of NAD from NADH.
e. They are toxic to monogastric animals.

PRACTICE ANSWERS

1. d   2. c   3. a   4. c   5. d

31

Postabsorptive nutrient utilization

Homeostatic mechanisms balance the supply and demand of nearly all nutrients

The furnace

The tricarboxylic acid (or Krebs) cycle is the major energy-yielding pathway of fuel utilization in the body

The fuels

1   The major metabolic fuels consist of glucose, amino acids, fatty acids, and ketone bodies; various storage and transport forms exist for these compounds

2   Glucose is the central fuel in the energy metabolism of most animals

3   Amino acids are important fuels in addition to being the building blocks of protein

4   Fatty acids are the major form of energy storage in the animal body

5   Ketone bodies are fat-derived, water-soluble metabolites that serve as glucose substitutes

Nutrient utilization during the absorptive phase

1   During the absorptive phase, the liver takes up glucose and converts it into glycogen and triglyceride

2   The conversion of glucose to fatty acids is an irreversible process

3   Transport of fatty acids out of the liver is through chylomicron-like particles known as very low density lipoproteins

4   Amino acids can be classified into groups on the basis of metabolic characteristics

5   Amino acids are extensively modified during absorption

6   Many amino acids are removed by the liver on "first pass," never reaching the systemic circulation

7   Some amino acids taken up by the liver are used for protein synthesis

8   Most amino acids taken up by the liver are converted to carbohydrates

9   Not all amino acids are subject to hepatic destruction

10   Metabolism at the tissue level is coordinated with hepatic metabolism and results in the deposition of fuel into storage tissues during the absorptive period

11   Insulin promotes the synthesis of protein and the deposition of glycogen in muscle

12   Insulin-stimulated uptake of amino acids by muscle results in a net increase in muscle protein synthesis

13   During the absorptive phase, triglyceride accumulation in adipose tissue occurs by two mechanisms: uptake from very low density lipoproteins, and direct lipid synthesis from glucose

Nutrient utilization during the postabsorptive phase

1   Hepatic metabolism switches from glucose utilization to glucose production during the postabsorptive phase

2   Fuel mobilization in peripheral tissues occurs when the blood insulin concentration declines

3   Muscle reacts to a metabolic demand for glucose by mobilizing amino acids to support hepatic gluconeogenesis

4   Muscle release of amino acids is related to reduced glucose and amino acid uptake

5   The complex pattern of muscle amino acid catabolism and release is necessary to accommodate the liver's limited capacity for uptake of branched-chain amino acids and facilitate the removal of amino nitrogen from the muscle

6   The reaction of adipose tissue during the postabsorptive phase is to mobilize fatty acids

Nutrient utilization during prolonged periods of energy malnutrition or complete food deprivation

1   During prolonged periods of fasting or undernutrition, glucose and amino acids are conserved by extensive utilization of fats and ketone bodies for energy production

2   A large portion of the fatty acids released from adipose tissue is taken up directly by the liver

3   Hepatic ketone body formation is promoted by low glucose availability, a high glucagon-to-insulin ratio, and a ready supply of fatty acids

4   Glucagon plays an important role in the excessive production of ketone bodies during diabetes mellitus

5 Fatty acids cannot be used for glucose synthesis

6 Ketone bodies are formed in the mitochondria from acetyl CoA

7 Hepatic very low density lipoproteins may be synthesized from adipose-derived fatty acid as well as from newly synthesized fatty acid

8 Hormonal conditions direct the distribution of very low density lipoprotein fatty acids in the body

9 Changes in growth hormone concentrations may aid in shifting peripheral fuel utilization from glucose and amino acids to ketone bodies and fatty acids

The special fuel considerations of ruminants

Ruminants exist in a perpetual state of gluconeogenesis because of their unique digestive process

---

The rate of absorption of nutrients from the gut is not constant; instead, it fluctuates greatly with food intake. Meals are digested at a rate dependent on their chemical composition, irrespective of the nutrient needs of the animal. The nature of digestion dictates that nutrient absorption from the gut is rapid during digestion and then ceases during interdigestive periods. In other words, the gut is not a storehouse for nutrients, and digestion is not modulated by the nutritional demands of the animal. The nutrient needs of the animal are not well matched to the wide fluctuations that occur in nutrient absorption from the gut. To the contrary, there is a vital need for a constant, steady supply of fuel-providing nutrients to maintain the basal metabolic functions of the body. In addition, the periods when the metabolic needs of the animal are greatly elevated often do not coincide with the times of rapid absorption of nutrients from the gut. Therefore, the animal must have a sophisticated system for maintaining the supply of nutrients, particularly energy-supplying nutrients, and buffering both the short- and long-term "feast or famine" effects associated with the absorptive and postabsorptive periods of digestion.

Homeostatic mechanisms balance the supply and demand of nearly all nutrients

This chapter focuses on supply regulation of the major energy-supplying nutrients; however, other nutrients, including vitamins and minerals, also are subject to homeostatic regulatory mechanisms. Although many of these mechanisms directly involve the digestive system, space does not permit them all to be discussed in this book. Descriptions of the homeostatic mechanisms regulating the supply of minerals and vitamins can be found in some of the references listed at the end of the chapter.

Energy-supplying nutrients are referred to as *metabolic fuels*, and the physiologic mechanisms for maintaining the supply of fuels and matching it to demand are known as *fuel homeostasis*. Fuel homeostasis is maintained by several mechanisms: the insulin-glucagon axis, the hypothalamic-pituitary axis, and the central nervous system. This chapter discusses some of the ways in which fuel is stored during the absorptive period of digestion and subsequently mobilized when needed to supply energy needs. The reader should review Chapter 1 and should read the section

on insulin and glucagon in Chapter 33 before reading this chapter.

THE FURNACE

The tricarboxylic acid (or Krebs) cycle is the major energy-yielding pathway of fuel utilization in the body

The Krebs cycle and the major pathways leading into it are briefly outlined in Figure 31–1. It is assumed that most readers have previously studied the *Krebs cycle, glycolysis,* and β-oxidation of fats in a basic course of biochemistry. Often in such courses, however, one becomes so intent on memorizing enzyme names and chemical changes in metabolites that the physiologic significance of the pathways is lost. For the purposes of this discussion, it is important only to follow the flow of the major carbon-containing nutrients into and out of the various pathways. The only specific metabolic steps that are emphasized are those points at which the flow of fuels is directed or regulated. The reader should note that the Krebs cycle and associated pathways of intermediary metabolism are sites not only of fuel utilization and energy production but also of transformation from one fuel type to another. These transformations are important in the overall scheme of fuel homeostasis.

THE FUELS

The major metabolic fuels consist of glucose, amino acids, fatty acids, and ketone bodies; various storage and transport forms exist for these compounds

Glucose, the digestion product of carbohydrate, is the basic metabolic fuel during periods of adequate nutrition in omnivorous monogastric animals, such as dogs and rats. Although there are other important fuels in the body, glucose has special significance, because under most conditions, it is the only fuel that is consumed by the central nervous system. Therefore, maintaining a steady supply of glucose for brain metabolism is of paramount importance to the body. It is not surprising that an elegant system of homeostasis exists to regulate the availability of glucose to the brain and other tissues. Discussion of this system of

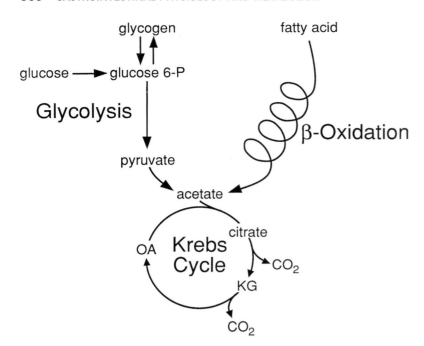

FIGURE 31–1. The relationship of the three major oxidative, catabolic pathways. OA, oxaloacetic acid; KG, α-ketoglutarate.

maintaining glucose availability is a major objective of this chapter.

Glucose is the central fuel in the energy metabolism of most animals

Glucose can be stored in the body as *glycogen,* a highly branched starch found in liver and skeletal muscle. Glycogen is the only direct storage form of glucose in the body, although glucose can be synthesized from other compounds. Directing glucose to and from glycogen depots is a major function of fuel homeostasis. When glucose is released from glycogen, the process is referred to as *glycogenolysis.*

The major means by which glucose is used as fuel is through the Embden-Meyerhof pathway, also referred to as *glycolysis.* Glycolysis is the series of biochemical steps that initiate the oxidation of glucose. Glycolysis leads directly into the *Krebs cycle,* the site of complete fuel oxidation and the major energy-yielding metabolic pathway of the body. For the study of fuel homeostasis, it should be appreciated that the process of glycolysis is, on an overall basis, reversible, meaning that glucose can be produced from the compounds that constitute the end products of glycolysis. Because of the close link between glycolysis and the Krebs cycle, any of the Krebs cycle intermediates can potentially move "backward" into the glycolytic pathway to produce glucose. The synthesis of glucose from end products of glycolysis and intermediates of the Krebs cycle, referred to as *gluconeogenesis,* is a critical part of fuel homeostasis. Although Krebs cycle activity occurs in virtually all tissues except red blood cells, the process of gluconeogenesis occurs only in the liver and, to a limited extent, kidney.

Another pathway for glucose oxidation is the *pentose-phosphate pathway.* This is a quantitatively minor pathway that does not have great impact on fuel homeostasis. However, it is an important metabolic pathway in erythrocytes, which have an absolute need for glucose, although these cells' overall need for energy is small compared with the rest of the body.

Amino acids are important fuels in addition to being the building blocks of protein

Amino acids are important fuels. Whereas these monomers are the building blocks of proteins, they are also carbon-containing compounds that can provide energy to the body. In addition, they are important substrates for gluconeogenesis, indicating that they (most amino acids) can be converted to glucose when the available glucose supply is short. Although it is sometimes said that there is no storage site of amino acids in the body, the protein of skeletal muscle could well be considered to have an amino acid storage function in addition to its locomotor functions.

Fatty acids are the major form of energy storage in the animal body

Fatty acids are stored in adipose tissue in the form of *triglycerides* (also called *triacylglycerols*), which consist of three fatty-acid molecules linked to a glycerol molecule by ester bonds (see Fig. 29–24). Triglycerides are an ideal form of energy storage for animals. They are highly reduced molecules (there is little oxygen compared with the amount of carbon and hydrogen), which means they are a concentrated energy source, having more than twice the caloric value per gram than carbohydrates or amino acids. In addition, adipose tissue contains little water compared with protein or glycogen, the storage forms of the other two potential fuels. Thus, adipose tissue is undiluted by bulky water, allowing it to be a concentrated form of energy storage that permits animals to carry with them a maximal amount of energy at a minimal amount of weight. Fats, however, have a metabolic disadvantage; they are not water-soluble. Therefore, special transport systems are needed to enable fats to be distributed among the tissues through the blood and lymph systems. In addition, fatty acids cannot be converted to glucose, so they cannot, under usual circumstances, contribute to the energy supply of the central nervous system. However, fatty acids can be converted to *ketone bodies.*

Ketone bodies are fat-derived, water-soluble metabolites that serve as glucose substitutes

Although glucose cannot be formed from fat, the fat-derived ketone bodies do have some glucose-like attributes. For example, ketone bodies can pass the blood-brain barrier, and during prolonged periods of dietary energy deprivation, they can provide a large portion of the energy supply to the central nervous system, at least in some species. It does appear, however, that ketone bodies cannot totally replace glucose in this function and that a small amount of glucose is always needed by the central nervous system.

In monogastric species, ketone bodies are formed exclusively in the liver and are used by a wide variety of tissues. Some tissues, including cardiac muscle, use ketone bodies in preference to glucose. In ruminants, the ketone body β-hydroxybutyrate is formed from butyrate in the rumen epithelium. Thus, in ruminants, ketone bodies are not only products of fatty-acid metabolism but also products of normal digestion. Elevated serum concentrations of ketone bodies are characteristic of several diseases associated with abnormalities of fuel homeostasis. This fact might lead one to conclude that ketone bodies are abnormal, or even toxic, metabolites. In fact, when present in physiologic concentrations, ketone bodies are important fuels that occupy an integral part of the scheme of fuel homeostasis. The chemical structure of the three major ketone bodies is illustrated in Figure 31–2.

NUTRIENT UTILIZATION DURING THE ABSORPTIVE PHASE

As absorption takes place, metabolic events in the liver and peripheral organs are coordinated to direct nutrients into storage molecules and storage sites. The general scheme of metabolism during the absorptive phase is illustrated in Figure 31–3.

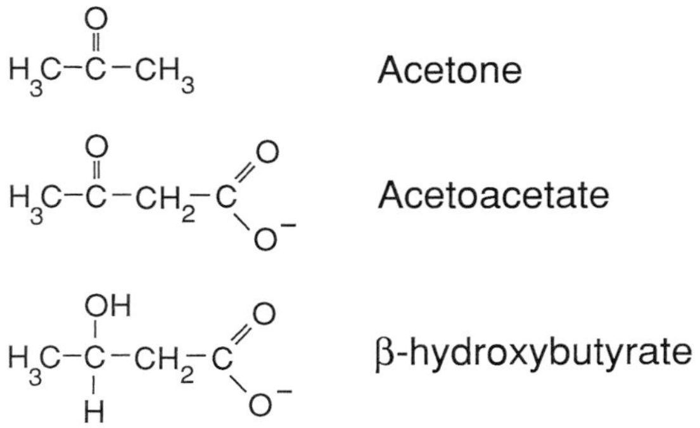

FIGURE 31–2. The physiologic ketone bodies.

During the absorptive phase, the liver takes up glucose and converts it into glycogen and triglyceride

When a meal is ingested, insulin secretion begins even before maximal absorption of glucose is achieved. This secretion is stimulated by the action of gastric inhibitory peptide (see Chapter 26) and perhaps other enteric hormones. Early insulin secretion ensures that the liver and other tissues will be "primed" and ready for the arrival of glucose from the gut. A large portion of the glucose absorbed postprandially is taken up by the liver, because the liver receives much of the total blood flow and has a high capacity for glucose uptake. Under the influence of insulin, glucose in the liver is diverted into glycogen synthesis. The net effect is that glucose from the gut is diverted into glycogen and stored there during absorptive periods, thus keeping blood glucose concentrations from becoming excessively high. Insulin exerts its stimulatory effect on hepatic glycogen synthesis by stimulating intracellular metabolic pathways that lead to the formation of glycogen. These effects are discussed further in reference to the counterbalancing effects of glucagon.

The amount of glycogen that can be stored in the liver is limited and, under normal conditions, probably never exceeds 10% of the total weight of the liver. In humans, this represents about 100 g of glycogen, and it is likely that a proportionately similar limit exists for the storage of glycogen in the livers of other species. This amount of glycogen does not account for all the glucose taken up by the liver during the digestion and absorption of a large carbohydrate meal; therefore, there must be some additional mechanism for the disposal of excess glucose. If there were no such alternatives for glucose disposal other than glycogen, blood glucose levels could rise out of control after glycogen concentrations had reached their maximum. Fatty-acid synthesis offers an alternative mechanism for glucose removal.

The conversion of glucose to fatty acids is an irreversible process

The synthesis of fatty acids from glucose begins with glycolysis. This pathway leads to the production of

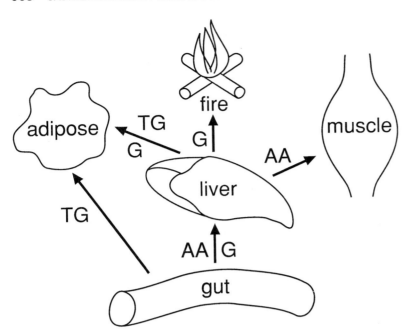

FIGURE 31–3. Metabolism during the absorptive period is characterized by the movement of potential fuels into depot sites and the utilization of glucose (G) as a fuel. AA, amino acid; TG, triglyceride.

two pyruvate molecules for each molecule of glucose consumed. Pyruvate can then enter the mitochondria to be activated to *acetyl coenzyme A* (acetyl CoA) for entry into the Krebs cycle. However, the Krebs cycle is for energy generation, and during the absorptive period, there is more than enough acetyl CoA and Krebs cycle activity to provide for energy needs; therefore, the excess acetyl CoA must be shunted away from the Krebs cycle. The excess acetyl CoA combines with *oxaloacetate* to form *citrate* in what is essentially the first reaction of the Krebs cycle. Instead of continuing through the Krebs cycle reactions, however, much of the citrate is transported out of the mitochondria into the cytosol during the absorptive period. Once in the cytosol, each citrate molecule contributes two carbons toward the synthesis of fatty acids. The remaining portion of the citrate molecule cycles back into the mitochondria for further use. Thus, because acetyl CoA cannot pass directly through the mitochondrial membrane, citrate serves as a carrier molecule to transport two-carbon acetate units, originally from glucose, out of the mitochondria for the synthesis of fatty acids in the cytosol (Fig. 31–4).

Several important steps in this conversion of glucose carbon to fatty acids are promoted by insulin and are discussed in greater detail later. It is important to recognize that the conversion of glucose to fatty acids is irreversible; thus, carbohydrate can form fat, but fat cannot form carbohydrate. The discussion here concerns hepatic metabolism, and the liver is an important site of fatty-acid synthesis in several species. Direct synthesis of fatty acids occurs also in adipose tissue. The relative importance of liver and adipose tissue as sites of fatty-acid synthesis varies with species, as discussed later.

Transport of fatty acids out of the liver is through chylomicron-like particles known as very low density lipoproteins

Once formed in the liver, fatty acids must be transported either to adipose tissue for storage or to other tissues, such as muscle, for direct utilization for energy production. Because fatty acids are insoluble in blood, some special transport mechanism for their distribution is necessary. This mechanism is through the hepatic formation of triglyceride-rich serum lipoproteins, also known as *very low density lipoprotein* or *VLDL*. The name *VLDL* is given because these triglyceride-rich lipoproteins are so much less dense compared with other lipoproteins that exist in blood serum. In the synthesis of VLDLs, fatty acids are first esterified to form triglycerides, and the triglycerides are wrapped in a coat of phospholipid, cholesterol, and specific proteins (Fig. 31–5). This is essentially the same mechanism by which fatty acids are transported out of the enterocytes after absorption from the gut. In the latter case, the lipoproteins are called chylomicrons. The VLDLs of the liver are smaller than chylomicrons but have a similar structure and function. The mechanisms by which VLDLs and chylomicrons deliver fatty acids to peripheral tissues are further discussed in relation to peripheral tissues.

Amino acids can be classified into groups on the basis of metabolic characteristics

The discussion of amino acid absorption and metabolism is complicated by the fact that not all amino

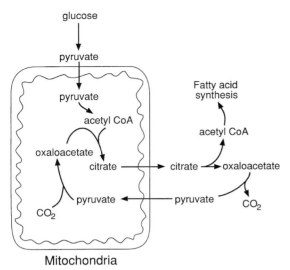

Mitochondria

FIGURE 31–4. The hepatic synthesis of fatty acid from carbohydrate requires the passage of carbohydrate carbons through the mitochondria. Citrate forms a shuttle to transport the carbons of acetyl coenzyme A (acetyl CoA) out of the mitochondria, because acetyl CoA cannot pass directly through the mitochondrial membrane. The formation of citrate from oxaloacetate and acetyl CoA is the first reaction of the Krebs cycle; thus, fatty-acid formation is an alternative to Krebs cycle oxidation when there is more than enough acetyl CoA to provide cellular energy through Krebs cycle activity.

acids are subject to the same reactions. For this discussion, the amino acids are divided into two groups, each containing two subgroups (Table 31–1). The major groups are the nutritionally dispensable amino acids and nutritionally indispensable amino acids. Within the dispensable amino acid group, glutamate, aspartate, and alanine are separated out as *transport amino acids*; within the indispensable amino acid group, leucine, isoleucine, and valine form a special subgroup known as the *branch-chain amino acids* (BCAAs). The transport amino acids are utilized in several reactions in which amino groups are transferred from molecule to molecule or organ to organ.

TABLE 31–1. Metabolic classification of amino acids

Indispensable amino acids		Dispensable amino acids	
BRANCH-CHAIN AMINO ACIDS	OTHERS	TRANSPORT AMINO ACIDS	OTHERS
Leucine	Arginine*	Alanine	Cysteine
Isoleucine	Histidine	Glutamine	Glycine
Valine	Lysine	Glutamic acid	Proline
	Methionine	Asparagine	Tyrosine†
	Phenylalanine	Aspartic acid	Serine
	Threonine		
	Tryptophan		

*Indispensable for cats, not required in the diets of many other species.
†Dietary adequacy depends on a supply of phenylalanine.

Amino acids are extensively modified during absorption

The profile of amino acids in the portal vein is considerably different from that of the diet, indicating that amino acid destruction and transformation occur during the absorptive process. Essentially all the glutamate and much of the aspartate in the diet are removed by the intestinal epithelial cells during absorption, so that the portal blood is nearly devoid of glutamate and contains little aspartate. Much of the nitrogen from glutamate and aspartate is transferred to pyruvate to form the amino acid alanine, which is present in high concentrations in portal blood. The metabolism of the transport amino acids in the intestinal epithelium is a good example of both the way in which amino groups can be gained and lost and how the metabolism of amino acids interfaces with the metabolism of carbohydrate. Glutamate and aspartate are similar to two Krebs cycle intermediates, α-ketoglutarate and oxaloacetate, differing only by the presence of an amino group or a keto-oxygen. Carbohydrates and amino acids having this relationship are said to be *analogues*; thus, α-ketoglutarate is the keto-analogue of glutamate, and pyruvate

FIGURE 31–5. Formation of very low density lipoprotein (VLDL). Fatty acids (FAs) for triglyceride (TG) formation may come either from synthesis from carbohydrate or amino acids or from adipose tissue FAs arriving at the liver in the form of nonesterified fatty acids (NEFAs). Note the similarity to chylomicron formation (see Fig.29–27). CH, cholesterol; PL, phospholipid; SER, smooth endoplasmic reticulum; RER, rough endoplasmic reticulum.

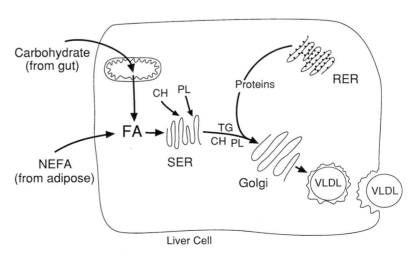

Liver Cell

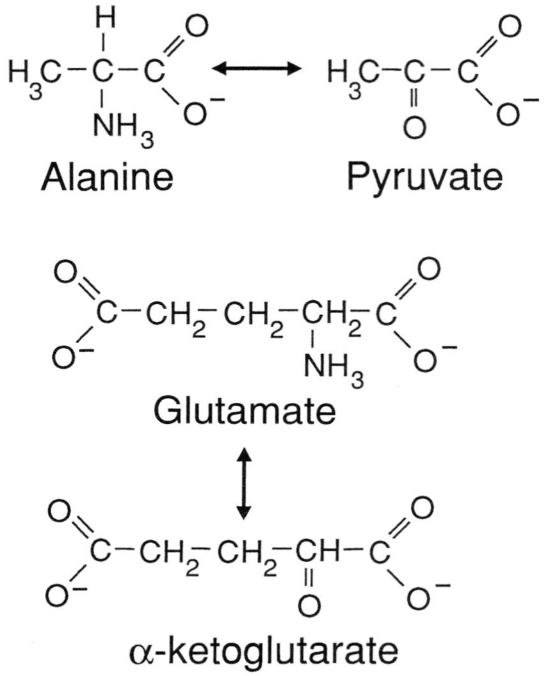

Alanine   Pyruvate

Glutamate

α-ketoglutarate

FIGURE 31–6. Example of amino acids and their keto-analogues. All amino acids can reversibly form keto-analogues.

is the keto-analogue of alanine (Fig. 31–6). All amino acids can form keto-analogues, and all keto-analogues can be readily converted back to their parent amino acids.

Many amino acids are removed by the liver on "first pass," never reaching the systemic circulation

The hepatic-portal circulation is arranged in such a way that all nutrients leaving the gut through the

blood pass through the liver before entering the systemic circulation (see Fig. 29–23). This arrangement places the liver in a "sentinel" position, from which it can modify the nutrient composition of portal blood before the blood is distributed to other tissues. The function of the liver in modifying portal blood composition is well illustrated in the case of amino acid absorption. A large portion of the amino acids absorbed into portal blood are removed as the blood passes the liver, so they never reach the general circulation. Figure 31–7 illustrates that in the dog, only about 23% of the amino acids reaching the liver during the absorptive period pass into the general circulation; the liver thus helps keep blood amino acid concentrations stable during periods of amino acid absorption. The blood amino acid concentration, like the blood glucose concentration, is usually kept relatively constant.

Some amino acids taken up by the liver are used for protein synthesis

The liver is an important site of protein synthesis, making its priority position for amino acid uptake seem reasonable. Figure 31–7 shows that approximately 20% of the portal blood amino acid supply is used for protein synthesis in the liver, although this proportion varies with dietary protein intake. Nearly all the serum proteins are synthesized in the liver, including such critical proteins as albumin and the blood-clotting factors. Although the liver-derived serum proteins serve many important functions, one function they do not serve is that of amino acid transport. The direct amino acid supply for protein synthesis in nonhepatic tissue comes from free amino acids in the blood, not from preformed serum proteins.

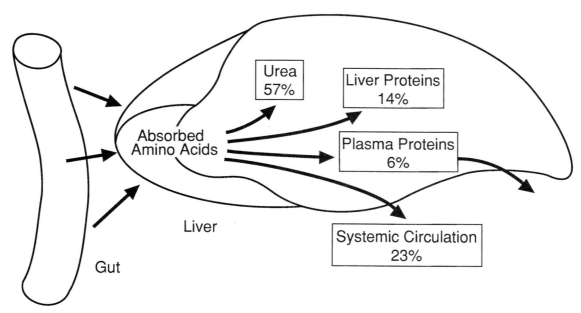

FIGURE 31–7. The fate of dietary amino acids reaching the canine liver.

Most amino acids taken up by the liver are converted to carbohydrates

Most amino acids entering the liver undergo *deamination*, which means that the amino groups are removed and the molecules converted to their keto-analogues. The keto-analogues enter the pathways of carbohydrate metabolism, from which they may be completely metabolized for energy, converted to glucose or glycogen, or shunted to fatty-acid synthesis. All these reactions proceed in the same manner as previously described for carbohydrate metabolism. The sites at which the various amino acids enter the carbohydrate pathways are illustrated in Figure 31–8.

Deamination of amino acids for the production of carbohydrate or energy may seem like a waste of expensive dietary protein; in some species, however, the deamination of amino acids is important for homeostasis of glucose and other fuels. The natural diets of the true carnivores, such as cats and mink, for example, contain a large portion of protein and little carbohydrate. Yet the glucose needs of these animals are no less than those of other animals, so it is extremely important that they synthesize glucose from amino acids. Ruminants are in a similar situation, because most of the carbohydrates they consume are digested by fermentative digestion and absorbed as volatile fatty acids rather than glucose. Ruminants, like carnivores, depend on amino acids for some of their glucose needs, although a large portion of ruminant glucose requirements may be met through conversion of propionate.

To allow carbohydrate production and the deamination of excess amino acids, the endocrine reactions to high-protein meals are somewhat different from those to meals containing substantial amounts of carbohydrate. During the digestion of high-protein meals, insulin and glucagon secretion does not occur in its usual reciprocal pattern. Insulin secretion is stimulated by amino acids as well as by glucose. Glucagon secretion, which is inhibited by glucose, is stimulated by amino acids as long as glucose concentrations are moderately low. This relationship means that during the digestion of a high-protein, low-carbohydrate meal, there is simultaneous secretion of insulin and glucagon. One of the effects of insulin is the greater cellular uptake of amino acids as well as glucose. Thus, the effect of insulin in this situation is to increase transport of amino acids into tissues.

If insulin secretion were the only action stimulated by amino acid absorption, however, the animal would risk insulin-stimulated hypoglycemia when it con-

FIGURE 31–8. The sites of entry of various amino acids into the scheme of carbohydrate metabolism. This figure illustrates the means by which glucose can be synthesized from amino acids in the process of gluconeogenesis. In the case of the dispensable amino acids, the reactions are reversible, allowing amino acid production from carbohydrate.

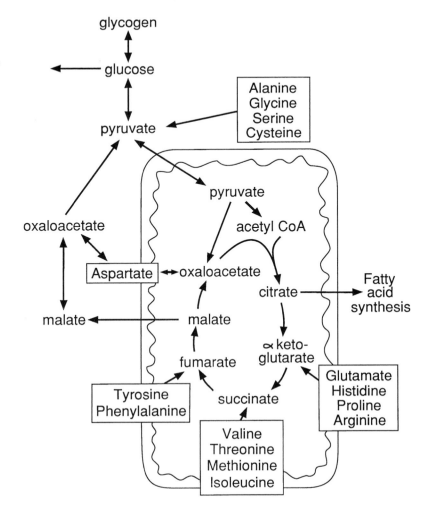

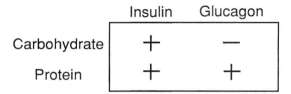

FIGURE 31–9. The influence of dietary carbohydrate and protein on insulin and glucagon secretion.

sumed a high-protein, low-carbohydrate diet. An important action of glucagon is to stimulate gluconeogenesis through the deamination of amino acids in the liver. This process ensures that adequate glucose will be available to counterbalance the effects of amino acid–stimulated insulin secretion. The relationship of insulin secretion and glucagon secretion during the absorption of diets with different carbohydrate and protein concentrations is illustrated in Figure 31–9.

Not all amino acids are subject to hepatic destruction

During the absorptive period, amino acids for peripheral (nonhepatic) protein synthesis must come from that portion of amino acids that escape hepatic destruction. As seen from Figure 31–7, this portion amounts to only about 23% of the amino acids absorbed from the gut. Although this may seem like a meager portion of amino acids to be allocated for protein synthesis by all body tissues except liver, several considerations make it seem more appropriate. First, amino acids are selectively taken up by the liver, so the distribution of individual amino acids in blood leaving the liver is not the same as that in blood reaching the liver. The indispensable amino acids, especially the BCAAs, are not avidly extracted by the liver, whereas some of the dispensable amino acids, alanine for example, are extensively taken up by hepatic tissue. The dispensable amino acids can be synthesized by protein-producing tissues; thus, the relatively low concentration of serum amino acids resulting from hepatic amino acid removal is not rate-limiting for tissue protein synthesis. Second, the proportion of amino acids taken up by the liver, and the fate of the amino acids that are taken up, is not constant but can be adjusted according to the body's protein needs. Low-protein diets lead to reductions in hepatic amino acid uptake, protein synthesis, and amino acid destruction by the liver.

Metabolism at the tissue level is coordinated with hepatic metabolism and results in the deposition of fuel into storage tissues during the absorptive period

The overall effects of hepatic metabolism during the absorption of a meal are the removal of glucose and amino acids and the synthesis of protein and fat. Complementary changes occur in peripheral tissues, so that additional glucose and amino acids are removed by skeletal muscle and adipose tissue. In addition, fatty acids secreted by the liver as VLDL triglyceride are deposited in adipose tissue, as are the triglycerides of chylomicrons.

Insulin promotes the synthesis of protein and the deposition of glycogen in muscle

The absorptive period is dominated by the effects of insulin. In skeletal muscle, the largest tissue mass of the body, insulin, promotes the uptake of glucose and amino acids, thus tending to moderate the increase in the blood concentration of these nutrients during absorption of a meal. The uptake of glucose by muscle is associated with glycogen synthesis, just as in the liver. Muscle glycogen, in contrast to liver glycogen, cannot be made directly available to augment blood glucose concentrations during periods of low glucose availability. Thus, muscle glycogen is primarily for metabolism in the muscle, although at certain times muscle glycogen can indirectly provide substrate for hepatic gluconeogenesis.

Insulin-stimulated uptake of amino acids by muscle results in a net increase in muscle protein synthesis

The term *net increase* is used in reference to muscle protein synthesis, because muscle protein is in a state of dynamic equilibrium, that is, a constant state of flux. Protein molecules are continuously being broken down and their amino acids added to an intracellular amino acid pool. Simultaneously, new proteins are constantly being made, deriving their amino acids from the same pool (Fig. 31–10). The size of the amino acid pool depends on the relative rates of entry and exit of amino acids. Amino acids enter the pool from the blood during the absorptive phase and at all times from the breakdown of protein. Exit of amino acids from the pool occurs because of protein synthesis and oxidative catabolism. In the absorptive phase of digestion, the amino acid pool is large, because amino acids are being taken up from the blood. In addition, few of the amino acids leaving the pool are directed toward oxidative catabolism, because there is plenty of available glucose for oxidation and energy generation. The result is that the amino acid pool is large, and a high proportion of amino acids is directed to protein synthesis. When the rate of protein synthesis exceeds the rate of protein breakdown, there is a net increase in the amount of muscle protein. Thus, during the absorptive phase, amino acids are stored in muscle protein, protein that has a functional role not only for locomotion and posture but also as amino acid storage.

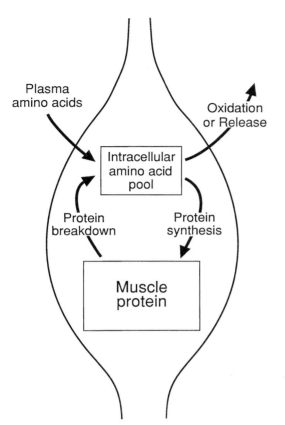

FIGURE 31–10. The intracellular amino acid pool. The size of the pool depends on the rates of amino acid uptake from plasma and muscle protein relative to the rates of amino acid loss owing to oxidation, export to plasma, and protein synthesis.

During the absorptive phase, triglyceride accumulation in adipose tissue occurs by two mechanisms: uptake from very low density lipoproteins, and direct lipid synthesis from glucose

Triglyceride fatty acids are transferred from chylomicrons and VLDLs to adipose tissue by the action of *lipoprotein lipase (LPL)*. This enzyme resides on endothelial surfaces of capillaries and, when activated, binds to chylomicrons and VLDLs, catalyzing the hydrolysis of fatty acids from their core triglycerides and allowing the transfer of those fatty acids to the surrounding tissues. The sensitivity of LPL to specific hormones varies in different tissues. Adipose tissue LPL is stimulated by insulin; thus, during the absorptive phase, fatty acids from the triglycerides of chylomicrons and VLDLs are selectively transferred to adipose tissue. Therefore, under the influence of insulin during the absorptive phase, excess carbohydrate and amino acids are converted to fatty acids in the liver, and those fatty acids are subsequently transported, through VLDL triglyceride, to the adipose tissue. Similarly, chylomicron triglyceride arising from intestinal fatty-acid absorption is also selectively transported to adipose tissue, under the influence of insulin.

Adipose tissue fatty acids may also arise from direct synthesis in addition to uptake from chylomicrons and VLDLs. Adipose tissue cells are metabolically active, and under the influence of insulin, they take up glucose. Within the adipocytes, glucose can be converted to fatty acids by the same metabolic mechanisms by which fatty acids were synthesized in the liver. In addition, acetate from fermentative digestion also can serve as a substrate for fatty-acid synthesis in adipose tissue (see later discussion of the special fuel considerations of ruminants). Thus, there are two major sites of fatty-acid synthesis in the body, the liver and adipose tissue. The relative importance of these sites varies with species.

NUTRIENT UTILIZATION DURING THE POSTABSORPTIVE PHASE

The *postabsorptive phase* is the relatively brief period (usually a few hours) between meals in well-fed animals. It is characterized by short-term changes that mobilize nutrients from storage pools to maintain fuel availability for metabolically active tissue. The general scheme of postabsorptive metabolism is illustrated in Figure 31–11.

Hepatic metabolism switches from glucose utilization to glucose production during the postabsorptive phase

As the absorption of a meal is completed, the rate of glucose absorption from the gut wanes, and the blood glucose concentration diminishes, removing the stimulus for insulin production and stimulating glucagon secretion. The primary target organ of glucagon is the liver, in which it creates marked metabolic changes. Through stimulation of specific cell surface receptors on hepatocytes, glucagon activates adenyl cyclase, leading to the phosphorylation of numerous cellular enzymes (see Chapter 1 for a more complete discussion of phosphorylation and dephosphorylation reactions). Some enzymes are activated by phosphorylation, whereas others are inactivated, and unless the overall scheme of substrate flow is considered, the whole phosphorylation-dephosphorylation system appears to be quite random and to make little sense. Considering the actions of the individual enzymes in light of their effect on the flow of energy substrate through the liver, however, reveals that the system is an elegant and incredibly well-orchestrated mechanism for the maintenance of fuel homeostasis.

Those enzymes that stimulate mobilization and utilization of fuels are activated by phosphorylation, whereas those stimulating storage of fuels are inactivated by phosphorylation. It must be understood that many enzymes of intermediary metabolism serve a passive role, catalyzing reactions that can go in either direction, depending on substrate concentrations. A relatively small number of regulatory enzymes usu-

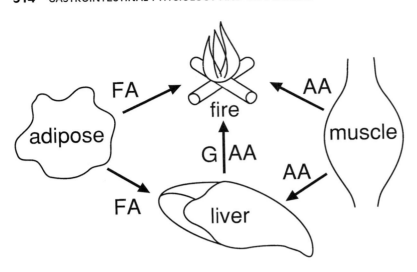

FIGURE 31–11. Postabsorptive metabolism is characterized by movement of fuels out of depot sites for immediate use. Glucose (G) arising either from glycogenolysis or gluconeogenesis is a major fuel, although some fatty acid (FA) is consumed also. Amino acid (AA) forms the substrate for gluconeogenesis.

ally stand at the head of metabolic pathways and determine the substrate concentrations to which the other, unregulated enzymes are exposed. Through its effect on several key regulatory enzymes, glucagon—a stimulator of phosphorylation—-places the liver in a fuel-mobilization state. In contrast, insulin—an inhibitor of phosphorylation—promotes a hepatic metabolic pattern that favors fuel storage, as discussed in the previous section on absorptive-phase metabolism.

The opposing actions of insulin and glucagon on hepatic metabolism are evident from their actions on

two key regulatory enzyme pairs: *glycogen synthase* and *glycogen phosphatase*, and *phosphofructokinase* and *fructose-1,6-bisphosphatase*. The first of these pairs regulates glycogen synthesis and breakdown, whereas the second regulates glycolysis and gluconeogenesis, respectively. The actions of these enzymes and their regulatory effects are illustrated in Figure 31–12. Glycogen synthase and phosphofructokinase are inhibited by phosphorylation and thus are stimulated by insulin. Glycogen phosphatase and fructose-1,6-bisphosphatase are stimulated by phosphorylation and, thus, stimulated by glucagon. The actions of insulin

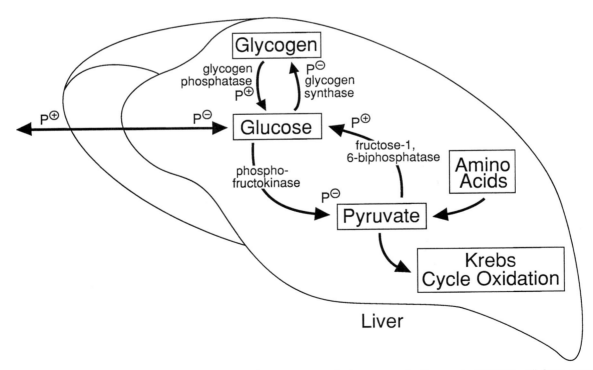

FIGURE 31–12. The effects of phosphorylation on four key enzymes of glucose production and utilization. All four enzymes are phosphorylated under the influence of cyclic adenosine monophosphate (AMP). Note, however, that the enzymes that favor glucose formation are stimulated by phosphorylation (P+), whereas those that favor glucose utilization and storage are inhibited by phosphorylation (P−).

and glucagon on these antagonistic enzyme pairs emphasize the importance of the insulin-to-glucagon ratio to which the liver is exposed. Neither hormone elicits an "all-or-none" reaction but, rather, alters the balance of opposing reactions by influencing the relative activity of antagonistic enzymes. Thus, the fuel mobilizing or fuel storing activity of the liver depends on which hormone is most dominant. For this reason, the ratio of insulin to glucagon appears to be more important to liver metabolism than the absolute concentration of either hormone.

Under the influence of glucagon, glycogen phosphatase is activated by phosphorylation, promoting glycogenolysis and the elevation of intracellular glucose concentrations. As glucose accumulates, it is prevented from cycling back into glycogen, because the major enzyme catalyzing that reaction, glycogen synthase, is blocked by phosphorylation. In addition, the flow of glucose into glycolysis is also blocked by phosphorylation inhibition of phosphofructokinase (see Fig. 31–12). Thus, the normal pathways for glucose utilization within the hepatocyte are all inhibited by glucagon, allowing glucose from glycogen breakdown to accumulate in the cells. Eventually, intracellular glucose escapes into the extracellular fluid and on into the blood. In this manner, hepatic glycogen is mobilized to elevate and maintain blood glucose concentrations when they begin to decline.

The liver stores of glycogen are relatively limited and cannot maintain blood glucose concentrations for long. Estimates in humans are that hepatic glycogen will serve blood glucose needs for 6 to 12 hours under conditions of light exertion and for only about 20 minutes under conditions of heavy exertion. Values for animals are probably similar. Therefore, there must be some means, in addition to glycogen mobilization, of maintaining the body's glucose supply during periods of exertion or when the period between meals is prolonged. Under these conditions of greater demand, glucose is provided by gluconeogenesis. Gluconeogenesis is promoted by the phosphorylation-stimulated enzyme fructose-1,6-bisphosphatase. This enzyme essentially puts the glycolytic pathway into reverse, leading to glucose production from the same molecules that are intermediates in its oxidative destruction. Important substrates are pyruvate and all the intermediates of the Krebs cycle.

At this point, it is important to remember that most of the Krebs cycle intermediates or pyruvate can be supplied by the deamination of amino acids. The entry point of the various amino acids into the scheme of carbohydrate metabolism is illustrated in Figure 31–8. Pyruvate and all the Krebs cycle intermediates can flow backward through the oxidative pathway (not all the reactions of gluconeogenesis are the exact reverse of the corresponding reactions in glycolysis, but the net result of gluconeogenesis is the reverse of glycolysis), resulting in the production of glucose. Thus, amino acids provide a large store of precursors for glucose formation through gluconeogenesis. The end result of glucagon stimulation is to promote the production of glucose through glycoge-

nolysis and gluconeogenesis, turning the liver into a glucose-synthesizing organ.

Fuel mobilization in peripheral tissues occurs when the blood insulin concentration declines

The pattern of metabolism in the peripheral tissues changes in the postabsorptive phase to support the liver's capacity to maintain fuel supplies.

Muscle reacts to a metabolic demand for glucose by mobilizing amino acids to support hepatic gluconeogenesis

Mobilization of amino acid from muscle appears to be stimulated, to a large extent, by a relative lack of insulin; thus, mobilization occurs when blood glucose concentrations are low. Amino acids mobilized from skeletal muscle come from the intracellular amino acid pool referred to earlier (see Fig. 31–10). However, the mobilizing reactions are complex, and the distribution of amino acids leaving the muscle does not reflect the distribution of amino acids in the intracellular pool, as explained later.

Muscle release of amino acids is related to reduced glucose and amino acid uptake

The postabsorptive decline in the serum insulin concentration has a twofold effect on muscle: the entry of amino acids from the serum into the intracellular amino acid pool is diminished, and in addition, the entry of glucose into muscle cells for energy production declines. Reduced amino acid entry results in conditions favoring net protein degradation to maintain the cellular amino acid pool size. Reduced glucose entry results in increased utilization of amino acids from the pool for energy production.

The pattern of utilization of amino acids for energy by muscle may, at first, seem unnecessarily complex, involving selective use and extensive transformation of amino acids. BCAAs serve as primary sources of energy in muscle cells during the postabsorptive phase, because these amino acids account for approximately one third of all muscle amino acid. Catabolism of BCAAs begins with deamination and the formation of the α-keto-acid of the BCAA. The α-keto-acids then enter the Krebs cycle for energy production. Deamination of the BCAA requires that some acceptor be available to receive the amino group, and this acceptor is ultimately pyruvate, resulting in the formation of alanine. The source of pyruvate can be muscle glycogen, blood glucose, or the metabolic products of BCAA α-keto-acids. When metabolism of BCAA α-keto-acids serves as the supply of pyruvate for alanine synthesis, the net reaction is conversion of BCAA to alanine (Fig. 31–13). Thus, the overall

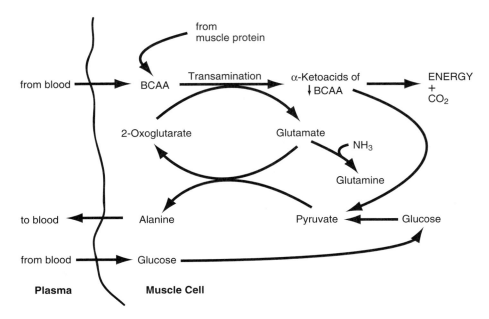

FIGURE 31-13. Catabolism of branch-chain amino acids (BCAAs) by muscle cells. The pyruvate for export of amino groups may be derived from glucose or the amino acids themselves.

metabolic activity in muscle during the postabsorptive phase is the destruction of BCAAs and the formation of alanine. The alanine formed is released from the muscle cells into the blood, from which it may be taken up by the liver for gluconeogenesis.

The complex pattern of muscle amino acid catabolism and release is necessary to accommodate the liver's limited capacity for uptake of branched-chain amino acids and facilitate the removal of amino nitrogen from the muscle

It might appear that a simpler system of amino acid transfer to the liver would suffice. Why are amino acids not just released from muscle cell amino acid pools into the blood and transported to the liver for glucose synthesis? The answer lies in the limited uptake capacity of the liver for BCAAs and the need to transport amino nitrogen out of the muscle. BCAAs, the predominant amino acids of skeletal muscle, are not taken up readily by the liver; thus, if BCAAs were not transformed to alanine, amino acid transfer to the liver would be limited.

In addition, alanine is a convenient means by which nitrogen from the deamination of muscle amino acid can be transported to the liver. This is important, because free amino groups liberated by the catabolism of amino acids in muscle, if not removed, could lead to the formation of toxic levels of ammonia. Ammonia is detoxified in the body by the formation of urea, but urea formation occurs only in the liver. Thus, alanine forms a gluconeogenic precursor that also transports nitrogen to the liver for urea synthesis. Figures 31-13 and 31-14 illustrate the role of alanine in the transport of amino acid nitrogen and carbon to

the liver for synthesis of urea and glucose, respectively.

The regulation of muscle protein mobilization is influenced to a large extent by the lack of insulin. However, the adrenocortical hormone cortisol has an important effect of stimulating protein breakdown and amino acid mobilization. Through the mobilization of muscle protein and stimulation of hepatic gluconeogenesis, cortisol exerts one of its major ef-

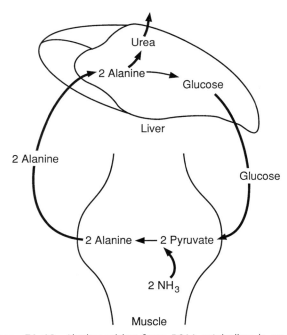

FIGURE 31-14. Alanine arising from BCAA catabolism in muscle is converted to glucose and urea in the liver. The glucose produced can potentially return to the muscle for alanine production. Thus, the cycle of alanine to glucose forms a shuttle to transport nitrogen from the muscle to the liver for urea synthesis.

fects, raising the blood glucose concentration. Under normal conditions, glucagon, the other major gluconeogenic hormone, exerts its effects on the liver and does not appear to have a direct effect on muscle.

The reaction of adipose tissue during the postabsorptive phase is to mobilize fatty acids

Fatty acids are released from adipose tissue because of the action of the phosphorylation-stimulated enzyme *hormone-sensitive lipase (HSL)*. This enzyme is stimulated by the relative lack of insulin in the postabsorptive period; insulin suppresses the action of HSL by promoting its dephosphorylation. Glucagon may have some adipose tissue activity in promoting triglyceride breakdown by stimulating the phosphorylation and activation of HSL. More likely, however, glucagon's effects are restricted to the liver, and the normal stimulation of HSL comes from epinephrine or norepinephrine; norepinephrine originates from sympathetic nerves in the adipose tissue. The exact means by which sympathetic nerve activity in adipose tissue is coordinated with body fuel availability is not well established, but the catecholamine hormones and neuroregulators appear to be the primary positive stimulus for breakdown of adipose triglyceride. However, the negative stimulus provided by the absence of insulin may be the most important regulator of adipose fat mobilization.

Stimulation of HSL in the postabsorptive state leads to the release of fatty acids from adipose tissue into the blood. Fatty acids in blood are reversibly bound to albumin, because they are not otherwise soluble in water. Albumin-bound fatty acids in blood are usually referred to as *nonesterified fatty acids (NEFAs)* to distinguish them from triglyceride fatty acids in chylomicrons and lipoproteins. NEFAs in blood may be used directly for energy by many tissues. However, a large portion of the fatty acids are taken up by the liver and used for either ketone body production or VLDL synthesis, as discussed in the next section.

NUTRIENT UTILIZATION DURING PROLONGED PERIODS OF ENERGY MALNUTRITION OR COMPLETE FOOD DEPRIVATION

During prolonged periods of fasting or undernutrition, glucose and amino acids are conserved by extensive utilization of fats and ketone bodies for energy production

From the previous discussion of postabsorptive metabolism, it can be appreciated that amino acids form an important depot for glucose precursors and energy-producing substrate. During prolonged fasting or undernutrition, however, it would not be advantageous for animals to rely heavily on their skeletal muscle for energy and glucose production, because doing so would soon lead to severe weakness as the skeletal muscle protein was consumed. Thus, protective mechanisms have developed by which skeletal muscle is preserved during periods of insufficient energy intake. In utilization of stored fuels, shifts away from glucose and toward adipose fat stores are necessary for protein sparing. The general scheme of metabolism during prolonged catabolic periods is illustrated in Figure 31–15.

A large portion of the fatty acids released from adipose tissue is taken up directly by the liver

During prolonged periods of undernutrition, low glucose availability leads to rapid mobilization of adipose fatty acids in the form of NEFAs. Although NEFAs are metabolized by many tissues, a large portion of them is extracted from the blood by the liver, which receives much of the total blood flow and has an efficient hepatic NEFA extraction mechanism. Once the NEFAs are in the hepatocytes, they may follow any of three potential metabolic paths. The first is complete oxidation for energy production;

FIGURE 31–15. During prolonged periods of food deprivation or energy deficiency, the ketone bodies (K), fatty acids (FA), and triglycerides (TG) become the major fuels. Glucose oxidation becomes minor, thus sparing muscle protein that otherwise would be needed for gluconeogenesis.

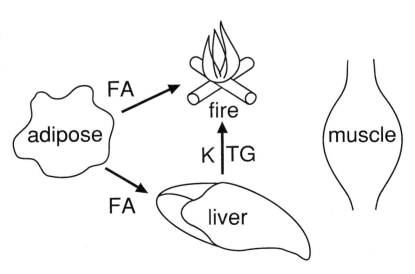

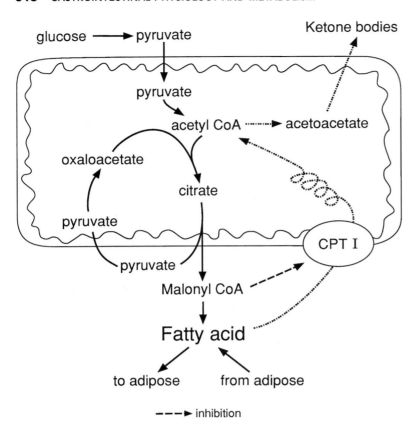

FIGURE 31-16. The liver is a site of both destruction and synthesis of fatty acids. To keep both processes from occurring simultaneously, fatty-acid destruction is inhibited during periods of fatty-acid synthesis. The pathway of fatty-acid synthesis is indicated by the *solid lines*, whereas that of fatty-acid destruction is indicated by the *irregular broken line*. Oxidative destruction is suppressed by the action of malonyl CoA, an intermediate in the synthesis of fatty acid. Malonyl CoA blocks the transport of fatty acids into the mitochondria at the translocation enzyme carnitine palmitoyltransferase I (CPT I).

however, the hepatic requirements for energy are such that only a small amount of the total fatty-acid supply during adipose mobilization needs to be used for complete oxidation. The second pathway is esterification with triglyceride production, and the third is the production of ketone bodies. Triglyceride synthesis is discussed later; here, ketone body production is the focus.

Hepatic ketone body formation is promoted by low glucose availability, a high glucagon-to-insulin ratio, and a ready supply of fatty acids

Ketone body formation occurs within the hepatic mitochondria, and the rate of ketone body synthesis is controlled by the regulated transport of fatty acids across the mitochondrial membrane (Fig. 31–16). Fatty acids enter mitochondria in combination with a molecule known as *carnitine,* and transport depends on an enzyme known as *carnitine palmitoyltransferase I (CPT I).* The activity of this enzyme, along with the availability of fatty acid, is the primary determinant of the rate of ketone body formation. CPT I activity is regulated in an interesting fashion, being inhibited by an intermediate of the fatty-acid synthesis pathway, *malonyl CoA.* Malonyl CoA concentrations are high when there is an excess of glucose, that is, when the liver is responding to insulin and glucose is being used for fatty-acid synthesis. When glucose supplies are low, or glucagon concentrations are high relative

to insulin levels, little fatty acid is synthesized in the liver. Thus, malonyl CoA concentrations are low and CPT I is fully active when the insulin-to-glucagon ratio is low.

Under conditions of active CPT I, most available fatty acid is transported into the mitochondria for ketone body synthesis. This well-orchestrated but somewhat complex regulatory system is important, because the liver can both produce and consume fatty acids. If there were not a way of "turning off" fatty-acid destruction during periods of synthesis, a futile cycle of synthesis and destruction would occur. The inhibition of CPT I by malonyl CoA provides a system that blocks the metabolic destruction of newly synthesized fatty acid while still providing a mechanism for the utilization of fatty acids derived from adipose tissue in times of insufficient energy supply. The overall pattern of metabolism results in a reciprocal relationship between glucose availability and ketone body production. Although ketone bodies are produced in the liver, they cannot be used there for energy production. Therefore, all ketone bodies are transported to peripheral tissues for utilization. When the concentration of ketone bodies in the blood becomes abnormally high, some are excreted in the urine.

Glucagon plays an important role in the excessive production of ketone bodies during diabetes mellitus

If untreated, diabetes mellitus in animals, especially dogs, leads to high concentrations of ketone bodies in the blood. Diabetes mellitus occurs because of a lack of insulin, but the hepatic production of ketone bodies occurs because of the unrestrained action of glucagon. Even though serum concentrations of glucose are high in diabetes mellitus, the inability of the pancreas to secrete insulin leads to a low insulin-to-glucagon ratio; thus, the liver is functioning solely under the direction of glucagon. Glucagon inhibits fatty-acid production from glucose, so malonyl CoA concentrations are low and CPT I activity is high. Because of the lack of insulin to suppress adipose HSL, blood NEFA concentrations are high. The combination of high NEFA availability and unrestrained CPT I activity results in rapid transport of fatty acids into the mitochondria with extensive ketone body production, even though blood glucose concentrations are high.

Fatty acids cannot be used for glucose synthesis

It is important to understand that the metabolism of fat within the mitochondria cannot contribute directly to gluconeogenesis. Once across the mitochondrial membrane, fatty acids undergo β-oxidation, which leads to the successive removal of two-carbon acetyl CoA units from the carbon chains of the fatty acids. The resulting acetyl CoA can enter the Krebs cycle through condensation with oxaloacetate. Because any of the Krebs cycle intermediates can lead to glucose production, it may appear at first that acetyl CoA from fatty-acid β-oxidation could lead to the production of glucose. However, this is not the case; there is no *net* production of oxaloacetate associated with the consumption of acetyl CoA by the Krebs cycle (Fig. 31–17). Existing oxaloacetate combines with acetyl CoA to form citrate in the initial step of the cycle. At the end of the cycle, the original oxaloacetate is reformed, as the two carbons from the acetyl CoA are converted to carbon dioxide. No new oxaloacetate can be produced by this process.

Ketone bodies are formed in the mitochondria from acetyl CoA

Not all mitochondrial acetyl CoA must enter the Krebs cycle. In fact, when fatty acids are rapidly entering the mitochondria, there is far more acetyl CoA available than necessary for Krebs cycle activity. It is this excess acetyl CoA, originating from fatty acids, from which the ketone bodies are synthesized (see Fig. 31–16). Ketone bodies are able to leave the mitochondria freely.

Ketone bodies affect fuel homeostasis in peripheral tissues, where they may serve as a substitute for glucose. In this way, they conserve available glucose and reduce the need for gluconeogenesis.

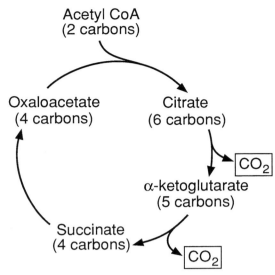

FIGURE 31–17. Oxidation of acetyl CoA (from acetate) by the Krebs cycle. The two carbons of acetyl CoA result in the formation of carbon dioxide; there is no net synthesis of oxaloacetate. Because it is oxaloacetate that forms the precursor for glucose synthesis, acetyl CoA (and thus acetate) cannot lead to glucose formation.

Hepatic very low density lipoproteins may be synthesized from adipose-derived fatty acid as well as from newly synthesized fatty acid

In the section on absorptive-phase metabolism, the hepatic production of VLDL is discussed. During the absorptive phase, triglyceride for VLDL synthesis comes from fatty acids synthesized from glucose. During catabolic periods, VLDLs may continue to be produced, but fatty acids derived from serum NEFAs are used for VLDL synthesis (see Fig. 31–5). This may initially appear to be an unnecessary and inefficient metabolic step. Why should fatty acids from adipose tissue be transported to the liver for VLDL formation when they can be directly metabolized for energy by the tissues? The need for VLDL synthesis occurs because of the need for a better transport system. The capacity of the serum to transport NEFA is limited, because NEFA must circulate bound to albumin, and the NEFA-binding capacity of albumin is finite and may become nearly saturated during periods of rapid adipose mobilization. VLDLs provide a transport system for fatty acids that does not depend on albumin and thus is not limited, as the serum is, by the amount of fatty acid that can be accommodated by albumin.

Hormonal conditions direct the distribution of very low density lipoprotein fatty acids in the body

During the absorptive phase, VLDLs are directed to adipose tissue by the action of adipose tissue LPL, an insulin-stimulated enzyme. LPL also exists in muscle tissue, but does not depend on insulin stimulation for activity. Thus, during periods of low glucose availability, adipose tissue LPL is inhibited because of a lack of insulin, but muscle tissue LPL is fully active. This situation leads to the selective direction of VLDL fatty acids to muscle tissue during times of adipose mobilization.

Changes in growth hormone concentrations may aid in shifting peripheral fuel utilization from glucose and amino acids to ketone bodies and fatty acids

The fat mobilization–induced changes in hepatic metabolism are effective in conserving protein only because of changes that occur in glucose and amino acid utilization in peripheral tissues. As ketone bodies, NEFA, and VLDL triglycerides become the major energy supplies, there is less tissue demand for glucose or amino acids as energy substrates. Endocrine alterations, in addition to low insulin concentrations, may aid in promoting this switch in peripheral fuel utilization. In several species, growth hormone concentrations rise during a prolonged period of energy deprivation. Growth hormone is antagonistic to insulin, thus promoting an increase in the serum glucose concentration even in the presence of normal or near-normal serum insulin levels. In addition, growth hormone may have some direct effect on conserving protein and mobilizing lipid.

THE SPECIAL FUEL CONSIDERATIONS OF RUMINANTS

Ruminants exist in a perpetual state of gluconeogenesis because of their unique digestive process

Most carbohydrate digestion in ruminants occurs in the forestomach through fermentative digestion. The result is that almost no digestible carbohydrate enters the intestine for glandular digestion and absorption as glucose. Therefore, ruminants exist in a constant state of potential glucose deficiency. In order to cope with this situation, ruminants have developed efficient systems of both production and conservation of glucose.

Essentially, all the glucose available to ruminants consuming most types of diets originates from gluconeogenesis. Quantitatively, the most important glucose precursor is the volatile fatty acid propionate. Propionate contributes to glucose synthesis after entering the Krebs cycle at the level of succinate. The reactions involved in the conversion of propionate to succinate are illustrated in Figure 31–18. Note that succinate is a four-carbon Krebs cycle intermediate that can lead to net formation of oxaloacetate, the entry metabolite for gluconeogenesis. The other volatile fatty acids, acetate and butyrate, also enter the Krebs cycle; however, like the long-chain fatty acids

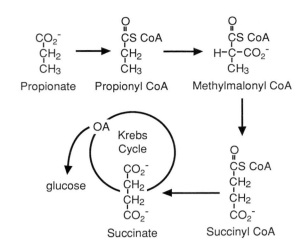

FIGURE 31–18. Gluconeogenesis from propionate involves its initial conversion to succinate. Succinate is a four-carbon Krebs cycle intermediate that can lead to net glucose synthesis.

from adipose tissue, acetate and butyrate enter the cycle as acetyl CoA. As previously discussed, acetyl CoA cannot lead to the net production of oxaloacetate or glucose. Therefore, of the ruminant's major energy sources—acetate, propionate, and butyrate—only propionate can support glucose production.

Nearly all propionate absorbed from the rumen is extracted from the portal blood by the liver, never entering the systemic circulation. Hepatic extraction of propionate determines that all propionate is used for gluconeogenesis. In addition to propionate, amino acids from intestinal absorption also provide substrate for gluconeogenesis. The use of dietary amino acid for gluconeogenesis is discussed earlier in relation to amino acid–stimulated release of glucagon in the section on absorptive-phase metabolism.

In addition to constant gluconeogenesis, ruminants also support their glucose needs by efficiently conserving glucose. Fatty acids, which in some animals, such as primates, rats, and dogs, are synthesized in the liver, are synthesized only in the adipose tissue of ruminants. Furthermore, glucose is essentially not used for fatty-acid synthesis. Rather, fatty acids are synthesized from acetate, which is the most abundant energy source in ruminants. The only glucose used by adipose tissue is for the synthesis of the glycerol backbone for triglycerides. In lactating animals, fatty acids produced in the udder for milk fat are synthesized from either acetate or ketone bodies, never from glucose.

Some important metabolic diseases of ruminants occur during periods when their system of glucose homeostasis is stressed. Dairy cows are especially vulnerable at peak lactation, because the synthesis of lactose, milk sugar, requires glucose. In high-producing cows, nearly all the glucose they produce goes to lactose synthesis, whereas the remainder of their tissues function on alternative fuels. Sheep experience a similar stress on glucose synthesis in late gestation. The energy needs of the fetus and placenta can be met only by glucose (or glucose-derived lactate) and amino acids. Sheep, in comparison with many other animals, have a high ratio of fetal mass to body size; thus, their fuel homeostatic mechanisms are particularly stressed by pregnancy. Failure of the glucose homeostatic mechanism frequently occurs under these circumstances, resulting in conditions known as lactational ketosis in dairy cows and pregnancy toxemia in ewes.

CLINICAL CORRELATIONS

Hepatic lipidosis in a cat

History You are asked to examine a 3-year-old intact female cat. She had been apparently normal, and in fact quite fat and happy, until 2 weeks ago, when she disappeared from her owner's apartment for 4 days. When she returned, she seemed depressed and would not eat. Over the next few days she became progressively more listless, almost somnolent.

Clinical and laboratory examination The cat has a normal pulse, temperature, and respiratory rate, but she is depressed and responds little to handling. The ocular sclera (whites of the eyes) appear icteric, or jaundiced. The latter physical sign leads you to suspect liver disease, so you submit blood samples for biochemical analysis. Analysis of blood taken from the jugular vein reveals a higher-than-normal concentration of bile acids and bilirubin, confirming a diagnosis of liver disease. A needle-aspiration biopsy of the liver reveals hepatocytes that are distended with large droplets of nonstaining material, probably fat.

Comment The presence of significant concentrations of bile acids in blood, other than in the hepatic-portal circulation, is evidence of reduced liver function. Recall that bile acids are absorbed from the ileum into the portal vein, in which they return to the liver. The normal liver extracts bile acids from portal blood efficiently, allowing only small amounts to escape into the systemic circulation; thus, elevated concentrations of bile acids in jugular blood indicate liver disease.

Hepatic lipidosis, or fatty liver, is a common disease of cats. It is brought on by a period of stress combined with either an unwillingness to eat or a lack of available food. In either situation, the cats begin to mobilize large quantities of fat to support their metabolic energy needs. Normally, it would be expected that much of the mobilized NEFA would be taken up by the liver and converted to VLDL for export to energy-using tissues. In cats that experience fatty liver, the hepatic influx of NEFA appears to overwhelm the liver's capacity to synthesize and secrete VLDL, so fat accumulates in the liver. When the fat accumulation becomes severe, hepatic function is compromised, and the cats become systemically ill. Their appetites become severely depressed, and thus, a downward spiral of events is created in which the hepatic lipidosis becomes more and more severe.

Treatment Treatment consists of reversing the state of negative energy balance by force-feeding. Various methods of force-feeding exist; the most practical consists of the placement of an indwelling gastric tube. The tube is often passed through the nostrils but may be placed by a number of different techniques, including direct intubation through the wall of the abdomen. The latter technique is facilitated by the use of a fiberoptic gastroscope. Once the cat is in positive energy balance, adipose mobilization ceases, and the liver eventually clears of fat. Tube feeding may have to continue for several days before the cat begins to eat on its own. Tube feeding has markedly improved the prognosis for this disease, although it is still a life-threatening condition.

Bibliography

Bauman DE, Currie WB: Partitioning of nutrients during pregnancy and lactation: A review of mechanisms involving homeostasis and homeorrhesis. J Dairy Sci 63:1514–1529, 1980.

Bender DA: Introduction to Nutrition and Metabolism, 2nd ed. Bristol, Pa.: Taylor & Francis, 1997.

Bondy PK, Rosenberg LE: Metabolic Control and Disease. Philadelphia: WB Saunders, 1979, pp 161–494.

Brody T: Nutritional Biochemistry, 2nd ed. San Diego: Academic Press, 1999.

Cahill GF: Starvation in man. Clin Endocrinol Metab 5:397–415, 1976.

DeGroot LJ (ed): Endocrinology. Philadelphia: WB Saunders, 1989, pp 2282–2293, 2367–2403.

Gillham B, Papachristodoulou DK, Thomas JH: Will's Biochemical Basis of Medicine, 3rd ed. Boston: Butterworth-Heinemann, 1996.

Herdt TH: Fuel homeostasis in the ruminant. Vet Clin North Am Food Anim Pract 4:213–231, 1988.

Kaneko JJ, Harvey JW, Bruss ML: Clinical Biochemistry of Domestic Animals, 5th ed. San Diego: Academic Press, 1997, pp 45–111.

Nordlie RC, Foster JD, Lange AJ: Regulation of glucose production by the liver. Annu Rev Nutr 19:379–406, 1999.

Thomas JH, Gillham B: Will's Biochemical Basis of Medicine, 2nd ed. London: Wright, 1989.

PRACTICE QUESTIONS

1. All of the following are metabolites that can be oxidized for fuel in the animal body. Which one is *not* important in the transport of energy between organs and organ systems?
    a. Triglyceride.
    b. Ketone bodies.
    c. Oxaloacetic acid.
    d. Nonesterified fatty acids.
    e. Amino acids.

2. Which of the following reactions is *not* characteristic of the absorptive phase of digestion?
    a. Hepatic synthesis of glycogen.
    b. Hepatic uptake of glucose.
    c. Destruction of dietary amino acid.
    d. Utilization of muscle-derived amino acid for gluconeogenesis.
    e. Hepatic synthesis of triglyceride from glucose.

3. Which of the following reactions in the liver could be expected to occur during both the digestive phase and a prolonged fast?
    a. Glycogen synthesis.
    b. Fatty-acid synthesis.
    c. Ketone body synthesis.
    d. Ketone body oxidation.
    e. Triglyceride synthesis from fatty acids.

4. Which of the following statements is true of both ketone bodies and nonesterified fatty acids?
    a. They are water-soluble.
    b. They provide energy for muscle metabolism.

c. They circulate in blood bound to albumin.
d. They can provide energy to the brain.
e. They are formed exclusively in the liver.

5. Which of the following amino acids is *not* extensively catabolized by the liver?
   a. Valine.
   b. Alanine.

c. Glutamine.
d. Asparagine.
e. Glycine.

PRACTICE ANSWERS

1. c   2. d   3. e   4. b   5. a

ENDOCRINOLOGY

Deborah Greco

George H. Stabenfeldt*

*Deceased.

32

The endocrine system

General concepts

1   Hormones are chemicals produced by specific tissues that are transported by the vascular system to affect other tissues at low concentrations
2   The endocrine and nervous systems are integrated in their control of physiologic processes

The synthesis of hormones

1   Protein hormones are initially synthesized as preprohormones and then cleaved in the rough endoplasmic reticulum to form prohormones and in the Golgi apparatus to form the active hormones, which are stored in granules before being released by exocytosis
2   Steroids are synthesized from cholesterol, which is synthesized by the liver; steroids are not stored but are released as they are synthesized

The transport of hormones in the blood

1   Protein hormones are hydrophilic and carried in the plasma in dissolved form
2   Steroids and thyroid hormones are lipophilic and carried in plasma in association with both specific and nonspecific binding proteins; the amount of unbound, active hormone is relatively small

Hormone-cell interaction

1   Protein hormones have specific receptors on target tissue plasma membranes, whereas steroids have specific receptors within the cytoplasm or nucleus

Postreceptor cell responses

1   Steroids interact directly with the cell nucleus through the formation of a complex with its cytosolic receptor, whereas protein hormones need a messenger because they cannot enter the cell

Metabolism of hormones

1   Steroid hormones are metabolized by conjugation with sulfates and glucuronides, which makes them water-soluble

Feedback control mechanisms

1   The most important control for hormones is the negative feedback system, in which increased hormone concentrations result in less production of the hormone, usually through an interaction with the hypothalamus or pituitary gland
2   Endocrine secretory patterns can be influenced by factors such as sleep or light and can produce circadian rhythms

The hypothalamus

1   The hypothalamus coordinates the activity of the pituitary gland through the secretion of peptides and amines

The pituitary gland

1   The neurohypophysis has cell bodies that originate in the hypothalamus, with cell endings that secrete oxytocin and vasopressin
2   Oxytocin and vasopressin are synthesized in cell bodies within the hypothalamus and are carried by axon flow to the posterior lobe, where they are released
3   The main effects of oxytocin are on the contraction of smooth muscle (mammary gland and uterus); the effects of vasopressin are primarily on the conservation of water (antidiuresis) and secondarily on blood pressure
4   Plasma osmolality controls the secretion of vasopressin
5   The anterior pituitary produces the following hormones: growth hormone, prolactin, thyroid-stimulating hormone, follicle-stimulating hormone, luteinizing hormone, and corticotropin
6   Adenohypophyseal activity is controlled by hypothalamic releasing hormones, which are released into the portal system, which in turn connects the median eminence of the hypothalamus and the anterior pituitary gland

GENERAL CONCEPTS

Hormones are chemicals produced by specific tissues that are transported by the vascular system to affect other tissues at low concentrations

The endocrine system has evolved to allow physiologic processes to be coordinated and regulated. The system uses chemical messengers called *hormones.*

Hormones have traditionally been defined as chemicals that are produced by specific endocrine organs, are transported by the vascular system, and are able to affect distant target organs in low concentration. Although this definition is useful from a veterinary medical point of view, it should be recognized that there are substances, such as prostaglandins and somatomedins, that are produced by many other tissues and yet are considered to be hormones.

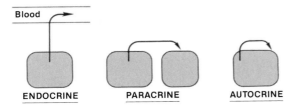

FIGURE 32–1. Types of cell communication via chemical mediators. (From Hedge GA, Colby HD, Goodman RL: Clinical Endocrine Physiology. Philadelphia: WB Saunders, 1987, p 29.)

Other types of control systems use chemical substances that are not transported in the vascular system to influence distant cell activity. These systems serve as means of local integration among or between cells. These systems are as follows:

1. *Paracrine effectors,* in which the messenger diffuses through the interstitial fluids, usually to influence adjacent cells; if the messenger acts on the cell of its origin, the substance is called an *autocrine* effector (Fig. 32–1).

2. *Neurotransmitters,* which affect communication between neurons, or between neurons and target cells; the substances are limited in the distance traveled and the area of the cell influenced (Fig. 32–2).

3. *Exocrine effectors,* such as hormones produced by the pancreas, are released into the gastrointestinal tract.

The endocrine and nervous systems are integrated in their control of physiologic processes

The endocrine system interacts with the other main regulatory system, the *nervous system,* which coordinates activities that require rapid control. An example of the close interaction of the two systems is the reflex in which suckling causes the release of milk. Suckling initiates the transmission of nerve impulses from the mammary gland to the hypothalamus (by way of the spinal tract). Neurosecretory neurons within the supraoptic and paraventricular nuclei are stimulated to synthesize oxytocin. Oxytocin is transported along axons of these nerves and is released from nerve endings in the posterior pituitary into the blood vascular system. Oxytocin is then carried to the mammary gland, where it causes contraction of myoepi-

thelial cells. These cells surround the smallest unit of milk-secreting cells, called an *alveolus.* This results in the movement of milk into the large cisternae adjacent to the teat and, subsequently, into the teat.

The interaction between the nervous and endocrine systems can be even more direct: for example, endocrine cells of the adrenal medulla are directly controlled by preganglionic neurons of the adrenal medulla, and the medullary hormones are released immediately in response to stressful stimuli. The endocrine and nervous systems also share transmitters; substances such as epinephrine, dopamine, histamine, and somatostatin are found in both endocrine and neural tissues.

The endocrine system is involved in control of physiologic functions, including *metabolism, growth,* and *reproduction.* Metabolism can be divided into two forms: *energy* and *mineral.* The hormones that control energy metabolism include insulin, glucagon, cortisol, epinephrine, thyroid hormone, and growth hormone. The hormones that control mineral metabolism include parathyroid hormone, calcitonin, angiotensin, and renin. The hormones that control growth include growth hormone, thyroid hormone, insulin, estrogen and androgens (both reproductive hormones), and a large number of growth factors. The hormones that control *reproduction* include estrogen, androgen, progesterone, luteinizing hormone (LH), follicle-stimulating hormone (FSH), prolactin (PRL), and oxytocin.

One of the important characteristics of the endocrine system is the *amplification* of the signal. The action of one steroid molecule to activate a gene can result in the formation of many messenger RNA (mRNA) molecules, and each of these can induce the formation of many enzyme molecules. Also, one protein molecule can influence the formation of many cyclic adenosine 3′,5′-monophosphate (cAMP) molecules, and each of these can activate many enzymes. Amplification is the basis for the sensitivity of the endocrine system, which allows small amounts of hormones in plasma (10^{-11} to 10^{-12} mol) to produce significant biologic effects. Hormone action also influences rates of existing enzyme reactions but not the initiation of new reactions. This implies that there are certain basal levels of enzyme activities even in the absence of hormones. Hormone action is relatively slow and prolonged, with the effects of hormones lasting minutes to days. This contrasts with the nervous system, in which the response is rapid and short (milliseconds to seconds).

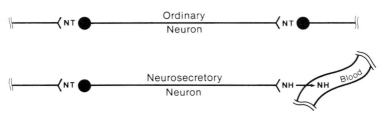

FIGURE 32–2. Comparison of functional arrangements of an ordinary neuron releasing its neurotransmitter *(NT)* into a synapse and a neurosecretory neuron releasing its neurohormone *(NH)* into a blood vessel. (From Hedge GA, Colby HD, Goodman RL: Clinical Endocrine Physiology. Philadelphia: WB Saunders, 1987, p 54.)

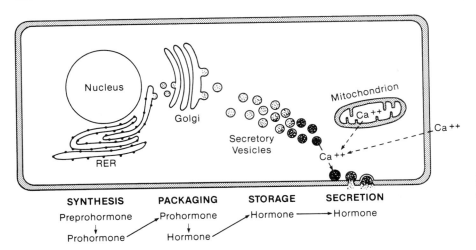

FIGURE 32–3. Subcellular components of peptide hormone synthesis and secretion. *RER*, rough endoplasmic reticulum. (From Hedge GA, Colby HD, Goodman RL: Clinical Endocrine Physiology. Philadelphia: WB Saunders, 1987, p 7.)

THE SYNTHESIS OF HORMONES

Protein hormones are initially synthesized as preprohormones and then cleaved in the rough endoplasmic reticulum to form prohormones and in the Golgi apparatus to form the active hormones, which are stored in granules before being released by exocytosis

The major classes of hormones include proteins (e.g., growth hormone, insulin, corticotropin [previously called adrenocorticotropic hormone, or ACTH]); peptides (e.g., oxytocin and vasopressin); amines (e.g., dopamine, melatonin, epinephrine); and steroids (e.g., cortisol, progesterone, vitamin D). The protein and peptide hormones are initially synthesized on ribosomes as larger precursor proteins, which are referred to as *preprohormones* (Fig. 32–3). Synthesis of protein hormones begins in ribosomes, with the "pre" portion immediately attaching to the rough endoplasmic reticulum (RER), which pulls the ribosomes into close apposition with the RER. During synthesis, the preprohormone is secreted into the interior of the RER. The presence of a peptidase within the wall of the RER allows the "pre" portion of the molecule to be rapidly removed and the prohormone to leave the RER in vesicles that have been pinched off from the RER. These vesicles then move to the Golgi apparatus, where they coalesce with Golgi membranes to form secretory granules. The prohormone is cleaved during this process, so that most of the hormone is in its final form within the Golgi apparatus, although some prohormone can also be found.

Protein hormones are stored in granules within the gland until needed for release. Although some of the hormone is secreted on a continuous basis, most is secreted through the process of exocytosis of granules in response to a specific signal. The process of exocytosis requires adenosine triphosphate and calcium. Increased cytoplasmic calcium results from intracellular release of calcium from mitochondria, or endoplasmic reticulum, or from the influx of extracellular calcium.

Steroids are synthesized from cholesterol, which is synthesized by the liver; steroids are not stored but are released as they are synthesized

Steroids represent a class of hormones that, unlike protein hormones, are lipophilic. In general, they belong to one of two categories: adrenocortical hormones (glucocorticoids, mineralocorticoids) and sex hormones (estrogen, progesterone, androgens). They have a common four-ring, 17-carbon skeleton that is derived from cholesterol (Fig. 32–4). Although the steroids can be synthesized de novo within the cell from the two-carbon molecule acetate, the majority of steroids are formed from cholesterol, which is synthesized by the liver (Fig. 32–5). Low-density lipoproteins enter steroid-producing cells through interaction with a membrane receptor. Cholesterol is released through the degradation of low-density lipoproteins by lysosomal enzymes. Cholesterol is either used immediately for steroid synthesis or stored in granules in an ester form within the cell. The first step in the synthesis of all steroid hormones from cholesterol

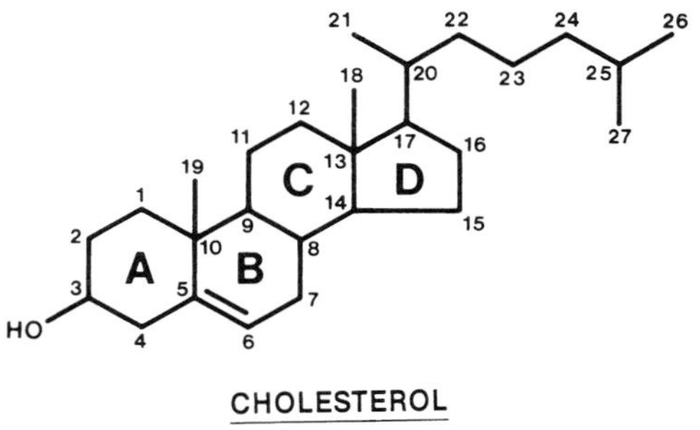

FIGURE 32–4. The ring structure and numbering system of the carbon atoms in steroid hormones, illustrated for the cholesterol molecule. (From Hedge GA, Colby HD, Goodman RL: Clinical Endocrine Physiology. Philadelphia: WB Saunders, 1987, p 9.)

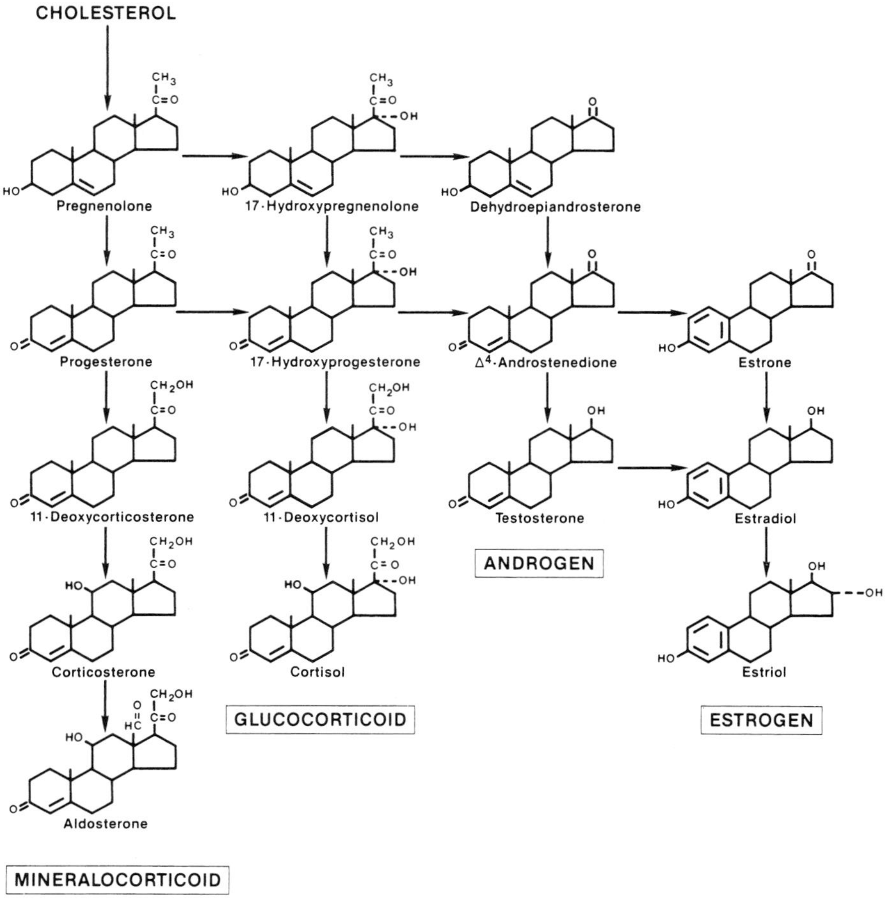

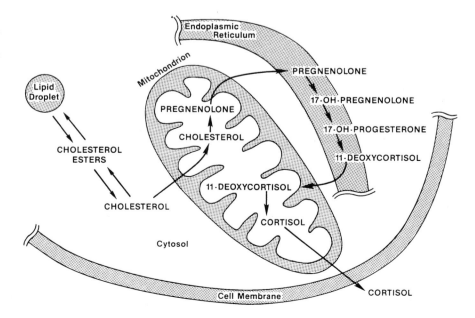

CHOLESTEROL

Pregnenolone 17-Hydroxypregnenolone Dehydroepiandrosterone

Progesterone 17-Hydroxyprogesterone Δ⁴-Androstenedione Estrone

11-Deoxycorticosterone 11-Deoxycortisol Testosterone Estradiol

ANDROGEN

Corticosterone Cortisol

GLUCOCORTICOID Estriol

ESTROGEN

Aldosterone

MINERALOCORTICOID

FIGURE 32-5. Pathways involved in the production of the major steroid hormones. (From Hedge GA, Colby HD, Goodman RL: Clinical Endocrine Physiology. Philadelphia: WB Saunders, 1987, p 12.)

involves cleavage of the side chain of cholesterol to form pregnenolone; this step occurs within the mitochondrion. Subsequent modifications of the steroid molecule may occur within the mitochondrion or may involve movement to other compartments of the cell

(Fig. 32–6). The control of movement of steroids among cell compartments during the synthesis process is not well understood.

The type of steroid hormone that is eventually synthesized is dependent on the presence of specific en-

FIGURE 32-6. Subcellular compartmentalization of cortisol biosynthesis. (From Hedge GA, Colby HD, Goodman RL: Clinical Endocrine Physiology. Philadelphia: WB Saunders, 1987, p 13.)

Endoplasmic Reticulum

Mitochondrion

PREGNENOLONE

Lipid Droplet

PREGNENOLONE

17-OH-PREGNENOLONE

CHOLESTEROL

17-OH-PROGESTERONE

CHOLESTEROL ESTERS

11-DEOXYCORTISOL

11-DEOXYCORTISOL

CHOLESTEROL

CORTISOL

Cytosol

Cell Membrane   CORTISOL

zymes within the particular cell. For example, only cells of the adrenal cortex contain enzymes (hydroxylases) that result in hydroxylation of the 11th and 21st carbon molecules, a process that is essential for the production of glucocorticoids and mineralocorticoids. The pattern for sex steroid biosynthesis is for pregnenolone to be modified in a sequence that involves progesterone, androgens, and, finally, estrogens. Cells that synthesize androgens (e.g., Leydig cells of the testis) have the enzymes required for the formation of pregnenolone and progesterone, as well as for the modification of progesterone to androgen, but lack the enzymes necessary to modify androgens into estrogens. Although the sex steroid–forming cells do not have enzymes that allow the formation of adrenocortical hormones, the adrenal cortex contains the enzyme systems necessary for the formation of both adrenocortical hormones and sex hormones, although the former are emphasized. As a result, the adrenal cortex normally produces small amounts of sex steroids and produces larger amounts in certain pathophysiologic conditions.

There is no provision for the storage of steroid hormones within the cell; they are secreted immediately after formation by simple diffusion across the cell membrane because of their lipophilic structure. Thus, synthesis and secretion of steroid hormones occur in a tightly coupled manner, whereby the rate of hormone secretion is controlled by the rate of synthesis. The only storage form of steroids within these cells involves that of the precursor molecule, cholesterol, as an ester.

THE TRANSPORT OF HORMONES IN THE BLOOD

Protein hormones are hydrophilic and carried in the plasma in dissolved form

This chapter is concerned mainly with hormones that are transported to target tissues in the vascular system. The means by which hormones are transported in the blood varies according to the solubility of the hormone. Protein and peptide hormones are hydrophilic and are carried in the plasma in dissolved form. The protein hormones may circulate in monomeric (single unit) or polymeric (multiple unit) form (e.g., insulin). Hormones that have subunits can appear in the circulation in subunit form, although this reduces the biologic potency of the molecule.

Steroids and thyroid hormones are lipophilic and carried in plasma in association with both specific and nonspecific binding proteins; the amount of unbound, active hormone is relatively small

The transport of steroid and thyroid hormones is more complicated than that of protein hormones, because the steroid and thyroid hormones are lipophilic and thus have limited solubility in aqueous solutions. These hormones are transported in the blood through association with various types of proteins. Some of the proteins that bind steroids have a high affinity for a particular steroid; for example, a globulin, transcortin, has a high affinity for cortisol and corticosterone but also serves as an important transport vehicle for progesterone, even though it has a lower affinity for this hormone. The carrier proteins that have high affinities have low capacity because of their low plasma concentration. In contrast, the general class of plasma proteins called *albumins* have low affinities for steroid hormones but have a high capacity for steroid transport because of their high concentration in plasma.

A hormone must be in the free, or unbound, form before it can penetrate a target cell and elicit biologic activity. This is accomplished by the establishment of an equilibrium between bound and free hormone levels in the plasma. The free form usually represents only about 1% of the total amount of hormone in the plasma (up to 10% of cortisol may be in the free form). The system is responsive to use of the free form, and the free form is replenished quickly by dissociation of bound hormone from the protein. The total amount of the hormone is usually measured, with the exception of thyroid hormone, in which attempts are usually made to estimate the amounts of bound and free. As indicated for steroid hormones, synthesis and release are tightly linked, and because metabolic clearance rates are usually constant, concentrations of steroids in plasma are usually a good reflection of the secretion rate. Under certain physiologic conditions, such as pregnancy in humans, metabolism of estrogens can change because of the increased production of estrogen-binding proteins.

HORMONE-CELL INTERACTION

Protein hormones have specific receptors on target tissue plasma membranes, whereas steroids have specific receptors within the cytoplasm or nucleus

A central question in endocrinology is how hormones and target cells of a particular tissue interact in a specific manner. The problem seems almost overwhelming for steroids because they are lipid-soluble and able to permeate all cells of the body. The solution is that target cells have receptors that are specific for a particular hormone. For steroids, the receptors are located in the cytoplasm or nucleus of the target cells, whereas receptors for protein and peptide hormones are located on the plasma membrane of the cell. In addition to specificity, receptors have a high affinity for their respective hormone. These characteristics of the receptor allow hormones to be in low concentration in the blood and yet effective in producing significant tissue response.

The greater the affinity of the receptor for the hormone, the longer the biologic response. Termination of the action of a hormone usually requires dissociation of the hormone from the receptor. This occurs most often as a result of a decrease in plasma concentrations of the hormone; the binding of receptor and hormone is noncovalent, and declining hormone concentrations favor a chemical equilibrium of dissociation over association. Termination of hormone action can also occur as a result of internalization of the receptor-hormone complex through the process of endocytosis. The hormone is degraded by lysosomal enzymes, whereas the receptor, protected because of its association with the vesicle membrane, can be recycled to the plasma membrane.

Receptors are present on cells in far greater numbers than are required for the elicitation of a biologic response. Occupancy by a hormone of considerably less than 50% of the receptors usually elicits a maximal biologic response. Even so, changes in receptor numbers that affect the sensitivity of the cell, although not its maximal responsiveness, can occur. Changes in receptor number affect the probability that an interaction will occur between receptor and hormone. Receptor synthesis can be stimulated by a hormone that is different from the hormone that interacts with the receptor. For example, predominant gonadotropin receptors on ovarian granulosa cells change from FSH to LH receptors late in the ovarian follicle phase because of the influence of FSH. This allows the control of the ovarian follicle to pass from FSH to LH, which facilitates ovulation and the formation of a corpus luteum. Conversely, receptor numbers can decrease in conjunction with continued interaction of receptor and hormone. This often occurs when an agonist that has great affinity for the receptor is administered or when amounts of hormone are pathologically elevated. The receptor numbers are down-regulated in this situation. The end result is that the animal becomes resistant to continued therapy with the hormone in question.

POSTRECEPTOR CELL RESPONSES

Steroids interact directly with the cell nucleus through the formation of a complex with its cytosolic receptor, whereas protein hormones need a messenger because they cannot enter the cell

The events that follow binding of the hormone and receptor depend on whether a steroid, protein, or peptide hormone is involved. With steroids, the hormone is able to interact within the cell because of its ability to penetrate the lipoprotein plasma membrane (Fig. 32–7). The interaction of receptor and steroid hormone results in activation of the subsequent comple translocation to the nucleus, where it interacts with specific sites on the chromatin. The result is the production of mRNA, which when translocated to the ribosomes directs synthesis of proteins that produce the desired biologic result.

Protein or peptide hormones require an intermediary to act in their behalf, because they are not able to penetrate the plasma membrane of the cell; the intermediary substance is known as a *second messenger* (Fig. 32–8). The best-documented second messenger is cAMP, which is produced by the activation of an enzyme, adenyl cyclase, through interaction of the hormone and receptor in the plasma membrane. The activation of adenyl cyclase and the production of cAMP result in the phosphorylation of protein kinases, which are responsible for the biologic response. Other second messengers include cytosolic calcium and its associated phosphodiesterase, calmodulin, as well as inositol triphosphate (IP_3) and diacylglycerol, both of which are products of phosphatidyl inositol metabolism. An important action of IP_3 is the stimulation of intracellular calcium release. One important response to diacylglycerol is the activation of phospholipase A and the formation of arachidonic acid, which leads to formation of members of the prosta-

FIGURE 32–7.   Subcellular mechanism of action of a lipophilic hormone (H) via an intracellular receptor (R). The H-R complex induces messenger RNA (mRNA) synthesis by binding to an acceptor site (A) on the chromatin. (From Hedge GA, Colby HD, Goodman RL: Clinical Endocrine Physiology. Philadelphia: WB Saunders, 1987, p 18.)

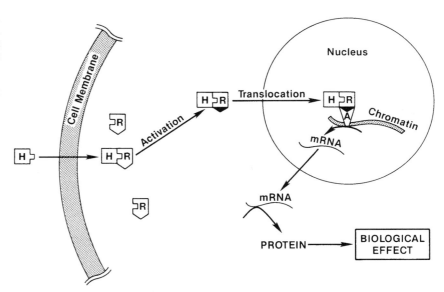

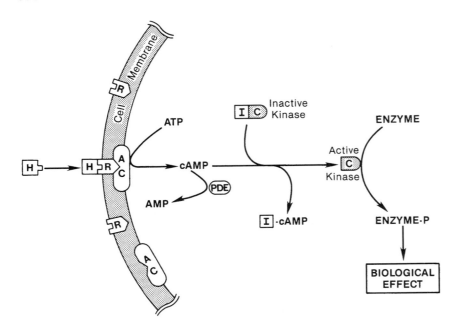

FIGURE 32–8. Subcellular mechanism of action of a hydrophilic hormone (H) via a membrane receptor (R), adenyl cyclase (AC), and cyclic adenosine monophosphate (cAMP). ATP, adenosine triphosphate; I and C, inhibitory and catalytic subunits of the kinase, respectively; PDE, phosphodiesterase. (From Hedge GA, Colby HD, Goodman RL: Clinical Endocrine Physiology. Philadelphia: WB Saunders, 1987, p 20.)

glandin family of molecules. The biologic response to a protein or peptide hormone–receptor interaction is more rapid than that to steroids; preexisting enzymes are activated, whereas the biologic response to steroid requires the synthesis of enzyme protein.

METABOLISM OF HORMONES

Steroid hormones are metabolized by conjugation with sulfates and glucuronides, which makes them water-soluble

Hormone activity is limited through the metabolism of hormones. The metabolism of steroids usually involves reduction of the molecule, followed by conjugation with sulfates and glucuronides, which increases the water solubility of the steroids, allowing them to be excreted in urine. The liver is the main organ responsible for this process. Iodine molecules are removed from thyroid hormones during metabolism. Protein hormones are cleaved by peptidases; this is preceded by reduction of disulfide bonds if that is a characteristic of the molecule. Although a metabolite is usually less biologically potent than the original molecule, there is some evidence that conjugates of steroids can have significant biologic activity. This raises the question of whether the conversion of hormones intracellularly, such as testosterone to dihydrotestosterone, represents metabolism, because dihydrotestosterone is more potent biologically than testosterone. Another example, the conversion of estradiol-17β to estrone by peripheral tissues, including adipose cells, is described as a form of metabolism; however, estrone is a natural, and relatively potent, estrogen.

Although there exist situations in which the rate of clearance of a hormone can change (e.g., decrease as a result of increased hormone-binding plasma proteins during pregnancy or increase as the result of decreased hormone-binding plasma proteins in conjunction with liver disease), metabolism of hormones is relatively constant, and the concentration of a hormone usually reflects the other determinant of hormone activity: the rate of synthesis of the hormone.

FEEDBACK CONTROL MECHANISMS

The most important feedback control for hormones is the negative feedback system, in which increased hormone concentrations result in less production of the hormone, usually through an interaction with the hypothalamus or pituitary gland

The effects of hormones are proportional to their concentrations in blood, and it follows that control of these concentrations is an important aspect in ensuring that physiologic function is normal. As indicated previously, the largest factor affecting hormone concentrations in blood is the secretion rate by a particular organ. There have evolved feedback loop control systems in which concentrations of hormones are monitored at the controlling point in order to either increase or decrease secretion of a hormone by an endocrine organ. The most common feedback system is negative feedback, in which continuous monitoring allows the system to counteract changes in hormone secretion or maintain a relatively constant environment.

An example of systems in which negative feedback control involves both the endocrine and the nervous system is shown in Figure 32–9. The hypothalamus, which controls secretion of tropic hormones in the anterior pituitary through the secretion of peptide-

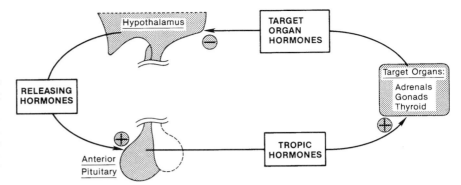

releasing hormones, has cells with a certain set-point by which they compare concentrations of hormone in the blood with the output of releasing hormones. If blood concentrations fall below the physiologic set-point, releasing hormone output increases; this occurrence, in turn, increases production of tropic hormones by the anterior pituitary gland and, subsequently, the secretion of the hormone by the target organ. Conversely, if the hormone concentration increases above acceptable physiologic limits, a shutdown of releasing hormone production occurs within the hypothalamus, tropic hormone secretion by the anterior pituitary decreases, and production of the hormone by the target organ decreases. This type of control system is not an all-or-none arrangement, because changes and adjustments are being made continuously in order to maintain an optimal concentration of hormone.

In the negative feedback system, an increase in secretion of hormone results in a decrease in tropic hormone secretion. It is also possible to have a negative feedback system in which an increase in a physiologic substance, such as glucose, causes an increase in a hormone: in this case, insulin, which plays an important role in glucose metabolism. This is considered to be a negative feedback system because blood glucose concentrations are being dampened, or returned, toward normal levels through the action of insulin.

Positive feedback systems also exist, although they are much less common than negative feedback systems. One example is the preovulatory release of LH, in which the pulsatile rate of LH secretion greatly increases during the late stages of ovarian follicle development because of increased estrogen production by the follicle. In this situation, there is a definitive end point: ovulation results in a decline in the stimulus, estrogen, although the duration of the LH surge is probably determined within the hypothalamus, and therefore the LH response to estrogen is modulated.

Endocrine secretory patterns can be influenced by factors such as sleep or light and can produce circadian rhythms

Endocrine secretion patterns can occur outside the control of negative feedback inhibition. Hormone patterns can change on an approximate 24-hour basis, a process referred to as a *diurnal* or *circadian rhythm*. *Circadian* is the preferred term, because *diurnal* refers to activity in the daytime; *nocturnal* should be used for the rhythms that are active at night. Most of the daily rhythms have some aspects of light, or lack of light, as a major influence in the rhythm. Rhythmic changes in hormone patterns that occur at shorter intervals, often in the range of an hour, are called *ultradian rhythms*.

THE HYPOTHALAMUS

The hypothalamus coordinates the activity of the pituitary gland through the secretion of peptides and amines

As indicated previously, the two major controlling systems are the nervous and the endocrine systems. The interface between these systems occurs, for the most part, in the hypothalamus. The hypothalamus is an area of the diencephalon that forms the floor of the third ventricle and includes the optic chiasma, tuber cinereum, mammillary bodies, and the median eminence. Often not included in this classification are the infundibulum and the neurohypophysis (stalk of the posterior lobe and the posterior lobe, respectively), although both tissues represent extensions of the hypothalamus into the pituitary gland. The hypothalamus produces peptides and amines that influence the pituitary gland to produce (1) tropic hormones (e.g., corticotropin), which in turn influence the production of hormones (e.g., cortisol) by peripheral target endocrine tissues, or (2) hormones that directly cause a biologic effect in tissues (e.g., PRL). The hypothalamus is also the center for the control of a large number of autonomic nervous system control pathways.

THE PITUITARY GLAND

The pituitary gland, or hypophysis cerebri, is composed of the adenohypophysis (pars distalis, or anterior lobe), the neurohypophysis (pars nervosa, or posterior lobe), the pars intermedia (intermediate lobe),

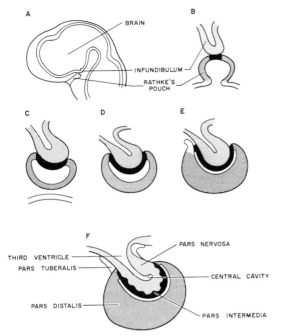

FIGURE 32–10. Diagrams showing progressive stages in the embryonic development of the pituitary gland. Rathke's pouch becomes detached from the oral epithelium at stage C. (*A,* from Villee CA, Walker WF Jr, Smith FE: General Zoology, 2nd ed. Philadelphia: WB Saunders, 1963. From Turner CD, Bagnara JT: General Endocrinology, 6th ed. Philadelphia: WB Saunders, 1977, p 81.)

and the pars tuberalis (Fig. 32–10). The adenohypophysis is formed from an area of the roof of the embryonic oral ectoderm called *Rathke's pouch,* which extends upward to meet the neurohypophysis, which extends downward as an outpouching of neural ectoderm from the floor of the third ventricle.

The neurohypophysis has cell bodies that originate in the hypothalamus, with cell endings that secrete oxytocin and vasopressin

The neurohypophysis is composed of axons whose neural origin is largely within the supraoptic and paraventricular nuclei of the hypothalamus. The neurohypophysis is an extension of the hypothalamus into the pituitary; that is, the cell bodies are in the hypothalamus. The axons form the stalk of the posterior lobe, and the nerve endings are in the lobe proper (Fig. 32–11).

The endocrine-secretory neurons that constitute the neurohypophysis differ from neurons involved in the transmission of neural signals in several ways: (1) neurosecretory neurons do not innervate other neurons, even though they are innervated; (2) the secretory product of neurosecretory neurons is secreted into the blood; and (3) the secretory product can act at distances greatly removed from the neuron. Also, in contrast to anterior pituitary hormones, which influence other tissues to produce hormones, posterior

lobe hormones can directly cause the desired tissue response.

The first indication of the physiologic activity of the neurohypophyseal lobe was the finding of Oliver and Schafer in 1895 that the injection of whole pituitary extracts caused a rise in blood pressure. This effect was soon found to be associated with the pars nervosa. This action represents the effects of one of the main neurohypophyseal hormones, vasopressin. The existence of the other main neurohypophyseal hormone, oxytocin, was first indicated in 1915, when Gaines showed that the injection of posterior pituitary gland extracts caused milk ejection. In 1941 Ely and Peterson showed that a denervated mammary gland could eject milk if the gland was perfused with blood that had been enriched with posterior pituitary extract. Both neurohypophyseal hormones were isolated and sequenced by du Vigneaud in 1954. These were some of the first proteins whose amino acid sequences were elucidated.

Oxytocin and vasopressin are synthesized in cell bodies within the hypothalamus and are carried by axon flow to the posterior lobe, where they are released

As indicated, the two important hormones produced by the neurohypophysis are vasopressin and oxytocin. Although it was previously thought that the two hormones were produced in separate nuclei, there is now evidence that both hormones are produced in both the supraoptic and the paraventricular nucleus. The cell bodies that synthesize the hormones are large and thus are called *magnocellular nuclei.* The synthesis of vasopressin and oxytocin, as described previously for protein and peptide hormones, involves first the production of a preprohormone, prepropressophysin for vasopressin and prepro-oxyphysin for oxytocin, at the level of the cell body within the hypothalamus

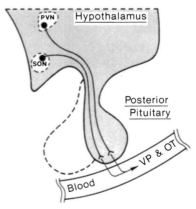

FIGURE 32–11. The hypothalamoneurohypophyseal system, which secretes vasopressin (VP) and oxytocin (OT). PVN, paraventricular nucleus; SON, supraoptic nucleus. (From Hedge GA, Colby HD, Goodman RL: Clinical Endocrine Physiology. Philadelphia: WB Saunders, 1987, p 56.)

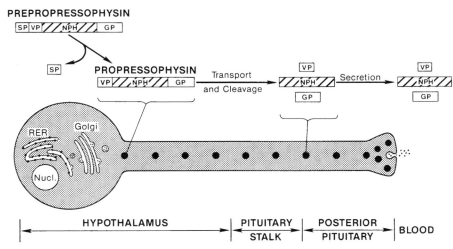

FIGURE 32–12. Diagram of a vasopressin-secreting neuron illustrating the subcellular components involved in synthesis and secretion. This process begins with the synthesis of prepropressophysin, which consists of (1) a signal peptide (SP); (2) vasopressin (VP); (3) neurophysin (NPH); and (4) a glycoprotein (GP). The production and release of oxytocin is identical except that no glycoprotein is involved. RER, rough endoplasmic reticulum; Nucl., nucleus. (From Hedge GA, Colby HD, Goodman RL: Clinical Endocrine Physiology. Philadelphia: WB Saunders, 1987, p 58.)

(Fig. 32–12). The "pre" portion of the molecule is cleaved before the molecules are packaged into granules. During passage of the granules down the axon, the prohormone is cleaved to produce either oxytocin or vasopressin; the remaining peptide fragments are called neurophysin I or neurophysin II, respectively. Neurophysin I, which is released into the blood vascular system along with oxytocin, has been quantified as an alternative means of following the release of oxytocin. At present, the physiologic function of the neurophysins is not known.

The release of the posterior lobe peptide hormones is initiated in the hypothalamus as a result of depolarization of the cell body because of stimulation by neural afferents. The action potential generated extends down the axon to the nerve terminal, where the secretory granules containing the hormone are stored. The depolarization of the nerve cell membrane allows the influx of calcium ions, which initiates the release of hormone through the process of exocytosis.

The main effects of oxytocin are on the contraction of smooth muscle (mammary gland and uterus); the effects of vasopressin are primarily on the conservation of water (antidiuresis) and secondarily on blood pressure

The main effects of oxytocin involve the contraction of the myoepithelial cells, which surround the alveoli in the mammary gland and the myometrium of the uterus. These actions are covered in Chapters 37 and 38.

The main activity of vasopressin belies its name because its main effect is antidiuretic, the enhancement of water retention by the kidney. As a consequence, the hormone is often called *antidiuretic hor-*

mone (ADH) (Fig. 32–13). Vasopressin is the most important hormone for the control of water balance. Vasopressin also has a pressor effect, which involves the contraction of smooth muscle of the vascular system and therefore has an effect on blood pressure. The main form of vasopressin in most species is arginine vasopressin, whereas in pigs it is lysine vasopressin, and in birds arginine vasotocin.

Plasma osmolality controls the secretion of vasopressin

The control of vasopressin secretion as a result of changes in plasma osmolality is through osmoreceptors located in the hypothalamus as well as through receptors located in the esophagus and stomach that immediately sense water intake (Fig. 32–14). An increase in osmolality of body fluids increases the rate of action potential firing in the osmoreceptors, which in turn activates hypothalamic cells that synthesize vasopressin. This negative feedback system is sensitive to changes in osmolality, and the solute-to-water ratio is maintained within 1% to 2% of the normal values. The regulation of the pressor effect of vasopressin—that is, through blood volume—is achieved by increasing the number of action potentials in stretch receptors located in the atria. A decrease in blood volume activates the stretch receptors, which inhibit activity of neurons, vagal in origin, that inhibit the osmoreceptor cells. Blood volume changes that decrease blood pressure also affect vasopressin release through activation of baroreceptors in the carotid sinus and aortic arch.

Diabetes insipidus (DI) is a disorder of water metabolism characterized by polyuria, urine of low specific gravity or osmolality, and polydipsia. It is caused

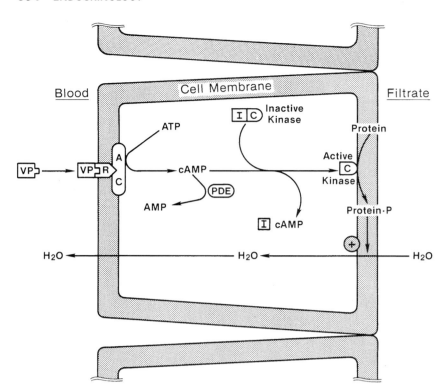

FIGURE 32-13. Antidiuretic mechanism of action of vasopressin (VP) on cells of the distal tubule and collecting ducts. AC, adenyl cyclase; AMP, adenosine monophosphate; ATP, adenosine triphosphate; cAMP, cyclic AMP; I and C, inhibitory and catalytic subunits of the kinase, respectively; PDE, phosphodiesterase; R, receptor. (From Hedge GA, Colby HD, Goodman RL: Clinical Endocrine Physiology. Philadelphia: WB Saunders, 1987, p 61.)

by defective secretion of ADH (central DI) or by the inability of the renal tubule to respond to ADH (nephrogenic DI). Deficiency of ADH can be partial or complete. Central DI is characterized by an absolute or relative lack of circulating ADH and is classified as primary (idiopathic and congenital) or secondary. Secondary central DI usually results from head trauma or neoplasia.

Central DI may appear at any age, in any breed of dogs and cats, and in either gender; however, young adults (6 months of age) are most commonly affected. The major clinical signs of DI are profound polyuria and polydipsia (more than 100 mL/kg/day; normal range is 40 to 70 mL/kg/day), nocturia, and incontinence, usually of several months' duration. The severity of the clinical signs varies, inasmuch as DI may result from a partial or complete defect in ADH secretion or action. Other, less consistent signs include weight loss (because these animals are constantly seeking water) and dehydration.

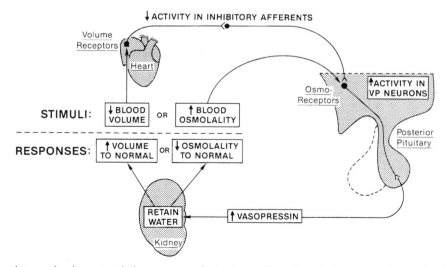

FIGURE 32-14. The major mechanisms regulating vasopressin (VP) secretion. A perturbation in either blood volume or osmolality modifies vasopressin secretion in order to restore these parameters to their normal values. However, this restoration requires appropriate water intake adjustments by thirst as well as by the modulation of water retention depicted. Also, the two responses indicated may be affected by simultaneous changes in sodium balance. (From Hedge GA, Colby HD, Goodman RL: Clinical Endocrine Physiology. Philadelphia: WB Saunders, 1987, p 63.)

Routine complete blood cell count and serum biochemical and electrolyte profiles are usually normal in animals with DI. Plasma osmolality is often high (>310 mOsm/L) in central or nephrogenic DI as a result of *dehydration*. Animals with primary polydipsia often exhibit low plasma osmolality (<290 mOsm/L) as a result of *overhydration*. When abnormalities, such as slightly increased hematocrit or hypernatremia, are present on initial evaluation, they are usually secondary to dehydration from water restriction by the pet owner. In DI, the urinalysis is unremarkable except for the finding of a persistently dilute urine (urine specific gravity, 1.004 to 1.012).

Diagnostic tests to confirm and differentiate central DI, nephrogenic DI, and psychogenic polydipsia include the modified water deprivation test or response to ADH supplementation. The modified water deprivation test is designed to determine whether endogenous ADH is released in response to dehydration and whether the kidneys can respond to ADH. The more common causes of polyuria and polydipsia should be ruled out before this procedure is performed. Failure to recognize renal failure before water deprivation may lead to an incorrect or inconclusive diagnosis or cause significant morbidity in the patient.

Hypersecretion of vasopressin in the absence of osmotic or volumetric stimulation is called the *syndrome of inappropriate antidiuretic hormone secretion*. Neoplastic processes are often involved in this syndrome; ectopic tumors, often located in the lung, are the neoplasms most commonly involved.

The anterior pituitary produces the following hormones: growth hormone, prolactin, thyroid-stimulating hormone, follicle-stimulating hormone, luteinizing hormone, and corticotropin

The adenohypophysis comprises the pars distalis and the pars intermedia. The major hormones produced by the anterior pituitary are growth hormone (GH; also called *somatotropin*); PRL; thyroid-stimulating hormone (TSH); FSH; LH; and corticotropin (Table 32-1). GH is produced by acidophilic somatotropes, and PRL is produced by lactotropes; both are classified as somatomammotropins. GH and PRL are single-chain proteins that contain two and three disulfide bonds, respectively. There is overlap of activity between GH and PRL; this overlap is based on the approximately 50% homology of their amino acid sequences. Of these two major somatomammotropins, GH is uniquely species-specific as to its activity.

TSH, produced by thyrotropes, and FSH and LH, produced by gonadotropes, are classified as glycoproteins because all three molecules have carbohydrate moieties. These hormones have α and β subunits that are linked by noncovalent binding. The α subunits are identical (and interchangeable) among the three glycoproteins. The β subunits, unique for each hormone, impart the specific action of each hormone.

TABLE 32-1. Six major hormones secreted by the anterior pituitary gland

Hormone	Abbreviation
Glycoproteins	
Follicle-stimulating hormone	FSH
Luteinizing hormone (interstitial cell–stimulating hormone)	LH (ICSH)
Thyroid-stimulating hormone (thyrotropin)	TSH
Somatotropins	
Growth hormone (somatotropin)	GH
Prolactin	PRL
Pro-opiomelanocortins	
β-Lipotropin	
Corticotropin	ACTH

Modified from Hedge GA, Colby HD, Goodman RL: Clinical Endocrine Physiology. Philadelphia: WB Saunders, 1987, p 71.

Other members of this family of hormones that are not of anterior pituitary origin include equine chorionic gonadotropin (also called *pregnant mare's serum gonadotropin*) and primate chorionic gonadotropin, which are produced by cells of the placental chorion.

Corticotropin and β-lipotropin belong to the pro-opiomelanocortin family in that they originate from a common prohormone (Fig. 32-15). Cells in both the pars distalis and pars intermedia synthesize pro-opiomelanocortin molecules. The emphasis on the type of hormone produced is different in the end product; corticotropin is produced by pars distalis corticotropes. In the pars intermedia, corticotropin is cleaved by corticotropes to form α-melanocyte–stimulating hormone (α-MSH), the predominant hormone of this lobe. The remaining peptide fragment is known as *corticotropin-like intermediate lobe peptide*; the physiologic activity of this peptide fragment is not known. In both the pars distalis and the pars intermedia, β-lipotropin is cleaved to form β-endorphins and γ-lipotropin. Endorphins have opioid activity and appear to modulate gonadotropin secretion.

Control of adenohypophyseal activity was not understood for a considerable length of time, first because the functional connection between the brain and the anterior pituitary gland was not understood. In the 1930s, Popa and Fielding, Budapest medical student and university professor, respectively, described the vascular system that connects the hypothalamus with the pituitary gland but were unable to determine the direction in which blood flowed. In about 1950, Geoffrey Harris drew the important conclusion that the linkage involved blood passage from the hypothalamus to the anterior pituitary gland through the portal blood system previously described by Popa and Fielding (Fig. 32-16). The dorsal hypophyseal artery, which supplies nutrients and oxygen to the adenohypophysis (the ventral hypophyseal artery supplies the neurohypophysis), terminates in the median eminence as a capillary plexus. Blood from these plexus is drained by two veins that empty into sinusoidal capillaries of the pars distalis, completing the portal venous system (one vein supplies the ven-

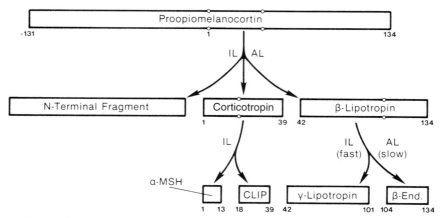

FIGURE 32–15. Cleavage of pro-opiomelanocortin to yield corticotropin and related peptides. By convention, the numbering of the amino acids begins with the first one of corticotropin and then increases positively toward the carboxy terminal and negatively toward the amino terminal. Cleavage occurs at pairs of basic amino acids indicated by the circles. AL, anterior lobe; α-MSH, α-melanocyte–stimulating hormone; β-End., β-endorphin; CLIP, corticotropin-like intermediate lobe peptide; IL, intermediate lobe. (From Hedge GA, Colby HD, Goodman RL: Clinical Endocrine Physiology. Philadelphia: WB Saunders, 1987, p 75.)

tral, central part of the pars distalis; the other supplies the dorsal, peripheral areas).

Adenohypophyseal activity is controlled by hypothalamic-releasing hormones, which are released into the portal system, which in turn connects the median eminence of the hypothalamus and the anterior pituitary gland

Whereas neurons that compose the neurohypophysis are influenced directly by neural input within the hypothalamus, the imposition of a vascular system between the hypothalamus and the adenohypophysis requires a different type of control system. The hypothalamus produces regulatory or hypophysiotropic hormones, which are transported to and released within the median eminence (comparable with posterior lobe hormones) (Fig. 32–17). These regulatory hormones then pass via the portal venous system to the adenohypophysis, where they stimulate the release of the various anterior pituitary hormones. The synthesis of adenohypophyseal regulatory hormones is controlled by both neural and hormonal inputs at the level of the hypothalamus. Some of the hypophyseal hormones have been found in other areas of the brain and extraneural sites, including the gastrointestinal tract and the pancreas.

The initial isolation and identification of the hypothalamic hormones required large amounts of tissue as well as expertise in biochemistry. The first identified hypothalamic hormone, which controls corticotropin release, was originally called *corticotropin-releasing factor* (now changed from *factor* to *hormone*).

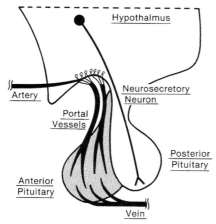

FIGURE 32–16. Diagram of the hypothalamopituitary unit, contrasting the vascular connection between the brain and the anterior pituitary gland with the neuronal connection between the brain and the posterior pituitary gland. (From Hedge GA, Colby HD, Goodman RL: Clinical Endocrine Physiology. Philadelphia: WB Saunders, 1987, p 70.)

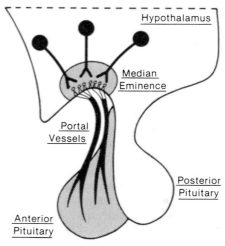

FIGURE 32–17. Hypothalamic neurosecretory neurons and hypothalamohypophyseal portal vessels. (From Hedge GA, Colby HD, Goodman RL: Clinical Endocrine Physiology. Philadelphia: WB Saunders, 1987, p 86.)

TABLE 32–2. Major hypophysiotropic hormones

Hormone	Abbreviation	Site of origin
Thyrotropin-releasing hormone	TRH	Paraventricular nucleus
Gonadotropin-releasing hormone	GnRH	Preoptic area of hypothalamus
Growth hormone–inhibiting hormone (somatostatin)	GHIH	Anterior hypothalamic area
Growth hormone–releasing hormone	GHRH	Arcuate nucleus
Corticotropin-releasing hormone	CRH	Paraventricular nucleus
Prolactin-releasing factor	PRF	?
Prolactin-inhibiting hormone (or dopamine)	PIH	Arcuate nucleus

Modified from Hedge GA, Colby HD, Goodman RL: Clinical Endocrine Physiology. Philadelphia: WB Saunders, 1987, p 87.

The initial work, done by Guillemin's group at the University of Houston in the early 1960s, required the collection, freezing, and transport of several hundred thousand sheep brains from abattoirs located in the western United States, as well as the subsequent dissection of the hypothalami. The hypothalamic hormones that have been characterized and the hormones they release include (1) corticotropin-releasing hormone, a 41–amino acid polypeptide that stimulates corticotropes to release all components of the pro-opiomelanocortin family of molecules; (2) gonadotropin-releasing hormone, a decapeptide that stimulates gonadotrope secretion of both FSH and LH; (3) thyrotropin-releasing hormone, a tripeptide that stimulates thyrotrope secretion of TSH; (4) dopamine, a catecholamine precursor of norepinephrine that inhibits lactotrope secretion of PRL and thyrotrope secretion of TSH; (5) somatostatin, a tetradecapeptide that inhibits somatotrope secretion of GH; and (6) growth hormone–releasing hormone, a 44–amino acid polypeptide that stimulates somatotrope secretion of GH (Table 32–2). Except for dopamine, all these hypophysiotropic hormones are peptides.

Previously, only four of the anterior pituitary hormones (FSH, LH, TSH, and corticotropin) were considered to be tropic; that is, their main effect was stimulation of hormone secretion by specific endocrine organs located peripheral to the pituitary gland. More recently, GH has been added to this list because GH stimulates the liver to produce somatomedins, which have a negative feedback effect on GH secretion. PRL remains as the only pars distalis hormone for which negative feedback inhibition has not been demonstrated through hormones produced by PRL-target tissues.

The most important regulation of secretion of the protein hormones by the pars distalis is by feedback inhibition. One feedback system involves negative feedback inhibition of the tropic pituitary hormone by interaction of the target organ hormone with the hypothalamus, as well as with the pituitary gland; this system is called a *long-loop feedback* system (Fig. 32–18). For example, cortisol is produced by the adrenal cortex, as a result of corticotropin stimulation, and cortisol, in turn, has a negative feedback effect on corticotropin production at the level of the hypothalamus and the anterior pituitary gland. *Short-loop feedback* systems have also been described; in these, an anterior pituitary hormone, such as corticotropin, has a direct negative feedback inhibition of hormone secretion—in this case, corticotropin-releasing hormone secretion—within the hypothalamus.

Even under conditions of negative feedback inhibition, the secretion of anterior pituitary hormones is not constant. For example, even though estrogens exert a continuous, potent negative feedback inhibition on gonadotropin secretion, gonadotropin secretion alternates between secretion and no secretion, with pulses of gonadotropins released into the blood vascular system. In the case of gonadotropins, the ovarian endocrine status influences the pulse rate and the amplitude of each pulse. Progesterone domination

FIGURE 32–18. Regulation of anterior pituitary hormone (APH) secretion by hypophysiotropic hormones (HH), short-loop negative feedback, and long-loop negative feedback by target organ hormones (TOH). Plus signs indicate stimulation, and minus signs indicate inhibition. (From Hedge GA, Colby HD, Goodman RL: Clinical Endocrine Physiology. Philadelphia: WB Saunders, 1987, p 78.)

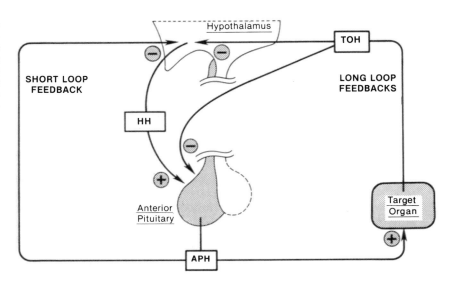

is associated with a decreased pulse rate and an increased pulse amplitude, whereas estrogen causes the opposite effect. The work of Irvine and Alexander has provided the best documentation of the precise relationship between secretory activity of hypothalamic regulatory and anterior pituitary hormones. Their data were obtained through analysis of hormones obtained from the intercavernal sinus, which collects venous blood from the pituitary gland of the horse.

Clinical syndromes of somatotropin deficiency and excess include pituitary dwarfism in the dog and acromegaly in the cat, respectively. Pituitary dwarfism results from destruction of the pituitary gland via a neoplastic, degenerative, or anomalous process. It may be associated with decreased production of other pituitary hormones, including TSH, ACTH, LH, FSH, and GH. Pituitary dwarfism is most common in German shepherd dogs aged 2 to 6 months. Other affected breeds include Carnelian bear dogs, spitz, toy pinschers, and Weimaraners. In German shepherd dogs, the disease is inherited as a simple autosomal recessive trait and occurs as a result of cystic Rathke's pouch. The first observable clinical signs of pituitary dwarfism are slow growth, noticed in the first 2 to 3 months of life, and mental retardation, usually manifested as difficulty in house-training. Physical examination findings may include proportionate dwarfism, retained puppy haircoat, hypotonic skin, truncal alopecia, cutaneous hyperpigmentation, infantile genitalia, and delayed dental eruption. Clinicopathologic features include eosinophilia, lymphocytosis, mild normocytic normochromic anemia, hypophosphatemia, and occasionally hypoglycemia resulting from secondary adrenal insufficiency. Differential diagnoses include other causes of stunted growth such as hypothyroid dwarfism, portosystemic shunt, diabetes mellitus, hyperadrenocorticism, malnutrition, and parasitism. Diagnosis is made by measuring serum growth hormone concentrations (assay no longer commercially available) or serum somatomedin C (insulin-like growth factor 1 [IGF-1]). The advantage of IGF-1 is that it is not species-specific. There is usually a subnormal response to exogenous TSH and ACTH stimulation tests; furthermore, endogenous TSH and ACTH are decreased in affected dogs as a result of panhypopituitarism.

Acromegaly, or hypersomatotropism, is the condition resulting from chronic excessive GH secretion in the adult animal. Canine acromegaly is an extremely rare disorder observed after the administration of progestational compounds for suppression of estrus in intact female dogs. The disease is caused by excessive secretion of GH from mammary cells under the influence of exogenous progesterone. Acromegaly in cats, as in humans, is caused by a GH-secreting tumor of the anterior pituitary gland. Such tumors in cats grow slowly and may be present for a long time before the onset of clinical signs. Feline acromegaly occurs in older (8- to 14-year-old) cats and occurs more commonly in males. Canine acromegaly occurs in intact female dogs given progestational compounds for estrus prevention.

Clinical signs of uncontrolled diabetes mellitus are often observed as the first manifestations of acromegaly; therefore, polydipsia, polyuria, and polyphagia are the most common presenting signs. Net weight gain of lean body mass in animals suffering from uncontrolled diabetes mellitus is a key sign of acromegaly. Organomegaly, including renomegaly (observed in both cats and humans suffering from acromegaly), hepatomegaly, and enlargement of endocrine organs, is also observed. Some dogs and cats show the classic enlargement of extremities, body size, jaw, tongue, and forehead that is characteristic of acromegaly in humans. Some of the most striking manifestations of acromegaly occur in the musculoskeletal system; they include an increase in muscle mass and growth of the acral segments of the body, including the paws, chin, and skull. Cardiovascular abnormalities, such as cardiomegaly (as determined radiographically and echocardiographically), systolic murmurs, and congestive heart failure, develop late in the course of the disease. Azotemia develops late in the course of the disease in approximately 50% of acromegalic cats. Neurologic signs of acromegaly in humans, such as peripheral neuropathies (paresthesias, carpal tunnel syndrome, sensory and motor defects), and parasellar manifestations, such as headache and visual field defects, are not generally detected in acromegalic small animals.

Impairments in glucose tolerance and insulin resistance that result in diabetes mellitus are observed in all cats and most dogs with acromegaly. Measurement of endogenous insulin reveals dramatically increased serum insulin concentrations. Despite severe insulin resistance and hyperglycemia, ketosis is rare in acromegalic animals. Feline acromegaly should be suspected in any diabetic cat (especially males) that has severe insulin resistance (insulin requirement > 20 U/cat/day). Hypercholesterolemia and mild increases in serum activities of liver enzymes are attributed to the diabetic state. Hyperphosphatemia without azotemia is also a common clinicopathologic finding, perhaps as a result of GH-stimulated bone growth. Urinalysis findings are unremarkable except for persistent proteinuria, probably as a result of systemic hypertension and glomerulosclerosis.

A definitive diagnosis of acromegaly requires documentation of increased plasma G or somatomedin C concentrations. Unfortunately, feline and canine GH assays are no longer commercially available.

Cushing's syndrome (hyperthyroidism) should be ruled out before measurement of GH. At this time, the most definitive test for the diagnosis of acromegaly in cats is computed tomography of the pituitary region. Computed tomographic findings, coupled with the exclusion of other disorders that cause insulin resistance (hyperthyroidism, hyperadrenocorticism), in cats that exhibit clinical signs of acromegaly should lead the clinician to a diagnosis of acromegaly.

CLINICAL CORRELATIONS

Equine Cushing's disease

History You are called to examine a 15-year-old mare whose owner complains that the mare has had stiffness in her legs for the past 9 months. The mare has been used as a brood mare and delivered a foal the past spring (and for the 7 previous years). She failed to conceive last spring, and now, in the early summer of the next year, she has yet to exhibit normal estrous cycles.

Clinical examination   As you gain a general perspective on the mare, you notice that she appears to have been clipped recently. She is not a show mare, and because it is early summer, you inquire why she has been clipped. The owner indicates that the mare has been slow to shed this spring, and she is tired of seeing the mare with a rough hair coat. The finding of a long hair coat out of season prompts you to ask about the water consumption of the mare; the owner indicates that the mare drank more water (and urinated accordingly) than would be expected. You examine the feet and find that the soles appear slightly "dropped"; you find a small abscess in the sole of one of the feet.

Comment   The main clue regarding the nature of the disease is the presence of a long hair coat out of season; this is the sine qua non of the disease. The usual complaints of owners of horses with Cushing's disease are related to chronic processes, such as pneumonia, laminitis, or weight loss, the latter often associated with parasitism and an inability to masticate properly because of tooth problems. It is relatively common for brood mares that are progressing into Cushing's disease to have a recent history of infertility after a successful brood mare career. Although the cause of infertility is not known, it is likely that a disturbance of gonadotropin secretion occurs in conjunction with disturbance of the pro-opiomelanocortin system.

The disease represents a classic case of loss of control of the intermediate lobe of the pituitary gland by the hypothalamus: in this case, the loss of dopaminergic control. Under normal conditions, melanotropes of the intermediate lobe process pro-opiomelanocortin to α-MSH and acetylated β-endorphin, residues 1 to 31, and non-opiate active carboxy-terminally shortened 1–26, or 1–27, endorphin. In the absence of dopamine, the melanotropes produce α-MSH, as well as β-endorphin, 1–31 (the active form) and small amounts of corticotropin; the latter stimulates glucocorticoid production by the adrenal cortex. The negative feedback control system fails in this situation, because the melanotropes do not have glucocorticoid receptors, even under normal conditions. The result is unchecked synthesis and secretion of melanotrope products, including corticotropin and unchecked glucocorticoid secretion. Activity of the corticotropes in the pars distalis is decreased because of negative feedback inhibition by the glucocorticoids. One of the long-term effects of excess glucocorticoid secretion is muscle wasting, a common finding in these animals. Also, some of the common manifestations of the disease are polydipsia and polyuria, which result from compression of the pars nervosa by the enlarging pars intermedia and reduction in ADH synthesis.

Although there is hyperplasia of the intermediate lobe in this disease, it has not been established whether this disease occurs because of autonomous hyperplasia of the intermediate lobe or, conversely, whether the hyperplasia occurs because of gradual loss of dopaminergic control by the hypothalamus. One theory is that chronic stress, such as that occurring with laminitis, could affect dopamine secretion by the hypothalamus, leading to loss of control of the intermediate lobe and the development of hyperplasia.

Treatment   At present, the only proven treatment is to provide the affected animals with the best possible husbandry. This care includes parasite control, floating of teeth, providing good nutrition, and taking proper care of the feet.

Bibliography

Dickson WM: Endocrine glands. In Swenson MJ (ed): Dukes' Physiology of Domestic Animals, 10th ed. Ithaca, New York: Cornell University Press, 1984, pp 761–797.
Feldman EC, Nelson RW: Canine and Feline Endocrinology and Reproduction. Philadelphia: WB Saunders, 1987.
Hedge GA, Colby HD, Goodman RL: Clinical Endocrine Physiology. Philadelphia: WB Saunders, 1987.
Martin R: Endocrine Physiology. New York: Oxford University Press, 1985.
McDonald LE, Pineda MH (eds): Veterinary Endocrinology and Reproduction, 4th ed. Philadelphia: Lea & Febiger, 1989.
Tepperman J, Tepperman M: Metabolic and Endocrine Physiology, 5th ed. Chicago: Year Book Medical, 1987.
Wilson JD, Foster DW: Williams Textbook of Endocrinology, 7th ed. Philadelphia: WB Saunders, 1985.

PRACTICE QUESTIONS

1. In general, hormones are classified as proteins, peptides, and steroids. Which one of the following hormones is a peptide?
   a. Growth hormone.
   b. Insulin.
   c. Vasopressin.
   d. Dopamine.
   e. Epinephrine.
   f. Melatonin.

2. In general, steroid hormones are classified as mineralocorticoid, glucocorticoid, and sex steroids. Which one of the following hormones is a glucocorticoid?
   a. Aldosterone.
   b. Corticosterone.
   c. Cortisol.
   d. Testosterone.
   e. Estrone.

3. Direct feedback control of corticotropin-releasing hormone by corticotropin is termed
   a. negative feedback.
   b. positive feedback.
   c. short-loop feedback.
   d. long-loop feedback.

4. Hormones from the pro-opiomelanocortin family are synthesized from precursor hormones produced in either the pars distalis or the pars intermedia. The two main hormones produced by these two lobes (in respective order) are
   a. α-MSH and endorphin.
   b. corticotropin and endorphin.
   c. α-MSH and corticotropin.
   d. corticotropin and α-MSH.
   e. corticotropin and α-lipotropin.

5. Increased hormonal activity that occurs during daylight hours is termed _____ rhythm.

a. circadian.
b. diurnal.
c. nocturnal.
d. ultradian.

PRACTICE ANSWERS

1. c   2. c   3. c   4. e   5. b

33

Endocrine glands and their function

The thyroid gland

1   The thyroid hormones are synthesized from two connected tyrosine molecules that contain three or four iodine molecules

2   Thyroid hormones are stored outside the cell and attached to thyroglobulin in the form of colloid

3   The release of thyroid hormones involves transport of thyroglobulin with attached thyroid hormones into the cell, cleavage of the thyroid hormones from thyroxine-binding globulin, and release into the interstitial tissues

4   Thyroid hormones are transported in the plasma attached to plasma proteins

5   The main routes of metabolism of thyroid hormones are through deiodination or the formation of glucuronides and sulfates via hepatic mechanisms

6   Thyroid hormones are the primary factors for the control of basal metabolism

7   The ingestion of compounds that inhibit the uptake or the organic binding of iodine blocks the ability of the thyroid to secrete thyroid hormones and causes goiter

The adrenal glands

1   The adrenal glands are composed of two organs: the outer gland (cortex) and the inner gland (medulla)

The adrenal cortex

1   The adrenal cortex has three zones: the zona glomerulosa, which secretes mineralocorticoids, and the zona fasciculata and the zona reticularis, which secrete glucocorticoids and sex steroids

2   Adrenal corticoids are synthesized from cholesterol; the critical difference in the activity of these corticoids is related to the hydroxyl group on C-17 of glucocorticoids

3   Adrenocortical hormones are carried in plasma in association with specific binding globulins (corticosteroid-binding globulin)

4   The metabolism of adrenocortical hormones involves the reduction of double bonds and conjugation of the steroids to glucuronides and sulfates

5   One of the most important functions of glucocorticoids is control of metabolism and, in particular, the stimulation of hepatic gluconeogenesis

6   Corticotropin is the pituitary hormone that regulates glucocorticoid synthesis by the adrenal cortex

7   One of the most important clinical uses of glucocorticoids is the suppression of the inflammatory response

The adrenal medulla

1   The synthesis of catecholamines is from tyrosine; the main catecholamine synthesized by the adrenal medulla is epinephrine

2   The primary actions of catecholamines are on metabolism, especially effects that increase the concentration of glucose

3   The main factors that stimulate catecholamine secretion are hypoglycemia and conditions that produce stress

Hormones of the pancreas

1   The synthesis of insulin is biphasic: an acute phase involves the release of preformed insulin, and a chronic phase involves the synthesis of protein

2   The metabolism of insulin involves splitting the A and B chains and reducing the chains to amino acids and peptides

3   The main metabolic functions of insulin are anabolic

4   The most important functions of glucagon are to decrease glycogen synthesis, increase glycogenolysis, and increase gluconeogenesis

5   Glucagon synthesis is stimulated by decreased glucose concentrations in the blood

6   The main functions of somatostatin are to inhibit the secretion of hormones produced by the pancreas (insulin, glucagon, pancreatic polypeptide)

Calcium and phosphate metabolism

1   Calcium is important for many intracellular reactions, including muscle contraction, nerve cell activity, the release of hormones through exocytosis, and the activation of enzymes

2   Phosphorus is important for the structure of bone and teeth; on a cellular basis, organic phosphate serves as part of the cell membrane and as part of a number of intracellular components

3   The most important body pool of calcium involved in homeostasis is the extracellular fluid component

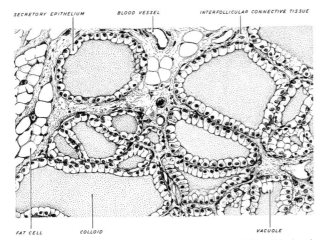

FIGURE 33–1. Histologic features of the normal thyroid gland of the rat. All normal thyroid glands are structurally similar, although slight variations occur with age, diet, habitation, and sexual status (neutered or intact). The normal animals of the colony to which this rat belonged were maintained on a high-protein ration, which probably accounts for the slight hypertrophic condition of the secretory epithelium. (From Turner CD, Bagnara JT: General Endocrinology, 6th ed. Philadelphia: WB Saunders, 1976, p 180.)

THE THYROID GLAND

In most mammals, the thyroid gland is located caudal to the trachea at the level of the first or second tracheal ring. The thyroid gland is composed of two lobes lying on either side of the trachea and connected by a narrow piece of tissue called the *isthmus*.

The thyroid gland is the most important endocrine gland for metabolic regulation. The glandular tissue has cells formed in a circular arrangement called a *follicle* (Fig. 33–1). The follicles are filled with a homogeneous-staining substance called *colloid*, which is the main storage form of the thyroid hormones. The follicular cells are cuboidal when the secretion is basal and are elongated when the cells are stimulated to release hormone. Another important endocrine cell, the *parafollicular*, or *C*, *cell* is located outside the follicles. This cell secretes *calcitonin*, a hormone important for the regulation of calcium. The activity of this hormone is discussed in the section on calcium metabolism.

The thyroid hormones are synthesized from two connected tyrosine molecules that contain three or four iodine molecules

The synthesis of thyroid hormone is unusual, because a large amount of the active hormone is stored as a colloid outside the follicle cells, within the lumen, or acinus, created by the circular arrangement of glandular cells. Two molecules are important for thyroid hormone synthesis: *tyrosine* and *iodine*. Tyrosine is a part of a large molecule (molecular weight, 660,000 D) called *thyroglobulin* that is formed within the follicle cell and secreted into the lumen of the follicle. Iodine is converted to iodide in the intestinal tract and then is transported to the thyroid, where the follicle cells effectively trap the iodide through an active transport process. This allows intracellular iodide concentrations to be 25 to 200 times higher than extracellular concentrations.

As iodide passes through the apical wall of the cell, it attaches to the ring structures of the tyrosine molecules, which are part of the thyroglobulin amino acid sequence. The tyrosyl ring can accommodate two iodide molecules; if one iodide molecule attaches, it is called *monoiodotyrosine,* and if two attach, it is called *diiodotyrosine.* The coupling of two iodinated tyrosine molecules results in the formation of the main thyroid hormones; two diiodotyrosine molecules form *tetraiodothyronine* (T_4) and one monoiodotyrosine and one diiodotyrosine molecule form *triiodothyronine* (T_3) (Fig. 33–2). A key enzyme in the biosynthesis of thyroid hormones is *thyroperoxidase* (which works in concert with an oxidant, hydrogen peroxide). Thyroperoxidase catalyzes the iodination of the tyrosyl residues of thyroxine-binding globulin (TBG) and the formation of T_3 and T_4. In addition to the unusual molecular storage form of the hormone, thyroid hormones are also unique in that they are the only hormones that contain a halide (i.e., iodine).

Thyroid hormones are stored outside the cell and attached to thyroglobulin in the form of colloid

Once thyroid hormones are synthesized, they remain in the extracellular acinar lumen until release. This

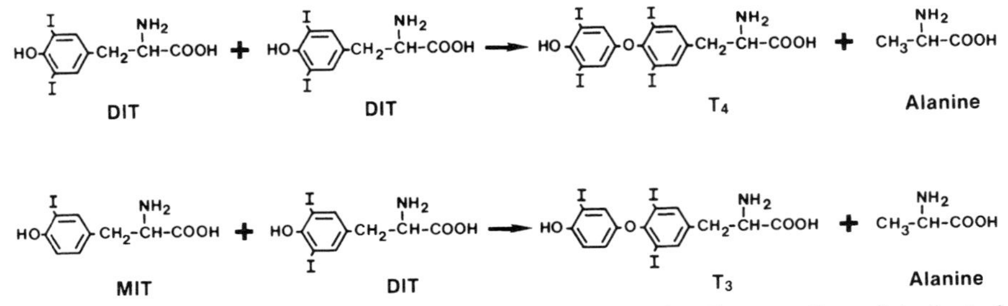

FIGURE 33–2. Production of tetraiodothyronine (T_4) and triiodothyronine (T_3) by the coupling of iodinated tyrosyl residues with thyroglobulin molecule. DIT, diiodotyrosine; MIT, monoiodotyrosine. (From Hedge GA, Colby HD, Goodman RL: Clinical Endocrine Physiology. Philadelphia: WB Saunders, 1987, p 106.)

extracellular storage of hormone within an endocrine gland is a unique storage arrangement. It allows the thyroid gland to have a large reserve of hormone. From a teleologic standpoint, thyroid hormone is the most important hormone of metabolism; it allows mammals to withstand periods of iodine deprivation without an immediate effect on the production of thyroid hormones.

The release of thyroid hormones involves transport of thyroglobulin with attached thyroid hormones into the cell, cleavage of the thyroid hormones from thyroxine-binding globulin, and release into the interstitial tissues

In order for thyroid hormones to be released from the thyroid gland, thyroglobulin with its attached monoiodotyrosine, diiodotyrosine, T_3, and T_4 molecules must be translocated into the follicle cell, and the hormones must be cleaved from thyroglobulin (Fig. 33–3). Key enzymes in this transfer are found in the lysosomes. On entering the cell, the TBG molecules fuse with lysosomes, and lysosomal enzymes cleave both the iodinated tyrosine molecules and the iodinated thyronines from the thyroglobulin molecule. The thyronines are released through the basal cell membrane (they freely pass through the cell membrane); monoiodotyrosine and diiodotyrosine are deiodinated by an enzyme called *iodotyrosine dehalogenase*; and both the iodide and the remaining tyrosine molecules are recycled to form new hormone in association with thyroglobulin.

The majority of T_3 formation occurs outside the thyroid gland by deiodination of T_4. Tissues that have the highest concentration of deiodinating enzymes are those of the liver and kidneys, although muscle tissue produces more T_3 on the basis of relative size. The enzyme that is involved in the removal of iodide from the outer phenolic ring of T_4 in the formation of T_3 is called *5'-monodeiodinase* (Fig. 33–4). Another type of T_3 in which an iodide molecule is removed from the inner phenolic ring of T_4, a compound called *reverse T_3*, is also formed. Reverse T_3 has little of the biologic effects of thyroid hormones and is formed only by the action of extrathyroidal deiodinating enzymes and not by activity of the thyroid gland.

Thyroid hormones are transported in the plasma attached to plasma proteins

As indicated in Chapter 32, lipid-soluble hormones are transported in the vascular system through association with specific binding plasma proteins. There is considerable species variation in the proteins that bind thyroid hormones. The most important carrier protein is TBG, which has high affinity for T_4, although it also has low capacity because of its low concentration. TBG also is an important carrier protein for T_3. TBG has been reported in all domestic animals except the cat. Albumin is also involved in the transport of thyroid hormones; however, albumin has low affinity for T_3 and T_4 but high capacity because of its high concentration in plasma. In the absence of TBG, albumin is the most important carrier of thyroid hormones. All species have a third plasma protein, thyroxine-binding prealbumin, which is specific for T_4 and has a specificity and capacity that are intermediate between those of TBG and albumin. The term *prealbumin* refers to the migration of the protein during electrophoresis, not to synthesis of the molecule.

As with all lipid-soluble hormones that are transported in plasma, most of the T_3 and T_4 is bound;

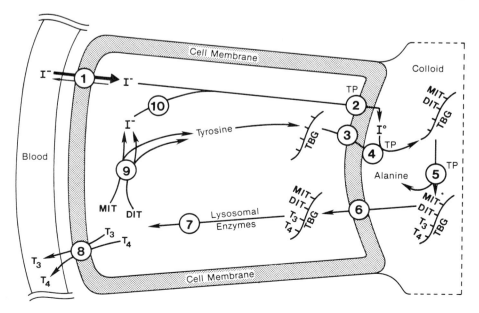

FIGURE 33–3. Depiction of follicular cell showing steps in the synthesis and release of triiodothyronine (T_3) and tetraiodothyronine (T_4). The numbers identify the major steps: (1) trapping of iodide; (2) oxidation of iodide; (3) exocytosis of thyroglobulin; (4) iodination of thyroglobulin; (5) coupling of iodotyrosines; (6) endocytosis of thyroglobulin; (7) hydrolysis of thyroglobulin; (8) release of T_3 and T_4; (9) deiodination of monoiodotyrosine (MIT) and diiodotyrosine (DIT); (10) recycling of iodide. TBG, thyroxine-binding globulin; TP, thyroperoxidase. (From Hedge GA, Colby HD, Goodman RL: Clinical Endocrine Physiology. Philadelphia: WB Saunders, 1987, p 105.)

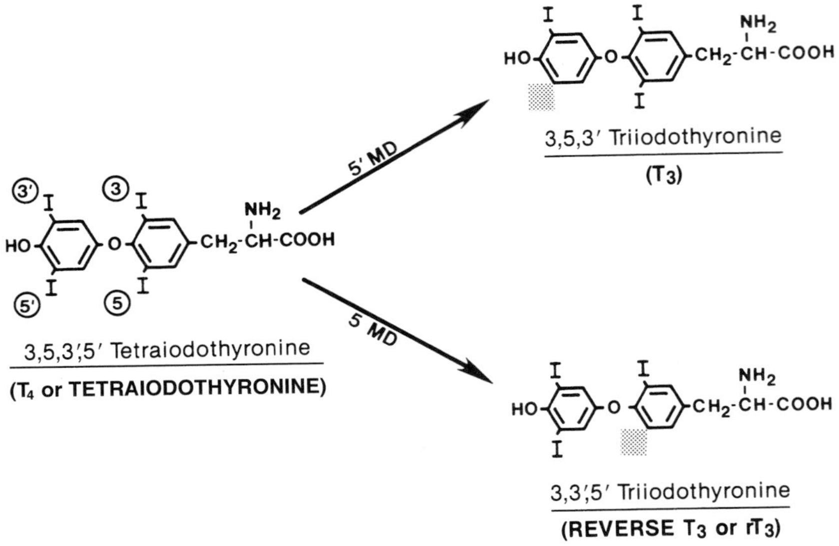

HO — ⟨ ⟩ — O — ⟨ ⟩ — CH_2-CH-COOH, NH_2

3,5,3′ Triiodothyronine
(T_3)

5′ MD

HO — ⟨ ⟩ — O — ⟨ ⟩ — CH_2-CH-COOH, NH_2

3,5,3′,5′ Tetraiodothyronine
(T_4 or TETRAIODOTHYRONINE)

5 MD

HO — ⟨ ⟩ — O — ⟨ ⟩ — CH_2-CH-COOH, NH_2

3,3′,5′ Triiodothyronine
(REVERSE T_3 or rT_3)

FIGURE 33–4. Structure and nomenclature of thyroxine and its conversion to the two triiodothyronines by 5′-monodeiodinase and 5-monodeiodinase (MD). Shaded squares indicate the sites of deiodination. (From Hedge GA, Colby HD, Goodman RL: Clinical Endocrine Physiology. Philadelphia: WB Saunders, 1987, p 103.)

little is free to interact with receptors on the cells of the target tissues. The amount of thyroid hormone that is free in plasma is remarkably low (e.g., in humans, 0.03% of T_4 and 0.3% of T_3). In dogs, the amount of free hormone is somewhat greater (a little less than 1.0% for T_4 and slightly more than 1.0% for T_3). This is because of less affinity between plasma-binding proteins and thyroid hormones in canine plasma than in human plasma. The equilibrium between free and bound hormone is easily shifted because of physiologic or pharmacologic situations, such as the increase in estrogen concentrations that occurs during pregnancy. Estrogens cause increased synthesis of TBG by the liver with a consequent shift toward the bound form. Adjustments to maintain a normal amount of free hormone occur rapidly with a decline in the rate of metabolism or with stimulation of thyroid hormone production through the release of thyroid-stimulating hormone (TSH).

The main routes of metabolism of thyroid hormones are through deiodination or the formation of glucuronides and sulfates via hepatic mechanisms

The main form of metabolism of thyroid hormones involves the removal of iodide molecules. Except for the T_3 formed from T_4, none of the deiodinated thyronine derivatives have any significant metabolic activity. The two enzymes involved in T_3 and reverse T_3 synthesis, 5′-deiodinase and 5-deiodinase, are also involved in the catabolism of thyroid hormones. Only these two enzymes are needed for catabolism, because they do not differentiate between the 3 and 5 positions of the phenolic rings of the thyronines. Skeletal muscle, liver, and kidney tissues are important tissues involved in the catabolism of thyroid hormones through deiodination. The formation of thyroid hormone conjugates represents another form of

inactivation; sulfates and glucuronides are formed mainly in the liver and kidneys. Conjugation is less common than deiodination as a means of metabolism of thyroid hormones. Another form of metabolism involves modification of the alanine moiety of the thyronines by either transamination or decarboxylation. The deiodinated and conjugated forms of the thyronines are eliminated primarily in the urine; unmetabolized thyronines are excreted with feces through bile secretion. Degradation of the conjugate forms in the feces results in the production of iodide molecules, which are reabsorbed as part of a cycle called the *enterohepatic cycle*. Humans are more efficient than dogs in recovery of iodide both intrathyroidally and enterohepatically.

One of the striking aspects of thyroid hormones is their long half-lives in humans; T_3 has a half-life of 1 day and T_4 of 6 to 7 days, whereas most other hormones have half-lives of seconds or minutes. One reason for these long half-lives is the large percentage of the circulating thyronines that are bound to the plasma proteins, which protects them from degradation. The difference in half-lives between T_3 and T_4 results from the tighter T_4 protein binding in comparison with T_3 and the resultant reduction in free circulating hormone. In contrast, the half-life for T_4 is relatively short in certain domestic species; dogs and cats exhibit a T_4 half-life of less than 24 hours.

Thyroid hormones are the primary factors for the control of basal metabolism

The mechanism of action of thyroid hormones at the cellular level is based on the fact that they can penetrate the cell membrane even though they are amino acids; in essence, they are lipophilic. Although it is thought that thyroid hormones interact directly with the nucleus to initiate the transcription of messenger

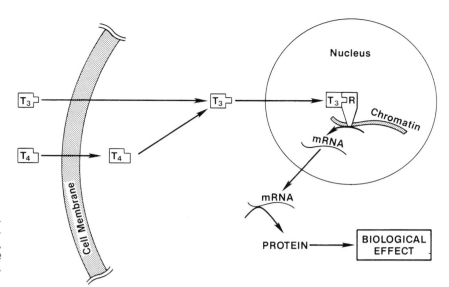

FIGURE 33–5. Proposed subcellular mechanism of thyroid hormone action. mRNA, messenger RNA; R, receptor. (From Hedge GA, Colby HD, Goodman RL: Clinical Endocrine Physiology. Philadelphia: WB Saunders, 1987, p 113.)

RNA (mRNA) (Fig. 33–5), the presence of T_3 receptors has been reported on mitochondria.

It is likely that thyroid hormones are the primary determinants of basal metabolism. However, it is difficult to define the precise physiologic effects of thyroid hormones. This is because many of the effects of thyroid hormones have been demonstrated through the creation of hypothyroid or hyperthyroid states. Nevertheless, it has long been recognized that thyroid hormones increase oxygen consumption of tissues and, as a result, heat production. This effect is known as the *calorigenic effect.* One site of action of the calorigenic effect of thyroid hormones is within the mitochondrion.

Thyroid hormones affect carbohydrate metabolism in several ways, including increasing intestinal glucose absorption and facilitating the movement of glucose into both fat and muscle. Furthermore, thyroid hormones facilitate insulin-mediated glucose uptake by cells. Glycogen formation is facilitated by small amounts of thyroid hormones; however, glycogenolysis occurs after larger dosages.

Thyroid hormones in concert with growth hormone are essential for normal growth and development. This is accomplished, in part, by the enhancement of amino acid uptake by tissues and enzyme systems that are involved in protein synthesis.

Whereas thyroid hormones affect all aspects of lipid metabolism, the emphasis is placed on lipolysis. One particular effect of thyroid hormones is the tendency to reduce plasma cholesterol levels. This appears to involve both increased cell uptake of low-density lipoproteins with associated cholesterol molecules and a tendency for increased degradation of both cholesterol and low-density lipoprotein. These effects on lipid metabolism are usually seen in pathophysiologic situations involving hypersecretion of thyroid hormone or in thyroid deficiency states in which hypercholesterolemia is a hallmark of thyroid deficiency. In this same context, the effects of thyroid hormones on metabolic processes, including carbohydrate, pro-

tein, and lipid metabolism, are often described as catabolic.

Thyroid hormones have noteworthy effects on the nervous and cardiovascular systems. The effects of the sympathetic nervous system are enhanced by the presence of thyroid hormones. This is thought to occur through thyroid stimulation of β-adrenergic receptors in tissues that are targets for the catecholamines, such as epinephrine and norepinephrine. In the central nervous system, thyroid hormones are important for normal development of tissues in the fetus and neonate; retardation of mental activity occurs when thyroid hormone exposure is inadequate. In humans, persons with hypothyroid activity are mentally dull and lethargic, which suggests that normal central nervous system function in the adult is dependent on the presence of adequate amounts of thyroid hormone.

Thyroid hormones increase the heart rate and force of contraction, probably through their interaction with the catecholamines. This interaction is caused by an increase in tissue responsiveness through the induction of catecholaminergic β receptors by thyroid hormones. Blood pressure is elevated because of increased systolic pressure, with no change in diastolic pressure; the end result is an increase in cardiac output. These responses are most easily observed in situations of increased thyroid activity. Perhaps the conclusion regarding the effect of thyroid hormones on cardiovascular activity is that they are important for maintaining normal contractile activity of cardiac muscle, including the transmission of nerve impulses.

Thyroid hormone was used in classic experiments involving the metamorphosis of amphibian larvae. Thyroxine administration causes the differentiation of tadpoles into frogs, whereas thyroidectomy results in development into large tadpoles. Thyroid-induced metamorphosis is limited to amphibians, but thyroid hormones are important for many (subtle) aspects of differentiation in other classes of animals.

Thyroid hormone activity is usually defined in

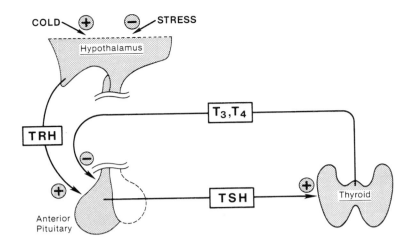

FIGURE 33–6. Hypothalamopituitary-thyroid axis. Plus signs indicate stimulation; minus signs, inhibition. T_3, triiodothyronine; T_4, tetraiodothyronine; TRH, thyrotropin-releasing hormone; TSH, thyroid-stimulating hormone. (From Hedge GA, Colby HD, Goodman RL: Clinical Endocrine Physiology. Philadelphia: WB Saunders, 1987, p 116.)

terms of tissue or organ responses to inadequate or excessive amounts of hormone. A more balanced view is that thyroid hormones are important for the normal metabolic activity of all tissues.

TSH, or thyrotropin, is the most important regulator of thyroid activity. It acts through the initiation of cyclic adenosine 3′,5′-monophosphate (cAMP) formation and the phosphorylation of protein kinases. TSH secretion is regulated by thyroid hormones by way of negative feedback inhibition of the synthesis of thyrotropin-releasing hormone at the level of the hypothalamus and by inhibition of the activity of TSH at the level of the pituitary gland (Fig. 33–6).

The ingestion of compounds that inhibit the uptake or the organic binding of iodine blocks the ability of the thyroid to secrete thyroid hormones, and causes goiter

An inability to secrete adequate amounts of thyroid hormone often leads to the enlargement of the thyroid gland, a condition known as *goiter*. In many places in the world, this condition is, or has been, caused by a deficiency of iodine in the diet. This has largely been corrected through the use of iodized salt. Certain plants—for example, cruciferous plants such as cabbage, kale, rutabaga, turnip, and rapeseed—contain a potent antithyroid compound called *progoitrin*, which is converted into goitrin within the digestive tract. Goitrin interferes with the organic binding of iodine. Many of the goitrogenic feeds also contain thiocyanates, which interfere with the trapping of iodine by the thyroid gland. The feeding of excess iodine can sometimes overcome the effects of thiocyanate but has less influence on overcoming the effects of goitrin. From studies of these phenomena has come the development of compounds for the treatment of hyperthyroidism; the most potent ones are the thiocarbamides, thiourea, and thiouracil. Other antithyroid drugs include sulfonamides, *p*-aminosalicylic acid, phenylbutazone, and chlorpromazine.

Hypothyroidism is most common in the dog, and the usual etiology of primary hypothyroidism is lymphocytic thyroiditis. Congenital hypothyroidism may be caused by thyroid dysgenesis, dyshormonogenesis, T_4 transport defects, goitrogens, or, in rare cases, iodine deficiency. Secondary hypothyroidism may be a secondary effect of pituitary tumors, radiation therapy, or ingestion of endogenous or exogenous glucocorticoids. Tertiary hypothyroidism can be acquired, as in the case of hypothalamic tumors, or can be congenital as a result of defective thyrotropin releasing hormone (TRH) or TRH receptor defects.

The signalment of hypothyroid dogs carries a distinct breed predisposition; high-risk breeds manifest symptoms as early as 2 to 3 years of age, and low-risk breeds manifest symptoms at a slightly older age (4 to 6 years). Breeds predisposed to hypothyroidism include golden retrievers, Doberman pinschers, dachshunds, Irish setters, miniature schnauzers, great Danes, miniature poodles, boxers, Shetland sheepdogs, Newfoundlands, chow chows, English bulldogs, Airedale terriers, cocker spaniels, Irish wolfhounds, giant schnauzers, Scottish deerhounds, and Afghan hounds.

Clinical signs of hypothyroidism are gradual and subtle in onset; lethargy and obesity are most common. Dermatologic evidence of hypothyroidism is the next most common clinical finding. Symmetric truncal or tail head alopecia is a classic finding in hypothyroid dogs. The skin is often thickened because of myxedematous accumulations in the dermis. Common haircoat changes seen in the hypothyroid dog include dull, dry hair, poor hair regrowth after clipping, and the presence or retention of puppy hair.

Cardiovascular signs of hypothyroidism include bradycardia, decreased cardiac contractility, and atherosclerosis, but these are uncommon presenting complaints. Neuromuscular signs such as myopathies and megaesophagus are also uncommon manifestations of canine hypothyroidism. Neuropathies, including bilateral or unilateral facial nerve paralysis, vestibular disease, and lower motor neuron disorders, are occasionally seen in hypothyroid dogs. Myxedema coma is an unusual finding in hypothyroid dogs and is secondary to myxedematous fluid accumulations in the brain and severe hyponatremia. Less common signs of hypothyroidism include reproductive disorders in female dogs, such as prolonged interestrous intervals, silent heat, and delivery of weak or stillborn puppies. Corneal lipid deposits and gastrointestinal problems such as constipation are occasionally observed in hypothyroid dogs.

Clinicopathologic findings such as anemia resulting from erythropoietin deficiency, decreased bone marrow activity, and decreased serum iron and iron binding capacity are observed in about 25% to 30% of hypothyroid dogs. Hypercholesterolemia is seen in approximately 75% of hypothyroid dogs because of altered lipid metabolism, decreased fecal excretion of cholesterol, and decreased conversion of lipids to bile acids. Hyponatremia, a common finding in human beings with hypothyroidism, is observed as a mild decrease in serum sodium in about 30% of hypothyroid dogs in one study. Hyponatremia is caused by an increase in total body water as a result of impaired renal excretion of water and by retention of water by hydrophilic deposits in tissues. An unusual clinicopathologic feature of hypothyroidism is increased serum creatine phosphokinase levels, possibly as a result of hypothyroid myopathy.

Diagnosis is based on measurement of serum basal total thyroxine (T$_4$) and triiodothyronine (T$_3$) concentrations, serum free T$_4$ and T$_3$ concentrations, and endogenous canine serum thyrotropin (TSH) levels (Table 33-1) and/or results of dynamic thyroid function tests, including the TRH and TSH stimulation tests. Variables that affect T$_4$ are numerous and include age, breed, environmental and body temperature, diurnal rhythm, obesity, and malnutrition. Specifically, affected greyhounds have approximately half

the normal total thyroxine (TT$_4$) and free thyroxine (unbound) (FT$_4$) concentrations of normal dogs. Obese dogs have mild increases in serum TT$_4$ concentrations. In puppies, the serum TT$_4$ concentration is two to five times higher than in adult dogs. Furthermore, there is an age-related decline in serum TT$_4$ concentrations and response to TSH stimulation in dogs. Euthyroid sick syndrome is characterized by a decrease in serum TT$_4$ and increase in reverse T$_3$. Concurrent illnesses such as diabetes mellitus, chronic renal failure, hepatic insufficiency, and infections, can cause euthyroid sick syndrome, resulting in decreases in serum TT$_4$ concentrations. Drugs such as anesthetics, phenobarbital, primidone, diazepam, trimethoprim-sulfa, quinidine, phenylbutazone, salicylates, and glucocorticoids can also decrease serum basal TT$_4$ concentrations.

Free thyroid hormone concentrations, or unbound thyroxine and triiodothyronine, are used in human medicine to differentiate between euthyroid sick syndrome and true hypothyroidism. In humans, the diagnostic accuracy of a single FT$_4$ measurement is approximately 90%. Measurement of FT$_4$ concentrations is achieved by equilibrium dialysis (gold standard) or analog immunoassays. Theoretically, FT$_4$ is not subject to spontaneous or drug-induced changes that occur with TT$_4$. Results of early studies, classifying dogs as hypothyroid on the basis of TSH stimulation tests, indicated that FT$_4$ measurements by equilibrium dialysis were 90% accurate, whereas other FT$_4$ assays (analog assays) were no better than TT$_4$. Glucocorticoids decrease both the FT$_4$ fraction and TT$_4$ in dogs.

With the advent of the endogenous canine TSH assay, veterinarians now have a method of assessing the thyroid-pituitary axis in dogs without dynamic testing. With thyroid gland failure, decreases in serum FT$_4$ and TT$_4$ are sensed by the pituitary gland, resulting in an increase in serum endogenous TSH concentration. Initial studies in dogs with experimentally induced hypothyroidism have been very encouraging. In human beings, when endogenous TSH concentrations are increased and FT$_4$ concentrations are decreased, diagnostic accuracy for primary hypothyroidism approaches 100%. As FT$_4$ concentration falls, there is a logarithmic increase in serum endogenous TSH concentration, which makes the TSH assay the most sensitive test for the detection of early hypothyroidism. However, nonthyroidal disease can affect endogenous TSH concentrations as much as FT$_4$ and TT$_4$ concentrations can; therefore, the use of endogenous TSH *alone* is not recommended as a method of assessing thyroid function.

The antithyroglobulin autoantibody test (ATAA) has become available and appears promising, on the basis of initial study results. The presence of antithyroglobulin antibodies theoretically presages the onset of hypothyroidism in dogs with autoimmune thyroiditis. It is hoped that this test will identify dogs with hereditary thyroid disease before breeding. However, no large studies of dogs with naturally occurring thyroid disease have been performed to evaluate this assay.

TABLE 33-1. Serum T$_4$ and T$_3$ values by radioimmunoassay

Species	T$_4$ (mg/dL)	T$_3$ (ng/dL)
Equine		
M ± SD	1.63 ± 0.51	77.1 ± 45.75
Range	0.95–2.38	31–153
Bovine		
M ± SD	6.22 ± 2.03	92.50 ± 53.61
Range	3.60–8.9	41–170
Caprine		
M ± SD	3.45 ± 0.47	145.9 ± 29.32
Range	3.0–4.23	88–190
Ovine		
M ± SD	4.41 ± 1.13	99.6 ± 27.34
Range	2.95–6.15	63–150
Porcine		
M ± SD	3.32 ± 0.80	89.8 ± 36.7
Range	1.70–4.68	43–140
Canine		
M ± SD	1.15 ± 0.38	96.2 ± 21.39
Range	0.70–2.18	63–130
Feline		
M ± SD	2.02 ± 0.61	64.7 ± 20.62
Range	1.18–2.95	39–112

N = 10 For all species listed.
T$_3$, triiodothyronines; T$_4$, tetraiodothyronine.
From McDonald LE, Pineda MH (eds): Veterinary Endocrinology and Reproduction, 4th ed. Philadelphia: Lea & Febiger, 1989, p 86.

For many years the TSH stimulation test was considered the gold standard for diagnosis of hypothyroidism in dogs. Unfortunately, this test does not differentiate between early hypothyroidism and euthyroid sick syndrome, nor does it identify dogs with secondary or tertiary hypothyroidism. Furthermore, exogenous bovine TSH is no longer commercially available. Other thyroid function tests include the TRH stimulation test, thyroid scan, and thyroid biopsy. However, each test has drawbacks (expense, inaccuracy, or invasiveness).

In summary, diagnosis of hypothyroidism is based on signalment, historical findings, physical examination findings, clinicopathologic features, and confirmation with a battery of thyroid function tests. The author uses TT_4 and endogenous TSH (eTSH) initially, followed by FT_4 by dialysis. If all measurements are abnormal, the dog is hypothyroid. If two of the three are abnormal, secondary hypothyroidism (low FT_4, low TSH) or early primary hypothyroidism (high TSH, low FT_4) is possible. If only one of the three thyroid measurements is abnormal, the dog should be reevaluated in 3 to 6 months.

Hyperthyroidism is the most common endocrinopathy of cats and is caused by adenomatous hyperplasia of the thyroid gland. Middle-aged to older cats are typically affected, and there is no predilection for breed or sex. Hyperthyroidism is characterized by hypermetabolism; therefore, polyphagia, weight loss, polydipsia, and polyuria are the most prominent features of the disease. Activation of the sympathetic nervous system is also seen; hyperactivity, tachycardia, pupillary dilatation, and behavioral changes are characteristic of the disease in cats. Long-standing hyperthyroidism leads to hypertrophic cardiomyopathy, high-output heart failure, and cachexia, which may lead to death.

Clinicopathologic features of hyperthyroidism include erythrocytosis and an excitement leukogram (neutrophilia, lymphocytosis) caused by increased circulating catecholamine concentrations. Increased catabolism of muscle tissue in hyperthyroid cats may result in increased levels of blood urea nitrogen (BUN) but not creatinine. In fact, glomerular filtration rate is increased in hyperthyroid cats, and this increase may mask underlying renal insufficiency. Although hyperthyroidism increases glomerular filtration rate, the effect of thyroid hormone excess on the urinalysis is variable. Most cats, however, have decreased urine specific gravity, particularly if they are exhibiting polyuria as a clinical sign. Increased metabolic rate results in liver hypermetabolism; therefore, serum activities of liver enzymes (alanine aminotransferase, aspartate aminotransferase) increase in 80% to 90% of hyperthyroid cats. Serum cholesterol decreases, not as a result of decreased synthesis, but rather as a result of increased hepatic clearance mediated by thyroid hormone excess.

Feline hyperthyroidism is diagnosed through measurement of TT_4; TT_3 measurement is generally noncontributory to a diagnosis. Because the disease has become more common and recognized in its early stages, FT_4 concentrations have been shown to be more diagnostic of early or "occult" hyperthyroidism. However, FT_4 concentrations should be interpreted in light of the TT_4 because nonthyroidal illness (chronic renal failure) can result in spurious elevations of FT_4 as well. Free triiodothyronine (FT_3) concentrations do not provide any further advantage over FT_4.

THE ADRENAL GLANDS

The adrenal glands are composed of two organs: the outer gland (cortex) and the inner gland (medulla)

The adrenal glands are two bilaterally symmetric endocrine organs located just anterior to the kidneys. Each gland is divided into two separate entities, a medulla and a cortex (Fig. 33–7), each of which produces different types of hormones. These adrenal tissues have different embryonic origins; the medulla arises from the neuroectoderm and produces amines such as norepinephrine and epinephrine. The cortex arises from the mesodermal coelomic epithelium and produces steroid hormones such as cortisol, corticosterone, sex steroids, and aldosterone. The utility of placing two such disparate tissues together is not apparent. The one common factor is that both sets of hormones are important for adaptation to adverse environmental conditions (i.e., stress).

Interest in the function of the adrenal cortex was heightened in the 1930s because of the research of Hans Selye. He published a series of papers on the effects of adrenalectomy and the ability of the surgically treated animal to defend itself against injury. Selye's hypothesis was termed the *general adaptation syndrome*, which he divided into three parts: the alarm reaction, the stage of resistance, and the stage of exhaustion. The critical aspect of this theory was that in addition to specific responses to injury, animals responded in nonspecific ways to combat injury, and the adrenal cortex was the most important organ in leading the nonspecific response. One example of the beneficial effects of glucocorticoids in a situation of injury is the mobilization of glucose, a readily usable source of energy for running away or healing injury. The adaptation of animals to stressful environments is often accompanied by enlargement of the adrenal cortex, such as in domestic chickens raised in crowded conditions and wild animals living in relatively high density.

THE ADRENAL CORTEX

The adrenal cortex has three zones: the zona glomerulosa, which secretes mineralocorticoids, and the zona fasciculata and the zona reticularis, which secrete glucocorticoids and sex steroids

The adrenal cortex is organized into three zones in mammals (see Fig. 33–7). The outer zone, the zona

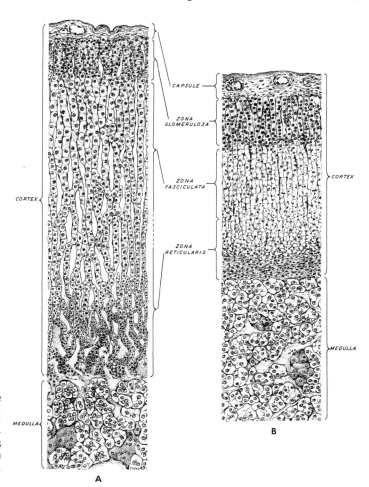

FIGURE 33–7. Depictions of comparable sections through the adrenal glands of *(A)* normal and *(B)* hypophysectomized rats. Because the functional capacity of the adrenal cortex is conditioned by the release of corticotropin, hypophysectomy results in tremendous shrinkage of the cortex. The medulla is not influenced by hypophysectomy. Both sections are drawn to scale. (From Turner CD, Bagnara JT: General Endocrinology, 6th ed. Philadelphia: WB Saunders, 1976, p 293.)

glomerulosa, is relatively narrow, and its cells are organized in a whorl-type arrangement. The middle zone, the zona fasciculata, is relatively wide, and its cells are organized in columns. In the cow and sheep, the zona fasciculata is further divided into inner and outer layers. The inner zone of the adrenal cortex, the zona reticularis, which is adjacent to the adrenal medulla, is intermediate in size, and cells are more randomly organized.

All the cells of the adrenal cortex have intracellular features characteristic of steroid hormone synthesis: an abundance of lipid droplets (containing cholesterol esters), mitochondria, and smooth endoplasmic reticulum. Human adrenal glands have an additional zone, the fetal zone, that is present during fetal life and for the first year of life. The fetal zone participates with the placenta in the production of estrogen during gestation. Immature mice and rabbits have an inner X zone that becomes the zona reticularis at puberty.

The adrenal cortex produces two major types of steroid hormones: the mineralocorticoids and the glucocorticoids. These are hormones that have distinctly different functions. The mineralocorticoids, produced by the zona glomerulosa, play an important role in electrolyte balance and, as a result, are important in

the regulation of blood pressure. The major mineralocorticoid is aldosterone. The glucocorticoids, produced by the zona fasciculata (which accounts for the majority of glucocorticoid production) and reticularis, are important in the regulation of all aspects of metabolism, either directly or through an interaction with other hormones. The major glucocorticoid is cortisol.

Adrenal corticoids are synthesized from cholesterol; the critical difference in the activity of these corticoids is related to the hydroxyl group on C-17 of glucocorticoids

The synthesis of adrenal steroids involves the classical pathways for steroid biosynthesis. As indicated previously, cholesterol is the major starting material for the synthesis of steroid hormones. Cholesterol is readily available to the steroid-synthesizing cells, because it is stored in large quantities in ester form within lipid droplets in these cells. One of the initial steps in steroid formation is the hydrolysis of the ester. The first step in steroid synthesis involves an enzyme that cleaves the carbon side chain from the steroid molecule, leaving a C-21 steroid known as

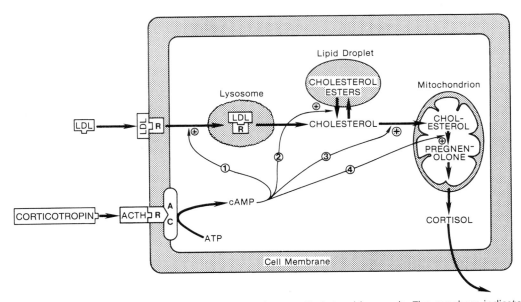

FIGURE 33–8. Mechanism of action of corticotropin (ACTH) on adrenocortical steroidogenesis. The numbers indicate the processes stimulated (indicated by plus signs) by corticotropin as follows: (1) stimulation of the uptake of low-density lipoproteins (LDL), which are further processed to free cholesterol; (2) stimulation of the hydrolysis of stored cholesterol esters to generate free cholesterol; (3) stimulation of the transport of cholesterol into mitochondria, where cleavage of the cholesterol side chain occurs; and (4) promotion of the binding of cholesterol to the enzyme. AC, adenyl cyclase; ATP, adenosine triphosphate; cAMP, cyclic adenosine monophosphate; R, receptor. (From Hedge GA, Colby HD, Goodman RL: Clinical Endocrine Physiology. Philadelphia: WB Saunders, 1987, p 146.)

pregnenolone. This step occurs within the mitochondrion (Fig. 33–8). The synthesis of all steroid hormones, regardless of their form, utilizes pregnenolone in the synthetic pathway (see Fig. 32–5).

The critical aspect of adrenal corticoid synthesis, which differentiates adrenal corticoids from the progesterone family of steroids, is a hydroxylation step at C-21 (directed by a C-21 hydroxylase). The difference between the mineralocorticoids (aldosterone) and the glucocorticoids (cortisol) is a hydroxyl group on C-17, which is part of the glucocorticoid molecule. As expected, cells of the zona fasciculata and reticularis have the hydroxylating enzyme for C-17 (17α-hydroxylase), whereas cells of the zona glomerulosa do not have this enzyme. Both aldosterone and cortisol have hydroxyl groups on C-11. Because of the marked difference in biologic activity of the mineralocorticoids and glucocorticoids, it is useful to view the zona glomerulosa as an endocrine organ that is distinct from the zona fasciculata and zona reticularis.

Two intermediate compounds in the synthesis of aldosterone have significant adrenocortical activity. 11-Deoxycorticosterone has significant mineralocorticoid activity, although it is secreted in relatively small amounts. Corticosterone, the immediate precursor to aldosterone, is a relatively important glucocorticoid in animals, although its potency is less than that of cortisol.

In adrenal cortical cells, there exist biosynthetic pathways that allow some synthesis of androgens and estrogens. Although the amount of sex steroids produced by the adrenal cortex under normal conditions is low, significant amounts can be synthesized under pathologic conditions.

Adrenocortical hormones are carried in plasma in association with specific binding globulins (corticosteroid-binding globulin)

Steroid hormones, as indicated previously, are lipids and depend on binding to plasma proteins for transport in the blood. A specific globulin that has a high affinity for cortisol has been identified: *corticosteroid-binding globulin,* or *transcortin.* Of the cortisol carried in plasma, 75% is bound to transcortin and 15% to albumin, leaving 10% in the unbound, or free, state. This amount of free hormone is large in comparison to thyroid hormones: less than 0.1% of T_4 is free. The transport of aldosterone is mainly associated with albumin (50%), and only 10% is associated with transcortin, leaving a very large amount (40%) in the free state.

Changes in physiologic or pathophysiologic states can influence the amount of binding proteins present in plasma. Estrogen produced in increasing amounts by the fetoplacental unit during pregnancy results in an increase in hepatic synthesis of transcortin, whereas liver dysfunction can result in lower concentrations of transcortin. The large pool of hormone present in the bound state during pregnancy gives animals a good reserve from which to make appropriate adjustments in the amount of free hormone available for influencing biologic activity. Because the total amount of glucocorticoid is determined in the assay of plasma concentrations, the veterinary clinician needs to be aware that total concentrations not only reflect secretion rate but also can be influenced by the amount of glucocorticoid-binding plasma proteins.

The metabolism of adrenocortical hormones involves the reduction of double bonds and conjugation of the steroids to glucuronides and sulfates

The clearance half-life of cortisol is about 60 minutes, and that of aldosterone is about 20 minutes. This difference is attributable to the observed difference in protein binding of these hormones within the plasma. In general, metabolism of mineralocorticoid and glucocorticoid hormones involves the reduction of double bonds and ketone configurations, which reduces the biologic activity of the molecules. The liver, an organ important for modification of these hormones, is also an important site for the conjugation of these steroids with sulfates and glucuronides; this reduces their biologic potency and renders them water-soluble for passage in the urine.

One of the most important functions of glucocorticoids is control of metabolism and, in particular, the stimulation of hepatic gluconeogenesis

The mechanism of action of adrenal hormones is similar to that of other lipophilic hormones: they are able to penetrate the cell membrane and interact in the cytoplasm with specific cytosolic receptors. This complex is transferred to the nucleus with a resultant transcription of certain genes and the synthesis of specific proteins that affect the biologic action of the adrenal hormones.

As emphasized previously, adrenocortical hormones are classified as either glucocorticoid or mineralocorticoid in their activity. Before the biologic actions of each class are discussed, it is important to realize that there is overlap of activity (Table 33–2). For example, whereas cortisol is the dominant gluco-

TABLE 33–2. Relative glucocorticoid and mineralocorticoid potencies of various steroids

Steroid	Glucocorticoid potency (relative to cortisol)	Mineralocorticoid potency
Cortisol	1	1
Aldosterone	0.1	400
Corticosterone	0.2	2
11-Deoxycorticosterone	<0.1	20
Dexamethasone	30	2
Fludrocortisone	10	400
Prednisone	4	0.7
Triamcinolone	5	<0.1

From Hedge GA, Colby HD, Goodman RL: Clinical Endocrine Physiology. Philadelphia: WB Saunders, 1987, p 136.

corticoid hormone, it also has mineralocorticoid effects, although at a reduced potency.

The glucocorticoid hormones are important mediators of intermediary metabolism. One of the important specific effects of glucocorticoids is the stimulation of hepatic gluconeogenesis, which involves the conversion of amino acids to carbohydrates. The net result is an increase in hepatic glycogen and a tendency to increase blood glucose levels. These effects on glycogen metabolism are observed mainly in animals that suffer from excessive glucocorticoid secretion (hyperadrenocorticism) or that have an insulin deficiency. The effect of glucocorticoids on carbohydrate metabolism is permissive; that is, their presence is required for the gluconeogenic and glycogenolytic actions of glucagon and epinephrine, respectively.

Whereas glucocorticoids and insulin have similar effects on liver glycogen metabolism, their effects on the peripheral use of glucose are different. Glucocorticoids inhibit glucose uptake and metabolism in the peripheral tissues, particularly in muscle and adipose cells. This effect has been termed the *anti-insulin effect.* The chronic administration of glucocorticoids can lead to the development of a syndrome called *steroid diabetes* because of the hyperglycemic effect produced at the level of the liver, whereby use of glucose decreases in the peripheral tissues because of insulin antagonism.

Whereas the actions of glucocorticoids on fat metabolism tend to be complex, the direct effect on adipose tissue is to increase the rate of lipolysis and to redistribute fat into the liver and abdomen. In fact, this fat redistribution leads to the classic "potbelly" appearance of animals and human beings with hyperadrenocorticism.

Protein synthesis is inhibited by glucocorticoids; in fact, protein catabolism is enhanced, with an accompanying release of amino acids. This process supports hepatic gluconeogenesis. Two tissues, cardiac and brain, are spared from the effect of glucocorticoids on protein catabolism. Chronic administration of glucocorticoids results in muscle wasting and the weakening of bone. The mobilization and incorporation of amino acids into glycogen results in an increase in urinary excretion of nitrogen and a negative nitrogen balance.

Glucocorticoids play a role in water diuresis (i.e., the enhancement of water excretion). Whereas glucocorticoids inhibit vasopressin activity in the distal tubule, the most important effect is to increase the glomerular filtration rate. A summary of the effects of glucocorticoids is shown in Table 33–3.

Corticotropin is the pituitary hormone that regulates glucocorticoid synthesis by the adrenal cortex

The control of the secretion of the glucocorticoids by the zona fasciculata and zona reticularis is by the tropic hormone (corticotropin) (Fig. 33–9). A negative

TABLE 33–3. Glucocorticoid effects and target tissues

Effect	Site of action
Stimulates gluconeogenesis	Liver
Increases hepatic glycogen	Liver
Increases blood glucose	Liver
Facilitates lipolysis	Adipose tissue
Is catabolic (negative nitrogen balance)	Muscle, liver
Inhibits corticotropin secretion	Hypothalamus, anterior pituitary gland
Facilitates water excretion	Kidney
Blocks inflammatory response	Multiple sites
Suppresses immune system	Macrophages, lymphocytes
Stimulates gastric acid secretion	Stomach

From Hedge GA, Colby HD, Goodman RL: Clinical Endocrine Physiology. Philadelphia: WB Saunders, 1987, p 137.

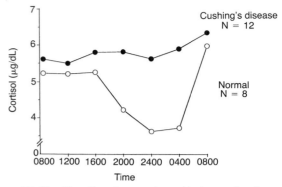

FIGURE 33–10. Circadian changes in cortisol secretion in normal horses *(open circles)*, in comparison with no circadian change in horses with equine Cushing's disease. (From Dybdal N: Studies on equine Cushing's disease [PhD thesis]. Davis: University of California, Davis, 1990.)

feedback system exists, whereby glucocorticoids inhibit the release of hypothalamic corticotropin-releasing hormone, and this, in turn, results in decreased corticotropin secretion by the pituitary gland. There is some evidence that glucocorticoids also have a negative feedback effect at the level of the pituitary gland. The potency of a glucocorticoid in negative feedback inhibition of corticotropin is directly related to its glucocorticoid potency; for example, cortisol has more potent negative feedback effects than does corticosterone, the former having more potent glucocorticoid effects than the latter.

The negative feedback control system that exists for the secretion of glucocorticoids does not result in the maintenance of uniform hormone concentrations in blood throughout the day. Sleep and activity patterns are superimposed on the negative feedback system so that there occurs a predictable circadian rhythm in which concentrations of glucocorticoids are lowest late at night and highest in the early morning hours (Fig. 33–10).

Another factor that can modify the negative feedback control of glucocorticoids is stress. Stress can result from physical or psychological stimuli that are harmful to the individual. The effects of stress, like the factors that influence circadian rhythms of glucocorticoid secretion, are mediated through the central nervous system. The glucocorticoid response to stress is immediate: concentrations of cortisol increase rapidly to reach, within minutes, values that are severalfold higher than normal. The glucocorticoid response is proportional to the severity of the stress; that is, lower levels of stress result in less cortisol production than do higher levels of stress.

One of the most important clinical uses of glucocorticoids is the suppression of the inflammatory response

Glucocorticoids have valuable clinical effects, particularly the inhibition of the inflammatory response, including the prevention of capillary dilatation, extravasation of fluid into tissue spaces, leukocyte migration, fibrin deposition, and connective tissue synthesis. Whereas the process of inflammation is important for the walling off and destruction of systemic noxious agents, the end response is often the replacement of

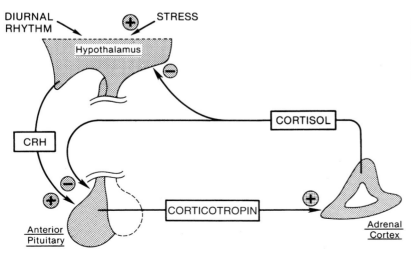

FIGURE 33–9. Regulation of cortisol secretion by the hypothalamopituitary axis. Plus signs indicate stimulation; minus signs indicate inhibition. CRH, corticotropin-releasing hormone. (From Hedge GA, Colby HD, Goodman RL: Clinical Endocrine Physiology. Philadelphia: WB Saunders, 1987, p 143.)

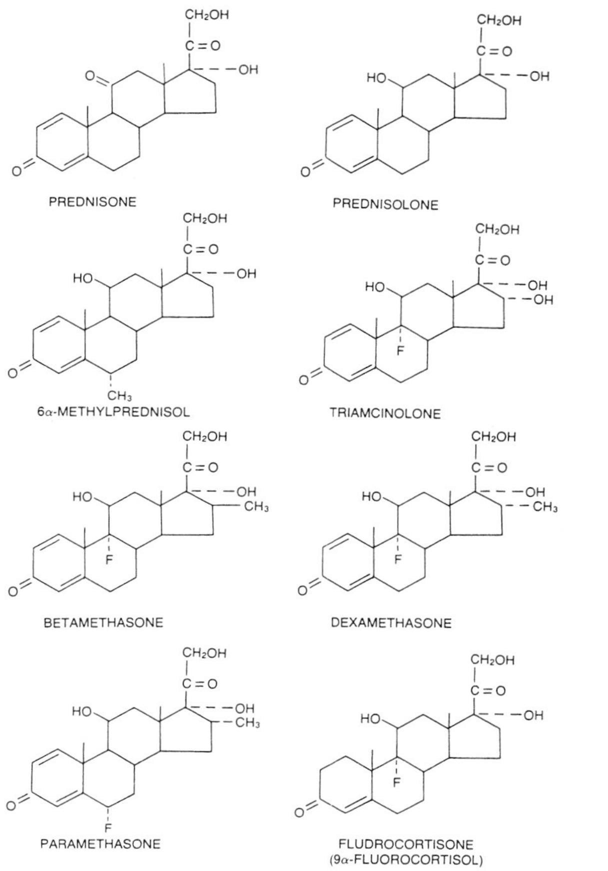

FIGURE 33–11. The chemical structures of some clinically useful glucocorticoid analogues. (From Martin CR: Endocrine Physiology. London: Oxford University Press, 1985, p 246.)

functional tissue with fibrous connective tissue, with a resultant loss of function. For example, inflammatory processes in the mammary gland often result in the isolation of the injurious agent by the laying down of connective tissue as a part of the defense mechanism; however, the gland may lose much of its functional capacity as a result. Administration of glucocorticoids, in conjunction with antibiotic therapy, can help reduce the loss of functional tissue by inhibiting the development of connective tissue. The chemical structures of some of the synthetic glucocorticoids used in clinical practice are shown in Figure 33–11.

One of the ways in which glucocorticoids inhibit the inflammatory response is through the inhibition of the formation of substances that promote inflammation. Glucocorticoids inhibit the synthesis of inflammatory mediators, such as prostaglandins, thromboxanes, and leukotrienes, that arise as a result of arachidonic acid metabolism. This effect is mediated through the stabilization of lysosomal membranes and the prevention of phospholipase A_2 activation. Glucocorticoids are also used to inhibit allergic reactions. This action occurs through the inhibition of the release of certain biogenic amines, such as histamine, from the granules of mast cells.

Hyperadrenocorticism (Cushing's syndrome) in the

dog may be caused by a pituitary tumor, pituitary hyperplasia, adrenal tumors, adrenal hyperplasia, or nonendocrine tumors (usually of the lung), or it may be iatrogenic. Approximately 85% of dogs with hyperadrenocorticism have pituitary gland–dependent disease, whereas 15% exhibit adrenal tumors. Hyperadrenocorticism is a disease of middle-aged and older dogs (aged 7 to 12 years). Breeds commonly affected by pituitary-dependent hyperadrenocorticism include miniature poodles, dachshunds, boxers, Boston terriers, and beagles. Adrenal tumors are seen more frequently in large-breed dogs, and there is a predilection for females (ratio, 3:1). Hyperadrenocorticism is a rare endocrine disorder of cats and is usually pituitary in origin in that species.

The most common clinical signs associated with canine hyperadrenocorticism are polydipsia, polyuria, polyphagia, heat intolerance, lethargy, abdominal enlargement or "potbelly," panting, obesity, muscle weakness, and recurrent urinary tract infections. Dermatologic manifestations of canine hyperadrenocorticism can include alopecia (especially truncal), thin skin, phlebectasias, comedones, bruising, cutaneous hyperpigmentation, calcinosis cutis, pyoderma, dermal atrophy (especially around scars), seborrhea, and secondary demodicosis. Thin skin is the hallmark of feline hyperadrenocorticism. Cats with Cushing's syndrome develop such severe thinning of the epidermis that they may incur open wounds just by grooming themselves.

Attempts to diagnose hyperadrenocorticism can be challenging. Uncommon clinical manifestations of hyperadrenocorticism in dogs can include signs such as hypertension, congestive heart failure, bronchial calcification, pulmonary thromboembolism, polyneuropathy, polymyopathy, pseudomyotonia, behavioral changes, and blindness. Evidence of increased collagenase activity caused by hypercortisolemia may result in nonhealing corneal ulceration and bilateral cranial cruciate rupture (in small dogs). Unusual reproductive signs may include testicular atrophy, prostatomegaly in castrated male dogs, clitoral hypertrophy, and perianal adenoma in females or castrated males.

Serum chemistry abnormalities associated with hypercortisolemia in dogs include increased serum activities of alkaline phosphatase and alanine aminotransferase, hypercholesterolemia, hyperglycemia, and decreased BUN. The hemogram is often characterized by evidence of erythroid regeneration (nucleated red blood cells) and a classic "stress leukogram." Basophilia is occasionally observed. Many dogs with hyperadrenocorticism have evidence of urinary tract infection without pyuria. Proteinuria resulting from glomerulosclerosis is also common. Urine specific gravity is usually decreased and may be hyposthenuric. Thyroid status is often affected in animals with hyperadrenocorticism, as evidenced by (1) decreases in TT_4 and TT_3 that are caused by euthyroid sick syndrome and (2) a response to TSH stimulation that is attenuated as a result of overcrowding of pituitary thyrotrophs by adrenocorticotrophs. Overt diabetes mellitus may result from the insulin antagonism caused by hypercortisolemia in about 15% of dogs with hyperadrenocorticism and 85% of cats with hyperadrenocorticism. Conversely, hyperadrenocorticism can be a cause of insulin resistance and poor glycemic control in diabetic animals.

The diagnosis of hyperadrenocorticism should be based on suggestive clinical signs and supporting minimal database abnormalities (e.g., high serum cholesterol, increased serum alkaline phosphatase activity) and confirmed by an appropriate screening test. If screening test results are inconclusive, the dog should be retested at a later date (3 to 6 months) rather than be subjected to treatment without a definitive diagnosis.

Screening tests for hyperadrenocorticism, such as the low-dose dexamethasone suppression (LDDS) test and the corticotropin stimulation test, work on the principle of suppression or stimulation of the pituitary-adrenal axis. In the case of the LDDS test, dexamethasone is administered at a low dosage to cause negative feedback to the pituitary gland. In a normal animal, this negative feedback results in a decrease in endogenous corticotropin secretion and a resultant decrease in circulating cortisol concentrations. Dexamethasone is the only synthetic corticosteroid that does not cross-react with the cortisol assay. The corticotropin stimulation is used to determine the extent of adrenal enlargement. Adrenal glands that are enlarged because of chronic pituitary stimulation by corticotropin or that are neoplastic show an exaggerated response to exogenous corticotropin.

The LDDS test has traditionally been the screening test of choice for canine hyperadrenocorticism. It is sensitive (92% to 95%); only 5% to 8% of dogs with pituitary dependent hyperadrenocorticism exhibit

TABLE 33–4. Mineralocorticoid effects and target tissues

Effect	Site of action
Stimulates Na+ reabsorption	Kidney, salivary glands, sweat glands
Stimulates K+ excretion	Kidney, salivary glands, sweat glands
Stimulates H+ excretion	Kidney

From Hedge GA, Colby HD, Goodman RL: Clinical Endocrine Physiology. Philadelphia: WB Saunders, 1987, p 139.

suppressed cortisol concentrations at 8 hours (i.e., 5% to 10% false-negative results). In addition, 30% of dogs with pituitary-dependent hyperadrenocorticism exhibit suppression at 3 or 4 hours, followed by "escape" of suppression at 8 hours; this pattern is diagnostic for pituitary-dependent disease and makes further testing unnecessary. The major disadvantage of the LDDS test is the lack of specificity in dogs with nonadrenal illness. It is recommended that a dog be allowed to recover from the nonadrenal illness before being assessed for hyperadrenocorticism with the LDDS test.

MINERALOCORTICOIDS

The mineralocorticoids, produced in the outer zone (zona glomerulosa) of the adrenal cortex, have surprisingly different functions in comparison with glucocorticoids; the functions are surprising because both types of hormones are produced by tissues that are part of the same gland. As indicated previously, electrolyte balance and blood pressure homeostasis represent the principal physiologic effects of mineralocorticoids (Table 33–4). These actions are carried out at the

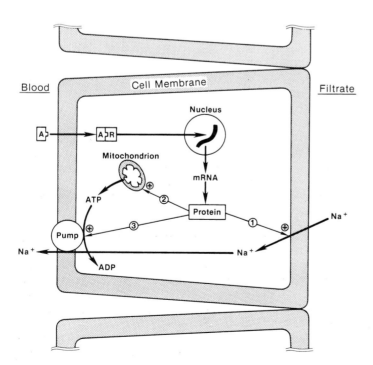

FIGURE 33–12. Mechanisms of action of aldosterone on sodium transport in the renal tubular cell. The numbered arrows indicate the three putative sites of action of aldosterone: (1) increasing the permeability of the luminal membrane to sodium; (2) increasing mitochondrial ATP production; and (3) increasing Na+,K+-ATPase activity in the contraluminal membrane. Plus signs indicate stimulation. A, aldosterone; ADP, adenosine diphosphate; ATP, adenosine triphosphate; mRNA, messenger RNA; R, receptor. (From Hedge GA, Colby HD, Goodman RL: Clinical Endocrine Physiology. Philadelphia: WB Saunders, 1987, p 140.)

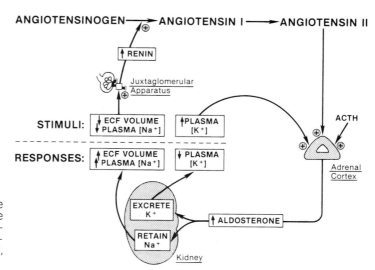

FIGURE 33-13. Regulation of aldosterone secretion by the zona glomerulosa of the adrenal cortex. Plus signs indicate stimulation. ACTH, adrenocorticotropic hormone; ECF, extracellular fluid. (From Hedge GA, Colby HD, Goodman RL: Clinical Endocrine Physiology. Philadelphia: WB Saunders, 1987, p 147.)

level of the distal tubules in the kidney. The effect of the mineralocorticoids is to promote retention of sodium and secretion of potassium and hydrogen. The cellular response to mineralocorticoids is to synthesize a protein that increases the permeability of the luminal cell surface to sodium influx from the renal filtrate and increases Na^+,K^+-ATPase activity in the contraluminal cell surface, which allows movement of sodium out of the cell into the interstitial tissue (Fig. 33-12).

The control of secretion of potassium by mineralocorticoids is passive in the sense that potassium is retained in the renal filtrate to maintain the osmolality of urine. There is, however, evidence that mineralocorticoids have an effect on sodium secretion that is independent of sodium retention. The secretion of potassium continues to be influenced by mineralocorticoids after mineralocorticoid administration, whereas sodium retention decreases within a few days.

In situations of excessive mineralocorticoid production, the effects of increased sodium retention are to increase the extracellular fluid volume and to cause hypertension; conversely, low blood pressure (hypotension) occurs as a result of inadequate secretion of mineralocorticoids. Hypersecretion of mineralocorticoids can also lead to excessive hydrogen ion loss and metabolic alkalosis, whereas hyposecretion can result in increased retention of hydrogen ion and metabolic acidosis.

The regulation of mineralocorticoid secretion, in contrast to glucocorticoid secretion, is not controlled by tropic hormones from the pituitary gland (Fig. 33-13). In the case of mineralocorticoids, the main controlling factors are produced in the target organ, i.e., the kidney. Cells in the juxtaglomerular apparatus of the kidney produce an enzyme, renin, in response to decreases in blood pressure. Renin acts on angiotensinogen, an α_2 globulin produced by the liver and present in the circulation, and this results in the production of angiotensin I, a decapeptide. Angiotensin I is further hydrolyzed to angiotensin II, an octapeptide, by angiotensin-converting enzyme. Angiotensin

II stimulates the zona glomerulosa to produce mineralocorticoids. Angiotensin II also increases peripheral resistance of the blood vascular system by causing vasoconstriction of smooth muscle of the blood vessels. Angiotensin II, if present on a long-term basis, also increases the size of the zona glomerulosa.

There is evidence that cells of the macula densa, groups of specialized cells that are located at the origin of the distal tubule of the kidney (Fig. 33-14), exert control on the renin-angiotensin system. This is done through the sensing of changes in sodium concentrations in tissue fluids. Sodium increase results in decreased renin release, and sodium decrease results in increased renin release. In either case, the change produced tends to restore the mineralocorticoid concentrations to normal. In addition to the effect of sodium, the macula densa may control changes in the renin-angiotensin system through the sensing of changes in chloride ion concentrations in tissue fluids.

Another major regulatory factor in the control of mineralocorticoid secretion is the blood potassium

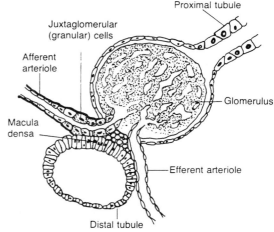

FIGURE 33-14. Diagrammatic representation of juxtaglomerular apparatus. (From Martin CR: Endocrine Physiology. London: Oxford University Press, 1985, p 338.)

concentration. An increase in potassium concentration stimulates the zona glomerulosa to secrete mineralocorticoids, whereas a decline in potassium has the opposite effect. This stimulation is independent of the renin-angiotensin system.

It has been thought that corticotropin has little to do with control of the zona glomerulosa. This viewpoint resulted from experimental studies, in which hypophysectomy has little effect on the zona glomerulosa. More recently, it was shown that cells of the zona glomerulosa have receptors for corticotropin, and corticotropin may play some role, albeit minor, in the control of mineralocorticoid secretion.

In contrast to the sodium-conserving effect of mineralocorticoids, a 28-amino acid peptide called *atrial natriuretic peptide* has been identified. It reduces sodium retention by the kidneys. Atrial natriuretic peptide also causes peripheral vasodilation and, as a consequence, a lowering of blood pressure. Atrial natriuretic peptide may also inhibit the production of mineralocorticoids and renin. As indicated in its name, atrial natriuretic peptide is produced by cells of the cardiac atria, but it is also produced in other sites, including the brain.

Hypoadrenocorticism, caused by lack of mineralocorticoids and glucocorticoids, is most commonly diagnosed in young female dogs and usually has an immune-mediated etiology. Certain breeds, such as Leonbergers, standard poodles, and Portuguese water dogs, are at increased risk for the disease; however, hypoadrenocorticism may be diagnosed in any breed. Historical findings compatible with hypoadrenocorticism include intermittent vomiting, diarrhea, weight loss, lethargy, anorexia, and weakness. These symptoms often resolve with fluid therapy and/or corticosteroid treatment. Physical examination of animals in an acute hypoadrenal crisis reveals weak pulse, bradycardia, prolonged capillary refill time, severe mental slowness, and profound muscle weakness. Clinical features of hypoadrenocorticism that should raise suspicion include a normal or slow heart rate in the presence of circulatory shock and the "waxing and waning" course of disease before collapse.

Electrolyte abnormalities consisting of severe hyponatremia and hypochloremia associated with hyperkalemia are the hallmarks of hypoadrenocorticism. Azotemia and hyperphosphatemia also accompany primary hypoadrenocorticism, which makes it difficult to differentiate it from acute renal failure. Azotemia may be prerenal as a result of dehydration and hypovolemia, or increase in BUN may be caused by gastrointestinal hemorrhage. Hematologic abnormalities consist of eosinophilia and lymphocytosis, or eosinophil and lymphocyte counts may be normal in the presence of severe metabolic stress. The anemia of hypoadrenocorticism has classically been attributed to lack of glucocorticoid effects on the bone marrow. However, more recent studies have suggested that hemorrhagic gastroenteritis contributes significantly to the anemia. Although hypoglycemia is more common with secondary or atypical hypoadrenocorticism, it is rarely seen with typical hypoadrenocorticism.

Urine specific gravity is frequently low, and this finding is attributed to medullary washout (inadequate medullary gradient caused by sodium depletion) and decreased medullary blood flow. Dilute urine in the presence of azotemia and hyperkalemia may easily be mistaken for acute renal failure. Hormonal assays are necessary to confirm the presence or absence of adrenal disease and to differentiate between hypoadrenocorticism and renal failure.

Diagnosis of primary hypoadrenocorticism is based on clinical signs, classic electrolyte imbalances, and confirmation with a corticotropin response test. The baseline cortisol sample should be collected with the initial blood work and synthetic corticotropin (cosyntropin [Cortrosyn], 0.25 mg) should be administered intravenously during the initial fluid therapy. A 1-hour, post-corticotropin sample may then be drawn, and glucocorticoids may be administered after the 1-hour sample is taken. Intramuscular injection of corticotropin (gel or synthetic) may not be absorbed in animals in circulatory shock; therefore, intravenous administration of synthetic corticotropin is preferred. If glucocorticoids must be administered before the measurement of cortisol, dexamethasone sodium phosphate is preferred because it does not interfere with the cortisol assay. Endogenous plasma corticotropin may be measured to determine whether the hypoadrenocorticism is primary or secondary.

Dogs and cats with primary hypoadrenocorticism exhibit a subnormal response to corticotropin administration. Both the baseline and the post-corticotropin cortisol concentrations are usually low or undetectable. Endogenous plasma corticotropin concentrations are dramatically increased in animals with primary hypoadrenocorticism as a result of loss of negative feedback to the pituitary gland, which is caused by decreased serum cortisol concentrations. In the case of secondary hypoadrenocorticism, which is caused by a pituitary deficiency of corticotropin, the endogenous corticotropin concentrations are typically decreased (<20 pg/mL). The response to exogenous corticotropin is diminished, but not as dramatically as for primary hypoadrenocorticism. Baseline and post-corticotropin cortisol concentrations may be in the normal range.

THE ADRENAL MEDULLA

The adrenal medulla, as its name indicates, occupies the central portion of the adrenal gland (see Fig. 33-7). A stimulatory effect of adrenal medullary extracts on cardiac activity was first recognized by Oliver and Schafer in 1894. Thereafter, the main hormone of the adrenal medulla, epinephrine, became the first hormone to be isolated (by Abel in 1898), crystallized (by Takamine and Aldrich in 1901), and synthesized (by Stolz in 1904). Theories on the importance of the adrenal medulla include that of Cannon, who in 1932 proposed the flight-or-fight hypothesis, in which the adrenal medulla is activated to aid in combating situations of extreme stress. Others advocated the tonus

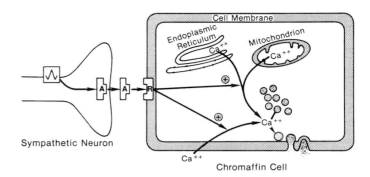

FIGURE 33–15. Stimulus-secretion coupling in the adrenal chromaffin cell. Note that cytosolic calcium may be derived from intracellular or extracellular sources. Circled plus signs indicate stimulation. A, acetylcholine; R, receptor. (From Hedge GA, Colby HD, Goodman RL: Clinical Endocrine Physiology. Philadelphia: WB Saunders, 1987, p 303.)

theory, which stated that cells of the adrenal medulla are constantly in a state of readiness. In fact, the adrenal medulla has a constant output of catecholamines that can be accentuated dramatically if the need arises.

It was recognized early in this research that cells of the adrenal medulla are the equivalent of postganglionic cells of the sympathetic nervous system. Therefore, it was assumed that epinephrine was the mediator of postganglionic activity of the sympathetic nervous system. It was later recognized that another catecholamine, norepinephrine, is the neurotransmitter of the sympathetic nervous system. Both epinephrine and norepinephrine are released when preganglionic nerve fibers to the adrenal medulla are stimulated; in fact, most of the norepinephrine found in plasma originates from the adrenal medulla. However, epinephrine is the major catecholamine secreted by the adrenal medulla of most mammals. Exceptions to this generalization include the dominance of norepinephrine over epinephrine in whales and chickens and in the fetal tissues of all species.

The synthesis of catecholamines is from tyrosine; the main catecholamine synthesized by the adrenal medulla is epinephrine

The cells of the adrenal medulla that synthesize catecholamines are classified as chromaffin cells. This classification is based on the histochemical reaction of the cells when exposed to potassium dichromate: that is, a darkening of the cells as a result of the formation of colored pigments in conjunction with the oxidation of the catecholamines. The cells that produce epinephrine are different from those that synthesize norepinephrine; accordingly, the type of chromaffin granule present is different for each cell type. In cattle, the epinephrine-secreting cells tend to be on the outer edge of the medulla. Acetylcholine release from the preganglionic nerve fibers initiates the synthesis of the catecholamines by the medullary cells (Fig. 33–15). Acetylcholine also stimulates the release of catecholamines from chromaffin granules, a phenomenon called *stimulus-secretion coupling*.

The synthesis of the catecholamines begins with either of the amino acids phenylalanine or tyrosine. However, tyrosine is a naturally occurring amino acid, and most of the synthesis of catecholamines begins with this amino acid (Fig. 33–16). The initial step in the biosynthetic pathway begins with the conversion of tyrosine to dihydroxyphenylalanine (DOPA). Tyrosine hydroxylase, the enzyme responsible for the conversion of tyrosine, is the rate-limiting enzyme in the formation of catecholamines. The end products of tyrosine metabolism, including DOPA, dopamine, norepinephrine, and epinephrine, inhibit the activity of tyrosine hydroxylase. DOPA is converted to dopamine through the enzymatic activity of aromatic-L-amino acid decarboxylase (DOPA decar-

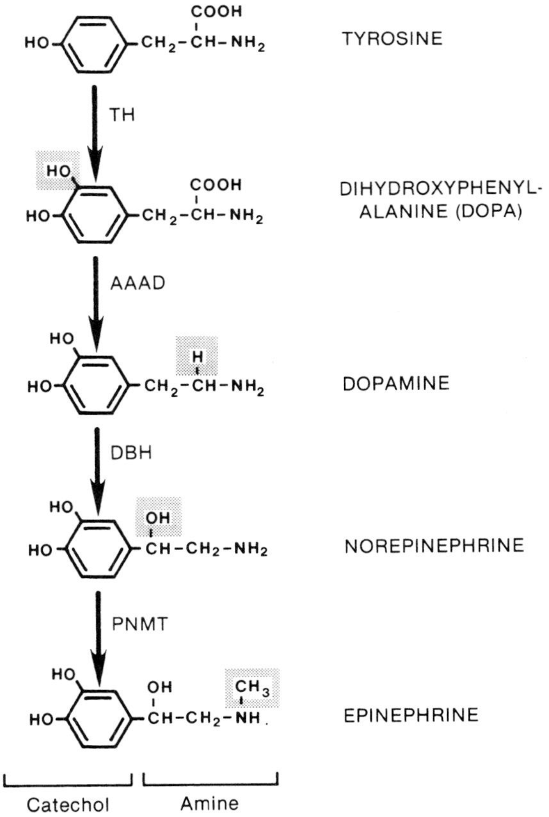

FIGURE 33–16. Pathway of catecholamine synthesis in the adrenal medulla. Shaded areas denote the structural changes occurring at each step. AAAD, aromatic-l-amino acid decarboxylase; DBH, dopamine-β-hydroxylase; PNMT, phenylethanolamine-N-methyltransferase; TH, tyrosine hydroxylase. (From Hedge GA, Colby HD, Goodman RL: Clinical Endocrine Physiology. Philadelphia: WB Saunders, 1987, p 298.)

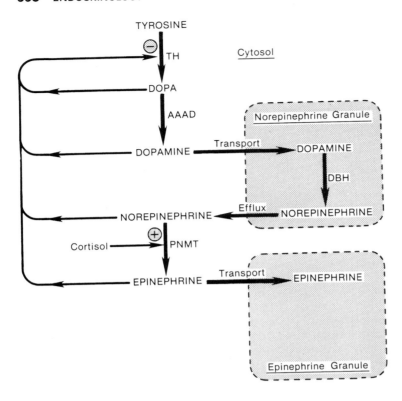

FIGURE 33-17. Regulation of catecholamine biosynthesis in the adrenal medulla. Plus sign indicates stimulation; minus sign indicates inhibition. AAAD, aromatic-l-amino acid decarboxylase; DBH, dopamine-β-hydroxylase; DOPA, dihydroxyphenylalanine; PNMT, phenylethanolamine-N-methyltransferase; TH, tyrosine hydroxylase. (From Hedge GA, Colby HD, Goodman RL: Clinical Endocrine Physiology. Philadelphia: WB Saunders, 1987, p 300.)

boxylase). To this point, the biochemical transformations have occurred in the cytosol. The conversion of dopamine to norepinephrine occurs within the chromaffin granule, because the key enzyme, dopamine-β-hydroxylase, is localized within the granule (Fig. 33-17).

If the cell secretes norepinephrine, the biochemical pathway is ended, and the hormone remains in the norepinephrine granule, ready for secretion. If the cell secretes epinephrine, norepinephrine moves back into the cytosol, where it is converted to epinephrine through the activity of phenylethanolamine-N-methyltransferase. Epinephrine then moves into an epinephrine granule for storage before its release. The metabolism of catecholamines is rapid (2 minutes for norepinephrine, less for epinephrine) and is accomplished mainly by the liver and kidneys.

The importance of the anatomic association of the adrenal cortex and medulla may be related to the fact that cortisol is important for the activity of the enzyme phenylethanolamine-N-methyltransferase. The chromaffin cells are located close to the venous sinuses that drain the adrenal cortex and therefore are exposed to venous effluent that contains high concentrations of cortisol.

The primary actions of catecholamines are on metabolism, especially effects that increase the concentration of glucose

The actions of the catecholamines involve the regulation of intermediary metabolism as well as responses that allow animals to adjust to situations involving acute stress. The actions of catecholamines are mediated through adrenergic receptors located on target tissues (Fig. 33-18). There are two major types of receptors, α and β, which are subdivided into α_1, α_2, β_1, and β_2. The α receptors control catecholamine release from sympathetic nerve endings, α_1 affecting postsynaptic nerve endings and α_2 affecting presynaptic terminals. The β_1 receptors affect mainly the heart, and β_2 receptors affect smooth muscle contraction and intermediary metabolism. Whereas all adrenergic receptors are responsive to both epinephrine and norepinephrine, the responses to the two catecholamines are different. In addition, the receptor types on various tissues vary in number, which, together with the different responses of adrenergic receptors on tissues, results in variable adrenergic responses' being produced by a particular catecholamine.

The metabolic effects of catecholamines are mediated mainly by β_2 receptors. Because epinephrine is 10 times more potent than norepinephrine with β_2 receptors, epinephrine plays a much more important role in the control of intermediary metabolism than does norepinephrine. The effects of epinephrine on glucose metabolism are similar to those of glucagon and opposite to those of insulin. Epinephrine increases blood glucose concentrations, with the effect mainly in the liver; that is, epinephrine promotes both hepatic glycogenolysis and gluconeogenesis. Epinephrine also stimulates glycogenolysis in skeletal muscle, which in this situation is in contrast with the action of glucagon. Because glucose-6-phosphatase is not present in skeletal muscle, lactate is produced

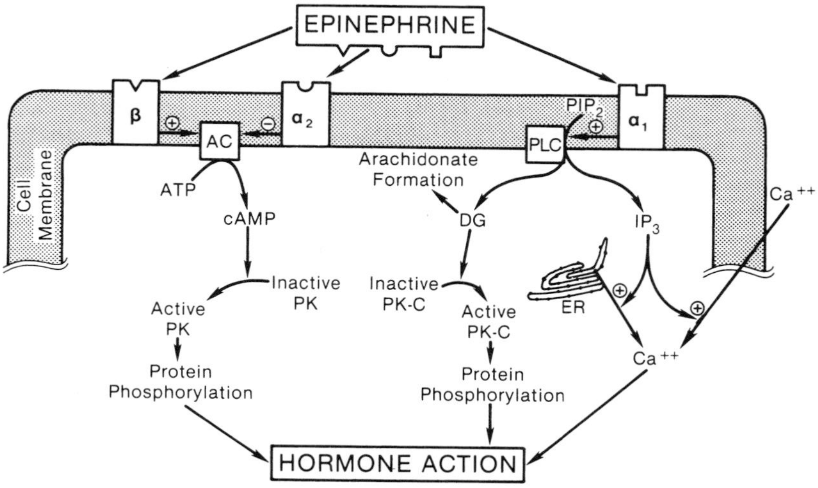

FIGURE 33-18. Mechanisms of action of epinephrine in target cells mediated by β, α_2, and α_1 adrenergic receptors. Plus signs indicate stimulation; the minus sign indicates inhibition. AC, adenyl cyclase; ATP, adenosine triphosphate; cAMP, cyclic adenosine monophosphate; DG, diacylglycerol; ER, endoplasmic reticulum; IP_3, inositol 1,4,5-triphosphate; PIP_2, phosphatidyl inositol 4,5-bisphosphate; PK, protein kinase; PK-C, protein kinase C; PLC, phospholipase C. (From Hedge GA, Colby HD, Goodman RL: Clinical Endocrine Physiology. Philadelphia: WB Saunders, 1987, p 305.)

instead of glucose; the liver takes up lactate and converts it to glucose. Additional effects on glucose metabolism include the inhibition of insulin secretion (through α receptors) and stimulation of glucagon secretion by the pancreas; both actions increase blood glucose concentrations.

Epinephrine promotes lipolysis through interaction with two receptors on adipose cells. Activation of a lipase enzyme results in an increase in free fatty acids in the blood. Glucocorticoids potentiate the effect of epinephrine on lipolysis.

Catecholamines stimulate cardiac function. Both epinephrine and norepinephrine interact with β_1 receptors to increase both the force of contraction and the heart rate, the latter resulting from the promotion of a shorter period of diastolic depolarization. Whereas both catecholamines promote arteriolar constriction through interaction with α receptors, epinephrine, through its high affinity for β_2 receptors, causes the dilation of blood vessels both in the heart and in skeletal muscle. The end result is that total peripheral resistance is decreased by the action of epinephrine with a concomitant decline in diastolic pressure; however, blood pressure is changed little, and cardiac output increases because of the increase in heart rate. The action of epinephrine to increase cardiac output is an obvious beneficial effect in situations that are described as "flight or fight."

Catecholamines affect smooth muscle. Epinephrine causes relaxation of bronchial smooth muscle, particularly in situations in which the muscle is in a contracted state. As the action is mediated through β_2 receptors, norepinephrine has little effect on bronchial smooth muscle. Epinephrine causes relaxation of the smooth muscle of the gastrointestinal tract through interaction with β_2 receptors. Catecholamine stimulation of α receptors results in contraction of uterine smooth muscle, and stimulation of β_2 receptors results in relaxation. Because of its dominant effect on β_2 receptors, epinephrine causes relaxation of the uterus, whereas both epinephrine and norepinephrine interact with α receptors to cause contraction.

The effects of the catecholamines on bladder smooth muscle are dependent on different locations of α and β receptors; α receptors are located within the neck of the bladder, and β receptors are located within the body of the bladder. Epinephrine relaxes the body and contracts the neck of the bladder; norepinephrine contracts the neck of the bladder. The net effect is retention of urine.

Although the parasympathetic nervous system is the principal system involved in penile erection, the sympathetic nervous system may also play a role. Epinephrine promotes erection through vasodilation of the blood vasculature mediated by β receptors. Higher concentrations of epinephrine (and norepinephrine) can cause ejaculation through α receptor interaction and vasoconstriction.

In the eye, epinephrine causes relaxation of the lens through stimulation of β receptors on the ciliary muscles. It causes dilation of the pupil through stimulation of α receptors, with resultant contraction of the radial muscle of the iris.

The effects of epinephrine on the central nervous system are excitatory. Drugs that affect the central nervous system probably do so by modulation of catecholamine concentrations, whereby sedation is associated with lower values of epinephrine. Other effects of catecholamine include the promotion of sweating and piloerection. Epinephrine also increases renin production by the renal juxtaglomerular cells. A summary of the effects of catecholamines is shown in Table 33-5.

The main factors that stimulate catecholamine secretion are hypoglycemia and conditions that produce stress

Any factor that increases sympathetic nervous system stimulation of the adrenal medulla results in the immediate secretion of catecholamines. The main physiologic factor that influences catecholamine secretion is hypoglycemia. In this situation, epinephrine secretion is stimulated by decreases in blood glucose con-

TABLE 33–5. **Responses of target tissues to catecholamines**

Target tissue	Receptor type	Response
Liver	β_2	Glycogenolysis, lipolysis, gluconeogenesis
Adipose tissue	β_2	Lipolysis
Skeletal muscle	β_2	Glycogenolysis
Pancreas	α_2	Decreased insulin secretion
	β_2	Increased insulin secretion
Cardiovascular system	β_1	Increased heart rate, increased contractility, increased conduction velocity
	α_2	Vasoconstriction
	β_2	Vasodilation in skeletal muscle arterioles, coronary arteries, and all veins
Bronchial muscle	β_2	Relaxation
Gastrointestinal tract	β_2	Decreased contractility
Urinary bladder	α_2	Sphincter contraction
	β_2	Detrusor relaxation
Uterus	α_2	Contraction
	β_2	Relaxation
Male sex organs	α_2	Ejaculation, detumescence
	β_2	Erection?
Eye	α_1	Radial muscle contraction
	β_2	Ciliary muscle relaxation
Central nervous system	α_2	Stimulation
Skin	α_2	Piloerection, sweat production
Renin secretion	β_1	Stimulation

From Hedge GA, Colby HD, Goodman RL: Clinical Endocrine Physiology. Philadelphia: WB Saunders, 1987, p 305.

centrations that are within normal physiologic limits. In contrast, other parts of the sympathetic nervous system are depressed by decreases in blood glucose levels. Factors that elicit a massive release of catecholamines are categorized as stressful, particularly those that are acute. Catecholamines are especially important for the maintenance of blood pressure in conjunction with severe blood loss; decreased blood pressure stimulates epinephrine secretion. Catecholamines are also important for adaptation to cold exposure in terms of increased heat production; decreased temperature increases epinephrine secretion. The response to acute stress can be particularly marked, because each preganglionic sympathetic neuron that supplies the adrenal medulla affects a number of chromaffin cells; that is, the signal is greatly amplified.

HORMONES OF THE PANCREAS

The pancreas has important endocrine and nonendocrine functions. The nonendocrine functions occur as a result of activity of the exocrine part of the pancreas and are concerned with gastrointestinal function. The endocrine portion of the pancreas is organized as discrete islets (islets of Langerhans) (Fig. 33–19) that contain four cell types, each of which produces a different hormone. The most numerous of the islet cells are β cells, which produce insulin; α cells produce glucagon, D cells produce somatostatin, and F or PP cells produce pancreatic polypeptide (Fig. 33–20). Although these hormones have different functions, they are all involved in the control of metabolism and, more particularly, in glucose homeostasis.

Insulin

The first studies that associated the pancreas with carbohydrate metabolism were done by von Mering and Minkowski in 1889, when they showed that pancreatectomy of dogs resulted in signs that were similar to those characteristic of diabetes mellitus. Later, Banting and Best were able to show that injection of pancreatic extracts could alleviate the signs of diabetes mellitus in dogs and humans. Able was the first to crystallize insulin, and its structure was elucidated by Sanger in 1960.

Insulin is a protein consisting of two chains, designated A (21 amino acids) and B (30 amino acids), that are connected by two disulfide bridges. The monomer form of the hormone is thought to be the active form; insulin also exists in dimer and hexamer forms, the latter being complexed with two zinc molecules. Although there are some differences in amino acid composition among species, the differences are small; for example, cattle, sheep, horses, dogs, and whales differ only in positions 8, 9, and 10 of the A chain. As a result, the biologic activities of insulin are not highly species-specific. Of the domestic species, feline insulin is most similar to bovine insulin, and canine insulin

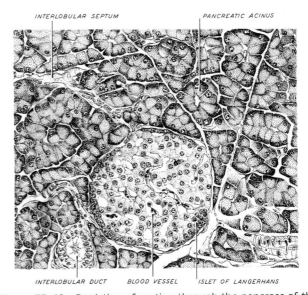

INTERLOBULAR SEPTUM PANCREATIC ACINUS

INTERLOBULAR DUCT   BLOOD VESSEL   ISLET OF LANGERHANS

FIGURE 33–19. Depiction of section through the pancreas of the rat. The islet of Langerhans is a gland of internal secretion, whereas the surrounding acinar tissue forms an exocrine gland. (From Turner CD, Bagnara JT: General Endocrinology, 6th ed. Philadelphia: WB Saunders, 1976, p 259.)

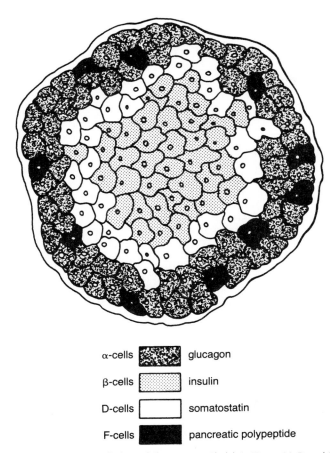

α-cells		glucagon
β-cells		insulin
D-cells		somatostatin
F-cells		pancreatic polypeptide

FIGURE 33–20. Depiction of the pancreatic islet. (From McDonald LE: Veterinary Endocrinology and Reproduction, 4th ed. Philadelphia: Lea & Febiger, 1989, p 188.)

is similar to human insulin and identical to porcine insulin in its amino acid structure.

THE SYNTHESIS OF INSULIN IS BIPHASIC: AN ACUTE PHASE INVOLVES THE RELEASE OF PREFORMED INSULIN, AND A CHRONIC PHASE INVOLVES THE SYNTHESIS OF PROTEIN

The synthesis of insulin, similar to that of other peptide hormones, begins with the formation of a linear polypeptide preproinsulin within the rough endoplas-

mic reticulum. A small peptide fragment is removed to form proinsulin. Proinsulin is coiled, and the end fragments are joined by disulfide bonds. Proinsulin is transferred to the Golgi apparatus, where it is further processed and packaged into granules that contain both insulin and the connecting or C peptide (33 amino acids in length).

The secretion of insulin follows biphasic kinetics in response to appropriate stimuli (Fig. 33–21). The initial, acute release of insulin involves the exocytosis of preformed insulin from secretion granules. After the acute phase, a chronic phase of secretion occurs that involves the synthesis of protein and, hence, probably the synthesis of insulin.

THE METABOLISM OF INSULIN INVOLVES SPLITTING THE A AND B CHAINS AND REDUCING THE CHAINS TO AMINO ACIDS AND PEPTIDES

Insulin is metabolized mainly by the liver and kidneys. Enzymes that are present reduce the disulfide bonds that link the A and B chains, and the chains are then subjected to protease activity, which reduces them to peptides and amino acids. The half-life of insulin is about 10 minutes.

THE MAIN METABOLIC FUNCTIONS OF INSULIN ARE ANABOLIC

Insulin acts at a number of sites within the metabolic pathways of carbohydrates, fats, and proteins (Fig. 33–22). It is important to realize that the liver is an especially important target organ, in part because the pancreatic venous effluent passes directly to the liver. The net effect of the actions of insulin is to lower blood concentrations of glucose, fatty acids, and amino acids and to promote intracellular conversion of these compounds to their storage forms (i.e., glycogen, triglycerides, and protein, respectively) (Table 33–6). Glucose does not readily penetrate cell membranes except in a few tissues, such as brain, liver, and red and white blood cells, all of which must have continual access to glucose. The presence of insulin is critical to the movement of glucose through the plasma membrane into the cell.

Insulin has profound effects on carbohydrate me-

FIGURE 33–21. Kinetics of insulin secretion by the β cell in response to a continued glucose stimulus. (From Hedge GA, Colby HD, Goodman RL: Clinical Endocrine Physiology. Philadelphia: WB Saunders, 1987, p 270.)

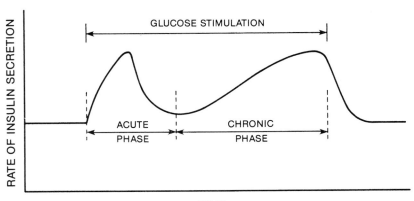

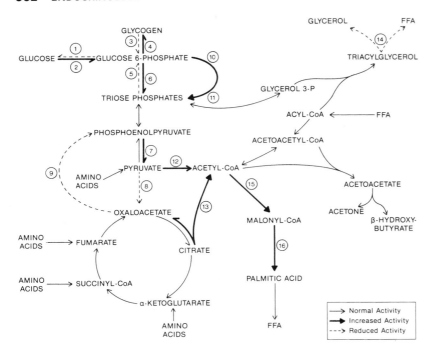

FIGURE 33–22. Metabolic pathways affected by insulin. The numbers correspond to each of the following enzymes: (1) glucose-6-phosphatase; (2) glucokinase; (3) phosphorylase; (4) glycogen synthase; (5) fructose-1,6-bisphosphate aldolase; (6) 6-phosphofructokinase; (7) pyruvate kinase; (8) pyruvate carboxylase; (9) phosphoenolpyruvate carboxykinase; (10) glucose-6-phosphate-dehydrogenase; (11) 6-phosphogluconate dehydrogenase; (12) pyruvate dehydrogenase; (13) adenosine triphosphate (ATP)–citrate lyase; (14) hormone-sensitive lipase; (15) acetyl–coenzyme A (CoA) carboxylase; (16) fatty acid synthase. FFA, free fatty acid. (From Hedge GA, Colby HD, Goodman RL: Clinical Endocrine Physiology. Philadelphia: WB Saunders, 1987, p 271.)

tabolism. Insulin facilitates the use of glucose: namely, glycolysis, which involves the oxidation of glucose to pyruvate and lactate through the induction of enzymes, such as glucokinase, phosphofructokinase, and pyruvate kinase. Insulin promotes glycogen production in the liver, in adipose tissue, and in skeletal muscle by increasing glycogen synthetase activity with a concomitant decrease in glycogen phosphorylase activity. Gluconeogenesis is decreased by insulin because of the promotion of protein synthesis in peripheral tissues, thereby decreasing the amount of amino acids available for gluconeogenesis. In addition, insulin decreases the activities of hepatic enzymes (fructose 1,6-bisphosphate aldolase, pyruvate carboxylase, phosphoenolpyruvate carboxylase, and glucose-6-phosphatase) that are involved in the conversion of amino acids to glucose.

In adipose tissue, insulin promotes the synthesis of triglycerides. Insulin facilitates the intracellular use of glucose, which results in increased levels of pyruvate, a precursor of acetyl–coenzyme A (CoA) (in turn, a precursor of fatty acids) and increased glycerol 3-phosphate for the esterification of fatty acids. Insulin activates the enzymes pyruvate dehydrogenase and acetyl-CoA carboxylase, which promote the synthesis of fatty acids from acetyl-CoA. Insulin also increases the activity of lipoprotein lipase located in the endothelium of capillaries of extrahepatic tissues, which promotes the movement of fatty acids into adipose tissue. Finally, insulin decreases lipolysis in adipose tissue.

With protein metabolism, insulin promotes uptake of amino acids by most tissues, including skeletal muscle, but not liver. Insulin promotes protein synthesis and inhibits protein degradation. Therefore, insulin promotes the maintenance of a positive nitrogen balance. With insulin deficiency, protein catabolism increases, with increased amounts of amino acids available for hepatic gluconeogenesis and a resultant increase in the blood glucose concentrations.

The most important factor in the control of insulin secretion is the concentration of blood glucose. Increased concentrations of blood glucose initiate the synthesis and release of insulin by the β cells of the pancreatic islets (Fig. 33–23). There are two theories regarding the mechanism of cellular induction of insulin synthesis and release. One is that it exists within the plasma membrane, whereby glucose interacts with a membrane receptor protein that directs intracellular events toward the synthesis and release of insulin. The other is that it occurs at the intracellular level, whereby the metabolism of glucose produces the signal for insulin synthesis and release. Glucose control of insulin secretion is a positive feedback sys-

TABLE 33–6 Sites of action and effects of insulin on cabohydrate, lipid, and protein metabolism

Process affected	Site of action		
	LIVER	MUSCLE	ADIPOSE
Carbohydrate metabolism			
↑ Glucose transport		X	X
↑ Glycogen synthesis	X	X	X
↓ Glycogenolysis	X	X	X
↓ Gluconeogenesis	X		
Lipid metabolism			
↑ Lipogenesis	X		X
↓ Lipolysis	X		X
Protein metabolism			
↑ Amino acid uptake		X	
↑ Protein synthesis		X	
↓ Protein degradation		X	
↓ Gluconeogenesis	X		

From Hedge GA, Colby HD, Goodman RL: Clinical Endocrine Physiology. Philadelphia: WB Saunders, 1987, p 272.

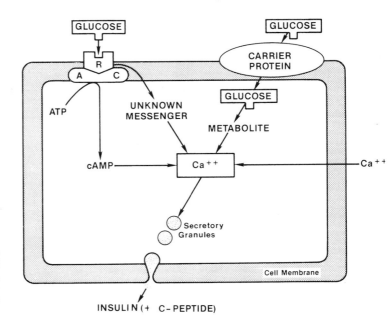

FIGURE 33–23. Proposed mechanisms of action of glucose on insulin secretion by the β cell. AC, adenyl cyclase; ATP, adenosine triphosphate; R, receptor. (From Hedge GA, Colby HD, Goodman RL: Clinical Endocrine Physiology. Philadelphia: WB Saunders, 1987, p 269.)

tem in which increased concentrations of glucose lead to increased concentrations of insulin.

Because the oral administration of glucose produces a larger insulin response than does systemic administration, factors from the intestinal tract were thought to affect insulin secretion. It is now known that a number of gastrointestinal hormones, including gastrin, cholecystokinin, secretin, and gastric inhibitory peptide, stimulate insulin secretion. The presence of amino acids and fatty acids in the intestinal tract also stimulates the release of insulin, although with less potency than that of glucose (Table 33–7).

Hormones other than those from the gastrointestinal tract are important for the control of insulin secretion. Glucagon from the α cells of the pancreas has a direct stimulatory effect on the β cells to secrete insulin. Conversely, somatostatin inhibits the secretion of insulin. Both hormones work through the adenyl cyclase system, glucagon being stimulatory and somatostatin being inhibitory. Catecholamines tend to de-

crease insulin secretion through an interaction with the α-adrenergic receptors on the β cells. Whereas epinephrine is the main circulating catecholamine that affects insulin secretion, norepinephrine also influences insulin secretion, because the pancreas has adrenergic innervation by the autonomic nervous system. The pancreas also has cholinergic innervation by the autonomic nervous system, and, in contrast to adrenergic stimulation, cholinergic activity increases insulin secretion through the release of acetylcholine.

A lack or deficiency of insulin produces a syndrome called *diabetes mellitus.* Blood glucose concentrations increase because of a variety of factors: (1) decreased uptake of glucose by body tissues, (2) increased glycogenolysis, and (3) increased gluconeogenesis. The latter occurs as a result of increased hepatic gluconeogenesis caused by the increased availability of amino acids, which occurs as a result of increased protein catabolism. Glucose appears in the urine when the capacity of the kidney for reabsorption is exceeded; the resulting osmotic effect leads to diuresis or polyuria. As mentioned previously, increased metabolism of triglycerides leads to increased concentrations of fatty acids in the blood and the formation of ketone bodies by the liver. Insulin deficiency increases lipolysis and, as a result, increases the level of free fatty acids in blood. The fatty acids are oxidized by the liver to form acetyl-CoA, which can be further converted to acetoacetate, β-hydroxybutyrate, and acetone, collectively called *ketone bodies* (see Fig. 33–21). The ketone bodies are acidic anions, and their presence produces acidosis because of the depletion of bicarbonate ions.

Glucagon

Glucagon is a protein hormone produced by the α cells of the islets of Langerhans. It has a close relationship with insulin in the control of glucose metabolism.

TABLE 33–7. Factors affecting insulin secretion

Stimuli
    Glucose
    Amino acids
    Fatty acids
    Gastrin
    Pancreozymin-cholecystokinin
    Secretin
    Gastric inhibitory polypeptide
    Glucagon
    Acetylcholine
Inhibitors
    Somatostatin
    Epinephrine
    Norepinephrine

From Hedge GA, Colby HD, Goodman RL: Clinical Endocrine Physiology. Philadelphia: WB Saunders, 1987, p 276.

Glucagon is a polypeptide consisting of a single chain composed of 29 amino acids. There is considerable homology in amino acid composition among species. There are other sites of production of glucagon besides the pancreas; the stomach produces a molecule called *gut glucagon* that is identical to the pancreatic glucagon molecule, and the small intestine produces an immunologically similar molecule called *glicentin*. Like other polypeptide hormones, glucagon is first synthesized in the endoplasmic reticulum as part of a precursor molecule, packaged in the Golgi apparatus, and final processing occurs in the secretory granules. Glucagon is released by exocytosis. Glucagon is metabolized mainly by the liver and kidneys. It has a half-life in plasma of about 5 minutes.

THE MOST IMPORTANT FUNCTIONS OF GLUCAGON ARE TO DECREASE GLYCOGEN SYNTHESIS, INCREASE GLYCOGENOLYSIS, AND INCREASE GLUCONEOGENESIS

The physiologic actions of glucagon are opposite those of insulin; most of the effect of glucagon is centered on the liver. Glucagon increases cAMP production in the liver, which leads to decreased glycogen synthesis, increased glycogenolysis, and increased gluconeogenesis, the last being related to the effects of glucagon on protein metabolism (Fig. 33–24). The net result is an increase in glucose concentrations in the blood.

Changes in glucagon secretion counterbalance the effects of insulin in association with the daily ingestion of food and the intervals between food intake periods. After the consumption of food, the initial response of the metabolic system is increased insulin secretion, which results in conservation of energy through the formation of storage forms of carbohydrates, fats, and proteins. Glucagon secretion, which begins with the ingestion of food, increases as the interval from food ingestion lengthens and blood glucose concentrations begin to decline. This secretion allows the individual to mobilize energy stores for the maintenance of glucose homeostasis (i.e., to prevent postprandial hypoglycemia) (Fig. 33–25).

GLUCAGON SYNTHESIS IS STIMULATED BY DECREASED GLUCOSE CONCENTRATIONS IN THE BLOOD

The main factor that regulates glucagon secretion is plasma glucose concentration. In contrast to insulin synthesis, decreased glucose concentrations stimulate glucagon synthesis and release, a relationship that represents a negative feedback system. It must be remembered that glucagon regulation works in tandem with insulin regulation in order to maintain glucose concentrations within the physiologic range. In fact, if glucagon were not secreted to maintain blood glucose concentrations, the individual would die of hypoglycemic shock. Because the α cells require insulin for glucose entry into the cells (as do most cells), in clinical syndromes involving insulin insufficiency (diabetes mellitus), glucose entry into the α cells is reduced, and plasma glucagon concentrations are paradoxically elevated. Glucagon promotes lipolysis and an increase in fatty acids, which has a negative feedback effect on glucagon secretion.

Protein ingestion represents an exception to the rule of opposite responses of glucagon and insulin. The release of both insulin and glucagon in response to protein ingestion appears logical; increased insulin secretion, in response to increased plasma amino acid levels, leads to lower glucose concentrations, and increased glucagon would counteract this through increased hepatic gluconeogenesis, resulting in maintenance of blood glucose within normal limits. The complementary responses of insulin and glucagon allow growth to occur in animals fed a diet of protein and fat only.

Intestinal hormones, with the exception of secretin, stimulate both glucagon and insulin secretion. A similar (inhibitory) response to somatostatin is observed

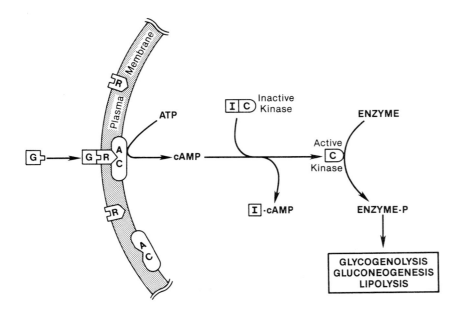

FIGURE 33–24. Mechanism of action of glucagon (G) on its target cells. AC, adenyl cyclase; ATP, adenosine triphosphate; cAMP, cyclic adenosine monophosphate; I and C, inhibitory and catalytic subunits of the kinase, respectively; R, receptor. (From Hedge GA, Colby HD, Goodman RL: Clinical Endocrine Physiology. Philadelphia: WB Saunders, 1987, p 286.)

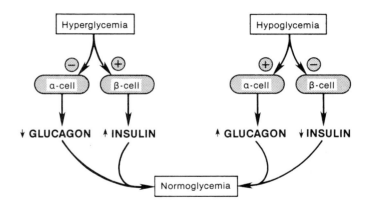

FIGURE 33–25. Effects of hyperglycemia and hypoglycemia on the secretion of insulin and glucagon by the pancreatic β cells and α cells, respectively. Plus signs indicate stimulation; minus signs indicate inhibition. (From Hedge GA, Colby HD, Goodman RL: Clinical Endocrine Physiology. Philadelphia: WB Saunders, 1987, p 288.)

for both glucagon and insulin. Both sympathetic and parasympathetic stimulation of the autonomic nervous system induce secretion of glucagon (Fig. 33–26).

In some birds, there is a predominance of glucagon in the pancreas, which suggests that glucagon may have a more important role in carbohydrate metabolism of avian species than in mammals.

Somatostatin

As indicated in Chapter 32, somatostatin was first described in the brain as a 14–amino acid peptide that inhibits growth hormone secretion by the pars distalis. The molecule has since been identified in a number of tissues, including other areas of the brain, the gastrointestinal tract, and the D cells of the pancreatic islets. Its synthesis and secretion are similar to those observed for other protein hormones. The metabolism of somatostatin is rapid (about 5 minutes) and occurs mainly in the liver and kidneys.

THE MAIN FUNCTIONS OF SOMATOSTATIN ARE TO INHIBIT THE SECRETION OF HORMONES PRODUCED BY THE PANCREAS (INSULIN, GLUCAGON, PANCREATIC POLYPEPTIDE)

The actions of somatostatin can be classified as inhibitory. Pancreatic somatostatin inhibits the digestive

processes by decreasing nutritive absorption and digestion. The motility and secretory activity of the gastrointestinal tract are decreased by somatostatin. One of the most important physiologic functions of pancreatic somatostatin is the regulation of the endocrine cells of the pancreas (Fig. 33–27). Somatostatin inhibits secretion of all endocrine cell types of the islets of Langerhans, including the D cells. The α cells are more affected by the inhibitory action of somatostatin than are β cells; therefore, glucagon secretion is more affected by somatostatin than is insulin secretion.

Somatostatin secretion is increased by nutrients, such as glucose and amino acids, and by the neurotransmitters of the autonomic nervous system: epinephrine, norepinephrine, and acetylcholine. Of the hormones produced by the pancreas, only glucagon stimulates somatostatin secretion.

Pancreatic Polypeptide

Pancreatic polypeptide, a 36–amino acid polypeptide, is produced by the F cells of the pancreas (see Fig. 33–20). In contrast to somatostatin secretion, pancreatic polypeptide secretion is limited to the pancreas.

The effects of pancreatic polypeptide are directed

FIGURE 33–26. Regulation of insulin and glucagon secretion by the autonomic nervous system. Plus signs indicate stimulation; minus signs indicate inhibition. NS, nervous system. (From Hedge GA, Colby HD, Goodman RL: Clinical Endocrine Physiology. Philadelphia: WB Saunders, 1987, p 277.)

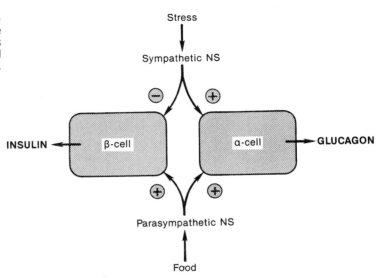

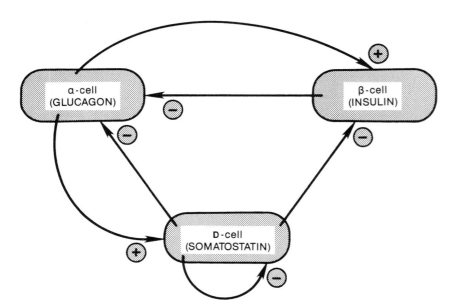

FIGURE 33–27. Possible cell-to-cell interactions in the pancreatic islets. Plus signs indicate stimulation; minus signs indicate inhibition. (From Hedge GA, Colby HD, Goodman RL: Clinical Endocrine Physiology. Philadelphia: WB Saunders, 1987, p 292.)

toward the gastrointestinal tract. The secretion of pancreatic enzymes and the contraction of the gallbladder are inhibited by the actions of this hormone. Both gut motility and gastric emptying are increased by the action of pancreatic polypeptide.

The secretion of pancreatic polypeptide is stimulated by intestinal hormones, including cholecystokinin, secretin, and gastrin. Stimulation of the vagus nerve also promotes pancreatic polypeptide secretion. The ingestion of protein is stimulatory for secretion, whereas carbohydrates and fats have little effect. As indicated previously, somatostatin inhibits pancreatic polypeptide secretion.

▬ CALCIUM AND PHOSPHATE METABOLISM

▬ Calcium is important for intracellular reactions, including muscle contraction, nerve cell activity, the release of hormones through exocytosis, and the activation of enzymes

The control of calcium and phosphate metabolism is important because these ions play a major role in physiologic processes. Calcium homeostasis is tightly controlled; adjustments are made within a range of 5% of normal. Calcium is important for a number of intracellular reactions, including muscle contraction, nerve cell activity, the release of hormones through the process of exocytosis, and the activation of a number of enzymes. Calcium is important for coagulation of blood and for maintaining the stability of cell membranes and the linkage between cells. On a less acute basis, calcium is important for the structural integrity of bone and teeth.

▬ Phosphate is important for the structure of bone and teeth; on a cellular basis, organic phosphate serves as part of the cell membrane and as part of a number of intracellular components

Phosphate concentrations are controlled by the same systems that control calcium concentrations. Inorganic phosphate in blood serves as the source of phosphate, which is important for the structure of bone and teeth. Inorganic phosphate also functions as an important hydrogen ion buffering system in blood. Organic phosphate is an important part of the cell, including the plasma membrane and intracellular components, such as nucleic acids, adenosine triphosphate, and adenosine monophosphate.

▬ The most important body pool of calcium involved in homeostasis is the extracellular fluid component

The great majority (99%) of calcium in the body is in bone in the form of hydroxyapatite crystals, which contain calcium, phosphate, and water. The next largest pool of calcium is intracellular calcium. As stated previously, calcium is important for the response of cells in carrying out their physiologic activities, including the secretion of hormones. In the inactive cell state, calcium concentrations are relatively low in the cytosol; calcium is bound to proteins or contained within the mitochondria or granules of the endoplasmic reticulum. Increased intracellular calcium concentrations are indicative of increased cell activity.

The smallest pool of calcium, which resides in the extracellular fluid, is the most important pool for physiologic control of calcium concentrations in the blood. This component comprises interstitial calcium, blood calcium, and a small (0.5%) but important part of the bone calcium pool, which exists as amorphous crystals or in solution. The soluble bone calcium pool allows access to the large reserve of calcium that resides in bone.

The regulation of calcium levels involves control of the movement of calcium between the extracellular fluid and three body organs: bone, gastrointestinal tract, and kidneys. The exchange of calcium ions between the extracellular and intracellular fluid occurs in conjunction with the control of intracellular metabolism, with little effect on plasma concentrations of calcium.

The absorption of calcium from the gastrointestinal tract is by passive diffusion and active transport. The passive diffusion of calcium across the intestinal mucosa occurs in the presence of high concentrations and, as such, is not an important aspect of calcium absorption. Active transport involves the movement of calcium into the intestinal cell down a concentration gradient, which is facilitated by carrier proteins located on the luminal side of the mucosal cell. Calcium is moved through the serosal side of the mucosal cell into the interstitial fluid through a calcium pump system. The active transport system adjusts according to the amount of calcium in the diet, becoming more active when calcium concentrations in the diet are lower and less active when calcium concentrations are higher. Calcium excretion into the gastrointestinal tract is not affected by calcium uptake, and this can exacerbate conditions involving hypocalcemia. The gastrointestinal tract serves as the source of calcium for the body, even though both absorption and excretion of calcium occur through the tract. As discussed later, vitamin D plays an important role in the absorption of calcium from the gastrointestinal tract.

The kidneys serve as the route of excretion of calcium. Most of the calcium that passes into the kidneys is reabsorbed, with a net loss of only about 2%. This amount is matched by net absorption of calcium by the gastrointestinal tract. Most of the calcium filtered by the kidneys is reabsorbed in the proximal tubules; the next largest amount is absorbed by the distal tubules, and a lesser amount, by the ascending loop of Henle. The distal tubules are under hormonal control and therefore are the sites of regulation of calcium in the kidneys.

The most important regulation of calcium metabolism between bone and extracellular fluid involves the soluble portion of bone. Amorphous crystals and soluble calcium, which form the source of ready exchange of ions with the blood, are located between the osteoblasts, which line the blood vessel channels, and the osteocytes, which are deeper in the bone (Fig. 33–28). These two cell types have cytoplasmic projections that interact intimately through the presence of tight cell junctions. In order for labile bone calcium to reach the blood, calcium must cross the membrane barrier created by the osteoblasts and osteocytes. Movement of calcium from stable bone into the extracellular fluid also occurs, but it has little impact on the acute regulation of calcium concentrations. The process of remodeling bone, which occurs on a continuous basis, involves the breakdown of hydroxyapatite crystals by osteoclasts; a laying down of organic matrix by osteoblasts in the tunnels made by the osteoclasts; and, finally, the mineralization of the organic matrix by hydroxyapatite crystals. If an animal is subjected to prolonged changes involving calcium metabolism, the slowness of bone calcium exchange can have a significant impact on calcium metabolism.

PARATHYROID HORMONE

The main organ involved in the control of calcium and phosphate metabolism is the parathyroid gland (Fig. 33–29). Most domestic animals have four pairs of parathyroid glands that are generally located at the poles of the two lobes of the thyroid gland; the pig has only one pair of parathyroid glands, and they lie anterior to the thyroid. The cranial pair of parathyroid glands in dogs and cats are at the craniolateral poles of the thyroid, and those of ruminants and horses are anterior to the thyroid. The caudal pair of parathyroid glands in dogs, cats, and ruminants are located within the medial surface of the thyroid, whereas in the horse they lie near the bifurcation of the carotid trunk. The parathyroid cells that are in the active process

FIGURE 33–28. Structure of the osteon, the functional unit of bone, depicted in cross section at two magnifications. (From Hedge GA, Colby HD, Goodman RL: Clinical Endocrine Physiology. Philadelphia: WB Saunders, 1987, p 360.)

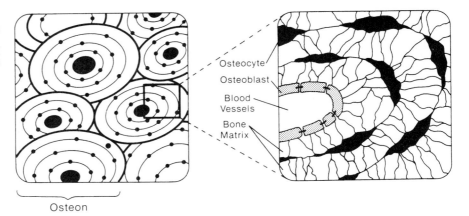

Osteocyte
Osteoblast
Blood Vessels
Bone Matrix

Osteon

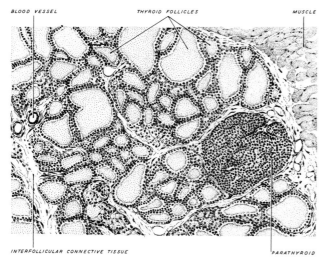

BLOOD VESSEL   *THYROID FOLLICLES*   *MUSCLE*

INTERFOLLICULAR CONNECTIVE TISSUE   *PARATHYROID*

FIGURE 33–29. Depiction of a section of the thyroid and parathyroid glands of the rat as seen under low power of the microscope. Notice that the parathyroid gland lies near the surface of the thyroid gland and is surrounded on three sides by the thyroid follicles. (From Turner CD, Bagnara JT: General Endocrinology, 6th ed. Philadelphia: WB Saunders, 1976, p 226.)

of hormone secretion are called *chief cells,* whereas inactive, or degenerate, cells are called *oxyphil cells.*

The synthesis of parathyroid hormone (PTH) is similar to the synthesis of other protein hormones; a prepro-PTH of 115 amino acids is synthesized in the rough endoplasmic reticulum and then cleaved by 25 amino acids to form pro-PTH. A 6–amino acid "pro" portion is removed by the Golgi apparatus; the resulting PTH has 84 amino acids. PTH is secreted by the process of exocytosis. PTH is rapidly metabolized by the liver and kidneys and has a relatively short half-life (5 to 10 minutes) in blood.

The effect of PTH is to increase calcium and decrease phosphate concentrations in extracellular fluids. PTH has direct effects on bone and kidney metabolism of calcium and indirect effects on gastrointestinal metabolism of calcium. The initial effect of PTH on bone is to promote the transfer of calcium across the osteoblast-osteocyte membrane. This level of action occurs without the movement of phosphate and therefore has no effect on phosphate concentrations in blood. PTH has additional effects on stable bone, which results in the resorption of the bone. This effect involves increased osteoclast activity and an inhibition of osteoblast activity. The effect of PTH on stable bone results in the release of both calcium and phosphate.

PTH acts on the distal convoluted tubules of the kidneys to increase absorption of calcium and decrease renal phosphate reabsorption through an effect on the proximal tubules. PTH is involved also in the activation of vitamin D at the kidney level. PTH mediates the absorption of calcium from the gut indirectly through its effect on vitamin D.

PTH secretion is controlled by free (ionized) calcium concentrations in blood; decreases in calcium levels stimulate PTH secretion, and increases in calcium turn off secretion (Fig. 33–30). Both actions are mediated by an effect on cAMP metabolism. Epinephrine stimulates PTH secretion through stimulation of gb-adrenergic receptors. Magnesium affects PTH secretion in the same manner as calcium, but its physiologic impact is much less. Sleep affects the secretion of PTH; values are highest immediately after waking.

CALCITONIN

Calcitonin, a hormone produced by cells in the thyroid gland, also affects calcium metabolism. Cells of the type involved in the synthesis of calcitonin—parafollicular, or C, cells—are scattered throughout the thyroid gland and are distinctly different from the cells that synthesize thyroid hormones. During the

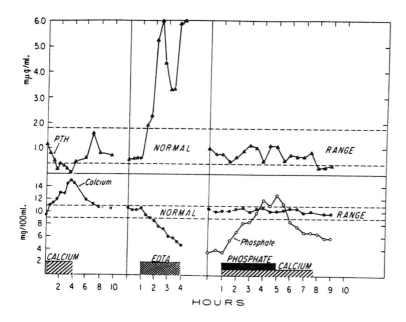

FIGURE 33–30. Changes in plasma immunoreactive parathyroid hormone (PTH) levels in response to hypercalcemia induced by calcium infusion; in response to hypocalcemia produced by ethylene-diaminetetraacetic acid (EDTA) infusion; and in response to hyperphosphatemia with normocalcemia in a cow. (From Capen CC: The calcium regulating hormones: Parathyroid hormone, calcitonin, and cholecalciferol. In McDonald LE, Pineda MH [eds]: Veterinary Endocrinology and Reproduction. Philadelphia: Lea & Febiger, 1989, p 105.)

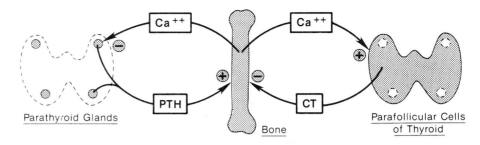

FIGURE 33–31. Negative feedback loops controlling parathyroid hormone (PTH) and calcitonin (CT) secretion. Plus signs indicate stimulation; minus signs indicate inhibition. (From Hedge GA, Colby HD, Goodman RL: Clinical Endocrine Physiology. Philadelphia: WB Saunders, 1987, p 363.)

early studies of calcitonin in animal classes such as fish, amphibians, reptiles, and birds, which have separate thyroid and ultimobranchial glands, it was found that all the calcitonin activity was in the ultimobranchial glands. Therefore, the calcitonin cells represent ultimobranchial gland tissue that has been incorporated into the thyroid during embryonic development.

Calcitonin, synthesized as a preprohormone, has 32 amino acids; a ring structure at the amino terminus contains a disulfide link that bridges between amino acids 1 and 7. The processing of the molecule is interesting because calcitonin is located in the middle of procalcitonin, so that an additional enzyme cleavage is required for the formation of the active molecule. The secretion of calcitonin is by exocytosis from granules.

Calcitonin acts as a counterbalance to PTH, because it causes hypocalcemia and hypophosphatemia. The effect of calcitonin on mineral metabolism is mainly on bone (Fig. 33–31). Calcitonin decreases the movement of calcium from the labile bone calcium pool (behind the osteoblast-osteocyte barrier) to the extracellular fluid and decreases bone resorption through an inhibitory effect on osteoclasts. Whereas the inhibition of bone resorption explains one aspect of the hypophosphatemic effects of calcitonin, calcitonin

also increases movement of phosphate from the extracellular fluid into bone. Calcitonin decreases gastrointestinal activity directly by inhibiting gastric acid secretion and indirectly by inhibiting gastrin secretion. The importance of this in a physiologic sense is not known. Calcitonin also increases renal excretion of calcium and phosphate.

The control of secretion of calcitonin is by calcium; increased concentrations cause increased secretion of calcitonin. The physiologic control of calcium metabolism by calcitonin operates in situations of hypercalcemia with increased secretion of calcitonin and concomitant inhibition of PTH secretion. During hypocalcemic conditions (Fig. 33–32), calcitonin synthesis is inhibited, and PTH becomes responsible for reestablishing normal calcium concentrations in the extracellular fluids. Gastrointestinal hormones, including gastrin, cholecystokinin, secretin, and glucagon, stimulate the secretion of calcitonin, gastrin being the most potent. These hormones limit postprandial hypercalcemia.

VITAMIN D

Vitamin D is important for the absorption of calcium from the gut. It is a steroid-like molecule, and because it is produced in one tissue and transported by the

FIGURE 33–32. Synthesis and metabolism of vitamin D. The position of hydroxylation of 25-OH-vitamin D in the kidney is controlled by parathyroid hormone (PTH), phosphate (PO_4), and 1,25-$(OH)_2$-vitamin D. Shading indicates structural change at each step; the dashed line indicates the position of cleavage of 7-dehydrocholesterol to produce vitamin D. Enzymes: (1) 25-hydroxylase, (2) 1α-hydroxylase, (3) 24-hydroxylase. Plus signs indicate stimulation; minus signs indicate inhibition. (From Hedge GA, Colby HD, Goodman RL: Clinical Endocrine Physiology. Philadelphia: WB Saunders, 1987, p 367.)

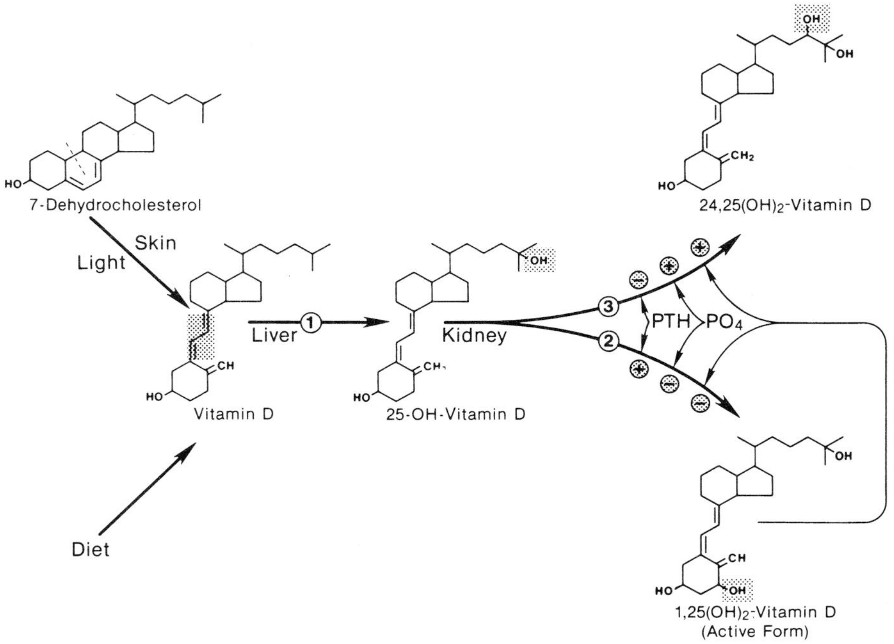

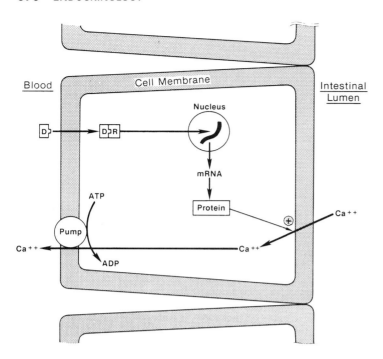

FIGURE 33–33. Mechanism of action of 1,25-(OH)₂-vitamin D (D) to increase calcium absorption in the intestine. Plus sign indicates stimulation. R, receptor. (From Hedge GA, Colby HD, Goodman RL: Clinical Endocrine Physiology. Philadelphia: WB Saunders, 1987, p 369.)

blood to a distant site of action, it should probably be called a hormone instead of a vitamin. All the vitamin D produced by the body is produced in the skin. Epithelial cells of the skin synthesize the immediate precursor of vitamin D, 7-dehydrocholesterol, from acetate. Exposure of the skin to ultraviolet light results in cleavage of the C-9 and C-10 bonds of 7-dehydrocholesterol, which results in the formation of vitamin D (Fig. 33–32). The vitamin D molecule, as such, is inactive, and must be transformed by both the liver and kidney before the molecule is biologically activated. The liver first hydroxylates the molecule at the C-25 position, and the kidney subsequently hydroxylates the molecule at C-1 to produce the active compound, 1,25-(OH)₂-vitamin D (1,25-vitamin D).

Control of the C-1 hydroxylase in the kidney by PTH is the most important control linkage for the synthesis of 1,25-vitamin D. Decreases in calcium concentrations stimulate PTH secretion, which in turn favors the synthesis of active vitamin D and increased intestinal absorption of calcium. Phosphate also regulates vitamin D metabolism. Increased serum phosphate concentrations stimulate an enzyme that promotes hydroxylation of C-24 (instead of C-1) by the kidney, which leads to the formation of 24,25-(OH)₂-vitamin D, an inactive molecule. The active molecule, 1,25-vitamin D, also regulates itself by decreasing C-1 hydroxylase and increasing C-24 hydroxylase activity; decreased amounts of active vitamin D is the result.

Because of its lipid nature, 1,25-vitamin D is transported by binding to proteins in the plasma. Most of vitamin D is carried in association with a specific α globulin called *transcalciferin,* a molecule synthesized by the liver.

The most important effects of vitamin D concern increased absorption of calcium by the gastrointestinal tract. Vitamin D stimulates the synthesis of protein within the mucosal cells, which aids the rate-limiting step in calcium absorption: movement of calcium into the mucosal cell (Fig. 33–33). Because the intestinal effect of vitamin D depends on the activation of protein synthesis by mucosal cells, the effect on calcium absorption (Fig. 33–34) usually requires several hours. Although the stimulation of protein synthesis relates mostly to active transport of calcium, vitamin D also stimulates passive transfer of calcium. Vitamin D also has effects on bone, promoting the movement of calcium ions from the labile pool into extracellular fluids and the resorption of bone, as well as enhancing the effects of PTH on bone metabolism of calcium.

The control of 1,25-vitamin D synthesis is by PTH and phosphate. A decrease in calcium concentrations results in increased PTH secretion and increased formation of 1,25-vitamin D through enhancement of C-1 hydroxylation. This action leads to the correction of hypocalcemia by increasing absorption of calcium by the gut. A decline in phosphate concentrations results in decreased inhibition of the C-1 hydroxylation, which indirectly results in increased 1,25-vitamin D production and increased absorption of phosphate. There is some evidence that hormones associated with pregnancy, such as growth hormone and prolactin, increase 1,25-vitamin D production by stimulating C-1 hydroxylation.

In the overall control of calcium metabolism, PTH is primarily responsible for the maintenance of calcium homeostasis. The primary target tissue for PTH in calcium homeostasis is the labile pool in bone; changes in renal absorption of calcium are also important. In the case of long-term calcium deficit in the diet, both PTH and 1,25-vitamin D are important for correction of the deficit. Decreased dietary calcium leads to decreased concentrations of calcium in the extracellular fluids and the release of PTH. PTH affects resorption of calcium by the kidneys, but, of most importance for long-term correction of the problem, it causes increased 1,25-vitamin D secretion with increased absorption of dietary calcium. PTH also con-

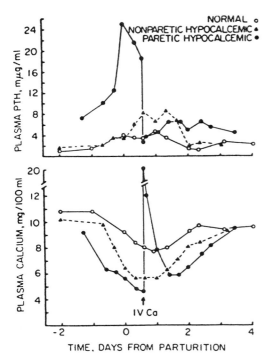

FIGURE 33–34. Development of varying degrees of hypocalcemia in cows near parturition, with corresponding increases in plasma parathyroid hormone (PTH) levels. The cow developing severe hypocalcemia (<5 mg/100 mL) had a considerably greater increase in plasma PTH levels than the moderate rise detected in the nonparetic hypocalcemic and the normal cow. Note that PTH levels declined rapidly after treatment of the paretic cow with intravenous calcium. (From Mayer CP: The roles of parathyroid hormone and thyrocalcitonin in parturient paresis. In Anderson JJB [ed]: Parturient Hypocalcemia. New York: Academic Press, 1970, p 179.)

tributes to the overall calcium pool through its effect on stable bone: that is, the promotion of resorption.

Hypercalcemia has a variety of causes, including malignancy, hyperparathyroidism, fungal disease, osteoporosis, hypoadrenocorticism, chronic renal disease, and hypervitaminosis D. The initial signs of hypercalcemia are polydipsia and polyuria that result from impaired response of distal renal tubules to antidiuretic hormone. Listlessness, depression, and muscle weakness result from depressed excitability of neuromuscular tissue. Mild gastrointestinal signs of hypercalcemia include inappetence, vomiting, and constipation. Persistent mild elevations in serum calcium (12 to 14 mg/dL) can cause uroliths and signs of urinary tract disease such as hematuria and stranguria. On the other hand, severe hypercalcemia (>14 mg/dL) can progress rapidly to acute renal failure when the calcium-phosphorus product (Ca [in milligrams per deciliter] × PO_4 [in milligrams per deciliter]) exceeds 60 to 80 because of mineralization of renal tissue.

The diagnostic approach to hypercalcemia consists of ruling out the most common cause: hypercalcemia of malignancy. A thorough history and physical examination, including lymph node and rectal examination (for anal sac adenocarcinoma), complete blood cell count, urinalysis, serum chemistry profile, and chest and abdominal radiographs, are necessary to search for underlying neoplastic processes. If lymphoma is not detected on the minimum database, a bone marrow examination and survey skeletal radiographs may be necessary. Once a diagnosis of neoplasia has been excluded, the next primary differential for hypercalcemia is chronic renal failure. This is the most difficult differential to exclude because other causes of hypercalcemia may result in renal damage because of soft tissue mineralization of the kidneys. Therefore, an animal with hypercalcemia, azotemia, and hyperphosphatemia could suffer from primary hyperparathyroidism, primary renal failure with secondary renal hyperparathyroidism, or vitamin D intoxication. Furthermore, patients with hypercalcemia secondary to renal disease may also exhibit elevations in intact PTH. Diagnosis of primary hyperparathyroidism is based on the findings of hypercalcemia (preferably ionized), hypophosphatemia (unless azotemic), high normal to elevated serum PTH concentrations, and a mass in the cervical region. Intact PTH, demonstrated by a sandwich assay validated for use in the dog and cat, should be measured. A normal PTH concentration in the presence of elevated total and/or ionized calcium is considered inappropriate for the calcium level and would be considered diagnostic for primary hyperparathyroidism. For suspected cases of hypercalcemia of malignancy in which the diagnostic approach has failed to identify a neoplastic process, PTH-related protein (PTH-rp) concentrations may be measured.

The classic biochemical findings in animals with hypoparathyroidism are hypocalcemia (both total and ionized) and hyperphosphatemia. Other causes of hypocalcemia include iatrogenic (post-thyroidectomy) hypoparathyroidism, chronic and acute renal failure, acute pancreatitis, hypoalbuminemia, puerperal tetany (eclampsia), ethylene glycol intoxication, intestinal malabsorption, and nutritional secondary hyperparathyroidism. Early signs of hypocalcemia are nonspecific and include anorexia, facial rubbing, nervousness, and a stiff, stilted gait. Later signs progress to paresthesias, hyperventilation, and, finally, generalized tetany and/or seizures.

Primary hypoparathyroidism is diagnosed by means of an intact PTH assay. Serum or plasma PTH concentrations should be measured on a freshly drawn morning sample in a fasting animal. Handling of the sample is crucial to appropriate diagnosis because PTH may degrade if subjected to warm temperatures. *Intact PTH* refers to the entire 85–amino acid sequence of PTH; this is measured in a double-antibody "sandwich" assay in most endocrine laboratories that perform PTH measurement. For the diagnosis of primary hypoparathyroidism, the sample should be analyzed for both ionized calcium and intact PTH. Low ionized calcium and undetectable intact PTH concentrations are diagnostic for hypoparathyroidism.

CLINICAL CORRELATIONS

Diabetes mellitus

History You are presented with a 10-year-old, intact, female poodle whose owner is upset because the dog urinates in the house. In addition, the owner has noticed that the animal drinks larger amounts of water than it has in the past. Although the owner indicates the dog has a good appetite, it appears to have lost weight over the past few months.

Clinical examination During the examination you check the dog's breath and detect a sweet odor. Among the organ systems you check are the eyes, and you find developing cataract formation. Because you have seen this dog many times before, you check its weight and find that it has lost 2 pounds since its last admittance a year ago. You are able to run a blood glucose determination in your hospital and tell the owner that the glucose concentration is 278 mg/dL.

Comment The findings in diabetes mellitus are all attributable to inadequate availability of insulin. Glycogen synthesis decreases in tissues, whereas glycogenolysis and gluconeogenesis increase, the latter two contributing to the high concentrations of glucose found in blood. When glucose concentrations exceed the reabsorption capacity in the tubular cells of the kidney, glucose appears in the urine. The loss of glucose in urine causes an osmotic diuresis (polyuria), and the dog compensates for this by drinking additional amounts of water. The sweetness of the breath is caused by the presence of ketone bodies. These form as the result of decreased triglyceride synthesis in adipose tissue, which stimulates lipase activity and the release of free fatty acids. These fatty acids are metabolized to ketone bodies (acetoacetate, acetone, β-hydroxybutyrate) by the liver in a situation of excess fatty acids. The end result is both a ketonemia and a ketonuria. Protein metabolism shifts toward catabolism during diabetes mellitus with decreased protein synthesis and increased protein degradation by muscle cells. This process increases the circulating concentrations of amino acids that are available to the liver for gluconeogenesis. The end result is nitrogen loss and a decrease in the muscle mass of the animal. The changes noted in the lenses of the eyes represent only one of a number of changes that occur in the presence of diabetes mellitus as a result of glycosylation of proteins, including lens proteins and hemoglobin.

Treatment Insulin administration is essential in the treatment of insulin-dependent diabetes mellitus. During the initial stages of treatment, considerable care must be taken to ensure that the dosage is correct. The goal of treatment is to maintain glucose concentrations between a low of 80 mg/dL and a high of 200 mg/dL with one or two insulin injections every 24 hours. Too much insulin has the potential for producing a hypoglycemic coma. Two other important aspects of treatment include feeding the animal a diet high in soluble fiber in conjunction with insulin administration and adequate exercise. Finally, the owner needs to be educated and prepared for the necessity of his or her intensive involvement in the management of the disease.

Bibliography

Dickson WM: Endocrine glands. In Swenson MJ (ed): Dukes' Physiology of Domestic Animals, 10th ed. Ithaca, New York: Cornell University Press, 1984, pp 761–797.

Feldman EC, Nelson RW: Canine and Feline Endocrinology and Reproduction. Philadelphia: WB Saunders, 1987.

Hedge GA, Colby HD, Goodman RL: Clinical Endocrine Physiology. Philadelphia: WB Saunders, 1987.

Martin R: Endocrine Physiology. New York: Oxford University Press, 1985.

McDonald LE, Pineda MH (eds): Veterinary Endocrinology and Reproduction, 4th ed. Philadelphia: Lea & Febiger, 1989.

Tepperman J, Tepperman HM: Metabolic and Endocrine Physiology, 5th ed. Chicago: Year Book Medical, 1987.

Wilson JD, Foster DW: Williams Textbook of Endocrinology, 7th ed. Philadelphia: WB Saunders, 1985.

PRACTICE QUESTIONS

1. The other main hormone secreted by the thyroid gland, in addition to tetraiodothyronine and triiodothyronine, is
   a. calcitonin.
   b. insulin.
   c. parathyroid hormone.
   d. glucagon.
   e. somatostatin.

2. The most important function of mineralocorticoids is
   a. control of carbohydrate metabolism.
   b. control of glucose metabolism.
   c. control of electrolyte metabolism.
   d. control of protein metabolism.

3. The pancreas has four types of cells, each of which produce a specific hormone. For example, the α cells of the pancreas produce
   a. insulin.
   b. glucagon.
   c. somatostatin.
   d. pancreatic polypeptide.

4. Two hormones play an important role in calcium homeostasis. The two hormones, _____ and _____, cause an increase and a decrease in calcium concentrations, respectively:
   a. calcitonin; glucagon.
   b. somatostatin; calcitonin.
   c. calcitonin; parathyroid hormone.
   d. parathyroid hormone; calcitonin.
   e. parathyroid hormone; glucagon.

5. The main functions of the catecholamines are to allow rapid body responses to acute stimuli, which include the mobilization of glucose. The catecholamines are secreted by the sympathetic portion of the autonomic nervous system. The _____ hormone is the main neurotransmitter of the sympathetic nervous system, whereas _____ is the main hormone produced by the postganglionic fibers of the adrenal medulla.
   a. serotonin; epinephrine.
   b. epinephrine; serotonin.
   c. epinephrine; norepinephrine.
   d. norepinephrine; epinephrine.
   e. serotonin; melatonin.

PRACTICE ANSWERS

1. a   2. c   3. b   4. d   5. d

REPRODUCTION AND LACTATION

George H. Stabenfeldt

Autumn P. Davidson

Chapter 39 by Steven P. Brinsko

34

Control of gonadal
and gamete development

Development of the reproductive system

1 The organization of the gonads is under genetic control

2 The sexual organization of the genitalia and brain depends on the presence, or absence, of testosterone

Hypothalamopituitary control of reproduction

1 The hypothalamus and anterior pituitary (adenohypophysis) secrete protein and peptide hormones, which control gonadal activity

2 The adenohypophysis (pars distalis) produces follicle-stimulating hormone, luteinizing hormone, and prolactin, all of which control reproductive processes

Modification of gonadotropin release

Ovarian follicle development

1 Gamete development occurs initially without gonadotropin support and subsequently with pulsatile gonadotropin secretion

2 In the preantral follicle, gonadotropin receptors for luteinizing hormone develop on the theca, which results in androgen synthesis; follicle-stimulating hormone direction of the granulosa causes it to transform the androgens to estrogens

3 Late in the ovarian follicular phase, luteinizing hormone receptors develop on the granulosa, which permits the preovulatory surge of luteinizing hormone to cause ovulation

— DEVELOPMENT OF THE REPRODUCTIVE SYSTEM

— The organization of the gonads is under genetic control

The initial development of the embryonic ovary involves the migration of germ cells into the genital ridge from the yolk sac. These primordial germ cells populate sex cords that have formed in the cortical region of the embryonic gonad from the proliferation of cells from the *coelomic epithelium* (so-called *germinal epithelium)* of the *genital ridge.* The sex cords contribute cells, known initially as *follicle cells* and subsequently as *granulosa cells,* that immediately surround the oocyte. The mesenchyme of the genital ridge contributes cells that will become the theca. The entire structure is called a *follicle,* which includes oocyte, granulosa, and theca cells.

No direct connections are formed between the oocytes and the tubes destined to become the oviducts, which are derived from *müllerian ducts.* The final result is that oocytes are released through the surface of the ovary by rupture of tissue elements that surround the ovary; this process is called *ovulation.* A specialized end of the oviduct, the fimbria, develops to enable the oocyte to be removed efficiently from the surface of the ovary. In some animals, oocytes are funneled to the fimbria through the use of a bursa, which tends to encompass the ovary; oocytes are directed to a relatively small opening in the bursa.

The development of the embryonic testis (Fig. 34–1) is similar to that of the ovary: germ cells migrate into the genital ridge and populate sex cords that have formed from an invagination of the surface (coelomic) epithelium. *Sertoli cells* (male counterparts of granulosa cells) develop from the sex cords, and *Leydig's cells* (male counterparts of thecal cells) develop from the mesenchyme of the genital ridge. One fundamental difference from ovarian development is that the invagination of the sex cords in the male continues into the medulla of the embryonic gonad, where connections are made with medullary cords from the mesonephros (primitive kidney). The duct of the mesonephros (wolffian duct) becomes the epididymis, vas deferens, and urethra, which has a direct connection to the seminiferous tubules. Thus, male germ cells pass to the exterior of the animal through a closed tubular system.

— The sexual organization of the genitalia and brain depends on the presence, or absence, of testosterone

The development of the genital tubular system and the external genitalia is under the control of the devel-

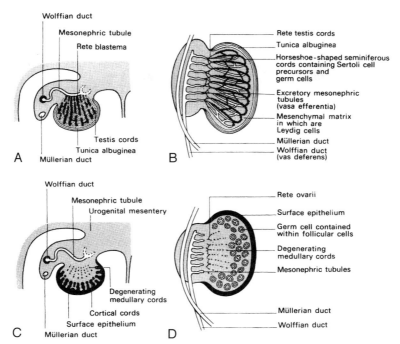

FIGURE 34–1. Testicular development during the 8th *(A)* and the 16th to 20th weeks *(B)* of human fetal life. *A,* The primitive sex cords proliferate in the medulla and establish contact with the rete testis. The tunica albuginea (fibrous connective tissue) separates the testis cords from the coelomic epithelium and eventually forms the capsule of the testis. *B,* Note the horseshoe shape of the seminiferous cords and their continuity with the rete testis cords. The vasa efferentia, derived from the excretory mesonephric tubules, connect the seminiferous cords with the wolffian duct (see text). Comparable diagrams of ovarian development around the 7th *(C)* and the 20th to 24th weeks *(D)* of development. *C,* Any primitive medullary sex cords degenerate and are replaced by the well-vascularized ovarian stroma. The cortex proliferates, and mesenchymal condensations later develop around the arriving primordial germ cells. *D,* In the absence of medullary cords and a true persistent rete ovarii, no communication is established with the mesonephric tubules. Hence, in the adult, ova are shed from the surface of the ovary and are not transported by tubules to the oviduct. (From Johnson M, Everitt B [eds]: Essential Reproduction, 3rd ed. London: Blackwell Scientific, 1988, p 9.)

oping gonad. If the individual is female—that is, the developing gonad is an ovary—the müllerian duct develops into oviduct, uterus, cervix, and vagina, whereas the wolffian duct regresses; the absence of testosterone is important for both changes (Fig. 34–2). If the individual is male, the rete testis produces müllerian-inhibiting factor, which causes regression of the müllerian ducts. The wolffian duct is maintained in the male because of the influence of androgens produced by the testis. To summarize, the müllerian ducts are "permanent" structures, and the wolffian ducts are "temporary" structures unless acted on by the presence of male hormones. The presence of an enzyme, 5α-reductase, is important for the effect of the androgens, because testosterone must be converted intracellularly into dihydrotestosterone for masculinization of the tissues to occur. The use of 5α-reductase inhibitors (used to treat prostatic disease in humans) in breeding stud dogs is discouraged, as disorders of sexual development in resultant fetuses can occur.

Development of the external genitalia follows the development and direction of the gonads. If the individual's genotype is female, folds of tissue called *labia* form the *vulva,* and a *clitoris* develops. If the individ-

ual is male, androgens from the testis direct formation of the *penis* (male counterpart of the clitoris) and the *scrotum* (male counterpart of the labia). Again, the absence or presence of androgens is an important factor influencing the formation of external genitalia.

The final organization of the individual with regard to gender comes with sexual differentiation of the hypothalamus. Exposure of the hypothalamus to androgens at around the time of birth causes the hypothalamus to be organized as male. A paradoxical finding is that conversion (aromatization) of androgens to estrogens is essential for maleness, mediated by enzymes in the neural tissue. In the absence of androgens, the hypothalamus is organized as female.

The fundamental concept of organization of the reproductive system with regard to genotype is that the female system is organized in the absence of testes. If the individual is to be male, there must be active intervention by the testes through the production of androgens and appropriate tissue enzymes in two circumstances: (1) within the internal genitalia for conversion to more potent androgens, and (2) within the hypothalamus for conversion to estrogens.

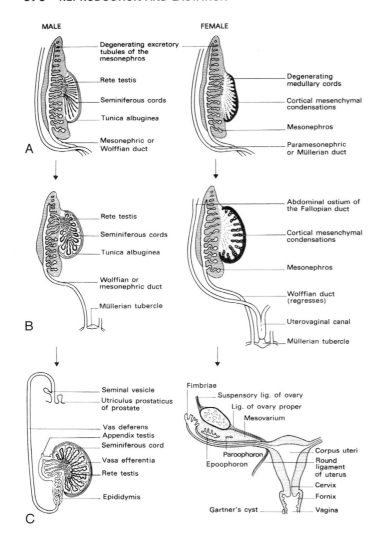

FIGURE 34–2. Differentiation of the internal genitalia in the human male and female at the sixth week of gestation *(A)*, the fourth month of gestation *(B)*, and the time of descent of testis and ovary *(C)*. Note that the müllerian and wolffian ducts are present in both sexes early on; the müllerian ducts eventually regress in the male and persist in the female, and the wolffian ducts regress in the female and persist in the male. The appendix testis and utriculus prostaticus in the male and epoöphoron, paroöphoron, and Gartner's cyst in the female are remnants of the degenerated müllerian and wolffian ducts, respectively. *lig.*, ligament. (From Johnson M, Everitt B [eds]: Essential Reproduction, 3rd ed. London: Blackwell Scientific, 1988, p 10.)

HYPOTHALAMOPITUITARY CONTROL OF REPRODUCTION

The hypothalamus and anterior pituitary (adenohypophysis) secrete protein and peptide hormones, which control gonadal activity

Gonadal activity is under the control of both the *hypothalamus* and the *anterior pituitary gland* (Fig. 34–3). The hypothalamus is a relatively small structure that lies midcentral in the base of the brain. It is divided into halves by the third ventricle and, in actuality, forms the ventral and lateral walls of the third ventricle. The hypothalamus has clusters of neurons, collectively called *nuclei,* that secrete peptide hormones important for controlling pituitary activity. As described in more detail later, these peptides move to the pituitary either directly by passage through the axons of neurons or by a blood vascular portal system. The pituitary responds to the hypothalamic peptides to produce hormones that are important for the control of the gonads.

The adenohypophysis (pars distalis) produces follicle-stimulating hormone, luteinizing hormone, and prolactin, all of which control reproductive processes

The pituitary gland is composed of three parts: an anterior lobe called the *adenohypophysis,* or *pars distalis;* an intermediate lobe called the *pars intermedia;* and a posterior lobe called the *neurohypophysis,* or *pars nervosa.* The lobes are of different embryologic origins; the pars distalis is derived from the endoectoderm (derived, in turn, from a small diverticulum off the dorsal pharynx, called Rathke's pouch), and the pars intermedia and pars nervosa are derived from neuroectoderm. The adenohypophysis produces protein hormones that are important for the control of reproduction: namely, two gonadotropins, *follicle-stimulating hormone* (FSH) and *luteinizing hormone* (LH), and a third hormone called *prolactin;* other pituitary hormones include *growth hormone* (GH), *adrenocorticotropic hormone* (ACTH), and *thyroid-stimulating hormone* (TSH). FSH and LH are synergistic in the

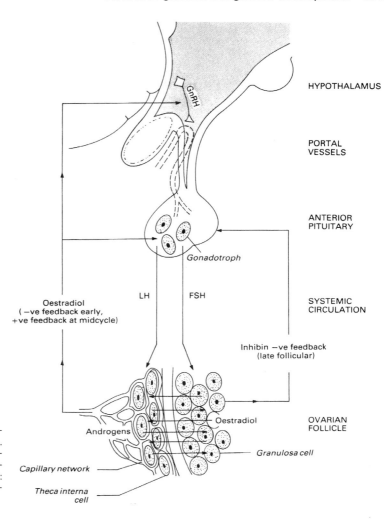

FIGURE 34–3. Summary of hypothalamic-pituitary-ovarian interactions during the follicular phase of the cycle. *FSH*, follicle-stimulating hormone; *GnRH*, gonadotropin-releasing hormone; *LH*, luteinizing hormone; *-ve*, negative; *+ve*, positive. (From Johnson M, Everitt B [eds]: Essential Reproduction, 3rd ed. London: Blackwell Scientific, 1988, p 151.)

development and ovulation of ovarian follicles; FSH plays a more dominant role during the growth of follicles, and LH plays a more dominant role during the final stages of follicle maturation through ovulation. The gonadotropins, as well as TSH, are called *glycoproteins*, because their molecules contain carbohydrate moieties that contribute to their function. *Oxytocin*, which is released by the neurohypophysis, is the hormone of importance for reproduction.

Besides being an important center for the control of reproduction, the hypothalamus regulates appetite and temperature and integrates the activity of the autonomic nervous system. Because of a common embryologic origin, the hypothalamus has a direct connection to the neurohypophysis. This connection is through the neural stalk, which contains axons that originate from neuronal cell bodies located in the hypothalamus. Two sets of neurons within the hypothalamus, the *supraoptic* and *paraventricular nuclei*, are responsible for the synthesis of *vasopressin* and oxytocin, respectively. These small peptide hormones are coupled to larger peptide molecules, called *neurophysins*, and are transported from the site of synthesis in

the hypothalamus (neuronal cell bodies) through axons to the site of storage and eventual release—that is, the neurohypophysis.

The connection of the hypothalamus to the adenohypophysis does not involve the direct passage of axons through the *neural stalk*. A *venous portal system* connects the median eminence within the hypothalamus to the adenohypophysis. Hypothalamic substances that control the adenohypophysis are carried from the median eminence of the hypothalamus to the pituitary by a venous portal system. For example, *gonadotropin-releasing hormone* (GnRH), a peptide, is produced in the medial preoptic nucleus, and dopamine, an amino acid, is produced in the arcuate nucleus. Axons transport both substances from the hypothalamus to the *median eminence*, where they are released into the venous portal system. The synthesis of GnRH, like that of oxytocin and vasopressin, involves the production of a larger precursor molecule, with a C-terminal region of 56 amino acids, called *GnRH-associated peptide* (GAP). Although GAP can stimulate the release of FSH and LH, GnRH is still thought to be the critical hormone for gonadotropin release. An even more important function of GAP may be its ability to inhibit prolactin secretion.

MODIFICATION OF GONADOTROPIN RELEASE

The main secretory pattern of gonadotropins is *pulsatile*; the pattern is driven by pulsatile secretion of GnRH from the hypothalamus (Fig. 34–4). The importance of this mode of delivery is shown by the fact that if GnRH is administered in a continuous (pharmacologic) manner, the system can be down-regulated. Continual occupancy of GnRH receptors on gonadotrophs by GnRH interrupts the intracellular signal for the synthesis and release of gonadotropins. Successful induction of a fertile estrus in bitches can be performed by administering canine analogue GnRH; however, the dose must be diminished as estrus approaches, or down-regulation will occur.

In general, the *pulse generator system* for gonadotropin secretion is increased in the *follicular phase* and decreased in the *luteal phase* of the estrous cycle (Fig. 34–5). Estrogen decreases the pulse amplitude, and progesterone decreases the pulse frequency of gonadotropin secretion. This means that during the follicular phase, pulse frequency increases because of the absence of progesterone, and pulse amplitude decreases because of the presence of estrogen. This combination of increased pulse frequency and decreased pulse amplitude is important for nurturing the final growth phase of the developing antral follicle.

The hypothalamus and adenohypophysis are capable of responding to a sustained increase in estrogen secretion by increased secretion of gonadotropins, a relationship that is termed *positive feedback*. The sudden sustained increase in estrogen concentrations, which occurs over one to several days during final

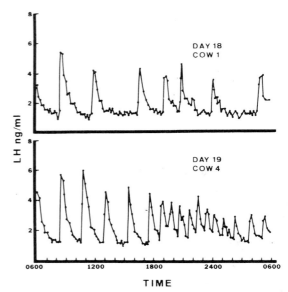

FIGURE 34–5. Pattern of plasma luteinizing hormone (LH) concentration on day 18 or 19 of the estrous cycle in two cows. (From Rahe CH, Owens RE, Fleeger JL, et al: Pattern of plasma luteinizing hormone in the cyclic cow: Dependence upon the period of the cycle. Endocrinology 107:498, 1980.)

antral follicle development, causes an increase in gonadotropin secretion by increasing the frequency of pulsatile release of GnRH and, as a result, gonadotropin secretion. In essence, the frequency of pulsatile release of gonadotropins overcomes the metabolic clearance rate. The purpose of the gonadotropin surge is to induce changes within the follicle that lead to its rupture (ovulation). The duration of the gonadotropin surge is relatively short (usually 12 to 24 hours), possibly because the main factor driving the response, estrogen, declines in concentration as the follicles respond to the preovulatory gonadotropin surge. This particular physiologic mechanism for initiating the onset of ovulation is effective, because the follicle is able to signal its stage of maturity to the hypothalamus and adenohypophysis by a product (estrogen) that is produced in increasing amounts with increasing follicle maturity.

The secretion of gonadotropins is modified by the ovarian steroid hormones *estrogen* and *progesterone*. With time, the effect of these hormones is suppressive for gonadotropin secretion. Estrogens, in particular, cause *negative feedback inhibition* of gonadotropin secretion, which is characterized by its sensitivity (effective at low concentrations) and its rapid onset (within a few hours). The substantial increase in gonadotropin concentrations that occurs after ovariectomy is caused largely by the removal of estrogens.

Because progesterone affects gonadotropin pulse frequency, it is thought that its modulatory effect is at the level of the hypothalamus. Estrogens are thought to affect gonadotropin secretion through an effect on both the pituitary gland and the hypothalamus. Although there are differences in the site of action among species, it appears that the hypothalamic site for negative feedback inhibition of gonado-

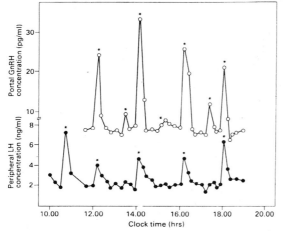

FIGURE 34–4. Concentrations of gonadotropin-releasing hormone (GnRH) in portal plasma *(open circles)* and luteinizing hormone (LH) in jugular venous plasma *(solid circles)* of four ovariectomized ewes. *Asterisks* indicate secretory episodes (pulses) of GnRH and LH. (From Johnson M, Everitt B [eds]: Essential Reproduction, 3rd ed. London: Blackwell Scientific, 1988, p 110.)

tropins by both progesterone and estrogen is in an area immediately above the median eminence, known as the *arcuate nucleus.* The hypothalamic site for positive feedback stimulation of gonadotropin release by estrogen is probably further anterior—that is, in the preoptic anterior hypothalamic region.

The secretion of gonadotropins can be modified by peptide and protein hormones produced by both the hypothalamus and ovary. β-Endorphin, an opioid peptide produced from the hypothalamic precursor molecule pro-opiomelanocortin, can inhibit LH secretion when pharmacologically administered systemically. Its role in the physiologic modulation of gonadotropin secretion, however, remains to be identified. Another hormone, inhibin, a protein produced by the granulosa cells of the developing follicle, also inhibits gonadotropin secretion, particularly FSH, during the final stages of follicle development. As described in the section on folliculogenesis, this depression of FSH secretion may be important to the animal for controlling the number of follicles that are brought to final maturation.

Control of gonadotropin secretion in the male is similar to that in the female; pulses of GnRH, arising in the hypothalamus, affect pulsatile secretion of the gonadotropins. This, in turn, causes the secretion of testosterone, also in pulsatile form, from the testes. One major difference between the sexes is that the need for positive feedback release of gonadotropins in males does not exist; gametes are produced and released on a continuous basis within a tubular system that opens to the exterior. This negates any need for a surge release of gonadotropins, as is required in the female to rupture the ovarian surface for the release of oocytes.

Prolactin is the third adenohypophysis-produced hormone that is important in the reproductive process, mainly because of its effect on the mammary gland and lactation in mammals. Although the secretion of prolactin is pulsatile, the control of secretion has more emphasis on inhibition than does stimulation of secretion. This concept is supported by the finding that prolactin secretion increases if the pituitary gland is disconnected from the hypothalamus by either cutting the pituitary stalk or transplanting the pituitary gland to another site (e.g., kidney capsule). Thus, most attention has been given to factors that inhibit prolactin secretion. The catecholamine *dopamine,* which is produced by neurons in the ventral hypothalamus (arcuate nucleus), is a potent inhibitor of prolactin secretion (Fig. 34–6). Other factors that inhibit prolactin secretion are γ-aminobutyric acid (GABA) and GAP. Dopamine agonists, such as the ergot-type compound *bromocriptine,* can be used to suppress prolactin secretion in cases of *hyperprolactinemia.* Cabergoline, a potent prolactin inhibitor, can be used to shorten interestrous intervals in female dogs and cause luteolysis in female dogs and female cats during the latter half of pregnancy. The negative feedback control of prolactin is shown in Figure 34–6.

One of the first known prolactin-releasing factors was thyrotropin-releasing hormone (TRH). The physi-

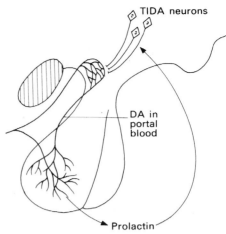

FIGURE 34–6. Diagrammatic summary of the proposed negative feedback relationship between prolactin and dopamine (DA). Prolactin is believed to accelerate dopamine turnover in the arcuate nucleus neurons (tuberoinfundibular dopamine [TIDA] neurons), and the amine is then released into the portal capillaries to gain access to the lactotropes. Hyperprolactinemia could be caused by either a failure of prolactin inhibitory factor activity at the dopamine receptor level in the anterior pituitary or a reduction of TIDA neuron activity in the hypothalamus. (From Johnson M, Everitt B [eds]: Essential Reproduction, 3rd ed. London: Blackwell Scientific, 1988, p 138.)

ologic relevance of TRH in prolactin secretion is still unknown in spite of the fact that receptors for TRH have been identified on lactotropes within the adenohypophysis. *Vasoactive intestinal peptide* (VIP), a potent stimulator of prolactin secretion, may play a physiologic role in prolactin secretion through inhibition of dopamine synthesis within the hypothalamus. Estrogens can increase prolactin secretion by lactotropes by decreasing lactotrope sensitivity to dopamine and increasing the number of TRH receptors. Of interest is that female dogs undergoing ovariohysterectomy with a cesarean section usually maintain the ability to lactate effectively afterward.

OVARIAN FOLLICLE DEVELOPMENT

Gamete development occurs initially without gonadotropin support and subsequently with pulsatile gonadotropin secretion

Oocyte proliferation, which occurs by *mitotic division* during fetal development, ends at about the time of birth in most mammalian species. Oocytes begin the process of reduction of chromosome numbers to the haploid state by *meiosis* shortly after birth under the influence of *meiosis-initiating factor,* thought to be produced by the *rete ovarii.* The process is soon interrupted at *the diplotene,* or *dictyate,* stage of meiosis I by the meiosis-inhibiting factor, which is probably produced by the developing follicle cells. Oocytes remain in this stage until the follicle begins its final development, an interval that can be as long as 50 years or more in humans. The *follicle,* at this point, is delineated by an outer basement membrane *(membrana propria),* which is secreted by the follicle cells.

The initial development of the follicle involves growth of the oocyte. This growth is accompanied by intense synthetic activity; a large amount of RNA is synthesized. At the same time, follicle cells begin to divide and form a granulosa that is several cells thick. The granulosa cells then secrete another boundary substance, the zona pellucida, that lies within the granulosa and that immediately surrounds the oocyte. Granulosa cells maintain contact with the oocyte through the zona pellucida by means of the development of cytoplasmic processes. Interaction among granulosa cells is facilitated by the development of gap junctions. This form of communication is important, because the granulosa is without blood supply; blood vessels are excluded at the level of the membrana propria. The thecal layer of the follicle forms around the membrana propria to complete the layers of the follicle. Follicles at this stage are called *primary,* or *preantral, follicles.*

Factors that control initial follicle growth are not known. External factors, such as gonadotropins, are not required, because preantral follicles can develop in hypophysectomized animals. In species such as cattle and horses (perhaps sheep and goats, also) in which several dominant follicles develop during the estrous cycle, it is likely that a few follicles begin to develop each day. In animals in which a cohort of follicles develops synchronously (pigs, cats, dogs), there appears to be less of a tendency to have competing follicle growth waves during the luteal phase (pig) and a tendency to have only one cohort of follicles during the preovulatory period (cat and dog). Thus, the development of a cohort of follicles may limit follicle development from the primordial state, at least during the period of active follicle development leading to ovulation. It is obvious that initial follicle growth is under genetic control, and the pattern reflects the needs of the particular species.

In the preantral follicle, gonadotropin receptors for luteinizing hormone develop on the theca, which results in androgen synthesis; follicle-stimulating hormone direction of the granulosa causes it to transform the androgens to estrogens

In order for follicles to progress beyond the preantral stage, the granulosa and theca need to develop *receptors* for gonadotropins. FSH and LH receptors develop on the granulosa and theca, respectively. The onset of the antral follicle is marked by the appearance of fluid that begins to divide the granulosa. The follicular fluid, a secretory product of the granulosa, coalesces to form an increasingly larger fluid cavity *(antrum)* within the granulosa. In later development of the antral follicle, the oocyte remains surrounded by a layer of granulosa cells called the *cumulus oooph-*

orus, which are attached to the wall of the follicle by a small stalk of granulosa cells.

The proximity of the granulosa and theca cells allows cooperative estrogen synthesis. The *theca* produces *androgens* (testosterone and androstenedione) under the influence of LH, which diffuses across the membrana propria into the *granulosa,* where the androgens are transformed into *estrogen* (estradiol-17). At this time of development, the granulosa is incapable of forming androgens, the precursors of estrogen biosynthesis, and the theca has limited capacity for producing estrogens. This concept of cooperative effort, called the *two-cell mechanism* for estrogen secretion, is generally accepted as being the way most follicular estrogen is produced. These estrogens have a positive feedback effect upon the granulosa; they stimulate the cells to undergo mitotic division, and thus the follicle grows in size as the granulosa proliferates in response to its own secretory product (estrogen).

One effect of estrogen is the formation of additional receptors for FSH as follicle development proceeds. In this situation, the antral follicle becomes increasingly sensitive to FSH as it develops and is able to grow under a relatively steady state of FSH secretion.

Late in the ovarian follicular phase, luteinizing hormone receptors develop on the granulosa, which permits the preovulatory surge of luteinizing hormone to cause ovulation

Late in antral follicle development, FSH and estrogens initiate the formation of LH receptors on the granulosa, whereas FSH receptors begin to diminish. Increasing secretion of estrogen by the antral follicle finally results in the initiation of the *preovulatory surge of gonadotropins.* Thus, in the last stages of development, the follicle falls progressively under the control of LH as it makes its last growth spurt to the point of ovulation.

CLINICAL CORRELATIONS

Androgen insensitivity

History   You are called to examine a mare that has recently been brought to a brood mare farm after a successful racing career. It is late spring, yet the mare has shown estrous behavior only on an intermittent basis.

Clinical examination   As you approach the mare you notice that she is large. The genital examination reveals a normal vulva, but when you introduce the speculum it can be inserted only about 5 to 6 inches. Digital examination of the genital tract through the vulva results in a finding of complete blockage at the level of the vestibulovaginal conjunction with no evidence for the presence of the external os of the cervix. Upon doing an examination per rectum, you find the vagina, cervix, uterus, and oviducts to be absent; the gonads are symmetric in shape without the usual indentation caused by the ovulation fossa that is characteristic of equine ovaries.

Comment You tell the shocked owner that you are suspicious that the animal is not, in fact, a mare, but a male masquerading as a female. One of the easiest ways to confirm the diagnosis is to have a testosterone analysis done on plasma. If the gonads are testes, they still retain the ability to secrete significant amounts of testosterone even though they are retained (cryptorchid, in a sense) within the abdominal cavity. You could also have a chromosomal analysis to verify that the animal has an XY sex chromosome complement. In this case, it is likely that the testes were able to secrete the *müllerian-inhibiting factor*, which resulted in regression of the tubular system of the genital tract that forms the female system (i.e., oviducts, uterus, cervix, and vagina). But why, asks the owner, did the external genitalia not turn out to be male? There is evidence, in cases such as this, that the tissues of the external genitalia lacked critical receptors for androgens; thus, the external genitalia were female in type. The rule of sexual development is that the female state develops in the absence of testicular input, the latter including müllerian-inhibiting factor and testosterone. In this case, the lack of sexual differentiation also appeared to involve the hypothalamus, because the "mare" did not exhibit male behavior in spite of relatively high testosterone concentrations.

Treatment There is obviously no treatment for this syndrome. It would be unethical to take her back to the track and race her once again as a female, when the owner knows that "she" is a male.

Bibliography

Austin CR, Short RV (eds): Reproduction in Mammals, vols 1–6. Cambridge, United Kingdom: Cambridge University Press, 1986.

Cain JL, Lasley GR, Cain GR, et al: Induction of ovulation in bitches with pulsatile or continuous infusion of GnRH. J Reprod Fertil Suppl 39:143–147, 1989.

Concannon PW, Morton DB, Weir BJ (eds): Dog and cat reproduction, contraception and artificial insemination. J Reprod Fertil Suppl Vol 39, 1989.

Cupps PT (ed): Reproduction in Domestic Animals, 4th ed. New York: Academic Press, 1991.

Feldman EC, Nelson RW: Canine and Feline Endocrinology and Reproduction. Philadelphia: WB Saunders, 1996.

Hafez EWE (ed): Reproduction in Farm Animals, 5th ed. Philadelphia: Lea & Febiger, 1987.

Jochle W, Arbeiter K, Post R, et al: Effects on pseudopregnancy, pregnancy and interoestrous intervals of pharmacological suppression of prolactin secretion in female dogs and cats. J Reprod Fertil Suppl 39:199–207, 1989.

Johnson M, Everitt B (eds): Essential Reproduction, 3rd ed. London: Blackwell Scientific, 1988.

Knobil E, Neill JD, Ewing LL, et al (eds): The Physiology of Reproduction, vols 1, 2. New York: Raven Press, 1988.

McDonald LE, Pineda MH (eds): Veterinary Endocrinology and Reproduction, 4th ed. Philadelphia: Lea & Febiger, 1989.

PRACTICE QUESTIONS

1. Which of the following statements is true?
   a. Müllerian ducts develop in the female because of the presence of estrogen.
   b. Müllerian ducts develop in the female because of a müllerian-stimulating factor.
   c. Wolffian ducts develop in the male because of a wolffian-stimulating factor.
   d. Wolffian ducts develop in the male because of the presence of androgen.

2. The most potent factor involved in the organization of the internal and external parts of the genital tract is
   a. müllerian-inhibiting factor.
   b. müllerian-stimulating factor.
   c. estrogen.
   d. androgen.

3. Which of the following groups of hormones is transported to the anterior pituitary by the hypothalamohypophyseal portal system?
   a. Oxytocin, GnRH, and dopamine.
   b. GnRH, dopamine, and vasopressin.
   c. Dopamine, vasopressin, and oxytocin.
   d. Dopamine and GnRH.

4. Which of the following groups of hormones controls the synthesis and release of hypophyseal hormones involved in reproductive processes?
   a. Oxytocin, GnRH, VIP, and dopamine.
   b. GnRH, dopamine, VIP, and vasopressin.
   c. Dopamine, vasopressin, VIP, and oxytocin.
   d. GAP, dopamine, VIP, and GnRH.
   e. GAP, GnRH, VIP, and oxytocin.

5. Which of the following factors is responsible for causing oocytes to remain in a diplotene or dictyate state?
   a. Müllerian-inhibiting factor.
   b. Müllerian-stimulating factor.
   c. Meiosis-inhibiting factor.
   d. Meiosis-stimulating factor.
   e. Wolffian-inhibiting factor.
   f. Wolffian-stimulating factor.

PRACTICE ANSWERS

1. d   2. d   3. d   4. c   5. c

Control of ovulation and the corpus luteum

Ovulation

1 Ovulatory follicles are selected at the onset of luteolysis (large domestic animals)

2 Ovulation is caused by an estrogen-induced pre-ovulatory surge of gonadotropins

Corpus luteum

1 The corpus luteum secretes progesterone, which is essential for pregnancy

2 Luteinizing hormone is important for the maintenance of the corpus luteum

3 Regression of the corpus luteum in nonpregnant large domestic animals is controlled by uterine secretion of prostaglandin $F_{2\alpha}$

4 Changes in luteal life span in large domestic animals occur because of changes in prostaglandin $F_{2\alpha}$ synthesis by the uterus

Ovarian cycles

1 In spontaneously ovulating animals, ovarian cycles have two phases: follicular and luteal; animals that require copulation for ovulation can have only a follicular phase

2 The luteal phase is modified by copulation in some species

▬ OVULATION

▬ Ovulatory follicles are selected at the onset of luteolysis (large domestic animals)

Until the advent of ultrasonography, it was difficult to identify growth patterns of follicles in domestic animals, especially those of follicles that develop during the luteal phase of the cycle. With ultrasonography, it has been possible to define follicular growth and regression during the luteal phase of the cycle in the cow and mare. In cattle, the predominant pattern is for several dominant (large) antral follicles to develop sequentially during the cycle (Fig. 35–1). The follicular cycles are distinct to the extent that follicle regression usually begins (as indicated by follicle size) before the onset of the growth of the next follicle. The first dominant follicle regresses approximately in the middle of the luteal phase, and a second dominant follicle begins growth immediately. Whether the second dominant follicle is the ovulatory follicle, or whether a third develops, depends on the stage of the follicle at the time of regression of the *corpus luteum* (CL). If the second dominant follicle has begun to regress at the time of CL regression, a third follicle develops. Thus, the selected ovulatory follicle is, by chance, the dominant follicle that is still in a developmental stage when regression of the CL is initiated.

The duration required for the development of the antral follicle to the point of ovulation has been estimated by various techniques to be about 10 days in domestic animals and perhaps slightly longer in some primates.

From ultrasonographic and endocrinologic studies, it appears that there are two different phases in final antral follicle development in large domestic animals: a relatively slow one that lasts for 4 to 5 days, followed by a second phase of accelerated growth, again lasting 4 to 5 days, that terminates in ovulation (Fig. 35–2). Because the final growth phase of follicle development can be initiated during the luteal phase, it is apparent that the initiation of this phase can occur under the influence of a relatively slow pulse rate of gonadotropin release that occurs during the luteal phase. The rapidly growing follicle requires exposure to a faster gonadotropin pulse rate by the third or fourth day in order for one or more follicles to complete the normal growth pattern through ovulation. This situation usually occurs in conjunction with the onset of CL regression, which passively allows an increase in pulsatile rate of gonadotropin secretion (see Fig. 34–4).

One of the ways in which the dominant follicle maintains its status is to produce substances that inhibit the development of other antral follicles. One of the substances is *inhibin*, a peptide hormone produced by the granulosa, which inhibits the secretion of folli-

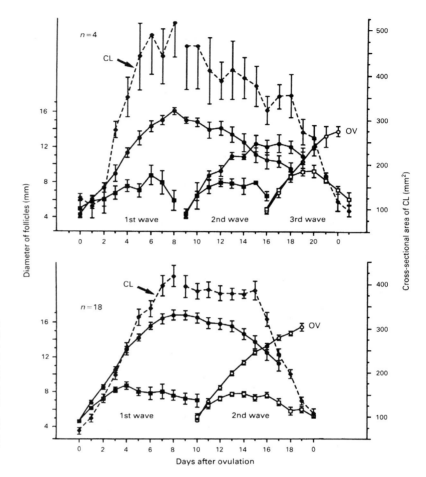

FIGURE 35-1. Mean (± standard error of the mean) profiles of diameters of dominant follicles and the largest subordinate follicle and the cross-sectional luteinized area of the corpus luteum (CL) for the interovulatory intervals with three and two follicular waves in cattle. Regression (P < 0.05) of the corpus luteum began between days 18 and 20 for three-wave intervals and between days 15 and 16 for two-wave intervals. OV, ovulation. (From Ginther OJ, Knopf L, Kastelic JP: Temporal associations among ovarian events in cattle during oestrous cycles with two and three follicular waves. J Reprod Fertil 87:223, 1989.)

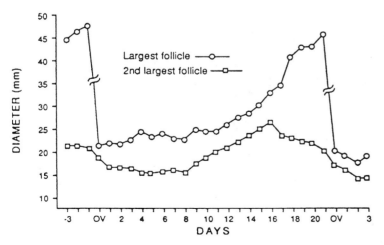

FIGURE 35-2. Development of the dominant and second largest follicle during the estrous cycle of the mare. Note the divergence in diameter between the largest and second-largest follicles 1 day after ovulation. (From Pierson RA, Ginther OJ: Follicular population dynamics during the estrous cycle of the mare. Anim Reprod Sci 14:219, 1987.)

cle-stimulating hormone (FSH). The dominant follicle is able to compensate for the lower FSH concentrations and continue to grow because of the numbers of FSH receptors it has in comparison with competitor follicles. Follicle development is dynamic once the rapid growth phase is achieved; the follicle must be acted upon through proper gonadotropin stimulation within a few days, or the result is death of the follicle. If the rapidly growing antral follicle is not exposed to the proper gonadotropin environment, *atresia* (regression) of the follicle begins almost immediately. Follicles that regress are invaded by inflammatory cells, and the area previously occupied by the antral follicle is eventually filled by connective tissue; that is, the follicle is replaced by an ovarian scar.

Ovulation is caused by an estrogen-induced preovulatory surge of gonadotropins

The preovulatory surge of luteinizing hormone (LH), which begins about 24 hours before ovulation in most domestic species (including the cow, dog, goat, pig, and sheep), initiates the critical changes in the follicle that affect its endocrine organ status and result in release of the oocyte (Fig. 35–3). Two important cells, the oocyte and the granulosa cells, have been kept under control by the production of inhibitory substances that are probably of granulosa origin. One is an *oocyte-inhibiting factor*, which prevents the oocyte from resuming meiosis, and another is a *luteinizing-inhibiting factor*, which prevents the granulosa from being changed prematurely into luteal tissue. The impact of the LH surge blocks the production of both these factors. In most animals, the resumption of meiosis results in the first division of meiosis (meiosis I), or formation of the *first polar body*, which is complete before ovulation. In animals with the potential for relatively long reproductivity (e.g., cattle), the initiation of the meiotic process could begin as long as 10 or more years before its completion.

The effect of the LH surge on the granulosa is to allow the initiation of the process of luteinization, one that transforms the cells from estrogen to progesterone secretion. This process is under way before ovulation occurs. With the advent of the LH surge, estrogen secretion declines concomitantly with the onset of progesterone secretion.

Another function of the preovulatory surge release of LH is to cause the granulosa to produce substances, such as *relaxin* and *prostaglandin* $F_{2\alpha}$ ($PGF_{2\alpha}$), that affect the continuity of the connective tissue of the thecal layers of the follicle. These and other unknown substances disrupt the theca through the development of vesicles (within fibrocytes) that contain hydrolytic enzymes capable of breaking down the collagen matrix of connective tissue; the rupture of the follicle results from the disintegration of the connective tissue.

In summary, estrogen is used by the follicles (1) to stimulate the growth and development of the granu-

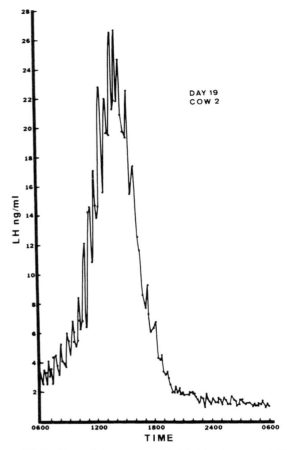

FIGURE 35–3. Preovulatory surge of luteinizing hormone (LH) on day 19 of the estrous cycle in a cow. (From Rahe CH, Owens RE, Fleeger JL, et al: Pattern of plasma luteinizing hormone in the cyclic cow: Dependence upon the period of the cycle. Endocrinology 107:498, 1980.)

losa and (2) to signal the hypothalamus and anterior pituitary gland as to the readiness of the follicles for ovulation.

CORPUS LUTEUM

The corpus luteum secretes progesterone, which is essential for pregnancy

The main function of the CL is the secretion of progesterone, which prepares the uterus for the initiation and maintenance of pregnancy.

The CL forms from the wall of the follicle, which is collapsed and folded after ovulation. With rupture of the follicle, there is a breakdown of the tissues that surround the granulosa, particularly the membrana propria, and vessels in the theca can hemorrhage into the cavity. The folds of tissue that protrude inward into the cavity contain granulosa and theca cells and, very important, the blood vascular system that will support cell growth and differentiation. Although the granulosa cell is the dominant cell of the CL, theca cells also contribute significantly to the composition of the structure. The process that granulosa cells undergo during the change from estrogen to progesterone secretion, *luteinization,* begins with the onset of the preovulatory LH surge and accelerates with ovulation.

In most domestic species, significant production of progesterone by the CL begins within 24 hours of ovulation. In some species, including the dog and primates, small amounts of progesterone are produced during the preovulatory LH surge; in the dog, this is important for the expression of sexual receptivity, which occurs as estrogen levels decline while progesterone levels increase.

Luteinizing hormone is important for the maintenance of the corpus luteum

For most domestic animals, LH is the important *luteotropin;* the CL is maintained in either nonpregnant or pregnant animals by a relatively slow pulsatile pattern of LH release (one pulse per 2 to 3 hours). In rodents, prolactin is the important luteotropin; daily biphasic release of prolactin is initiated by copulation, which is essential for the maintenance of the CL. Of the domestic species, prolactin has been implicated as a luteotropin in sheep and dogs.

Normal folliculogenesis, a prerequisite for ovulation, sets the stage for the subsequent development of the postovulatory CL. Thus, more clinical attention is paid to factors controlling the regression of the CL than to luteotropic factors.

Regression of the corpus luteum in nonpregnant large domestic animals is controlled by uterine secretion of prostaglandin F$_{2\alpha}$

Regression of the CL is important in large domestic nonpregnant animals in order that the animals reenter a potentially fertile state as soon as possible. The CL's life span after ovulation must be of sufficient duration to allow a newly developing conceptus to synthesize and release factors that allow the CL to be maintained; however, it must be relatively short so that a nonpregnant animal can return to a potentially fertile state. In large domestic animals, the duration of the luteal phase is about 14 days in the absence of pregnancy. This allows large domestic animals to complete cycles at relatively frequent intervals (i.e., approximately every 3 weeks).

Leo Loeb first showed (in 1923) the importance of the uterus for the regression of the CL through hysterectomy studies that extended the luteal phase in guinea pigs. He concluded that the uterus must produce a substance that terminated luteal activity. This information lay dormant for many years until hysterectomy studies in cattle, pigs, and sheep in the 1950s produced similar results: that is, a prolongation of the luteal phase of the estrous cycle. Through these

studies, there developed the concept that the uterus is responsible for control of the duration of the life span of the CL, at least in large domestic species (and guinea pigs).

It is now accepted that PGF$_{2\alpha}$, a 20-carbon unsaturated fatty acid, is the uterine substance that causes regression of the CL in large domestic animals, including cattle, goats, horses, pigs, and sheep; PGF$_{2\alpha}$ has no known natural role in CL regression in cats and dogs or in primates. PGF$_{2\alpha}$ and prostaglandin E therapy has been used clinically to cause luteolysis in the bitch and queen, for the treatment of pyometra, or to induce abortion. In large domestic species, regression of the CL is initiated by uterine synthesis and release of PGF$_{2\alpha}$ (likely of endometrial origin) at about 14 days after ovulation. The mode of transfer of PGF$_{2\alpha}$ from the uterus to the ovary is thought to occur by either *local countercurrent transfer* or *general systemic transfer.* Countercurrent transfer involves the movement of molecules across the blood vascular system from higher concentrations in the venous effluent (utero-ovarian vein) to an area of lower concentration (ovarian artery) (Fig. 35–4). Systemic transfer involves passage of the molecules through the general circulatory system. In some species (cow and ewe), PGF$_{2\alpha}$ synthesis from a uterine horn influences the life span of the CL only in the ipsilateral ovary. In other species (sow and perhaps mare), PGF$_{2\alpha}$ synthesis from one horn is sufficient to cause regression of CL in both ovaries. This effect probably occurs because of greater production of PGF$_{2\alpha}$ by uterine tissue, as well as a difference in the rate of metabolism of PGF$_{2\alpha}$. PGF$_{2\alpha}$ is rapidly metabolized systemically; more than 90% is changed by one passage through the lungs. Thus, the system involving the use of PGF$_{2\alpha}$ as the luteolytic agent in large domestic species requires that PGF$_{2\alpha}$ be conserved through a special

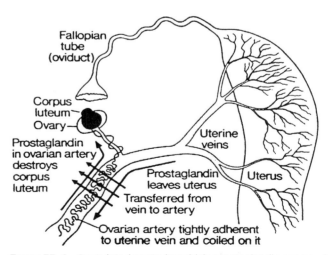

FIGURE 35–4. Postulated route by which prostaglandin secreted by the progesterone-primed uterus is able to enter the ovarian artery and destroy the corpus luteum in sheep. (From Baird DT: The ovary. In Austin CR, Short RV [eds]: Hormonal Control of Reproduction. Reproduction in Mammals, vol 3. Cambridge, United Kingdom: Cambridge University Press, 1984.)

transfer system or that it be produced in relatively large amounts.

The pattern of synthesis and release of $PGF_{2\alpha}$ is essential to its luteolytic effect. For example, $PGF_{2\alpha}$ synthesis and release must be pulsatile, whereby pulses occur at about 6-hour intervals, in order for luteolysis to be affected (Fig. 35–5). There has developed the concept that a minimum of four to five pulses within 24 hours is necessary to effect complete luteolysis. If pulse intervals increase significantly before complete luteolysis (e.g., to 12 hours), the CL can recover and continue to function, even if at a lower level of steroid synthetic activity. The uterus must be exposed to estrogen and progesterone in order to synthesize and release $PGF_{2\alpha}$. Although the initiation of $PGF_{2\alpha}$ synthesis that leads to luteolysis is not completely understood, one possible explanation is that estrogen (from an antral follicle) causes the initial synthesis and release of $PGF_{2\alpha}$. In sheep, it is thought that an interplay occurs between the uterus and ovary after the initial $PGF_{2\alpha}$ pulse. $PGF_{2\alpha}$ affects the CL to cause both a reduction in progesterone production and the release of *luteal oxytocin.* Oxytocin then interacts with receptors within the uterus to initiate an-

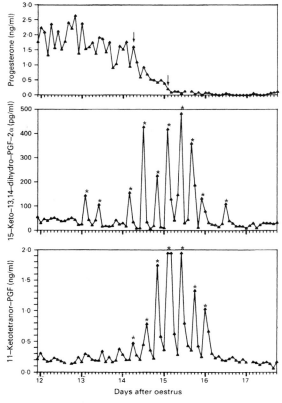

FIGURE 35–5. Concentrations of progesterone, 15-keto-13,14-dihydro-$PGF_{2\alpha}$, and 11-ketotetranor-PGF metabolites in a nonpregnant ewe. Values identified as significant pulses of either $PGF_{2\alpha}$ metabolite are indicated by an *asterisk.* The times of initiation and completion of functional luteolysis are indicated by *arrows.* PGF, prostaglandin F. (From Zarco L, Stabenfeldt GH, Basu S, et al: Modification of prostaglandin $PGF_{2\alpha}$ synthesis and release in the ewe during the initial establishment of pregnancy. J Reprod Fertil 83:527, 1988.)

other round of $PGF_{2\alpha}$ synthesis. $PGF_{2\alpha}$ synthesis ceases within 6 to 12 hours after progesterone concentrations have become basal—that is, with the completion of luteolysis. A system for early reinitiation of the cycle is not present in nonpregnant dogs and cats in terms of regression of CLs; the luteal phases are about 70 and 35 days, respectively. Bitches experiencing infertility as a result of frequent estrous cycles may have pathologically shortened diestrus or anestrus.

Changes in luteal life span in large domestic animals occur because of changes in prostaglandin $F_{2\alpha}$ synthesis by the uterus

Significant changes in the length of the life span of the CL in nonpregnant large domestic species occur only because of changes within the uterus. As discussed in Chapter 37, the presence of an embryo results in the blockage of $PGF_{2\alpha}$ synthesis and a continuance in luteal activity. Luteal phases are also commonly prolonged in mares in the absence of uterine infection. This deficit in $PGF_{2\alpha}$ in mares appears to be caused by a genetic propensity toward inadequate synthesis and release. The absence of a uterine horn can result also in a lengthened luteal phase in animals in which the ipsilateral horn controls the CL (local control). In this situation (e.g., in the cow), if ovulation occurs in the ovary ipsilateral to the missing horn, the luteal phase is prolonged because of the necessity of the ipsilateral uterine horn for controlling the life span of the CL.

In nonpregnant large domestic animals, inflammatory responses of the endometrium resulting from bacterial contamination can result in significant synthesis and release of $PGF_{2\alpha}$, leading to premature luteolysis and a shortening of the estrous cycle. It should be emphasized that luteal activity is almost always normal in the absence of uterine abnormality in large domestic species. Thus, short estrous cycles in large domestic animals are pathognomonic for uterine infection.

OVARIAN CYCLES

In spontaneously ovulating animals, ovarian cycles have two phases: follicular and luteal; animals that require copulation for ovulation can have only a follicular phase

An *ovarian cycle* in a nonpregnant animal is defined as the interval between successive ovulations. The cycle is composed of two phases: an initial *follicular phase* and a subsequent *luteal phase;* ovulation separates the phases. In most domestic animals and primates, the ovulatory process is governed by internal mechanisms; estrogen from the antral follicle initiates the ovulatory release of gonadotropins. These animals are called *spontaneous* ovulators.

There are fundamental differences between animals with regard to the relationship of the follicular and luteal phases of the cycle. In higher primates, there is complete separation of follicular and luteal phases; no significant follicle growth occurs until luteolysis is complete. In large domestic animals, significant follicle growth does occur during the luteal phase of the cycle. For example, in the cow, a large antral follicle is present at the time of the onset of luteolysis, and in the mare, follicle growth can even result in ovulation of follicles during the luteal phase (about 5% of cycles). Thus, in large domestic animals, much of the follicle growth extends into the luteal phase. This situation results in shorter cycles in large domestic animals than in primates (17 to 21 days vs. 28 days); the interval of luteolysis to ovulation is shorter in large domestic animals (5 to 10 days) than in primates (12 to 13 days). The period of antral follicle growth leading to ovulation is, however, not appreciably different; the final progression of antral follicle growth requires about 10 days in large domestic animals and about 12 to 13 days in primates.

Animals that require copulation for ovulation are known as *induced ovulators*. They include cats, rabbits, ferrets, mink, camels, llamas, and alpacas. Copulation replaces estrogen as the stimulus that induces the ovulatory release of gonadotropins. However, these animals require exposure to elevated estrogen concentrations before they can respond to copulation by the release of gonadotropins.

Induced ovulators have follicle growth patterns (in the absence of coitus) in which cohorts of follicles develop, are maintained in a mature state for a few days, and then regress. Follicle growth patterns can be distinctly separated, as in the cat, wherein follicles develop and regress over a 6- to 7-day period, with a minimum of 8 to 9 days between follicle growth waves. Follicle waves can also have some overlap, as in llamas and alpacas (Fig. 35–6), or can closely overlap, as in the rabbit.

The luteal phase is modified by copulation in some species

In rodent species, the luteal phase of the ovarian cycle is extended by copulation. The life span of the CL is only 1 to 2 days in the absence of copulation. Copulation initiates the release of prolactin, which results in prolongation of luteal activity for up to 10 to 11 days in the absence of pregnancy. This phenomenon is often called *pseudopregnancy*. In the canine, spontaneous regression of the CL, marking the end of diestrus, occurs in association with increased levels of prolactin, causing clinical pseudopregnancy. Nonpregnant bitches can nest, lactate, and nurture objects during this time.

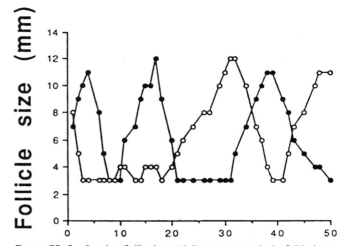

FIGURE 35–6. Ovarian follicular activity over a period of 50 days in a llama, indicating follicle growth alternating between the left *(open circles)* and right *(solid circles)* ovaries. (From Bravo PW, Fowler ME, Stabenfeldt GH, et al: Ovarian follicular dynamics in the llama. Biol Reprod 43:579, 1990.)

CLINICAL CORRELATIONS

Persistent luteal phase in the mare

History You have been called to examine a mare that foaled this spring but was not bred at the foal "heat" because of a retained placenta. It has been 40 days since the foal "heat," and the owner wants to know why the mare has not returned to estrus.

Clinical examination The main clinical findings are a cervix that is found (through speculum examination) to be relatively small and tightly constricted and (through palpation per rectum) to have considerable tone. Rectal palpation also reveals a uterus that has considerable tone. The ovaries are normal in size; in fact, one ovary has a 35-mm follicle. This prompts you to ask the owner whether the mare has been vigorously teased by a stallion for the detection of estrus. The owner brings the teasing stallion to the mare to demonstrate the farm's teasing technique, and, as predicted, the mare vigorously rejects the stallion.

Comment A history of a mare that has been previously in estrus and has not returned to estrus within 30 days usually indicates the presence of a persistent CL. The CL persists because of inadequate PGF$_{2\alpha}$ synthesis and release, which normally occurs approximately 14 days after ovulation and causes regression of the CL in the absence of pregnancy. The incidence of the syndrome is perhaps as high as 15% to 20%. The CL can remain active for as long as 3 months before the mare is able to synthesize and release PGF$_{2\alpha}$ in amounts sufficient to cause regression of the CL. It is difficult to palpate a persistent CL per rectum because it tends to shrink into the interior of the ovary. The structure may be visualized by ultrasonography, but this is not always possible. The appearance of the cervix and the tone of the cervix and uterus suggest that the genital tubular system is under the influence of progesterone; these findings, together with the history, support a tentative diagnosis. A tentative diagnosis can also be made if the mare returns to estrus within a few days after the administration of PGF$_{2\alpha}$. A definitive diagnosis can be made by progesterone analysis of blood; values are often 1 to 2 ng/mL in this syndrome, in contrast to 3 ng/mL or more in mares with normal estrous cycle CLs.

The clinical finding that can be confusing in this syndrome is the presence of a large follicle in the absence of estrus. Ovarian follicles develop in this syndrome, and sometimes ovulation even occurs. However, mares do not show sexual receptivity in the presence of large follicles if luteal-phase concentrations of progesterone are present. One possibility that should be considered in a differential diagnosis is that ovarian activity has stopped (i.e., the mare has become anestrous). Although this does not occur often in foaling mares, mares that foal early can be deleteriously affected by the relatively short photoperiod that is present. In this case, the clinical signs do not support the diagnosis of anestrus.

Treatment The administration of PGF$_{2\alpha}$, or one of its analogues, usually initiates regression of the persistent CL and results in the appearance of estrus within a few days. The early return to estrus is based on the fact that ovarian follicles tend to develop on a continuous basis throughout the persistent luteal-phase syndrome. Regression of the CL allows the current dominant follicle to continue to develop and produce estrogen, which brings the mare into estrus. One caveat: If a large follicle, e.g., 40 to 45 mm, is present at the time of treatment, the follicle may ovulate before the mare manifests estrus, and the treatment will be judged as failing. In this case, the animal needs to be monitored daily; if ovulation occurs within a few days of treatment, the animal may need to be inseminated artificially if breed rules allow.

Bibliography

Austin CR, Short RV (eds): Reproduction in Mammals, vols 1–6. Cambridge, United Kingdom: Cambridge University Press, 1986.
Concannon PW, Morton DB, Weir BJ (eds): Dog and cat reproduction, contraception and artificial insemination. J Reprod Fertil Suppl vol 39, 1989.
Cupps PT (ed): Reproduction in Domestic Animals, 4th ed. New York: Academic Press, 1991.
Feldman EC, Nelson RW (eds): Canine and Feline Endocrinology and Reproduction. Philadelphia: WB Saunders, 1996.
Hafez EWE (ed): Reproduction in Farm Animals, 5th ed. Philadelphia: Lea & Febiger, 1987.
Johnson M, Everitt B (eds): Essential Reproduction, 3rd ed. London: Blackwell Scientific, 1988.
Knobil E, Neill JD, Ewing LL, et al (eds): The Physiology of Reproduction, vols 1, 2. New York: Raven Press, 1988.
McDonald LE, Pineda MH (eds): Veterinary Endocrinology and Reproduction, 4th ed. Philadelphia: Lea & Febiger, 1989.

PRACTICE QUESTIONS

1. The main hormone secreted by the dominant follicle that allows the follicle to maintain its dominant state is
    a. estrogen.
    b. inhibin.
    c. oocyte inhibiting factor.
    d. progesterone.

2. The factor that is most important in determining whether a luteal-phase dominant follicle will go on to ovulation is
    a. inadequate pituitary stimulation.
    b. regression of the CL.
    c. atresia of the follicle.

3. The initiation of the preovulatory LH surge that leads to ovulation in spontaneous ovulators results from
    a. estrogen.
    b. inhibin.
    c. progesterone.
    d. FSH.
    e. prolactin.

4. The substance responsible for the regression of the CL in large domestic animals is
    a. estrogen.
    b. inhibin.
    c. oxytocin.
    d. prolactin.
    e. PGF$_{2\alpha}$.

5. Ovarian follicle patterns in animals that are induced ovulators—that is, those that require copulation for the induction of ovulation—are as follows:
    a. Ovarian follicle waves greatly overlap.
    b. Ovarian follicle waves slightly overlap.
    c. Ovarian follicle waves are distinctly separated.
    d. All of the above.

PRACTICE ANSWERS

1. b   2. c   3. a   4. e   5. d

36

Reproductive cycles

Reproductive cycles

1 The two types of reproductive cycles are estrous and menstrual

Puberty and reproductive senescence

1 Puberty is the time when animals first release mature germ cells

2 Reproductive senescence in primates occurs because of ovarian inadequacy, not inadequacy of gonadotropin secretion

Sexual behavior

1 Sexual receptivity is keyed by the hormones estrogen and gonadotropin-releasing hormone in the female and by testosterone in the male

External factors controlling reproductive cycles

1 Photoperiod, lactation, nutrition, and animal interaction are important factors that affect reproduction

2 Inadequate nutrition results in ovarian inactivity, especially in cattle

REPRODUCTIVE CYCLES

The two types of reproductive cycles are estrous and menstrual

Two types of reproductive cycles are recognized: *estrous* and *menstrual;* the term *ovarian cycle* represents the interval between two successive ovulations. These terms have developed in order to use certain external characteristics for accurately identifying a particular stage of the reproductive cycle and, of most importance, relating it to the time of ovulation.

In domestic animals, which have limited periods of *estrus (sexual receptivity),* the term *estrous cycle* is appropriate, and the onset of proestrus defines the start of the cycle (Fig. 36–1). In primates, which are sexually receptive during most of the reproductive cycle, the term *menstrual cycle* is appropriate; the onset of *menstruation* (vaginal discharge of blood-tinged fluids and tissues) is designated as the start of the cycle (Fig. 36–2). The first day of the cycle for both estrous and menstrual cycles in many species begins shortly after the end of the luteal phase. In the dog, a normal anestrous period, lasting approximately 3 months, separates diestrus and proestrus (the stages of the cycle are described later).

In domestic animals, except for the dog and pig, proestrus usually begins within 48 hours after the end of the luteal phase; proestrus in the pig does not occur for 5 to 6 days. In primates, menstruation usually begins within 24 hours of the end of the luteal phase. Even though both cycles begin at the same time in relation to the luteal phase (shortly after), the time of ovulation differs. This is because, as discussed

in Chapter 35, luteal and follicular phases are separated in primates, and ovulation occurs at a minimum of 12 to 13 days after the onset of menses. In most domestic animals, the follicular phase overlaps the luteal phase; as a result, ovulation occurs relatively earlier in the estrous cycle. Ovulation is easier to predict in domestic animals than in primates because estrus is usually tightly coupled to the preovulatory release of gonadotropins and ovulation. The onset of follicular development in primates can be delayed for a variety of reasons, including stress; thus, the time of ovulation is less predictable for primates than for domestic animals.

The estrous cycle has been classically divided into stages that represent either behavioral or gonadal events (see Fig. 36–1). The terms, originally developed for the guinea pig, rat, and mouse, are as follows: *proestrus* is the period of follicle development, which occurs after luteal regression and ends at estrus; *estrus* is the period of sexual receptivity; *metestrus* is the period of initial development of the corpus luteum (CL); and *diestrus* is the period of the mature phase of the CL.

The classical terminology per se is not particularly useful for domestic animals. The common terms used for domestic animals involve either *behavioral* or *gonadal* activity. The cycle can be described in a behavioral manner by indicating whether animals are in *estrus (sexually receptive)* or not, including the stages of proestrus, metestrus, and diestrus. The cycle can also be described with reference to the activity of the gonads if differentiation of follicles and the CL is possible. Animals can be in the *follicular phase* (proestrus and estrus) or the *luteal phase* (metestrus and diestrus).

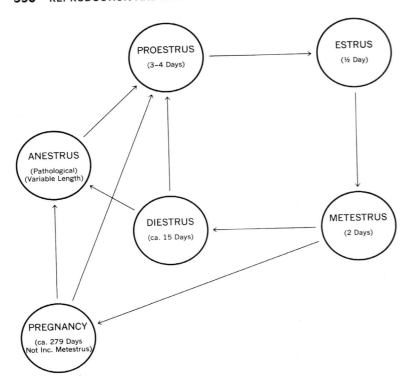

FIGURE 36–1. Various stages of the ovarian cycle of the cow. (From McDonald LE, Pineda MH [eds]: Veterinary Endocrinology and Reproduction, 4th ed. Philadelphia: Lea & Febiger, 1989.)

Because the equine CL is relatively difficult to identify by palpation per rectum, horses are usually classified by sexual behavior, in estrus or nonestrus. The behavioral classification is used also in other domestic species, including the goat, pig, and sheep, because of the difficulty of determining their ovarian status. The ovarian status of cattle can be determined accurately by palpation per rectum, and cows are usually classified by ovarian status: follicular or luteal. The ovarian status of the dog and cat can be determined by measuring serum progesterone levels. If a CL can be identified, ovarian activity can be judged normal in the particular animal, because the CL represents the culmination of follicle growth and ovulation.

PUBERTY AND REPRODUCTIVE SENESCENCE

Puberty is the time when animals first release mature germ cells

In order for females to begin reproductive cycles, they must undergo a process called *puberty*. The term

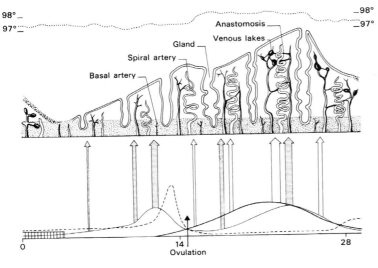

FIGURE 36–2. Changes in human endometrium during the menstrual cycle. Underlying steroid changes are indicated below, and basal body temperature is indicated above. Thickness of *arrows* (estrogens, *stippled*; progestogens, *white*) indicates strength of action. LH, luteinizing hormone. (From Johnson M, Everitt B [eds]: Essential Reproduction, 3rd ed. London: Blackwell Scientific, 1988, p 176.)

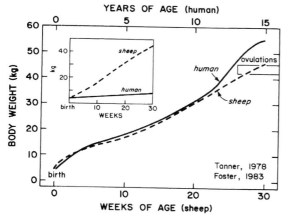

FIGURE 36–3. Body weight from birth through the initiation of ovulation for sheep (mean) and human beings (50th percentile). Inset shows absolute growth during the first 30 weeks. (From Foster DL, Karsch FJ, Olster DH, et al: Determinants of puberty in a seasonal breeder. Recent Prog Horm Res 42:331, 1986.)

puberty is used to define the onset of reproductive life. For the female, although the onset of sexual activity (in domestic animals) or first menstrual bleeding (in primates) is often used as the onset of puberty, the most precise definition is the time of first ovulation. For all species there is a critical requirement for the attainment of a certain size in order for puberty to be initiated; for example, in cattle, it is approximately 275 kg, and in sheep, approximately 40 kg (Fig. 36–3). If this critical requirement is not met because of inadequate nutrition, puberty is delayed. The ages at puberty for domestic animals are as follows: 6 to 12 months for cats, 8 to 12 months for cows, 6 to 12 months for dogs, 7 to 8 months for goats, 12 to 18 months for horses, and 7 to 8 months for sheep. Typically, bitches have attained 75% of their adult size before puberty occurs.

The physiologic mechanisms involving control of puberty in domestic animals are best known in sheep. One of the fundamental concepts of the onset of puberty involves an increase in the synthesis and release of gonadotropin-releasing hormone (GnRH) from the hypothalamus, which drives gonadotropin secretion (in pulsatile form) and follicle growth. Before puberty, GnRH and gonadotropin secretion are kept in check, because the hypothalamus is highly sensitive to *negative feedback inhibition by estrogens.* One of the keys to puberty in lambs is a maturation of the hypothalamus, which results in reduced sensitivity to negative feedback by estrogen. Puberty onset is not delayed as a result of lack of responsiveness of the prepubertal gonads, because ovarian follicle development can be elicited by gonadotropin administration.

Changes in *photoperiod* (daylight exposure) are important for allowing lambs to enter puberty. It has been shown that lambs must have some exposure to a long photoperiod during their prepubertal development; the period can be as short as 1 to 2 weeks (under experimental conditions). Termination of the long photoperiod, which occurs with the summer

solstice, allows the sensitivity of the hypothalamus to decrease in response to negative estrogen feedback. The minimal interval from the end of the long photoperiod exposure to the onset of puberty is 10 weeks under experimental conditions. This aspect agrees well with the timing of spontaneous puberty, in which the first ovulation often occurs in the latter part of September, or about 13 weeks after the summer solstice. This concept of the initiation of puberty does not involve decreasing photoperiod per se; the emphasis is on a turning point that involves the cessation of exposure to a long photoperiod.

With appropriate growth and photoperiod exposure, the secretion of gonadotropins in lambs causes significant follicle growth. This growth is maintained because of decreased sensitivity of the hypothalamus to estrogens produced by growing follicles. The first endocrine event of puberty in the ewe lamb is the appearance of a preovulatory-type surge of gonadotropins, presumably induced by estrogens produced by developing follicles (Fig. 36–4). The gonadotropin surge results in the production of a luteal structure, through luteinization of one or more follicles, that has a short life span (3 to 4 days). After the demise of the initial luteal structure, another gonadotropin surge occurs, which leads to ovulation and the formation of a CL, which usually has a longer life span. At this time, cyclical ovarian activity is finally initiated in the ewe lamb.

Photoperiod can have a suppressive effect on the timing of puberty in animals whose ovarian cycles are controlled by light. Kittens born in the spring may be large enough to enter puberty by late autumn, but puberty could be delayed a few months if the kittens are exposed to the natural photoperiod.

Photoperiod influences the timing of puberty onset in macaque monkeys, depending on the physiologic maturity of the individual. The first ovulation, or puberty onset, can occur during the late autumn or early winter, at about 30 months of age (20% of animals) or 12 months later at about 42 months of age (80% of animals). The animals undergoing puberty at about 30 months have an earlier maturation of the neuroendocrine system, wherein significant gonado-

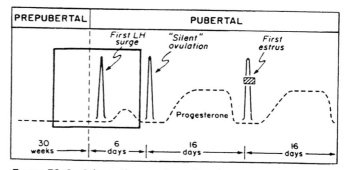

FIGURE 36–4. Schematic overview of major events during the transition into adulthood in the female sheep. LH, luteinizing hormone. (From Foster D, Ryan K: Mechanisms governing onset of ovarian cyclicity at puberty in the lamb. Ann Biol Anim Biochem Biophys 19:1369, 1979.)

tropin secretion begins during the previous spring. Thus, there is a window of opportunity for the onset of puberty in macaques that must be entered within the favorable photoperiod of decreasing light if puberty is to occur at an earlier time; nutrition and growth are likely determinants of the earlier time of onset of puberty.

The onset of puberty usually results in the establishment of cyclical ovarian activity within a relatively short period (within a few weeks to a month in lambs). Ewe lambs can initiate normal ovarian activity at the onset of puberty, which can lead to pregnancy (if the lambs are mated) at the first estrus, or they can have false starts with the establishment of limited luteal phases and cessation of ovarian activity for several weeks to a month before ovarian activity resumes. In general, the onset of ovarian cycles starts later and ends earlier for ewe lambs than for adults of the same breed. The earlier cessation of ovarian activity is caused by an earlier response to negative estrogen feedback.

The initiation of cyclical ovarian activity in pubertal primates takes longer; the first significant follicle growth usually ends in ovulatory failure. In macaque monkeys, 3 to 6 months is usually required after the onset of menarche, or first vaginal bleeding, before the occurrence of the first ovulation of puberty. In humans, follicle growth without ovulation can occur for up to a year before the establishment of normal ovarian cycles, including ovulation and CL formation.

For male lambs, the onset of puberty is first keyed when lambs begin to lose their sensitivity to estrogen feedback inhibition, usually by about 15 weeks of age. For many males, this occurs during the period of increasing, or long, photoperiod, which is in contrast to the pubertal process in the ewe lamb. Spermatogenesis (process of sperm production resulting in the presence of mature sperm) usually begins at this time, but because of the length of the process, lambs are usually not capable of successful breeding until they are more than 30 weeks of age, or in concert with the onset of puberty in ewe lambs. Thus, puberty is a relatively gradual phenomenon in male sheep, in comparison with the abrupt process in females.

Because adult ewes experience the same double gonadotropin surge at the onset of the breeding season, it has been suggested that adult animals recapitulate puberty each year as they enter the breeding season. Studies in adult ewes, however, indicate that *refractoriness* to the long photoperiod experienced by animals during the spring and summer is the most critical aspect for the establishment of ovarian activity. Thus, the idea that the renewal of ovarian activity in sheep recapitulates puberty appears not to be accurate, at least in some aspects.

Reproductive senescence in primates occurs because of ovarian inadequacy, not inadequacy of gonadotropin secretion

The end to ovarian activity that occurs in primates is called *menopause.* In humans, for example, it usually occurs between the ages of 45 and 50 years. Menopause occurs because of the depletion of oocytes, which has occurred throughout the reproductive life of the individual; in essence, it represents ovarian failure. It is not clear whether follicles fail to develop from their primordial state because of an absolute or relative reduction in follicle numbers, or whether the absence of gonadotropin receptors prohibits follicles from entering the gonadotropin-dependent stage of growth. The initiation of menopause often involves cyclical irregularity as a result of failure of follicle development and ovulation. Gonadotropin secretion can be increased or normal, because of the lack of estrogen and, therefore, lack of negative feedback on gonadotropin secretion. In the end, ovarian follicle activity ceases, estrogen concentrations decline, and in the absence of negative feedback inhibition, gonadotropin concentrations increase dramatically.

Reproductive senescence is not recognized in domestic animals. This may be in part because some domestic species have lives that are shortened for economic or humane reasons. Nevertheless, it seems clear that a phenomenon such as menopause does not occur in domestic animals. One effect of age that can be noted is in the dog, in which estrous cycle intervals gradually increase from the norm of 7.5 months to 12 to 15 months toward the end of the life span. In addition, litter size diminishes and increased neonatal mortality occurs with increasing age of the dam.

SEXUAL BEHAVIOR

Sexual receptivity is keyed by the hormones estrogen and gonadotropin-releasing hormone in the female and by testosterone in the male

As indicated previously, the establishment of sexual behavior depends on exposure, or lack of exposure, of the hypothalamus to testosterone during the early neonatal period. In essence, testosterone (converted to estrogen) causes masculinization of the sexual centers in the hypothalamus; in the absence of testosterone, the hypothalamus becomes feminized. An area within the hypothalamus, the *medial preoptic area,* has been identified in the rat as an area that is modified structurally by exposure to testosterone.

There exist several principles regarding the effects of hormones on sexual behavior of domestic animals. First, the magnitude of change in hormone concentration that affects sexual behavior is small; for example, in the cat, an increase in estradiol 17 (concentrations from 10 to 20 pg/mL of plasma) results in signs of proestrus. Second, synergism between hormones is often important for sexual receptiveness; for example, in the dog, it is important that estrogen priming be followed by progesterone. Third, the sequence of exposure to hormones can be important; for example, progesterone priming is required before estrogen exposure for manifestation of estrus in the ewe.

Estrogen, from the developing antral follicle, is the

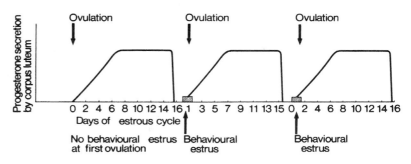

FIGURE 36-5. The estrous cycle of the ewe, showing how the first ovulation of the season is unaccompanied by estrus. Note the short time interval between regression of the corpus luteum and the next ovulation. (From Short RV: Oestrous and menstrual cycles. In Austin CR, Short RV [eds]: Hormonal Control of Reproduction. Reproduction in Mammals, vol 3. Cambridge, United Kingdom: Cambridge University Press, 1984.)

one hormone required for sexual receptivity in all domestic animals. Progesterone derived from either the granulosa of the preovulatory follicle, or the CL, is also important for estrus in some animals.

In sheep, estrus occurs in response to estrogen only if the animal has been exposed previously to progesterone (through the presence of a previous CL). Estrus usually begins within a short period after the end of the luteal phase (i.e., 24 to 36 hours), because of the presence of large antral follicles at luteolysis; thus, the period from last exposure to progesterone and the onset of estrus is short (Fig. 36–5). The requirement for progesterone for sexual receptivity means that the first follicular phase of the breeding season, which leads to ovulation in the ewe, is not accompanied by estrus. Most adult ewes manifest estrus after the first luteal phase. Ewe lambs often require the exposure of two or more luteal phases before they manifest estrus.

Of the domestic species, dogs are unusual in that sexual receptivity is keyed by progesterone, produced initially by the granulosa during the preovulatory luteinizing hormone surge and subsequently by the developing CL. Prior exposure to estrogen makes the female attractive to males but does not produce sexual receptivity; estrus requires the additional exposure to progesterone. Estrus is often maintained for up to a week in the presence of a developing luteal phase. In other domestic species, progesterone inhibits estrous activity.

The importance of prior progesterone priming for estrus manifestation has been suggested for dairy cattle by the finding of a reduced incidence of estrus at the first postpartum ovulation (days 15 to 20). Complete progesterone withdrawal occurs in the cow immediately before delivery, and animals would not have been exposed to progesterone for 2 to 3 weeks in this situation. Sows also have a reduced incidence of estrus at the first ovulation, which usually does not occur until after weaning, usually not until at least 45 days after parturition. Other domestic species (e.g., cats, goats, and horses) show estrus with the first ovulation of the season with no apparent requirement for progesterone priming.

Testosterone is important for *libido* in female primates. The theca layer from degenerating follicles forms an active interstitium that secretes the androgens androstenedione and testosterone. Androgens are also essential for the maintenance of libido in males. Occasionally, castrated males, particularly horses, are able to maintain libido in spite of the

lower concentrations of androgens (of adrenal origin) that are present after castration. These animals can sometimes be differentiated from those with retained testicles (*cryptorchids*) by testosterone analysis of plasma; however, serum testosterone level in intact males varies by the minute. A GnRH stimulation test more accurately identifies remaining testicular tissues (2.2 µg/kg intravenously; samples drawn before and 1 to 3 hours after GnRH administration).

There is both experimental and circumstantial evidence to indicate that GnRH plays a role in sexual receptivity. The administration of GnRH to ovariectomized rats produced sexual (lordotic) responses, and in prepubertal gilts, GnRH administration resulted in the occurrence of estrus within 24 hours. The circumstantial evidence is that the onset of sexual receptivity in animals is tightly coupled to the onset of the preovulatory gonadotropin surge (Fig. 36–6). Because the preovulatory gonadotropin surge is the result of an increased rate of pulsatile release of gonadotropins driven by increased GnRH synthesis and release, it is

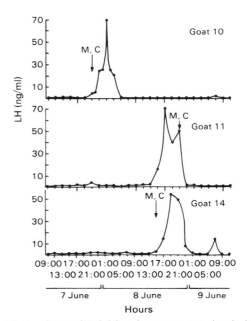

FIGURE 36-6. Plasma luteinizing hormone (LH) levels in three nannies exhibiting an ovulatory surge during the 50-hour period of intensive sampling (7 to 9 June). M, marked; C, copulation. (From BonDurant RH, Darien BJ, Munro CJ, et al: Photoperiod induction of fertile oestrus and changes in LH and progesterone concentrations in yearling goats [Capra hircus]. J Reprod Fertil 63:1, 1981.)

likely that this increased GnRH secretory activity affects sexual centers within the hypothalamus for the promotion of sexual receptivity. This allows the onset of the ovulatory process, triggered by the gonadotropin surge, to be tightly coupled with sexual receptivity.

EXTERNAL FACTORS CONTROLLING REPRODUCTIVE CYCLES

Photoperiod, lactation, nutrition, and animal interaction are important factors that affect reproduction

PHOTOPERIOD

Photoperiod controls the occurrence of reproductive cycles in a number of domestic species, including cats, goats, horses, and sheep. The result is that these animals have an annual period in which they have continuous (cyclical) ovarian activity and another period of no ovarian activity; the latter period is termed *anestrus*. The responses to photoperiod are different among these species; cats and horses are positively affected with increasing light, and goats and sheep are positively affected by decreasing photoperiod (Fig. 36–7).

A positive response to a change in the photoperiod usually occurs relatively soon after the occurrence of the summer or winter solstice: that is, within 1 to 2 months. A negative response to a change in photoperiod usually requires a longer duration for an effect: that is, 2 to 4 months to suppress ovarian activity after the occurrence of the particular solstice. The net result is that in the absence of pregnancy, cyclical ovarian activity usually occupies more than half the year for these four seasonally breeding species.

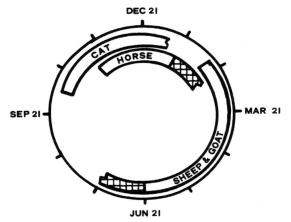

FIGURE 36–7. A diagrammatic representation of the effect of photoperiod on ovarian activity in the typical cat, horse, sheep, and goat. The bars represent periods of ovarian inactivity (anestrum). The transitional periods for the horse, sheep, and goat are shown by the hatched portions of the bars. (From Stabenfeldt GH, Edqvist L-E: Female reproductive processes. In Swenson MJ [ed]: Dukes' Physiology of Domestic Animals, 10th ed. Ithaca, New York: Cornell University Press, 1984.)

In cats, cyclical ovarian activity can occur from late January through October in the Northern Hemisphere. In horses, the usual period of ovarian activity is March through October. Conversely, sheep and goats have ovarian activity from late July through February or March (depending on the breed). As indicated previously, progesterone priming immediately before follicle development is required for sexual receptivity in sheep. The full length of the reproductive season of sheep is not manifested externally because, first, the first ovulation is not preceded by the presence of a CL and, second, the last follicle phase may be delayed because of a negative photoperiod, the priming effects of progesterone being lost before follicle growth.

The main translator of photoperiod is the *pineal gland*, which produces *melatonin* in response to darkness. The central nervous system pathway involved with the translation of light includes the *retina*, the *suprachiasmatic nucleus*, the *superior cervical ganglion*, and the *pineal gland*. Whereas melatonin was traditionally described as antigonadal, this is obviously not true, because both short and long phases of darkness, with resultant short and long durations of melatonin secretion, can have a positive effect on reproductive cycles. In sheep, however, exposure to increasing darkness may be important only for maintaining ovarian activity. The onset of ovarian activity is thought to occur in response to the development of refractoriness to the long photoperiod. The development of *photorefractoriness* to a long photoperiod as a requisite to ovarian cyclicity is consonant with the fact that sheep can begin cyclical ovarian activity even before the summer solstice.

Of the seasonal breeders, the cat is the most sensitive to photoperiod change; estrus, in conjunction with the presence of mature, antral follicles, can occur as early as January 15. It is likely that initial follicle activity begins at least 10 days before the first expression of estrus, or 15 days after the winter solstice. Thus, a total photoperiod change of as little as 15 minutes can be perceived and translated by the cat into ovarian activity.

The suppressive effects of photoperiod can be overcome by exposure to artificial lighting regimens. This is relatively easy in the case of cats and horses, in which environments with photoperiods are compatible with ovarian activity (i.e., at least 12 hours of light per day). If the photoperiod is established before the end of ovarian activity in the autumn, cyclical ovarian activity continues through the time associated with anestrus. If mares are allowed to become anestrous in the autumn, it can take a minimum of 2 months of exposure to increased light to reestablish ovarian activity. The usual time for placing mares under lights is December 1 in the Northern Hemisphere; cyclical ovarian activity is expected by early February.

It is usually not possible to place sheep and goats in light-tight barns to increase their exposure to dark in order to overcome the suppressive effects of increasing light. One development in this regard has been the oral or systemic (implant) administration of melatonin in sheep during the spring. This exposure to melatonin has resulted in an early onset of ovarian activity and increased the number of multiple ovulations above that normally observed at the beginning of the breeding season.

LACTATION

Lactation can have suppressive effects on ovarian activity. In pigs, suppression of ovarian activity is complete; sows do not manifest estrus until after piglets are weaned. In cats, ovarian activity can be suppressed throughout lactation, although they occasionally manifest estrus during the latter part of lactation. Ovarian activity tends to be suppressed in lactating beef cows; the first estrus and ovulation do not occur before postpartum day 45. The suckling process appears important to ovarian suppression; in dairy cows, ovarian activity is not suppressed by lactation unless a large nutritional deficit is involved.

Goats and sheep usually begin lactation during a photoperiod that is increasingly suppressive for ovarian activity, and therefore the reestablishment of ovarian activity in these species is confounded by the photoperiod. Ewes delivering in the autumn ovulated as early as postpartum day 12 (average, postpartum day 23), which indicates that lactation has little suppressive effect on ovarian activity in sheep. Mares usually ovulate by postpartum days 10 to 15, and lactation has no suppressive effect on ovarian activity during this ovulatory interval.

One of the concepts of *lactational suppression of ovarian activity* involves the importance of suckling with its related stimulation of prolactin synthesis. Prolactin synthesis is inhibited by factors such as dopamine and GnRH-associated peptide; thus, these factors must be suppressed. The sensory input from suckling suppresses the production of these prolactin-inhibiting factors. Because both dopamine and GnRH-associated peptide are essential links in the synthesis of gonadotropins, their reduced output results in reduced ovarian activity through decreased gonadotropin synthesis and release.

PHEROMONES

Pheromones are chemical compounds that allow communication among animals through the olfactory system. When sexual behavior is affected, the compounds are called *sex pheromones.* Pheromones arise from several tissue sources; the most prominent ones in animals are sebaceous glands, the reproductive tract, and the urinary tract.

Some of the first experiments that demonstrated the potency of male odors to influence reproductive behavior were conducted with mice. One phenomenon, called the *Whitten effect,* involved the synchronization of estrus in female mice through the sudden introduction of a male (or male odor through bedding); a large number of animals exhibited cycles within 3 days of introduction of the male. The effect of the pheromones in this case is to stimulate the

synthesis and release of gonadotropins. Another phenomenon, called the *Bruce effect,* involves the blockage of pregnancy development by the introduction of a different (strange) male into proximity with a recently bred female. The effect of the odor of the strange male is to block the release of prolactin, the hormone responsible for the maintenance of the CL in association with pregnancy in rodents. Regression of the CL in this case produces fetal loss. Thus, it is possible for pheromones to strongly affect reproductive cycles.

Pheromones are important for the attraction of the male to the female at the time of sexual receptivity. Sexual attractiveness of the female evolves from the pheromones that she emits on a limited, cyclical basis in association with estrus. For example, methyl-*p*-hydroxybenzoate, isolated from the vaginal secretions of dogs in proestrus and estrus, has produced intense anogenital interest by males when applied to anestrous females. Females are also influenced by male odors; for example, sows in estrus assume a breeding *(rigidity)* stance when exposed to the urine of males. Androgens can serve as pheromones, or they can influence the production of substances within the kidney that influence female sexual behavior. The attractiveness of the female to the male involves a change in perception of the male by the female as the result of a changing physiologic state within the female, not because of changes that are occurring in the male.

The classical way for males to delineate their territory has been for them to mark the area with urine. In general, pheromones that affect sexual behavior tend to have a musk type of odor. The classic pheromone used by humans is perfume, which is derived from civetone, a cyclical 17-carbon compound obtained from the civet cat.

The Whitten effect has been used to manipulate the estrous cycles of animals. Male sheep are introduced into a flock of ewes before the breeding season to either advance or ensure ovarian cycle at the beginning of the breeding season. Whereas it was previously thought the effect of the introduction of a male was short-lived—that is, a gonadotropin response could be obtained only within the first few days from ewes that had antral follicles—it is now clear that the interaction of rams with ewes over extended periods of the anestrus results in earlier ovarian activity.

As discussed, pheromones can account for some of the effect of the male. More recent studies, however, have shown that *sight* of the male by the female as well as *physical contact* are important factors that influence gonadotropin secretion and thus ovarian activity.

The Whitten effect has also been used to influence the onset of puberty in pigs. The introduction of males into groups of gilts beginning several weeks before the expected time of puberty (180 to 200 days after birth) has been used to ensure or advance the onset of puberty. The *dormitory effect,* well-recognized synchronization of menstrual cycles in women who are roommates, occurs in bitches kenneled together as well.

Inadequate nutrition results in ovarian inactivity, especially in cattle

In dairy cattle, genetically selected for high productivity, the ability to produce up to 100 pounds of milk per day is a remarkable achievement. It is almost impossible for dairy cows to consume enough feed during the first part of the lactation cycle to maintain their body weight, and they are often in a negative nutritional balance for up to 100 days after parturition. Because animals must have an adequate level of nutrition to initiate ovarian activity, ovarian activity is suppressed until a positive energy balance is established. If a dairy cow is to produce large quantities of milk, enough time is needed for nutrition to catch up with milk production.

Inadequate nutrition can affect ovarian activity in the postpartum period. A management practice that is sometimes used to enhance production efficiency is to maintain beef cows on a marginal plane of nutrition during the winter. This approach is for the purpose of forcing animals to use fat that has been developed and stored during the grazing season. If pregnant beef cows are not returned to a positive nutritional balance by the last month of pregnancy, the reestablishment of ovarian cycles, which usually occurs between postpartum days 45 and 60, will be delayed. Another situation that can affect ovarian activity involves pregnant beef heifers. These animals often need extra nutrition in the postpartum period in order to reestablish ovarian activity, because they have requirements for growth as well as for lactation.

CLINICAL CORRELATIONS

Sexual attractiveness in the spayed bitch

History You are called by a veterinary colleague who has seen a bitch owned by one of her important clients. The client is upset because the dog is attracting males in spite of recently having undergone an ovariohysterectomy. You inquire whether the dog allows intromission by males. Although the answer is no, the owner is sure that a portion of an ovary was left in situ. Your colleague is sure she removed the ovaries during the surgical procedure. You are asked to examine the dog as a favor to your colleague.

Clinical examination The dog has a vulva that is slightly swollen with a small amount of discharge present. An examination of a vaginal smear reveals some cornified epithelial cells but mainly an increased number of neutrophils. You indicate to the owner that you believe the male dogs are being attracted by the presence of an infection in the urogenital tract; the owner needs more convincing. You decide to obtain a reproductive endocrine panel (estrogen and progesterone) and a urinalysis from the dog. The values for both estrogen and progesterone are low and thus are not supportive of the presence of ovarian tissue. The presence of white blood cells and bacteria in the urine suggests a urinary tract infection.

Comment It is common for bitches with genitourinary infections to attract male dogs, presumably because of the odors generated by the infection. One of the most important points of differentiation as to cause (i.e., bladder infection vs. the presence of an ovarian remnant) is to know about the sexual behavior of the animal. The bitch allows intromission by a male only if she has been exposed to progesterone after priming with estrogen. This situation occurs only if an ovarian follicle is present and has begun to luteinize after the preovulatory luteinizing hormone surge. If the animal in question had allowed intromission, the presence of an ovarian remnant would be likely. Because of the failure of the bitch to allow intromission, you indicate that the animal almost certainly lacks ovarian tissue. With regard to the endocrine analysis, if the animal was completely ovariectomized, both values will be low. This finding per se does not rule out the presence of ovarian tissue, but if the sample is obtained when the animal is showing the "sexual behavior," it can be stated with assurance that the behavior is not caused by hormones or, by extension, activity of ovarian tissue.

Treatment The bladder infection is treated, and the owner is instructed to keep the female away from males until the infection is cleared.

Bibliography

Austin CR, Short RV (eds): Reproduction in Mammals, vols 1–6. Cambridge, United Kingdom: Cambridge University Press, 1986.

Beach FA: Coital behavior in dogs. Behavior 36:544–548, 1970.

Concannon PW, Morton DB, Weir BJ (eds): Dog and cat reproduction, contraception and artificial insemination. J Reprod Fertil Suppl vol 39, 1989.

Cupps PT (ed): Reproduction in Domestic Animals, 4th ed. New York: Academic Press, 1991.

Feldman EC, Nelson RW: Canine and Feline Endocrinology and Reproduction. Philadelphia: WB Saunders, 1996.

Hafez EWE (ed): Reproduction in Farm Animals, 5th ed. Philadelphia: Lea & Febiger, 1987.

Johnson M, Everitt B (eds): Essential Reproduction, 3rd ed. London: Blackwell Scientific, 1988.

Knobil E, Neill JD, Ewing LL, et al (eds): The Physiology of Reproduction, vols 1, 2. New York: Raven Press, 1988.

McDonald LE, Pineda MH (eds): Veterinary Endocrinology and Reproduction, 4th ed. Philadelphia: Lea & Febiger, 1989.

PRACTICE QUESTIONS

1. The first estrous cycle of the cow after parturition follows which sequence?
   a. Anestrus, diestrus, estrus, metestrus, proestrus.
   b. Anestrus, estrus, diestrus, metestrus, proestrus.
   c. Anestrus, metestrus, diestrus, estrus, proestrus.
   d. Anestrus, proestrus, estrus, diestrus, proestrus.
   e. Anestrus, proestrus, estrus, metestrus, diestrus.

2. The usual situation in large domestic animals is for one or more dominant follicles to be present at the time of luteal regression, with sexual receptivity manifested within 1 to 2 days after luteal regression; the one large animal that is the exception to this generalization is the
   a. cow.
   b. doe.
   c. ewe.
   d. mare.

e. sow.

3. The hormones that form the foundation for sexual receptivity are
   a. estrogen and prostaglandin $F_{2\alpha}$ ($PGF_{2\alpha}$).
   b. progesterone and estrogen.
   c. estrogen and GnRH.
   d. progesterone and $PGF_{2\alpha}$.
   e. $PGF_{2\alpha}$ and GnRH.

4. Decreasing light turns off cyclical ovarian activity after a number of months, whereas increasing light reverses the process after a number of months, including the development of a transitional period. This description fits which domestic species?
   a. Cat.
   b. Cow.
   c. Dog.
   d. Goat.
   e. Horse.
   f. Pig.
   g. Sheep.

5. What response occurs as a result of the Whitten effect in animals, a situation in which the introduction of a male into a group of noncyclical animals results in the reestablishment of ovarian activity?

a. Increased estrogen secretion.
b. Increased progesterone secretion.
c. Increased prolactin secretion.
d. Increased follicle-stimulating hormone secretion.
e. Increased luteinizing hormone secretion.
f. Increased follicle-stimulating hormone and luteinizing hormone secretion.

6. One of the domestic species requires progesterone priming, before estrogen, to manifest estrus. Hence, this species does not manifest estrus with the first ovarian cycle in the postpartum period. The animal is the
   a. cat.
   b. dog.
   c. goat.
   d. horse.
   e. pig.
   f. sheep.

PRACTICE ANSWERS

1. e   2. e   3. c   4. a, e   5. f   6. f

37

Pregnancy and parturition

Pregnancy

1 The development of an embryo involves fusion of an oocyte and a spermatozoon within the oviduct

2 Extension of the life span of the corpus luteum in large domestic species and cats is essential for pregnancy maintenance

3 The placenta acts as an endocrine organ

Parturition

1 Fetal cortisol initiates delivery through increased secretion of estrogen and, as a result, prostaglandin $F_{2\alpha}$

PREGNANCY

The development of an embryo involves fusion of an oocyte and a spermatozoon within the oviduct

The development of a new individual requires the transfer of male gametes to the female genital tract for fertilization of the female gametes. *Spermatozoa,* which have been concentrated and stored in the epididymis, gradually change from *oxidative* (aerobic) to *glycolytic* (anaerobic) *metabolism* as they progress through the epididymis. In this state, spermatozoa are in a situation of reduced metabolism. Mature sperm are able to metabolize only a special sugar, *fructose,* within the reproductive tract. Lactose, glucose, dextrose, and fructose have all been used in commercially available semen extenders.

Sperm are usually ejaculated into the vagina; some domestic species (dog, horse, and pig) ejaculate directly onto the cervix and into the uterus. The movement of sperm through the cervix is aided by estrogen-induced changes in cervical mucus, which result in the formation of channels that facilitate movement of sperm. This has been emphasized particularly in primates, in which the thinning of mucus occurs just before ovulation, a factor that can be used to predict the time of ovulation.

The environment of the female genital system is generally inhospitable to the survival of sperm; for example, white blood cells are quickly attracted to the uterine lumen because sperm cells are foreign to the female genital tract. Special reservoirs have evolved in the female tract to aid in the survival of sperm during transport; these include the cervix and oviduct, the latter involving areas at the uterotubule junction and within the ampulla. The reservoirs are progressively filled (in a caudal-to-cranial direction in the tract), which takes hours. Finally, the reservoir within the ampulla is able to release a few sperm on a continuous basis, so that fertilization can occur shortly after the arrival of oocytes within the oviduct.

The first studies in *sperm transport* emphasized the rapidity of the process; sperm were reported to pass from the vagina to the fimbriated end of the oviduct within minutes. It is now known that sperm undergoing so-called fast transport are not involved in fertilization; in fact, they are damaged by the rapid transport.

Sperm need to undergo changes within the female genital tract that are a prerequisite for fertilization; the process is called *capacitation.* One of the effects of capacitation is the removal of glycoproteins from the sperm cell surface.

The glycoproteins, perhaps present for protective purposes, interfere with fertilization. This change allows sperm to undergo the *acrosome reaction* when they come in contact with oocytes. The acrosome reaction involves the release of hydrolytic enzymes from the acrosomal cap; this may be important for penetration of the sperm through the granulosa and zona pellucida to the oocyte plasma membrane. *Hyaluronidase* causes breakdown of hyaluronic acid, an important component of the intercellular matrix of granulosa cells that surround the oocyte. *Acrosin,* a proteolytic enzyme, digests the acellular coating around the oocyte. Both enzymatic events allow the sperm to penetrate to the oocyte. The acrosome reaction also changes the surface of the sperm, which allows it to fuse with the oocyte. The acrosomal reaction results in tail movements that feature a flagellar beat that tends to drive sperm in a forward direction.

Because of the changes that spermatozoa must undergo within the female reproductive tract before fertilization, the deposition of sperm before ovulation is the preferred timing for maximal fertility. An exception to this preference is when sperm with reduced longevity, such as chilled-extended semen or frozen semen, are used. In these instances, deposition of semen into the female reproductive tract should occur close to the time of ova maturation associated with fertilization. Females are usually sexually receptive for at least 24 hours before ovulation and, in the natural setting (free interaction between sexes), insemination usually occurs a number of hours before the occurrence of ovulation. Even in induced ovulators, such as cats, the interval from copulation to ovulation is usually 24 hours or more. In essence, the system has evolved to have ready-to-fertilize sperm at the fertilization site when oocytes arrive. This is in concert with the finding that the life span of male gametes tends to be twice that of female gametes.

The presentation of male gametes before female gametes in the oviduct implies that oocytes are ready for fertilization upon arrival in the ampulla; this is probably true for a majority of animals. A prerequisite for fertilization of the oocyte is that it must undergo the first meiotic division before fertilization. Although this occurs in a number of species before ovulation, in the horse and dog the first meiotic division does not occur until after ovulation (in the dog, not for at least 48 hours). In this situation, spermatozoa often wait for oocytes to mature in the oviduct before fertilization can occur. One means of adaptation to delayed completion of meiosis is that spermatozoa have a relatively longer life span in the dog and horse than in other domestic species.

Once fertilization has occurred, the *embryo* usually develops to the *morula,* or early *blastocyst,* stage within the oviduct before moving into the uterus. This period, usually 4 to 5 days, affords the uterus time to finish its inflammatory response concerning the removal of spermatozoa and allows the endometrial glands time to secrete nutrients under the influence of progesterone from the developing corpus luteum (CL); the nutrients are essential for the development of embryos during their preimplantation stage.

An interesting finding in the mare is the ability to distinguish fertilized from unfertilized oocytes; unfertilized oocytes from previous cycles are retained within the oviduct, whereas recently fertilized oocytes (embryos) move through the oviduct to the uterus. It is likely that all animals recognize pregnancy by the presence of one or more embryos at the early oviductal stage. However, this recognition does not necessarily result in prolongation of the CL and the continued production of progesterone, which is essential for the maintenance of pregnancy. In the bitch, it has been shown that despite ovulation and ova maturation's spanning several hours, embryonic ages are synchronized by some mechanism inherent to the bitch's reproductive tract.

Extension of the life span of the corpus luteum in large domestic species and cats is essential for pregnancy maintenance

For the domestic animals (cattle, goats, horses, pigs, sheep) whose luteal activity is controlled by the uterus, modification of *uterine prostaglandin $F_{2\alpha}$* ($PGF_{2\alpha}$) synthesis and release is critical for the establishment of pregnancy. It seems clear that the embryo produces substances that modify uterine production of $PGF_{2\alpha}$. *Estrogen synthesis* by the embryo is one way in which the endometrium may be informed of the presence of an embryo. A specific protein of embryonic origin called *trophoblastin,* produced before day 14 of pregnancy (or postovulation) in both sheep and cattle, is of interest for the establishment of pregnancy from an immunologic point of view; it has a close structural relationship to the molecule *interferon.* Movement of the embryo or embryos in the tract is also important for pregnancy recognition. In the mare, the embryo moves throughout both horns before implantation in the uterine lining at day 16. In pigs, a minimal number of embryos need to be present (i.e., about 4), presumably to occupy a sufficiently large area of the endometrium. In litter-bearing animals, transuterine migration is also used to maximize the opportunity for fetal development; this procedure aids the recognition of the pregnancy process. The end result is either suppression of $PGF_{2\alpha}$ synthesis, as seen in the cow (Fig. 37–1), or modification of the secretion mode (i.e., continuous instead of pulsatile),

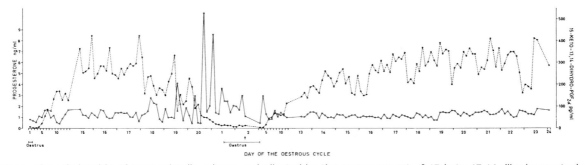

FIGURE 37–1. The relationship of prostaglandin release, as indicated by the measurement of 15-keto-13,14-dihydroprostaglandin $F_{2\alpha}$, and progesterone production by the corpus luteum during a nonfertile cycle and after a conception in the same cow. (From Kindahl H, Edqvist L-E, Bane A: Blood levels of progesterone and 15-keto-13,14-dihydroprostaglandin F-2_α during the normal oestrous cycle and early pregnancy of heifers. Acta Endocrinol 82:134, 1976.)

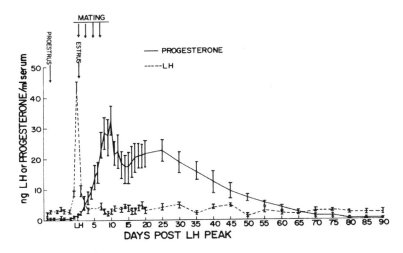

Figure 37-2. Luteinizing hormone (LH) and progesterone concentrations during pregnancy in nine dogs. Vertical bars represent the standard error of the mean. (From Smith MS, McDonald LE: Serum levels of luteinizing hormone and progesterone during the estrous cycle, pseudopregnancy and pregnancy in the dog. Endocrinology 94:404, 1974. Copyright © by The Endocrine Society.)

as in sheep. It seems clear that the absence of pulsatile secretion of $PGF_{2\alpha}$ is critical for the extension of the life span of the CL and the establishment of pregnancy in large domestic species.

In the cat, the CL lasts for 35 to 40 days after ovulation, regardless of the presence of pregnancy, and thus early modification of luteal activity is not essential for the establishment of pregnancy. Implantation occurs at about day 13, which allows the fetoplacental unit to influence and extend luteal activity that is compatible with pregnancy maintenance. The luteotropic hormone that is responsible for luteal maintenance in the cat is not known. One hormone that probably synergizes with progesterone for the support of pregnancy is *relaxin,* a placental hormone that is produced in the queen, beginning at about day 20 of pregnancy (Fig. 37–2).

In the dog, the luteal phase is not extended during pregnancy; the luteal phase in the nonpregnant animal is often slightly longer (70 days) than in pregnant bitches (56 to 58 days). Nevertheless, enhancement of luteal activity occurs through a placental luteotropin, probably relaxin; progesterone secretion is enhanced beginning at about day 20 of pregnancy or a few days after implantation. Early in the luteal phase, luteal function in the bitch is likely autonomous. During the second half of the luteal phase, luteinizing hormone (LH) and prolactin are probably luteotrophs.

The rescue of the CL at the onset of pregnancy in primates involves the production of a luteotropin called *chorionic gonadotropin* (CG; for humans, hCG), which is produced by trophoblastic cells (*syncytiotrophoblasts*) of the embryo (Fig. 37–3). In order for trophoblast tissue to produce CG, it must have intimate contact with the interstitium of the endometrium. This contact occurs by *interstitial* implantation, in which the embryo penetrates the endometrium approximately 8 to 9 days after fertilization in humans and nonhuman primates. Secretion of CG begins 24 to 48 hours after implantation with immediate enhancement of luteal progesterone production. Rescue of the CL in human pregnancy occurs as late as 4 to 5 days before the end of the luteal phase.

In primates, as indicated, interstitial implantation

is essential for the development of pregnancy. Implantation is less invasive in the dog and cat; this type is termed *eccentric.* In the large domestic species, there is little invasion of the endometrium per se; implantation occurs within special endometrial protrusions called *caruncles* in ruminants and by relatively minor *villus* invasion of the endometrium in horses and pigs. Domestic animals are more dependent on uterine secretions for the support of pregnancy than are primates. For cattle and horses, the first indications of implantation begin about days 25 to 30 after fertilization, and it is likely that another 7 to 10 days pass

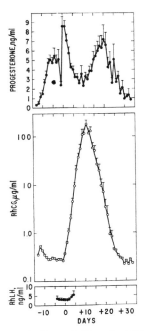

Figure 37-3. Summarization of 15 early pregnancies in normal rhesus monkeys normalized to the day of corpus luteum rescue (day 0). Points are means plus or minus standard error. Note the temporal relationship between luteal progesterone production (before day +10) and chorionic gonadotropin output. RhCG, rhesus chorionic gonadotropin; RhLH, rhesus luteinizing hormone. (From Knobil E: On the regulation of the primate corpus luteum. Biol Reprod 8:246, 1973.)

before a significant amount of embryonic nutrition is obtained through the implantation site. Subclinical uterine infections or an inadequate number of endometrial glands can interfere with the establishment of pregnancy in the species with a long interval between fertilization and implantation. The cervix forms an important barrier to contamination of the uterine lumen in both nonpregnant and pregnant animals; in the latter, the cervix becomes sealed.

The placenta acts as an endocrine organ

Besides the essential role of providing nutrients and oxygen for embryonic metabolism, the placenta functions as an endocrine organ. One of the most important functions of the placenta is the *production of progesterone.* In primates, this function is established early in gestation, and it is likely that the placenta can maintain pregnancy within 2 to 3 weeks after implantation. Placental production of sufficient progesterone to maintain pregnancy occurs later in domestic animals (in sheep, day 50 of a 150-day gestation; in horses, day 70 of a 340-day gestation; in cats, day 45 of a 65-day gestation); in some species, the placenta never produces enough progesterone to support pregnancy (cattle, goats, pigs).

The *production of estrogen,* in contrast to that of progesterone, requires interaction between the fetus and the placenta. The primate placenta is unable to produce estrogen from progesterone even though the steroids are minimally separated in the biochemical synthetic pathway (see Fig. 37–5). The placenta does not possess the enzymes necessary for the conversion of progesterone to androgens. Therefore, a system has evolved in which the placenta supplies *pregnenolone,* the immediate precursor of progesterone, to the fetus, and the *fetal zone of the adrenal cortex* transforms pregnenolone to an androgen, *dehydroepiandrosterone.* This is returned to the placenta, which is able to convert *dehydroepiandrosterone* to an estrogen. In humans, the primary estrogen of pregnancy is *estriol.* Because the fetus is involved in the production of estriol, the well-being of the fetus can be judged by determining estriol concentrations in the plasma of the mother.

The production of estrogen in the mare also involves an interaction between the placenta and fetus (Fig. 37–4). The work of R. L. Pashen and W. R. Allen showed that the fetal gonads replace the fetal adrenal glands in primates as the key fetal endocrine organ involved in the cooperative synthesis of estrogen. The interstitial cells of the gonads appear to be the interactive cells, and fetal gonads enlarge to a size greater than that of the maternal gonads during the latter part of gestation. The production of estrogens during pregnancy in other domestic species, occurring relatively late in gestation, may involve the development of placental enzymes that allow progesterone to be metabolized to estrogens without the direct intervention of a fetal endocrine organ (fetal cortisol, however, is important for the induction of these placental enzymes, particularly in sheep; see the section on parturition).

The protein hormones that are produced during pregnancy tend to be of placental origin. For example, *relaxin* is a hormone produced by the placenta in the cat, dog, and horse beginning at about days 20, 20, and 70, respectively. Besides its importance for preparing the soft tissues of the pelvic canal for passage of the fetus at birth (see the section on parturition), relaxin may be important for the support of pregnancy through a synergistic action with progesterone. In exception to the general rule of protein hormone production by the placenta, relaxin is produced by the CL in the pig, cow, and primates during pregnancy, with prepartum release occurring in conjunction with luteolysis.

The only CG identified in domestic animals to date is equine CG (eCG; formerly called *pregnant mares' serum gonadotropin* by its discoverer, Harold Cole) (see Fig. 37–4). The eCG is produced by trophoblast cells that initially form as a band on the chorion (*chorionic girdle*), detach themselves around day 35 of gestation, penetrate the endometrium, and form associations

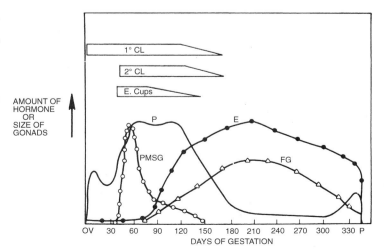

FIGURE 37–4. Summary of the temporal relationships among changes in hormonal concentrations and morphologic changes throughout the gestation period of the mare. 1° CL, primary corpus luteum; 2° CL, secondary corpora lutea; E, estrogens; E. Cups, endometrial cups; FG, fetal gonads; P, progesterone; PMSG, pregnant mare serum gonadotropin (equine chorionic gonadotropin). (From Daels PF, Hughes JP, Stabenfeldt GH: Reproduction in horses. In Cupps PT [ed]: Reproduction in Domestic Animals, 4th ed. New York: Academic Press, 1991, p 423.)

of cells called *endometrial cups.* The eCG enhances progesterone production by the primary CL of pregnancy and aids in the formation of additional (secondary) corpora lutea through the luteinization, or ovulation, of preformed follicles. The essentiality of eCG for pregnancy maintenance is not known, because the primary CL is adequate for maintaining pregnancy.

Placental lactogen is another placental protein hormone. Its production increases in primates as CG secretion wanes during pregnancy. Placental lactogen has been found in goats and sheep, with secretion increasing during the latter part of pregnancy. The hormone appears to have both *somatotropic* and *lactogenic effects,* on the basis of growth hormone and prolactin-like properties. In dairy cattle, for example, placental lactogen may be important for mammary gland alveolar development, setting the stage for the next period of lactation. Another hormone whose production is increased during gestation, *prolactin,* also is important for alveolar development during the prepartum period. Prolactin is not a hormone of placental origin; prolactin increases during the latter part of gestation as a result of the effect of estrogen on its release from the adenohypophysis.

━ PARTURITION

▬ Fetal cortisol initiates delivery through increased secretion of estrogen and, as a result, prostaglandin F₂α

During pregnancy, the uterus progressively enlarges and stretches because of the growing fetus. Progesterone plays an important role in maintaining the quiescence of the myometrium as well as in promoting a tightly contracted cervix. During the latter part of pregnancy, estrogen begins to influence uterine muscle by stimulating the production of *contractile protein* and the formation of *gap junctions;* the former increases the contractile potential of the uterus, and the latter facilitates the contractile process through increased communication among smooth muscle cells. Thus, important changes that set the stage for parturition begin weeks before the actual process begins. In the end, the uterus is converted from a quiescent to a contractile organ and, of importance, the cervix relaxes and opens to allow the fetus to be delivered.

The most important question about parturition concerns what initiates the process. In domestic animals, it is clear that maturation of the fetus eventually brings about changes that initiate the delivery process. The key organ system of the fetus responsible for initiating the process is the *fetal adrenal cortex;* the hypothalamus and adenohypophysis play important supporting roles. This concept came from the work by Liggins and Kennedy, who showed that destruction of the anterior pituitary of the sheep fetus resulted in prolongation of gestation; Drost subsequently found the same results after fetal adrenalectomy. Critical changes in *cortisol secretion* by the fetus eventually

result in the synthesis and release of PGF₂α from the uterus, which produces contraction of muscles and relaxation of the cervix. The following details of the initiation of parturition pertain in particular to ruminants. It is unclear whether elevated cortisol levels contribute to the initiation of parturition in the dog.

The maturation of the fetal adrenal cortex is of critical importance in the initiation of parturition. It is likely that the adrenal cortex becomes progressively sensitive to fetal adrenocorticotropic hormone (ACTH) (Fig. 37–5). The time of adrenal maturation is under fetal genetic control, as shown by studies conducted at the University of California, Davis on fetal lambs of different breeds in the same uterus (produced by embryo transfer) in which the prepartum initiation of cortisol production occurred at times that were characteristic (and different) for the breed. Fetal cortisol induces placental enzymes (17-hydroxylase and C17-20 lyase) that direct steroid synthesis away from progesterone to estrogen. This process occurs at different times before parturition in domestic species: for example, beginning at prepartum days 25 to 30 in cattle, 7 to 10 in pigs, and 2 to 3 in sheep. The end result of increased estrogen secretion is the secretion of *prostaglandins,* particularly PGF₂α. PGF₂α is the pivotal hormone for the initiation of parturition; once its secretion begins, the acute phase of delivery is activated. The role of oxytocin in the initiation of

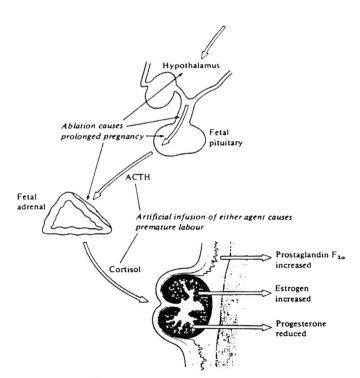

FIGURE 37–5. Diagrammatic summary explaining how the fetal lamb controls the onset of labor. Experimental procedures that lengthen or shorten pregnancy are shown. ACTH, adrenocorticotropic hormone. (Redrawn from Liggins CG: The foetal role in the initiation of parturition in the ewe. In Wolstenholme GEW, O'Connor M [eds]: Foetal Autonomy. London: Churchill Livingstone, 1969.)

delivery is not certain; it probably complements $PGF_{2\alpha}$ once the delivery process has started.

The synthesis of $PGF_{2\alpha}$ is thought to come about through increased availability of the substrate *arachidonic acid,* which is the main rate-limiting step in the synthesis of $PGF_{2\alpha}$. Estrogens are proposed to influence the system by making available the enzyme *phospholipase A,* a membrane-bound lysosomal enzyme that initiates the subsequent hydrolysis of phospholipids and release of arachidonic acid. This probably results from an increasing estrogen-to-progesterone ratio, whereby progesterone initially stabilizes and then estrogens destabilize lysosomal membranes. The end result is increased availability of arachidonic acid for the synthesis of $PGF_{2\alpha}$. The onset of $PGF_{2\alpha}$ synthesis results in the immediate release of the hormone, because $PGF_{2\alpha}$ is not stored. The critical effect of $PGF_{2\alpha}$ on the myometrium is to release intracellular calcium ion, which binds to *actin* and *myosin* to initiate the contractile process. Prostaglandins, both prostaglandin E and $PGF_{2\alpha}$, also have important effects on the cervix, which allow it to relax and dilate, allowing the passage of the fetus. The end result is a direct effect of $PGF_{2\alpha}$ on the intracellular matrix of the cervix, in which there is a loss of collagen with a concomitant increase in *glycosaminoglycans,* the latter affecting the aggregation of collagen fibers.

In some animals, such as the cow, goat, dog, and cat, $PGF_{2\alpha}$ synthesis and release initiates regression of the CL beginning 24 to 36 hours before delivery; complete withdrawal of progesterone occurs 12 to 24 hours before delivery. Although the withdrawal of progesterone in these species is essential for delivery,

it should be pointed out that progesterone withdrawal per se does not initiate delivery; it is the release of $PGF_{2\alpha}$ that both causes luteolysis and drives myometrial contractions.

In the mare, as in primates, delivery occurs even though progesterone concentrations remain elevated during the process. In this situation, $PGF_{2\alpha}$ is able to overcome the suppressive effects of progesterone on myometrial activity.

Oxytocin is also important for the delivery process (Fig. 37–6). Estrogen induces *oxytocin receptor* formation in the myometrium. Data indicate that significant amounts of oxytocin are released only with the entry of the fetus into the birth canal. Oxytocin release occurs through the so-called *Ferguson reflex.* The afferent stimulation for the reflex is by passage of impulses through sensory nerves in the spinal cord to the appropriate nuclei in the hypothalamus; the efferent pathway involves transport of oxytocin from the neurohypophysis by the blood vascular system. Oxytocin is synergistic with $PGF_{2\alpha}$ in promoting contraction of the uterus.

One hormone important for the preparation of parturition is relaxin. This hormone was first identified as responsible for the separation of the pubic symphysis through relaxation of the interpubic ligament. Relaxin causes the ligaments and associated muscles surrounding the pelvic canal to relax, which allows the fetus to expand the pelvic canal to its fullest potential. In the mare, a well-defined area of muscle softening can be discerned on the midline from the top of the croup through the ventral commissure of the vulva. In the cow, muscles posterior to the hip become re-

FIGURE 37–6. The neuroendocrine reflex (Ferguson reflex) underlying oxytocin synthesis and secretion. (From Johnson M, Everitt B [eds]: Essential Reproduction, 3rd ed. London: Blackwell Scientific, 1988, p 299.)

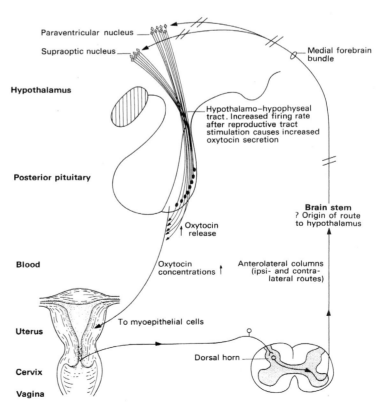

laxed to the point that they undulate as the animal walks in the final 24 hours before parturition. In the cow and pig, the CL is the source of relaxin. In both these species, the prepartum release of $PGF_{2\alpha}$ causes luteolysis with a concomitant decline in progesterone production and the release of preformed relaxin. In other domestic species, such as cats, dogs, and horses, the source of relaxin is the placenta. In these species, significant relaxin production begins during the first part of gestation, and values are sustained through parturition. A relaxin assay has been developed for the diagnosis of pregnancy in the dog with good accuracy when performed 25 days or more after conception. It may be that relaxin is important in these species for the maintenance of pregnancy in synergism with progesterone (see Fig. 37–2).

The *first stage of parturition* involves presentation of the fetus at the internal os of the cervix. This likely comes about because of increased myometrial activity resulting from $PGF_{2\alpha}$ release. Once the cervix opens and the fetus passes into the pelvic canal, myometrial contractions become less important for delivery of the fetus; abdominal press, accomplished by closure of the epiglottis and contraction of maternal abdominal muscles, becomes the main force involved in the delivery process. The actual delivery process is called the *second stage of parturition.*

The *third stage of parturition* involves the delivery of the fetal membranes. In litter-bearing animals, such as the cat, dog, and pig, the placental membranes are delivered often with, or immediately after, the appearance of each fetus. In single-bearing species, the placenta may be delivered immediately or within a few hours. Studies of mares at the University of California, Davis, have shown that major, sustained surges of $PGF_{2\alpha}$ occur in the immediate postpartum period and are important for expulsion of placental membranes and reduction of uterine size through myometrial contraction. $PGF_{2\alpha}$ is likely the most important contributor to uterine size reduction in the immediate postpartum period for all domestic species. This can be inferred from the episodes of discomfort that parturient animals undergo during the hours immediately after delivery.

The neonate must make a major physiologic adjustment to life outside the uterus. The major change involves the vascular system, particularly with regard to the respiratory system. During fetal life, blood bypasses the lungs (except for the perfusion of lung tissue in support of development) by two routes: through the atria by way of the *foramen ovale* and from the pulmonary artery to the aorta through the *ductus arteriosus.* The foramen ovale is closed functionally at birth by a flap of tissue in the left ventricle through the development of pressures within the left ventricle that exceed those within the right ventricle. Although the ductus arteriosus immediately constricts at birth, it requires months before it is completely closed. This course of closure is also true for the *ductus venosus,* which serves as a hepatic shunt during fetal life. The rapid conversion from a fluid to a gaseous environment, as occurs at birth, is a truly remarkable adaptation.

CLINICAL CORRELATIONS

Prolonged gestation

History You are called to examine a purebred Holstein cow that is 12 days overdue in comparison with the herd gestation average of 280 days. She was artificially inseminated, was found to be pregnant 35 days later, and has not been observed in estrus since insemination. You inquire about the presence of bulls on the dairy, but there are none.

Clinical examination The cow has a greatly enlarged abdomen. On palpation of the uterus per rectum, you find the presence of a large calf. The cow certainly appears to be term as far as the size of the calf. You are puzzled, though, by the lack of colostrum in the udder.

Comment The history and physical examination findings are compatible with an animal that has a fetus that is defective in terms of the initiation of parturition. A normal fetal hypothalamic-pituitary-adrenocortical system is essential for the production of cortisol, which initiates the delivery process. In the cow, this can begin 3 to 4 weeks before parturition, whereby fetal cortisol directs the increased production of estrogen; this, in turn, eventually initiates $PGF_{2\alpha}$ synthesis and release. The deficit could be the result of a malformation of the adrenal gland, pituitary gland, or hypothalamus. In one syndrome described for Holsteins, the critical defect was a lack of corticotropin-producing cells in the pituitary, which led to inadequate stimulation of the adrenal cortex and inadequate fetal cortisol production. The lack of lactogenesis reflects the fact that the endocrine changes that begin 3 to 4 weeks before parturition as a prelude to delivery are also important for lactogenesis, and in their absence, colostral formation is delayed.

Treatment The animal can respond to glucocorticoids; delivery usually occurs 2 to 3 days later. The placenta is normal in this situation, and the systemic administration of glucocorticoids substitutes for fetal cortisol in initiating the endocrine events that lead to parturition. Lactogenesis is usually initiated by glucocorticoid treatment, although the process is usually less advanced than that expected at normal delivery. Because the calf continues to grow in utero in this syndrome, it is often too large to be delivered vaginally, and a cesarean section may have to be performed 2 to 3 days after treatment in concert with dilation of the cervix.

You need to tell the owner that the calf will probably not survive because of inadequate adrenal secretion. If the calf were an extremely valuable bull prospect, one could administer both glucocorticoids and mineralocorticoids for a number of months with the hope the animal would eventually be able to take over its own adrenal support (this actually occurred in one case at the University of California, Davis). It would be questionable, however, to initiate treatment of the calf because the disease is an autosomal recessive inherited condition.

Bibliography

Austin CR, Short RV (eds): Reproduction in Mammals, vols 1–6. Cambridge, United Kingdom: Cambridge University Press, 1986.

Concannon PW, Morton DB, Weir BJ (eds): Dog and cat reproduction, contraception and artificial insemination. J Reprod Fertil Suppl vol 39, 1989.

Cupps PT (ed): Reproduction in Domestic Animals, 4th ed. New York: Academic Press, 1991.

Feldman EC, Nelson RW: Canine and Feline Endocrinology and Reproduction. Philadelphia: WB Saunders, 1996.

Hafez EWE (ed): Reproduction in Farm Animals, 5th ed. Philadelphia: Lea & Febiger, 1987.

Johnson M, Everitt B (eds): Essential Reproduction, 3rd ed. London: Blackwell Scientific, 1988.

Knobil E, Neill JD, Ewing LL, et al (eds): The Physiology of Reproduction, vols 1, 2. New York: Raven Press, 1988.

McDonald LE, Pineda MH (eds): Veterinary Endocrinology and Reproduction, 4th ed. Philadelphia: Lea & Febiger, 1989.

Olson PN, Nett TM, Bowen RA, et al: Endocrine regulation of the corpus luteum of the bitch as a potential target for altering fertility. J Reprod Fertil Suppl 39:27–40, 1989.

Silva LDM, Verstegen JP: Comparisons between three different extenders for canine intrauterine insemination with frozen-thawed spermatozoa. Theriogenology 44:571–579, 1995.

PRACTICE QUESTIONS

1. Active rescue of luteal activity by means of suppression of pulsatile prostaglandin synthesis and release by the production of embryonic signals must occur in which of the following species in order for a developing pregnancy to have the early progestational support that is essential for pregnancy maintenance? (Select more than one letter.)
   a. Cattle.
   b. Dog.
   c. Goat.
   d. Horse.
   e. Pig.
   f. Sheep.

2. In primates, it has been established that estrogen production during much of pregnancy is a cooperative venture between fetal adrenal glands and the placenta. The domestic species studied most extensively in this regard is the horse. In this species, the main two interactive organs involved in the synthesis of estrogen during pregnancy are
   a. the placenta and the fetal adrenal glands.
   b. the placenta and the fetal gonads.
   c. the placenta and the fetal liver.
   d. the placenta and the fetal hypothalamus.
   e. the placenta and the fetal pituitary.

3. Which of the following hormones initiates the final process that eventually leads to parturition?
   a. Maternal estrogen.
   b. Maternal progesterone.
   c. Fetal cortisol.
   d. Maternal relaxin.
   e. Maternal prostaglandin.
   f. Maternal oxytocin.

4. The hormone that initiates the myometrial contractile process that acutely initiates parturition is
   a. maternal estrogen.
   b. maternal progesterone.
   c. fetal cortisol.
   d. maternal relaxin.
   e. maternal prostaglandin.
   f. maternal oxytocin.

5. The hormone released by the passage of the fetus into the pelvic canal through the cervix is
   a. maternal estrogen.
   b. maternal progesterone.
   c. fetal cortisol.
   d. maternal relaxin.
   e. maternal prostaglandin.
   f. maternal oxytocin.

PRACTICE ANSWERS

1. a, c, d, e, f   2. b   3. c   4. e   5. f

38

The mammary gland

Anatomic aspects of the mammary gland

1 The milk-secreting cells of the mammary gland develop through the proliferation of epithelium into hollow structures called *alveoli*

2 Most of the milk that accumulates before suckling or milking is stored in the alveoli even though animals have enlarged milk-storage areas, called *cisterns*

3 A suspensory system involving the udder of the cow allows the animal to carry a large amount of milk

Control of mammogenesis

1 The initial development of the mammary gland is programmed by embryonic mesenchyme

2 Proliferation of the mammary duct system begins at puberty with ducts under the control of estrogens, growth hormone, and adrenal steroids and alveoli under the control of progesterone and prolactin

Colostrum

1 Prepartum milk secretion (without removal) results in the formation of colostrum

2 The ingestion of colostrum is important because of the passive immunity that it confers through the presence of high concentrations of immunoglobulins

3 The time during which immunoglobulins can be absorbed through the gut is limited to the first 24 to 36 hours of life

4 Lipids (particularly vitamin A) and proteins (caseins and albumins) are highly concentrated in colostrum; concentrations of carbohydrates (lactose) are low

Lactogenesis

1 Prolactin, inhibited by dopamine and stimulated by vasoactive intestinal peptide and growth hormone, is central to lactogenesis

2 The release of fat into milk from the alveolar cell involves constriction of the plasma membrane around the fat droplet; fats are dispersed in milk in droplet form

3 Milk proteins and lactose are released from alveolar cells by the process of exocytosis

4 Efficient milk removal requires the release of oxytocin, which causes contraction of muscle cells that surround the alveoli (myoepithelial cells) and movement of milk into the ducts and cisterns

5 Carbohydrate stores are increased in neonates born as singles or twins, whereas carbohydrate stores are low in neonates born in litters; the former can stand a longer interval to first suckling than can the latter

Composition of milk

1 Fats are the most important energy source in milk

2 Lactose, composed of glucose and galactose, is the main carbohydrate of mammalian milk

3 The main proteins in milk are called caseins and are found in curd

The Lactation Cycle

1 Milk production peaks 1 month after parturition in dairy cattle, followed by a slow decline in production; milking usually stops at 305 days after parturition, permitting preparation for the next lactation

2 Lactation can be induced by hormone administration (estrogen and progesterone) and enhanced by growth hormone and increased photoperiod exposure

Diseases associated with the mammary gland

1 Common diseases that affect the mammary gland directly are mastitis (prevalent in dairy cattle) and neoplasia (prevalent in intact bitches)

2 The mammary gland is involved with neonatal isoerythrolysis as a result of the passive transfer of red blood cell–agglutinating antibodies to the neonatal foal or kitten via nursing; eclampsia is hypocalcemia associated with lactation, most common in cows at the onset of the milking period and bitches in the perinatal period

Animals that belong to the class Mammalia are characterized as having bodies that are basically covered with hair, delivering live young instead of eggs (the monotremes are an exception), and, pertinent to this chapter, nurturing their young through the use of structures called *mammary glands.* The ability of mammals to nurture their young through milk secretion by mammary glands during the early part of postfetal life has given these animals survival advantages. Because the reproductive strategy of mammals involves the production of far fewer young than does that of reptiles, amphibians, and birds, mammary glands have allowed mammals to be much more efficient in the nurture of their young. Egg-laying classes of animals, such as fish, reptiles, and amphibians, depend on favorable environmental factors for the nurture of their young; the offspring are often vulnerable to the vagaries of nature. Mammalian young do not require teeth for the *suckling* process and thus can be delivered in a relatively mature state, although with immature maxillae and mandibles, which facilitates the delivery of the head. The development of teeth coincides with the need to consume food other than milk.

ANATOMIC ASPECTS OF THE MAMMARY GLAND

The milk-secreting cells of the mammary gland develop through the proliferation of epithelium into hollow structures called *alveoli*

Embryonic ectoderm is the source of the mammary glands. The mammary ectoderm is first represented by parallel linear thickenings on the ventral belly wall. The continuity of the ridge that is formed is broken into the appropriate number of *mammary buds* from which the functional part of the mammary gland is later derived.

The *parenchyma,* or milk-secreting cells, of the mammary gland develops through the proliferation of epithelial cells that arise from the primary mammary cord. The epithelial cells eventually form hollow, circular structures called *alveoli,* which are the fundamental milk-secreting units of the mammary gland (Fig. 38–1). In concert with this development, an enlarged area of epithelium, the *nipple,* which is the external connection to the internal milk-secreting system, develops on the surface. In males, although nipples often develop, the underlying primary mammary cord does not develop into glandular tissue.

Most of the milk that accumulates before suckling or milking is stored in the alveoli even though animals have enlarged milk-storage areas, called *cisterns*

Duct systems connect alveoli with the nipple, or teat, enabling milk to pass from the area of formation to the area of delivery (nipple). The ducts may come together so that there is only one final duct per gland, which has one opening through the nipple or teat, such as occurs in cattle, goats, and sheep. Two main ducts and associated openings occur in the mare and sow, whereas the cat and dog can have 10 or more openings in the nipple, each opening representing separate glands (Fig. 38–2). Both the cow and goat have specialized areas for holding milk, called *cisterns,* which are located in the ventral part of the gland and into which all main ducts empty (Fig. 38–3). This has enabled the cow, for example, to synthesize and store larger amounts of milk than would otherwise be possible. In spite of this adaptation, it is important to realize that a majority of the milk present

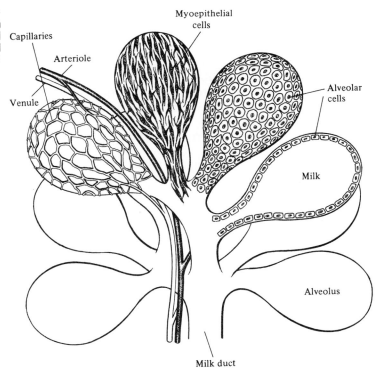

FIGURE 38–1. Diagram of a cluster of alveoli in the mammary gland of a goat. (From Cowie AT: Lactation. In Austin CR, Short RV [eds]: Hormonal Control of Reproduction, vol 3: Reproduction in Mammals, 2nd ed. Cambridge, United Kingdom: Cambridge University Press, 1984, pp 195–231.)

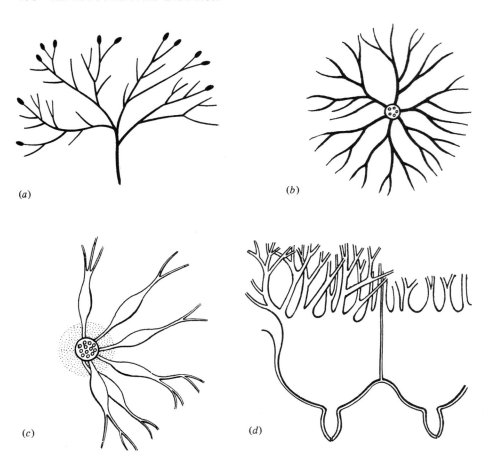

FIGURE 38-2. Diagram showing four different arrangements of the mammary duct system. (From Cowie AT: Lactation. In Austin CR, Short RV [eds]: Hormonal Control of Reproduction, vol 3: Reproduction in Mammals, 2nd ed. Cambridge, United Kingdom: Cambridge University Press, 1984, pp 195–231.)

at the time of milking is stored in the duct system of the mammary glands.

Mammary glands develop typically as paired structures. The number of pairs varies in domestic animals; for example, goats, horses, and sheep have one pair; cattle have two; sows have seven to nine; and dogs and cats have 7 to 10. The position of mammary glands varies in animals: it is thoracic in primates; it extends the length of the thorax and abdomen in cats, dogs, and pigs; and it is inguinal in cattle, goats, and horses. In domestic species, such as cattle, goats, horses, and sheep, pairs of mammary glands are closely apposed to each other; the resulting structure is called an *udder*. In the cow, for example, two pairs of glands (four quarters) compose the udder.

A suspensory system involving the udder of the cow allows the animal to carry a large amount of milk

One of the important anatomic adaptations of the udder that allows dairy cows to carry large amounts of milk is the development of a suspension system for the udder. This system is formed by the median suspensory ligament (formed between pairs of mammary glands) composed of elastic connective tissue that originates from the abdominal tunic. The lateral (nonelastic) suspensory ligament, which originates from prepubic and subpubic ligaments, enters the glands laterally at various levels to become part of the interstitial connective tissue framework of the udder. It is not unusual for heavily productive dairy cows to have 25 kilograms of milk in their udders immediately before milking. If the suspensory support system were not in place, the mammary gland system would soon break down because of the weight of the milk.

CONTROL OF MAMMOGENESIS

The initial development of the mammary gland is programmed by embryonic mesenchyme

The fetal development of the mammary gland is under both genetic and endocrine control. The initial development of the mammary bud is under control of embryonic mesenchyme (connective tissue). If mammary mesenchyme is transplanted to another area, mammary bud formation will occur at the site of transplantation. Although little is known about fetal mammary development, it is not thought to be driven by hormones. It is possible, however, for a neonate to have actively secreting mammary glands that have been caused by exogenous administration of certain hormones to the mother.

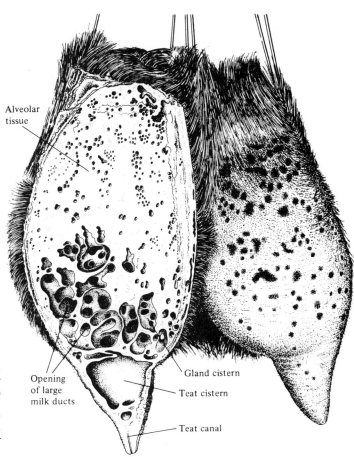

FIGURE 38–3. Depiction of the udder of a goat in which a section of the left mammary gland shows the dense alveolar tissues, the gland cistern with the large ducts opening into it, the teat cistern, and the teat canal. (From Cowie AT: Lactation. In Austin CR, Short RV [eds]: Hormonal Control of Reproduction, vol 3: Reproduction in Mammals, 2nd ed. Cambridge, United Kingdom: Cambridge University Press, 1984, pp 195–231.)

Proliferation of the mammary duct system begins at puberty with ducts under the control of estrogens, growth hormone, and adrenal steroids and alveoli under the control of progesterone and prolactin

Development of the mammary gland in postfetal life usually starts in concert with puberty. Cyclic ovarian activity results in the production of estrogen and progesterone. Estrogen, with growth hormone and adrenal steroids, is responsible for proliferation of the duct system. The development of alveoli from the terminal ends of the ducts requires the addition of progesterone and prolactin (Fig. 38–4).

Although the development of the mammary gland begins with the onset of puberty, the gland remains relatively undeveloped until the occurrence of pregnancy. In most domestic animals, udder development usually becomes evident by the middle of pregnancy; the secretion of milk often begins during the last trimester (mainly because of increasing prolactin secretion) and results in the formation of colostrum (colostrum is discussed later). By the end of pregnancy, the mammary gland has been transformed from a structure involving mostly stromal (connective tissue) elements to a structure filled with alveolar cells that are actively synthesizing and secreting milk.

Groups of adjacent alveoli form lobules that are further associated into larger structures called *lobes*. Connective tissue bands delineate the lobules and the lobes (Fig. 38–5).

COLOSTRUM

Prepartum milk secretion (without removal) results in the formation of colostrum

The milk formed before parturition is called *colostrum.* Its formation represents a secretory process in which lactogenesis occurs in the absence of milk removal. *Lactation,* however, cannot fully develop until parturition. This is because of the inhibitory effects of progesterone and estrogen on milk secretion; the inhibitory factors are removed at or just before delivery.

The ingestion of colostrum is important because of the passive immunity that it confers through the presence of high concentrations of immunoglobulins

When colostrum is formed before parturition, certain substances are concentrated in the process. Ingestion

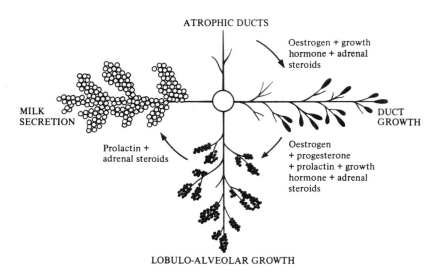

FIGURE 38–4. The hormones involved in the growth of the mammary gland and in the initiation of milk secretion in the hypophysectomized-ovariectomized-adrenalectomized rat. (From Cowie AT: Lactation. In Austin CR, Short RV [eds]: Hormonal Control of Reproduction, vol 3: Reproduction in Mammals, 2nd ed. Cambridge, United Kingdom: Cambridge University Press, 1984, pp 195–231.)

of colostrum is important for the well-being of the neonate. In addition to nutrition, colostrum has an important function in temporary, or passive, protection against infectious agents. *Immunoglobulins* (e.g., immunoglobulin A) are produced in the mammary gland by plasma cells (derived from B lymphocytes originating in the gut) as a result of exposure of the mother to certain microorganisms. The immunoglobulins gain access to the milk system through the migration of the plasma cells from adjacent tissue sites. The immunoglobulins are highly concentrated in colostrum, and through the consumption of colostrum, the neonate can receive passive immunity against pathogens encountered by the mother. This allows the young to receive immediate protection from environmental organisms. The neonates of all domestic animals acquire antibodies through the ingestion of colostrum. In contrast, in other species, including humans, rabbits, and guinea pigs, a significant amount of antibody is passed to the fetus through the placenta.

The time during which immunoglobulins can be absorbed through the gut is limited to the first 24 to 36 hours of life

Neonates usually have a limited time (24 to 36 hours) in which immunoglobulins (proteins) can be absorbed through the gut. Thus, the feeding of colostrum within this time period is important to ensure the presence of immunoglobulins in the newborn. Other antimicrobial factors found in milk that are important for protection against the development of enteric bacterial flora include lysozymes, lactoferrin, and the lactoperoxidase system.

Lipids (particularly vitamin A) and proteins (caseins and albumins) are highly concentrated in colostrum; concentrations of carbohydrates (lactose) are low

Colostrum is a rich source of nutrients, especially *vitamin A*, in addition to immunoglobulins. Placental transfer of vitamin A is limited in domestic animals;

calves and piglets have particularly low levels of vitamin A at birth. This deficiency is corrected by the ingestion of colostrum. Lipids and proteins, including *caseins* and *albumins,* are also present in relatively high concentration in colostrum. One exception is *lactose,* whose synthesis is significantly inhibited by progesterone until about the time of delivery. Nevertheless, at the moment of delivery, the milk supply is nutritive (high protein, fat, and vitamin A content) and protective (immunoglobulins) (Table 38–1).

LACTOGENESIS

Prolactin, inhibited by dopamine and stimulated by vasoactive intestinal peptide and growth hormone, is central to lactogenesis

Prolactin plays an important role in the secretion of milk, or *lactogenesis.* Prolactin is released in conjunction with manipulation of the teat through either the

TABLE 38–1. Amounts of selected components of bovine colostrum as percentage of level in normal milk

Constituent	Days after parturition		
	0	3	5
Dry matter	220	100	100
Lactose	45	90	100
Lipids	150	90	100
Minerals	120	100	100
Proteins			
Casein	210	110	110
Albumin	500	120	105
Globulin	3500	300	200
Vitamins			
A	600	120	100
Carotene	1200	250	125
E	500	200	125
Thiamine	150	150	150
Riboflavin	320	130	110
Pantothenic acid	45	110	105

From Jacobson NL, McGilland AD: The Mammary Gland and Lactation. In Swenson MJ (ed): Dukes' Physiology of Domestic Animals, 10th ed. Ithaca, New York: Cornell University Press, 1984.

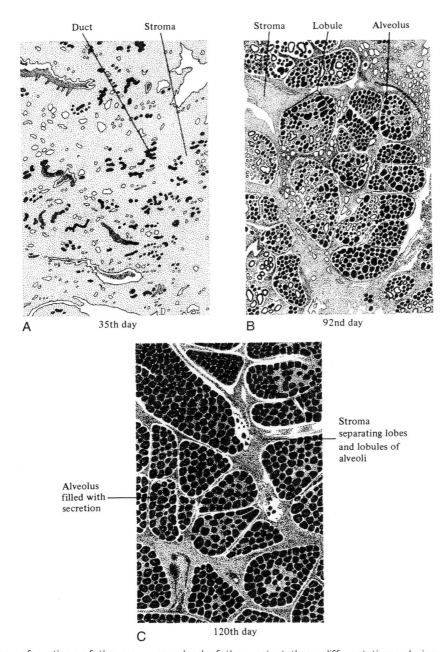

FIGURE 38–5. Drawings of sections of the mammary gland of the goat at three different times during pregnancy (which lasts approximately 150 days). *A,* Note the small collections of ducts scattered throughout the stroma on the 35th day. *B,* On the 92nd day, the lobules of alveoli are forming in groups known as lobes; secretion is present in some of the alveolar lumina and there is still considerable stromal tissue. *C,* On the 120th day, the lobules of alveoli are almost fully developed; the alveoli are full of secretion, and the stromal tissue is reduced to thin bands separating lobules and thicker strands between lobes. *(A–C, From Falconer IR [ed]: Lactation. London: Butterworths, 1970.)*

milking or the suckling process. Sensory stimuli are carried into the hypothalamus, wherein the synthesis of *dopamine,* a major inhibitor of prolactin secretion, is blocked, and neurons in the *paraventricular nucleus* are stimulated to produce *vasoactive intestinal peptide,* a stimulator of prolactin release (Fig. 38–6). A short-lived surge of prolactin secretion occurs immediately after the onset of milk removal; peak values are usually reached within 30 minutes after the initial stimulus. It is apparent that major surges of prolactin do not have to be elicited on an hourly basis to maintain lactation, because 12-hour release intervals, as occur in association with the milking of dairy cows, are sufficient to maintain lactogenesis. Prolactin responses, as judged by the amount of hormone release after mammary gland stimulation, decrease as the lactation period progresses.

Another major hormone required for milk production in ruminants is *growth hormone* (GH). There is now considerable interest in the use of GH to promote additional milk production from cows through exogenous administration of the hormone.

The release of fat into milk from the alveolar cell involves constriction of the plasma membrane around the fat droplet; fats are dispersed in milk in droplet form

The synthesis and release of milk by alveolar epithelial cells is a remarkable physiologic process (Fig.

38–7). Alveolar cells synthesize fats, proteins, and carbohydrates, and these products are extruded into the lumen of the alveolus. Fat droplets first accumulate in the basal cytoplasm of the cell and then move to the apex, where the droplet extrudes into the alveolar lumen. The cell membrane constricts about the base of the fat droplet, so that fat is dispersed in milk in small droplets, surrounded by cell membranes; the droplet often contains portions of cell cytoplasm.

Milk proteins and lactose are released from alveolar cells by the process of exocytosis

Milk proteins are synthesized on the endoplasmic reticulum; the casein molecules move into the Golgi apparatus, where they are phosphorylated and formed into micelles within the Golgi vesicles. Lactose is also synthesized within the Golgi vesicles and is released in conjunction with milk proteins. The process of extrusion of proteins and carbohydrates is different from that of fat; the Golgi vesicles fuse with the cell membrane, and the release of proteins and carbohydrates occurs by *exocytosis.* Although it is not certain how often cells go through a cycle of synthesis and extrusion, it probably occurs twice daily, particularly in dairy cows that are milked two times per day.

In order for lactogenesis to be maintained, milk must be removed from the mammary gland by suck-

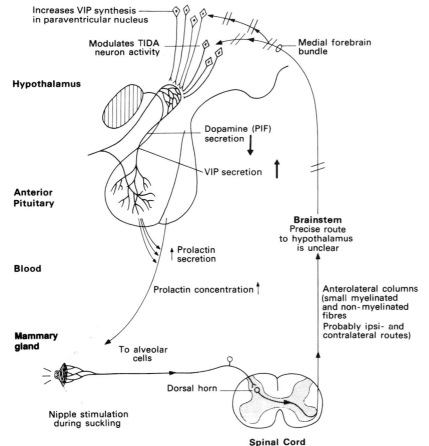

FIGURE 38–6. Somatosensory pathways in the suckling-induced reflex release of prolactin. The exact route taken by sensory information between brainstem and hypothalamus is speculative. Although tuberoinfundibular (TIDA) dopamine neuron activity is modulated as a result of the arrival of this somatosensory-derived input (prolactin inhibiting factor [PIF]), the increased secretory activity of neurons containing vasoactive intestinal protein (VIP) in the paraventricular nucleus is probably also crucial in driving prolactin secretion during suckling. (Adapted from Johnson M, Everitt B: Essential Reproduction, 3rd ed. London: Blackwell Scientific, 1988.)

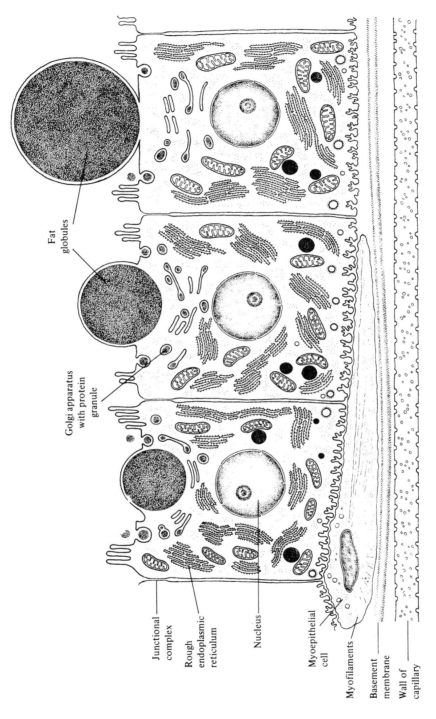

Fat
globules

Golgi apparatus
with protein
granule

Junctional
complex

Rough
endoplasmic
reticulum

Nucleus

Myoepithelial
cell

Myofilaments

Basement
membrane

Wall of
capillary

FIGURE 38–7. Diagram of the ultrastructure of three alveolar cells and a myoepithelial cell. (From Cowie AT: Lactation. In Austin CR, Short RV [eds]: Hormonal Control of Reproduction, vol 3: Reproduction in Mammals, 2nd ed. Cambridge, United Kingdom: Cambridge University Press, 1984, pp 195–231.)

ling or milking. If milk is not removed within about 16 hours in dairy cows, the synthesis of milk begins to be suppressed. As indicated previously, most of the milk in the udder of a dairy cow at the time of milking is located in the ducts and alveoli. The movement of milk into the gland cistern at suckling or milking would be slow, and less milk would be obtained during the milking of a cow, if the drainage of milk were a passive process.

Efficient milk removal requires the release of oxytocin, which causes contraction of muscle cells that surround the alveoli (myoepithelial cells) and movement of milk into the ducts and cisterns

To facilitate the process of milk removal, *myoepithelial cells* surround the alveoli and ducts (see Figs. 38–1 and 38–7). The myoepithelial cells are particularly responsive to *oxytocin* and, in fact, contract when exposed to the hormone. The synthesis and release of oxytocin from the posterior pituitary gland is elicited by a neuroendocrine reflex involving tactile stimulation of the udder by suckling by the young or the manual stimulation of washing before milking. The sensory stimuli from the udder are carried through the spinal cord into the hypothalamus. Neurons in the paraventricular and supraoptic nuclei are stimu-

lated to synthesize oxytocin and release it from nerve terminals that impinge on the median eminence (Fig. 38–8). Other sensory stimuli that elicit oxytocin release include auditory, visual, or olfactory stimuli that occur near or within the milking parlor. Traditional societies used various deceptions to get earlier breeds of cattle to release their milk. They often allowed the calf to suckle one teat while they milked the other glands. They also knew about the *Ferguson reflex*, if not in name, whereby stimulation of the cervix (and release of oxytocin) was effected by blowing air into the vagina by the use of hollow tubes.

The release of oxytocin occurs within seconds after the stimulus arrives in the hypothalamus; increased pressure within the mammary gland is evident within a minute of stimulation as milk is forced out of the alveoli and ducts because of contraction of the myoepithelial cells. The term used in mammals to describe this phenomenon is *letdown* of milk. Increased pressure within the udder is often obvious within a minute of the stimulation. The release of oxytocin lasts only a few minutes, and it is important that the milking process begin soon after the letdown of milk is complete (Fig. 38–9). The milking process, as done by machine or by hand, is often completed within 4 to 5 minutes.

It is interesting to compare stimuli that release oxytocin, which initiates the passive part of lactogenesis, with stimuli that release prolactin, which directly influences lactogenesis. Any sensory stimulus that a

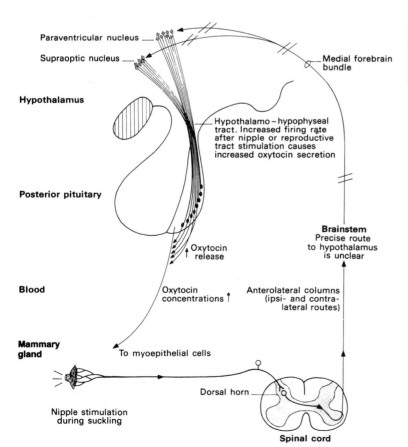

FIGURE 38–8. Somatosensory pathways in the suckling-induced reflex release of oxytocin. The actual pathway of sensory input in the hypothalamus is unknown, but it probably involves the medial forebrain bundle. (Adapted from Johnson M, Everitt B: Essential Reproduction, 3rd ed. London: Blackwell Scientific, 1988.)

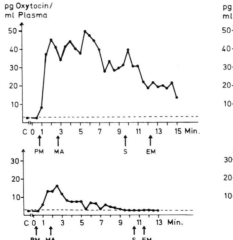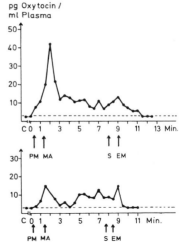

FIGURE 38–9. Oxytocin in the blood of cows before, during, and after milking. Abscissae show time in minutes. C, control level; EM, end of machine milking; PM, preparation for milking; MA, application of teat cups; S, stripping. (From Cowie AT: Lactation. In Austin CR, Short RV [eds]: Hormonal Control of Reproduction, vol 3: Reproduction in Mammals, 2nd ed. Cambridge, United Kingdom: Cambridge University Press, 1984, pp 195–231.)

cow associates with milking has the potential for releasing oxytocin. The neuroendocrine reflex is elicited in the expectation of milk removal because of the environment (milking parlor) to which the animal is exposed. Prolactin, in contrast, is released only by tactile stimulation of the udder. The latter makes sense, because there is no need to stimulate milk synthesis and release unless the evidence for milk removal (udder stimulation) is strong.

Carbohydrate stores are increased in neonates born as singles or twins, whereas carbohydrate stores are low in neonates born in litters; the former can stand a longer interval to first suckling than can the latter

In domestic animals that have one or two offspring, such as cattle, horses, sheep, and goats, the young have to be able to stand in order to suckle. In this situation, neonates have reasonably good carbohydrate stores, and suckling may be delayed for 1 to 2 hours without adverse effect as the young gain the ability to stand and locate the mammary gland. Young that are part of litters (cats, dogs, and pigs) are usually nestled toward the mammary glands immediately and often begin suckling within 30 minutes. This is important for animals born in litters, because they tend to be blind and nonambulatory at birth and susceptible to hypoglycemia, especially piglets, and suckling delays are often detrimental to their survival.

The suckling interval during the neonatal period varies considerably among domestic animals. Species nursing litters, such as cats, dogs, and pigs, often nurse at intervals of 1 hour or less. Goats, horses, and sheep nurse at slightly longer intervals, often up to 2 hours. Rabbits are an exception regarding the time interval between suckling periods; their young nurse at 24-hour intervals. As can be imagined, baby rabbits exhibit marked abdominal distension after each suckling period.

COMPOSITION OF MILK

Fats are the most important energy source in milk

Of the components of milk, fat is the most important energy source. Milk fat is composed of a number of lipids, including monoglycerides, diglycerides, triglycerides, free fatty acids, phospholipids, and steroids; *triglycerides* are the main component of milk fat. The types of lipid synthesized are complex; great variations in both chain length and saturation of fatty acids have been observed on the basis of species. The amount of fat produced varies greatly both within and among species (Table 38–2). Marine mammal milk has a high fat content, with values of about 40% to 50% in seals, 40% in dolphins, and 30% in whales. In this situation, the high energy content of the milk through fat helps offset the heat loss of the young.

In the milk of domestic animals, sheep, swine, dogs, and cats, fat content ranges from 7% to 10%. In dairy cattle it ranges from 3.5% to 5.5%; in goats, it is similar to that of cows (3.5%), and in mares, it is lower (1.6%). During earlier times, milk was sold on a butterfat basis, and breeds that had a relatively high butterfat content of milk (e.g., the Jersey, with 5% butterfat) found more acceptance in dairy operations than is currently the case. Small farms produced

TABLE 38–2. **Composition of milk from various species (percentage)**

Species	Fat	Protein	Lactose	Ash
Cat	7.1	10.1	4.2	0.5
Cow	3.5	3.1	4.9	0.7
Dog	9.5	9.3	3.1	1.2
Goat	3.5	3.1	4.6	0.8
Horse	1.6	2.4	6.1	0.5

Adapted from Jacobson NL, McGilliard AD: The Mammary Gland and Lactation. In Swenson MJ (ed): Dukes' Physiology of Domestic Animals, 10th ed. Ithaca, New York: Cornell University Press, 1984.

mainly cream (for butter manufacture); the fat-concentrated portion of milk was produced by use of a separator that separated cream on the basis of specific gravity and centrifugal force. Because milk is now sold on a solids, not fat, basis, breeds that produce more milk (and protein) are favored, even though the fat content of the favored breed, Holstein-Friesian, is lower (3.5%).

Lactose, composed of glucose and galactose, is the main carbohydrate of mammalian milk

Lactose is the main carbohydrate of most mammals. It is composed of glucose and galactose. Blood glucose is the main precursor molecule for lactose, with propionate an important precursor for glucose in ruminants. Lactose is formed under the direction of *lactose synthetase,* an enzyme composed of α-*lactalbumin* (a milk protein) and *galactosyl transferase.* Lactose synthesis is held in abeyance until immediately before term, because progesterone is inhibitory for the formation of α-lactalbumin. Prolactin, on the other hand, is stimulatory for the formation of lactose synthetase. Animals must have the enzyme *lactase* present in the jejunum in order for lactose to be cleaved (to glucose and galactose) and used. Lactase is present in most mammalian young but is sometimes not present in adult animals, including humans. In the absence of lactase, lactose can have an osmotic effect in the gastrointestinal tract, which can lead to diarrhea.

The main proteins in milk are called caseins and are found in curd

The main proteins produced by the alveolar cells are called *caseins.* Caseins can be removed (as a curd) from milk through a process called *curdling* or *coagulation;* other milk proteins, such as albumins and globulins, remain in the fluid part of the milk (whey).

THE LACTATION CYCLE

The time required for changeover from colostrum to normal milk secretion varies with each species. In cattle, *colostral milk* tends to be stringy and yellow for several days after parturition. The complex bovine udder needs time for all areas to be flushed of colostrum. The milk of cattle is withheld from commercial milk production for humans for several days because of its unacceptable aesthetics, not because of the quality of the milk.

Milk production peaks 1 month after parturition in dairy cattle, followed by a slow decline in production; milking usually stops at 305 days after parturition, permitting preparation for the next lactation

Milk production tends to increase for the first 3 to 4 weeks of lactation and then begins to decline slowly

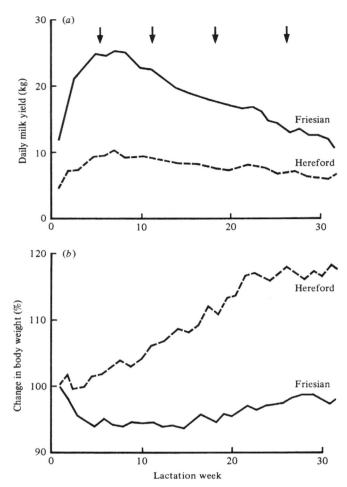

FIGURE 38–10. Average daily milk yield *(top)* and average percentage change in body weight *(bottom)* in seven low-yielding cows *(broken line)* and eight high-yielding cows *(solid line).* Arrows indicate times of blood sampling. (Courtesy of Dr. I. C. Hart. From Cowie AT: Lactation. In Austin CR, Short RV [eds]: Hormonal Control of Reproduction, vol 3: Reproduction in Mammals, 2nd ed. Cambridge, United Kingdom: Cambridge University Press, 1984, pp 195–231.)

(Fig. 38–10). Animals are usually "dried up" after 305-day lactational periods; pounds of milk and butterfat production rates are calculated on this basis. Animals are forced to stop lactating in order to prepare for the next lactation. The usual procedure is to stop milking the animals. The back pressure of milk within the alveoli gradually inhibits the secretion of milk by the alveolar epithelial cells, with a resultant regression of the alveolar cells and small ducts. The process, called *involution,* often requires at least a month, with a 6-week period usually desired as the minimal interval from drying off to the onset of the next lactational period. Within a period of 1 to 2 months, the secretory (alveoli) and excretory (duct) systems regress and are once again replaced. The process by which epithelial structures regress and yet retain coding for the renewal of duct and alveolar systems is truly remarkable.

Lactation can be induced by hormone administration (estrogen and progesterone) and enhanced by growth hormone and increased photoperiod exposure

The *induction of lactation* by hormone treatment is sometimes desired, especially in animals with high lactation records but poor reproductive performance. The use of a combined treatment of estrogen and progesterone over a relatively short period of time (1 week) has induced alveolar development sufficiently to result in milk production. Although the amount of milk produced is less than normal, the cows can be maintained in the milking string while efforts to get them pregnant continue. In order to induce lactogenesis by hormonal means, animals should not be lactating at the time of treatment, and their mammary glands should be free of infection.

GH, which is important to the normal lactational process, can be used for the enhancement of lactation when administered over a rather wide range of concentrations (Fig. 38–11). The ability to synthesize the hormone is relatively recent; its availability has increased interest in its use for increasing the amount of milk produced by dairy cows. In general, GH acts on the postabsorptive use of nutrients so that protein metabolism, fat metabolism, and carbohydrate metabolism in the whole body are changed, and the nutrients are directed toward milk synthesis. If cows are in early lactation and in a negative energy balance, GH administration results in the mobilization of body fats that are used for milk formation. If cows are in positive energy balance, GH has no effect on the metabolism of body fat. Initially, GH treatment decreases the energy balance of cows; however, this is adjusted by a voluntary increase in feed consumption. In spite of the increased feed consumption, GH administration increases the gross efficiency of lactation

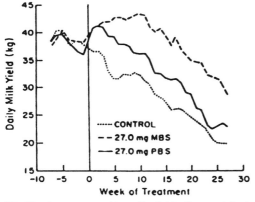

FIGURE 38–11. Average weekly milk yield of cows injected daily with diluent (control), 27 mg of methionyl bovine somatotropin (MBS), or 27 mg of pituitary bovine somatotropin (PBS). Treatments began at week 0 at an average of 84 ± 10 days after parturition. (From Tucker HA: Lactation and its hormonal control. In Knobil E, Neill J, Ewing LL, et al [eds]: The Physiology of Reproduction, vol 2. New York: Raven Press, 1988, pp 2235–2263.)

by as much as 19%. In essence, the effects of exogenous GH do not depend on gross alterations in nutrient digestibility or on body maintenance requirements. The use of GH may be economically viable, with the increased milk production justifying the expense of the hormone.

An interesting controversy has arisen from the fact that cows treated with GH do not produce "organically" derived milk, in spite of the fact that synthetic GH is almost identical to endogenously derived GH. Although there is no evidence that increased concentrations of GH occur in the milk as a result of its administration, some consider the resultant milk to be abnormal.

The results with GH are in contrast to those of the studies in which thyroid hormone administration, in the form of *iodinated casein* (thyroprotein), was used to increase lactation in cows. Although the administration of thyroprotein increased lactation, extra feed was necessary to prevent excessive body weight loss, and milk production declined abruptly when thyroprotein was removed from the diet. In essence, the use of thyroprotein does not affect the efficiency of the lactational process as GH does. In dogs, one differential diagnosis for gynecomastia is profound hypothyroidism, causing elevation in thyrotropin-releasing hormone levels, which in turn stimulates prolactin secretion.

Another interesting finding of the 1980s concerning the manipulation of lactation was that the milk yield in cows can be increased by exposing them to increased light. Cows under a *photoperiod regimen* of 16 hours of light (8 hours of dark) produced 6% to 10% more milk than did animals under the reverse photoperiod regimen (8 hours of light and 16 hours of dark) (Fig. 38–12). Although the mechanism by which light affects lactation is not known, it probably involves prolactin secretion, at least to some extent, in that increased light exposure results in increased prolactin secretion. Similarly, the queen's estrous cycle is affected by photoperiod, mediated by melatonin and prolactin levels. Melatonin and prolactin secretion may play a role in ovarian function in the cat, with lower levels of both hormones present during estrus than during the interestrous period. There exist protocols for improving lactation in postpartum bitches by means of low-dose oxytocin and metoclopramide (a dopamine agonist).

DISEASES ASSOCIATED WITH THE MAMMARY GLAND

Common diseases that affect the mammary gland directly are mastitis (prevalent in dairy cattle) and neoplasia (prevalent in intact bitches)

The most important problems involved in the production of milk are those caused by inflammation of the gland *(mastitis).* One fundamental cause of mastitis is injury to the teat canal from the repeated stretching

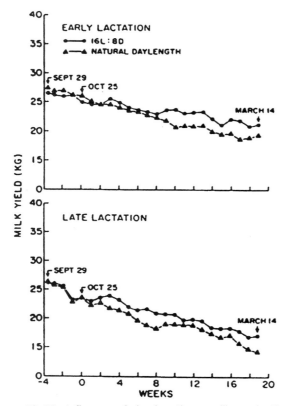

FIGURE 38–12. Influence of day length on milk production of Holstein cows. Between September 29 and October 24, cows 37 to 74 days (early lactation) or 94 to 204 days (late lactation) after parturition were exposed to natural photoperiods of 12 hours of light per day and standardized diets. Between October 25 and March 14, cows were exposed to natural photoperiod (9 to 12 hours of light daily) or to 16 hours of fluorescent lighting superimposed on the natural photoperiod. L, light; D, dark. (From Tucker HA: Lactation and its hormonal control. In Knobil E, Neill J, Ewing LL, et al [eds]: The Physiology of Reproduction, vol 2. New York: Raven Press, 1988, pp 2235–2263.)

that occurs with the milking process. Organisms that ordinarily would be excluded from the gland are able to make their way past the barrier located within the teat canal, and with repeated microorganism exposure, an infection is established.

One of the adverse consequences of mastitis is the formation of connective tissue within the udder as a result of the attempt of the gland to wall off the infection. The presence of connective tissue limits the area into which ducts and alveoli can proliferate, thus reducing the milk-producing potential of the gland. The mammary gland is an example of an organ (the eye is another example) in which the elicitation of an inflammatory response is often detrimental to the function of the organ. Thus, therapies directed toward the treatment of mastitis often combine anti-inflammatory and antibacterial agents.

Another process that disturbs the structure of the mammary gland is *neoplasia*. Of the domestic animals, the dog is most susceptible to the occurrence of mammary tumors. The exposure of the mammae to the ovarian hormones estrogen and progesterone greatly increases the chance of neoplasia. The incidence of mammary tumors is relatively low among dogs who are ovariectomized before the first estrous cycle, but it increases progressively through exposure to two ovarian cycles; ovariectomy performed after the third or fourth cycle has little effect on the incidence of neoplasia. Many owners have wanted their dogs to have one or two cycles before they are ovariectomized. It is important for veterinarians to point out the beneficial aspects of ovariectomy before the onset of puberty because of the incidence of mammary neoplasia, as well as the usual benefits of fertility and behavioral control.

— **The mammary gland is involved with neonatal isoerythrolysis as a result of the passive transfer of red blood cell–agglutinating antibodies to the neonatal foal or kitten via nursing; eclampsia is hypocalcemia associated with lactation, most common in cows at the onset of the milking period and bitches in the perinatal period**

An immunologic disease associated with the mammary gland involves the transfer of *red blood cell–agglutinating antibodies* to the fetus through the milk. The situation is most common in the horse, in which fetal red blood cells pass into the maternal system and elicit antibody formation against the fetal red blood cells. These antibodies tend to be concentrated in the colostrum along with other immunoglobulins. At birth, the foal is able to absorb the red blood cell–agglutinating antibodies (as well as other beneficial immunoglobulins) for up to 48 hours. Affected foals often go into a hemolytic crisis between 24 and 48 hours after delivery and can die unless given vigorous therapy, including blood transfusions. If fetal red blood cell antibody formation is suspected in a mare, the disease can be handled by muzzling the foal while with the dam at birth through 48 hours and bottle feeding with colostrum saved (frozen) from other preparturient mares. A similar condition has been reported in kittens born to queens sensitized by a previous litter with dissimilar blood type.

A disease that is associated with the mammary gland and that is life-threatening to the dam is *hypocalcemia*. At parturition, the acceleration of lactogenesis causes a great increase in the movement of calcium from the blood into the milk. Both cows and dogs are particularly susceptible; some dams are unable to respond immediately to the calcium drain from the blood by the mobilization of calcium. As a result, the animals lose their ability to maintain normal muscle activity, are often unable to stand, and become prostrate with the appearance of being comatose. The syndrome occurs in cows at parturition and in dogs during the last weeks of pregnancy or the first few weeks after parturition, when lactation reaches its peak. Inappropriate prenatal nutrition, often with excessive calcium supplementation, sets bitches up for this condition by inhibiting normal parathyroid gland development, which is necessary for meeting the demands for mobilization of calcium by lactation. The systemic administration of calcium to hypocalcemic cows often produces a dramatic recovery within 10 to 20 minutes.

CLINICAL CORRELATIONS

Neonatal isoerythrolysis

History   You are called to examine a mare, 7 months pregnant, that has a previous history of having conceived and delivered a normal foal after her first pregnancy; the foal was subsequently suckled and was sold as a weanling. The mare had no trouble conceiving and carrying the next two pregnancies, but the foals died within 2 days of birth even though they were healthy and vigorous at birth. The previous owner became discouraged because of these deaths and, as a result, sold the mare to the current owner at a bargain price.

Clinical examination   You perform a general physical examination of the mare and find all organ systems to be normal. Palpation of the uterus per rectum reveals the presence of a viable fetus that appears to be of the correct size for a pregnancy of the purported duration. Both the external genitalia and the mammary glands are normal in appearance.

Comment   From the history, and from the fact that the mare appears to be undergoing a normal pregnancy, you conclude that there is nothing wrong with the reproductive process per se. The fact that the previous two foals were healthy at birth and yet weakened rapidly and died within 2 days indicates that something likely happened to them after delivery. In mares, the most likely cause of this syndrome is neonatal isoerythrolysis. In this situation, the mare becomes exposed to the red blood cells of the fetus during the initial pregnancy (or this could occur initially at subsequent pregnancies). If fetal red blood cells enter the circulation of the dam, she responds by making antibodies to the red blood cells because of the presence of foreign antigen on the fetal red blood cells that were inherited from the sire. In the mare, these antibodies do not pass through the placental barrier, so the fetus is protected from these antibodies during pregnancy. The antibodies do pass into the colostrum and are concentrated during the process of colostrum formation.

Treatment   The foal needs to be prevented from suckling the mare for the first 2 to 3 days of life. During the first 1 to 2 days, the foal is able to absorb large protein molecules, including the important immunoglobulins that enable the foal to ward off infections, as well as, in this case, antibodies against fetal red cell antigens. The gut epithelium closes to the passage of large protein molecules by 36 to 48 hours of life; at this time, or shortly thereafter, the foal can be allowed to suckle without risk of absorbing the antibodies. The key is to prevent the foal from suckling during the first 2 to 3 days of life. The mare needs to be monitored closely before parturition so that the foal can be muzzled shortly after delivery. The foal does need nourishment during the first 2 to 3 days of life; thus, it is important that the foal be fed colostrum obtained from other mares (usually maintained frozen). Blood typing of stallions and mares is now conducted to anticipate this disorder.

Bibliography

Cowie T: Lactation. In Austin CR, Short RV (eds): Hormonal Control of Reproduction, vol 3: Reproduction in Mammals, 2nd ed. Cambridge, United Kingdom: Cambridge University Press, 1984, pp 195–231.

Feldman EC, Nelson RW: Hypothyroidism. In Canine and Feline Endocrinology and Reproduction, 2nd ed. Philadelphia: WB Saunders, 1996, pp 68–117.

Jacobson NL, McGilliard AD: The mammary gland and lactation. In Swenson MJ (ed): Dukes' Physiology of Domestic Animals, 10th ed. Ithaca, New York: Cornell University Press, 1984, pp 863–880.

Leyva H, Madley T, Stabenfeldt GH: Effect of light manipulation on ovarian activity and melatonin and prolactin secretion in the domestic cat. J Reprod Fertil Suppl 39:125–133, 1989.

McNeilly AS: Suckling and the control of gonadotropin secretion. In Knobil E, Neill J, Ewing LL, et al (eds): The Physiology of Reproduction, vol 2. New York: Raven Press, 1988, pp 2323–2340.

Tucker HA: Lactation and its hormonal control. In Knobil E, Neill J, Ewing LL, et al (eds): The Physiology of Reproduction, vol 2. New York: Raven Press, 1988, pp 2235–2263.

Wakerley JB, Clarke G, Summerlee AJS: Milk ejection and its control. In Knobil E, Neill J, Ewing LL, et al (eds): The Physiology of Reproduction, vol 2. New York: Raven Press, 1988, pp 2283–2321.

PRACTICE QUESTIONS

1. The development of the duct system in the mammary gland is under the control of estrogens, growth hormone, and adrenal steroids. If the duct system is to develop functional milk-secreting units, called alveoli, which of the following hormones is/are essential to this development?
   a. Progesterone.
   b. Prolactin.
   c. Relaxin.
   d. Prolactin and progesterone.
   e. Prolactin and relaxin.
   f. Progesterone and relaxin.

2. The hormone that is most important for the maintenance of lactation (lactogenesis) is
   a. estrogen.
   b. oxytocin.
   c. progesterone.
   d. prolactin.
   e. relaxin.

3. Sensory inputs, including sound, sight, and smell, but not necessarily touch, elicit the release of what important hormone required for the lactation process in the cow?
   a. Estrogen.
   b. Oxytocin.
   c. Progesterone.
   d. Prolactin.
   e. Relaxin.

4. The contraction of what anatomic structure is of fundamental importance for the release of milk from the udder of the cow?
   a. Alveoli.
   b. Duct.

c. Myoepithelial cell.
d. Duct cistern.
e. Teat cistern.

5. The most important energy source in milk is
   a. carbohydrates.
   b. lactose.

c. lipids.
d. proteins.

PRACTICE ANSWERS

1. d   2. d   3. b   4. c   5. c

Reproductive physiology of the male

Functional anatomy
1   The male reproductive system consists of many individual organs acting in concert to produce spermatozoa and to deliver them to the female's reproductive tract
2   Emission is the release of spermatozoa and accessory gland fluids into the pelvic urethra, whereas ejaculation is the forceful expulsion of semen from the urethra
Spermatogenesis
1   Spermatogenesis is a lengthy orchestrated process in which diploid stem cells divide by mitosis to maintain their own numbers and to cyclically produce progeny that undergo meiotic division and differentiation into haploid germ cells

The hypothalamic-pituitary-testicular axis
1   The reproductive system of the male is regulated by the hypothalamus, which is hormonally linked to the anterior pituitary and testes by luteinizing hormone and follicle-stimulating hormone
Puberty
1   Puberty is not synonymous with sexual maturity
2   Puberty results from a continuous process of endocrine changes that are initiated shortly after birth
Anabolic steroids
1   Anabolic steroids are androgen derivatives that exert negative feedback on the hypothalamic-pituitary-testicular axis

▬ FUNCTIONAL ANATOMY

▬ The male reproductive system consists of many individual organs acting in concert to produce spermatozoa and to deliver them to the female's reproductive tract

The male reproductive system is made up of a number of individual organs acting in concert to produce spermatozoa and deliver them to the reproductive tract of the female. This concerted effort involves both the neuroendocrine (hypothalamus and anterior pituitary glands) and the genital system. The genital organs consist of two testes, each suspended within the scrotum by a spermatic cord and external cremaster muscle; two epididymides; two deferent ducts; accessory sex glands; and the penis. The accessory sex glands include paired ampullae, paired seminal vesicles (vesicular glands), a prostate gland, and paired bulbourethral glands (Cowper glands). The presence of individual accessory glands, the testicular orientation, the type of penis, and the site of semen deposition in the female are dependent on the species (Table 39–1).

The scrotum, along with the cremaster muscles and the vascular anatomy of the testicular arteries and veins, protects and thermoregulates the testes. Present in all domestic animals, the scrotum essentially is a skin pouch with a subcutaneous fibroelastic and muscular layer called the *tunica dartos*. The vascular arrangement of the testicular artery surrounded by the plexus of testicular veins (pampiniform plexus) provides a countercurrent heat exchange mechanism that is vital to testicular thermoregulation. Contraction and relaxation of the tunica dartos and cremaster muscles occur with changes in ambient temperature as well as in response to other tactile stimuli. The scrotum of some species, such as the horse, contains numerous sweat and sebaceous glands that further contribute to the thermoregulatory mechanism.

The testis is the pivotal organ of the male reproductive system. It must be remembered, however, that all testicular functions are profoundly influenced by the neuroendocrine system. The testis is responsible for steroidogenesis, primarily the production of androgens, as well as the generation of haploid germ cells by spermatogenesis. These two functions occur in the Leydig cells and the seminiferous tubules, respectively.

Functionally, the testis is considered to have three compartments. The *interstitial tissue* compartment, containing the Leydig cells, surrounds the seminiferous tubules and bathes them with testosterone-rich fluid. The other two compartments reside within the seminiferous tubules. The *basal* compartment contains

TABLE 39–1. **Male reproductive parameters**

	Bull, Buck and Ram	Stallion	Boar	Dog	Tom	Llama
Testis orientation	Vertical cauda down	Horizontal	Perineal cauda up	Horizontal	Perineal cauda up	Perineal cauda up
Ampullae	+	+	±	±	−	±
Seminal vesicle	+	+	+	−	−	−
Bulbourethra	+	+	+ +	−	+	+
Prostate	+	+	+	+	+	+
Penis type	Fibroelastic sigmoid	Vascular	Fibroelastic sigmoid	Vascular	Vascular	Fibroelastic sigmoid
Semen deposition	Vagina	Uterus	Cervix	Vagina	Vagina	Cervix/uterus

spermatogonia, which divide through mitosis, whereas the *adluminal* compartment represents a special environment where spermatocytes undergo meiosis and continue their meiotic divisions to differentiate into spermatids and finally into spermatozoa. Within the seminiferous tubules, the Sertoli cells, which provide support and nourishment to the developing germ cells, extend from the basal compartment into the adluminal compartment. Tight-junctional complexes between the Sertoli cells separate the basal and adluminal compartments and form the major component of the blood-testis barrier, which functionally prevents many compounds found in the blood and interstitial fluid from entering the adluminal compartment.

In domestic mammals, normal testicular function, especially normal spermatogenesis, is temperature dependent and requires an environment that is lower than core body temperature. Hence, in normal domestic males, the testes are located outside the abdominal cavity, in the scrotum. Failure of one or both of the testes to descend into the scrotum is known as *cryptorchidism*. Although the cryptorchid testis is still capable of producing androgens, it is incapable of producing normal spermatozoa. Consequently, a bilaterally cryptorchid male would be sterile. The cryptorchid testis is more prone to torsion of the spermatic cord and 10 times more likely to be neoplastic. Cryptorchidism appears to be genetic, although the exact mechanism is not completely understood and may vary among species. It is most common in boars, dogs, and stallions and least common in bulls, rams, and bucks. Descent of the testes into the scrotum normally occurs in domestic animals during the following time periods:

Horse: 9 to 11 months of gestation
Cattle: 3.5 to 4 months of gestation
Sheep: 80 days of gestation
Pig: 90 days of gestation
Dog: 5 days after birth
Cat: 2 to 5 days after birth
Llama: usually present at birth

For the majority of domestic species, passage of the testes through the internal rings by 2 weeks after birth is necessary for a final scrotal position to occur. Many animals may have testes in the inguinal region

at birth, and the testes may remain there for weeks or months before descending into the scrotum. In the dog, testicular descent is uncommon after 14 weeks of age and does not occur after 6 months of age. In the stallion, although it is considered abnormal, descent of inguinally retained testes has been known to occur as late as 2 to 3 years of age.

The seminiferous tubules empty their contents into the rete testis, which subsequently transports the spermatozoa and seminiferous tubular fluid into the epididymis. The epididymis is a single tortuous duct of considerable length (from 2 m in the cat to 80 m in the stallion) that is anatomically divided into three segments: head, or caput; body, or corpus; and tail, or cauda. The epididymis not only is a conduit for spermatozoa but also provides a special environment in which spermatozoa are concentrated, undergo maturation, and acquire fertilizing capacity. Spermatozoa that enter the caput from the rete testis are immotile and incapable of fertilization. Only after they undergo migration and maturation through the caput and corpus are both motility and the capacity for fertilization achieved. The cauda epididymis and the deferent duct, into which the cauda empties, serve as a storage depot for mature spermatozoa; together, these are known as the *extragonadal sperm reserves*. The spermatozoal transit time through the caput and corpus epididymis is not altered by ejaculation and is similar (2 to 5 days) for domestic species. Storage time in the cauda epididymis is more variable among species (3 to 13 days) and can be reduced by several days in sexually active males. Animals that rest sexually for 7 to 10 days have a maximum number of spermatozoa in the cauda epididymis, and this reserve is reduced by at least 25% with daily or every other day ejaculation.

The deferent ducts, or vasa deferentia, pass through the inguinal rings into the abdomen and connect the cauda epididymis with the pelvic urethra. In most species, the terminal portion of the deferent ducts enlarges to form prominent ampullae such as those found in the bull and the stallion. In other species, the ampullae either are absent or are anatomically indistinct from the vasa deferentia. The ampullae serve as an additional storage depot for spermatozoa, and in some species, such as the bull, stallion, and dog, ampullary glands add to the ejaculate. Along with spermatozoa, ejaculated semen is composed primarily of accessory gland secretions that add volume, nutrients, buffers, and a number of other substances whose exact functions are unknown. The contribution to the ejaculate by each of the accessory glands varies with the species and is responsible for the variation in concentration, volume, and character between ejaculates. The seminal vesicles lie lateral to the ampullae near the neck of the bladder. In the bull, ram, and buck, these organs are firm and lobulated with a narrow lumen, whereas in the stallion and boar, they are more sac-like. The dog and tom lack seminal vesicles but have relatively prominent prostate glands, especially the dog. The prostate gland is present in all domestic males and is intimately associated with the pelvic urethra, but it varies in size and appearance among species. The bulbourethral glands of the tom are nearly as large as the prostate, but these glands are absent in the dog. In the stallion and bull, the bulbourethral glands are small, round to ovoid structures that lie adjacent to the pelvic urethra near the ischial arch, whereas those of the boar are large and cylindric. The male llama lacks seminal vesicles, and both the bulbourethral and prostate glands are small.

The copulatory organ of the male is the penis. It is more or less cylindric in all species and extends from the ischial arch to near the umbilicus on the ventral abdominal wall, except in the tom and the llama, in which the penis points posteriorly in the relaxed state. The body of the penis is surrounded by a thick fibrous capsule (the tunica albuginea) that encloses numerous cavernous spaces (the corpus cavernosum penis) as well as the corpus spongiosum penis, which immediately surrounds the urethra. Erection is a psychosomatic event that involves mutually occurring actions of the vascular, neurologic, and endocrine systems. Contraction of the ischiocavernosus muscle during erection results in occlusion of venous outflow. At the same time, the parasympathetically mediated relaxation of corpus cavernosum and corpus spongiosum results in these cavernous spaces becoming engorged with blood, and the penis becomes elongated and turgid.

Emission is the release of spermatozoa and accessory gland fluids into the pelvic urethra, whereas ejaculation is the forceful expulsion of semen from the urethra

Emission is the release of spermatozoa and accessory gland fluids into the pelvic urethra as a result of sympathetically mediated thoracolumbar reflex contraction of the smooth muscle in the ductus deferens and accessory glands. *Ejaculation* is the forceful expulsion of semen from the urethra and is prompted by a parasympathetically mediated sacral reflex that induces rhythmic contractions of the bulbospongiosus, ischiocavernosus, and urethralis muscles. After ejaculation, a sacral sympathetically mediated increase in the smooth muscle tone of the cavernous spaces increases the outflow of blood, and contraction of the retractor penis muscle withdraws the penis into the prepuce.

SPERMATOGENESIS

Spermatogenesis is a lengthy orchestrated process in which diploid stem cells divide by mitosis to maintain their own numbers and to cyclically produce progeny that undergo meiotic division and differentiation into haploid germ cells

Spermatogenesis is a lengthy orchestrated process in which diploid stem cells at the base of the seminiferous tubules (spermatogonia) divide through mitosis to maintain their own numbers and to cyclically produce progeny that undergo further meiotic division and differentiation into haploid spermatids, which are released as spermatozoa (Fig. 39–1). Spermatogenesis is generally divided into three major events: spermatocytogenesis, meiosis, and spermiogenesis. Spermatocytogenesis accomplishes two important functions. First, the mitotic divisions of type A spermatogonia produce other spermatogonia that are not yet committed to the immediate spermatozoal production process, thus maintaining a population of stem cells. These stem cell divisions are responsible for the ability of the male to continuously produce spermatozoa throughout his adult life. Second, type A spermatogonia become type B spermatogonia, which further divide through mitosis to produce primary spermatocytes. The primary spermatocytes enter into the pool of meiotically dividing cells and ultimately produce spermatozoa.

Meiosis occurs only during the processes of oogenesis and spermatogenesis, in which the haploid condition results after two cell divisions with only one chromosomal duplication. During meiosis, homologous chromosomes pair, and this facilitates the exchange of genetic material between chromosomes. At the first meiotic division, the homologous chromosomes segregate into the two resulting cells, creating a haploid condition. In the male, the resultant haploid cells are the secondary spermatocytes with duplicated chromatids. In less than 1 day after their formation, secondary spermatocytes divide to form spermatids that contain one chromatid from each of the haploid chromosomes.

The newly formed spermatids continue to differentiate without dividing to form mature spermatids through the process of spermiogenesis. Spermiogenesis occurs just before spermatids are released as spermatozoa at the luminal surface of the seminiferous tubule (spermiation). The major features of spermiogenesis include formation of the acrosome from the Golgi apparatus, condensation and elongation of the nucleus, formation of the flagellum, and extensive shedding of cytoplasm. The spermiated spermato-

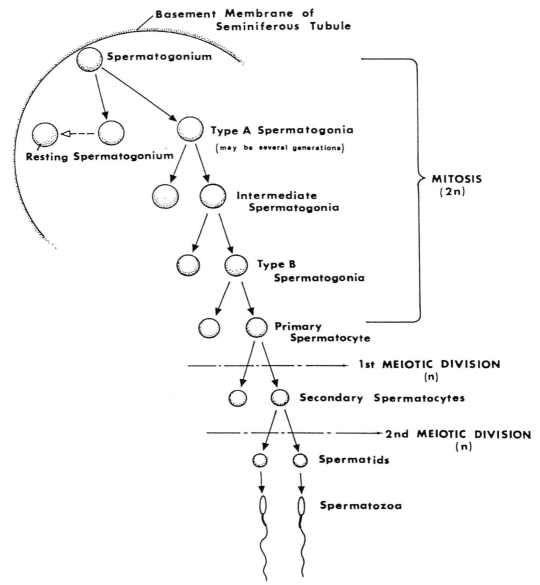

FIGURE 39-1. Diagram of spermatogenesis. (From McDonald LE, Pineda MH [eds]: Veterinary Endocrinology and Reproduction. Philadelphia: Lea & Febiger, 1989.)

zoon consists of a head, middle piece, and tail. The head contains the genetic material to be combined with that of the oocyte during fertilization. Overlying the head is the acrosome, which contains hydrolytic enzymes necessary for penetration of the oocyte. The middle piece contains mitochondria, which provide the energy for microtubules extending into the tail to slide back and forth, past each other, thus producing tail movement. Taking epididymal transit time into account, the interval from type A spermatogonia to ejaculated spermatozoa is approximately 60 to 70 days for the ram and the bull and 50 to 60 days for the boar, the dog, and the stallion. Therefore, the interval from an event that may adversely affect the testis or epididymis to a decline in seminal quality may be as short as a few days to as long as 2 months. Similarly, at least 60 days would likely be required

for an ejaculate to return to normal after a toxic insult to the testis.

In theory, 16 primary spermatocytes and 64 spermatozoa develop from one type A spermatogonium in the bull and the ram. However, a percentage of potential sperm production is lost to degeneration during the normal course of spermatogenesis. In humans, approximately 40% of the sperm production potential is lost during the latter stages of meiosis. Daily sperm production is the number of spermatozoa produced per day by the testes. It is highly correlated with testicular size and is not affected by frequency of use for breeding. Because of the influence of testicular size, there is a wide range in daily sperm production among domestic species. For example, daily sperm production has been calculated to be 0.37×10^9 in the dog and 16.2×10^9 in the boar. Within a species, both individual and breed variation in testicular size can also influence daily sperm production.

THE HYPOTHALAMIC-PITUITARY-TESTICULAR AXIS

The reproductive system of the male is regulated by the hypothalamus, which is hormonally linked to the anterior pituitary and testes by luteinizing hormone and follicle-stimulating hormone

The reproductive system of male mammals is regulated by intricate feedback mechanisms involving the hypothalamus, anterior pituitary, and testes (Fig. 39–2). The hypothalamus synthesizes and secretes the decapeptide gonadotropin-releasing hormone (GnRH). Secreted in a pulsatile manner, GnRH acts directly on gonadotropic cells in the anterior pituitary. On stimulation by GnRH, these gonadotropes synthesize and secrete the gonadotropins follicle-stimulating hormone (FSH) and luteinizing hormone (LH). Both FSH and LH are heterodimeric glycoproteins made up of two noncovalently linked polypeptides. The α subunit protein is common to both FSH and LH, whereas the β subunit is specific for each. Individual gonadotropes have the ability to synthesize and secrete FSH, LH, or both. The release of FSH and LH is dependent on the pulsatile pattern of GnRH secretion. Irregular, low-amplitude GnRH pulses result in FSH release, whereas high-frequency GnRH pulses induce the release of LH.

Within the testis, LH binds to membrane receptors on the Leydig cells and stimulates them to convert cholesterol to testosterone. Synthesized androgens diffuse into blood and lymph, where they are bound to androgen-binding protein produced by the Sertoli cells. High local concentrations of androgens within the testis are considered essential for normal spermatogenesis to occur. Androgen-binding protein enhances the accumulation of testosterone and dihydrotestosterone in high concentrations within the seminiferous tubules and the interstitium of the testis. Within the testis, the target cells for testosterone are the peritubular myoid cells and the Sertoli cells, which envelope and support the developing sperm cells. Androgen-binding protein also facilitates the transport of androgens from the testis to the epididymis, where these hormones influence epididymal transit and the further maturation of spermatozoa.

Studies have demonstrated that FSH specifically targets receptors on the Sertoli cells within the seminiferous tubules. FSH and testosterone stimulate a variety of Sertoli cell functions, including the synthesis and secretion of androgen-binding protein, inhibin, activin, estrogen, and several products such as transferrin that are involved in the transfer of nutrients to germ cells; meiosis; spermatocyte maturation; spermiation; and Leydig cell function. Sertoli and Leydig cells appear to interact in a paracrine fashion.

Steroid production of Leydig cells can be stimulated by a product released by Sertoli cells, the secretion of which is enhanced by FSH. A potential candidate for such a substance is inhibin, which is produced by Sertoli cells in response to FSH and stimulates steroidogenesis in Leydig cells. Inhibin, along with testosterone, is involved in the complex feedback regulation of pituitary function. Gonadal steroids are known to suppress FSH release, but inhibin appears to be the most potent inhibitor of FSH secretion from the pituitary. Testosterone, dihydrotestosterone, and estrogen regulate LH synthesis and secretion through negative feedback exerted at the level of hypothalamus or the anterior pituitary gland. Because FSH and LH are necessary for high testicular concentrations of substances responsible for normal spermatogenesis, exogenous administration of testosterone or inhibin to enhance fertility would be contraindicated since they would impede the secretion of those factors responsible for maintaining an optimal spermatogenic environment.

PUBERTY

Puberty is not synonymous with sexual maturity

Puberty in the male is when he is first able to produce sufficient numbers of sperm to impregnate a female. For practical reasons, for bulls, boars, rams, and stallions, this could be defined as the age when the ejaculate contains 50×10^6 spermatozoa, of which 10% or more are motile. It must be remembered that puberty is not synonymous with sexual maturity, which can occur months to years later, depending on the species.

Puberty results from a continuous process of endocrine changes that are initiated shortly after birth

The pituitary gland, gonads, and steroid-dependent target tissues are capable of responding to stimulatory hormones before puberty; therefore, the hypothalamus is considered to play a pivotal role in the initiation of puberty. Puberty appears to be the end result of a continuous process of endocrine changes that are initiated shortly after birth. Some investigators theorize that puberty occurs when the animal's hypothalamic-pituitary complex becomes desensitized to the feedback inhibition of gonadal steroids. This desensitization would apparently allow increased discharge of GnRH from the hypothalamus and a greater response of the pituitary to GnRH. Although numerous factors can influence the modulation by the central nervous system of the endocrine system, the major factors that affect age at puberty in domestic animals are breed, energy intake, and season of birth.

The hypothalamic-pituitary-gonadal system in humans differentiates and functions during fetal life and

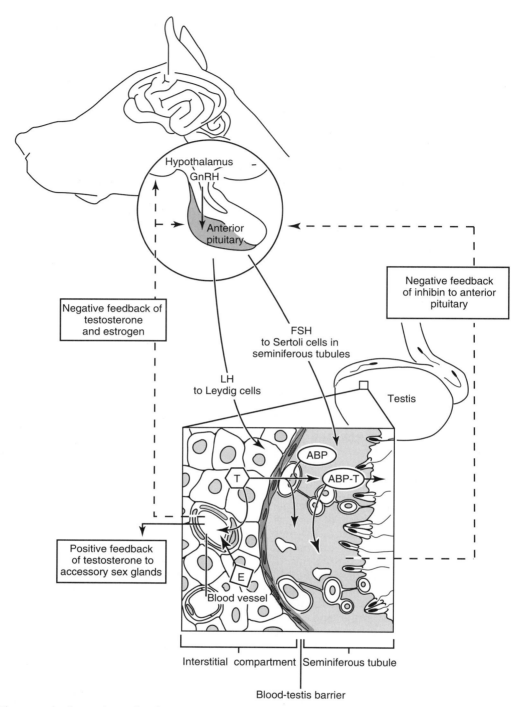

FIGURE 39–2. The reproductive system of male mammals is regulated by intricate feedback mechanisms that involve the hypothalamus, anterior pituitary, and testes. ABP, androgen-binding protein; ABP-T, androgen-binding protein–testosterone; E, estrogen; FSH, follicle-stimulating hormone; GnRH, gonadotropin-releasing hormone; LH, luteinizing hormone; T, testosterone.

briefly during infancy; it then is suppressed during childhood and is reactivated during puberty after almost a decade of low activity. Inhibition of the hypothalamic-pituitary-gonadal system in prepubertal children is mediated through the suppression of GnRH synthesis and pulsatile secretion. Progressive pulsatile stimulation of the pituitary by GnRH and the gonads by LH and FSH is required for the initiation and progression of puberty. Prepubertal children

secrete small amounts of FSH and LH from the pituitary, indicating that the hypothalamic-pituitary-gonadal axis is functional but at a low level. This low level of gonadotropin secretion rapidly decreases when sex steroids are administered. Therefore, there appears to be a highly sensitive negative feedback mechanism in young prepubertal children, and a similar mechanism is likely to exist in prepubertal domestic animals.

ANABOLIC STEROIDS

Anabolic steroids are androgen derivatives that exert negative feedback on the hypothalamic-pituitary-testicular axis

The use of anabolic steroids has become widespread in human and animal athletes, as many attempt to increase performance. Testimonials from veterinarians, physicians, human athletes, and trainers indicate that improvements in the athlete's mental attitude, stamina, and physical strength are attained after anabolic steroids are administered. What is of major concern is the fact that many individuals receiving anabolic steroids are peripubescent or prepubescent. Anabolic steroids are androgen derivatives that have been altered to maximize their anabolic action and to minimize their androgenic side effects. It is not yet possible, however, to produce anabolic steroids that are devoid of androgenic activity, and many of the undesirable side effects of these drugs are caused by their androgenic activity. The adverse reproductive side effects observed with anabolic steroid use are similar to those associated with testosterone administration. Sustained testosterone or anabolic steroid administration affects pituitary function and leads to long-lasting impairment of testicular endocrine function. Potential side effects of the use of anabolic steroids in young animals may lead to incomplete development of the hypothalamic-pituitary-gonadal axis. The long-term side effects of anabolic steroid use on reproductive parameters in sexually immature animals are not yet known.

A high percentage of colts and stallions in training or racing receive androgenic drugs, including anabolic steroids, and these horses have smaller testicles than similar horses not receiving such drugs. Only two anabolic steroids—stanozolol and boldenone undecylenate—are approved by the Food and Drug Administration for use in horses. Neither of these is approved for use in stallions. The administration of anabolic steroids to stallions has been shown to reduce seminal quality, daily sperm output, daily sperm production, and testicular size. These effects most likely result from a negative feedback mechanism on gonadotropin release from the pituitary. Alterations in seminal parameters are also observed, including depression of sperm concentration, sperm motility, and total number of sperm per ejaculate. Histologic examination of the testes demonstrates a reduction in the number of developing germ cells other than type A spermatogonia. In addition, the mean diameter of Leydig cells is decreased, and changes indicative of testicular degeneration, including marked cytoplasmic vacuolization, shrunken tubules and Leydig cells, and phagocytosis of spermatids by multinucleated giant cells, have been observed. These adverse effects on the testes tend to be more severe in younger stallions. Repeated implantation of anabolic steroids in prepubertal bulls also results in decreased testicular size. Effects on testicular growth are dependent on the type of anabolic steroid administered, the age of the patient, and the dosage and duration of therapy.

Human studies, which did not directly investigate the effects of anabolic steroids on spermatogenesis, also found reduced levels of circulating gonadotropins, testosterone, or both. Individuals using high doses of testosterone and anabolic steroids for only 3 months still had hypogonadotropic hypogonadism 3 weeks after the cessation of drug use. The presence of atrophic testicles and low LH, FSH, and testosterone levels after drug withdrawal indicates that long-term androgenic or anabolic steroid use affects pituitary function and leads to long-lasting impairment of testicular endocrine function.

Questions regarding the possibility of permanent sterility or testicular atrophy with long-term anabolic steroid use have not been answered for adults, and even less is known about the effects in prepubertal or peripubertal individuals. Indirect evidence suggests that prepubertal individuals may be at a higher risk for permanent derangements from anabolic steroid use than adults. Therefore, the use of anabolic steroids in males intended for breeding should be strongly discouraged.

CLINICAL CORRELATIONS

Infertility in a stallion

History   You are asked to perform a breeding soundness examination on a 3-year-old quarter horse stallion who was mated with 10 mares last year and impregnated only 1 mare. The stallion is in demand because of his bloodlines and the fact that his muscular and mature appearance contributed to his winning a number of shows as a yearling. All of the mares mated to this young stallion have been shown to be free of reproductive abnormalities. You ask whether the horse has had any illness or febrile episodes or has been on any medication recently. The answer to all these queries is no.

Clinical examination   The stallion demonstrates normal libido when exposed to a mare in estrus, and two ejaculates are obtained 1 hour apart by means of an artificial vagina. Examination of both semen samples reveals poor spermatozoal concentration, low sperm numbers, and a high percentage of morphologically abnormal spermatozoa and immature germ cells. The stallion has a normal penis and prepuce, but his testes are small and soft. You ask if the stallion has ever received anabolic steroids, and with some reluctance the owner admits that the trainer did give anabolic steroids to the horse in preparation for the yearling futurity and for shows thereafter.

Comment   The use of anabolic steroids in performance animals is not uncommon. Even so, many owners and trainers are reluctant to admit to their use. Many colts are given these drugs to give them a competitive edge in the show ring or on the racetrack so that they will later be in demand as sires. Unfortunately, because they are testosterone derivatives, the negative feedback effects of anabolic steroids adversely affect the fertility of these animals, sometimes permanently. It is not known how severe or long-standing the adverse effects will be if anabolic steroids are given in the peripubertal period. The fact that this animal's testes are so small and soft indicates that he apparently received high doses of anabolic steroids for a prolonged period of time during the development of the hypothalamic-pituitary-testicular axis, and the effects are most likely irreversible. It must be noted that as a 3-year-old, the horse is not yet sexually mature, and in the future he may still be able to produce sufficient numbers of normal spermatozoa to impregnate a small number of mares per season but certainly not a full book.

Treatment   Other than time, there is no known treatment that will reverse the detrimental side effects caused by anabolic steroid use in adult males. Even less is known about the long-term effects in young animals.

BIBLIOGRAPHY

Amann RP, Schanbacher BD: Physiology of male reproduction. J Anim Sci 57(suppl 2):380–403, 1983.

Knobil E, Neill JD, Ewing LL, et al (eds): The Physiology of Reproduction, vols 1 and 2. New York: Raven Press, 1988.

Robaire B, Pryor JL, Trasler JM: Handbook of Andrology. Lawrence, KS: Allen Press, 1995.

Roberts SJ: Veterinary Obstetrics and Genital Diseases Theriogenology, 3rd ed. Woodstock, VT: David & Charles, 1986.

Yen SC, Jaffe RB: Reproductive Endocrinology: Physiology, Pathophysiology, and Clinical Management, 3rd ed. Philadelphia: WB Saunders, 1991.

PRACTICE QUESTIONS

1. For most domestic species, the duration of spermatogenesis is approximately
   a. 120 days.
   b. 10 days.
   c. 60 days.
   d. 6 months.
   e. 21 days.

2. Normal spermatogenesis in domestic mammals requires a testicular temperature that is
   a. higher than core body temperature.
   b. lower than core body temperature.
   c. the same as core body temperature.
   d. above freezing but below boiling.
   e. conducive to testosterone metabolism.

3. Normal spermatogenesis requires an intratesticular testosterone concentration that is
   a. the same as circulating levels.
   b. lower than circulating levels.
   c. static and unchanging.
   d. much higher than circulating levels.
   e. able to change rapidly with the maturational stage of the spermatozoon.

4. Puberty in the male
   a. occurs at about the same time for all species.
   b. is influenced only by the age of the animal.
   c. is synonymous with sexual maturity.
   d. is defined as when he is first able to produce sufficient numbers of sperm to impregnate a female.
   e. is independent of GnRH secretion.

5. Anabolic steroids are testosterone derivatives and therefore
   a. should be helpful in treating infertile males.
   b. have no effect on male fertility.
   c. enhance testicular function.
   d. are only approved for use in stallions.
   e. should not be used in males intended for breeding because of negative feedback effects.

PRACTICE ANSWERS

1. c   2. b   3. d   4. d   5. e

RENAL PHYSIOLOGY

Jill W. Verlander

40

Glomerular filtration

1 Introduction to the physiology of the kidney
2 The glomerulus filters the blood
3 The structure of the glomerulus provides for its filtration properties
4 The glomerular filtration rate is determined by the mean net filtration pressure, the permeability of the filtration barrier, and the area available for filtration

5 The filtration barrier is selectively permeable
6 Changes in the glomerular filtration rate are moderated by systemic and intrinsic factors
7 The glomerular filtration rate is measured by determining the rate of clearance of the plasma

▬ INTRODUCTION TO THE PHYSIOLOGY OF THE KIDNEY

The kidney is a remarkable organ charged with a diverse set of responsibilities in maintaining homeostasis. In mammals, the two kidneys receive approximately 25% of the cardiac output. The kidneys filter this blood in order to excrete metabolic waste, and they retrieve the filtered materials that are needed by the body, including low-molecular-weight proteins, water, and a variety of electrolytes. The kidneys recognize when water and specific electrolytes are deficient or excessive, and they respond by altering the rate of reabsorption or secretion of these substances. They contribute substantially to the maintenance of acid-base homeostasis. In addition, the kidneys produce hormones that play vital roles in the control of systemic blood pressure and red blood cell production. The kidneys accomplish these tasks by means of an extensive variety of cell types, each endowed with an individual set of functions and designed to respond as needed to a complex battery of direct and indirect signals. These cells are arranged in a particular pattern to form the functional unit of the kidney, the nephron. The nephron is composed of the glomerulus, where the blood is filtered, and various distinct segments of the renal tubule, where filtered substances are absorbed from and plasma components are secreted into the tubular fluid. In the renal cortex, the nephrons join with the collecting duct system, which traverses the kidney and ends with the inner medullary collecting duct, where the final alterations of the tubular fluid take place in the formation of urine. Figure 40–1 provides an overview of the anatomic arrangement of nephrons within the kidney and a brief outline of the major functions of the various segments of the nephron.

The specific functions of the kidney are discussed in this chapter. Most of the experimental evidence for what is believed about renal physiology has been obtained from the rat and rabbit, and our understanding of renal physiology will continue to be modified as more information is gathered.

▬ THE GLOMERULUS FILTERS THE BLOOD

The first step in the complex series of processes performed by the kidney is the filtration of the blood. Filtration takes place in the glomerulus, which is a network of capillaries with a structure specifically designed to retain cellular components and medium- to high-molecular-weight proteins within the vascular system while extruding a fluid that is nearly identical to the plasma in its electrolyte and water composition. This fluid is the glomerular filtrate, and the process of formation is glomerular filtration.

The rate of glomerular filtration is a parameter of renal function that is frequently assessed in clinical practice. The glomerular filtration rate (GFR) is expressed as milliliters of glomerular filtrate formed per minute for every kilogram of body weight. To understand GFR, it may help to think of these numbers in more tangible terms. An average-size beagle of 10 kg body weight with a typical GFR of 3.7 mL/minute/kg would produce approximately 37 mL of glomerular filtrate per minute, or 53.3 L (a little more than 14 gallons) of glomerular filtrate per day, nearly 27 times the beagle's extracellular fluid volume.

▬ THE STRUCTURE OF THE GLOMERULUS PROVIDES FOR ITS FILTRATION PROPERTIES

In order to understand the factors that determine GFR, it is necessary to be familiar with the ultrastruc-

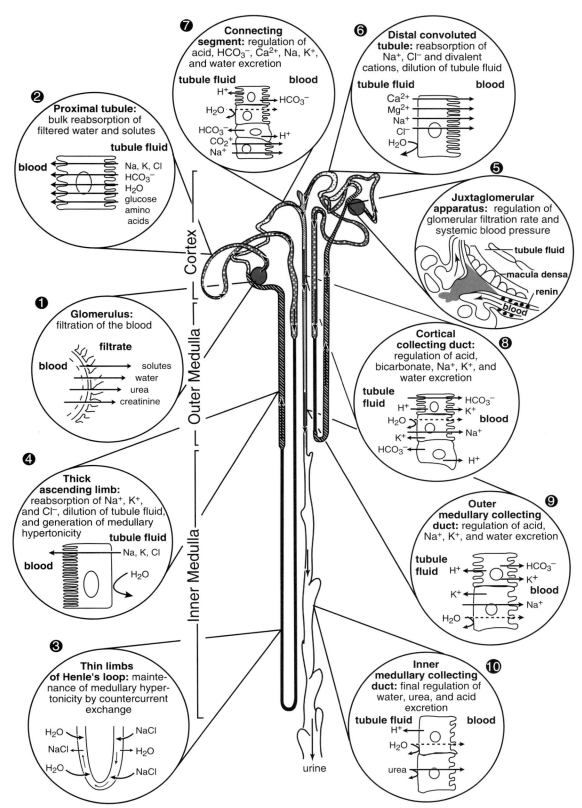

FIGURE 40–1. Schematic illustration of juxtamedullary and superficial nephrons and summary of the functions of the segments of the nephron and collecting duct. The glomerulus of a juxtamedullary nephron is located deep in the cortex near the corticomedullary junction. The thin limb (TL) of Henle's loop extends deep into the inner medulla. The glomerulus of a superficial nephron is located in the outer cortex, and Henle's loop extends only into the outer medulla. *Arrows* indicate the direction of tubule fluid flow. Segments are numbered in sequential order of modification of the tubule fluid, beginning with the glomerulus. CCD, cortical collecting duct; CNT, connecting segment; CTAL, cortical thick ascending limb; DCT, distal convoluted tubule; IMCD, inner medullary collecting duct; MTAL, medullary thick ascending limb; OMCD, outer medullary collecting duct; PCT, proximal convoluted tubule; PST, proximal straight tubule. (Modified from Madsen KM: Anatomy of the kidney. In Tisher CC, Wilcox CS [eds]: Nephrology for the House Officer. Baltimore: Williams & Wilkins, 1989.)

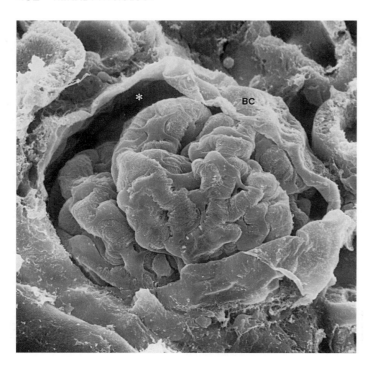

FIGURE 40–2. Scanning electron micrograph of rat glomerulus. The glomerular tuft is a complex network of capillaries that is encased in visceral epithelial cells and Bowman's capsule (BC). Between the visceral epithelial cells and BC is Bowman's space *(asterisk),* where the glomerular filtrate is collected and delivered to the proximal tubule. Magnification, ×600.

ture of the glomerulus. The glomerular tuft (Figs. 40–2 and 40–3) is composed of a network of capillaries. In mammals, blood from the renal artery is delivered to the afferent arteriole, which divides into numerous glomerular capillaries. The capillaries coalesce to form the efferent arteriole, which conducts the blood away from the glomerulus, to be returned eventually to the systemic circulation through the renal vein. In birds there are three pairs of renal arteries: anterior, middle, and posterior. Avian kidneys contain both mammalian-type and reptilian-type nephrons; in glomeruli of reptilian-type nephrons, the capillaries have few branches.

The glomerular tuft is encased within a layer of epithelial cells known as *Bowman's capsule.* The area between the glomerular tuft and Bowman's capsule

is known as *Bowman's space* and is the site of collection of the glomerular filtrate, which is funneled directly into the first segment of the proximal tubule.

The structure of the glomerular capillaries is important in determining the rate and selectivity of glomerular filtration. The wall of the capillary consists of three layers: the capillary endothelium, the basement membrane, and the visceral epithelium (Fig. 40–4). The capillary endothelium is composed of a single layer of cells whose cytoplasmic extensions are pierced by numerous fenestrae (windows). The endothelial fenestrae provide channels for the passage of water and noncellular components from the blood to the second layer of the glomerular capillary wall, the *glomerular basement membrane.* This is an acellular structure composed of various glycoproteins, including type IV and type V collagens, proteoglycans, laminin, fibronectin, and entactin. The glomerular basement membrane is arranged in three layers, presumably created during development by the fusion of the basement membranes of the endothelial and epithelial cell layers. The three layers are named according to both their density with regard to an electron beam and their relative position. As shown in Figure 40–4, the lamina densa (dense layer) is relatively dark, because it is relatively resistant to the passage of electrons when viewed with a transmission electron microscope. The lamina densa is composed of tightly packed glycoprotein fibrils. It is sandwiched between the lamina rara interna (inside thin layer) on the endothelial side of the glomerular basement membrane and the lamina rara externa (outside thin layer) on the epithelial side of the glomerular basement membrane. The laminae rarae are composed of a loose network of glycoprotein fibrils.

The third compartment of the glomerular capillary

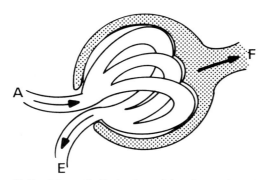

FIGURE 40–3. Schematic illustration of the glomerulus. The afferent arteriole (A) carries blood to the glomerulus and subdivides into numerous glomerular capillaries. Water and solutes cross the glomerular capillary wall into Bowman's space, forming the glomerular filtrate (F, *stippled area),* which flows into the proximal tubule. The glomerular capillaries coalesce, and the filtered blood leaves the glomerulus through the efferent arteriole (E).

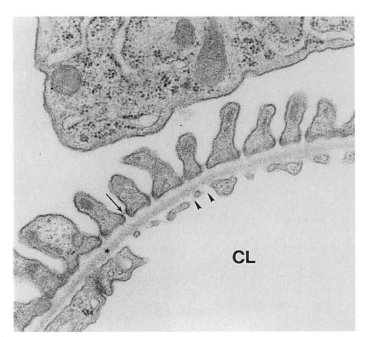

FIGURE 40–4. Transmission electron micrograph of rat glomerular capillary wall. The three main layers of the capillary wall are viewed in cross section. A single layer of glomerular capillary endothelial cells lines the capillary lumen (CL). Numerous fenestrae *(arrowheads)* pierce the endothelial cells. On the outside of the capillary is a single layer of visceral epithelial cells. At the top of the micrograph is a portion of the cell body of a visceral epithelial cell. The secondary foot processes are aligned along the capillary wall, and the spaces between them are spanned by the slit diaphragm *(arrow)*. Between the endothelial and epithelial cell layers is the glomerular basement membrane, consisting of the electron-lucent lamina rara interna adjacent to the endothelial cells, the lamina densa *(asterisk)*, and the lamina rara externa adjacent to the visceral epithelial cells. Magnification, ×19,000.

wall is the visceral epithelium, which is a layer of intricate, interlocking cells called *podocytes.* Numerous long, narrow extensions, called *primary* and *secondary foot processes,* interdigitate with foot processes from other podocytes and wrap around the individual capillaries (Fig. 40–5). Spanning the space between adjacent foot processes is the epithelial slit diaphragm (see Fig. 40–4).

THE GLOMERULAR FILTRATION RATE IS DETERMINED BY THE MEAN NET FILTRATION PRESSURE, THE PERMEABILITY OF THE FILTRATION BARRIER, AND THE AREA AVAILABLE FOR FILTRATION

The glomerular capillary wall creates a barrier to the forces favoring and opposing filtration of the blood. The forces favoring filtration—that is, movement of water and solutes across the glomerular capillary wall—are the hydrostatic pressure of the blood within the capillary and the oncotic pressure of the fluid within Bowman's space (the ultrafiltrate). Normally, the oncotic pressure of the ultrafiltrate is inconsequential, because medium- to high-molecular-weight proteins are not filtered. Therefore, the main driving force for filtration is the glomerular capillary hydrostatic pressure (P_{gc}). Forces opposing filtration are the plasma oncotic pressure within the glomerular capillary (π_b) and the hydrostatic pressure in Bowman's space (P_t). The direction and magnitude of these forces are illustrated in Figure 40–6.

The net filtration pressure (P_f) at any point along the glomerular capillary is the difference between the capillary hydrostatic pressure favoring filtration and the capillary oncotic pressure plus hydrostatic pressure of the ultrafiltrate opposing filtration. This relationship is expressed mathematically as follows:

$$P_f = P_{gc} - (\pi_b + P_t).$$

As blood travels through the glomerular capillary, a large proportion of the fluid component of the plasma is forced across the capillary wall, whereas the plasma proteins are retained in the capillary lumen. Therefore, the plasma oncotic pressure increases significantly along the capillary bed. At the same time, the loss of plasma volume along the capillary bed causes a decrease in the hydrostatic pressure in the capillary, although this change is small because of the resistance created by the efferent arteriole. The result is that the net filtration pressure tends to decrease along the capillary bed.

The GFR is the product of the mean net filtration pressure, and the P_f is the permeability of the filtration barrier, and the surface area available for filtration. The permeability of the filtration barrier is determined by the structural and chemical characteristics of the glomerular capillary wall. The product of the filtration barrier permeability and its surface area is the ultrafiltration coefficient K_f. Thus, the combined effects of the determinants of GFR are mathematically represented by the following equation:

$$GFR = P_f \cdot K_f$$

The filtration barrier is selectively permeable

In addition to determining the hydraulic permeability of the filtration barrier, the structural and chemical characteristics of the glomerular capillary wall establish the selective permeability (permselectivity) of the filtration barrier. The permselectivity of the filtration

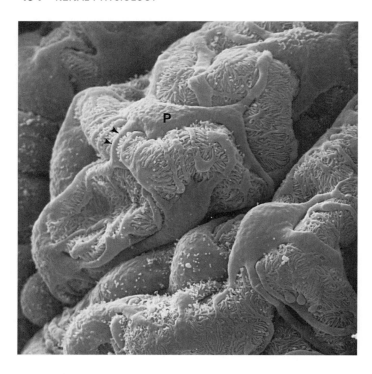

FIGURE 40–5. Scanning electron micrograph of the surface of rat glomerular capillaries viewed from Bowman's space. The cell bodies (P) of visceral epithelial cells, or podocytes, nestle between the capillary loops. The primary foot processes *(arrowheads)* radiate outward and wrap around the capillaries. Secondary foot processes extend from the primary foot processes and interdigitate with secondary foot processes from other podocytes. Magnification, ×1500.

barrier is responsible for differences in the rate of filtration of blood components. Normally, all cellular components and plasma proteins the size of albumin molecules or larger are retained within the blood stream, whereas water and solutes are freely filtered. In general, substances with a molecular radius of 4 nm or more are not filtered, whereas molecules with a radius of 2 nm or less are filtered without restriction.

However, characteristics other than size affect the ability of blood components to cross the filtration barrier. The net electrical charge of a molecule has a dramatic effect on its rate of filtration. It has been demonstrated that the cationic (positively charged) form of a variety of substances is more freely filtered than is the neutral form, which is more freely filtered than is the anionic (negatively charged) form of the

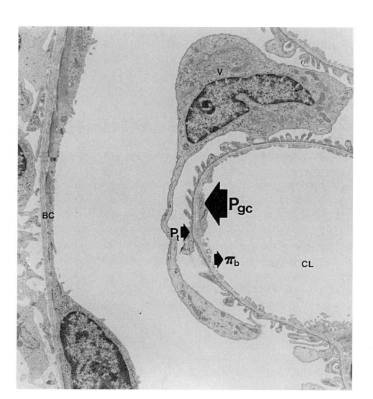

FIGURE 40–6. Transmission electron micrograph of a rat glomerular capillary and Bowman's capsule (BC) illustrating the forces favoring and opposing filtration. The main force favoring filtration is the hydrostatic pressure of the glomerular capillary (P_{gc}). The forces opposing filtration are the hydrostatic pressure of Bowman's space (P_t) and the oncotic pressure of the blood (π_b). CL, capillary lumen; V, visceral epithelial cell. Magnification, ×2400.

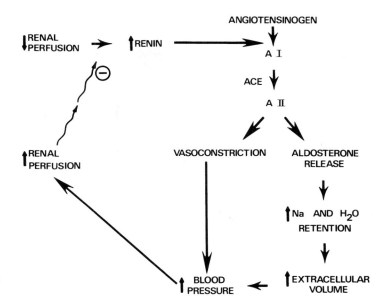

FIGURE 40–7. Schematic illustration of the renin-angiotensin-aldosterone system. Circled minus sign represents inhibition. A I, angiotensin I; ACE, angiotensin-converting enzyme; A II, angiotensin II.

same molecule. For example, the cationic form of albumin is excreted at a rate approximately 300 times that of native albumin, which has a net negative charge. These differences are thought to be caused by the presence of a charge-selective barrier in the glomerular capillary wall created by negatively charged residues of glycoproteins incorporated in the glomerular basement membrane and coating the endothelial and epithelial cells. These fixed negative charges are believed to repel negatively charged plasma proteins and thus reduce their passage across the filtration barrier. The shape and deformability of the molecule also play a role in its ability to cross the filtration barrier. Neutral dextran, a long, flexible molecule, crosses the filtration barrier approximately seven times as easily as horseradish peroxidase, a globular protein with a similar molecular radius and net charge.

Changes in the glomerular filtration rate are moderated by systemic and intrinsic factors

The kidney normally maintains the GFR at a relatively constant level despite changes in systemic blood pressure and renal blood flow. The GFR is maintained within the physiologic range by renal modulation of systemic blood pressure and intravascular volume and by intrinsic control of renal blood flow, glomerular capillary pressure, and K_f. Renal effects on systemic blood pressure and volume are mediated primarily through humoral factors, particularly the renin-angiotensin-aldosterone system. Intrinsic control of glomerular capillary perfusion is mediated by two autoregulatory systems that control the resistance to flow in the afferent and efferent arterioles: the *myogenic reflex* and *tubuloglomerular feedback.*

The renin-angiotensin-aldosterone system is an im-

portant mechanism of control of GFR and renal blood flow. Renin is a hormone produced by specialized cells of the wall of the afferent arteriole, the *granular extraglomerular mesangial cells,* which are specialized *juxtaglomerular cells.* Renin release is stimulated by a decrease in renal perfusion pressure, most commonly caused by systemic hypotension. Renin catalyzes the transformation of angiotensinogen produced by the liver to angiotensin I. Angiotensin I is converted to the more active angiotensin II by angiotensin-converting enzyme, which is located primarily in the vascular endothelium of the lung. Angiotensin-converting enzyme is also present in the vascular endothelium of the kidneys and other organs, and thus the conversion of angiotensin I to angiotensin II may occur in these extrapulmonary sites as well.

Angiotensin II is a potent vasoconstrictor that acts directly to increase systemic blood pressure and renal perfusion pressure. In addition, angiotensin II stimulates the release of the mineralocorticoid aldosterone from the adrenal gland and the release of vasopressin from the pituitary. In the collecting duct, aldosterone enhances sodium and water reabsorption, and vasopressin enhances urea and water reabsorption. The augmented solute and water uptake increases intravascular volume and thereby improves renal perfusion. Renin release is suppressed by both the improvement in renal perfusion and the elevated levels of plasma angiotensin II, creating a negative feedback system that maintains renal perfusion and GFR within the physiologic range (Fig. 40–7).

Increased levels of angiotensin II also stimulate production and release of at least two vasodilative renal prostaglandins: prostaglandin E_2 and prostaglandin I_2 (prostacyclin). This response is an important moderator of the renin-angiotensin-aldosterone system. The intrarenal production of these vasodilators counteracts the vasoconstrictive effect of angiotensin II on the intrarenal vasculature and helps to maintain renal vascular resistance at normal or near-normal levels.

Without this protective effect, generalized vasoconstriction would result in reduced renal blood flow and GFR, despite an elevation of blood pressure.

Within the kidney itself, there appears to be direct control of glomerular capillary perfusion by two systems previously mentioned: the myogenic reflex and tubuloglomerular feedback.

A mechanism of autoregulation of renal blood flow and GFR was proposed after the observation that glomerular arterioles respond to changes in arteriolar wall tension. This response is called the *myogenic reflex,* and the result is almost immediate arteriolar constriction after an increase in arteriolar wall tension. Conversely, a decrease in arteriolar wall tension results in virtually immediate arteriolar dilation. Arteriolar dilation and constriction respectively decrease and increase the resistance to blood flow in the afferent arteriole. These changes in vascular resistance contribute to maintenance of GFR and renal blood flow at a constant level, despite marked alterations in the blood pressure in the renal artery. This reflex has been shown to be independent of renal innervation but may be influenced by chemical mediators, such as nitric oxide.

The second intrinsic control mechanism to consider is a system known as *tubuloglomerular feedback.* In order to grasp this concept, it is important to review the anatomic arrangement of an individual nephron (see Fig. 40–1). Specifically, recall that the distal tubule is closely associated with the glomerulus of the same nephron. An anatomically distinct cluster of epithelial cells, known as the *macula densa,* is located in the distal portion of the thick ascending limb of the loop of Henle. The macula densa is situated between the afferent and efferent arterioles and adjacent to the extraglomerular mesangial region. These four structures together are known as the *juxtaglomerular apparatus,* and they appear to be closely related functionally as well as structurally.

The basic observation supporting the concept of a tubuloglomerular feedback mechanism was made by means of micropuncture of individual nephrons. These experiments demonstrated that an increase in the tubular fluid flow rate at the macula densa results in a decrease in the filtration rate of the glomerulus of that nephron. In theory, such a system would check the single-nephron GRF in order to avoid exceeding the capacity of the tubule to reabsorb fluid or solute and thus would prevent excessive fluid and solute loss. Although it is generally accepted that this tubuloglomerular feedback mechanism exists, the actual signal that precipitates the negative feedback is controversial; different researchers have proposed increased delivery of fluid, solute, or chloride to the macula densa. Whatever the signal, the result is increased resistance to flow in the afferent arteriole, decreased glomerular capillary perfusion pressure, reduced K_f, and reduced single-nephron GFR. The mechanism by which the signal at the macula densa is translated into these effects may involve differential effects of vasoconstrictors and vasodilators on the afferent and efferent arterioles as well as mesangial cell contraction.

Futhermore, it is now evident that the endothelium contributes to local control of renal vascular tone by producing potent vasoconstrictors and vasodilators. Endothelium-derived constricting factors include the potent vasoconstrictor endothelin thromboxane A_2 (a metabolite of arachidonic acid) and angiotensin II. Endothelium-derived relaxing factors include nitric oxide, prostaglandin I_2 (prostacyclin), and prostaglandin E_2. Of these, nitric oxide was the first vasodilative agent derived from endothelial cells to be identified, and thus in some of the scientific literature, *endothelium-derived relaxing factor* is used as a synonym for nitric oxide. The significance and interactions of the effects of these agents on renal blood flow and GFR in various physiologic and pathologic conditions remain to be defined.

In addition to controls exerted by the kidney itself, systemic factors can contribute to changes in GFR. These include systemic control of blood volume and vessel tone. Many hormones regulate blood volume. As mentioned previously, aldosterone and vasopressin (antidiuretic hormone) secretion enhance water and solute reabsorption by the kidney and thus increase blood volume. Atrial natriuretic peptide, a hormone produced in the cardiac atria, causes both natriuresis (sodium wasting) and diuresis (water wasting) and thereby reduces blood volume.

Systemic factors that affect vessel tone also affect systemic blood pressure, renal perfusion, and ultrafiltration. Vasopressin and circulating catecholamines can cause systemic vasoconstriction and increase blood pressure. β-adrenergic stimulation can activate the renin-angiotensin system, and α-adrenergic stimulation can cause renal vasoconstriction, causing both a reduction and a redistribution of renal blood flow. In addition to altering renal perfusion, vasoconstrictors can affect the other determinant of GFR, the ultrafiltration coefficient K_f. Vasoconstrictors may cause contraction of the mesangial cells within the glomerulus and reduce the area available for filtration. Because K_f is the product of the area available for filtration and the hydraulic permeability, mesangial cell contraction that occurs in vivo would lead to reductions in K_f and thus GFR.

Insulin-like growth factor and high dietary protein levels enhance GFR. Insulin-like growth factor increases GFR in kidneys of normal animals and after experimental renal ischemia. Furthermore, it has been demonstrated that high levels of dietary protein cause sustained increases in renal blood flow and GFR. These parameters are also transiently elevated after a single high-protein meal. The mechanisms and clinical implications of the effects of insulin-like growth factor and high dietary protein on renal function are not clearly understood at this time and continue to be explored.

In birds, the GFR is more variable than that of mammals, but the regulatory mechanisms are not well understood. Birds, unlike mammals, exhibit intermittent filtration in reptilian-type glomeruli; this occurs during dehydration and decreases the GFR. This may result from the release of arginine vasotocin, the avian analogue of mammalian arginine vasopressin, which has been shown to decrease GFR in birds by causing constriction of the afferent arteriole of reptilian-type nephrons. Although some authors report that a juxtaglomerular apparatus is present in avian kidneys, the macula densa is either absent or rudimentary; tubuloglomerular feedback has not yet been demonstrated.

The glomerular filtration rate is measured by determining the rate of clearance of the plasma

Both in an experimental setting and in clinical practice, GFR is one of the most important parameters of renal function. Determination of GFR relies on the concept of clearance: that is, the rate at which the plasma is cleared of a substance. The rate of clearance of a substance is measured by the rate of elimination divided by the plasma concentration of the substance, mathematically expressed by

$$C_x = (U_xV)/P_x,$$

where C_x is the volume of plasma cleared of substance X per unit time, U_x is the urine concentration of substance X, V is the volume of urine collected divided by the time period of the collection, and P_x is the plasma concentration of substance X.

The total rate of clearance of a substance is the sum of the rates of filtration and secretion minus the rate of reabsorption of the substance. In order to determine the filtration rate accurately, it is necessary to exclude the effects of secretion and reabsorption from the equation. This requirement is neatly satisfied by selecting inulin as the substance for the measurement of clearance. Inulin is a substance that is freely filtered by the glomerulus but is neither reabsorbed nor secreted by the renal tubular cells. Because of these properties, and because inulin is not produced by the body, the rate of its disappearance from the blood after intravascular injection is strictly related to the rate of glomerular filtration. Therefore, measurement of GFR can be expressed mathematically by the clearance equation, in which substance X is inulin:

$$GFR = C_{inulin} = (U_{inulin}V)/P_{inulin,}$$

where GFR is in milliliters per minute, C_{inulin} is the rate of clearance of inulin from the plasma in milliliters per minute, U_{inulin} is the inulin concentration in a urine sample collected over a period of time T in minutes, V is the volume of the urine collected over time T, and P_{inulin} is the mean plasma inulin concentration during time T. Although the standard method of determination of GFR is by the rate of clearance of inulin from the blood, GFR can be measured in a variety of ways. In clinical situations the most widely used measure of glomerular filtration is endogenous creatinine clearance. Creatinine is a byproduct of muscle metabolism that is handled by the kidney in a manner similar to its handling of inulin. It is freely filtered, is not reabsorbed by the tubule, and, at least

in the dog, is not secreted by the tubule. However, in some species, approximately 10% of the excreted creatinine is secreted by the tubule. Nevertheless, depending on the accuracy of the assay used for creatinine (colorimetric assays overestimate the concentration of creatinine in the blood, but not that in the urine), the endogenous creatinine clearance test provides a rough estimate of GFR. In practice, the measurement of endogenous creatinine clearance requires collecting the urine produced by a patient over a 24-hour period, either by using a metabolic cage that "catches" voided urine or by collecting the urine by catheterization if necessary. The volume of urine produced over 24 hours is recorded, and the creatinine concentration is measured. The mean plasma concentration of creatinine is represented either by the plasma concentration measured at the midpoint of the collection period or by the mean of the plasma concentration measured at the beginning and end of the collection period. These values are used in the clearance equation

$$C_{creatinine} = U_{creatinine}V/P_{creatinine}$$

and result in an approximation of GFR in milliliters per minute. In veterinary medicine, the GFR is better expressed on the basis of body weight or body surface area—that is, as milliliters per minute per kilogram or milliliters per minute per square meter—because of the large variation in size within individual species.

In birds, creatinine clearance cannot be used for determination of GFR; avian renal tubules can secrete creatinine when the plasma level is elevated, but at normal plasma levels, creatinine is reabsorbed by the tubules.

CLINICAL CORRELATIONS

Chronic renal failure

History   You examine a 15-year-old male Siamese cat. The owner reports that her cat is listless, inappetent, and thin. The cat has been drinking more water than usual lately, urinating large volumes, and vomiting frequently.

Clinical examination   The cat is very thin and moderately dehydrated. The mucous membranes are pale, and the kidneys feel small and slightly irregular. Her hematocrit is 22% (normal, 30% to 42%), serum creatinine level is 8.7 mg/dL (normal, 0.5 to 1.2 mg/dL), and urine specific gravity is 1.012.

Comment   The cat has chronic renal failure, which is seen frequently in geriatric patients in small animal practice. The serum creatinine level is elevated because progressive loss of glomerular function has severely reduced the GFR, and creatinine as well as other waste products is not cleared from the plasma. The urine is not concentrated in response to dehydration because tubular function is also compromised. The smallness of the kidneys is an indication of chronicity and is a result of gradual nephron loss and scarring. Anemia is common in chronic renal failure and results from many factors, one being decreased production of erythropoietin by the kidney.

Treatment In veterinary medicine, the treatment of chronic renal failure is usually supportive and symptomatic. This cat would probably benefit from rehydration with intravenous fluids, correction of electrolyte and acid-base disturbances as dictated by the serum chemistry profile, and a low-protein diet supplemented with the water-soluble vitamins. Anabolic steroids may help improve the anemia. Exogenous erythropoietin has become standard treatment in humans with anemia caused by chronic renal failure and is now being used in veterinary medicine as well.

Glomerulonephritis

History A client presents his 3-year-old spayed female Springer spaniel. He reports that the dog has not been eating well for several days and seems to tire easily.

Clinical examination The dog seems bright and alert and is in good flesh. The only abnormality detected by physical examination is slight pitting edema in the distal extremities. The left kidney is palpable and feels smooth and of normal size. A urinalysis yields normal results except for 3 + protein (normal, negative to trace amounts) and the presence of a few red blood cell casts. A complete blood cell count is normal, and the only abnormality on a serum chemistry profile is a serum albumin level of 1.5 g/dL (normal, 2.3 to 4.3 g/dL).

Comment This dog has acute glomerulonephritis. Proteinuria is indicative of glomerular disease, because normally the filtration barrier established by the glomerular capillary wall prevents the passage of proteins into the tubular fluid. When the glomerulus is damaged, it becomes leaky, and protein appears in the urine. The loss of albumin in this case appears to be marked, because the serum albumin level has dropped below normal levels. The peripheral edema is probably caused by the hypoalbuminemia, hence the lowered intracapillary oncotic pressure and leakage of fluid into the extravascular space.

In this case, acute glomerulonephritis is suspected because of the recent onset of clinical signs, the absence of renal failure, and the presence of red blood cell casts in the urine. Additional tests that are helpful in guiding and assessing therapy include a 24-hour urine collection to measure the severity of the protein loss and an endogenous creatinine clearance test done at the same time to determine whether the GFR has been altered. A renal biopsy is necessary to verify the type and severity of glomerular injury.

Treatment The treatment of glomerulonephritis varies. Occasionally, the precipitating cause can be determined and removed. Some cases resolve spontaneously; at other times, various combinations of immunosuppressive and anti-inflammatory agents are used to combat ongoing damage from immune complex deposition and glomerular inflammation. If either renal failure or pulmonary edema secondary to hypoalbuminemia is present, this problem must be treated to sustain the animal until the glomerular lesion is resolved or controlled if possible.

Bibliography

Brenner BM (ed): Brenner & Rector's The Kidney, 6th ed. Philadelphia: WB Saunders, 2000.

Seldin SW, Giebish G (eds): The Kidney: Physiology and Pathophysiology, 3rd ed. Philadelphia: Lippincott Williams & Wilkins, 2000.

Valtin H, Schafer JA: Renal Function: Mechanisms Preserving Fluid and Solute Balance in Health, 3rd ed. Boston: Little, Brown, 1995.

PRACTICE QUESTIONS

1. The major force favoring filtration across the glomerular capillary wall is
   a. the oncotic pressure of the plasma.
   b. the oncotic pressure of the glomerular filtrate.
   c. the hydrostatic pressure of the blood.
   d. the hydrostatic pressure of the glomerular filtrate.
   e. the ultrafiltration coefficient.

2. The glomerular filtration rate is
   a. the volume of blood filtered by the kidneys per minute per kilogram of body weight.
   b. the volume of plasma filtered by the kidneys per minute per kilogram of body weight.
   c. the volume of urine produced by the kidneys per minute per kilogram of body weight.
   d. the volume of glomerular filtrate formed by the kidneys per minute per kilogram of body weight.
   e. the volume of blood cleared of creatinine by the kidneys per minute per kilogram of body weight.

3. In clinical practice, the GFR is often estimated by determining the rate of creatinine clearance. The rate of creatinine clearance is
   a. the volume of plasma cleared of creatinine per minute per kilogram of body weight.
   b. the volume of glomerular filtrate formed per minute per kilogram of body weight.
   c. the weight of creatinine filtered from the blood per minute per kilogram of body weight.
   d. the weight of creatinine per volume of urine formed per minute per kilogram of body weight.
   e. the difference between the rate of plasma flow in the afferent and efferent arterioles.

4. The two major characteristics that determine whether a blood component is filtered or retained in the capillary lumen are its
   a. molecular radius and molecular weight.
   b. molecular radius and lipid solubility.
   c. molecular radius and plasma concentration.
   d. molecular radius and electrical charge.
   e. molecular weight and length.

5. The GFR is increased by
   a. a low-protein meal.
   b. afferent arteriolar constriction.
   c. tubuloglomerular feedback.
   d. release of atrial natriuretic peptide.
   e. activation of the renin-angiotensin-aldosterone system.

PRACTICE ANSWERS

1. c   2. d   3. a   4. d   5. e

41

Solute reabsorption

1 The renal tubule reabsorbs filtered substances

2 Renal tubule function may be assessed by determining fractional excretion and fractional reabsorption rates

3 The proximal tubule is responsible for the reabsorption of the bulk of filtered solutes

4 The proximal tubule secretes organic ions

5 The distal tubule segments reabsorb salts and dilute the tubule fluid

6 The collecting duct reabsorbs NaCl and can secrete or reabsorb K^+

7 The distal tubule and collecting duct respond to systemic signals to alter salt excretion as required

8 Aldosterone enhances Na^+ reabsorption and K^+ secretion

9 Ca^{2+} is reabsorbed in the distal nephron and connecting segment; Ca^{2+} reabsorption is regulated by parathyroid hormone, $1\alpha,25-(OH)_2$–vitamin D_3, and calcitonin

The renal tubule reabsorbs filtered substances

It is vital that the bulk of the ultrafiltrate formed in the glomerulus be reabsorbed by the remainder of the nephron rather than excreted in the urine. To illustrate the importance of reabsorption of the components of the ultrafiltrate, consider an example from the previous chapter, the 10-kg beagle that forms 53.3 L of glomerular filtrate each day. The ultrafiltrate contains virtually the same concentration of salts and glucose as does the plasma; therefore, without tubular reabsorption, the urinary loss of sodium, chloride, potassium, bicarbonate, and glucose alone would total more than 500 g of solute. In the absence of tubular reabsorption, the beagle would need to constantly replace these chemicals throughout the day by eating more than a pound of salts and drinking more than 50 L of water at the same rate as the urinary loss in order to stay in fluid and salt balance.

Fortunately, the renal tubule efficiently retrieves these and other constituents of the ultrafiltrate. Figure 41–1 illustrates the percentages of various filtered substances that remain in the tubule fluid at various points along the tubule. One hundred percent of the filtered glucose is rapidly reabsorbed by the proximal tubule; by the time the final urine is formed in the terminal collecting duct, approximately 99% of the filtered water and sodium has been retrieved.

Renal tubule function may be assessed by determining fractional excretion and fractional reabsorption rates

The percentage of a filtered substance that is ultimately excreted in the urine is called the *fractional excretion rate*. It is the net result of the tubular reabsorption and secretion of the filtered substance. Mathematically, the fractional excretion rate of a substance, X, is the ratio of the urinary concentration of X (U_X) to the plasma concentration of X (P_X) divided by the urinary/plasma ratio of a reference substance. Relating U_X/P_X to the U/P ratio of a reference substance

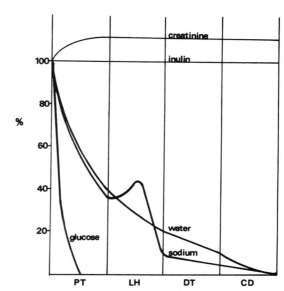

FIGURE 41–1. Illustration of the percentage of filtered substances [$(U_X/P_X) \times 100/(U_{inulin}/P_{inulin})$] remaining in the tubule fluid in various tubule segments. Creatinine is secreted by the proximal tubule and is excreted at a greater rate than the reference substance, inulin. CD, collecting duct; DT, distal tubule; LH, loop of Henle; PT, proximal tubule. (Modified from Sullivan LP, Grantham JJ [eds]: Physiology of the Kidney, 2nd ed. Philadelphia: Lea & Febiger, 1982.)

eliminates the confounding effect of water reabsorption on the urinary concentration of X. In experimental situations, the urinary and plasma concentrations of inulin during a constant inulin infusion may be used for reference. However, it is more practical in clinical situations to use creatinine as the reference substance. Therefore, the fractional excretion rate of X (FE_X) is determined by the equation

$$FE_X = U_X/P_X \div U_{creatinine}/P_{creatinine,}$$

where $U_{creatinine}$ and $P_{creatinine}$ are the urinary and plasma concentrations of creatinine, respectively. By multiplying Fe_X by 100, the fractional excretion rate is expressed as the percentage of filtered X that is excreted.

The fractional reabsorption rate of X (FR_X) represents the proportion of filtered X that is reabsorbed by the tubule. FR_X is mathematically determined by the equation

$$FR_X = 1 - FE_X$$

and can be expressed as a percentage by multiplying FR_X by 100.

The proximal tubule is responsible for the reabsorption of the bulk of filtered solutes

The rate of reabsorption and secretion of filtered substances varies among segments of the renal tubule. In general, the proximal tubule is responsible for reabsorption of the ultrafiltrate to a greater extent than is the remainder of the tubule. At least 60% of most filtered substances are reabsorbed before the tubular fluid leaves the proximal tubule.

The anatomic arrangement of the proximal tubule and its relationship to the peritubular capillary facilitate the movement of tubule fluid components into the blood through two pathways: the transcellular pathway and the paracellular pathway. The tubule fluid flows over the apical surface of the tubular epithelial cell. Substances transported through the transcellular pathway are taken up by the cell from the tubule fluid across the apical plasma membrane and are discharged into the interstitial fluid on the blood side of the cell, across the basolateral plasma membrane. Passage through the transcellular pathway occurs largely by carrier-mediated transport. The surface area available for transport of tubule fluid components into the cell is vast, because of extensive microprojections of the apical plasma membrane, called *microvilli*, which collectively create a beautiful membranous structure known as the *brush border* (Figs. 41–2 and 41–3). On the blood side of the cell, there are also complex infoldings of the basolateral plasma membrane; these enhance the surface area available for transport from the cell into the interstitial fluid, where the transported substance becomes available for uptake by the peritubular capillary.

The second route of transport in the proximal tubule is the paracellular pathway. Substances reabsorbed through the paracellular pathway move from the tubule fluid across the zonula occludens, a highly permeable structure that attaches the proximal tubule cells to each other and forms the boundary between the apical and basolateral plasma membrane domains (Fig. 41–4). Paracellular transport occurs by passive diffusion or by *solvent drag*, which is the entrainment of solute by the flow of water. Substances crossing the zonula occludens enter the lateral intercellular space, which is thought to communicate freely with the interstitial fluid; from there, reabsorbed substances can be taken up by the peritubular capillary.

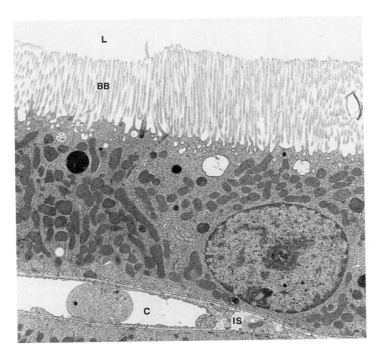

FIGURE 41–2. Transmission electron micrograph of cross section of rat proximal tubule. The brush border (BB) of the apical plasma membrane extends from the epithelial cells into the tubule lumen (L), where it is bathed by the tubule fluid. On the basal side of the cell is the interstitial space (IS) and the peritubular capillary (C). Magnification, ×3400.

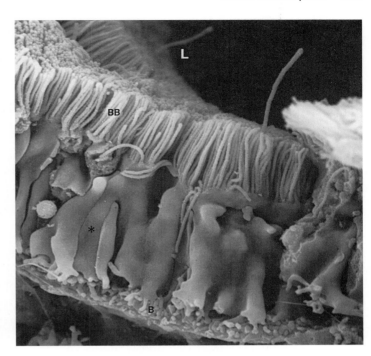

FIGURE 41–3. Scanning electron micrograph of rat proximal tubule, viewed from the lateral intercellular space. The lush brush border (BB) carpets the luminal aspect (L). Lateral cellular processes *(asterisk)* interdigitate with those of neighboring cells. The surface of the basal plasma membrane (B) is amplified by extensive membrane infoldings, creating numerous processes called *micropedici* ("tiny feet"). Magnification, ×4400.

Movement of water and solute from the interstitial fluid into the blood stream is favored by the location of the peritubular capillary and is driven by Starling's forces. In mammals, the peritubular capillary originates at the glomerular efferent arteriole, subdivides, and wraps closely around the basal aspect of the proximal tubule (Fig. 41–5). The plasma leaving the glomerulus has a high oncotic pressure as a result of the selective filtration of water and salts and the retention of proteins within the capillary lumen. Because of low resistance in the peritubular capillary, the hydrostatic pressure in the capillary is low. Both of these conditions—high peritubular plasma oncotic pressure and low peritubular capillary hydrostatic pressure—favor the movement of fluid and solute from the interstitium into the blood stream.

In birds, the effect of the peritubular blood supply on tubular reabsorption and secretion is complicated by the presence of a renal portal circulation. Renal portal veins anastomose with the efferent glomerular arterioles and supply peritubular blood to the reptilian nephrons and the proximal and distal tubules of mammalian-type nephrons; thus, these tubules, but not the loops of Henle of the mammalian-type nephrons, are supplied with a mixture of portal venous and arterial blood. Furthermore, the rate of flow to the renal portal supply varies and is controlled by a smooth muscle valve.

FIGURE 41–4. Transmission electron micrograph of apical region of rat proximal tubule viewed in cross section. The zonula occludens *(arrow)* joins adjacent proximal tubule cells. The zonula occludens divides the apical plasma membrane from the basolateral plasma membrane and separates the tubule fluid from the fluid of the lateral intercellular space. Also seen are coated pits *(arrowheads)* that contain the binding sites for substances reabsorbed by receptor-mediated endocytosis. Magnification, ×19,600.

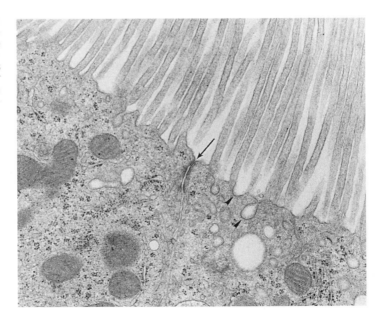

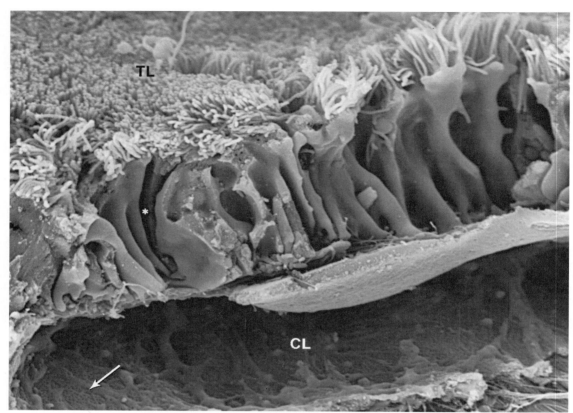

FIGURE 41–5. Scanning electron micrograph of rat proximal tubule and peritubular capillary. The peritubular capillary wraps around the basal aspect of the proximal tubule cells. Substances retrieved from the tubule lumen (TL) are delivered through either the transcellular pathway or the paracellular pathway into the fluid bathing the basolateral aspect of the epithelial cells. Water and solutes enter the interstitial space and diffuse into the peritubular capillary lumen (CL). The *asterisk* represents lateral intercellular space; the *arrow* represents fenestrae of peritubular capillary endothelium. Magnification, ×7000.

Reabsorption of solutes takes place by a number of transport mechanisms, including passive diffusion, solvent drag, and primary active transport (transport mechanisms are described in Chapter 1). In the proximal tubule, much of the transport of substances from the tubular fluid to the blood is driven by the active transport of Na^+ by a Na^+,K^+ pump (Na^+,K^+-ATPase) located in the basolateral plasma membrane (Fig. 41–6). Under optimal conditions, the Na^+,K^+-ATPase pump extrudes three Na^+ ions into the interstitial fluid and takes up two K^+ ions into the cell.

The normal operation of the Na^+,K^+-ATPase pump reduces the concentration of Na^+ within the cell and increases the concentration of K^+ within the cell. Subsequent outward diffusion of K^+ via K^+ channels polarizes the cell, so that the interior of the cell is electrically negative in relation to the exterior. Thus, an electrochemical gradient for Na^+ across the apical plasma membrane is established, encouraging the movement of Na^+ from the tubular fluid into the cell. The movement of Na^+ across the apical cell membrane is facilitated by a variety of specific transporters located in the membrane. The movement of Na^+ through most of these transporters is coupled to the movement of other solutes in the same direction as Na^+ (cotransport) or in the opposite direction (countertransport). Substances that are taken up from the

proximal tubular fluid into the cells by this mechanism (*secondary active transport*) include glucose, amino acids, phosphate, sulfate, and organic anions. The active uptake of these substances increases their intracellular concentration and allows them to move

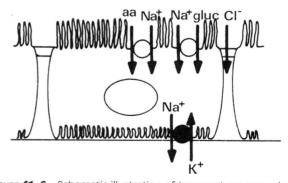

FIGURE 41–6. Schematic illustration of transport processes in the proximal tubule epithelial cell. Virtually all transport is believed to be driven by active reabsorption of Na^+ by the Na^+,K^+-ATPase located in the basolateral plasma membrane. Glucose (gluc) and amino acids (aa), as well as many other solutes, enter the cell by secondary active transport with Na^+, driven by the low intracellular Na^+ concentration resulting from the active transport of Na^+ out of the cell. Cl^- diffuses across the zonula occludens into the lateral intercellular spaces down its electrochemical gradient.

across the basolateral plasma membrane and into the blood by passive or facilitated diffusion.

The reabsorption of bicarbonate (HCO_3^-) by the proximal tubule is also driven by the Na^+ gradient, although indirectly. Na^+ and proton (H^+) counter transport across the apical plasma membrane occurs via an Na^+/H^+ exchanger and is driven by the chemical gradient for Na^+. Secreted H^+ combines in the tubular fluid with filtered HCO_3^- to form H_2O and CO_2, catalyzed by the enzyme carbonic anhydrase in the apical plasma membrane of proximal tubule cells. The CO_2 diffuses passively across the apical plasma membrane into the cell. There, cytoplasmic carbonic anhydrase catalyzes the hydroxylation of CO_2 with OH^- donated from H_2O, resulting in the formation of H^+ and HCO_3^- within the cell. The HCO_3^- moves across the basolateral plasma membrane and back into the blood primarily through an $Na^+,3\text{-}HCO_3^-$ cotransporter as well as a HCO_3^-/Cl^- antiporter. The H^+ is transported into the tubular fluid through the Na^+/H^+ antiporter, which completes the cycle. By this complex mechanism, illustrated in Figure 41–7, the proximal tubule reabsorbs 60% to 85% of the filtered HCO_3^-.

The passive reabsorption of Cl^- in the proximal tubule is also indirectly powered by the Na^+,K^+-ATPase pump. As Na^+, HCO_3^-, glucose, amino acids, and other solutes are selectively reabsorbed and water

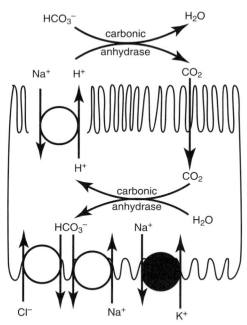

FIGURE 41–7. Schematic illustration of HCO_3^- reabsorption and acid secretion in the proximal tubule. The active reabsorption of Na^+ by the basolateral Na^+,K^+-ATPase drives the secretion of H^+ through the Na^+/H^+ exchanger in the apical plasma membrane. In the lumen, the secreted H^+ and filtered HCO_3^- form H_2O and CO_2 under the influence of apical membrane-associated carbonic anhydrase. The CO_2 readily diffuses across the apical plasma membrane into the cell and combines with intracellular H_2O to form H^+ and HCO_3^-. This process is catalyzed by cytoplasmic carbonic anhydrase. The H^+ is secreted into the tubule fluid, and the HCO_3^- is transported to the blood side of the cell through countertransport with Na^+ or possibly Cl^-.

is taken up along with these solutes, the concentration of Cl^- in the tubular fluid rises, establishing a chemical gradient for Cl^- movement in the direction of the blood side of the tubule. In addition, in the early proximal tubule, the selective uptake of Na^+ exceeds that of anions, resulting in a net transfer of positive charge to the blood side of the epithelium. This creates a small electrical gradient for anions in the direction of the blood. Thus, in the early proximal tubule, the chemical gradient and the electrical gradient favor the reabsorption of Cl^-. Because the zonula occludens is highly permeable to Cl^-, passive, paracellular transfer of Cl^- from the tubule lumen to the interstitial fluid occurs.

In the more distal portions of the proximal tubule, the tubule fluid becomes depleted of many of the substances necessary for Na^+ reabsorption by cotransport. There, the Na^+,K^+-ATPase pump continues to move Na^+ from the cell into the interstitial fluid, but mechanisms of Na^+ uptake other than cotransport predominate. These mechanisms include some form of electrically neutral NaCl uptake and passive reabsorption of Na^+ through the paracellular pathway. This paracellular transport of Na^+ is made possible by the chemical gradient for Cl^- established by the selective reabsorption of other solutes in the early proximal tubule. As Cl^- moves passively down its chemical gradient from the urine side to the blood side of the tubule epithelium, it carries Na^+ along with it, as a result of electrostatic attraction. The passage of Cl^- down its chemical gradient also abolishes the small lumen-negative charge and in fact establishes a small lumen-positive charge in the late proximal tubule, which further favors the passive transfer of Na^+ to the blood side of the epithelium.

Other filtered solutes, such as K^+ and Ca^{2+} ions, are present in the tubule fluid in low concentrations, and they are also reabsorbed by the proximal tubule epithelium. It is believed that the majority of K^+ and Ca^{2+} reabsorption in the proximal tubule occurs by passive mechanisms, including solvent drag and passive diffusion down the electrical gradient in the late proximal tubule. However, there is evidence for a small contribution to Ca^{2+} reabsorption by an active, transcellular pathway. Similarly, it has been suggested that active K^+ reabsorption occurs in the proximal tubule, but a mechanism for such transport has not yet been identified.

The proximal tubule is also responsible for the reabsorption of filtered peptides and low-molecular-weight proteins. A large proportion of filtered peptides are degraded to amino acids by peptidases present in the proximal tubule brush border and are reabsorbed by cotransport with Na^+ across the apical plasma membrane. There is also evidence that small peptides are themselves transported across the apical plasma membrane through cotransport with H^+, driven by the tubular fluid–to–blood proton gradient.

Low-molecular-weight proteins are also avidly reabsorbed by the proximal tubule, but by a different mechanism. These filtered proteins, such as insulin, glucagon, and parathyroid hormone, are taken up from the tubule fluid into proximal tubule cells by carrier-mediated endocytosis along the apical plasma membrane (see Fig. 41–4). The proteins are delivered by the endocytic vesicles to a system of intracellular organelles called *lysosomes* (Fig. 41–8). Proteolytic enzymes within the lysosomes degrade the reabsorbed proteins, and the resultant amino acids are transported into the interstitial fluid and returned to the blood.

The proximal tubule secretes organic ions

Another important function of the proximal tubule is the removal of a wide variety of organic ions from the blood and their secretion into the tubule fluid. This group of organic ions includes both endogenous waste products and exogenous drugs or toxins. Because many of these substances are protein-bound in the plasma, they are poorly filtered by the glomerulus. For this reason, tubular secretion plays a vital role in the clearance of these substances from the blood. The mechanism of secretion involves uptake of these substances from the blood into the tubule cell, followed by extrusion of the substance into the tubule fluid by a carrier-mediated process. Endogenous organic compounds secreted by the proximal tubule include bile salts, oxalate, urate, creatinine, prostaglandins, epinephrine, and hippurates. Also secreted by the proximal tubule are antibiotics, such as penicillin G and trimethoprim; diuretics, such as chlorothiazide and furosemide; the analgesic morphine and many of its derivatives; and the potent herbicide paraquat. The practical applications of this aspect of proximal tubule function are broad. Tubular secretion of endogenous organic ions, drugs, and toxins provides the basis for urine testing for hormones and foreign substances as a reflection of blood levels

that may be only transiently elevated. Tubular secretion of exogenous *p*-aminohippurate is used to estimate renal plasma flow. Tubular secretion of certain antibiotics is important in determining which antibiotics can reach high concentrations in the urine for more effective treatment of urinary tract infections. Similarly, secretion of diuretics such as furosemide by the proximal tubule enhances delivery of these drugs to their site of action in the thick ascending limb of the loop of Henle. Finally, tubular secretion of certain drugs determines in part their excretion rate and affects their appropriate dosage, which can be particularly important in patients with compromised renal function.

In birds, tubular secretion plays a larger role than in mammals. The end product of protein metabolism in mammals is urea, which is excreted primarily through glomerular filtration. However, in birds, the end product of protein metabolism is uric acid. Uric acid is produced by the liver and the kidney in birds, and the majority of its excretion is accomplished by tubular secretion. The importance of this process in the excretion of nitrogenous waste in birds is demonstrated by the finding that in starlings, the total amount of uric acid excreted by the kidney is more than five times the amount filtered. The principal site of uric acid secretion in the avian kidney is believed to be the proximal portion of reptilian-type nephrons.

The distal tubule segments reabsorb salts and dilute the tubule fluid

The structure of the tubule epithelium changes abruptly and dramatically at the end of the proximal tubule. The proximal tubule, with its large numbers of mitochondria, luxuriant brush border, and pronounced infoldings of the basolateral plasma membrane, is designed for high-volume transport of a large variety of substances by both active and passive mechanisms. The segments that follow the proximal tubule each have a unique and highly specific cell structure, reflecting their specialized functions. Immediately downstream from the straight portion of the proximal tubule is the thin limb of the loop of Henle, which is a low epithelium with few mitochondria and few membranous infoldings (Fig. 41–9). As might be expected, physiologic studies suggest that active transport of solutes in this segment is virtually nonexistent. The function of the thin limb is determined by its passive permeability properties and its spatial orientation within the inner medulla. These characteristics are essential to its role in water reabsorption and are discussed in a later section.

In the ascending limb of the loop of Henle, the low epithelium of the thin ascending limb abruptly changes to the tall epithelium of the thick ascending limb. The thick ascending limb is endowed with numerous mitochondria and basolateral plasma membrane infoldings, reflecting its high capacity for active solute transport (Fig. 41–10). The distal convoluted

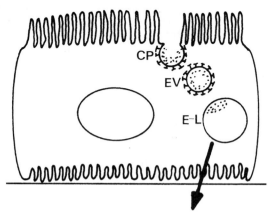

FIGURE 41–8. Schematic illustration of receptor-mediated endocytosis of filtered proteins in the proximal tubule. Filtered proteins bind with their receptors in the membrane of coated pits (CP) in the apical plasma membrane. The coated pits invaginate and form endocytic vesicles (EV) that transport the proteins to the endosomal-lysosomal system (E-L), from which the reabsorbed proteins or their degradation products are returned to the circulatory system.

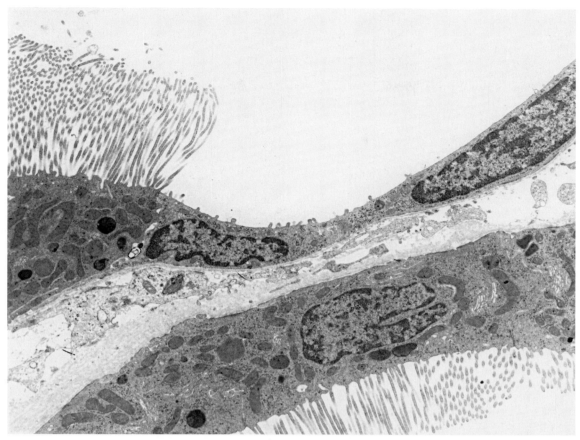

FIGURE 41–9. Transmission electron micrograph of rat kidney illustrating the transition from the proximal tubule to the thin descending limb of the loop of Henle. The tall epithelium of the proximal tubule with the extensive brush border and abundant mitochondria abruptly changes to the low epithelium of the thin limb of the loop of Henle. Epithelial cells of the thin limb have a smooth, simple plasma membrane surface and few mitochondria, which is consistent with the absence of active transport functions. Magnification, $\times 5900$.

tubule follows with an even taller epithelium and a dense array of mitochondria and leads into the connecting segment, which makes the transition from the distal nephron to the collecting duct system.

The distal tubule segments, which include the thick ascending limb of the loop of Henle and the distal convoluted tubule, reabsorb Na^+, K^+, Cl^-, and the divalent cations Ca^{2+} and Mg^{2+}. These segments are able to reabsorb solutes against a high gradient, and by the time the tubule fluid leaves the distal convoluted tubule, more than 90% of the filtered salts has been reabsorbed, and the osmolality of the tubule fluid is typically reduced to 100 mOsm/kg H_2O.

Salt reabsorption in the distal tubule segments is driven by the Na^+,K^+-ATPase pump in the basolateral plasma membrane, as in the proximal tubule, and the distal convoluted tubule has the highest Na^+,K^+-ATPase activity of any nephron segment. In the thick ascending limb of the loop of Henle, the basolateral Na^+,K^+-ATPase pump actively transports Na^+ from the cell into the interstitial fluid, creating an electrochemical gradient for Na^+ across the apical plasma membrane. This gradient drives an $Na^+,K^+,2Cl^-$ cotransporter in the apical plasma membrane, and these ions move from the tubule fluid into the cell by sec-

ondary active transport (Fig. 41–11). The Cl^- diffuses down its chemical gradient into the interstitial fluid via Cl^- channels in the basolateral plasma membrane. The K^+ moves extracellularly down its concentration gradient through K^+ channels across both the basolateral plasma membrane and the apical plasma membrane. The result of the Cl^- absorption and K^+ secretion is the development of a lumen-positive voltage (electrical potential) with regard to the interstitium, and this creates a lumen-to-blood electrical gradient for cations that then diffuse into the interstitial fluid through the paracellular pathway. The apical $Na^+,K^+,2Cl^-$ cotransporter in the thick ascending limb is inhibited by the loop diuretics, such as bumetanide and furosemide, which are commonly used in clinical veterinary medicine.

The distal convoluted tubule and connecting segment contain both an NaCl cotransporter and an Na^+ channel in the apical plasma membrane that permit transport of Na^+ from the tubule fluid down the chemical gradient for Na^+ generated by the basolateral Na^+,K^+-ATPase pump. The Cl^- that is transported into the cell via the apical cotransporter moves to the interstitial fluid via a basolateral Cl^- channel, driven by the electrical gradient. The activity of the

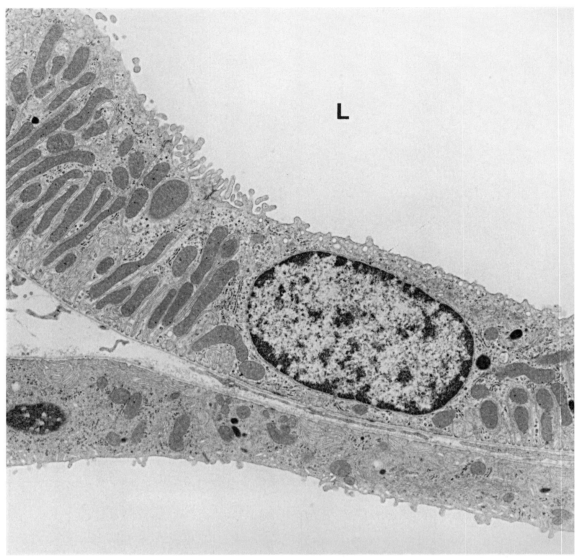

FIGURE *41–10.* Transmission electron micrograph of thick ascending limb of the loop of Henle in the rat. In accordance with its important role in active Na+ reabsorption, the thick ascending limb is a tall epithelium, with extensive basolateral plasma membrane infoldings and numerous mitochondria. A collecting duct is adjacent to the basolateral aspect of the thick limb. L, tubule lumen. Magnification, ×5600.

apical NaCl cotransporter is inhibited by thiazide diuretics.

Both the thick ascending limb and the distal convoluted tubule are impermeable to water. The avid reabsorption of salts without concurrent water reabsorption results in a hypotonic tubule fluid, and thus these segments are sometimes called the *diluting segments.* Dilution of the tubule fluid takes place regardless of the volume status of the animal, although in some species, antidiuretic hormone, which is released when an animal is in a volume-depleted state, dehydrated, or hypotensive, enhances salt reabsorption from the thick ascending limb. Although antidiuretic hormone stimulation of salt reabsorption in the thick ascending limb has the seemingly paradoxical effect of enhancing the dilution of the tubule fluid, this effect allows

maximal salt and water conservation because water reabsorption in the collecting ducts is also enhanced.

The dilution of the tubule fluid in these segments is an important component of fluid volume regulation by the kidney, allowing the kidney to excrete excess water without salt, thereby preventing water overload and plasma hypotonicity. The role of the thick ascending limb and the distal convoluted tubule in water balance is discussed further in Chapter 42.

The collecting duct reabsorbs NaCl and can secrete or reabsorb K+

The collecting duct system begins with the connecting segment, which is a transition region from the distal

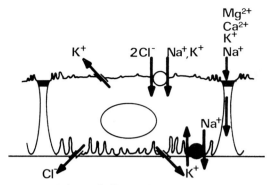

FIGURE 41–11. Schematic illustration of transport functions of the thick ascending limb. Na$^+$ is actively reabsorbed through the basolateral Na$^+$,K$^+$-ATPase. Na$^+$, K$^+$, and Cl$^-$ enter the cell from the luminal fluid through secondary active cotransport. Cl$^-$ diffuses down its concentration gradient across the basolateral plasma membrane through a Cl$^-$ channel. K$^+$ leaves the cell through both an apical and a basolateral K$^+$ channel. A lumen-to-blood gradient for cations is present in this segment, which drives reabsorption of Na$^+$, K$^+$, Ca^{2+}, and Mg^{2+} through the cation-selective paracellular pathway.

convoluted tubule to the initial collecting tubule. Depending on the species, the connecting segment is composed of several cell types, including distal convoluted tubule cells; connecting segment cells; intercalated cells, which have large numbers of intracytoplasmic vesicles as well as mitochondria; and principal cells, which have fewer mitochondria but extensive basolateral plasma membrane infoldings. It appears that each of these structurally distinct cell types has distinct physiologic functions.

The initial collecting tubules converge and empty into the collecting duct, which descends through the cortex and medulla to the papillary tip, where the tubule fluid (urine) discharges into the renal pelvis. Throughout most of the collecting duct system, there exist two main cell types: the intercalated cell and the principal cell (Fig. 41–12). The principal cell is the major cell type in the initial collecting duct, the cortical collecting duct, and the outer medullary collecting duct, accounting for approximately two thirds of the cells in most regions. The intercalated cell accounts for the remainder of the cortical and outer medullary collecting duct cells, and in some species (rat and human, at least) it persists even in the inner medullary collecting duct.

The principal cell is primarily responsible for NaCl reabsorption in the collecting duct. It has extensive basolateral plasma membrane infoldings, which contain Na$^+$,K$^+$-ATPase. As in other tubule segments already discussed, Na$^+$ is actively transported via this pump from the cell into the interstitial fluid, which establishes an electrochemical gradient for Na$^+$ uptake from the tubular fluid via Na$^+$ channels in the apical plasma membrane. This results in a lumen-negative electrical potential that can drive Cl$^-$ absorption passively through the paracellular pathway. At the same time, K$^+$ is pumped actively from the interstitial fluid into the cell by Na$^+$,K$^+$-ATPase, raising the intracellular K$^+$ concentration above that of the

interstitial fluid and the tubule fluid. Intracellular K$^+$ exits the cell down the chemical gradient via K$^+$ channels present in the apical and basolateral plasma membranes. However, under normal circumstances, net K$^+$ secretion occurs for two reasons: (1) the apical K$^+$ channel is more permeable than the basolateral K$^+$ channel, and (2) the lumen-negative electrical potential favors K$^+$ secretion (Fig. 41–13).

The collecting duct is also capable of K$^+$ reabsorption, and the intercalated cell appears to be responsible for this function. Potassium ions are actively transported from the cytoplasm across the apical plasma membrane of the intercalated cell in exchange for hydrogen ions by an Na$^+$,K$^+$-ATPase pump similar to that in the parietal cell of the stomach. This pump has an additional role in contributing to the acidification of the urine, which is discussed later.

The distal tubule and collecting duct respond to systemic signals to alter salt excretion as required

In the proximal tubule, filtered solutes and water are generally reabsorbed regardless of the animal's physiologic state. In contrast, the distal tubule and collecting duct control the ultimate rate of excretion of electrolytes and water in order to maintain homeostasis despite variations in dietary intake and extrarenal losses of salts and water. The specific responses of these segments to markedly alter the rate of reabsorption or secretion of Na$^+$, K$^+$, Ca^{2+}, and water result in large part from the action of several hormones, including aldosterone, atrial natriuretic peptide, antidiuretic hormone, parathyroid hormone, $1\alpha,25$-(OH)$_2$–vitamin D$_3$, and calcitonin. The effect of antidiuretic hormone in some species to enhance Na$^+$ reabsorption in the thick ascending limb of the loop of Henle has already been discussed. The hormone atrial natriuretic peptide is produced in the cardiac atria and enhances Na$^+$ excretion in the distal tubules and collecting ducts by inhibiting aldosterone release and also by direct effects on the collecting ducts. The role of the remainder of these hormones in regulating renal solute excretion is discussed later.

In birds, the mechanisms of regulation of salt excretion are complicated by the fact that the majority of nephrons are the reptilian type, which lack loops of Henle. The relative importance of the reptilian, loopless nephrons and the mammalian-type nephrons in regulation of salt balance has not been established. Furthermore, in many species of birds, particularly marine and desert species, sodium balance is regulated largely by secretion of NaCl by the nasal (supraorbital) gland, rather than by regulation of renal excretion. Finally, ureteral urine delivered to the cloaca moves in a retrograde manner into the digestive tract, where additional salt reabsorption occurs.

Aldosterone enhances Na$^+$ reabsorption and K$^+$ secretion

Aldosterone is a mineralocorticoid hormone that is secreted by the adrenal cortex. Aldosterone release is

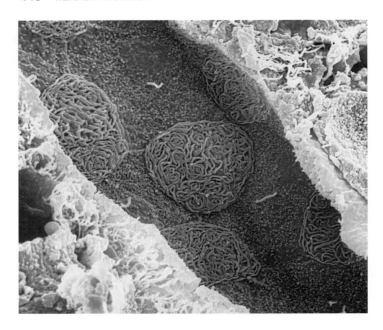

FIGURE 41–12. Scanning electron micrograph of outer medullary collecting duct in the rat, viewed from the luminal surface. Two cell types are evident: the principal cell, with short, small projections over the apical surface and a single central cilium, and the intercalated cell, with extensive, complex membrane folds (microplicae) over the apical surface. Magnification, ×2000.

stimulated by systemic hypotension through the renin-angiotensin system and acts on the connecting segment cells and the principal cells of the collecting duct to enhance Na+ reabsorption, which in turn enhances water reabsorption in order to correct perceived volume depletion. At the cellular level, aldosterone increases the permeability of the apical plasma membrane Na+ channels and stimulates Na+,K+-ATPase activity, thereby enhancing Na+ reabsorption. Chronic aldosterone stimulation even causes a structural adaptation in these cells: the proliferation of the basolateral plasma membrane, where Na+,K+-ATPase resides.

Aldosterone release is also stimulated by hyperkalemia (elevated plasma K+ level) and has an important role in regulating K+ homeostasis. The acute effect of aldosterone on K+ is to enhance its entry into aldosterone responsive cells by stimulation of

Na+,K+-ATPase activity, which lowers serum K+ levels but has little effect on renal K+ excretion. More chronic aldosterone stimulation of connecting segment cells and principal cells increases the number of K+ channels in the apical plasma membrane, thereby increasing the apical K+ permeability, which results in enhanced secretion of intracellular K+. Thus, the immediate effect of aldosterone is a redistribution of K+ from extracellular to intracellular compartments, but with continued aldosterone stimulation, renal elimination of K+ is augmented.

Although aldosterone appears to be necessary for a rapid response to an increased demand for Na+ reabsorption or K+ secretion, it has been shown that an adaptive response by the distal tubule and collecting duct is possible even in the absence of aldosterone. Chronic administration of a low-Na+–high-K+ diet to adrenalectomized (mineralocorticoid-deficient) rabbits causes proliferation of the basolateral plasma membrane of connecting segment cells and principal cells of the collecting duct, as well as an increase in Na+,K+-ATPase activity in these segments. The mechanism underlying this response is not known.

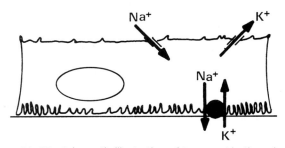

FIGURE 41–13. Schematic illustration of transport in the principal cell of the collecting duct. The extensive basal plasma membrane infoldings contain large amounts of Na+,K+-ATPase. Active transport of Na+ by this pump drives passive diffusion of Na+ from the tubule lumen into the cell through an Na+-selective channel in the apical plasma membrane. A K+-selective channel in the apical plasma membrane provides a route for passive diffusion of intracellular K+ into the tubule fluid. The hormone aldosterone enhances Na+,K+-ATPase activity and increases the Na+ and K+ permeability of the apical plasma membrane, thus enhancing Na+ reabsorption and K+ secretion in this segment.

Ca²⁺ is reabsorbed in the distal nephron and connecting segment; Ca²⁺ reabsorption is regulated by parathyroid hormone, 1α,25-(OH)₂–vitamin D₃, and calcitonin

The kidney reasorbs the majority of filtered Ca2+ and contributes significantly to the regulation of systemic Ca2+ balance. Approximately 65% of filtered Ca2+ is absorbed in the proximal tubule, where the majority of Ca2+ reabsorption is paracellular and passive, driven by electrical and chemical gradients. Approximately 20% of the filtered Ca2+ is reabsorbed in the thick ascending limb of the loop of Henle. Ca2+ reabsorption in this segment is believed to occur by passive, paracellular means, driven by electrochemical gradients, and by active, transcellular transport. The distal convoluted tubule and the connecting segment reabsorb an additional 10% of the filtered Ca^{2+}, primarily by active transcellular transport. The basolateral plasma membrane of cells in the distal tubule contains a Ca^{2+}-ATPase pump that actively extrudes intracellular Ca^{2+} into the interstitial fluid. Ca^{2+} is also transported across the basolateral plasma membrane by an Na^+/Ca^{2+} antiporter that exchanges extracellular Na^+ for intracellular Ca^{2+}. Ca^{2+} in the tubule fluid enters the cell across the apical plasma membrane via an Ca^{2+} channel, and diffusion to the basolateral side of the cell is facilitated by binding to a Ca^{2+}-binding protein, calbindin 28k. Finally, 1% to 2% of the filtered Ca^{2+} is reabsorbed in the collecting ducts; the mechanisms of Ca^{2+} transport in the collecting duct have not been determined.

Regulation of Ca^{2+} transport occurs in the distal convoluted tubule, the connecting segment, and the cortical thick ascending limb of the loop of Henle. Parathyroid hormone, calcitonin, and $1\alpha,25$-$(OH)_2$–vitamin D_3 have important roles in controlling renal Ca^{2+} excretion.

Hypocalcemia (low plasma Ca^{2+} level) stimulates parathyroid hormone release, which has an effect on bone, the intestines, and the kidneys to raise the plasma Ca^{2+} level. The response of the kidney occurs in the cortical thick ascending limb, the distal convoluted tubule, and the connecting segment. Parathyroid hormone is believed to increase the permeability of the apical plasma membrane of these segments by stimulating the activity of the apical Ca^{2+} channel, an effect that is mediated by increased production of cyclic adenosine 3',5'-monophosphate. Furthermore, at least in the distal convoluted tubule, parathyroid hormone increases the Cl^- conductance at the basolateral plasma membrane, which hyperpolarizes the cells (the interior becomes more electronegative) and thus increases the driving force for Ca^{2+} entry.

The hormone $1\alpha,25$-$(OH)_2$–vitamin D_3 is converted to its active form in the proximal convoluted tubules; this process is stimulated by parathyroid hormone. Receptors for vitamin D_3 are located predominantly in the distal tubule. There it increases the cellular content of the Ca^{2+}-binding protein calbindin 28k and thus contributes to enhanced Ca^{2+} reabsorption in the distal convoluted tubule.

Calcitonin reduces the serum Ca^{2+} concentration, largely as a result of deposition of Ca^{2+} in bone. Although pharmacologic doses of calcitonin may enhance renal Ca^{2+} excretion, physiologic doses reduce renal Ca^{2+} excretion. Calcitonin has been shown to enhance Ca^{2+} reabsorption in the thick ascending limb, the distal convoluted tubule, and the connecting segment; it is believed that calcitonin hyperpolarizes cells in these segments and thereby enhances Ca^{2+} entry from the tubule fluid. Calcitonin has additional effects on the proximal tubule, where it stimulates synthesis of $1\alpha,25$-$(OH)_2$–vitamin D_3 and also inhibits phosphate absorption.

CLINICAL CORRELATIONS

Glucosuria

History A client presents her 10-year-old female miniature schnauzer with the complaint of a dramatic increase in water consumption and urine volume over the previous 2 weeks.

Clinical examination No major abnormalities are found on physical examination. The dog appears alert and is moderately overweight. The urinalysis reveals 4+ glucose (normally negative for glucose), and the urine specific gravity is 1.030. The plasma glucose level is tested immediately and is 275 mg/dL (normal, 80 to 120 mg/dL).

Comment The dog is suffering from diabetes mellitus, which results from a relative or absolute deficiency of insulin secreted from the β cells of the pancreas. The insulin deficiency results in elevated plasma glucose levels. Glucose is freely filtered by the glomerulus and normally is entirely reabsorbed by the proximal tubule. As the plasma glucose level rises, the glucose concentration in the glomerular filtrate rises. When it exceeds the reabsorptive capacity of the proximal tubule (the renal threshold) of approximately 180 mg/dL, glucose appears in the urine. The glucose acts as an osmotic agent and increases the volume of urine excreted. The dog then drinks more water to replace the excessive fluid loss.

Treatment Treatment of diabetes mellitus in veterinary patients usually involves the administration of insulin injections two to three times each day, with adjustments of the dose in accordance with frequent evaluations of the plasma or urine glucose values. When the insulin dosage is appropriate, the plasma glucose level is normalized, the glucosuria disappears, and the urine volume and water consumption decrease.

Hypoadrenocorticism

History A concerned client presents her 1-year-old spayed female Samoyed with the complaint of severe weakness, inappetence, and vomiting since the previous day.

Clinical examination The dog appears to be lethargic, weak, and markedly dehydrated. The heart rate is normal, but pulses are weak. No other abnormalities are detected on physical examination. Samples of blood and urine are collected immediately for a complete blood count, serum chemistry profile, and urinalysis, and then an intravenous catheter is placed to start volume replacement therapy with a balanced electrolyte solution. The urinalysis is normal with a specific gravity of 1.025. Abdominal radiographs are normal, but the thoracic radiographs demonstrate a small cardiac silhouette and small thoracic vessels. The serum creatinine level is 2.5 mg/dL (normal, 0.6 to 1.2 mg/dL), the serum K^+ level is 6.5 mEq/L (normal, 3.6 to 5.6 mEq/L), the serum Na^+ level is 129 mEq/L (normal, 141 to 155 mEq/L), the serum Cl^- level is 97 mEq/L (normal, 103 to 115 mEq/L), and the serum HCO_3^- level is 12 mEq/L (normal, 18 to 24 mEq/L).

Comment The dog has hypoadrenocorticism. The metabolic disturbances result from a deficiency of the mineralocorticoid hormone aldosterone. In a normal animal, aldosterone stimulates Na^+,K^+-ATPase activity and enhances the apical plasma membrane Na^+ and K^+ permeability in the connecting segment and the collecting duct, thereby enhancing Na^+ reabsorption and K^+ secretion. In the absence of aldosterone, Na^+ conservation and K^+ secretion in these segments are impaired. Cl^- and water follow the path of Na^+ and also are excreted excessively by the kidney. Hyperkalemia (high serum K^+ level) has profound effects on excitable tissue, including nerve and muscle cells, and results in muscle weakness, decreased cardiac output, hypotension, and cardiac arrhythmias. The loss of Na^+ and water results in volume depletion and the decreased size of the heart and thoracic blood vessels and exacerbates the hypotension and poor tissue perfusion.

Poor perfusion of the kidneys is probably the major cause of the elevated serum creatinine level (azotemia), because inadequate renal blood flow and reduced glomerular capillary hydrostatic pressure prevent adequate glomerular filtration. This is called *prerenal* azotemia. In most cases of prerenal azotemia, the urine is maximally concentrated in an attempt to retain fluid and restore blood volume, but in hypoadrenocorticism, this response is often blunted, possibly by the hyponatremia (reduced serum Na^+ level) or by the absence of glucocorticoids, which have been shown to have a permissive effect on maximal urine concentration (see Chapter 42). The decreased serum bicarbonate level indicates metabolic acidosis, which is the result of both the diminished renal ability to secrete H^+ and reabsorb HCO_3^- (see Chapter 43) and the increased production of acid from poorly perfused tissue.

Treatment   Prompt treatment is important for the survival of the animal, because the hyperkalemia and acidosis can cause fatal cardiac arrhythmias. Volume repletion with normal saline and correction of the *base deficit* (low serum HCO_3^- level) often stabilizes the animal. Replacement therapy with mineralocorticoid hormones such as desoxycorticosterone acetate, desoxycorticosterone pivalate, or fludrocortisone acetate restores apical Na^+ channel and basolateral Na^+,K^+-ATPase activity and should be started as soon as possible. Frequently, glucocorticoid hormones are given early to treat shock even before the electrolyte status is known; they are beneficial for two reasons. Hypoadrenocorticism usually results in glucocorticoid deficiency, sometimes manifested by hypoglycemia, and replacement therapy is indicated. In addition, the mineralocorticoid activity in many of these preparations may be beneficial in correcting the hyperkalemia and hyponatremia.

A definitive diagnosis may be obtained by an adrenocorticotropic hormone challenge test, which maximally stimulates the release of cortisol from the adrenal gland and shows little or no response in animals with hypoadrenocorticism.

Chronic maintenance usually involves oral therapy with fludrocortisone acetate; the proper dosage is determined by periodic evaluations of the serum K^+ and Na^+ levels. Chronic replacement of glucocorticoids is also recommended.

Acknowledgment

The author thanks Dr. Charles S. Wingo for his contributions in many thoughtful discussions during the revision of this chapter.

Bibliography

Brenner BM (ed): Brenner & Rector's The Kidney, 6th ed. Philadelphia: WB Saunders, 2000.
Seldin SW, Giebish G (eds): The Kidney: Physiology and Pathophysiology, 3rd ed. Philadelphia: Lippincott Williams & Wilkins, 2000.
Valtin H, Schafer JA: Renal Function: Mechanisms Preserving Fluid and Solute Balance in Health, 3rd ed. Boston: Little, Brown, 1995.

PRACTICE QUESTIONS

1. Which segment of the renal tubule is responsible for the reabsorption of the bulk of filtered solutes?
   a. Proximal tubule.
   b. Thin limbs of the loop of Henle.
   c. Thick ascending limb of the loop of Henle.
   d. Distal convoluted tubule.
   e. Collecting duct.

2. The main driving force for the reabsorption of solutes from the tubule fluid is
   a. active transport of solutes across the apical plasma membrane.
   b. secondary active transport of solutes across the apical plasma membrane.
   c. active transport of Na^+ from the tubule epithelial cell across the basolateral plasma membrane by the electrogenic Na^+ channel.
   d. active transport of Na^+ from the tubule epithelial cell across the basolateral plasma membrane by the Na^+,K^+-ATPase pump.
   e. passive diffusion of solutes through the paracellular pathway.

3. The net rate of reabsorption of a solute in the proximal tubule fluid is determined by
   a. the rate of active transport of the solute.
   b. the rates of tubular reabsorption and secretion of the solute.
   c. the systemic requirements of the animal for the solute.
   d. the lipid permeability of the solute.
   e. the glomerular filtration rate.

4. The ultimate rate of excretion of K^+ in the urine is determined by
   a. the concentration of K^+ in the glomerular filtrate.
   b. the proximal tubule, which reabsorbs or secretes K^+ to meet the physiologic requirements of the animals.
   c. the thick ascending limb, where K^+ secretion is enhanced by high plasma K^+ concentrations.
   d. the distal convoluted tubule, which has K^+ pumps that are inserted in the apical or basolateral plasma membranes, depending on the need for reabsorption or secretion of K^+.
   e. the collecting duct, in which the principal cells are capable of K^+ secretion, and the intercalated cells are capable of K^+ reabsorption.

5. Which of the following are effects of aldosterone on Na^+ transport in the connecting segment and collecting duct?

a. Enhances the permeability of Na^+ channels in the apical plasma membrane, thereby enhancing Na^+ and water reabsorption.

b. Stimulates Na^+,K^+-ATPase activity in the basolateral plasma membrane, thereby enhancing Na^+ and water reabsorption.

c. Reduces the Na^+ permeability of the apical plasma membrane, thereby inhibiting Na^+ and water reabsorption.

d. Reduces Na^+,K^+-ATPase activity in the basolateral plasma membrane, thereby inhibiting Na^+ and water reabsorption.

e. Reduces the K^+ permeability of the apical plasma membrane, thereby inhibiting K^+ reabsorption.

PRACTICE ANSWERS

1. a   2. d   3. b   4. e   5. a, b

CHAPTER

42

Water balance

1　The renal tubules maintain water balance

2　The proximal tubule reabsorbs more than 60% of filtered water

3　The kidney can produce either concentrated or diluted urine

4　The hypertonic medullary interstitium allows the formation of concentrated urine

5　The juxtamedullary nephrons extend deep into the inner medulla

6　Medullary hypertonicity depends on solute reabsorption by the medullary thick ascending limb and collecting duct

7　The countercurrent mechanism increases medullary interstitial osmolality with little energy expenditure

8　Countercurrent exchange in the vasa recta results in the removal of water from the medullary interstitium without reducing medullary interstitial hypertonicity

9　Active NaCl reabsorption in the thick ascending limb and the distal convoluted tubule permits the formation of dilute urine

10　The collecting duct responds to antidiuretic hormone to determine the final urine osmolality

11　Cells in the inner medulla adapt to interstitial hyperosmolality by accumulation of organic osmolytes

The renal tubules maintain water balance

One of the most important functions of the kidney is the maintenance of the water content of the body and the tonicity of the plasma. Terrestrial animals must guard against desiccation, and thus their kidneys are designed to reabsorb most of the water in the glomerular filtrate. However, the kidney is also able to respond to a water overload by excreting hypotonic urine. Under normal conditions, a 10-kg beagle that produces 53.3 L of glomerular filtrate every day may reabsorb more than 99% of the water contained in the glomerular filtrate, excreting only 0.2 to 0.25 L of urine. During water deprivation, a normal dog is able to produce urine that has seven to eight times the osmolality of plasma, significantly higher than 2000 mOsm per kilogram of H_2O. After a water load, the same dog responds by excreting urine with an osmolality as low as 100 mOsm per kilogram of H_2O, approximately one third that of plasma. The means by which the kidney accomplishes these feats are discussed in this chapter.

The proximal tubule reabsorbs more than 60% of filtered water

As discussed in Chapter 41, the proximal tubule is responsible for the reabsorption of the majority of the

ultrafiltrate. Solutes are retrieved in this segment by both active and passive means. The Na^+,K^+-ATPase pump in the basolateral plasma membrane actively transports Na^+ and also drives carrier-mediated secondary active transport and passive diffusion. This pump also drives water reabsorption. As Na^+ is actively transported from the cell into the interstitial fluid, Na^+ and other solutes are removed from the tubule fluid by secondary active transport, and Cl^- diffuses passively from the tubule fluid into the lateral intercellular spaces. The reabsorption of these solutes dilutes the tubule fluid, creating a slight gradient favoring the movement of water into the cells and the intercellular spaces. Because the brush border of the proximal tubule provides a large surface area for reabsorption and the epithelium is highly permeable to water, the small gradient results in rapid movement of large volumes of water from the tubule fluid to the interstitial fluid. As discussed previously, the high oncotic pressure and low hydrostatic pressure of the peritubular capillaries favor the movement of reabsorbed water and solute from the interstitial fluid to the blood. During the course of a day, between 32 and 37 L of water are reabsorbed by the proximal tubules in the kidneys of the 10-kg beagle considered in previous chapters. However, because the water is reabsorbed nearly isotonically with salt, there is little change in the osmolality of the tubule fluid between Bowman's space and the beginning of the thin descending limb of the loop of Henle.

The kidney can produce either concentrated or diluted urine

An ingenious system has evolved in the mammalian kidney to allow the excretion of urine that is either concentrated or diluted in relation to plasma as circumstances warrant. This system can be divided into three main components: (1) the generation of a hypertonic medullary interstitium, which allows the formation of concentrated urine; (2) the dilution of the tubule fluid by the thick ascending limb and the distal convoluted tubule, which allows the formation of dilute urine; and (3) the variability in water permeability of the collecting duct in response to antidiuretic hormone (ADH), which determines the final concentration of the urine. The beauty of this system is that all the factors necessary for urine concentration and dilution are operative at any given time, so that the kidney can respond immediately to changes in ADH levels with corresponding changes in urine osmolality and water excretion.

The hypertonic medullary interstitium allows the formation of concentrated urine

The urine of terrestrial mammals usually has a concentration well above the osmolality of plasma. The excretion of concentrated wastes conserves water and, therefore, reduces the volume of water that must be consumed each day to prevent dehydration. Two of the three factors mentioned earlier are responsible for the formation of concentrated urine: (1) the generation of a hypertonic medullary interstitium and (2) enhanced water permeability in the collecting duct in the presence of ADH.

Two main factors are responsible for the hypertonicity of the medullary interstitium. The first is the reabsorption of osmotically active substances by tubules in the medulla. The second is the removal of water from the interstitium by the vasa recta.

The juxtamedullary nephrons extend deep into the inner medulla

The anatomic arrangement of the renal tubules in the medulla is crucial for the function of the urine-concentrating mechanism. The nephrons of the mammalian kidney may be subdivided into two populations, called *superficial* and *juxtamedullary nephrons,* on the basis of the location of their respective glomeruli (see Fig. 40–1). Superficial nephrons have short loops of Henle that extend only into the inner stripe of the outer medulla. Juxtamedullary nephrons have long loops of Henle that extend deep into the inner medulla. The juxtamedullary nephrons are particularly responsible for the kidney's ability to concentrate urine far above the osmolality of plasma.

As mentioned in previous chapters, avian kidneys contain both mammalian-type and reptilian-type nephrons. The reptilian-type nephrons have glomeruli that are located superficially in the renal cortex and have no loops of Henle. The mammalian-type nephrons have glomeruli that are situated more deeply in the cortex and have either short or long loops of Henle that extend into the medullary cone. These mammalian-type nephrons are believed to be at least partially responsible for the ability of birds, like mammals, to excrete urine that is hypertonic in relation to plasma. However, the percentage of mammalian-type nephrons in various bird species has not been correlated with the degree of concentrating ability.

Medullary hypertonicity depends on solute reabsorption by the medullary thick ascending limb and collecting duct

The thick ascending limb of the loop of Henle actively takes up NaCl but is impermeable to water. Therefore, as discussed in Chapter 41, this segment takes up salt relatively free of water and raises the osmolality of the interstitial fluid, thus generating medullary interstitial hypertonicity and an osmotic gradient.

The inner medullary collecting ducts also actively reabsorb NaCl, but their more important contribution to the medullary hypertonicity is the reabsorption of urea (Fig. 42–1). Although the cortical and outer medullary collecting ducts are impermeable to urea, the terminal portion of the inner medullary collecting duct (IMCD) is highly permeable to urea because of the presence of carrier-mediated passive urea transport. Urea permeability in the terminal IMCD is enhanced by ADH by enhancement of this facilitated urea transport process. Thus, urea is conserved in the tubule fluid until it reaches the terminal IMCD deep in the medulla. There, urea reabsorption into the interstitial fluid is moderated by ADH, so that when conditions demand enhanced conservation of water (increased concentration of urine), urea reabsorption is enhanced. Increased urea uptake enhances the osmotic gradient for water uptake. Because the thin limbs are permeable to urea, whereas the tubule segments that intervene between the thin ascending limb and the terminal IMCD are impermeable to urea, the urea that is reabsorbed from the terminal IMCD is recycled back to the IMCD. In mammals, this system of urea recycling enhances the efficiency of the urine-concentrating mechanism. In birds, however, urea is nearly absent in the medullary interstitium, and because of their low aqueous solubility, urates do not contribute appreciably to osmotic pressure. Thus, medullary hypertonicity in birds is dependent on single-solute (NaCl) recycling.

The countercurrent mechanism increases medullary interstitial osmolality with little energy expenditure

The countercurrent mechanism is responsible for the amplification of the medullary hypertonicity initiated

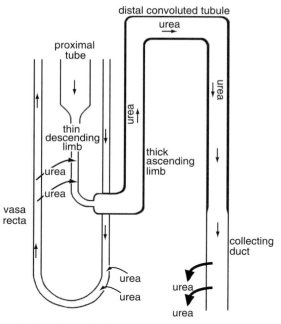

FIGURE 42–1. Schematic illustration of urea recycling in the kidney. Filtered urea is reabsorbed in the inner medullary collecting duct by carrier-mediated facilitated transport and diffuses down its concentration gradient into the vasa recta. It is believed that urea diffuses out of the fenestrated ascending vasa recta down its concentration gradient and returns to the tubule lumen by transport into the descending thin limbs of the loop of Henle. Urea uptake in the descending thin limbs and descending vasa recta is enhanced by the presence of urea transporters. The accumulation of urea in the medullary interstitium contributes to the osmotic pressure and is an important component of renal regulation of water balance.

by the active reabsorption of solutes by the thick ascending limb and the medullary collecting duct. This function is accomplished with a minimal expenditure of energy because of two characteristics: (1) the anatomic arrangement of the thin limbs of the loop of Henle and the vasa recta and (2) the differential water and salt permeabilities of the descending and ascending thin limbs.

The thin limbs of the loop of Henle in juxtamedullary nephrons extend deep into the inner medulla. The descending and ascending thin limbs are joined by a sharp, "hairpin" turn. The result is that the descending and ascending thin limbs are parallel and juxtaposed, with the tubule fluid flow in opposite directions. A similar arrangement exists for the vasa recta. This arrangement of parallel, adjacent conduits with opposite directions of flow enables an energy-efficient conservation of solute in the region, similar to heat conservation mechanisms present in the extremities of arctic animals (Fig. 42–2) and in heat pumps used for home heating. First, consider the contribution of the thin limbs of the loop of Henle to solute and water reabsorption (Fig. 42–3). The descending thin limb originates from the straight portion of the proximal tubule and is aligned with the thick ascending limb of the loop of Henle. The tubule fluid entering the thin limb is essentially isosmotic to

plasma. The surrounding interstitial fluid is hyperosmotic because of active reabsorption of sodium by the water-impermeable thick ascending limb. Therefore, a gradient for water and solutes is established between the tubule and interstitial fluid. Because the descending thin limb is highly permeable to water, but not to salt, the tubule fluid rapidly equilibrates with the interstitial fluid by the movement of water into the interstitium and the osmolality of the tubule fluid rises.

The osmolality of the medullary interstitial fluid is progressively higher in the deeper regions of the medulla. As the water-permeable descending thin limb reaches regions of higher and higher interstitial osmolality, the tubule fluid continues to equilibrate by the diffusion of water into the interstitium, and the osmolality of the tubule fluid progressively rises until it reaches its maximal concentration at the hairpin turn.

At this point, the thin limb begins to ascend through regions of progressively lower interstitial osmolality, and once again the tubule fluid equilibrates with the interstitial fluid. However, the ascending thin limb is impermeable to water and permeable to NaCl, so the equilibration occurs, not by movement of water into the tubule fluid, but by diffusion of NaCl from the tubule fluid into the interstitial fluid. The osmolality of the tubule fluid decreases, and the osmolality of the interstitium increases. This process continues until the point at which the ascending thin

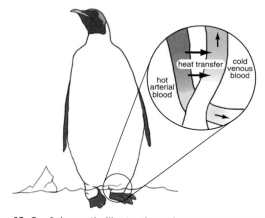

FIGURE 42–2. Schematic illustration of countercurrent blood flow for conservation of heat. In many cases, aquatic birds and aquatic mammals have a countercurrent arrangement of blood vessels in their extremities in order to conserve body heat despite constant exposure to cold ambient temperatures without the insulation provided by feathers or subcutaneous fat. Arteries carrying hot blood to the distal extremities, such as the penguin's foot, are closely intertwined with the veins returning cooled blood from the capillary bed. In this way, the arterial blood entering the foot warms the returning venous blood. This arrangement minimizes the loss of heat (energy) to the cold environment and cooling of the body core by the return of chilled venous blood. The countercurrent flow provides efficient energy conservation by creating a temperature gradient between the arterial and venous systems at every level. (Redrawn from Berl T, Schrier RW: Disorders of water metabolism. In Schrier RW [ed]: Renal and Electrolyte Disorders, 4th ed. Boston: Little, Brown, 1992, p 6.)

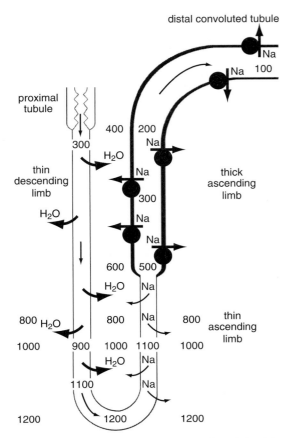

distal convoluted tubule

proximal tubule

400 200

300

thin descending limb

H₂O

H₂O

300

600 500

H₂O

800 H₂O

1000 900 1000 1100 1000

H₂O

1100

1200 1200 1200

Na
Na 100
Na
Na
Na
Na
Na
Na
Na
Na

thick ascending limb

800 800 thin ascending limb

Figure 42–3. Schematic illustration of the roles of the thin limbs of Henle's loop and the distal nephron to the generation and maintenance of a medullary interstitial concentration gradient and a dilute tubule fluid. The osmolality of the tubule fluid is approximately 300 mOsm per kilogram of H₂O when it leaves the proximal tubule and enters the environment of a progressively more concentrated medullary interstitium. Because the thin descending limb is impermeable to sodium but is permeable to water, the gradient between the tubule fluid and the interstitial fluid is reduced by diffusion of water into the interstitium, thus raising the osmolality of the tubule fluid. After the hairpin turn deep in the inner medulla, the concentrated tubule fluid enters regions of lower interstitial osmolality as it flows through the ascending thin limb of Henle's loop. Because this segment is impermeable to water but is permeable to sodium, the gradient between the tubule fluid is minimized by movement of sodium into the interstitium from the tubule fluid. The differential permeabilities of the descending and ascending thin limbs and the countercurrent arrangement preserve the medullary interstitial concentration gradient. The thick ascending limb of Henle's loop is impermeable to water and actively transports sodium into the interstitium, thus diluting the tubule fluid and generating the medullary concentration gradient. The process of dilution of the tubule fluid is continued in the distal convoluted tubule so that the osmolality of the tubule fluid delivered to the collecting duct system is approximately 100 mOsm per kilogram of H₂O, far less than that of plasma (295 to 300 mOsm per kilogram of H₂O).

limb leaves the inner medulla and merges with the thick ascending limb. At the transition to the thick ascending limb, the tubule fluid osmolality is only moderately hypertonic.

At this point, what has been accomplished? By passive means, the thin limbs have reabsorbed both water and salt. The water was reabsorbed from the

descending thin limb, and the salt was reabsorbed from the ascending thin limb. At the same time, the countercurrent flow in these two segments has helped to amplify the medullary hypertonicity.

Countercurrent exchange in the vasa recta results in the removal of water from the medullary interstitium without reducing medullary interstitial hypertonicity

The diffusion of water from the descending thin limb into the interstitium would tend to dilute the effect of salt transport into the interstitium and cause swelling of the inner medulla if it were not for the ability of the vasa recta to remove the reabsorbed fluid from the medullary interstitium. The walls of the vasa recta are permeable to water and salts. The relatively high plasma oncotic pressure in the vasa recta entering the medulla favors the movement of water into the capillary lumen, and NaCl is retained with the water. As the vessels descend in the inner medulla, the plasma osmolality equilibrates with that of the interstitial fluid by passive diffusion, rising as it nears the hairpin turn and then falling as it ascends out of the medulla (Fig. 42–4).

The previous paragraph may give the impression that there is no net effect on the interstitial fluid as a result of passive equilibration with the plasma in the vasa recta. However, two observations indicate that by the time the ascending vasa recta leave the medulla, there has been net movement of fluid into the capillary: first, the plasma oncotic pressure has fallen; second, the blood flow in the ascending vasa recta is approximately double that in the descending vasa recta. Thus, the countercurrent arrangement of the vasa recta, the passive equilibration of the plasma with the changing interstitial osmolalities in different regions of the medulla, and the relatively high initial plasma oncotic pressure allow the removal of both water and solute from the medullary interstitium, without dissipating the medullary hypertonicity.

Active NaCl reabsorption in the thick ascending limb and the distal convoluted tubule permits the formation of dilute urine

As discussed in Chapter 41, the thick ascending limb and the distal convoluted tubule actively reabsorb Na⁺, which drives Cl⁻ reabsorption secondarily. Because these segments are impermeable to water, active solute reabsorption results in a progressive decline in the osmolality of the tubule fluid. Thus, the thick ascending limb and distal convoluted tubule are often called the *diluting segments*. The result is that the tubule fluid delivered into the collecting duct system is hypotonic, regardless of the physiologic state of the animal.

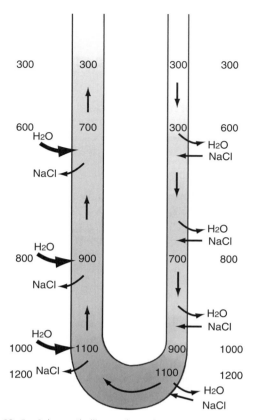

300   300   300   300

600   700   300   600
H₂O   H₂O
                         NaCl
NaCl

H₂O   H₂O
800   900   700   800   NaCl
NaCl

H₂O   H₂O
1000 1100   900   1000   NaCl

1200 NaCl   1100 1200
                         H₂O
                         NaCl

FIGURE 42–4. Schematic illustration of countercurrent exchange in the vasa recta. The walls of the vasa recta are permeable to both water and salt. Plasma entering the medulla in the descending vasa recta has an osmolality of approximately 300 mOsm per kilogram of H₂O, which rises as it traverses deeper regions of the medulla, where the interstitial osmolality is elevated. Similarly, after the hairpin turn, the plasma osmolality progressively decreases as the vessel ascends into regions of lower interstitial osmolality. In both arms of the vasa recta, the gradient between the plasma and interstitial osmolality is reduced by movement of water and solute in opposite directions. This system prevents the dissipation of the medullary concentration gradient. In addition, there is net removal of water from the interstitium by virtue of the relatively low hydrostatic pressure and relatively high oncotic pressure in the vasa recta.

─ The collecting duct responds to antidiuretic hormone to determine the final urine osmolality

The generation of medullary hypertonicity and the dilution of the tubule fluid in the distal nephron segments set the stage for the elimination of either concentrated or dilute urine, as warranted by the fluid volume status of the animal. The permeability

characteristics of the collecting duct under the influence of ADH (arginine vasotocin in birds) determine the osmolality of the excreted urine.

Under conditions of water overload, ADH is absent and the collecting duct is relatively impermeable to water. The tubule fluid delivered by the distal convoluted tubule remains hypotonic, because the water is confined within the collecting duct. Thus, in the absence of ADH, dilute urine is formed, excess water is excreted (Fig. 42–5), and normal plasma osmolality is maintained.

Under conditions perceived as dehydration or volume depletion, ADH is released from the pituitary. These conditions include factors such as dehydration or salt overload that raise the plasma osmolality as little as 3 to 5 mOsm per kilogram of H₂O. In addition to dehydration, other factors that lower the blood pressure stimulate ADH release. These factors include isosmotic volume depletion from vomiting, diarrhea, or hemorrhage; systemic vasodilation; and heart failure. In these circumstances, the goal is to reduce the plasma osmolality to normal or to restore fluid volume.

The effect of ADH is to markedly enhance the water permeability of the collecting duct. This is accomplished by the specific subcellular location of members of a group of water channel proteins named *aquaporins*. When ADH is absent, the water channel that has been identified in the collecting duct, aquaporin 2, is contained in cytoplasmic vesicles in the apical region of ADH-responsive cells: that is, principal cells and IMCD cells in the collecting duct. ADH secretion stimulates the insertion of aquaporin 2 into the apical plasma membrane of these cells, and water freely crosses the apical plasma membrane through these channels. In addition, ADH may activate aquaporin 2 already present in the plasma membrane. Forms of the clinical condition known as *nephrogenic diabetes insipidus,* which is characterized by renal unresponsiveness to ADH, have been shown to be caused by either abnormalities in or a deficiency of aquaporin 2 proteins. Another member of this water channel family, aquaporin 3, is believed to be present in the basolateral plasma membrane of collecting duct cells, regardless of ADH status, and allows the movement of water from inside the cell to the interstitial space.

Thus, when ADH is present, water rapidly flows from the dilute tubule fluid into the interstitium down the concentration gradient, producing structural alterations that include cell swelling and dilation of the intercellular spaces (Fig. 42–6). As the now water-permeable collecting duct traverses the inner medulla through regions of progressively higher in-

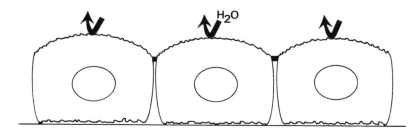

FIGURE 42–5. Schematic illustration of the collecting duct epithelium in the absence of antidiuretic hormone (ADH). When ADH is absent, the apical plasma membrane is impermeable to water, and dilute urine is excreted.

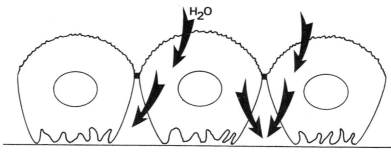

FIGURE 42–6.   Schematic illustration of the water permeability of the apical plasma membrane of the collecting duct epithelium in the presence of ADH. ADH stimulates the insertion of water channels into the apical plasma membrane, which enhances its water permeability. Water rushes into the cells and across the water-permeable basolateral plasma membrane into the lateral intercellular spaces, where solute concentrations are high in relation to the tubule fluid. Morphologic changes that have been observed include translocation of membrane containing the aquaporin 2 water channels from intracytoplasmic vesicles to the apical plasma membrane, cell swelling into the tubule lumen, and dilation of the lateral intercellular spaces.

terstitial fluid osmolality, the tubule fluid equilibrates by diffusion of water into the interstitium, and a highly concentrated tubule fluid, now urine, is eliminated.

In birds, salt and water reabsorption occur distal to the collecting ducts. Birds lack a urinary bladder, and urine from the kidneys travels via the ureters to the cloaca, where both salt and water are reabsorbed. Furthermore, cloacal urine passes in a retrograde manner into the digestive tract, where additional salt and water are reabsorbed.

Cells in the inner medulla adapt to interstitial hyperosmolality by accumulation of organic osmolytes

Cells in the inner medulla not only exist in a hypertonic environment but also regulate cell volume during changes in ambient osmolality. These cells accomplish this by accumulating organic osmolytes that maintain the intracellular osmotic pressure and prevent cell shrinking without marked increases in the concentration of intracellular electrolytes. These substances include sorbitol, betaine, inositol, and glycerophosphorylcholine. The intracellular concentrations of these osmolytes vary with the diuretic state of the animal, increasing during periods of urine concentration, when the medullary interstitial osmolality is maximized, and decreasing during diuresis, when medullary interstitial osmolality decreases. Changes in the intracellular content of these organic osmolytes when cells are exposed to changes in the ambient osmolality are the result of parallel changes in either the production (sorbitol) or transmembrane transport (betaine) of the osmolytes.

CLINICAL CORRELATIONS

Diabetes insipidus

History   A client presents her 6-month-old female Boston terrier with the complaint of excessive water consumption and urination.

Clinical examination   The physical examination reveals no abnormalities. The dog is alert and active. A urinalysis is normal, and the urine specific gravity is 1.002 (osmolality, 152 mOsm per kilogram of H_2O). The serum chemistry profile and a complete blood cell count are normal.

You admit the dog to your clinic for a modified water deprivation test. The urine fails to become concentrated despite a 5% loss of body weight. You administer vasopressin, and the urine specific gravity is 1.029 (osmolality, 852 mOsm per kilogram of H_2O) 1 hour later.

Comment   The dog has central diabetes insipidus, which is a deficiency of ADH. The urine is diluted by the thick ascending limb of the loop of Henle and the distal convoluted tubule. Solute-free water absorption in the collecting duct is dependent on the action of ADH. In the absence of ADH, excessive volumes of water are excreted, and the dog drinks voraciously to prevent dehydration.

Other causes of excretion of dilute urine (urine osmolality markedly lower than serum osmolality) are psychogenic polydipsia, hyperadrenocorticism, glucocorticoid therapy, hypercalcemia, hypokalemia, and nephrogenic diabetes insipidus. Most of these can be detected from a thorough history, physical examination, complete blood cell count, and serum chemistry profile. When only psychogenic polydipsia, central diabetes insipidus, and nephrogenic diabetes insipidus remain in the differential diagnosis, the diagnosis usually can be made by means of the modified water deprivation test. Animals with psychogenic polydipsia can secrete ADH and have normal kidneys; therefore, they concentrate their urine after water deprivation. Dogs with diabetes insipidus can concentrate their urine minimally or not at all after water deprivation. If the problem is insufficient ADH release (central diabetes insipidus), the urine concentration increases in response to exogenous ADH. If the kidney is unresponsive to ADH (nephrogenic diabetes insipidus), the urine concentration does not increase further in response to additional ADH.

Treatment   Treatment of central diabetes insipidus includes free access to water and daily administration of exogenous vasopressin by parenteral or intranasal routes.

Chronic renal insufficiency

History   You recommend routine dentistry for a 15-year-old male miniature schnauzer that appears to be in good health. Before the general anesthetic is to be administered, you obtain a complete blood cell count, serum chemistry profile, and urinalysis to detect any sub-clinical organ dysfunction.

Clinical examination The complete blood count and serum chemistry profile are normal. The urinalysis is normal with a specific gravity of 1.010 (osmolality, 352 mOsm per kilogram of H_2O). You ask the owner to submit a sample of the dog's urine from the first void of the day. The specific gravity of this sample is 1.012 (osmolality, 401 mOsm per kilogram of H_2O).

Comment Chronic renal insufficiency is common in geriatric patients and is probably responsible for the two urine specific gravity values in the "fixed range" of 1.008 to 1.012. These values correspond to osmolalities similar to or slightly higher than normal plasma osmolality. Additional evaluation would have to be performed to verify that this animal could neither dilute nor concentrate his urine significantly; however, in an animal of advanced age and in the absence of other clinical abnormalities, further evaluation is probably not indicated.

In chronic renal insufficiency, the loss of functional nephrons is first manifested by the inability to significantly alter the urine concentration in response to a water load or water deprivation. The residual nephrons are able initially to sustain adequate filtration rates to prevent azotemia (elevated serum creatinine and urea nitrogen levels), but the compensatory increase in flow rates in individual nephrons probably exceeds the capacity of the thick ascending limb and distal convoluted tubule to significantly dilute the tubule fluid. The residual nephrons are also unable to generate a steep medullary concentration gradient, and thus, the tubule fluid cannot be concentrated well above the level of the plasma osmolality. If there is progressive nephron loss, the glomerular filtration rate will continue to decline, and renal failure will ensue.

Treatment It is important to be aware that your patient has chronic renal insufficiency and is unable to respond efficiently to changes in fluid and salt intake. Water should be withheld only briefly, and caution should be exercised in supporting the animal with intravenous fluids during anesthesia while avoiding fluid overload.

There is evidence that a low-protein diet may retard the progression of chronic renal disease and delay the onset of renal failure, at least in some species. This question is a point of considerable controversy and is under intense study.

Acknowledgment

The author thanks Dr. Kirsten M. Madsen for her contributions in many thoughtful discussions during the revision of this chapter.

Bibliography

Brenner BM (ed): Brenner & Rector's The Kidney, 6th ed. Philadelphia: WB Saunders, 2000.
Seldin SW, Giebish G (eds): The Kidney: Physiology and Pathophysiology, 3rd ed. Philadelphia: Lippincott Williams & Wilkins, 2000.
Valtin H, Schafer JA: Renal Function: Mechanisms Preserving Fluid and Solute Balance in Health, 3rd ed. Boston: Little, Brown, 1995.

PRACTICE QUESTIONS

1. The bulk of filtered water is reabsorbed by which renal tubule segment?
   a. Proximal tubule.
   b. Thin limbs of the loop of Henle.
   c. Thick ascending limb of the loop of Henle.
   d. Cortical collecting duct.
   e. Inner medullary collecting duct.

2. The kidney is designed to respond rapidly to changing water requirements. The ability to efficiently alter the rate of water excretion by markedly concentrating or diluting the urine is the result of several factors. Which of the following does *not* contribute to this ability?
   a. Generation of hypertonic medullary interstitium.
   b. Countercurrent flow and differential salt and water permeabilities in the thin limbs of the loop of Henle.
   c. Dilution of the tubule fluid by the thick ascending limb and the distal convoluted tubule.
   d. Responsiveness of the collecting duct to ADH.
   e. ADH regulated countercurrent flow and enhanced water permeability in the vasa recta.

3. The hypertonic medullary interstitium (necessary for producing urine that is more concentrated than plasma) is generated in large part by
   a. active transport of Na^+ by the straight portion of the proximal tubule.
   b. active reabsorption of Na^+ by the water-impermeable ascending thin limb of the loop of Henle.
   c. active reabsorption of Na^+ by the water-impermeable thick ascending limb of the loop of Henle.
   d. increase in water channels in the apical plasma membrane of collecting duct cells under the influence of vasopressin.
   e. enhanced urea permeability of the ascending thin limb of the loop of Henle under the influence of vasopressin.

4. In dehydration, ADH is released, which reduces water excretion by
   a. enhancing water reabsorption in the proximal tubules by stimulating Na^+,K^+-ATPase.
   b. enhancing water reabsorption in the thick ascending limb by stimulating the insertion of water channels into the apical plasma membrane.
   c. enhancing water reabsorption in the collecting duct by stimulating Na^+,K^+-ATPase activity.
   d. enhancing water permeability in the collecting duct by stimulating the insertion of water channels into the apical plasma membrane.
   e. reducing the glomerular filtration rate by activation of tubuloglomerular feedback.

5. In clinical situations, the excretion of a dilute urine may be due to all but which of the following?
   a. Chronic renal disease.
   b. Glucocorticoid administration.
   c. ADH deficiency.
   d. Hypoadrenocorticism.
   e. Acute renal hypoperfusion.

PRACTICE ANSWERS

1. a   2. e   3. c   4. d   5. e

43

Acid-base balance

1 Buffers, lungs, and kidneys collaborate to maintain acid-base balance
2 The kidneys excrete acid by tubule secretion of H^+
3 Acid excretion by the renal tubules is achieved by acid secretion and buffering in the tubule fluid
4 The kidneys generate and excrete ammonium ion

5 The proximal tubule has a high capacity for H^+ secretion and HCO_3^- reabsorption
6 The collecting duct determines the final urine pH
7 The collecting duct can secrete protons and generate acidic urine
8 The collecting duct is capable of net bicarbonate secretion

Buffers, lungs, and kidneys collaborate to maintain acid-base balance

The normal blood pH is approximately 7.4, and it is necessary for normal function of cellular processes to maintain the pH close to this value. Three systems are at work to maintain acid-base homeostasis: intracellular and extracellular buffers, the respiratory system, and the kidneys. The first two of these are responsible for rapid correction of pH changes, whereas the kidneys are responsible for long-term acid-base homeostasis and the excretion of excess hydrogen ion.

The usual condition that must be corrected is the addition of excess acid, or hydrogen ion, to body fluids. Acid is constantly produced in the body as a byproduct of metabolism. The amount of acid produced varies, depending on changes in the diet; levels of exercise; functions of other physiologic processes; or, in birds, the phases of the egg-laying cycle. Therefore, the systems designed to maintain acid-base homeostasis must be able to adapt to changes in the acid load. Less often, certain disturbances result in an excess base load, which also must be eliminated.

Several intracellular and extracellular buffers titrate H^+ to maintain the pH within physiologic limits. These include hemoglobin and other proteins, carbonate in bone, and phosphate and bicarbonate. These buffers rapidly normalize the pH after acute alterations in the acid load, unless the buffering capacity is exceeded. In addition, during chronic metabolic acidosis, bone provides a reservoir of buffer that contributes to maintenance of systemic pH. In this condition, excess H^+ and low HCO_3^- in the extracellular fluid promote physicochemical as well as osteoclast-mediated dissolution of bone, releasing carbonate, which buffers the H^+ ion.

The respiratory system also can respond rapidly to maintain normal blood pH by altering the rate of removal of CO_2 from the blood. The enzyme carbonic anhydrase (CA), present in red blood cells and many other cells, catalyzes the reaction

$$CO_2 + H_2O \overset{CA}{\leftrightarrow} HCO_3^- + H^+$$

Removal of CO_2 from the blood by respiration shifts this reaction to the left, and the concentration of H^+ is consequently reduced (pH is raised). Thus, the lung provides an important avenue for stabilization of the blood pH, particularly in response to rapid changes in the acid load.

The kidney is the third line of defense of acid-base balance. Although the buffering and respiratory systems are able to stabilize the blood pH, the kidneys are responsible for the actual excretion of the majority of excess H^+.

The kidneys excrete acid by tubule secretion of H^+

Whereas the lungs alter blood pH by removing CO_2, the kidneys are capable of excretion of acid by tubular secretion of H^+, primarily in the proximal tubule and the collecting duct. These two segments operate by different mechanisms to excrete excess acid and to control blood pH precisely. The proximal tubule is primarily responsible for the bulk of acid secretion, whereas the collecting duct is primarily responsible for the control of net acid excretion and the final urine pH.

Acid excretion by the renal tubules is achieved by acid secretion and buffering in the tubule fluid

Efficient acid excretion is achieved in the kidney by the activity of enzymes and transporters that specifically promote the transport of H^+ from the epithelial cells into the tubule fluid, combined with the presence of buffers that minimize increases in H^+ concentration in the tubule fluid.

The majority of H^+ transported across the apical plasma membrane is handled by three transporters: a Na^+/H^+ exchanger, a H^+-ATPase pump, and a H^+,K^+-ATPase pump. The Na^+/H^+ antiporter exchanges intraluminal Na^+ for intracellular H^+ and is driven by the gradient for Na^+ generated by basolateral H^+,K^+-ATPase (secondary active transport). Na^+/H^+ exchange is the main route of H^+ secretion in the proximal tubule. The H^+-ATPase pump is an electrogenic proton pump that actively transports intracellular H^+ across the apical plasma membrane and contributes a net positive charge to the tubule fluid. The H^+,K^+-ATPase pump, which is similar to the gastric proton pump, actively secretes acid by the electrically neutral exchange of intracellular H^+ for K^+ in the tubule fluid. Although it has long been believed that the H^+-ATPase pump is responsible for the majority of H^+ secretion by intercalated cells of the collecting duct, there is evidence in some species that the H^+,K^+-ATPase pump may contribute equally to acidification in the collecting duct.

The buffers in the tubule fluid are vital for efficient acid excretion. The buffers accept secreted H^+ and minimize the decrease in tubule fluid pH that would otherwise result from rapid rates of H^+ secretion by the epithelial cells. In mammals, the most important buffers are bicarbonate and phosphate. In birds, urates also contribute to titration of secreted acid. The mechanisms of removal of acid by intraluminal buffers are illustrated in Figure 43–1.

In the proximal tubule, HCO_3^- is the most important intraluminal buffer, for two main reasons. The first is that the concentration of HCO_3^- in the tubule fluid is high. Although large amounts of HCO_3^- are reabsorbed in the proximal tubule, roughly proportional amounts of H_2O are reabsorbed, and the HCO_3^- concentration remains similar to that of the glomerular filtrate. Second, under the influence of apical plasma membrane–associated carbonic anhydrase, secreted H^+ combines with luminal HCO_3^- to form H_2O and CO_2, and accumulation of luminal H^+ is averted.

Filtered phosphate also contributes to the buffering capacity of the tubule fluid. Secreted H^+ titrates HPO_4^{2-} to form $H_2PO_4^-$. Because the titrated form is a charged molecule, it is lipid-insoluble, and therefore, in the absence of a phosphate transporter, it does not diffuse readily across the epithelium. Thus the secreted acid is retained in the tubule fluid. In birds, titration of urate to form uric acid, like titration of phosphate, contributes to the excretion of secreted protons. Furthermore, in addition to being lipid-insoluble, uric acid also has a low aqueous permeability, and thus a significant portion of acid is removed as uric acid precipitates.

The kidneys generate and excrete ammonium ion

Renal generation and excretion of ammonium ion (NH_4^+) is a major component in the maintenance of acid-base balance; the mechanisms of renal NH_4^+ excretion are illustrated in Figure 43–2. In proximal tubule cells, the amino acid glutamine is metabolized to produce NH_4^+. This process is called *ammoniagenesis*. The NH_4^+ that is formed in the cell enters the tubule fluid through secondary active transport by substitution for H^+ on the Na^+/H^+ exchanger. In addition, other products of glutamine metabolism are metabolized to produce new bicarbonate anions. Thus, the net result of the renal generation and excretion of NH_4^+ is acid excretion and bicarbonate production. Renal ammoniagenesis is enhanced by acidosis and is an important renal response to an increase in the acid load.

In the thick ascending limb of the loop of Henle, NH_4^+ in the lumen is reabsorbed by substitution for K^+ on the $Na^+,K^+,2Cl^-$ cotransporter. The NH_4^+ reabsorption in this segment has two significant effects: (1) it results in the accumulation of ammonia (NH_3) and NH_4^+ in the medullary interstitium and (2) it prevents NH_4^+ in the tubule fluid from reaching cortical distal nephron segments, where it would be reabsorbed into the blood and converted in the liver to urea and H^+.

The accumulation of NH_3 and NH_4^+ in the medullary interstitium is enhanced by a countercurrent mul-

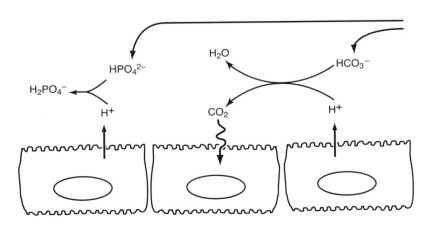

FIGURE 43–1. Schematic illustration of buffer mechanisms at work in tubule fluid. In the proximal tubule, buffering by filtered HCO_3^- predominates because of the relatively high concentration of HCO_3^-. In the cortical collecting duct, buffering by filtered, nonbicarbonate buffers, such as HPO_4^{2-}, predominates.

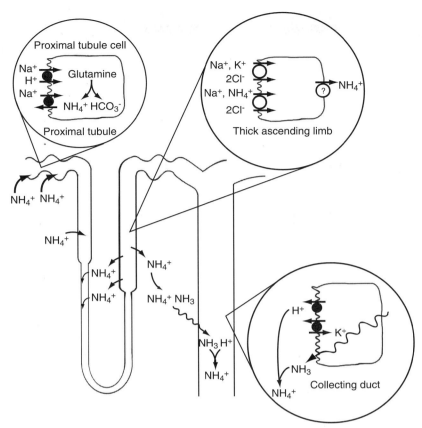

FIGURE 43–2. Schematic illustration of the roles of various nephron segments in ammonium excretion. In the proximal tubule, glutamine is catabolized to generate ammonium ion (NH_4^+) and bicarbonate. NH_4^+ is secreted into the lumen by substitution for H^+ on the Na/H exchanger in the apical plasma membrane. Ammonium ion recycles in the loop of Henle by reabsorption by the thick ascending limb, in which NH_4^+ is reabsorbed by substitution for K^+ on the $Na^+,K^+,2Cl^-$ transporter in the apical plasma membrane, which is followed by some form of facilitated transport across the basolateral plasma membrane. The elevation of the interstitial NH_4^+ concentration results in movement into the descending thin limbs of the loop of Henle and subsequent return to the thick ascending limb. This medullary recycling results in a high concentration of ammonia (NH_3) and NH_4^+ in the medullary interstitium and prevents its return to the cortex, where it would be reabsorbed into the blood. Ammonia readily diffuses into the collecting duct, where it is rapidly protonated, trapped in the lumen, and then excreted in the urine.

tiplication system in the loops of Henle, similar to that described in Chapter 42. This creates a steep concentration gradient for NH_3, which favors its movement into the medullary collecting duct. Ammonia diffuses across plasma membranes and into the luminal fluid, where it combines with H^+ to form NH_4^+. Because NH_4^+ is lipid-insoluble, it cannot diffuse back across the apical plasma membrane and is trapped within the tubule fluid.

The formation of NH_4^+ from intraluminal NH_3 and H^+ lowers the concentration of both NH_3 and H^+ in the tubule fluid. This contributes to the maintenance of a favorable gradient for the diffusion of NH_3 into the tubule fluid and reduces the magnitude of the electrochemical gradient for H^+ that is created by active proton secretion in the collecting duct.

The proximal tubule has a high capacity for H^+ secretion and HCO_3^- reabsorption

As described in Chapter 41, the proximal tubule normally reabsorbs the majority of the filtered HCO_3^-.

The mechanism of bicarbonate reabsorption in the proximal tubule is described in that chapter and is illustrated in Figure 41–7. In brief, apical membrane-bound carbonic anhydrase catalyzes the formation of H_2O and CO_2 from filtered HCO_3^- and secreted H^+. The CO_2 diffuses into the epithelial cell and combines with intracellular H_2O under the influence of cytoplasmic carbonic anhydrase to form HCO_3^- and H^+. HCO_3^- is transported across the basolateral plasma membrane and is reabsorbed into the blood, whereas H^+ is transported into the lumen, primarily by the Na^+/H^+ antiporter. There is also evidence that significant electrogenic H^+ secretion occurs across the apical plasma membrane of proximal tubule cells. The contribution of the H^+-ATPase pump to acid secretion in this segment may be as much as 35% of the total. Net HCO_3^- reabsorption and net H^+ secretion are essentially equivalent terms in this system.

Although the proximal tubule has a great capacity for HCO_3^- reabsorption (H^+ secretion), it cannot maintain a large pH gradient across the apical plasma membrane. The net secretion of H^+ in this segment is particularly dependent on the presence of the intraluminal buffers discussed earlier to combine with secreted H^+ and maintain the concentration of H^+ in the tubule fluid at a relatively constant level. As a result, although the majority of renal acid secretion (HCO_3^- reabsorption) occurs in the proximal tubule, the pH of the tubule fluid when it leaves this segment is similar to that of the glomerular filtrate. As mentioned, the buffer that is most important in the proximal tubule is HCO_3^-, primarily because of its high concentration in the glomerular filtrate and the rapid dispersion of CO_2 by intracellular diffusion and the formation of intracellular HCO_3^-.

The collecting duct determines the final urine pH

The rate of acid secretion by the collecting duct determines the final urine pH and the net acid excretion by the kidney. Although the proximal tubule has a large capacity for H^+ secretion (HCO_3^- reabsorption) and reabsorbs 80% to 90% of the filtered HCO_3^-, the pH of the tubule fluid is virtually unchanged when it leaves the proximal tubules. The segments intervening between the proximal tubule and the connecting segment have little acid-secreting ability, and so the tubule fluid that reaches the connecting segment has a H^+ concentration similar to that of the glomerular filtrate. However, the normal urine pH of carnivores ranges from 5.5 to 7.5, that of ruminants ranges from 6 to 9, and even greater extremes of pH in response to acidosis and alkalosis are possible. The collecting duct is responsible for this ability to excrete urine with a pH markedly different from that of plasma.

The collecting duct can secrete protons and generate acidic urine

In contrast to the proximal tubule, which is a high-capacity, low-gradient system of H^+ secretion, the collecting duct has a lower capacity for H^+ secretion but can generate a steep H^+ concentration gradient.

Acid secretion in most of the collecting duct system is a function of a specialized group of cells, the intercalated cells (see Fig. 41–12). The intercalated cells, which are rich in carbonic anhydrase, first appear in the connecting segment and, in some species, persist as far as the inner medullary collecting duct. In intercalated cells, intracellular H_2O combines with CO_2 to form intracellular H^+ and HCO_3^-, catalyzed by carbonic anhydrase. H^+ is secreted into the tubule fluid by the electrogenic proton pump, H^+-ATPase, or by the electrically neutral H^+,K^+-ATPase pump, both of which are present in the apical plasma membrane of intercalated cells. HCO_3^- is transported across the basolateral plasma membrane to the blood side of the cell by a Cl^-/HCO_3^- exchanger similar to the Cl^-/HCO_3^- exchanger in red blood cell membranes (Fig. 43–3). The acid-secreting intercalated cells are capable of altering the rate of H^+ secretion by altering the numbers of proton pumps in the apical

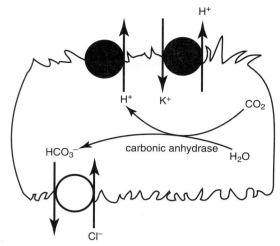

FIGURE 43–3. Schematic illustration of the mechanisms of H^+ secretion and HCO_3^- reabsorption in the acid-secreting intercalated cells of the collecting duct. Two means of active transport of H^+ across the apical plasma membrane are present: the electrogenic proton pump, H^+-ATPase, and the electrically neutral H^+,K^+-ATPase pump. The intracellular formation of H^+ and HCO_3^- from CO_2 and H_2O is catalyzed by the enzyme cytoplasmic carbonic anhydrase (CA). The basolateral plasma membrane contains a Cl^-/HCO_3^- exchanger that allows HCO_3^- reabsorption.

plasma membrane. This is accomplished by the insertion or removal of proton pump–containing membrane vesicles and results in structural changes that reflect the physiologic response (Fig. 43–4). Furthermore, it is evident that in some species the Cl^-/HCO_3^- exchanger is translocated from intracellular compartments to the basolateral plasma membrane in acidosis. In this way, the acid-secreting intercalated cells are able to respond to changes in the acid load and alter acid secretion accordingly.

The activity of the H^+,K^+-ATPase pump is enhanced by hypokalemia (low serum K^+ level), and it appears that in hypokalemia, the contribution of the H^+,K^+-ATPase pump to renal acidification is augmented. Mineralocorticoid hormones, such as aldosterone, also enhance acidification in the collecting duct. It has been postulated that this increase in H^+ secretion results from an increase in the numbers of proton transporters—either H^+-ATPase or H^+,K^+-ATPase, or both—in the apical plasma membrane of the acid-secreting intercalated cells, which is similar to the adaptive response seen in acidosis.

There is also evidence that the terminal segments of the collecting duct, in which few or no intercalated cells exist, are capable of acid secretion. A Na^+/H^+ exchanger, an electrogenic proton pump, and a H^+,K^+-ATPase pump all may participate in H^+ transport in this region, but the question of the importance and mechanism of acid secretion in these segments is currently unresolved.

The collecting duct is capable of net bicarbonate secretion

The proximal tubule reabsorbs HCO_3^- and secretes H^+, regardless of the plasma HCO_3^- concentration

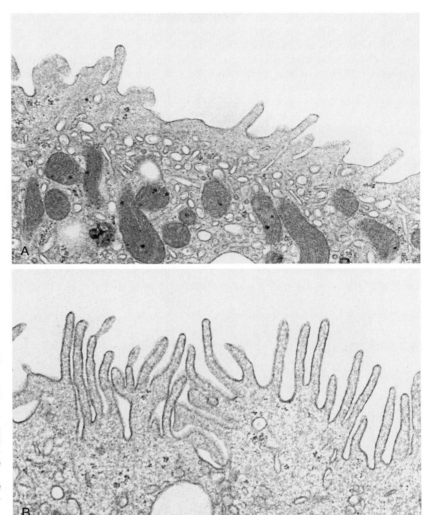

Figure 43–4. Transmission electron micrographs of an acid-secreting (type A) intercalated cell from rat cortical collecting duct. *A,* In a control animal, the apical plasma membrane contains few small membranous projections, and the apical cytoplasm is filled with numerous membrane vesicles. *B,* In a rat with acute respiratory acidosis, the apical surface is covered with numerous long membranous projections, and the number of apical cytoplasmic vesicular profiles is markedly reduced. This is the result of the insertion of membrane vesicles containing H^+ transporters into the apical plasma membrane in response to acidosis, thus enhancing the acid-secreting capacity of the cell. Magnification, ×11,300.

and the blood pH. In fact, as the plasma HCO_3^- concentration increases, the concentration of HCO_3^- in the glomerular filtrate increases, and the amount of HCO_3^- reabsorption by the proximal tubule epithelium also increases. Although the HCO_3^- reabsorptive capacity of the proximal tubule can be saturated, the amount of H^+ secretion and HCO_3^- reabsorption in this segment is generally determined by the concentration of intraluminal buffers rather than by the need for conserving or excreting acid or base.

However, the collecting duct is capable of net HCO_3^- secretion in response to alkalosis. Net HCO_3^- secretion has been shown to be a function of the connecting segment and the cortical collecting duct in rats and rabbits (Fig. 43–5). A distinct subset of intercalated cells (type B intercalated cells) is present in the cortical collecting duct segments in many species. These cells are capable of HCO_3^- secretion and are known to be rich in carbonic anhydrase and to contain a basolateral electrogenic proton pump. Furthermore, functional studies of the isolated perfused cortical collecting duct have demonstrated that the type B intercalated cell contains an apical Cl^-/HCO_3^- exchanger. In these ways, bicarbonate-secreting cells represent a mirror image of acid-secreting cells, with active H^+ reabsorption and exchange of Cl^- in the tubule fluid for intracellular HCO_3^- (Fig. 43–6).

Although information about these mechanisms is accumulating rapidly, little is known about the comparative physiology of renal control of acid-base balance. It is likely that considerable anatomic and functional differences exist among species, particularly among carnivores, which usually excrete acid urine,

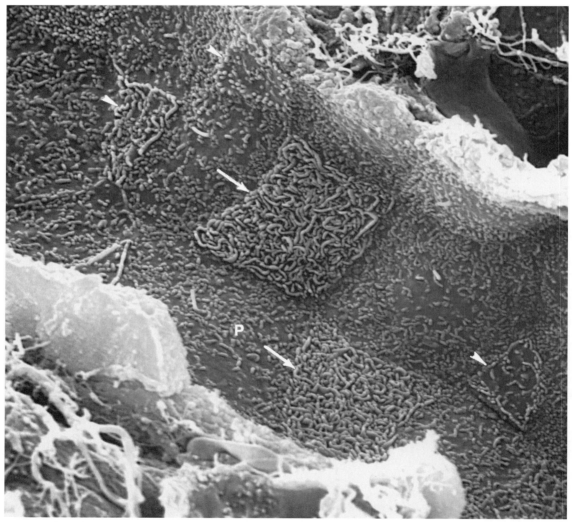

FIGURE 43–5. Scanning electron micrograph of rat cortical collecting duct viewed from the tubule lumen. Three cell types are evident. The principal cells *(P)* are large, with a single central cilium and few apical surface microprojections. The type A (acid-secreting) intercalated cells *(arrows)* have a large apical surface covered with extensive membrane folds (microplicae). The type B (bicarbonate-secreting) intercalated cells *(arrowheads)* have a small apical surface area covered with sparse microprojections, either microvilli or a mixture of microvilli and microplicae. Magnification, ×4000.

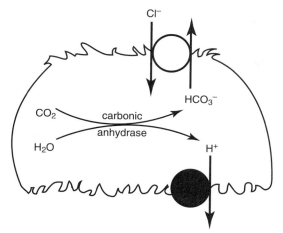

FIGURE 43-6. Schematic illustration of the proposed mechanism of HCO_3^- secretion (H^+ reabsorption) in the type B intercalated cell of the cortical collecting duct. These cells contain H^+-ATPase in the basolateral plasma membrane and are rich in cytoplasmic carbonic anhydrase. Functional evidence indicates that a Cl^-/HCO_3^- exchanger is present in the apical plasma membrane.

and among ruminants, which usually excrete neutral or alkaline urine.

CLINICAL CORRELATIONS

Respiratory acidosis with renal compensation

History   A 6-year-old male German shepherd is presented to you with the complaints of weakness, exercise intolerance, and inappetence that have become progressively worse over the past 6 weeks.

Clinical examination   The dog is recumbent and anxious. Respiration is labored, and the heart rate is rapid, but pulses are strong and regular. Crackles are heard over all lung fields. Thoracic radiographs reveal a diffuse, severe pulmonary interstitial and alveolar infiltrate with enlargement of the hilar lymph nodes. You obtain samples of blood and urine for a complete blood cell count, serum chemistry panel, urinalysis, and arterial blood gas measurement. The urine pH is 5.0, and the arterial blood gas results are as follows: pH, 7.37 (normal, 7.45); Po_2, 38 mm Hg (normal, 80 to 100 mm Hg); Pco_2, 70 mm Hg (normal, 31 to 35 mm Hg); and HCO_3^-, 37 mEq/L (normal, 18 to 24 mEq/L).

Comment   The dog has chronic respiratory acidosis caused by severe pulmonary infiltrates. The lung is unable to ventilate adequately, and the blood level of CO_2 rises, increasing the concentration of carbonic acid and lowering the blood pH. Although the increased level of CO_2 contributes slightly to an increase in blood HCO_3^- levels, the marked increase in the blood HCO_3^- levels in this case results from enhanced renal retention of HCO_3^- and secretion of H^+. Acidemia also enhances ammoniagenesis in the proximal tubule, thereby enhancing acid excretion in the form of ammonium ion and the generation of new bicarbonate. Respiratory acidosis activates the acid-secreting intercalated cells in the collecting duct, where HCO_3^- is reabsorbed and H^+ is secreted.

The blood HCO_3^- concentration rises and helps return the blood pH toward normal. A steep H^+ gradient is established in the collecting ducts, and acidic urine is excreted.

Treatment   Treatment necessitates diagnosis and correction of the pulmonary disease if possible. Bicarbonate therapy is not indicated, because the blood bicarbonate level is elevated already, and the blood pH is partially corrected. Oxygen therapy may be beneficial in supporting the animal until specific treatment is instituted.

Metabolic alkalosis with paradoxic aciduria

History   You are asked to examine a 3-year-old Holstein-Friesian cow that has been inappetent for 2 to 3 days. The cow recently calved and freshened normally, but milk production has dropped in the last 2 days, and the feces are loose.

Clinical examination   Physical examination reveals dehydration and an elevated heart rate. Percussion of the abdomen reveals an area of high-pitched resonance on the right side. A distended abomasum is palpable on rectal examination. You diagnose a right displaced abomasum and suspect abomasal torsion. Attempts to correct the displacement by rolling the cow fail. The cow is transported to your clinic for surgery, and samples are obtained for a complete blood cell count, serum chemistry profile, and urinalysis. The serum K^+ level is 2.7 mEq/L (normal, 4.0 to 5.1 mEq/L), serum Cl^- level is 77 mEq/L (normal, 85 to 103 mEq/L), and total CO_2 concentration (which is nearly equivalent to the serum HCO_3^- concentration) is 35 mEq/L (normal, 24 to 27 mEq/L). The urine pH is 6.0.

Comment   The cow has hypokalemic, hypochloremic, metabolic alkalosis secondary to abomasal displacement. The alkalosis was initiated by continued secretion of HCl by the abomasum and blunted HCO_3^- secretion by the intestine after the gastrointestinal obstruction. The hypokalemia is a result largely of intracellular movement of K^+ secondary to alkalosis and may not reflect a decrease in total body K^+ levels.

The expected renal response to alkalosis is the excretion of alkaline urine. However, in this case the volume contraction and hypochloremia prevent the formation of alkaline urine, and the result is *paradoxic aciduria*. As mentioned, the proximal tubule reabsorbs the filtered HCO_3^-, regardless of the plasma pH or serum HCO_3^- concentration. The volume depletion enhances Na^+ reabsorption primarily through the action of aldosterone, and Cl^- and H_2O reabsorption are enhanced as a secondary reaction to the increased Na^+ uptake.

Renal secretion of HCO_3^- is believed to result from apical exchange of Cl^- in the tubule fluid for intracellular HCO_3^-, probably in type B intercalated cells in the collecting duct. Because NaCl is avidly reabsorbed to combat volume depletion, little Cl^- remains for exchange with HCO_3^-, and net HCO_3^- secretion does not occur. Acid secretion in the collecting duct is known to increase in response to aldosterone and may be enhanced in this volume-depleted animal. Hypokalemia may contribute also to the excretion of acid urine in this case. Hypokalemia activates the acid-secreting intercalated cells in the collecting duct. It is possible that the activity of the apical H^+,K^+-ATPase pump, which exchanges luminal K^+ for intracellular H$^+$, is enhanced in these cells, and net acid secretion is thus favored by this mechanism as well.

Treatment Treatment involves vigorous volume replacement with intravenous normal saline with KCl added and surgical correction of the abomasal displacement.

Bibliography

Brenner BM (ed): Brenner & Rector's The Kidney, 6th ed. Philadelphia: WB Saunders, 2000.

Seldin SW, Giebish G (eds): The Kidney: Physiology and Pathophysiology, 3rd ed. Philadelphia: Lippincott Williams & Wilkins, 2000.

Valtin H, Schafer JA: Renal Function: Mechanisms Preserving Fluid and Solute Balance in Health, 3rd ed. Boston: Little, Brown, 1995.

PRACTICE QUESTIONS

1. In carnivores, the usual role of the kidney in maintaining acid-base homeostasis is to
   a. secrete excess bicarbonate.
   b. secrete excess ammonia.
   c. secrete excess acid.
   d. secrete excess carbon dioxide.
   e. secrete excess phosphate buffer.

2. The bulk of acid secretion (bicarbonate reabsorption) is accomplished by which renal tubule segment?
   a. Proximal tubule.
   b. Thin limbs of the loop of Henle.
   c. Thick ascending limb of the loop of Henle.
   d. Distal convoluted tubule.
   e. Collecting duct.

3. Which of the following factors does *not* contribute to efficient acid excretion (bicarbonate reabsorption) by the renal tubules?
   a. Vasopressin-responsive bicarbonate reabsorption.
   b. Intraluminal buffering by bicarbonate.
   c. Intraluminal buffering by ammonia and phosphate.
   d. Intracellular and membrane-associated carbonic anhydrase.
   e. Transmembrane proton transport by the Na$^+$/H$^+$ exchanger, the H$^+$-ATPase pump, and the H$^+$,K$^+$-ATPase pump.

4. Which of the following statements regarding mechanisms of acid-base regulation by the collecting duct is false?
   a. The cortical collecting duct responds to acidosis by increasing the net rate of acid secretion.
   b. The cortical collecting duct responds to alkalosis with net bicarbonate secretion.
   c. Proton and bicarbonate transport in the collecting duct are only slightly altered in response to systemic acid-base disturbances.
   d. The collecting duct ultimately determines the pH of the urine.
   e. The intercalated cells are largely responsible for acid secretion by the collecting duct.

5. Which of the following statements is correct?
   a. Aldosterone affects acid excretion by enhancing proton secretion by the proximal tubule.
   b. Aldosterone affects acid excretion by enhancing proton secretion by the collecting duct.
   c. Aldosterone affects acid excretion by enhancing bicarbonate secretion by the collecting duct.
   d. Aldosterone affects acid excretion by inhibiting bicarbonate reabsorption by the proximal tubule.
   e. Aldosterone has no effect on acid excretion.

PRACTICE ANSWERS

1. c   2. a   3. a   4. c   5. b

RESPIRATORY FUNCTION

N. Edward Robinson

Overview of respiratory function: ventilation of the lung

Respiratory function

1 The respiratory system's primary function is the transport of oxygen and carbon dioxide between the environment and the tissues

Ventilation

1 Ventilation is the movement of gas into and out of the lung

2 Ventilation requires muscular energy

3 The respiratory muscles generate work to stretch the lung and overcome the frictional resistance to airflow

4 Lung elasticity results from tissue and surface tension forces

5 The lung is mechanically connected to the thoracic cage by the pleural liquid

6 Airflow is opposed by frictional resistance in the airways

7 Smooth muscle contraction affects the diameters of the trachea, bronchi, and bronchioles

8 Dynamic compression can narrow the airways

9 The distribution of air depends on the local mechanical properties of the lung

10 In some species, air travels between adjacent regions of lung via collateral pathways

RESPIRATORY FUNCTION

The respiratory system's primary function is the transport of oxygen and carbon dioxide between the environment and the tissues

The respiratory system provides oxygen to support tissue metabolism and removes carbon dioxide. *Oxygen consumption* and *carbon dioxide production* vary with the metabolic rate, which is dependent on the animal's level of activity. Basal metabolism, the metabolism of the resting animal, is a function of metabolic body weight ($M^{0.75}$). Therefore, smaller species consume more oxygen per kilogram of body weight than do larger species. When animals exercise, their muscles need more oxygen, which leads to an increase in oxygen consumption. Oxygen consumption can increase up to a maximum known as $\dot{V}_{O_{2max}}$. Although $\dot{V}_{O_{2max}}$ generally increases with body size, there are some interesting deviations from this general relationship. Maximal oxygen consumption in the horse is threefold greater than maximal oxygen consumption in a cow of similar body weight, and dogs have higher maximal oxygen consumption than similarly sized goats. The more aerobic species, such as the dog and horse, have a higher $\dot{V}_{O_{2max}}$ per kilogram, because their skeletal muscle mitochondrial density is greater than that of the less aerobic species.

Gas exchange requirements vary with metabolism and may increase up to 30 times during strenuous exercise (Fig. 44–1). Surprisingly, these variations are normally accomplished with only a small energy cost. The energy cost of breathing increases in animals with respiratory disease, which leads to a decrease in the amount of energy available for exercise or weight gain. The owner then notices the poor performance of the animal. The respiratory system is also important in thermoregulation; metabolism of endogenous and exogenous substances; and protection of the animal against inhaled dusts, toxic gases, and infectious agents.

Figure 44–2 shows the processes involved in gas exchange, including *ventilation*; *distribution* of gas within the lung; *diffusion* at the alveolocapillary membrane; *transport* of oxygen in the blood from the lungs to the tissue capillaries and of carbon dioxide in the reverse direction; and *diffusion* of gases between blood and tissues.

VENTILATION

Ventilation is the movement of gas into and out of the lung

The oxygen requirements of metabolism are that an animal take a certain volume of air into its lungs,

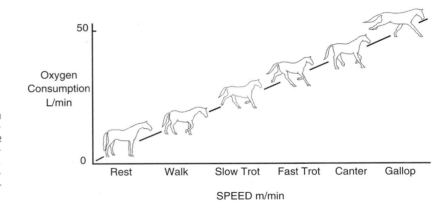

FIGURE 44–1. The effect of exercise on oxygen consumption in the horse. Oxygen consumption increases in a linear manner as the horse increases speed; the total increase is approximately 30-fold. (Modified from Hornicke H, Meixner R, Pollman U: Equine Exercise Physiology. Cambridge, United Kingdom: Granta Editions, 1983, p 7.)

especially its alveoli, each minute. The total volume of air breathed per minute, or *minute ventilation* ($\dot{V}_E$), is determined by the volume of each breath, or *tidal volume* (VT), multiplied by the number of breaths per minute, or *respiratory frequency.* The increase in $\dot{V}_E$, which must occur when an increase in metabolic rate demands more oxygen, can be brought about through an increase in VT, in respiratory frequency, or in both.

Air flows into the *alveoli* through the *nares, nasal cavity, pharynx, larynx, trachea, bronchi,* and *bronchioles.* These structures constitute the *conducting airways.* Because gas exchange does not occur in these pathways, they are also known as the *anatomic dead-space* (Fig. 44–3). A portion of each VT and, therefore, of $\dot{V}_E$, ventilates the anatomic dead-space. The portion of each breath that participates in gas exchange is known as *alveolar ventilation;* that ventilating dead-space is known as dead-space ventilation ($\dot{V}_D$). Minute ventilation is the sum of alveolar and dead-space ventilation:

$$\dot{V}_E = \dot{V}_A + \dot{V}_D$$

Alveolar ventilation is regulated by control mechanisms to match the oxygen uptake and carbon dioxide

elimination necessitated by metabolism. Thus, when an animal exercises, its alveolar ventilation increases in order to take in more oxygen and eliminate more carbon dioxide.

Dead-space ventilation can also occur within the alveoli. This *alveolar dead-space* is caused by ventilation of alveoli that are poorly perfused with blood, so that gas exchange cannot occur optimally (see Chapter 46). *Physiologic dead-space* is the sum of the anatomic and the alveolar dead-space. The fraction of each breath that ventilates the dead-space is known as the *dead-space/tidal volume ratio* (VD/VT). This VD/VT ratio varies considerably between species. In smaller species, such as dogs, it approximates 33%, whereas in some larger species, such as cattle and horses, it approximates 50% to 75%.

Because the volume of the anatomic dead space is relatively constant, changes in VT, respiratory frequency, or both can alter the relative amounts of air that ventilate the alveoli and dead-space. These changes in VT and respiratory frequency occur in animals during exercise and thermoregulation. For example, the small VT and rapid respiratory frequency characteristic of *panting* in dogs cause more

FIGURE 44–2. Diagrammatic representation of the processes involved in gas exchange. The lung is shown on the left, the heart in the center, and tissues on the right. The brain is shown at the top.

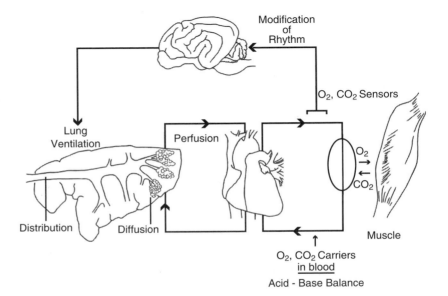

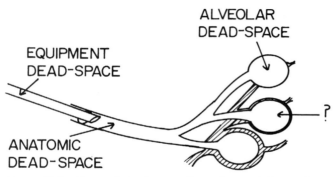

FIGURE 44-3. Types of dead-space. The volume of the trachea and bronchi constitutes the anatomic dead-space; equipment dead-space is created by an endotracheal tube; and alveolar dead-space is the volume of air ventilating poorly perfused alveoli. *Top,* An unperfused alveolus is shown; *bottom,* a normally perfused alveolus; *middle,* an alveolus with less than optimal perfusion for the amount of ventilation received.

air to ventilate the dead-space in order to cause water evaporation and heat loss. Cattle, pigs, and mules subjected to heat stress also increase respiratory rate and dead-space ventilation when trying to lose heat. In contrast to the effects of heat stress, cold-stressed animals have a higher metabolic rate, which is necessary to maintain body temperature in cold conditions. This leads to an increase in both oxygen consumption and carbon dioxide production, making it necessary for the animal to increase alveolar ventilation and decrease dead-space ventilation. The latter adaptations are accomplished by reducing the respiratory frequency and increasing VT.

The veterinarian needs to ensure that equipment used for anesthesia or respiratory therapy does not increase the dead-space. Excessively long endotracheal tubes or overly large face masks should be avoided.

Ventilation requires muscular energy

During *inhalation,* energy provided by muscles causes air to enter the lungs. During *exhalation,* much of the energy causing air to leave the lungs is provided by the *elastic force* stored in the stretched lung and thorax. Therefore, in most animals at rest, inhalation is an active process, whereas exhalation is passive. Horses are an exception to this general rule and have an active phase to exhalation even at rest. During exercise or in the presence of respiratory disease, exhalation is assisted by muscle contraction in most species.

The *diaphragm,* a domed musculotendinous sheet separating the abdomen and thorax and innervated by the *phrenic nerve,* is the primary inspiratory muscle. It consists of a costal portion arising from the xiphoid process and the costochondral junctions of the 8th to 12th ribs (8th to 14th ribs in Equidae), and a crural portion arising from the ventral surface of the first three to four lumbar vertebrae and extending toward the tendinous center of the diaphragm. The apex of the dome of the diaphragm extends rostrally to the

seventh or eighth intercostal space at the level of the base of the heart. During contraction, the dome of the diaphragm is pulled caudally and thereby enlarges the thoracic cavity. The tendinous center pushes against the abdominal contents, elevating intra-abdominal pressure, which displaces the caudal ribs outward, thus also tending to enlarge the thorax. It is the enlargement of the thorax that creates the negative (subatmospheric) pressure necessary to make air flow into the lungs.

The *external intercostal muscles,* which join the ribs, are also active during inhalation. The fibers of these muscle are directed caudoventrally from the caudal border of one rib to the cranial border of the next, so contraction moves the ribs rostrally and outward. The relative contributions of diaphragmatic and costal movement to ventilation under different metabolic demands are not well defined in animals. Because the cranial ribs support the forelimbs in quadrupeds, they probably participate less in ventilation than do the more caudal ribs. Other inspiratory muscles include those connecting the sternum and head. These muscles contract during strenuous breathing and move the sternum rostrally.

The subatmospheric pressure generated within the respiratory tract during inhalation tends to collapse the external nares, pharynx, and larynx. Contraction of *abductor muscles* attached to these structures is essential for preventing collapse. Abductor muscle contraction during inhalation can be observed as dilation of the external nares. *Laryngeal hemiplegia* in horses is a condition in which the abductor muscles on the left side of the larynx fail to contract during inhalation. During exercise these horses exhibit a sound known as "roaring." Roaring occurs as the result of the turbulent airflow that is generated upon inhalation as the vocal fold on the paralyzed side is sucked into the lumen of the larynx by the subatmospheric pressure.

The *abdominal muscles* and *internal intercostal muscles* are the expiratory muscles. Contraction of the abdominal muscles increases abdominal pressure, which forces the relaxed diaphragm forward and reduces the size of the thorax. The fibers of the internal intercostal muscles are directed cranioventrally from the cranial border of one rib to the caudal border of the next cranial rib, so that their contraction decreases the size of the thorax by moving the ribs caudally and ventrally. As the thorax gets smaller, the pressure therein increases and forces air out of the lungs.

During exercise, respiratory muscle activity increases in order to generate the increase in V̇E. In cursorial (running) mammals, ventilation is synchronized with gait in the canter and gallop, but not in the trot (Fig. 44–4). Inhalation occurs as the forelimbs are extended and the hind limbs are accelerating the animal forward. Exhalation occurs when the forelimbs are in contact with the ground.

The respiratory muscles generate work to stretch the lung and overcome the frictional resistance to airflow

At the end of a normal exhalation, some air (approximately 45 mL/kg) remains in the lung. This air vol-

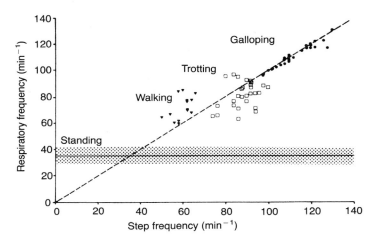

FIGURE 44–4. The relationship between gait and respiration in the horse. In the walk and trot, step and respiratory frequency are not correlated. At the gallop (and canter), respiratory and step frequency bear a 1:1 relationship. (From Hornicke H, Meixner R, Pollman U: Equine Exercise Physiology. Cambridge, United Kingdom: Granta Editions, 1983, p 7.)

ume is known as *functional residual capacity* (FRC). At FRC, the *pressure in the pleural cavity* (Ppl) that surrounds the lung is approximately 5 cm H_2O below atmospheric pressure (-5 cm H_2O). As previously mentioned, Ppl decreases during inhalation as the thorax enlarges and the respiratory muscles perform work to stretch the *elastic lung* and thorax and generate airflow through air passages that provide a *resistance to flow* (Fig. 44–5). The magnitude of the change in pleural pressure (ΔPpl) during each breath is determined by the change in lung volume (ΔV), by lung compliance (C), by airflow rate (V), and by *airway resistance* (R):

$$\Delta Ppl = (\Delta V/C) + R\dot{V}.$$

Resting animals breathe slowly and have low flow rates. In this situation, the primary work of the respiratory muscles is to overcome the elasticity of the lung. When the respiratory rate increases—for example, during exercise—flow rates increase, and more energy is used to generate flow against the frictional resistance of the airways.

Lung elasticity results from tissue and surface tension forces

At FRC, the slightly subatmospheric pressure in the pleural cavity keeps the lung inflated. If the thorax is opened and the lungs are exposed to atmospheric pressure, the lungs collapse to their minimal volume. At this volume, some air remains trapped within the alveoli behind closed peripheral airways, which causes a piece of such normal lung to float in water. The collapse of the lung when the thorax is opened is a result of the lung's inherent elasticity, which is generated by both elastic and collagen tissue and by surface tension forces.

The importance of surface tension can be demonstrated experimentally by inflating the lung with air or saline while concurrently measuring the pressure required for inflation, transpulmonary pressure (PL). Figure 44–6 represents the resulting lung pressure-

volume curve and demonstrates several important points:

1. A high pressure is required to initially inflate the lung with air from the gas-free state. This is because

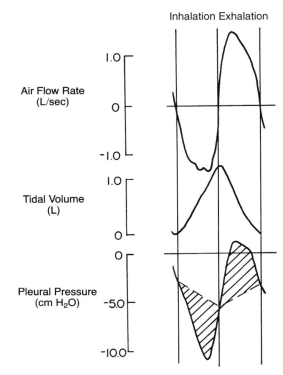

FIGURE 44–5. Air flow rate, tidal volume, and pleural pressure during inhalation *(left)* and exhalation *(right)*. During inhalation, pleural pressure decreases as the thorax enlarges, air flow rates increase, and the volume of air in the lung increases. At the end of inhalation, flow rates return to zero, and pleural pressure becomes less negative. During exhalation, pleural pressure increases as the thorax decreases in size, flow rates increase to a peak and then decrease again, and the volume of air in the lung decreases. The *broken line* shows the change in pleural pressure necessary to overcome the elasticity of the lung (proportional to volume). The *shaded area* represents the change in pleural pressure necessary to overcome the frictional resistance of the airways. The peaks of pleural pressure on both inhalation and exhalation coincide with peaks of flow.

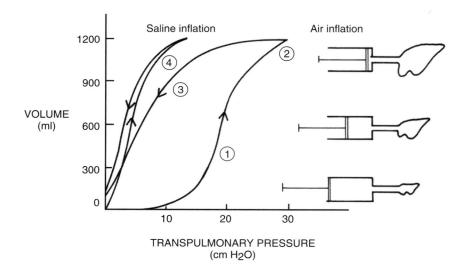

FIGURE 44–6. Pressure-volume curve of the lung during inflation with saline and with air. The pressure gradient across the lung (transpulmonary pressure) is shown on the abscissa and lung volume on the ordinate. During air inflation, the inflation and deflation curves are separated; that is, there is pressure-volume hysteresis. Hysteresis is abolished by inflating the lung with saline. The lung inflates more easily (i.e., it takes less pressure for a given volume) with saline than with air. Numbers correspond to numbers in the section "lung elasticity results from tissue and surface tension forces."

high pressure is required for the initial opening of the bronchioles. In life, the lung is gas-free only in the fetus and for a few seconds after birth until the first breath is taken. Usually, tidal breathing is initiated from FRC when the bronchioles are already open.

2. The lung reaches its elastic limits at PL of approximately 30 cm H_2O. The volume of air in the lung at this point is known as the *total lung capacity.*

3. The lung's elastic properties differ during inflation and deflation; less pressure is necessary to maintain a given volume during deflation than during inflation. This phenomenon, known as *pressure-volume hysteresis,* is a result of changes in surface tension forces, the same forces that made it necessary for the high pressure to initially inflate the lung.

4. When saline is used instead of air to inflate the lung, less pressure is required for inflation, and the pressure-volume hysteresis is abolished. These two phenomena occur because when the lung is inflated with saline, the air-liquid interface of the fluid film overlying the alveolar epithelium is abolished. Because surface tension forces arise from this interface, they too are eliminated when the lung is inflated with saline. A comparison of the pressure-volume curves when the lung is inflated with air and with saline (see Fig. 44–6) shows that surface forces are responsible for a considerable part of the elastic recoil of the lung.

Surface tension forces continually try to collapse the alveoli. Therefore, alveolar stability depends on the presence of a *pulmonary surfactant* that reduces the surface tension of the alveolar lining. Pulmonary surfactant is a mixture of lipids and proteins. The most plentiful lipid component, *dipalmitoyl phosphatidylcholine,* is responsible for the surface tension reduction. Surfactant is produced in *type II alveolar cells,* and its hydrophilic and hydrophobic portions cause it to seek the surface of the alveolar lining (Fig. 44–7). As lung volume decreases and the alveolar surface area shrinks, surfactant molecules become concen-

trated on the alveolar surface, reducing surface tension and promoting alveolar stability.

There are four important surfactant proteins. Two are hydrophobic and aid in surfactant secretion, maintenance of surface films, and reuptake of surfactant into type II cells. The two other proteins are hydrophilic; they also have antimicrobial properties.

Pulmonary surfactant is released into the alveolar spaces and tracheal fluid late in gestation (85% of the length of gestation in the sheep). Its appearance correlates with the rise in fetal plasma cortisol levels. Animals born prematurely have difficulty inflating their lungs because of inadequate surfactant. Synthetic surfactants can be used to treat premature newborns that lack adequate surfactant.

The slope of the lung-pressure volume curve is called *lung compliance.* Because the pressure-volume curve is not linear, compliance obviously varies with the state of lung inflation. It is usually measured over the range of VT and, when adjusted for differences in lung size, does not vary greatly among adult mammals. Consequently, most mammals generate similar changes in pleural pressure during breathing.

The lung is mechanically connected to the thoracic cage by the pleural liquid

The lung is covered by the visceral pleura, and the ribs are covered by the parietal pleura. These two pleural surfaces are maintained in close apposition by a thin layer of pleural fluid so that the lung and thoracic cage mechanically interact. When an animal exhales below FRC, the stiff thorax increasingly resists deformation, so that *residual volume,* the volume of air in the lung at the end of a maximal exhalation, is determined by the limits to which the rib cage can be compressed.

The thorax is generally more stiff—that is, it is less

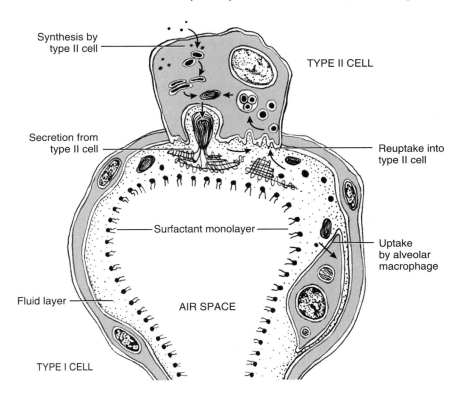

FIGURE 44–7. Diagram of an alveolus to show the movement of surfactant components through the type II cell and the alveolar liquid.

compliant—in large animals than in small animals; the stiff chest wall of the horse and cow is in contrast with the very compliant chest wall of small rodents. Neonates have a more compliant chest than do adults. Lung collapse, also known as *atelectasis*, is more likely to occur in species with compliant thoraces. For this reason, atelectasis is more common in newborn animals than in adults.

Airflow is opposed by frictional resistance in the airways

During breathing, air flows through the tubes of the *upper airway* (i.e., nose, pharynx, and larynx) and the *tracheobronchial tree*, which present *frictional resistance* to the movement of air. In the resting animal, the nasal cavity, pharynx, and larynx, which warm and humidify the air, provide approximately 60% of the frictional resistance to breathing (Fig. 44–8). Nasal resistance can be decreased—for example, during exercise—by dilation of the external nares and by vasoconstriction of the extensive vascular tissue in the nose. When airflow rates increase during exercise, or when the nasal cavity is obstructed, some species, such as the cow and dog, breathe through the mouth to bypass the high-resistance nasal cavity. Other species, such as the horse, are obligate nose breathers and are solely dependent on a decrease in nasal resistance to keep the work of breathing at a reasonable level. The horse accomplishes this by flaring its nostrils and by constricting blood vessels to shrink the nasal mucosa.

The tracheobronchial tree has up to 24 branches lined by a secretory, ciliated epithelium. The larger airways—*trachea* and *bronchi*—are supported by *cartilage* and supplied with secretory *bronchial glands*. The smaller airways in the lung are known as bronchioles. *Bronchioles* lack cartilage and a connective tissue sheath. Alveoli surround the intrapulmonary airways, and the alveolar septa attach to the outer layers of the airways so that the tension in the alveolar septa pulls the airways open and helps to maintain their patency.

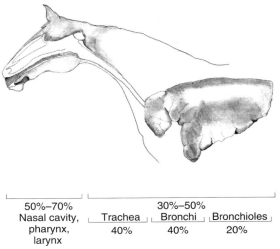

50%–70% Nasal cavity, pharynx, larynx	30%–50%		
	Trachea 40%	Bronchi 40%	Bronchioles 20%

FIGURE 44–8. The distribution of airway resistance in a horse.

The lungs have a total of six lobes, each supplied by a *lobar bronchus*, which gives rise to daughter bronchi. At each division of the bronchi, the diameters of the daughter airways are not equal. One daughter airway is much narrower than the parent, whereas the diameter of the other is similar to that of the parent. This *monopodial* system of branching continues through at least the first six generations of bronchi. At the level of the bronchioles, the diameters of parent and daughter bronchioles are the same. As a result of this branching pattern, the total *cross-sectional area* of the tracheobronchial tree through which air flows increases only a little between the trachea and the first four generations of bronchi, but it doubles at each division of the peripheral airways. Because the total cross-sectional area increases dramatically toward the periphery of the lung, the *velocity of airflow* diminishes progressively from the trachea toward the bronchioles. The high-velocity *turbulent airflow* in the trachea and bronchi produces the *lung sounds* heard through a stethoscope in a normal animal. *Laminar airflow* (low-velocity flow) in the bronchioles produces no sound. Also as a result of the branching pattern of the tracheobronchial tree, airways larger than 2 to 5 mm in diameter contribute up to 80% of the frictional resistance to breathing in the tracheobronchial tree; bronchioles contribute as little as 20%.

Resistance to airflow is determined by the radius and length of the airways. Airway length changes little, but radius can be altered by several passive and active forces. As the lung inflates, airways dilate passively. This occurs because the alveolar septa are attached to the airways, and as the alveoli inflate, tension increases in their septa, causing the attached airways to dilate (Fig. 44–9). Contraction of bronchial smooth muscle is the other major factor determining airway caliber.

Smooth muscle contraction affects the diameters of the trachea, bronchi, and bronchioles

There is *smooth muscle* in the walls of the airways from the trachea to the alveolar ducts. In the trachea, it forms the *trachealis muscle,* which connects the ends of tracheal cartilages. In the bronchi and the bronchioles, smooth muscle encircles the airways. Smooth muscle actively regulates airway diameter in response to neural and other stimuli. The *parasympathetic* nervous system supplies airway smooth muscle via the *vagus nerve* (Fig. 44–10). Activation of this system causes the release of *acetylcholine*, which binds to *muscarinic receptors* on airway smooth muscle, leading to muscle contraction and *bronchoconstriction.* When irritating materials such as dusts are inhaled, tracheobronchial *irritant receptors* are stimulated, which in turn activates the parasympathetic system, resulting in reflex bronchoconstriction.

Airway smooth muscle also contracts in response to many of the *inflammatory mediators,* particularly *histamine* and the *leukotrienes.* Some of these mediators act directly on the smooth muscle; others act in a reflexive manner through the parasympathetic system. They are responsible for the airway obstruction that occurs in diseases such as heaves in horses and asthma in cats.

Relaxation of smooth muscle, and therefore dilation of the airways, occurs during activation of β₂-adrenergic receptors by circulating catecholamines released

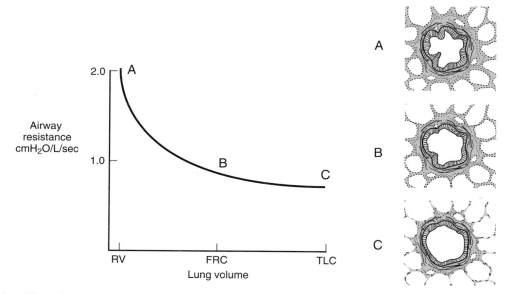

FIGURE 44–9. The effect of change in lung volume on airway resistance. The airway is represented by the large circle, to which are attached alveoli, the septa of which link the airway wall to the pleural surface. As the lung volume increases, the alveolar septa become stretched and thus dilate the airway and reduce resistance. FRC, functional residual capacity; RV, residual volume; TLC, total lung capacity.

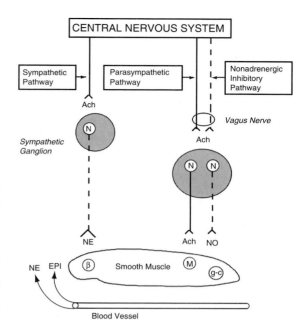

FIGURE 44–10. Diagrammatic representation of the efferent autonomic innervation of the tracheobronchial tree. Smooth muscle β-adrenergic receptors (β) are activated by circulating catecholamines such as epinephrine (EPI) or, in a few species, by release of norepinephrine (NE) from sympathetic nerves. Muscarinic receptors (M) are activated by acetylcholine (Ach) released from postganglionic parasympathetic nerve terminals. The nonadrenergic inhibitory nervous system that travels in the vagus nerve releases nitric oxide (NO) that activates guanyl cyclase (g-c) in the smooth muscle. N, neuron. (From Nadel JA, Barnes PJ, Holtzman MJ: Autonomic factors in hyperreactivity of airway smooth muscle. In Fishman AP, Macklem PT, Mead J, et al [eds]: Handbook of Physiology, Section 3, Vol 3, Part 2. Bethesda, Md.: American Physiology Society, 1986, p 694.)

from the adrenal medulla. Norepinephrine released from the sympathetic nervous system also causes airway dilation through β2-adrenergic receptors but to a lesser extent. Another bronchodilator system, the *nonadrenergic noncholinergic inhibitory nervous system,* exists in some species. The efferent fibers are in the vagus nerve, and neurotransmission involves *nitric oxide.*

Dynamic compression can narrow the airways

The airway walls are not rigid, and therefore the airways can be compressed or expanded by the pressure gradient across their walls. In the nasal cavity, pharynx, and larynx, which are surrounded by atmospheric pressure, *dynamic compression* of the airway occurs during inhalation when pressure within the airways is subatmospheric. Because of its bony support, the nasal cavity is less prone to compression than the more poorly supported nares, pharynx, and larynx. Contraction of the abductor muscles of the nares, pharynx, and larynx during inhalation is necessary to prevent collapse of these regions. Failure of the abductor muscles of the larynx to contract during inhalation allows the vocal folds to be sucked into the lumen of the airway and is responsible for the inspiratory noise and poor performance of horses suffering from laryngeal hemiplegia (roaring).

In the intrathoracic airways, dynamic collapse occurs during *forced exhalation,* when intrapleural pressure exceeds pressures within the intrathoracic airway lumen. *Cough* is a forced exhalation during which dynamic collapse narrows the airways. The high air velocity through the narrowed portion of the airway facilitates removal of foreign material. Toy breeds of dogs have a high incidence of collapsing trachea. In

this disease, the weakened intrathoracic trachea is dynamically collapsed during the forceful ventilation of exercise. Affected dogs make a "honking" expiratory noise as air is forced past the collapsed region of the trachea.

The distribution of air depends on the local mechanical properties of the lung

Optimal gas exchange requires bringing together air and blood at the alveolus: that is, the matching of ventilation and blood flow. Obviously, gas exchange cannot occur if an alveolus receives blood but no ventilation, or vice versa. Ideally, each region of lung should receive approximately equal amounts of ventilation, but this never occurs in either animals or people. Uneven distribution of ventilation can be caused by local decreases in lung compliance (e.g., in pneumonia) or local airway obstructions (e.g., by mucus or bronchospasm) (Fig. 44–11).

The distribution of ventilation is very uneven in recumbent large animals, especially in the supine and laterally recumbent positions. This is because the lowermost regions of the lung are compressed to such an extent that they receive little or no ventilation. This can cause severe derangements of gas exchange in anesthetized horses.

In some species, air travels between adjacent regions of lung via collateral pathways

The lungs of mammalian species differ in the degree to which they are subdivided by connective tissue into *secondary lobules.* In the lungs of pigs and cattle, there is complete separation of lobules, and in dogs

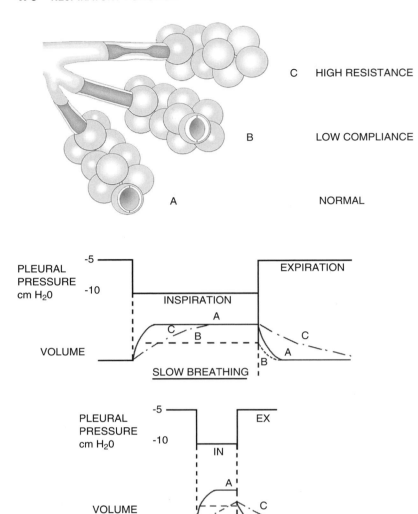

FIGURE 44-11. The effects of mechanical properties of the lung on airway resistance. Alveolus A is normal, alveolus B has low compliance, and alveolus C has high resistance as a result of a partially obstructed airway. Step changes in pleural pressure are applied to these three schematic alveoli, and the changes in volume are shown during slow breathing and during more rapid breathing. During rapid breathing, alveolus C does not have time to fill, so ventilation becomes more unevenly distributed.

and cats there is no separation. In horses and sheep, there is partial separation. The *connective tissue septa* prevent *collateral ventilation* (i.e., movement of air between adjacent lobules) in cattle and pigs. Collateral ventilation is extensive in dogs and intermediate in horses. Collateral ventilation provides air to alveoli when their main parent bronchus is obstructed. The differences in collateral ventilation mean that gas exchange abnormalities that follow airway obstruction are more serious in pigs and cattle than in dogs.

CLINICAL CORRELATIONS

Lung fibrosis in the dog

History   A 3-year-old English setter in respiratory distress is presented at a teaching hospital. The owner first noticed reluctance of the dog to exercise 3 weeks ago. Since that time, the animal has had progressive difficulty in breathing. It appears hungry but cannot eat because it gets out of breath.

Clinical examination   Inspection reveals a thin dog breathing through its mouth. The respiratory rate is elevated, but the dog seems to be moving little air despite strong inspiratory efforts during which the intercostal spaces sink in. Exhalation presents no difficulty; the ribs collapse rapidly, and there is no accentuated abdominal effort.

Examination reveals slightly blue-colored mucous membranes. Lung sounds are not remarkable. All other systems are normal.

Radiographs of the thorax show diffuse miliary density (whiteness) over the parts of the lung that are normally air-filled. The bronchi are normal. An elevated change in pleural pressure during breathing, normal airway resistance, and decreased static lung compliance are the key findings on lung function testing. VT is greatly reduced.

Comment   The history and clinical signs point to a respiratory problem. The elevated change in pleural pressure during breathing confirms the increased effort necessary to breathe. This could be caused by (1) increased air movement resulting from an increased metabolic rate, (2) airway obstruction, or (3) a decrease in lung compliance (stiffening of the lung). The increased density in the normally air-filled elastic part of the lungs, coupled with the normal air passages, suggests a decrease in lung compliance rather than airway obstruction. This was confirmed when measurements of lung function revealed a normal airway resistance and decreased lung compliance.

The retraction of intercostal spaces indicates that the stiff lung is resisting expansion. Exhalation is no problem, because the lung has an increased tendency to collapse and the airways are normal.

This dog has a diffuse disease of the exchange area of the lung, which, by decreasing compliance, increases the work of breathing. The blue tinge to the mucous membranes indicates desaturation of hemoglobin as a result of impaired oxygen exchange in the diseased lung. A biopsy reveals diffuse fibrosis around mineral particles in the walls of the alveoli. The prognosis for the dog is grave.

Chronic airway disease in the horse

History A 10-year-old horse is presented with a 2-year history of coughing and a progressive loss of exercise tolerance. Recently, the horse's problem has become so severe that it has difficulty breathing while resting in its stall. The cough is frequent. The horse has a normal appetite; however, it is losing weight even though the teeth are normal and the horse is on a parasite control program.

Clinical examination Inspection reveals a thin horse with flared nostrils and an anxious expression. The respiratory rate is elevated, and respiratory movements are accentuated. During inhalation, the intercostal spaces are pulled in between the ribs. The initial part of exhalation is characterized by a rapid relaxation of the rib cage. This is followed by a prolonged contraction of the abdominal muscles, which is terminated immediately before the next inhalation. During the prolonged contraction of the abdominal muscles, wheezes can be heard when you place your ear close to the nostrils.

The horse has an elevated pulse rate. The mucous membranes of the gums have a bluish tinge. Auscultation of the thorax reveals increased breath sounds over all the lung fields and musical wheezes audible at end exhalation. Excessive mucus pooled in the airway is viewed through a bronchoscope advanced into the trachea.

Because the horse is being examined at a teaching hospital, there are facilities for measurement of lung function. The change in pleural pressure (ΔPpl) during each breath is 25 cm H_2O (normal, 5 cm H_2O), and airway resistance is 3 cm H_2O/L/second (normal, 1 cm H_2O/L/second). Administration of atropine intravenously decreases ΔPpl to 7 cm H_2O and airway resistance to 1.5 cm H_2O/L/second. The horse looks less distressed, and wheezes are reduced after atropine therapy.

Comment The respiratory distress, cough, and lack of exercise tolerance point to a respiratory problem. The increased effort of breathing documented by the elevated ΔPpl could be caused by airway obstruction, a decrease in lung compliance, or increased breathing resulting from increased metabolic rate. The latter cause is eliminated, because the horse is resting in the clinic. The mucus in the airway and elevated airway resistance confirm airway obstruction. Musical wheezes at the end of exhalation typify airway disease and are the result of increased

air turbulence or vibration of mucus and the airway walls. Airway obstruction is caused in part by bronchospasm resulting from parasympathetic activity, because it is reversed by atropine, a parasympathetic antagonist. Atropine does not return resistance to normal, so there is also considerable obstruction by mucus and swelling of the airway wall.

The flared nostrils are an effort to reduce the work of breathing by dilating the upper airway. The blue-tinged mucous membranes indicate desaturation of hemoglobin because of impaired oxygen uptake in the diseased lungs.

Retraction of the intercostal muscles during inhalation indicates a major decrease in pleural pressure as the respiratory muscles work to inflate the lung and pull air through the obstructed airways. The prolonged contraction of abdominal muscles, or heaving, represents an effort by the horse to force air out through obstructed airways. Weight loss is probably a result of the increased work of breathing. Coughing is an effort by the horse to expel the excessive mucus.

Treatment This horse has chronic airway disease (heaves, chronic obstructive lung disease), a result of stabling in a dusty barn and eating poorly cured moldy hay. Heaves is the result of an allergic response to antigens in the hay and barn dust. The best treatment for the horse is to keep it out at pasture and supplement its diet with pelleted feed rather than hay.

Bibliography

Guyton AC, Hall JE: Pulmonary ventilation. In Textbook of Medical Physiology, 9th ed. Philadelphia: WB Saunders, 1996, pp 477–489.

Leff AR, Schumacker PT: Respiratory Physiology: Basics and Applications. Philadelphia: WB Saunders, 1993, pp 3–46.

Leith DE: Comparative mammalian respiratory mechanics. Physiologist 19:485–510, 1976.

Lekeux P, Art T: The respiratory system: Anatomy, physiology and adaptations to exercise and training. In Hodgson DR, Rose RJ (eds): The Athletic Horse. Philadelphia: WB Saunders, 1994, pp 79–127.

Murray JF: The Normal Lung. Philadelphia: WB Saunders, 1986, pp 83–119, 121–162.

Robinson NE: Some functional consequences of species differences in lung anatomy. Adv Vet Sci Comp Med 26:1–33, 1982.

Slonim NB, Hamilton LH: Respiratory Physiology, 5th ed. St. Louis: CV Mosby, 1987, pp 48–96.

PRACTICE QUESTIONS

1. Which of the following lists includes only structures that compose the anatomic dead-space?

a. Respiratory bronchioles, alveoli, trachea, nasal cavity.

b. Pharynx, bronchi, alveolar ducts, larynx.

c. Capillaries, respiratory bronchioles, trachea, ronchi.

d. Pharynx, nasal cavity, trachea, bronchi.

e. Capillaries, respiratory bronchioles, alveolar ducts, alveoli.

2. A horse has a tidal volume (V_T) of 5 L, respiratory rate of 12 breaths per minute, and VD/VT ratio of 0.5. Calculate minute ventilation ($\dot{V}_E$) and alveolar ventilation ($\dot{V}_A$).

a. $\dot{V}_E$ = 60 L/min; $\dot{V}_A$ = 2.5 L/min.
b. $\dot{V}_E$ = 30 L/min; $\dot{V}_A$ = 30 L/min.
c. $\dot{V}_E$ = 60 L/min; $\dot{V}_A$ = 30 L/min.
d. $\dot{V}_E$ = 2.5 L/min; $\dot{V}_A$ = 1.25 L/min.
e. $\dot{V}_E$ = 5.0 L/min; $\dot{V}_A$ = 2.5 L/min.

3. Which of the following occur during inhalation?
a. Diaphragm contracts, pleural pressure increases, alveolar pressure decreases.
b. Diaphragm relaxes, external intercostal muscles contract, pleural pressure increases.
c. Diaphragm relaxes, pleural pressure decreases, internal intercostal muscles relax.
d. External and internal intercostal muscles contract, pleural and alveolar pressure increases.
e. Diaphragm and external intercostal muscles contract, pleural and alveolar pressures decrease.

4. Lung compliance
a. has the units of pressure per volume (cm H_2O/L).
b. is greater at functional residual capacity than at total lung capacity.
c. is less when the lung is inflated with saline than when the lung is inflated with air.
d. is greater in small mammals than in large mammals, even when adjusted for differences in lung size.
e. is the only determinant of the change in pleural pressure during breathing.

5. Pulmonary surfactant

a. can be deficient in premature newborns.
b. is produced in type II alveolar cells.
c. is in part composed of dipalmitoyl phosphatidylcholine.
d. decreases surface tension of the fluid lining the alveoli.
e. all of the above.

6. Which of the following increases the frictional resistance to breathing?
a. Intravenous administration of a β-adrenergic agonist.
b. Contraction of the abductor muscles of the larynx.
c. A decrease in lung volume from FRC to residual volume.
d. Relaxation of the trachealis muscle.
e. Inhibition of the release of histamine from mast cells.

7. The distribution of ventilation within the lung is influenced by
a. regional variations in lung inflation.
b. regional variations in airway resistance.
c. regional variations in lung compliance.
d. collateral ventilation.
e. all of the above.

PRACTICE ANSWERS

1. d   2. c   3. e   4. b   5. e   6. c   7. e

Pulmonary blood flow

Pulmonary circulation

1 The structure of the pulmonary arteries varies among species
2 Functionally, pulmonary blood vessels can be classified as alveolar and extra-alveolar vessels
3 The pulmonary blood vessels offer a low resistance to flow
4 The distribution of pulmonary blood flow within the lung is influenced by several factors
5 Passive changes in vascular resistance result from changes in vascular transmural pressure

6 Neural and humoral factors cause contraction of the muscular pulmonary arteries
7 Alveolar hypoxia is a potent constrictor of small pulmonary arteries
8 During exercise, the pulmonary circulation must accommodate a large increase in blood flow

Bronchial circulation

1 The bronchial circulation provides a blood supply to airways, large vessels, and, in some species, the visceral pleura

The lung receives blood flow from two circulatory systems: the pulmonary circulation and the bronchial circulation. The *pulmonary circulation* receives the total output of the *right ventricle*, perfuses the *alveolar capillaries*, and participates in gas exchange. The *bronchial circulation*, a branch of the systemic circulation, provides blood supply to airways and other structures within the lung.

■ PULMONARY CIRCULATION

The pulmonary circulation differs from the systemic circulation in that all the blood passes through only one organ: the lung. When cardiac output increases, as occurs during exercise, the pulmonary circulation must be able to accommodate this increase in blood flow without a large increase in the work of the right ventricle. In addition, control mechanisms must exist to regulate the distribution of blood within the lung so that blood preferentially perfuses the well-oxygenated regions of the lung. The ability to regulate blood flow depends on the presence of pulmonary arterial smooth muscle, the quantity of which varies among species.

■ The structure of the pulmonary arteries varies among species

The main pulmonary arteries that accompany the bronchi are elastic, but the smaller arteries adjacent to the bronchioles and the alveolar ducts are muscular. The adult pig and the cow have a thick *medial muscle layer* in the smaller pulmonary arteries; the

horse has less muscle, and the sheep and dog have only a thin muscle layer. The amount of smooth muscle in the media of pulmonary arteries determines the *reactivity* of the vasculature to alveolar hypoxia and other neural and humoral stimuli (see later discussion).

The terminal branches of the pulmonary arteries, the *pulmonary arterioles*, consist of endothelium and an elastic lamina. Pulmonary arterioles lead into pulmonary capillaries, which form an extensive branching network of vessels within the *alveolar septum*, almost covering the alveolar surface. Not all capillaries are perfused in the resting animal. As a result, vessels that are unperfused in the resting animal can be recruited when pulmonary blood flow increases (e.g., during exercise). *Pulmonary veins* with thin walls conduct blood from capillaries to the *left atrium* and also form a reservoir of blood for the *left ventricle*. The reservoir of blood in the pulmonary veins can be used to initiate a change in cardiac output (e.g., at the start of a sudden burst of exercise).

■ Functionally, pulmonary blood vessels can be classified as alveolar and extra-alveolar vessels

Alveolar vessels are the thin-walled capillaries that perfuse the alveolar septum (Fig. 45–1). They are so called because they are exposed almost directly to the pressure changes that occur in the alveoli during breathing. *Extra-alveolar vessels* include the pulmonary arteries, veins, arterioles, and venules. They generally occur together with bronchi in a loose connective tissue sheath called the *bronchovascular bundle*. This

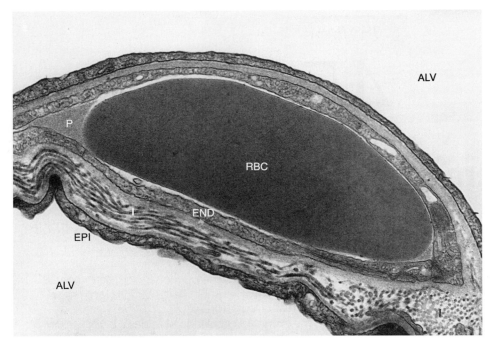

FIGURE 45–1. Transmission electron micrograph of a capillary in the alveolar septum of a horse lung. A red blood cell (RBC) is shown bathed by plasma (P) in a capillary surrounded by endothelium (END). Alveoli (ALV) are on both sides of the septum and separated from the capillary by the epithelium (EPI) and a layer of interstitium (I). The interstitium is much thicker on one side of the capillary than on the other. Fluid exchange between the capillary and the interstitium occurs primarily on the thicker side. (Courtesy of W. S. Tyler, Department of Anatomy, University of California, Davis.)

bronchovascular bundle is bounded by a limiting membrane to which alveolar septa are attached (Fig. 45–2). The behavior of extra-alveolar vessels is determined by pressure changes within the connective tissue space of the bronchovascular bundle rather than by changes in alveolar pressure.

The pulmonary blood vessels offer a low resistance to flow

Pulmonary vascular pressures can be measured by advancing a catheter through the jugular vein into the right ventricle and pulmonary artery. Even though the pulmonary circulation receives the total output of the right ventricle, pulmonary arterial pressures are much less than systemic pressures. Pulmonary arterial systolic, diastolic, and mean pressures average 25, 10, and 15 mm Hg, respectively, in mammals at sea level. If the catheter is advanced until it becomes wedged in a pulmonary artery, the occluded vessel becomes an extension of the catheter, allowing estimation of *pulmonary venous pressure,* also known as *pulmonary wedge pressure.* Pulmonary wedge pressure (average, 5 mm Hg) is only slightly greater than *left atrial pressure* (average, 3 to 4 mm Hg). The small difference in pressure between the pulmonary artery and left atrium indicates that the pulmonary circulation offers little *vascular resistance* to blood flow. Pulmonary vascular resistance (PVR) is calculated as follows:

$$PVR = (Ppa - Pla)/\dot{Q},$$

where Ppa is mean pulmonary arterial pressure, Pla is left atrial pressure, and $\dot{Q}$ is cardiac output.

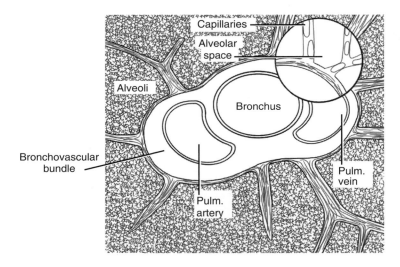

FIGURE 45–2. Diagrammatic representation of the extra-alveolar vessels (pulmonary [Pulm.] artery and vein) in the bronchovascular bundle and the alveolar vessels (capillaries) in the alveolar septum.

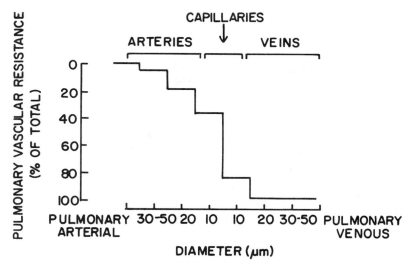

FIGURE 45-3. The distribution of vascular resistance in the pulmonary circulation, as determined by micropuncture studies. Unlike the resistance in the systemic circulation, a major portion of the resistance to blood flow in the pulmonary circulation is in the capillary bed. (From Bhattacharya J, Staub NC: Direct measurement of microvascular pressures in the isolated perfused dog lung. Science 210:327–328, 1980. Copyright 1980 by the American Association for the Advancement of Science.)

Although pulmonary vascular resistance is low in the normal resting animal, it decreases even further when pulmonary blood flow or pulmonary arterial pressure increases, as occurs during exercise. Recruitment of previously unperfused vessels and distention of all vessels cause the resistance decrease.

Micropuncture studies have shown that approximately half the vascular resistance in the pulmonary circulation is precapillary and that the capillaries themselves provide a considerable portion of resistance to blood flow (Fig. 45–3). Unlike the arterioles in the systemic circulation, arterioles in the pulmonary circulation neither provide large resistance nor dampen the arterial pulsations; consequently, pulmonary capillary blood flow is *pulsatile.* The pulmonary veins provide little resistance to blood flow.

The distribution of pulmonary blood flow within the lung is influenced by several factors

The understanding of the distribution of blood flow within the lung was based for many years on experiments performed on isolated perfused dog lungs suspended vertically to mimic the position of lungs in humans. Such experiments and measurements in humans indicated that there is a *vertical gradient of perfusion:* blood flow per unit lung volume increasing from the top to the bottom of the lung. Elegant models that considered pulmonary arterial, pulmonary venous, and alveolar pressure were proposed to explain gravity-dependent distribution of blood flow.

Although this description of gravitational zones has traditionally provided a good theoretical basis for understanding the effects of pressures on blood flow, its applicability to quadrupeds is now in doubt. Gravity is probably not the major factor determining distribution of blood flow in quadrupeds, particularly during exercise. There appears to be gravity-independent preferential distribution of blood flow to the dorsal region of the lung of standing quadrupeds (Fig. 45–4).

This distribution is accentuated by exercise and may even persist in animals under anesthesia.

Passive changes in vascular resistance result from changes in vascular transmural pressure

The diameter of blood vessels is a function of the pressure difference between the inside and the outside of the vessel, called the *transmural pressure.* When the pulmonary blood vessels contain an increased volume of blood—for example, during exercise—pressure within the vessels increases. This leads to an increase in transmural pressure, which causes the vessels to dilate. Transmural pressure can also increase if the pressure surrounding the vessel decreases. This occurs in large pulmonary arteries and veins as the lung inflates. These vessels are contained in the bronchovascular bundle, which is enlarged by the traction of the surrounding alveolar septa during lung inflation (see Chapter 44). Consequently, pres-

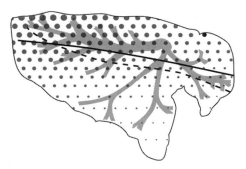

FIGURE 45-4. Graphic representation of the distribution of pulmonary blood flow in the horse's lung. Relative blood flow is indicated by the size of the dots. Blood flow distribution in a dorsal-caudal direction at rest and during exercise is shown by the solid and broken lines, respectively. (Compiled from data in Hlastala MP, Bernard SL, Erikson HH, et al: Pulmonary blood flow distribution in standing horses is not dominated by gravity. J Applied Physiol 81:1051–1061, 1996.)

sure in the perivascular connective tissue of the bronchovascular bundle decreases. This leads to an increase in transmural pressure, and these extra-alveolar vessels therefore dilate.

The overall changes in pulmonary vascular resistance during lung inflation and deflation reflect opposing effects on alveolar and extra-alveolar vessels. When the lung deflates to residual volume, pulmonary vascular resistance is high, because extra-alveolar vessels are narrowed. As the lung inflates to functional residual capacity, resistance decreases, primarily because of dilation of extra-alveolar vessels. Further inflation above functional residual capacity increases vascular resistance, primarily because alveolar capillaries are flattened by the high tension in the stretched alveolar septa (Fig. 45–5). Capillaries become progressively more elliptical and therefore offer more resistance to flow.

Neural and humoral factors cause contraction of the muscular pulmonary arteries

A variety of neural and humoral factors can contract or relax pulmonary vascular smooth muscle and thereby alter the resistance to blood flow. The magnitude of the response of vessels to these stimuli is determined to a large degree by the amount of smooth muscle in the small pulmonary arteries, which varies with species (Fig. 45–6). The increase in

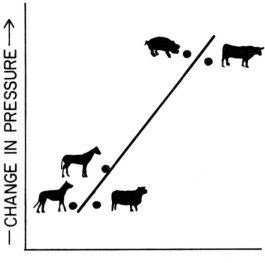

FIGURE 45–6. The relationship between the amount of muscle in the media of small pulmonary arteries and the change in pulmonary arterial pressure when animals are exposed to a hypoxic environment. Animals with thicker muscle layers, such as the cow and pig, have a greater vascular response to hypoxia than do animals with a small amount of muscle in the small pulmonary arteries, such as the dog and sheep. The horse has an intermediate response.

pulmonary vascular pressure in response to alveolar hypoxia and other stimuli is greater in calves than in sheep because of the greater amount of smooth muscle in calf pulmonary arteries.

Although pulmonary arteries have both *sympathetic* and *parasympathetic* innervation, the functional role of this *autonomic innervation* is unclear. In normal animals, sympathetic stimulation results in vasoconstriction through the activation of α-adrenergic receptors on smooth muscle by norepinephrine. Activation of these receptors causes smooth muscle contraction that leads to vasoconstriction of the pulmonary vessels. These actions are thought to occur during times of stress when this sympathetic stimulation may stiffen the pulmonary vascular bed, thus increasing pulsatility and improving perfusion to underperfused regions of the lung. Activation of the parasympathetic system, which releases acetylcholine, has little effect on pulmonary vascular resistance in normal animals.

The response of the pulmonary vasculature to a variety of chemical mediators is shown in Table 45–1. Responses may vary among species and with the initial degree of *vascular tone*. Some mediators such as acetylcholine and bradykinin relax smooth muscle and cause vasodilation by releasing *nitric oxide* or *vasodilator prostaglandins* from the endothelium. Release of nitric oxide also occurs in response to the increased shear stress across the endothelium when blood flow increases. The increased release of nitric oxide may be responsible, in part, for the dilation of the pulmonary circulation during exercise. Catecholamines, bradykinin, and prostaglandins are metabo-

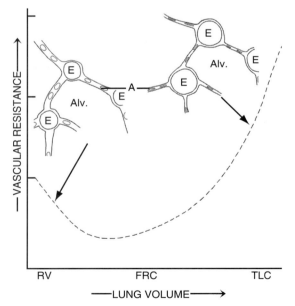

FIGURE 45–5. The change in vascular resistance that occurs with an increase in lung volume. The diagram shows alveolar (A) and extra-alveolar (E) vessels. At residual volume (RV), the extra-alveolar vessels are narrowed, but the alveolar vessels are distended. At total lung capacity (TLC), the extra-alveolar vessels are distended, but the alveolar vessels are flattened because of the tension in the alveolar septum. Minimal vascular resistance occurs close to functional residual capacity (FRC). Alv., alveolus.

TABLE 45–1. Pulmonary vascular response to chemical mediators

Agent	Action
Angiotensin II	Vasoconstriction
Histamine (H_1, H_2)	Usually vasoconstriction through H_1 receptors; if vascular tone elevated, vasodilation through H_2 receptors; acts on both arteries and veins
Serotonin (5-HT_2)	Vasoconstriction through 5-HT_2 receptors; action restricted to pulmonary arteries
Norepinephrine and phenylephrine	Vasoconstriction through α_1 and α_2 receptors
Epinephrine	Vasoconstriction or vasodilation depending on resting vascular tone and predominance of α or β receptors
Isoproterenol	Vasodilation through β receptors
Acetylcholine	Vasodilation through release of nitric oxide when endothelium intact. Vasoconstriction when endothelium removed
Bradykinin	Variable, usually vasodilation; acts through release of vasoactive prostaglandings and nitric oxide
Arachidonic acid	Usually vasoconstriction
Prostacyclin (prostaglandin I_2 [PGI_2])	Vasodilation
Thromboxane	Vasoconstriction
Leukotrienes	Usually vasoconstriction

lized by the vascular endothelium, and so their effects may be modified by endothelial damage.

Alveolar hypoxia is a potent constrictor of small pulmonary arteries

The air in poorly ventilated alveoli has a low partial pressure of oxygen, and it is of limited benefit to the animal to keep sending blood to such alveoli. To correct this problem, *alveolar hypoxia* results in vasoconstriction of pulmonary arteries. This *hypoxic vasoconstriction* reduces blood flow to poorly ventilated alveoli and redistributes pulmonary blood flow toward better ventilated regions of lung. Although the vasoconstrictor response to hypoxia is present in all species, the magnitude of the response varies greatly. Among domestic mammals, the response is most vigorous in cattle and pigs, less vigorous in horses, and trivial in sheep and dogs (see Fig. 45–6). The response to hypoxia is also minimal in the llama, which normally lives under hypoxic conditions at high altitude.

The ability of local alveolar hypoxia to cause a local reduction in blood flow has been clearly demonstrated in several species. Under conditions of *atelectasis*, when there is no ventilation to the collapsed region of lung, local blood flow is greatly reduced by a combination of vessel closure as the lung collapses and vasoconstriction in response to the local hypoxia. Hypoxic vasoconstriction is beneficial when there is localized alveolar hypoxia, but when hypoxia is generalized, as occurs when animals live at high altitude or have diffuse lung disease, the vasoconstric-

tion can have serious consequences. In cattle grazing at high altitude, the hypoxia of altitude causes vigorous generalized pulmonary hypoxic vasoconstriction (Fig. 45–7). This leads to an increase in pulmonary arterial pressure, which increases the work of the right ventricle and leads to *right-sided heart failure*. The clinical syndrome is known as *brisket disease*, because *edema* fluid accumulates in the brisket. There are genetically determined differences in the response to hypoxia; Holsteins respond most vigorously and are therefore highly susceptible to brisket disease. In those species, in which the acute hypoxic constrictor response is most vigorous, chronic hypoxia results in sustained pulmonary hypertension. This is caused by an increase in the quantity of smooth muscle in the media of the small pulmonary arteries. When animals have generalized hypoxic vasoconstriction as a result of lung disease, the resultant right-sided heart failure is known as *cor pulmonale*.

Hypoxic vasoconstriction can be demonstrated in isolated perfused lungs and, therefore, does not require intact innervation. In the smooth muscle of pulmonary arteries, hypoxia closes voltage-gated potassium channels. This increases positivity within the cell and promotes depolarization. The depolarization leads to an influx of calcium, which causes smooth muscle contraction. Many vasoactive agents, such as *histamine, catecholamines, angiotensin,* and *arachidonic acid metabolites*, were previously suggested as being involved in hypoxic vasoconstriction. Their role appears to be modulation of the degree of constriction.

During exercise, the pulmonary circulation must accommodate a large increase in blood flow

In order to transport the extra oxygen required for muscular effort, cardiac output increases six- to eight-fold during strenuous exercise. This increase in blood flow must pass through the pulmonary circulation, where it collects oxygen. In order to accommodate the increase in blood flow during exercise, the pulmonary blood vessels dilate; that is, pulmonary vascular resistance decreases. This dilation is in part passive as a result of the increase in intravascular pressure, which is a result of the increased blood flow. In addition, flow-induced release of nitric oxide from the endothelium also causes relaxation of smooth muscle and vessel dilation.

In most species, pulmonary arterial pressure during exercise is about 35 mm Hg, but in the horse it increases to more than 90 mm Hg. The latter increase is attributable in large part to a very high left atrial pressure (50 mm Hg), which is probably necessary for rapid left ventricular filling when the heart rate exceeds 200 beats per minute. These high exercise-associated intravascular pressures cause leakage of erythrocytes from the pulmonary capillaries when horses exercise strenuously, a phenomenon known as *exercise-induced pulmonary hemorrhage.*

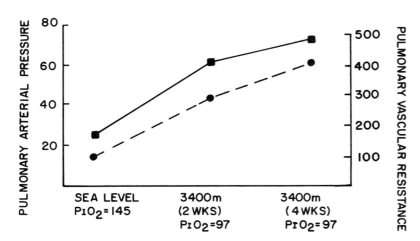

FIGURE 45-7. The change in mean pulmonary arterial pressure *(squares, solid line)* and pulmonary vascular resistance *(circles, broken line)* in calves transported from sea level to 3400 m for a 4-week sojourn. Both vascular resistance and arterial pressure increase when the calves are exposed to the hypoxia of altitude. Pressure and resistance continue to increase while at this altitude because of the proliferation of smooth muscle in the small pulmonary arteries. Pressure units are in millimeters of mercury (mm Hg); resistance units are in dyne·sec/cm⁵; inspired oxygen tension (PIO_2) units are in millimeters of mercury. (From data in Ruiz AV, Bisgard GE, Will JA: Hemodynamic response to hypoxia and hyperoxia in calves at sea level and altitude. Pflugers Arch 344:275–286, 1973.)

BRONCHIAL CIRCULATION

The bronchial circulation provides a blood supply to airways, large vessels, and, in some species, the visceral pleura

The *bronchial circulation,* which receives approximately 2% of the output of the left ventricle, originates from two sources: the *bronchoesophageal artery* and a branch of the bicarotid trunk, the right apical *bronchial artery.* The former supplies the *airways* and the *interlobular septa* of most of the lung; the latter supplies the airways of the right apical lobe. Bronchial arteries follow the tracheobronchial tree to the terminal bronchioles and form a *peribronchial plexus* in the connective tissue along the length of the airways. Branches from this plexus penetrate the smooth muscle layer of the bronchial wall and form a *subepithelial vascular plexus* that serves to warm inhaled air. Branches are also given off to form the *vasa vasorum* (nutrient blood vessels) of pulmonary vessels. At the level of the terminal bronchiole, bronchial vessels *anastomose* with the pulmonary circulation. There are few anastomoses between bronchial and pulmonary arteries; most anastomoses are present at the capillary or venular level. The extensiveness of the bronchial blood supply to the pleura varies among species. In cattle, sheep, pigs, and horses, the bronchial artery provides blood flow to the *visceral pleura*; in dogs, cats, and monkeys, it does not. The bronchial blood flow to the large extrapulmonary airways drains into the azygos vein; venous drainage of the intrapulmonary bronchial circulation enters the pulmonary circulation.

Although the bronchial circulation provides *nutrient blood flow* to many lung structures, the lung does not die if the bronchial circulation is obstructed. The extensive anastomoses between bronchial and pulmonary vessels provide pulmonary blood flow to bronchial vessels. Similarly, when the pulmonary circulation is obstructed, the bronchial circulation proliferates and maintains blood flow to the lung. The bronchial circulation also proliferates when the airways are inflamed.

Inflow pressure to the bronchial circulation is systemic arterial pressure, but outflow pressure varies, depending on whether venous drainage is through the azygos vein or pulmonary circulation. Changes in pressure in both the systemic and pulmonary vascular beds affect the magnitude of bronchial blood flow. Increasing systemic pressure increases flow, but increasing pulmonary vascular pressures (downstream pressure) reduces and may even reverse flow. Under hypoxic conditions, bronchial arteries dilate; in contrast, pulmonary arteries constrict under these conditions.

CLINICAL CORRELATIONS

Brisket disease in a heifer

History A 2-year-old Hereford heifer was kept during the winter on a farm in the foothills of the Rocky Mountains outside Denver, Colorado. In the late spring, the heifer was transported to Climax, Colorado (altitude, 3400 m), for summer grazing. After 6 weeks, the owners noticed that the animal was having some difficulty breathing, was reluctant to move around the pasture, and had developed an enlarged pendulous brisket and also some swelling between the jaws.

Clinical examination Inspection of the heifer reveals a lethargic animal in poor condition. The respiratory and heart rates are elevated, and air seems to be moving well through the nostrils. The most noticeable observation is an enlarged and pendulous brisket. The swelling extends up the neck, and there is also a pendulous area between the jaws. The jugular veins are distended.

Palpation of the swollen brisket reveals that it is heavy; when it is squeezed, the imprints of the fingers remain for some time. The swelling between the mandibles behaves in a similar manner when palpated. The mucous membranes of the heifer are a normal color, and the lung sounds are not remarkable.

Comment The swelling in the brisket and between the mandibles, which pits on palpation, is evidence of accumulation of interstitial edema in the dependent areas of the heifer, in which there is loose connective tissue. Accumulation of edema in these regions is an indication of the increase in systemic venous pressure, which is also causing jugular distention. Both are caused by right-sided heart failure. The most likely cause of right-sided heart failure in a heifer grazing at high altitude is diffuse vasoconstriction of the pulmonary circulation as a result of chronic hypoxia (inspired oxygen tension at 3400 m elevation is 97 mm Hg, in comparison with 150 mm Hg at sea level). The smooth muscle in the pulmonary arteries contracts in response to hypoxia; if this response is maintained for several weeks, the amount of smooth muscle in the pulmonary arteries increases. Furthermore, the animal produces extra erythrocytes in an attempt to transport more oxygen. These extra erythrocytes increase the hematocrit and make the blood more viscous and difficult to pump through the lung. Maintenance of cardiac output in the presence of the elevated pulmonary vascular resistance and increased blood viscosity leads to right-sided heart failure. If this animal is returned to lowland pasture, it will recover. The vasospasm in the pulmonary circulation and the hematocrit diminish once the hypoxic stimulus is removed. For immediate treatment, this animal could be given oxygen to relieve the hypoxic stimulus. This would cause a reduction in pulmonary arterial pressure, but not to normal levels, because of the increased amount of smooth muscle now present in the pulmonary arteries.

Bibliography

Deffebach ME, Charan NB, Lakshminaryan S, et al: State of art. The bronchial circulation: Small, but a vital attribute of the lung. Am Rev Respir Dis 135:463–481, 1987.

Guyton AC, Hall JE: Pulmonary circulation; pulmonary edema; pleural fluid. In Textbook of Medical Physiology, 9th ed. Philadelphia: WB Saunders, 1996, pp 491–499.

Leff AR, Schumacker PT: Respiratory Physiology: Basics and Applications. Philadelphia: WB Saunders, 1993, pp 56–68.

Lekeux P, Art T: The respiratory system: Anatomy, physiology and adaptations to exercise and training. In Hodgson DR, Rose RJ (eds): The Athletic Horse. Philadelphia: WB Saunders, 1994, pp 79–127.

Murray JF: The Normal Lung. Philadelphia: WB Saunders, 1986, pp 139–162.

Robinson NE: Some functional consequences of species differences in lung anatomy. Adv Vet Sci Comp Med 26:1–33, 1982.

Slonim NB, Hamilton LH: Respiratory Physiology, 5th ed. St. Louis: CV Mosby, 1987, pp 109–122.

West JB: Respiratory Physiology: The Essentials, 3rd ed. Baltimore: Williams & Wilkins, 1985, pp 31–46.

PRACTICE QUESTIONS

1. Which of the following statements accurately describes the pulmonary circulation?
   a. It receives the total output of the right ventricle except under conditions of alveolar hypoxia, when vasoconstriction reduces pulmonary blood flow.
   b. The medial layer of the main pulmonary arteries is composed of a thick layer of smooth muscle.
   c. The pulmonary veins return blood to the right atrium.
   d. Unlike systemic capillaries, the pulmonary capillaries provide a percentage of the total resistance to blood flow.
   e. All of the above.

2. During exercise, cardiac output can increase fivefold, but pulmonary arterial pressure may not even double. This occurs because
   a. pulmonary vascular resistance decreases during exercise.
   b. unperfused capillaries are recruited during exercise.
   c. previously perfused vessels are distended during exercise.
   d. factors that dilate the pulmonary arteries are released by the endothelium during exercise.
   e. all of the above.

3. Which of the following will cause the greatest increase in pulmonary arterial pressure?
   a. Exposure of a cow to the hypoxia of high altitude.
   b. A twofold increase in pulmonary blood flow.
   c. Stimulation of the vagus nerve (parasympathetic system) in a sheep.
   d. Inhalation of a tidal volume in a horse.
   e. None of the above will increase arterial pressure.

4. The bronchial circulation
   a. receives the total output of the right ventricle.
   b. drains into the pulmonary circulation and azygos vein.
   c. vasoconstricts in response to hypoxia.
   d. supplies nutrient blood flow only to bronchi and no other structures.
   e. has a bronchial arterial pressure of the same magnitude as pulmonary arterial pressure.

5. In quadrupeds, pulmonary blood flow
   a. is distributed within the lung as would be predicted by the action of gravity.
   b. is distributed primarily to the ventral part of the lung during exercise.
   c. is distributed so that the dorsal-caudal regions of the lung receive the most blood flow.
   d. is distributed uniformly among the alveoli.
   e. is distributed uniformly when the animal is anesthetized.

PRACTICE ANSWERS

1. d   2. e   3. a   4. b   5. c

46

Gas exchange

1 The composition of a gas mixture can be described by the fractional composition or partial pressure

2 Alveolar gas composition is determined by the rate of delivery of fresh gas and the exchange of oxygen and carbon dioxide

3 Exchange of oxygen and carbon dioxide between the alveolus and pulmonary capillary blood occurs by diffusion

4 The exchange of gases between the tissues and blood also occurs by diffusion

5 The amount of alveolar ventilation in relation to pulmonary capillary blood flow—the $\dot{V}/\dot{Q}$ ratio—determines the adequacy of pulmonary gas exchange

6 The composition of the systemic arterial blood is determined by the composition of the capillary blood that drains each alveolus

7 Right-to-left vascular shunts allow blood to bypass ventilated lung

8 Part of each breath ventilates dead-space and does not participate in gas exchange

9 Arterial oxygen (P_{ao_2}) and carbon dioxide (P_{aco_2}) tensions are measured to evaluate gas exchange

The composition of a gas mixture can be described by the fractional composition or partial pressure

Before a discussion of gas exchange, the measurement of gas composition and the forces causing gas movement within the lungs, blood, and tissues must be understood. For convenience, physiologists use many abbreviations when describing gas exchange. A glossary of these abbreviations appears in Table 46–1. Air contains 21% oxygen (the *fraction* of oxygen in inspired air, F_{io_2}, is 0.21). High in the Andes Mountains, the air still contains 21% oxygen, but mammals develop hypoxia at those altitudes. Clearly, therefore, it is not just the fraction of oxygen that is important for gas exchange; the hypoxia at high altitude is a result of the low barometric pressure. At this lower barometric pressure, the oxygen molecules are less densely packed, and therefore the partial pressure of oxygen in the air is decreased. It is this partial pressure (also called *tension*) and, of more importance, the partial pressure difference between two parts of the body, that results in gas transfer.

The oxygen tension (P_{o_2}) of a dry gas mixture is determined by barometric pressure (PB) multiplied by the fraction of oxygen (F_{o_2}) in the gas mixture, or

$$P_{o_2} = PB \cdot F_{o_2}.$$

In the atmosphere, F_{io_2} is 0.21, so P_{o_2} in dry air at sea level (PB = 760 mm Hg) is approximately 160 mm Hg:

$$P_{o_2} = 760 \cdot 0.21 = 160 \text{ mm Hg}.$$

P_{o_2} decreases at higher altitudes, because barometric pressure decreases.

During inhalation, air is warmed to body temperature and humidified in the larger air passages. The concentration of other gases is reduced by the presence of water vapor molecules; therefore, P_{o_2} de-

TABLE 46–1. Glossary of Abbreviations Used in Gas Exchange

AaD_{o_2}	Alveolar-to-arterial oxygen tension difference
F_{io_2}	Fraction of oxygen in inspired air
F_{o_2}	Fraction of oxygen in the gas mixture
P_{aco_2}	Arterial carbon dioxide tension
P_{Aco_2}	Alveolar carbon dioxide tension
P_{ao_2}	Arterial oxygen tension
P_{Ao_2}	Alveolar oxygen tension
PB	Barometric pressure
P_{capco_2}	Capillary carbon dioxide tension
P_{capo_2}	Capillary oxygen tension
P_{co_2}	Carbon dioxide tension
P_{H_2O}	Partial pressure of water vapor at body temperature
P_{Io_2}	Inspired oxygen tension
P_{o_2}	Oxygen tension
P_{vco_2}	Carbon dioxide tension of venous blood
P_{vo_2}	Oxygen tension of venous blood
$\dot{Q}$	Perfusion
R	Respiratory exchange ratio
$\dot{V}$	Ventilation
$\dot{V}A$	Amount of alveolar ventilation
$\dot{V}_{co_2}$	Rate of carbon dioxide production
$\dot{V}_{o_2}$	Rate of oxygen movement between the alveolus and the blood
$\dot{V}/\dot{Q}$ ratio	Ratio of alveolar ventilation to pulmonary capillary blood flow

creases. The P_{O_2} of humidified gas is calculated as follows:

$$P_{O_2} = (PB - PH_2O) \cdot FI_{O_2},$$

where PH_2O is the partial pressure of water vapor at body temperature. The PH_2O is determined by the temperature and percentage saturation of the air with water. In a mammal with a body temperature of 38.2°C, PH_2O in saturated air equals 50 mm Hg; therefore, the P_{O_2} of warmed, completely humidified gas in the conducting airways is approximately 149 mm Hg:

$$P_{O_2} = (760 - 50) \cdot 0.21 = 149 \text{ mm Hg}$$

Alveolar gas composition is determined by the rate of delivery of fresh gas and the exchange of oxygen and carbon dioxide

P_{O_2} is lower in the alveolus than in inspired air, because oxygen and carbon dioxide exchange occurs continually. *Alveolar oxygen tension* (PA_{O_2}) fluctuates around an average value during breathing, increasing during inhalation and decreasing during exhalation. The average oxygen tension in the alveoli of the lung can be calculated from the *alveolar gas equation*, a simplified version of which is as follows:

$$PA_{O_2} = [(PB - PH_2O) \cdot FI_{O_2}] - PA_{CO_2}/R$$

where R, the *respiratory exchange ratio*, is the ratio of the rate of carbon dioxide production to that of oxygen consumption. The respiratory exchange ratio is determined by the substrates being metabolized by the animal. This equation demonstrates that alveolar oxygen tension is determined by the inspired oxygen tension and the exchange of oxygen for carbon dioxide. Assuming an average R of 0.8 and an *alveolar carbon dioxide tension* (PA_{CO_2}) of 40 mm Hg, PA_{O_2} averages approximately 100 mm Hg at sea level, where PB is 760 mm Hg.

Because there is only a negligible amount of carbon dioxide in the inspired air, PA_{CO_2} is determined by the rate of carbon dioxide production ($\dot{V}_{CO_2}$) in relation to the amount of *alveolar ventilation* ($\dot{V}A$):

$$PA_{CO_2} = K \cdot \dot{V}_{CO_2}/\dot{V}A$$

where $K = PB - PH_2O$. It is obvious from this equation that if $\dot{V}_{CO_2}$ increases, as occurs during exercise, $\dot{V}A$ must also increase if PA_{CO_2} is to remain constant. If $\dot{V}A$ does not increase sufficiently, PA_{CO_2} rises. Similarly, if $\dot{V}_{CO_2}$ remains constant and $\dot{V}A$ halves, PA_{CO_2} doubles. The alveolar gas equation also shows that whenever PA_{CO_2} increases, PA_{O_2} decreases, and vice versa.

Alveolar hypoventilation, a decrease in alveolar ventilation in relation to carbon dioxide production, elevates PA_{CO_2} and decreases PA_{O_2}. Figure 46–1 shows the causes of alveolar hypoventilation. It occurs (1) when the central nervous system is depressed by drugs or injury, (2) when there is damage to the peripheral nerves, (3) when there is damage to the thorax and respiratory muscles, and (4) when there is severe airway obstruction (such as in exercising horses with laryngeal hemiplegia) or severe lung disease that decreases lung compliance. The converse of alveolar hypoventilation, *alveolar hyperventilation,* causes a decrease in PA_{CO_2} because ventilation is increased in relation to carbon dioxide production. Therefore, according to the alveolar gas equation, as PA_{CO_2} decreases, PA_{O_2} increases. Hyperventilation occurs when the need to ventilate is increased by stimuli such as hypoxia, increased production of hydrogen ions, or an increase in body temperature.

A modified form of the alveolar gas equation can be used to determine PA_{O_2} for clinical purposes:

$$PA_{O_2} = [(PB - PH_2O) \cdot FI_{O_2}] - Pa_{CO_2}/R$$

In this equation, arterial carbon dioxide tension (Pa_{CO_2}) is substituted for alveolar carbon dioxide tension (PA_{CO_2}).

FIGURE 46–1. Diagrammatic representation of the brain, peripheral nerves, thorax, airways, and lung to show the causes of alveolar hypoventilation. CNS, central nervous system.

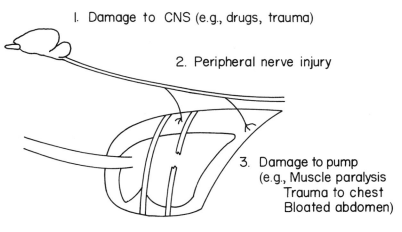

1. Damage to CNS (e.g., drugs, trauma)

2. Peripheral nerve injury

3. Damage to pump
(e.g., Muscle paralysis
Trauma to chest
Bloated abdomen)

4. Lung resisting inflation
(e.g., Airway obstruction
Decreased lung compliance)

Exchange of oxygen and carbon dioxide between the alveolus and pulmonary capillary blood occurs by diffusion

Diffusion is the passive movement of gases down a concentration (partial pressure) gradient. The rate of gas movement between the alveolus and the blood ($\dot{V}O_2$) is determined by the physical properties of the gas (D), the *surface area* available for *diffusion* (A), the *thickness* of the *air-blood barrier* (x), and the *driving pressure* gradient of the gas between the alveolus and capillary blood ($PAO_2 - PcapO_2$):

$$\dot{V}O_2 = D \cdot A \cdot (PAO_2 - PcapO_2)/x$$

D is determined by several factors, including the molecular weight and solubility of the gas. The alveolar surface area available for diffusion is that occupied by perfused pulmonary capillaries. During exercise, more capillaries become perfused by blood, and so the surface area available for diffusion increases.

In the lung, the barrier separating air and blood is less than 1.0 μm thick (Fig. 46–2). However, although thin, this barrier includes a layer of liquid and surfactant lining the alveolar surface; an epithelial layer, usually formed by type I epithelial cells; a basement membrane; variable-thickness interstitium; and a layer of endothelium. In addition to moving gases through this air-blood barrier, diffusion also moves gases within the plasma, allowing oxygen to gain access to erythrocytes and hemoglobin.

Blood entering the alveolar capillary from the pulmonary arterioles is known as *mixed venous blood* because it is blood that has returned to the right side of the heart in veins from all parts of the systemic circulation. The *driving pressure* for gas diffusion is the difference in oxygen tension between the alveolus and the capillary blood. PAO_2 averages 100 mm Hg; in a resting animal, blood entering the alveolar capillary—that is, mixed venous blood—has an oxygen tension ($P\bar{v}O_2$) of approximately 40 mm Hg. The driving pressure gradient of 60 mm Hg ($100 - 40$) causes rapid diffusion of oxygen into the capillary, where it combines with *hemoglobin*. Hemoglobin takes up oxygen from the plasma and helps maintain the gradient for oxygen diffusion.

Normally, equilibration between alveolar and capillary oxygen tensions occurs within 0.25 second, approximately one third of the time the blood is in the capillary (Fig. 46–3). During strenuous exercise, muscles extract a lot of oxygen from the blood, and so the venous blood returning to the lung contains little oxygen. In addition, during exercise, the cardiac output is high and the *velocity of blood flow* through the capillaries is rapid. More oxygen must therefore be transferred in less time than in the resting animal. Under these strenuous conditions, diffusion equilibrium may not occur, and the oxygen tension of blood leaving the lung and entering the systemic arteries (PaO_2) may decrease during intense exercise. This exercise-associated hypoxemia is observed in racing thoroughbred horses.

In a diseased lung, diffusion of oxygen may be impeded as a result of inflammation and edema, which may thicken the air-blood barrier or reduce the surface area available for gas exchange. In these situations, the therapeutic administration of oxygen can increase PAO_2 and thereby provide a greater driving pressure to deliver oxygen into the blood.

The carbon dioxide tension of venous blood returning to the lungs averages 46 mm Hg, and alveolar carbon dioxide tension ($PACO_2$) is 40 mm Hg. Thus the driving pressure for diffusion is only 6 mm Hg. Despite this small driving pressure, the amount of carbon dioxide that diffuses per minute between the capillaries and the alveoli is similar to the diffusion rate of oxygen. The 20-fold greater solubility of carbon dioxide in comparison with oxygen makes up for the small driving pressure gradient. For the same reason, carbon dioxide diffusion between the blood and the alveoli is rarely affected by lung disease.

The exchange of gases between the tissues and blood also occurs by diffusion

The PaO_2 of blood entering the tissue capillaries is 85 to 100 mm Hg, and the $PaCO_2$ is 40 mm Hg. As blood passes through the capillaries, it is exposed to the tissues that are consuming oxygen and producing carbon dioxide. *Tissue oxygen tension* is determined by the rate of delivery of oxygen in relation to its rate of consumption, but it averages 40 mm Hg. Similarly, tissue carbon dioxide tension is determined by the

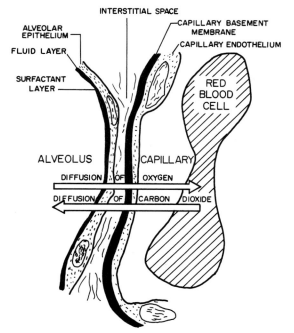

FIGURE 46–2. Diagrammatic representation of the air-blood barrier within the lung, showing the pathway for diffusion of oxygen and carbon dioxide between the alveolus and the erythrocyte within the pulmonary capillary.

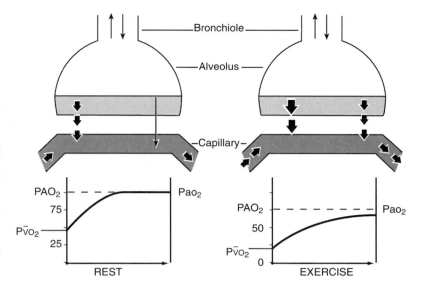

FIGURE 46–3. Schematic representation of an alveolus and pulmonary capillary, showing the increase in oxygen tension that occurs as blood passes through the capillaries. The shaded area within the alveolus represents mixing of gases by diffusion. The size of the arrows between the alveolus and the capillary represents the magnitude of the oxygen fluxes. In the resting animal, mixed venous oxygen tension ($P\bar{v}_{O_2}$) is approximately 40 mm Hg, and blood and air equilibrate rapidly. In the exercising animal, mixed venous oxygen tension is low, and even though oxygen fluxes are high, the blood has not equilibrated with the alveolar oxygen tension before it leaves the alveolus. PA_{O_2}, alveolar oxygen tension; Pa_{O_2}, arterial oxygen tension.

rate of tissue production in relation to the rate of removal by the blood, but it averages 46 mm Hg. As a result of the partial pressure differences between the tissues and capillaries, oxygen diffuses into the tissues and carbon dioxide diffuses into the blood until the partial pressures of blood and tissue are equal. Tissues with a high oxygen demand have more capillaries per gram of tissue. This provides a larger surface for diffusion and also means that the maximal distance between the tissue and the nearest capillary is less than in the poorly vascularized tissues (Fig. 46–4). During *exercise*, muscle blood flow increases, in part, as a result of *recruitment of capillaries* that are not perfused in the resting animal. Capillary recruitment brings blood closer to the metabolizing tissues and slows the rate of blood flow, which allows more time for diffusion equilibrium. In addition, exercise lowers the P_{O_2} and increases the carbon dioxide tension

(P_{CO_2}) of the muscle and, therefore, increases the driving pressure gradients for diffusion.

The amount of alveolar ventilation in relation to pulmonary capillary blood flow—the V̇/Q̇ ratio—determines the adequacy of pulmonary gas exchange

In the alveoli, gas exchange is accomplished by the close approximation of air and blood. Ideally, each of the millions of alveoli should receive air and blood in amounts that are optimal for gas exchange; that is, ventilation ($\dot{V}$) and perfusion ($\dot{Q}$) should be matched. In reality, this never occurs. Even in the young healthy animal, there is some *V̇/Q̇ mismatching*, in part as a result of gravitational forces acting on the

FIGURE 46–4. Effect of increasing capillary density on tissue oxygen tension (P_{O_2}). Oxygen tension is shown as a function of the distance from the capillary (Cap). *Left,* Point *A* has an oxygen tension of approximately 10 mm Hg, whereas, *right,* point *A* has an oxygen tension of approximately 50 mm Hg, because it is now closer to a second tissue capillary.

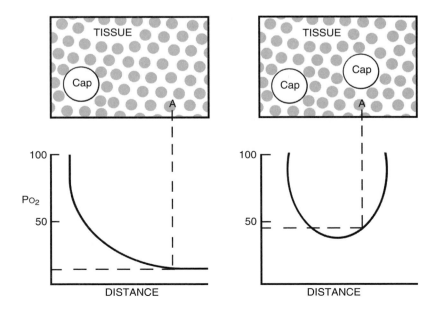

lung. In disease, this $\dot{V}/\dot{Q}$ mismatching becomes more extreme and leads to *hypoxemia*, a low PaO_2.

Figure 46–5 shows schematic alveoli and capillaries with a variety of $\dot{V}/\dot{Q}$ ratios. The alveolus in the center is ideal: it receives ventilation and blood flow with a $\dot{V}/\dot{Q}$ ratio of 0.8. Venous blood arrives with a PvO_2 and a carbon dioxide ($PvCO_2$) tension each of 46 mm Hg, is exposed to alveolar gas tensions (PAO_2 and $PACO_2$), and leaves with an end-capillary oxygen tension ($PcapO_2$) of 100 mm Hg and a capillary carbon dioxide tension ($PcapCO_2$) of 40 mm Hg. The units toward the bottom have a low $\dot{V}/\dot{Q}$ ratio and are relatively overperfused and underventilated. The oxygen tension of blood leaving these units is low, and the carbon dioxide tension is high. Low $\dot{V}/\dot{Q}$ units occur commonly in lung disease because ventilation is reduced by airway obstruction or by localized stiffening of the lung by inflammatory processes. The alveoli toward the top of Figure 46–5 have a high $\dot{V}/\dot{Q}$ ratio; ventilation is high in relation to blood flow. This can occur when pulmonary blood flow to part of the lung is reduced by vascular obstruction or by pulmonary hypotension. The blood leaving such units has a higher oxygen tension and a lower carbon dioxide tension than does blood from the units with a $\dot{V}/\dot{Q}$ ratio of 0.8.

Extending the concepts demonstrated in Figure 46–5 to the whole lung with its multitude of alveoli requires computer simulation and the investigation of the frequency distribution of $\dot{V}/\dot{Q}$ ratios within the lung. In the normal animal, the majority of alveoli have $\dot{V}/\dot{Q}$ ratios close to 1.0 (Fig. 46–6).

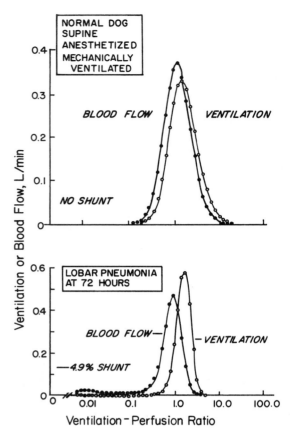

FIGURE 46–6. The distribution of ventilation and blood flow as a function of the ventilation/perfusion ratio. In the normal dog *(top)*, most of the blood flow and ventilation are received by gas exchange units with a ventilation/perfusion ratio close to 1.0. No blood flow and no ventilation are received by units with extremely high or extremely low ventilation/perfusion ratios. In the dog with pneumonia *(bottom)*, a considerable portion of the blood flow is received by units with low ventilation/perfusion ratios: that is, units with little ventilation. The amount of blood passing through right-to-left shunts is also increased in pneumonia. (From Wagner PD, Laravuso RB, Goldzimmer E, et al: Distributions of ventilation-perfusion ratios in dogs with normal and abnormal lungs. J Appl Physiol 38:1099–1109, 1975.)

The composition of the systemic arterial blood is determined by the composition of the capillary blood that drains each alveolus

Blood that returns from the lungs to the left ventricle for distribution to the tissues comes from capillaries associated with millions of alveoli, each of which may have a slightly different $\dot{V}/\dot{Q}$ ratio. The content of oxygen and carbon dioxide in blood that leaves each alveolus varies because of these differing $\dot{V}/\dot{Q}$ ratios. Thus the composition of arterial blood is determined by distribution of $\dot{V}/\dot{Q}$ ratios in the lung.

Lung disease accentuates $\dot{V}/\dot{Q}$ mismatching because of obstruction of airways, flooding of alveoli with exudates, and local obstructions to blood flow. This mismatching has a major effect on oxygen exchange but little effect on the exchange of carbon dioxide. In the case of oxygen, overventilation of

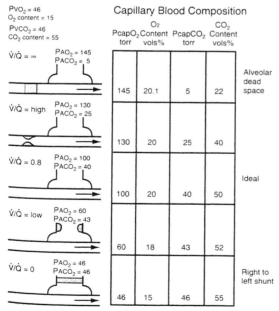

FIGURE 46–5. Diagrammatic representation of an alveolus and a capillary, showing the effect of differing ventilation/perfusion ($\dot{V}/\dot{Q}$) ratios on the partial pressure and gas content of blood leaving the alveolus. In the case of $\dot{V}/\dot{Q} = \infty$ (top), there is no bulk flow of blood past the alveolus, so capillary blood does not contribute to the arterial blood that leaves the left ventricle. See text for explanation and Table 46–1 for abbreviation definitions.

some alveoli does not compensate for underventilation of others. Because of the shape of the *oxyhemoglobin dissociation curve* (see Chapter 47) the overventilated (high $\dot{V}/\dot{Q}$) alveoli with a high PA_{O_2} cannot add enough oxygen to the blood to compensate for the deficiency that arises from the underventilated (low $\dot{V}/\dot{Q}$) alveoli with a low PA_{O_2}. Hypoxemia, therefore, occurs to varying degrees in most lung diseases. However, in contrast to oxygen, carbon dioxide is very soluble, and because its dissociation curve (see Chapter 47) is linear, the overventilated alveoli can compensate for those that are underventilated. For this reason, *hypercarbia*, or *hypercapnia* (an increased carbon dioxide tension in arterial blood), rarely occurs in the presence of lung disease.

As the degree of $\dot{V}/\dot{Q}$ mismatching increases and oxygen exchange becomes less efficient, the difference between the average alveolar tension and the arterial oxygen tension increases. Normally, this *alveolar-to-arterial oxygen tension difference* (AaD_{O_2}) averages 5 to 10 mm Hg, because there is a degree of $\dot{V}/\dot{Q}$ inequality even in normal lungs and because venous blood draining the bronchial and coronary circulations mixes with the oxygenated blood draining the alveoli. The AaD_{O_2} increases when animals are anesthetized or when they have lung disease, because many poorly ventilated regions of the lung continue to receive blood flow; that is, the number of units with low $\dot{V}/\dot{Q}$ increases (see Fig. 46-6).

Right-to-left vascular shunts allow blood to bypass ventilated lung

In a *right-to-left shunt*, blood from the right ventricle bypasses ventilated lung and returns to the left atrium (see Fig. 46-5, *bottom*). Such blood does not pick up oxygen and, when it leaves the lung, has the same composition as the venous blood that entered the lung. Right-to-left shunts have a $\dot{V}/\dot{Q}$ ratio of zero and are formed when alveoli are collapsed (*atelectasis*), are unventilated because of complete *airway obstruction*, or are filled with exudates, as in *acute pneumonia*. Right-to-left shunts can also result from complex congenital cardiac defects, such as *tetralogy of Fallot*, which allow blood to flow directly from the right to the left chambers of the heart, bypassing the lungs. Such large right-to-left shunts cause a major impairment of oxygen exchange. In normal animals, the venous blood (low P_{O_2}) from the bronchial and coronary veins joins the oxygenated blood leaving the lungs. This is equivalent to a right-to-left shunt and constitutes 5% of cardiac output.

Part of each breath ventilates dead-space and does not participate in gas exchange

Dead-space ventilation consists of the gas that does not participate in gas exchange. This includes both the anatomic (see Chapter 44) and *alveolar dead-space*. The latter consists of alveoli that receive ventilation but no blood flow; that is, they have a $\dot{V}/\dot{Q}$ ratio of infinity (see Fig. 46-5, *top*). Alveolar dead-space can form when the pulmonary arterial pressure is so low that many capillaries are unperfused or when the vessels are obstructed by thrombi.

Arterial oxygen (Pa_{O_2}) and carbon dioxide (Pa_{CO_2}) tensions are measured to evaluate gas exchange

To evaluate pulmonary gas exchange, blood that has just passed through the lung (i.e., systemic arterial blood) must be sampled. Venous blood samples are inadequate for evaluating gas exchange, because they reflect blood flow and metabolism in the tissues. Arterial blood gas tensions are the end result of the individual processes involved in gas exchange and thus are affected by the composition of inspired air, alveolar ventilation, alveolocapillary diffusion, and ventilation-perfusion matching.

Domestic animals breathe air containing 21% oxygen ($FI_{O_2} = 0.21$), but during anesthesia or oxygen therapy, FI_{O_2} is increased by the administration of oxygen, resulting in an increase in inspired oxygen tension (PI_{O_2}). More commonly, however, PI_{O_2} varies because of changes in PB. The daily fluctuations in PB caused by atmospheric conditions cause only trivial changes in PI_{O_2}, but the decrease in PB that occurs at higher altitudes results in a major decrease in PI_{O_2}. As a consequence of the decrease in PI_{O_2}, there is a decrease in PA_{O_2} and thus a decrease in Pa_{O_2} as animals ascend in altitude. Altitude-induced changes in Pa_{O_2} must always be considered when blood gas tensions are evaluated.

Adequacy of alveolar ventilation is assessed by examination of Pa_{CO_2}. It is elevated above the normal value of 40 mm Hg when animals hypoventilate and is decreased during hyperventilation. At the same time, hypoventilation decreases PA_{O_2} and Pa_{O_2}, and hyperventilation increases these tensions.

Diffusion abnormalities and $\dot{V}/\dot{Q}$ mismatching impair the transfer of oxygen from the alveolus to arterial blood, increase the AaD_{O_2}, and reduce Pa_{O_2}. Pa_{CO_2} is rarely elevated by these problems, because of the solubility of carbon dioxide and because the hypoxemia stimulates ventilation, keeping Pa_{CO_2} normal or even reducing it below normal.

In animals with normal lungs, increasing FI_{O_2} elevates Pa_{O_2}. As $\dot{V}/\dot{Q}$ mismatching becomes more extreme, increasing FI_{O_2} increases Pa_{O_2} only modestly, especially in the presence of right-to-left shunts. Concurrently, the alveolar-arterial oxygen difference widens. Because of greater mismatching of ventilation and blood flow, Pa_{O_2} tends to be lower in newborn animals than in adults.

CLINICAL CORRELATIONS

Hypoventilation in a bulldog

History A 5-year-old bulldog is presented to you because it refuses to exercise. Normally the dog is willing to go for short slow walks. Over the past 6 months, the dog has been making an increasing amount of noise when it breathes. When it is awake, it makes a rattling sound during inhalation; when it sleeps, it snores loudly and wakes frequently, standing up, turning around, and then lying down again. On one occasion the owner tried to get the dog to run, but the dog collapsed, making a loud noise in its throat as it struggled to inhale.

Clinical examination The bulldog is in good condition, but even as you walk into the room, you notice the loud rattling noises being made by the dog during breathing. You also observe that the mucous membranes of the pendulous lips have a bluish tinge. The dog is standing when you walk into the room, but while you are talking to the owner, the dog lies down and apparently goes to sleep. At this point, the noises of breathing become much louder.

Examination of the dog reveals no abnormalities in the heart or the digestive tract, but examination of the respiratory tract reveals multiple abnormalities. The external nares of the dog are extremely small, and it is difficult to introduce a speculum to examine the nasal cavity. When the dog's mouth is opened, an excessive amount of loosely folded tissue is observed in the pharynx, and it is impossible to move this aside in order to examine the larynx. Listening to the lungs is not helpful, because all the sounds being generated by the loose vibrating tissue in the upper airway are transmitted to the lungs. Radiographs, however, reveal no abnormalities in the lungs, but the trachea is quite narrow. An arterial blood sample is taken for measurement of carbon dioxide and oxygen tensions. Pa_{O_2} is 50 mm Hg, and Pa_{CO_2} is 75 mm Hg.

Comment This bulldog's condition represents an extreme form of the brachycephalic syndrome, which is seen in short-nosed dogs, particularly in bulldogs. The syndrome usually includes stenosis (narrowing) of the external nares and obstruction of the pharynx by pendulous folds of excessive soft tissue. In some of these dogs, the trachea is also very narrow. These dogs have difficulty breathing, particularly during inhalation, when the subatmospheric pressure within the upper airway sucks the loose folds of tissue into the airway lumen. This can result in total obstruction to ventilation. In general, these dogs make a lot of noise during inhalation as the loose folds of tissue vibrate. Exhalation presents less difficulty, because the higher-than-atmospheric pressure in the pharynx tends to push back the loose tissue and open the airway. Over a period of time, the chronic, excessively subatmospheric pressure during inhalation can cause deformity of the larynx.

The upper airway obstruction in this bulldog is limiting ventilation so severely that the dog is suffering from alveolar hypoventilation. This is indicated by the elevated Pa_{CO_2}. An elevation in Pa_{CO_2} occurs when alveolar ventilation is not sufficient to remove the carbon dioxide being produced by the body. The accumulating carbon dioxide in the alveolus and the lack of ventilation also depress the alveolar oxygen tension (PA_{O_2}), and this leads to a depression in the arterial oxygen tension, as in this dog. The hypoxemia then leads to hemoglobin desaturation, which accounts for the bluish color (cyanosis) to the mucous membranes of the dog.

Treatment The treatment for this dog is surgical removal of some of the excessive tissues of the upper airway and enlargement of the external nares. This will alle-

viate some of the obstruction and may improve ventilation. However, with the narrowing of the trachea observed in this dog, it is unlikely that the dog will ever be able to exercise to a significant degree, although its condition may be improved sufficiently that it can make a suitable pet.

Hypoxemia in an anesthetized Clydesdale horse

History A 2-year-old, 750-kg Clydesdale horse is presented for removal of a testicle that has been retained in the abdomen, a procedure that requires anesthesia. You know that anesthesia of heavy draft horses can lead to gas exchange problems, and therefore you have an anesthesia machine available to provide ventilation and to supplement the horse with extra oxygen. The horse is anesthetized with a short-acting intravenously administered barbiturate, an endotracheal tube is inserted, and the horse is connected to the anesthesia machine and allowed to breathe oxygen containing 2% to 3% halothane for anesthesia. Ventilation is not assisted.

Thirty minutes after the induction of anesthesia, the veterinary technician takes an arterial blood sample to monitor the horse's gas exchange. Pa_{O_2} is 70 mm Hg, and Pa_{CO_2} is 65 mm Hg. Are you happy with the results of the blood gas analysis? If not, what can be done to improve gas exchange?

Comment The elevation of Pa_{CO_2} from the normal value of 40 mm Hg to 65 mm Hg shows that the horse is suffering from alveolar hypoventilation; that is, the ventilation received by the alveoli is insufficient to remove the carbon dioxide being produced by the horse. This is probably a result of depression of the central nervous system by the anesthetic gases, so that the drive to breathe is reduced. In addition, the positioning of the horse on its back for removal of the retained testicle causes the heavy viscera to push on the diaphragm, making it difficult for the horse to ventilate. Alveolar hypoventilation in an anesthetized animal can be corrected by the use of positive-pressure ventilation. You have a ventilator as part of the anesthesia machine and choose to ventilate the horse to return the Pa_{CO_2} to acceptable levels.

The Pa_{O_2} of 70 mm Hg shows that the horse has considerable problems in exchanging oxygen. Although a Pa_{O_2} of 70 mm Hg is sufficient to almost saturate hemoglobin and would not be considered particularly low in an animal breathing air, it is very low in an animal breathing 100% oxygen. When animals breathe oxygen, the alveolar oxygen tension is over 600 mm Hg:

$$PA_{O_2} = (PB - PH_2O) \cdot FI_{O_2} - Pa_{CO_2}$$
$$= (760 - 50) \cdot 1.0 - 65$$
$$= 645 \text{ mm Hg}.$$

If the lung is functioning ideally, arterial oxygen should also be close to 600 mm Hg. In this horse, arterial oxygen tension is only 75 mm Hg, so there is an alveolar-arterial oxygen tension difference of close to 570 mm Hg.

This huge alveolar-arterial oxygen tension difference is not unusual in large anesthetized mammals. The positioning of the horse on its back with the consequent weight of the viscera pushing forward on the diaphragm and compressing the lungs can lead to severe $\dot{V}/\dot{Q}$ inequalities. Parts of the dependent lung are unable to ventilate, although they continue to receive blood flow and, therefore, become right-to-left shunts. These right-to-left shunts result in severe arterial hypoxemia. As long as the Pa_{O_2} is sufficient to saturate hemoglobin, the horse is in no danger. The dangerous point is during recovery from anesthesia. The horse must be supplemented with oxygen until it is sufficiently conscious to be able to rest on its sternum unaided and eventually to stand. Returning to these postures eliminates right-to-left shunts, restores the $\dot{V}/\dot{Q}$ distribution to normal, and improves gas exchange.

Bibliography

Guyton AC, Hall JE: Physical principles of gas exchange: Diffusion of oxygen carbon dioxide through the respiratory membrane. In Textbook of Medical Physiology, 9th ed. Philadelphia: WB Saunders, 1996, pp 501–512.

Leff AR, Schumacker PT: Respiratory Physiology: Basics and Applications. Philadelphia: WB Saunders, 1993, pp 82–92, 93–110.

Lekeux P, Art T: The respiratory system: Anatomy, physiology and adaptations to exercise and training. In Hodgson DR, Rose RJ (eds): The Athletic Horse. Philadelphia: WB Saunders, 1994, pp 79–127.

Murray JF: The Normal Lung. Philadelphia: WB Saunders, 1986, pp 163–172, 183–210.

Slonim NB, Hamilton LH: Respiratory Physiology, 5th ed. St. Louis: CV Mosby, 1987, pp 97–108, 123–134.

West JB: Respiratory Physiology: The Essentials, 3rd ed. Baltimore: Williams & Wilkins, 1985, pp 21–30, 49–66.

PRACTICE QUESTIONS

1. Calculate the alveolar oxygen tension (PA_{O_2}) of an anesthetized cow when the barometric pressure is 750 mm Hg, PH_2O at body temperature = 50 mm Hg, Pa_{CO_2} = 80 mm Hg. The cow is breathing a mixture of 50% oxygen and 50% nitrogen. Assume the respiratory exchange ratio is 1.0.
   a. 270 mm Hg.
   b. 620 mm Hg.
   c. 275 mm Hg.
   d. 195 mm Hg.
   e. 670 mm Hg.

2. Which of the following will decrease the rate of oxygen transfer between the alveolar air and the pulmonary capillary blood?
   a. Increasing PA_{O_2} from 100 to 500 mm Hg.
   b. Perfusing previously unperfused pulmonary capillaries.
   c. Decreasing the mixed venous oxygen tension from 40 to 10 mm Hg.
   d. Destruction of alveolar septa and pulmonary capillaries by a disease known as *alveolar emphysema*.
   e. None of the above.

3. During exercise, recruitment of muscle capillaries that are unperfused in the resting animal results in all of the following except
   a. an increase in the velocity of capillary blood flow.
   b. an increase in the surface area for gas diffusion between tissues and blood.
   c. a decrease in distance between tissue capillaries.
   d. maintenance of tissue P_{O_2} in the presence of increased demand for oxygen.
   e. a shorter distance for gas diffusion.

4. Which of the following could potentially result in more low $\dot{V}/\dot{Q}$ regions within the lung?
   a. Atelectasis of one lobe of a dog lung.
   b. Obstruction of both pulmonary arteries.
   c. Doubling the ventilation to the right cranial lobe while its blood flow remains constant.
   d. Vasoconstriction of the pulmonary arteries of the left lung in a cow.
   e. None of the above.

5. Which of the following statements is correct?
   a. Right-to-left shunts represent an extremely high $\dot{V}/\dot{Q}$ ratio.
   b. Right-to-left shunts are not a cause of elevated alveolar-arterial oxygen difference.
   c. An increase in the alveolar dead-space can result from an increase in the number of high $\dot{V}/\dot{Q}$ units in the lung.
   d. The shape of the oxyhemoglobin dissociation curve means that low $\dot{V}/\dot{Q}$ units in the lung are not a cause of hypoxemia (low Pa_{O_2}).
   e. Totally occluding the right pulmonary artery increases the right-to-left shunt fraction by 50%.

6. A horse has difficulty inhaling, especially during exercise. Arterial blood gas tensions at rest are as follows: Pa_{O_2} = 55 mm Hg, Pa_{CO_2} = 70 mm Hg. After you give the horse oxygen to breathe, Pa_{O_2} increases to 550 mm Hg, and Pa_{CO_2} remains unchanged. The cause of these gas tensions is
   a. right-to-left shunt through a complex cardiac defect.
   b. alveolar hyperventilation.
   c. a large number of alveoli with high $\dot{V}/\dot{Q}$ ratios.
   d. alveolar hypoventilation.
   e. none of the above.

PRACTICE ANSWERS

1. a   2. d   3. a   4. a   5. c   6. d

47

Gas transport in the blood

Oxygen transport

1 A small amount of oxygen is transported in solution in plasma, but most is in combination with hemoglobin

2 A molecule of hemoglobin can reversibly combine with four molecules of oxygen

3 The binding of oxygen and hemoglobin is determined by P_{O_2}

4 The oxyhemoglobin dissociation curve can be displayed with percentage saturation of hemoglobin as a function of P_{O_2}

5 The position of the oxyhemoglobin dissociation curve is not fixed but varies with blood temperature, pH, P_{CO_2}, and the intracellular concentration of certain organic phosphates

6 As hemoglobin is depleted of oxygen, its color changes from bright red to bluish red

7 Carbon monoxide has 200 times the affinity of oxygen for hemoglobin

8 Methemoglobinemia occurs in certain toxic states, notably nitrite poisoning

Carbon dioxide transport

1 Carbon dioxide is transported in the blood both in solution in plasma and in chemical combination

Gas transport during exercise

1 Oxygen demands of exercise are met by increases in blood flow, in hemoglobin levels, and in oxygen extraction from blood

▬ OXYGEN TRANSPORT

▬ A small amount of oxygen is transported in solution in plasma, but most is in combination with hemoglobin

Oxygen is poorly soluble in water and, therefore, in plasma. Because of this low solubility, most animals need an oxygen-carrying pigment in order to transport sufficient oxygen to the tissues. The only animals that can exist without hemoglobin live deep in the ocean in the cold parts of the world. The depth at which they live results in a high ambient pressure and hence a high P_{O_2}. In addition, the cold environment results in a low metabolic rate and, therefore, little need for oxygen. The high P_{O_2} and low oxygen demand enable them to exist without an oxygen-carrying pigment. All land-dwelling animals with which veterinarians deal have such a pigment, and in mammals and birds, that pigment is *hemoglobin.*

When blood in the pulmonary capillaries flows past the alveoli, oxygen diffuses from the alveoli into the blood until the partial pressures equilibrate: that is, there is no further driving pressure difference. Because oxygen is poorly soluble in water, only a very small amount dissolves in the plasma, and hemoglobin is necessary for delivery of sufficient oxygen to the tissues. Without hemoglobin, which transports the majority of the oxygen, the cardiac output would

have to be inordinately high to maintain the oxygen supply to the body organs.

Even though the amount of oxygen dissolved in plasma is small, it increases directly as the partial pressure of oxygen increases; 0.003 mL of oxygen dissolves in each 100 mL (1 dL) of plasma at an oxygen tension (P_{O_2}) of 1 mm Hg (Fig. 47–1). The pulmonary capillary blood equilibrates with the alveolar oxygen tension ($P_{A_{O_2}}$) of 100 mm Hg; therefore, 0.3 mL of oxygen dissolves in each deciliter of blood. If an animal breathes pure oxygen so that the $P_{A_{O_2}}$ increases to 600 mm Hg, 1.8 mL of oxygen dissolves in each deciliter of plasma.

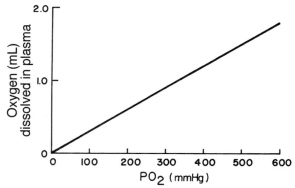

FIGURE 47–1. The amount of oxygen (in milliliters) dissolved in plasma as a function of oxygen tension (P_{O_2}).

A molecule of hemoglobin can reversibly combine with four molecules of oxygen

Mammalian hemoglobin consists of four units, each containing one *heme* and its associated protein. Heme is a *protoporphyrin* consisting of four *pyrroles* with a *ferrous* iron at the center. The ferrous iron combines reversibly with oxygen in proportion to P_{O_2}. The hemoglobin molecule is spheroid, an *amino acid side chain* being attached to each heme. The type and sequence of amino acids that compose these side chains affect the affinity of hemoglobin for oxygen and define the different types of mammalian hemoglobin. Adult hemoglobin contains two α and two β *amino acid chains*; fetal hemoglobin contains two α and two γ chains. Closely related species, such as humans and anthropoid apes, have similar amino acid sequences on the side chains, whereas more divergent species have a greater number of differences in amino acid sequences.

Each hemoglobin molecule can reversibly bind up to four molecules of oxygen, one with each heme. The reversible combination of oxygen with hemoglobin is shown in the *oxyhemoglobin dissociation curve* (Fig. 47–2). The binding of oxygen is a four-step process, and the *oxygen affinity* of a particular heme is influenced by the oxygenation of the others. This means that when the first heme unit is oxygenated, oxygen affinity of the second heme unit is increased, and so on. These *heme-heme interactions* are responsible for the *sigmoid* shape of the oxyhemoglobin dissociation curve.

The binding of oxygen and hemoglobin is determined by P_{O_2}

Figure 47–2 shows that the *oxygen content* of blood—that is, the amount of oxygen combined with

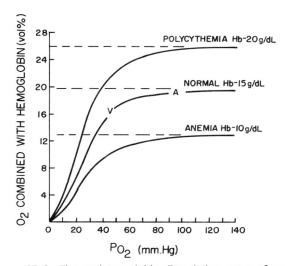

FIGURE 47–2. The oxyhemoglobin dissociation curve of normal (hemoglobin [Hb] = 15 g/dL), anemic (Hb = 10 g/dL), and polycythemic (Hb = 20 g/dL) blood. The amount of oxygen combined with hemoglobin (i.e., the oxygen content) is plotted as a function of oxygen tension (P_{O_2}). A, arterial; V, venous.

hemoglobin—is determined by P_{O_2}. At a P_{O_2} of more than approximately 70 mm Hg, the oxyhemoglobin dissociation curve is virtually flat, which indicates that further increases in P_{O_2} add little oxygen to hemoglobin. At this point, the hemoglobin is said to be saturated with oxygen. The fact that hemoglobin becomes virtually saturated with oxygen at a P_{O_2} of more than 70 mm Hg is important for animals that ascend to moderate altitude, where the barometric pressure results in a low PI_{O_2} (inspired oxygen tension).

One gram of saturated hemoglobin can hold 1.36 to 1.39 mL of oxygen; therefore, average mammalian blood with 10 to 15 g of hemoglobin per deciliter has an *oxygen capacity* of 13.6 to 21 mL of oxygen per deciliter (volume percentage) when hemoglobin is saturated with oxygen. The oxygen capacity of the blood is the maximal amount of oxygen that can be carried in the blood at any given time. *Anemia*, a reduction in the number of circulating erythrocytes with a consequent reduction in the amount of hemoglobin in the blood, decreases oxygen capacity. When the hemoglobin content of blood increases, oxygen capacity increases also. The latter occurs during exercise; contraction of the spleen forces more erythrocytes into the circulation. More erythrocytes than normal in the blood is known as *polycythemia*, and they increase the oxygen capacity of the blood. Splenic contraction is an especially rich source of erythrocytes in the exercising horse.

When the P_{O_2} is less than 60 mm Hg, the oxyhemoglobin dissociation curve has a steep slope. This is in the range of *tissue P_{O_2}* at which oxygen is unloaded from the blood. Tissue P_{O_2} varies in accordance with the blood flow/metabolism ratio, but average tissue P_{O_2} is 40 mm Hg. Blood exposed to such a P_{O_2} loses 25% of its oxygen to the tissues. In rapidly metabolizing tissues in which tissue P_{O_2} is lower, more oxygen is unloaded from the blood. The oxygen remaining in combination with hemoglobin forms a reserve that can be drawn upon in emergencies.

Oxygen content is a term that describes the amount of oxygen bound to hemoglobin. When hemoglobin is saturated with oxygen, oxygen content and oxygen capacity are equal. When oxygen leaves the blood in the tissues, oxygen content decreases, but the oxygen capacity remains the same.

The oxyhemoglobin dissociation curve can be displayed with percentage saturation of hemoglobin as a function of P_{O_2}

Percentage saturation of hemoglobin is the ratio of oxygen content to oxygen capacity. Hemoglobin is more than 95% saturated with oxygen when it leaves the lungs of an animal at sea level. Percentage saturation of mixed venous blood is 75; venous oxygen tension ($P\bar{v}_{O_2}$) is 40 mm Hg. Although all mammals have similarly shaped oxyhemoglobin dissociation curves, the position of the curve with regard to P_{O_2}

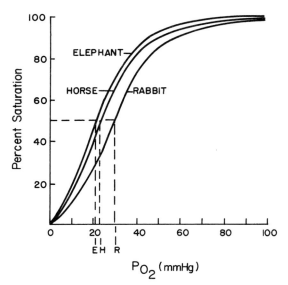

FIGURE 47–3. The oxyhemoglobin dissociation curve of three species of mammal. Percentage saturation of hemoglobin is plotted as a function of oxygen tension (P_{O_2}). Although the curves have similar shapes in all mammals, they are not superimposed. The differences between the curves can be expressed by the partial pressure at which hemoglobin is 50% saturated with oxygen (P_{50}). P_{50} for each species is indicated as E (elephant), H (horse), and R (rabbit).

varies (Fig. 47–3). This can be described by measurement of P_{50}, the partial pressure at which hemoglobin is 50% saturated with oxygen. A higher P_{50} is generally found in small mammals and allows unloading of oxygen at a high P_{O_2} to satisfy their higher metabolic demands.

The position of the oxyhemoglobin dissociation curve is not fixed but varies with blood temperature, pH, P_{CO_2}, and the intracellular concentration of certain organic phosphates

An increase in tissue metabolism produces heat, which elevates blood temperature and shifts the oxyhemoglobin dissociation curve to the right (increases P_{50}). Such a shift facilitates dissociation of oxygen from hemoglobin and releases oxygen to the tissues. Conversely, excessive cooling of the blood, as occurs in hypothermia, shifts the dissociation curve to the left, and so tissue P_{O_2} must be lower than usual to release oxygen from hemoglobin.

The shift in the oxyhemoglobin dissociation curve resulting from a change in the carbon dioxide tension (P_{CO_2}) is called the *Bohr shift*. This shift results in part from the combination of carbon dioxide with hemoglobin but mostly from the production of H+, which decreases the pH. A change in pH alters the oxygen binding by changing the structure of hemoglobin. As a result, a higher, more alkaline pH shifts the oxyhemoglobin dissociation curve to the left, and a lower, more acidic pH shifts the curve to the right

(Fig. 47–4). The Bohr effect is not constant among species; a given change in pH produces a greater shift in the dissociation curve for small mammals than for large mammals, supposedly ensuring the delivery of oxygen during high rates of metabolic activity, when carbon dioxide production is greatest.

A solution of mammalian hemoglobin generally has a lower affinity for oxygen than does whole blood until *organic phosphates*, such as diphosphoglycerate (DPG) and adenosine triphosphate (ATP), are added to the solution. In erythrocytes, DPG has a molar content equivalent to that of hemoglobin, much higher than in other cells. This DPG regulates the combination of oxygen with hemoglobin. When concentrations of DPG are high, as occurs under anaerobic conditions, the oxyhemoglobin dissociation curve is shifted to the right (P_{50} increases) and the unloading of oxygen is facilitated. In contrast, a reduction in DPG levels, as can occur in stored blood, shifts the dissociation curve to the left. Not all hemoglobins bind DPG equally. Ruminant hemoglobin in general is unresponsive to DPG, and elephant hemoglobin binds DPG weakly.

As hemoglobin is depleted of oxygen, its color changes from bright red to bluish red

The change in the color of hemoglobin from bright red to the bluish red known as *cyanosis* can be observed in the mucous membranes of animals when the blood in the underlying capillaries is hypoxic. Cyanosis can result from deficient oxygen uptake in the lungs, but it can also result from reduced blood flow to the peripheral tissues. The latter can occur when animals are in cardiovascular failure.

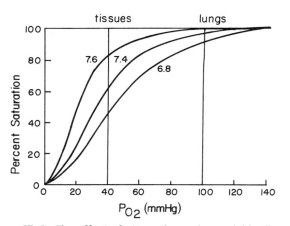

FIGURE 47–4. The effect of pH on the oxyhemoglobin dissociation curve. A decrease in pH shifts the dissociation curve to the right and therefore assists in unloading oxygen at the tissues. The shift in the dissociation curve has much less effect on the percentage saturation of hemoglobin when oxygen is being loaded into the blood in the lungs (i.e., $P_{O_2} = 100$ mm Hg) than when oxygen is being unloaded in the tissues (i.e., $P_{O_2} = 40$ mm Hg).

Carbon monoxide has 200 times the affinity of oxygen for hemoglobin

Carbon monoxide and oxygen bind to the same sites on hemoglobin, but carbon monoxide is bound much more avidly. As a result of the high affinity of carbon monoxide for hemoglobin, exposure to carbon monoxide levels of less than 1% in air can eventually saturate hemoglobin and displace oxygen, leading to death. Fortunately, such low levels of carbon monoxide must be breathed for some time in order to deliver sufficient carbon monoxide to saturate all the blood hemoglobin, and so toxic effects are not immediate. Carbon monoxide not only reduces the oxygen content of the blood but also displaces the oxyhemoglobin dissociation curve to the left. This shift indicates that with the onset of carbon monoxide poisoning, hemoglobin has a higher affinity for the remaining bound oxygen; thus, the release of oxygen into the tissues occurs at a tissue P_{O_2} much lower than normal. Treatment of carbon monoxide poisoning requires removal of the source of carbon monoxide and administration of oxygen to displace the carbon monoxide from hemoglobin.

Methemoglobinemia occurs in certain toxic states, notably nitrite poisoning

When the normal ferrous iron of hemoglobin is oxidized by *nitrites* and other toxins to ferric iron, brown-colored *methemoglobin* is formed. Methemoglobin does not bind oxygen; thus, the oxygen capacity of the blood is reduced. Nitrite can be ingested directly from spoiled feeds, but ruminants more commonly form nitrite in the rumen after ingestion of nitrate-rich feeds such as Sudan grass or mangel tops.

CARBON DIOXIDE TRANSPORT

Carbon dioxide is transported in the blood both in solution in plasma and in chemical combination

Unlike oxygen, which is bound only to hemoglobin, *carbon dioxide* is transported in several forms (Fig.

47–5). Carbon dioxide is produced in the tissue; therefore, tissue P_{CO_2} is higher than the P_{CO_2} of the blood arriving in the capillaries. Carbon dioxide diffuses down a concentration gradient from the tissues into the blood. When the blood leaves the tissues, P_{CO_2} has risen from 40 to approximately 46 mm Hg, exact values being dependent on the ratio of blood flow to metabolism.

Approximately 5% of the carbon dioxide entering the blood is transported in solution. The majority of carbon dioxide diffuses into the erythrocyte, where it undergoes one of two chemical reactions. Most of the carbon dioxide combines with water and forms *carbonic acid*, which then dissociates into *bicarbonate* and *hydrogen ion*:

$$H_2O + CO_2 \leftrightarrow H_2CO_3 \leftrightarrow H^+ + HCO_3^-$$

This reaction also occurs in plasma, but in the erythrocyte, the presence of *carbonic anhydrase* accelerates the hydration of carbon dioxide several hundred–fold. Ionization of carbonic acid occurs rapidly, and H^+ and HCO_3^- accumulate within the erythrocyte. The reversible reaction is kept moving to the right, because H^+ is *buffered* by hemoglobin. Most of the HCO_3^- that is produced in the erythrocyte diffuses out along a concentration gradient into the plasma. Chloride ion diffuses into the erythrocyte to maintain the *Gibbs-Donnan equilibrium.*

The addition of carbon dioxide to capillary blood is facilitated by the deoxygenation of hemoglobin occurring in the tissues. Deoxyhemoglobin is a weaker acid than oxyhemoglobin and, therefore, a better buffer. Thus, it combines more readily with H^+ and facilitates the formation of HCO_3^- from carbon dioxide.

The *carbamino compounds* are the second form in which carbon dioxide is transported in the blood. Carbamino compounds are formed by coupling of carbon dioxide to the -NH groups of proteins, particularly hemoglobin. Although carbamino compounds account for only 15% to 20% of the total carbon dioxide content of the blood, they are responsible for 20% to 30% of the carbon dioxide exchange between the tissues and the lungs.

When venous blood reaches the lungs, carbon diox-

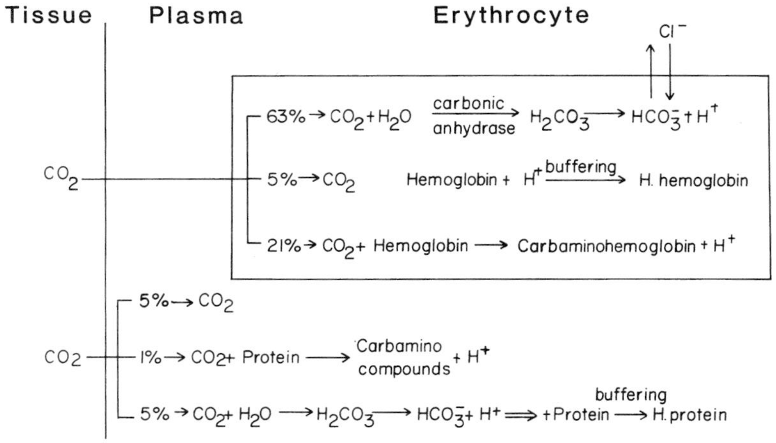

FIGURE 47–5. The forms of carbon dioxide transport in the blood. All reactions displayed in this diagram can be reversed when the blood reaches the lung and carbon dioxide diffuses into the alveolus.

ide diffuses into the alveoli from plasma and erythrocytes, thus causing the reactions shown in Figure 47–5 to move to the left. Simultaneously, the oxygenation of hemoglobin releases hydrogen ions, which combine with bicarbonate to form carbonic acid and, thus, carbon dioxide.

The blood *content of carbon dioxide* as a function of P_{CO_2} is depicted in the carbon dioxide equilibrium curves shown in Figure 47–6. Curves are shown for oxygenated blood ($P_{O_2} = 100$), for partially deoxygenated blood ($P_{O_2} = 50$), and for deoxygenated blood ($P_{O_2} = 0$). The curves are almost linear and have no plateau in the physiologic range; carbon dioxide can be added to the blood as long as the buffering capacity is available. The higher carbon dioxide content of deoxygenated blood resulting from the higher buffering capacity of deoxyhemoglobin is clearly visible. This effect of oxygenation on carbon dioxide content is termed the *Haldane effect*.

GAS TRANSPORT DURING EXERCISE

Oxygen demands of exercise are met by increases in blood flow, in hemoglobin levels, and in oxygen extraction from blood

The demands for gas transport in the blood are not constant but vary with metabolism. Strenuous exercise represents the most extreme demand placed on the gas transport mechanisms. In the galloping horse, oxygen consumption can increase 30-fold. Figure 47–7 shows how this extra demand for oxygen is met. Part of the demand is provided by an increase in *cardiac output*, which causes the amount of blood flowing through the lungs per minute to increase. This allows an increased uptake of oxygen from the lungs. The cardiac output also is redistributed, with an increased fraction of output going to the exercising muscles. The increase in cardiac output and redistribution increases muscle blood flow by 20-fold.

The horse also meets the increased oxygen demand with an increase in the number of circulating erythro-

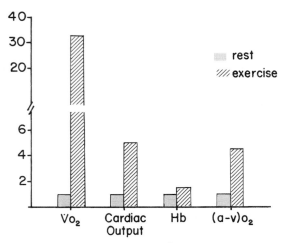

FIGURE 47–7. Oxygen consumption ($\dot{V}_{O_2}$), cardiac output, hemoglobin level (Hb), and arteriovenous oxygen difference [(a-v)$_{O_2}$] in a horse at rest and during strenuous exercise at a gallop. The 30-fold increase in $\dot{V}_{O_2}$ is accomplished by a fivefold increase in cardiac output, a 50% increase in Hb, and a fourfold increase in (a-v)$_{O_2}$.

cytes and, therefore, an increased amount of hemoglobin. Contraction of the spleen forces stored erythrocytes into the circulation and can increase the hematocrit from 35% to 50%. This provides almost 50% more binding sites for oxygen, which raises the oxygen capacity of the blood. The usefulness of an increase in hematocrit is limited, because it increases blood viscosity, which tends to slow the flow of blood through the capillaries and increase the work of the heart. The increase in muscle blood flow and hematocrit together increase the delivery of oxygen to the muscle. An exercising muscle extracts a larger percentage of the oxygen from the blood than does a muscle at rest. This is accomplished as follows: (1) the diffusion gradient for oxygen is increased by the decrease in muscle P_{O_2}, which results from the increase in metabolic rate; and (2) the affinity of hemoglobin for oxygen is decreased by the higher temperature of the exercising muscle and by the lower pH that results from release of carbon dioxide and hydrogen ions from the muscle. As a result of the increased extraction of oxygen, the arteriovenous oxygen content difference is increased.

Muscle itself contains an oxygen-binding pigment, myoglobin, that provides a small store of oxygen. However, myoglobin's main function is the transfer of oxygen within the muscle cell. Myoglobin, like hemoglobin, is an iron-containing pigment, but unlike hemoglobin, it contains only one heme group. As a result, the dissociation curve is not sigmoid but is a rectangular hyperbola. The affinity of myoglobin for oxygen is high, with 75% saturation at a P_{O_2} of 20 mm Hg and the steepest slope of the dissociation curve at P_{O_2} equaling 5 mm Hg. As a result of these dissociation characteristics, myoglobin releases oxygen only when intracellular P_{O_2} is low. Myoglobin is more plentiful in slow-twitch aerobic muscle fibers than in fast-twitch fibers, and the amount of myoglobin is increased by exercise training.

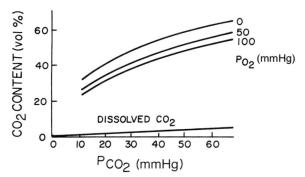

FIGURE 47–6. Carbon dioxide equilibration curves showing the amount of carbon dioxide contained in the blood (CO_2 content) as a function of carbon dioxide tension (P_{CO_2}). Curves are shown for dissolved carbon dioxide and for total carbon dioxide content at a variety of oxygen tensions (P_{O_2}).

Thus, in exercise the increased demand for oxygen is met by increases in blood flow, hematocrit, oxygen extraction from blood, and, to a small degree, by oxygen release from myoglobin. These mechanisms are available whenever unusual demands for gas exchange arise. In anemia, for example, oxygen capacity is reduced, but oxygen delivery to the tissues can be preserved somewhat by an increase in cardiac output and increased extraction of oxygen from the hemoglobin.

The respiratory system's role in acid-base balance is discussed in Chapter 51.

CLINICAL CORRELATIONS

Flea infestation in a cat

History A cat is presented to you because the owner notices that the cat seems extremely weak and recently has been staggering when it walks around the house. The cat's appetite is good, and, apart from the weakness, the owner thinks the cat is normal.

Clinical examination Inspection of the animal, which is resting quietly on the examination table, shows that it is in reasonable condition. The respiratory rate does not appear to be elevated, and from a distance there are no obvious signs of disease. When you place your hands on the cat's back, you immediately notice a gritty-feeling material within the fur of the cat. Further examination of the skin shows accumulations of this red-brown material deep within the coat, and you notice many fleas scurrying around when the coat is parted. When you moisten some of the gritty material, it produces a red liquid. The cat's mucous membranes are almost white, and the examination of the mucous membranes produces sufficient struggling that the cat begins to breathe rapidly. The cat's pulse rate is extremely elevated, but the lung sounds are normal. On physical examination, all of the body systems appear to be normal. A blood sample is taken. The packed cell volume (hematocrit) is 10 (normal levels are 30 to 45).

Comment This cat has a severe infestation of fleas. The gritty material in the fur is flea feces, which contains blood products that become red when wet. The infestation is further confirmed by the observation of many fleas in the coat. By their blood-sucking method of feeding, fleas can produce anemia when they are present in large numbers, as was the case with this cat. If the flea infestation develops gradually, the anemia is slow in onset, and the host animal may show few clinical signs until the infestation and anemia become severe. The anemia is confirmed in this case by the paleness of the mucous membranes and by the low hematocrit. The rapid heart rate of the cat is a response to the anemia. In order to deliver sufficient oxygen to the tissues, the cardiac output has had to be increased by increasing the heart rate. When the cat is stressed by your examination, it shows signs of respiratory distress, because there is inadequate oxygen delivery to the tissues; this causes production of lactic acid as a result of anaerobic metabolism. The resultant decrease in pH stimulates the chemoreceptors, causing the signs of respiratory distress.

Treatment You treat the cat in two ways. First, you administer blood to increase the cat's hematocrit and provide it with sufficient oxygen-carrying capacity until it can generate new erythrocytes. You also treat the flea infestation and instruct the owner on how to remove the fleas from the house.

Several weeks later the owner returns with the cat and notes that she has had no further problems. Occasionally, she notes a flea on the cat's coat and treats the cat immediately with flea medication. She is also diligent about regular vacuuming to remove fleas from the house.

Atrial fibrillation in a horse

History The owner of a 3-year-old Standardbred gelding is concerned because the horse is no longer able to complete its training program. Up until a week ago, the horse had been running well during its daily bouts of training. In the past 2 days, the horse has been extremely reluctant to exercise and, if pushed to do so, begins to stagger and appears weak in the rear legs.

Clinical examination Inspection of the horse reveals a normal-appearing Standardbred in excellent condition. It is standing in its box stall, eating, and looks alert when you enter the stall. Clinical examination reveals normal-colored mucous membranes, no abnormality of lung sounds, and no abnormalities in the gastrointestinal, urinary, or nervous system. When you take the pulse, you note that it is irregular in both amplitude and rate. Several pulses follow one another rapidly, and then there are prolonged pauses. There is no consistent pattern to the irregularity. Auscultation of the heart reveals a similar irregularity in the heart sounds.

You take a blood sample for measurement of the hematocrit, which is normal. You also obtain an electrocardiogram, which reveals a continuous pattern of multiple P waves with occasional and irregularly occurring QRS complexes.

Comment The history, heart rhythm, and electrocardiographic findings in this horse are typical of atrial fibrillation. The multiple P waves observed on the electrocardiogram are a result of circuitous depolarization of the atria. In atrial fibrillation, the atria contract and relax in an uncoordinated manner. The atrioventricular node is activated at intervals that vary considerably from cycle to cycle; hence, there is no constant interval between ventricular contractions. The variable time between ventricular contractions allows for variable degrees of ventricular filling and, therefore, results in uneven stroke volume; consequently, the pulse varies in amplitude as well as frequency.

The irregular ventricular rhythm may be sufficient to maintain cardiac output in the resting animal, but during exercise the cardiac output cannot be maintained. As a result, oxygen delivery to the muscles is inadequate to sustain exercise. This is an example of failure of oxygen delivery as a result of inadequate blood flow.

Treatment Treatment for atrial fibrillation in the horse is the administration of quinidine sulfate, which has a negative inotropic effect on the myocardium and slows atrioventricular conduction time. This allows the reestablishment of normal atrial and ventricular rhythm. The horse's heart rate returns to normal within 5 days and remains so for the following week, at which time training is reinstituted. Several months later the owner reports that the horse is still doing well.

Bibliography

Bartels H: Comparative physiology of oxygen transport in mammals. Lancet 2:599–604, 1964.

Guyton AC, Hall JE: Transport of oxygen carbon dioxide in the blood and body fluids. In Textbook of Medical Physiology, 9th ed. Philadelphia: WB Saunders, 1996, pp 513–523.

Kitchen H, Brett I: Embryonic and fetal hemoglobin in animals. Ann N Y Acad Sci 241:653–671, 1974.

Leff AR, Schumacker PT: Respiratory Physiology: Basics and Applications. Philadelphia: WB Saunders, 1983, pp 69–81.

Lekeux P, Art T: The respiratory system: Anatomy, physiology and adaptations to exercise and training. In Hodgson DR, Rose RJ (eds): The Athletic Horse. Philadelphia: WB Saunders, 1994, pp 79–127.

Murray JF: The Normal Lung. Philadelphia: WB Saunders, 1986, pp 172–182.

Prosser CL: Respiratory functions of blood. In Prosser CL (ed): Comparative Animal Physiology, 3rd ed. Philadelphia: WB Saunders, 1973, pp 317–361.

Slonim NB, Hamilton LH: Respiratory Physiology, 5th ed. St. Louis: CV Mosby, 1987, pp 135–153.

PRACTICE QUESTIONS

1. If 1 g of hemoglobin has an oxygen capacity of 1.36 mL of oxygen, what is the oxygen content of blood containing 10 g of hemoglobin when the blood P_{O_2} is 70 mm Hg?
   a. 13.6 mL/dL (vol %).
   b. 9.5 mL/dL (vol %).
   c. 6.8 mL/dL (vol %).
   d. 21 mL/dL (vol %).
   e. Cannot be calculated from the information provided.

2. An increase in pH of blood will
   a. shift the oxyhemoglobin dissociation curve to the right.
   b. decrease P_{50}.
   c. decrease the affinity of hemoglobin for oxygen.
   d. decrease the oxygen capacity of the blood.
   e. do all of the above.

3. Which of the following decreases oxygen content but does *not* alter Pa_{O_2} or percentage saturation of hemoglobin?
   a. Ascent to an altitude of 3500 meters.
   b. Polycythemia.
   c. Breathing 50% oxygen.
   d. Anemia.
   e. Development of a large right-to-left shunt.

4. All of the following shift the oxyhemoglobin dissociation curve to the right except
   a. an increase in pH.
   b. an increase in P_{CO_2}.
   c. an increase in 2,3-DPG.
   d. an increase in temperature.

5. Quantitatively, the most important form of carbon dioxide transport is
   a. HCO_3^- produced in plasma.
   b. carbon dioxide dissolved in plasma.
   c. HCO_3^- produced in the erythrocyte.
   d. carbon dioxide dissolved in the erythrocyte.
   e. carbon dioxide combined with plasma proteins.

6. Oxygenation of hemoglobin in the lungs assists with the release of carbon dioxide from the blood because
   a. oxygen combines with the -NH groups on hemoglobin and displaces carbon dioxide from carbamino compounds.
   b. oxygen combines with HCO_3^- and produces carbon dioxide.
   c. oxygen facilitates the movement of chloride ions out of the erythrocyte.
   d. oxygen combines with hemoglobin, making it a better buffer, which retains H^+.
   e. of none of the above.

PRACTICE ANSWERS

1. e   2. b   3. d   4. a   5. c   6. e

48

Control of ventilation

1 Respiration is regulated to meet the metabolic demands for delivery of oxygen and removal of carbon dioxide

Central control of respiration

1 Respiratory rhythmicity originates in the medulla and is modified by higher brain centers and inputs from peripheral receptors

Pulmonary and airway receptors

1 Pulmonary stretch receptors, irritant receptors, and juxtacapillary receptors can influence the rhythm of breathing
2 Muscle spindle stretch receptors monitor the effort exerted by respiratory muscles

Chemoreceptors

1 Hypoxia, acidosis, and hypercapnia are all potent stimuli for ventilation
2 Peripheral chemoreceptors are the only receptors monitoring blood oxygen levels
3 The ventilatory response to carbon dioxide is mediated through a medullary chemoreceptor
4 Ascent to high altitude is accompanied by a decrease in inspired oxygen tension and, consequently, by hypoxemia, which leads to an increase in ventilation
5 During exercise, ventilation must increase because the tissues demand more oxygen and produce more carbon dioxide

---

▬ Respiration is regulated to meet the metabolic demands for delivery of oxygen and removal of carbon dioxide

During its daily activities, an animal varies its level of activity and can breathe air of varying composition and purity. To allow the respiratory system to respond to these different challenges, control mechanisms monitor the chemical composition of the blood, the effort being exerted by the respiratory muscles on the lungs, and the presence of foreign materials in the respiratory tract. This information is integrated with the other nonrespiratory activities, such as thermoregulation, vocalization, parturition, and eructation, to produce a pattern of breathing that maintains gas exchange.

A *feedback control diagram* for the respiratory system is shown in Figure 48–1. The *central controller* generates the signals that regulate the activity of the respi-

ratory muscles, which by contracting give rise to alveolar ventilation. Changes in alveolar ventilation affect blood gas tensions and pH, which are monitored by the *chemoreceptors*. These receptors send signals back to the central controller so that necessary adjustments can be made to ventilation. *Mechanoreceptors* in various parts of the respiratory system monitor the degree of stretch of the lungs and changes in the airways and vasculature. Stretch receptors *(proprioceptors)* in respiratory muscles monitor the effort of breathing.

▬ CENTRAL CONTROL OF RESPIRATION

▬ Respiratory rhythmicity originates in the medulla and is modified by higher brain centers and inputs from peripheral receptors

Some of the early attempts to understand the brain's role in the regulation of breathing involved experi-

---

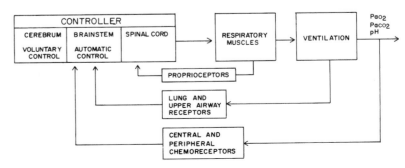

FIGURE 48–1. Feedback control diagram for the regulation of ventilation. The controller, which includes centers in the cerebrum and brainstem, drives the respiratory muscles that bring about ventilation. Changes in ventilation can cause changes in blood gas tensions (P_{O_2}, P_{CO_2}) and pH that are monitored by central and peripheral chemoreceptors. Receptors in the lung detect the stretch in the lung tissues and the presence of materials in the lungs and airways. Proprioceptors in the respiratory muscles monitor the amount of effort being applied by the muscles. Pa_{O_2}, arterial oxygen tension; Pa_{CO_2}, arterial carbon dioxide tension.

ments in brainstem transection to identify the regions of brain involved in maintenance of rhythmic breathing. Transection between the *spinal cord* and *medulla* arrests breathing, which indicates that the *rhythmicity of breathing* originates in the brain, not in the spinal cord or respiratory muscles. The effects of sectioning at different levels of the midbrain vary depending on whether the vagus is intact or cut. The results of these types of experiments have been interpreted as showing that respiratory rhythmicity originates in the medulla but is fine-tuned by afferent information received from the vagus and by higher centers in the brain: of most importance, the *pons.*

More recently, electrical recordings have identified three groups of neurons in the pons and medulla that fire synchronously with breathing (Fig. 48–2). The *pontine respiratory group* (also known as the *pneumotaxic center)* lies in the dorsal lateral pons, receives input from vagal reflexes related to lung volume, and modulates respiratory frequency. Within the medulla, two groups of neurons fire in association with respiration (see Fig. 48–2). The *dorsal respiratory group* is located in the ventral lateral portion of the *nucleus tractus solitarius*. The *ventral respiratory group* is located in the *nucleus ambiguus* and *retroambiguus.* The neurons of the dorsal respiratory group neurons fire primarily during inhalation, and those of the ventral respiratory group fire during both inhalation and exhalation. The axons from the dorsal respiratory group project through *bulbospinal pathways* to inspiratory spinal motoneurons (primarily those supplying the diaphragm) and to the ventral respiratory group. Axons from the ventral respiratory group project to spinal motoneurons of both expiratory muscles and accessory inspiratory muscles.

The origin of rhythmic breathing is currently unknown. Pacemaker neurons have been identified in the ventral respiratory group, but their role in normal breathing is unclear. Normal respiration (eupnea) seems to result from rhythmic inhibition of inspiratory activity. During inhalation there is an increase in activity in the inspiratory neurons. This increase in activity is further amplified by an increase in the chemical respiratory drive, such as hypoxia. Termination of inspiration can be a result of vagal inputs from pulmonary stretch receptors or from a central pontine off-switch. After vagotomy, the pontine off-switch terminates inhalation after a fixed time for inhalation, which is independent of chemical drive. When the vagus is intact and, therefore, signals from pulmonary stretch receptors are relayed to the brain, there is a complex interaction between the time for inhalation and the tidal volume. This interaction leads to a larger tidal volume and more rapid respiratory frequency when the chemical drive to breathe is increased.

When inhalation is terminated, inspiratory neurons are inhibited, and so exhalation occurs passively as a result of the elastic recoil of the lung and chest wall. There is activity in some inspiratory neurons early in exhalation that lead to inspiratory muscle activity, which provides a "brake" on exhalation and regulates the rate of expiratory air flow. Later in exhalation, the braking is removed. During this latter part of exhalation, expiratory muscles may be activated. When respiratory drive is low, this second phase of exhalation is initiated later than when drive is increased.

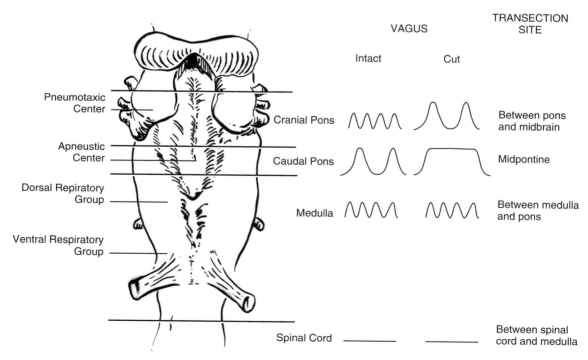

FIGURE 48–2. The ventral surface of the brainstem, including the pons, medulla, and spinal cord, showing centers involved in the regulation of respiration. The effect of sectioning the brain at the levels designated by the horizontal lines with the vagus intact or cut is shown on the right side of the diagram.

The "automatic" breathing just described is frequently overridden by demands from higher brain centers. Vocalization, parturition, swallowing, defecation, and many other activities require the active participation of the respiratory system.

PULMONARY AND AIRWAY RECEPTORS

Pulmonary stretch receptors, irritant receptors, and juxtacapillary receptors can influence the rhythm of breathing

Three types of receptors with vagal afferent nerves have been identified within the lung: *slowly adapting stretch receptors* and *irritant receptors,* both of which have *myelinated afferent nerves,* and C fibers with *unmyelinated axons.* Slowly adapting stretch receptors are nerve endings associated with smooth muscle in the trachea and main bronchi, but to a lesser degree in the smaller intrapulmonary airways. They are stimulated by deformation of the wall of larger airways, for example, when intrathoracic airways are stretched during lung inflation. Because firing rates from these receptors increase progressively as the lung inflates, they are thought to be responsible for the inhibition of breathing caused by lung inflation *(Hering-Breuer reflex).* Termination of input from these receptors by vagotomy leads to a slowing of respiration and an increase in tidal volume. Slowly adapting stretch receptors may be responsible in part for adjustments in the rate and depth of respiration to minimize the work of the respiratory muscles.

Rapidly adapting stretch, or irritant, receptors are thought to be unmyelinated nerve endings ramifying between epithelial cells in the larynx, trachea, large bronchi, and intrapulmonary airways. They are stimulated by mechanical deformation of the airways, such as the deformation that occurs during lung inflation, bronchoconstriction, and mechanical irritation of the airway surface. Irritant gases, dusts, histamine release, and a variety of other stimuli can also cause these receptors to respond. Stimulation of rapidly adapting irritant receptors leads to *cough, bronchoconstriction, mucus secretion,* and rapid shallow breathing (hyperpnea), all of which are protective responses to clear irritant materials from the respiratory system. These receptors may initiate the *sighs* that are thought to redistribute pulmonary surfactant over the alveolar surface.

C fibers ramify in the pulmonary interstitium close to pulmonary capillaries *(juxtacapillary receptors),* where they may monitor blood composition or the degree of distention of the interstitium. Similar fibers also occur in the walls of the airways. C fibers may be responsible for the hyperpnea that follows injury of the lung by allergic, infectious, or vascular diseases.

In addition to intrapulmonary receptors, there are *receptors in the upper airway.* Stimulation of receptors in the nasal cavity causes sniffing and sneezing, whereas stimulation of laryngeal and pharyngeal receptors may cause cough, apnea, or bronchoconstriction.

Muscle spindle stretch receptors monitor the effort exerted by respiratory muscles

The density of *muscle spindle stretch receptors* varies greatly in different respiratory muscles, and the effects of stimulating these receptors can vary with the anatomic location of the muscle group. The diaphragm has few muscle receptors, but intercostal muscles are well supplied with *tendon organs* and muscle spindles. In a reflexive manner, muscle receptors control the strength of respiratory muscle contraction and adjust the strength of contraction when ventilation is impeded by, for example, airway obstruction.

CHEMORECEPTORS

Hypoxia, acidosis, and hypercapnia are all potent stimuli for ventilation

Chemoreceptors monitor oxygen, carbon dioxide, and hydrogen ion concentration at several sites in the body and provide some tonic drive to respiration during normal breathing. As blood composition departs from normal, small changes in arterial carbon dioxide tension (Pa_{CO_2}) and hydrogen ion concentration produce major changes in ventilation, whereas hypoxemia has little effect on ventilation until the decrease in arterial oxygen tension (Pa_{O_2}) is large.

Peripheral chemoreceptors are the only receptors monitoring blood oxygen levels

Chemoreceptors are located at several sites in the body. Peripheral chemoreceptors are the *carotid and aortic bodies,* and their removal eliminates the respiratory response to hypoxia. The response to carbon dioxide levels persists, because they are also detected by a *central chemoreceptor.* Changes in hydrogen ion concentrations are detected by both the peripheral and central chemoreceptors.

The carotid bodies are located close to the bifurcation of the internal and external carotid arteries, and the aortic bodies are located around the aortic arch. The latter appear to be most active in the fetus and of little importance in the adult. Carotid bodies are small structures with high blood flow per kilogram. The aortic bodies are supplied by the *vagus nerve,* and the carotid bodies are supplied by a branch of the *glossopharyngeal nerve.* Fibers within the nerves supplying the peripheral chemoreceptors are primarily afferent except for a few parasympathetic and sympathetic efferent fibers to blood vessels.

Carotid bodies contain several cell types. Type I cells, or *glomus cells,* synapse with afferent nerves that transmit information back to the brain. These glomus cells contain a variety of neurotransmitters, including *catecholamines,* especially *dopamine.* Glomus cells are

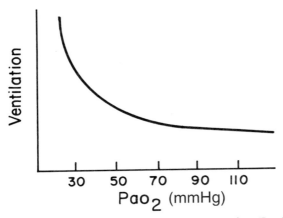

FIGURE 48-3. The effect of arterial oxygen tension (Pa_{O_2}) on ventilation.

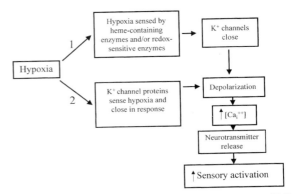

FIGURE 48-4. Hypothesized mechanisms of chemosensitivity in the carotid body. (1) Hypoxia is sensed by enzymes in the glomus cell, leading to closure of potassium channels, depolarization, and neurotransmitter release. (2) Hypoxia is sensed directly by potassium channels, causing their closure. (Modified from Prabhakar NR: Oxygen sensing by the carotid body chemoreceptors. J Appl Physiol 88:2287–2295, 2000.)

probably responsible for the *chemosensitivity* of the carotid bodies. Alternatively, they may modify the chemosensitivity of the afferent nerve terminals. Type II cells, or *sustentacular cells*, support the axons and blood vessels that ramify within the carotid body.

When the carotid bodies are perfused with blood that has a low oxygen tension (P_{O_2}), high carbon dioxide tension (P_{CO_2}), or low pH, firing rates in the carotid sinus nerve afferent fibers increase. As P_{CO_2} increases and pH decreases, there is an almost linear increase in ventilation. The response to P_{O_2} is nonlinear. Modest increases in firing rate and ventilation occur as P_{O_2} decreases from unphysiologic levels of 500 to 70 mm Hg. Further decreases cause a more rapid increase in ventilation, particularly at a P_{O_2} of less than 60 mm Hg, which is the P_{O_2} level at which hemoglobin begins to desaturate (Fig. 48–3). Ventilation does not increase in response to either modest anemia or carbon monoxide poisoning, conditions that decrease the oxygen content of blood but not Pa_{O_2}. For this reason, it is thought that P_{O_2} is more important than oxygen content as a stimulus to the carotid bodies.

Possible mechanism of chemosensitivity of the carotid bodies are shown in Figure 48–4. Glomus cells are depolarized by hypoxemia. Depolarization involves potassium channels and leads to an increase in intracellular calcium. The latter causes release of neurotransmitters, primarily dopamine and acetylcholine that activate the afferent nerve terminals. Hypercapnia (elevated P_{CO_2}) and changes in blood pH also may release neurotransmitters by decreasing the pH in the glomus cells.

The ventilatory response to carbon dioxide is mediated through a medullary chemoreceptor

By probing with carbon dioxide or acetazolamide (an inhibitor of carbonic anhydrase), chemosensitive tissue has been located along the ventral medulla, near the nucleus tractus solitarius, in the region of the

ventral respiratory group of neurons, and in regions of the brain not known to have a function in control of breathing. These chemosensitive neurons (the central chemoreceptor) apparently respond to changes in the pH of the *interstitial tissue fluid* in which they are bathed. A decrease in pH increases ventilation, and an increase in pH decreases ventilation. The brain interstitial fluid, which bathes the central chemoreceptors, communicates directly with cerebrospinal fluid (CSF). Because of this, changes in ventilation can be induced by changes in the composition of arterial blood (Fig. 48–5) and by changes in the hydrogen ion concentration of CSF.

The central chemosensitive neurons are separated from blood by the *blood-brain barrier*, which is freely permeable for CO_2 but less permeable for H^+ and HCO_3^-. An increase in blood P_{CO_2} causes a rapid increase in P_{CO_2} in the brain interstitial fluid. Carbonic acid forms and dissociates into H^+ and HCO_3^-; because the interstitial fluid is poorly buffered, the pH

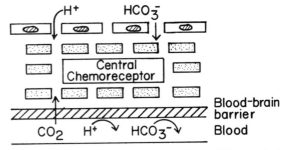

FIGURE 48-5. Diagrammatic representation of the central chemoreceptor separated from blood by the blood-brain barrier, which allows passage of carbon dioxide but is less permeable for hydrogen ion and bicarbonate. The central chemoreceptor is bathed by brain interstitial fluid, which is in communication with the cerebrospinal fluid.

around the chemosensitive neurons decreases, and this stimulates ventilation. Similarly, infusing H⁺ into the CSF decreases the interstitial fluid pH and increases ventilation.

An acute increase in the blood H⁺ concentration is not reflected immediately by a decrease in the pH of either the interstitial fluid or CSF, because the blood-brain barrier is relatively impermeable for H⁺. Therefore, acute increases in blood H⁺ concentration are detected by the peripheral chemoreceptors. However, changes in the brain interstitial fluid pH may follow those in the blood within 10 to 40 minutes.

The composition of CSF and hence brain interstitial fluid has a major effect on the response of the central chemoreceptor. If the HCO_3^- concentration of the CSF decreases, as occurs in *metabolic acidosis*, the buffering capacity of the CSF is reduced. An increase in P_{CO_2} then causes a greater decrease in the pH of the CSF than would occur in the presence of a normal buffering capacity, and so the ventilatory response to CO_2 is more vigorous than normal (Fig. 48–6). Conversely, in *metabolic alkalosis*, the HCO_3^- concentration in CSF increases, and the response to CO_2 is depressed. The CSF composition is regulated by the active transport of ions at the *choroid plexus*. In metabolic acidosis and alkalosis, changes in the HCO_3^- concentration in CSF tend to follow changes in the blood HCO_3^- concentration, but with a phase lag of several hours.

Ascent to high altitude is accompanied by a decrease in inspired oxygen tension and, consequently, by hypoxemia, which leads to an increase in ventilation

The ventilatory response to the hypoxia of altitude varies, depending on whether it lasts for less than an hour or for several days. The acute hypoxia experienced on first ascending to high altitude causes hyperventilation mediated through the peripheral chemoreceptors. However, hyperventilation decreases Pa_{CO_2}, which dampens the response to hypoxia by increasing the pH of the brain interstitial fluid that

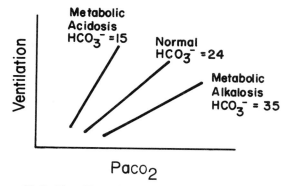

FIGURE 48–6. The effect of arterial carbon dioxide tension (Pa_{CO_2}) on ventilation in a normal animal and in animals with metabolic acidosis and alkalosis. A decrease in the bicarbonate level (mEq/L) increases the ventilatory response to carbon dioxide.

bathes the central chemoreceptor. After several hours to days, ventilation increases further and remains somewhat elevated for hours to days after the hypoxic stimulus is removed. In part, this short-term *acclimatization* can be explained by changes in the pH of CSF. The blood alkalosis caused by the hypoxia-induced hyperventilation leads to an increase in renal excretion of HCO_3^- that is followed by a decrease in the concentration of HCO_3^- in the brain interstitium. This reduces the buffering capacity, and hence the pH of the fluid bathing the central chemoreceptor decreases, which allows a further increase in ventilation despite the low P_{CO_2}.

During exercise, ventilation must increase because the tissues demand more oxygen and produce more carbon dioxide

The increase in ventilation after the onset of exercise is initially rapid, then progresses more slowly, and, provided the workload remains constant, reaches a steady state after about 4 minutes. Although the ventilatory response to exercise has been well described, the reasons for the increase in ventilation are still not well understood.

The primary chemical stimuli for ventilation—Pa_{O_2}, Pa_{CO_2}, and pH—do not change in most animals during moderate aerobic exercise. This shows that the increase in ventilation is well matched to the needs of the tissues and also that factors other than chemical drive increase ventilation during exercise. These other factors have been proposed to be (1) reflexes originating from motion of the exercising limbs, (2) factors related to the increase in cardiac output, (3) thermoregulatory factors, and (4) psychogenic factors that anticipate the onset of exercise. Current exercise control theory favors "central command neurons" that may be coupled to the neurons that regulate breathing. These command neurons control the responses of the respiratory and cardiovascular systems that are necessary to maintain oxygen delivery and carbon dioxide removal during exercise.

Once the *anaerobic threshold* is exceeded, it is easier to explain the increased ventilation. The production of *lactic acid* decreases blood pH. The latter stimulates an increase in ventilation, which leads to a decrease in Pa_{CO_2}. In the horse, the increase in ventilation that can occur during exercise may be limited by the fact that respiratory rate is linked, one breath per stride, with stride frequency. During strenuous anaerobic exercise, the horse's arterial pH decreases progressively, although ventilation remains constant. When exercise ceases, there is a further increase in ventilation, presumably because the restrictions imposed by locomotion are removed.

CLINICAL CORRELATIONS

Hypoxemia with hyperventilation in an 8-month-old Samoyed

History An 8-month-old Samoyed is brought to you because it is reluctant to exercise. Ever since the owner obtained the puppy, she has noticed that its behavior is not puppy-like; it tires easily and prefers to sleep rather than to play.

Clinical examination   The puppy is not well grown. Even though the owner thinks it has been growing, for a Samoyed of 8 months of age the dog is rather small. When it is standing quietly in the examination room, the dog breathes normally, but when you call it and it runs toward you, its respiratory rate increases and it begins to pant. At this point, you notice that the dog's tongue and gums have a distinct bluish tinge.

Before examining the dog further, you are already suspicious of a congenital cardiac anomaly. You arrive at this suspicion because of the dog's age, its history, and the fact that it became cyanotic with only a small amount of exercise.

Palpation of the dog shows that even though it is small, it is not thin. The major abnormalities are the cyanosis of the mucous membranes, an extremely elevated heart rate, and loud abnormal cardiac sounds. A murmur is audible over the tricuspid valve area during systole. The murmur is loud enough to produce a palpable vibration on the chest wall. You explain your suspicions of a cardiac defect to the owner, and together you decide to request some angiographic studies to determine the nature of the defect.

Before angiographic studies, an arterial blood gas sample is taken to determine the suitability of the dog for anesthesia. Pao_2 is 61 mm Hg, and Paco_2 is 23 mm Hg.

Angiography is performed successfully. A catheter is floated into the right atrium of the dog, and dye is injected at this site. Some of the dye passes into the right ventricle, but a large portion passes from the right atrium into the left atrium and out into the systemic circulation.

Comment   The blood gas results are fairly typical of an animal with a major oxygen exchange problem; in the case of this dog, there is a right-to-left vascular shunt through a cardiac defect. A large amount of the mixed venous blood returning to the heart is bypassing the lungs, resulting in the low Pao_2. The Pao_2 is low enough to cause a major increase in ventilation by stimulating the peripheral chemoreceptors. This increase in ventilation causes excessive elimination of carbon dioxide, resulting in the reduced Paco_2. Perhaps ventilation could have increased further, but the low Paco_2 acting on the central chemoreceptor slows down the increase.

The angiographic studies are indicative of a patent foramen ovale. Normally this would not result in right-to-left shunting of blood, because the pressure in the left atrium is usually higher than that in the right atrium. However, this dog probably also has abnormalities of the tricuspid valve that cause a partial obstruction. This is sufficient to increase the pressure in the right atrium and cause blood to flow from right to left through the foramen ovale.

Treatment   The cardiac defect will need to be corrected surgically if the dog is to have any chance of life.

Hypoventilation in an anesthetized Saint Bernard

History   A 2-year-old Saint Bernard is brought to you for treatment of a fractured femur. You elect to place an intramedullary pin in the femur, for which procedure the dog will require anesthesia. The dog is anesthetized with a barbiturate, an endotracheal tube is placed, and the dog is allowed to breathe oxygen containing 2% halothane. It is not ventilated but is allowed to breathe the anesthetic mixture spontaneously. The veterinary technician observing the dog notices that the gas reservoir bag on the anesthesia machine is not moving much when the dog breathes. Therefore, she draws an arterial blood gas sample for measurement of blood gases. Measurement reveals a Pao_2 equal to 480 mm Hg and a Paco_2 equal to 90 mm Hg.

Comment   This is an example of alveolar hypoventilation. Carbon dioxide is being eliminated by the lungs less quickly than it is produced by the tissues, and so the Paco_2 is elevated above the normal value of 40 mm Hg. The lung's ability to exchange oxygen is not impaired; the measured oxygen tension is acceptable for a dog breathing oxygen. Hypoventilation is a common occurrence in anesthetized animals, particularly when anesthesia is induced with a barbiturate drug. Perhaps the dog was slightly overdosed with barbiturate, resulting in the severe hypoventilation observed in this case. Hypoventilation occurs because the ventilatory response to carbon dioxide is depressed by anesthesia, and, therefore, it takes a larger increase in Paco_2 than normal to trigger an increase in ventilation.

Treatment   The dog needs more alveolar ventilation in order to decrease Paco_2 and prevent respiratory acidosis. The additional ventilation can be supplied by squeezing the re-breathing bag on the anesthetic machine. Once the dog recovers from anesthesia, its own respiratory control mechanisms will regulate alveolar ventilation and return Paco_2 to normal.

Bibliography

Berger AJ, Mitchell RA, Severinghaus JW: Regulation of respiration. N Engl J Med 297:92–97, 138–143, 194–201, 1977.

Guyton AC, Hall JE: Regulation of respiration. In Textbook of Medical Physiology, 9th ed. Philadelphia: WB Saunders, 1996, pp 525–535.

Leff AR, Schumacker PT: Respiratory Physiology: Basics and Applications. Philadelphia: WB Saunders, 1993, pp 111–122.

Murray JF: The Normal Lung. Philadelphia: WB Saunders, 1986, pp 233–260, 268–272.

Slonim NB, Hamilton LH: Respiratory Physiology, 5th ed. St. Louis: CV Mosby, 1987, pp 172–197.

PRACTICE QUESTIONS

1. The rhythmicity of breathing is thought to originate solely in
   a. the ventral respiratory group of medullary neurons.
   b. the apneustic center.
   c. the pons.
   d. rapidly adapting pulmonary stretch receptors.
   e. none of the above.

2. Which of the following receptors have afferent nerve fibers in the glossopharyngeal nerve?
   a. Carotid bodies
   b. Slowly adapting pulmonary stretch receptors
   c. Aortic bodies
   d. Intercostal stretch receptors
   e. Rapidly adapting pulmonary stretch receptors

3. Which of the following statements correctly describes the carotid bodies?
    a. Carotid bodies can increase ventilation in response to low Pa_{O_2}, but not in response to an increase in Pa_{CO_2}.
    b. Carotid bodies have a low blood flow/metabolism ratio.
    c. Chemoreception is thought to occur in the sustentacular cells.
    d. Carotid bodies are located near the bifurcation of the internal and external carotid arteries.
    e. All of the above

4. The duration of inhalation
    a. is independent of chemical drive.
    b. is independent of chemical drive only after vagotomy.
    c. is determined by the ventral respiratory group of neurons.
    d. is shortened by vagotomy.

5. The ventilatory response to a change in Pa_{CO_2}
    a. is mediated through a change in pH of interstitial fluid bathing the central chemoreceptors.
    b. is accentuated in metabolic acidosis, because there is less buffering of the interstitial fluid around the central chemoreceptors.
    c. is modified during exercise, so Pa_{CO_2} remains constant despite a large increase in carbon dioxide production.
    d. can occur in the absence of the peripheral chemoreceptors.
    e. All of the above

6. Which of the following receptors are thought to initiate a cough in response to mechanical deformation of the airway?
    a. Juxtacapillary receptors
    b. Rapidly adapting stretch receptors
    c. Slowly adapting stretch receptors
    d. Intercostal tendon organs
    e. None of the above

PRACTICE ANSWERS

1. e   2. a   3. d   4. b   5. e   6. b

49

Nonrespiratory functions of the lung

Defense mechanisms of the respiratory system

1 The extensive, delicate gas exchange surface of an animal's lung is protected by a variety of specific and nonspecific defense mechanisms

2 Particle deposition onto the mucociliary system is dependent on particle size and occurs by impaction, sedimentation, and diffusion

3 The respiratory tract is lined by a mucociliary blanket consisting of a ciliated epithelium overlaid with a layer of mucus

4 Alveolar macrophages scavenge particles deposited on the alveolar surface

5 Cytokines and chemokines coordinate the defense mechanisms of the lung

Pulmonary fluid exchange

1 The lung continuously produces lymph as a result of the net fluid movement from the pulmonary microvasculature into the pulmonary interstitium

2 The small volume of pleural fluid originates by filtration from capillaries in the visceral and parietal pleura

Metabolic functions of the lung

1 The lung removes many hormones and toxins from the blood and inactivates many others

---

▬ DEFENSE MECHANISMS OF THE RESPIRATORY SYSTEM

▬ The extensive, delicate gas exchange surface of an animal's lung is protected by a variety of specific and nonspecific defense mechanisms

When an animal is grazing in a rural environment, the air contains few potentially harmful particles and few pollutant gases. If, however, the animal is intensively housed or is being transported, the air may be rife with organic dust that can contain particles of plant and animal origin, infectious agents such as bacteria and viruses, allergens such as spores and pollen, and other agents such as endotoxin. In addition, there may be pollutant gases such as ammonia, diesel fumes, oxides of nitrogen, and ozone. The respiratory system has a variety of defense mechanisms to protect it against potentially injurious substances. Nonspecific defenses protect against many inhaled substances. Specific defenses involve the immune system and are directed against specific injurious agents, such as a bacterium. Respiratory defense mechanisms, which may provide adequate protection to an animal in its pastoral environment, are frequently overwhelmed by the stresses of intensive housing and transportation. When these stresses are severe—for example, the stress produced by transportation—the animal can acquire an acute infectious disease such

as pneumonia or pleuritis. Stresses that are less severe but more prolonged lead to chronic airway diseases, such as heaves in horses.

▬ Particle deposition onto the mucociliary system is dependent on particle size and occurs by impaction, sedimentation, and diffusion

Harmful material is inhaled as *aerosols* suspended in air, as coarser particles, or as gases. Particles and aerosols are removed from the air when they contact the moist epithelial surface of the tracheobronchial tree (Fig. 49–1). The distance that particles and aerosols travel into the tracheobronchial tree depends on particle size. Larger particles, greater than 5 μm in diameter, contact the airway wall by *inertial impaction*. Inertial impaction occurs at the bends in the large airways, because large particles traveling at high velocity have so much momentum that they fail to negotiate the turns. Sites of inertial impaction are provided with *lymphoid tissue*, such as *tonsils* and *bronchus-associated lymphoid tissue*. As airflow rates diminish deeper in the lung, particles 1.0 to 5.0 μm in diameter settle onto the walls of the airways (*sedimentation*). The smallest particles reach the peripheral airways and alveoli, where they either contact the epithelial surface by *diffusion* or are exhaled again.

The deposition of particles within the respiratory

Particle Deposition

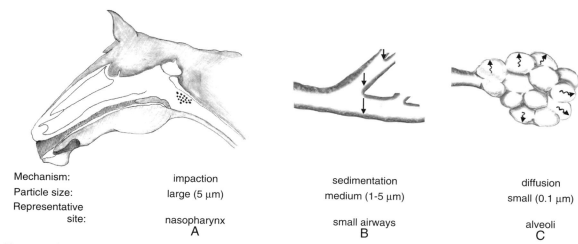

Mechanism:	impaction	sedimentation	diffusion
Particle size:	large (5 μm)	medium (1-5 μm)	small (0.1 μm)
Representative site:	nasopharynx	small airways	alveoli
	A	B	C

FIGURE 49–1. Mechanisms of particle deposition in the tracheobronchial tree. Large particles *(A)* are deposited by impaction in the bends in the larger airways; medium-sized particles *(B)* are deposited in the smaller airways by sedimentation; and small particles *(C)* contact the walls of the alveoli by diffusion.

tract is influenced by the pattern of breathing. Slow, deep breathing transports particles deep into the lung, whereas rapid, shallow breathing enhances inertial deposition in the larger airways. Bronchoconstriction enhances deposition of particles in more central airways, whereas bronchodilation favors more peripheral distribution.

The deposition of toxic gases depends on their solubility and concentration. Very soluble gases, such as SO_2, in low concentrations are removed by the nose, but in higher concentrations they can penetrate deeper into the lung. Less soluble gases may reach down to the alveoli. Toxic gases stimulate a variety of protective mechanisms, such as bronchospasm, mucus hypersecretion, coughing, and sneezing.

The respiratory tract is lined by a mucociliary blanket consisting of a ciliated epithelium overlaid with a layer of mucus

Particles deposited on the epithelial surface of the respiratory tract are transported on the *mucociliary escalator* to the pharynx, where they are then swallowed. The mucociliary system consists of *sol* and *gel mucus* layers overlying epithelial cells (Fig. 49–2). The low-viscosity sol layer, in which the *cilia* beat, bathes the surface of the epithelial cells. On its forward stroke, the extended cilium catches the overlying viscous gel layer, in which inhaled particles are entrapped, and propels it up the tracheobronchial system or through the nasal cavity. Differential rates of mucus transport are necessary in small and larger airways to prevent the accumulation of mucus in the trachea. Clearance rates and the beating frequency of cilia are slower in bronchioles than in bronchi and trachea. Gravity plays an important role in mucociliary clearance. If a horse is prevented from lowering

its head, bacterial numbers increase in the trachea and eventually lead to pneumonia. This may explain why transportation over long distances is the greatest risk factor for development of pneumonia in horses.

Respiratory tract mucus originates from several sites (see Fig. 49–2). In *respiratory bronchioles*, the nonciliated *Clara cells* are a source of the fluid that lines the airways. In the larger airways, *goblet cells* produce mucous secretions. In the *bronchi*, submucosal *bronchial glands* produce both serous and mucous secretions. Secretion is under autonomic regulation. Throughout the respiratory tract, transepithelial movement of water and ions can change the composi-

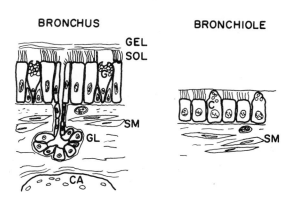

FIGURE 49–2. Diagram of the epithelium and submucosa of a bronchus and bronchiole. In the bronchus, the epithelium is pseudostratified columnar and includes goblet cells (G), ciliated cells, and basal cells that do not reach the surface of the epithelium. A bronchial gland (GL) is shown in the submucosa with its duct passing through the smooth muscle (SM). Cartilage (CA) underlies the mucosal layer. The cilia beat within a sol layer over which is a layer of gel-type mucus. In the bronchiole, the epithelium is cuboidal and is a mixture of ciliated cells and secretory Clara (C) cells. Smooth muscle is shown in the submucosa. Bronchioles normally do not have submucosal glands or goblet cells, and there is no cartilage in their walls.

tion of the mucus layer. Ion and fluid exchange is assisted by *microvilli* on the surface of epithelial cells.

Changes in the amount, composition, and viscosity of mucus occur in response to many stimuli and can be the cause or the result of respiratory disease. A change in the depth or viscosity of the sol layer impairs ciliary function, and changes in the viscoelastic properties of the gel layer alter clearance rates.

Coughing is part of the clearance mechanism of the respiratory tract and is initiated by stimulation of subepithelial irritant, or stretch, receptors, which are most numerous in the larger bronchi. Receptors can be stimulated by mechanical deformation resulting from either material on the epithelial surface or bronchoconstriction. The cough reflex becomes hyperresponsive when the air passages are inflamed and/or respiratory tract epithelium is injured (e.g., by viral infections).

Alveolar macrophages scavenge particles deposited on the alveolar surface

Macrophages constitute the majority of cells in the alveolar lining fluids. Macrophages originate in bone marrow as *monocytes* and differentiate during their passage from the blood into the alveolus, where their turnover time is in the order of days. *Complement, opsonins,* and *lysozyme* in respiratory tract secretions assist macrophages in the killing and removal of viable particulates, such as bacteria. Once phagocytized, particles are destroyed by the macrophage or transported out of the lung. Some macrophages enter the mucociliary system directly from the alveolus; others traverse the alveolar wall and enter the lymphoid tissues associated with the airways. In the lymphoid tissue, macrophages are antigen-presenting cells and thus play a critical role in orchestrating the lung's immune responses.

Macrophages have adapted to the high oxygen levels of the alveolus, and their role as phagocytes is depressed by hypoxia. Macrophage function is also suppressed by endogenous glucocorticoids that are released from the adrenal glands at times of stress and by synthetic corticosteroids that are used to relieve inflammation (e.g., in cases of arthritis). Stress-induced suppression of macrophage function is a contributor to respiratory disease in animals transported for long distances. In addition, excessive administration of synthetic corticosteroids can make animals more susceptible to bacterial infections of the lung. Viral infections also suppress macrophage function; this occurs approximately 7 days after virus inoculation (Fig. 49–3). This contributes to the secondary bacterial infections that commonly follow viral respiratory disease.

Alveolar macrophages are a first line of defense. When large numbers of particles are inhaled, the macrophage is assisted by other phagocytes from the blood, particularly *polymorphonuclear leukocytes,* especially neutrophils. Toxic *oxygen radicals* and *proteolytic*

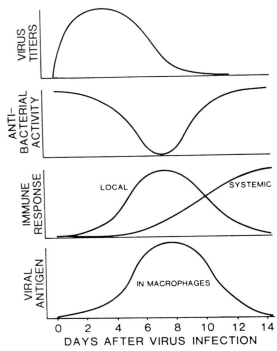

FIGURE 49–3. The effects of viral infection on antibacterial activity of alveolar macrophages. Antibacterial activity is depressed 7 days after experimental viral infection. At this time, the viral antigen is located in the macrophages, which are damaged by the local immune response to the virus. (From Jakab GT: Viral-bacterial interactions in respiratory tract infections: A review of the mechanisms of virus-induced suppression of pulmonary antibacterial defenses. In Loan RW [ed]: Bovine Respiratory Disease: A Symposium. College Station: Texas A&M University Press, 1984, p 238.)

enzymes are released by phagocytic cells to break down invading bacteria, but they may also damage the lung tissue in the process. Protease inhibitors (such as α_1-antitrypsin) and antioxidants (such as glutathione peroxidase) protect the lung from its own defense mechanisms.

Cytokines and chemokines coordinate the defense mechanisms of the lung

When the lung is injured, most commonly by infectious agents such as gram-negative bacteria, the inflammatory process is elicited. *Cytokines* and *chemokines* are two similar groups of proteins that are produced and released by monocytes, injured epithelial and endothelial cells, and various other cells involved in the inflammatory process. The roles of cytokines and chemokines are mainly to attract inflammatory cells to the site of injury and to provide a means for communication between the cells involved in the inflammatory process.

For example, physical injury to the lung epithelium or the presence of bacteria in the lung causes the release of cytokines tumor necrosis factor (TNF) and interleukin (IL)–1 from macrophages. These cytokines act to draw neutrophils into the injured area of the lung. In addition, TNF and IL-1 can cause epithelial cells, such as *alveolar type-II cells,* and endothelial cells to produce the *chemokine* IL-8, which prolongs the inflammatory response, and is also a potent chemoattractant of inflammatory cells. Injured bronchial epithelial cells are also capable of producing IL-1, IL-6, granulocyte-macrophage colony-stimulating factor (GM-CSF), and IL-8, all of which have roles in the cascade of inflammation. Other cytokines—IL-4, IL-5, IL-9, and IL-13—are involved in allergic inflammation.

PULMONARY FLUID EXCHANGE

The lung continuously produces lymph as a result of the net fluid movement from the pulmonary microvasculature into the pulmonary interstitium

Figure 49–4 represents a capillary in the alveolar septum. Fluid filtration normally occurs between the capillary and the interstitial tissue on the thick side of the alveolar septum, where a layer of interstitium is interposed between the endothelium and the epithelial basement membrane. On the thin side of the septum, interstitial tissue is absent because the capillary endothelium shares a basement membrane with the alveolar epithelium. Fluid movement out of the capillary is thought to occur between endothelial cells, but these gaps are too small to allow passage of macromolecules. The latter probably pass through endothelial cells in vesicles, which may fuse to form transendothelial channels. Another possibility is that these large molecules pass through gaps between cells that appear when the endothelia contract and become more permeable under the influence of mediators such as histamine. The alveolar epithelium is less permeable than the capillary endothelium, and so fluid does not leak into the alveoli unless the epithelium is damaged or unless there is considerable fluid accumulation in the interstitium.

The movement of fluid across the endothelium is governed by forces described in *Starling's equation:*

$$Qf = Kf \cdot [(Pmv - Pif) - \sigma(\pi mv - \pi if)],$$

where Qf is the amount of fluid flowing per minute;

Kf is the capillary filtration coefficient; Pmv is microvascular hydrostatic pressure; Pif is interstitial fluid hydrostatic pressure; πmv and πif are microvascular and interstitial colloid osmotic (oncotic) pressures, respectively; and σ is the *colloid reflection coefficient* (see also Chapter 22). Figure 49–4 shows average values for vascular and interstitial pressures.

When values shown in Figure 49–4 are inserted into Starling's equation, the net force favors fluid filtration from the capillaries to the interstitium of the lung. The fluid that is continuously filtered from capillaries moves through the interstitium toward the perivascular and peribronchial tissues, where *lymphatic vessels* are located. Fluid transport out of the lung along lymphatic vessels is aided by lymphatic vasomotion, valves, and the pumping action of the lungs during breathing.

The movement of fluid between the capillaries and the interstitium varies with changes in vascular permeability and with hydrostatic and oncotic pressures. Increases in capillary hydrostatic pressure occur during exercise and in animals with left-sided heart failure. They result in an increase in fluid filtration from the capillaries into the interstitium. The lymphatic vessels remove this filtered fluid and can accommodate quite large increases in fluid flux. Excess fluid accumulates around the bronchi and large blood vessels. The compliant peribronchial and perivascular spaces provide these intrapulmonary repositories for fluid accumulation. Fluid does not accumulate in the alveoli and cause clinically evident *pulmonary edema* unless there is a large increase in the amount of fluid being filtered from the capillaries. Alveolar flooding occurs once the peribronchial capacity is exceeded. The fluid probably enters the air spaces across the alveolar epithelial cells or at the level of the bronchioles. The foaming fluid typical of clinical pulmonary edema results from the mixing of air, edema fluid, and surfactant within the airways.

Increased fluid filtration and pulmonary edema can also be a result of a decrease in plasma oncotic pressure, which is a result of hypoproteinemia. Hypoproteinemia can be caused either by starvation or by the overvigorous administration of intravenous fluids that dilute the plasma proteins. Increased *vascular permeability* occurs in many inflammatory lung diseases, such as pneumonia. This results from the ef-

FIGURE 49–4. Diagrammatic representation of a capillary in the alveolar septum. *Top,* The capillary endothelium and alveolar epithelium share a basement membrane. *Bottom,* The endothelium and epithelium are separated by a layer of interstitial tissue. Values for capillary and interstitial hydrostatic pressures (Pcap and Pif) and capillary and interstitial fluid oncotic pressures (πcap and πif) are shown.

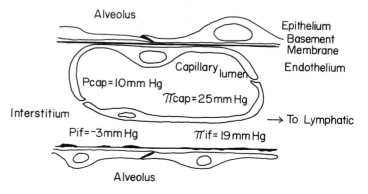

fects of neutrophil products, probably oxygen radicals, on the endothelium. Protein-rich fluid leaks into the interstitium, elevating interstitial fluid oncotic pressure and causing osmotic attraction of water into the interstitium from the vasculature.

The small volume of pleural fluid originates by filtration from capillaries in the visceral and parietal pleura

The pleural space contains a small volume of fluid that provides lubrication between the pleural surfaces. The protein content of pleural fluid is normally low (1.5 g/dL), but the net Starling forces favor filtration of fluid into the *pleural space*. Fluid is removed by lymphatic vessels that communicate directly with the pleural space through holes (*stomata*) in the surface of the parietal pleura. Fluid accumulates in the pleural cavity when capillary pressures increase or when vascular permeability is increased by inflammation of the pleura (pleuritis). If fibrin accumulates in the pleural space, lymphatic vessels may be obstructed, and drainage of the pleural space may be impaired. As a result, large volumes of fluid can accumulate between the lungs and chest wall, impeding ventilation and necessitating drainage by the use of tubes.

METABOLIC FUNCTIONS OF THE LUNG

The lung removes many hormones and toxins from the blood and inactivates many others

Because it receives the total cardiac output, the pulmonary capillary bed with its vast endothelial surface is ideally placed to cleanse the blood of substances produced in other parts of the body. The endothelial cell surface, which is enlarged by projections and by depressions known as *caveolae*, is the site of many enzymes involved in the uptake and metabolism of *vasoactive substances*. Serotonin is almost totally removed by uptake into endothelial cells, where it is degraded by monoamine oxidase. Norepinephrine is also removed to some degree, but acetylcholine, epinephrine, and histamine are not removed. The peptides bradykinin and angiotensin are metabolized by angiotensin-converting enzyme located on the endothelial surface. Bradykinin is inactivated, whereas angiotensin I is converted into angiotensin II. The lung degrades the majority of prostaglandin E_2 and prostaglandin F_2, but prostacyclin is unaffected. Leukotrienes are broken down by neutrophils, which are numerous in the pulmonary circulation. Many exogenous toxic substances are also removed from the blood by the pulmonary endothelium. This process can at times cause severe lung injury. For example, the toxins from *Crotalaria* species of plants can cause smooth muscle hypertrophy in the pulmonary arterioles, which leads to pulmonary hypertension.

CLINICAL CORRELATIONS

Pleuritis in a thoroughbred horse

History At your practice in California, you are asked to examine a 3-year-old thoroughbred, which on the previous day had arrived by truck from a racetrack in New York. On arrival, the horse appeared depressed. This morning it refused to eat and drink and is breathing rapidly. The owner reports that in New York the horse was at a racetrack where there was much through-traffic of young horses, many of which were coughing.

Clinical examination On arrival at the farm, you meet an anxious owner who leads you to a stall, where the thoroughbred is standing with its elbows slightly abducted, its head lowered, its nostrils flared, and an anxious look in its eye. The grain and hay from the morning's feed are untouched. The horse has a respiratory rate of 65 (normal is 12 to 20). On further questioning, the owner reports that the horse looked much as it does now when it arrived from New York, but he thought that this was just because it was tired from the truck ride. The trucker reported that the horse drank little when it was offered water on its 3-day trip across country and had only nibbled at its hay. It was in the truck with four other younger horses. The condition of these horses is unknown.

You examine the horse and find that it is febrile, and its pulse rate and respiratory rate are greatly elevated. The horse becomes anxious when approached and particularly when hands are laid on the thoracic cage. The horse's mucous membranes are a dull red. Auscultation of the abdomen reveals little in the way of gastrointestinal sounds, and there is no evidence of feces in the stall. You listen to the respiratory system and note louder, harsher sounds than normal in the trachea and in the dorsal part of the lung. However, the ventral part of the lung is notably silent.

You elect to take thoracic radiographs and notice that there is a fluid accumulation in the ventral half of the thorax, obscuring the cardiac shadow and much of the lung. In the dorsal part of the thorax, the lung tissue has a number of radiographic densities that have a fluffy appearance, suggesting they are in the alveolar spaces. A cannula is placed in the pleural cavity to drain the pleural fluid, which is foul-smelling and purulent. Ten liters are removed, and radiographs then reveal that the alveolar densities extend into the ventral part of the thorax.

Bacterial cultures of the pleural fluid grow an anaerobic organism (*Bacteroides fragilis*), which is probably responsible for the foul smell of the pleural fluid. A complete blood cell count reveals a decreased number of circulating neutrophils and a large number of immature forms of neutrophils. This is an indication that the neutrophil resources of the body are being depleted and the bone marrow is putting out immature forms. Presumably, the neutrophils are being sequestered within the lung and pleural cavity.

Comment The history and clinical findings in this horse are fairly typical of a case of pleuropneumonia. In New York, the horse was exposed to other animals that were coughing, probably as a result of a viral infection, such as equine influenza or equine rhinopneumonitis. Respiratory viruses generally impair the defense mechanisms of the lung in two ways. First, they denude the tracheobronchial epithelium of cilia and, therefore, reduce mucociliary clearance of the airways. Second, they impair macrophage function. This combination of events results in the deposition of bacteria in the lung and failure of the lung to remove them by either the ciliary system or the macrophages. As a result, the bacteria multiply. The stress of shipping makes the situation even worse. Stress probably resulted in the release of corticosteroids from the adrenal gland, and this further suppressed the defense mechanisms of the lung. Failure to drink leads to dehydration, which can make mucus more difficult to clear. Keeping the horse's head elevated during transport also impairs mucociliary function. As a result of these events, the horse acquired a bacterial infection of the lung, which resulted in the migration of large numbers of neutrophils into the alveoli. This resulted in the fluffy densities on the radiograph.

When the infection spread to the pleural cavity, neutrophils migrated to this region also. The release of neutrophil products designed to kill bacteria caused extensive damage to the membranes of the alveolar epithelium, pulmonary capillaries, and pleural capillaries. The protein that leaked into the alveolar spaces, interstitium of the lung, and pleural cavity raised the osmotic pressure within these regions. This resulted in the movement of fluid from the vascular space into the alveolar spaces, interstitium, and pleural cavity. Within the pleural cavity, the fluid accumulates ventrally because of gravity, and it is probably this accumulation of fluid that results in the inaudibility of lung sounds in the ventral part of the thorax.

Treatment The chest tube is left in the pleural cavity so that the fluid can be drained repeatedly. The horse is given high levels of antibiotics and a prostaglandin synthetase inhibitor, flunixin, which should reduce the inflammation and make the horse more comfortable. However, in view of the degree of alveolar involvement, the presence of an anaerobic organism, and the large amount of fluid in the pleural cavity, the prognosis for this horse is not good.

Mitral insufficiency in a dog

History A 12-year-old cocker spaniel is brought to a veterinary hospital because of a recent deterioration in its condition. The dog has been a faithful pet and has always enjoyed exercising with its owner, but over the past few months, the owner has noticed an increasing reluctance to exercise. The dog has also coughed, especially when it gets up from resting. In the past few days, the dog has refused to leave the house and has eaten little. The owner has noticed that the cough is much more frequent than previously and seems to be moist.

Clinical examination You have examined this dog on many occasions, and it has always been friendly, but when you walk into the examination room, the dog greets you with only a modest tail wag. It stands with its head down and its tongue hanging out; it is panting. It walks reluctantly toward you when you call it. The dog was formerly fat but is now in about normal flesh, so over the past few months it has lost some weight.

You lift the dog onto the examination table and begin by looking at the mucous membranes, which appear normal in color. The dog's temperature is normal. The dog is panting, which makes auscultation of the chest difficult, but on the occasions when the dog breathes without panting, you notice some increased sounds in the

trachea and in all the lung fields, which sound like fluid bubbling within the air spaces of the lungs. The heart rate is dramatically increased, and there is a loud murmur audible over the mitral area during systole. You tell the owner that you suspect that the dog has a heart problem, which is leading to the accumulation of fluid in the lungs. You take chest radiographs and an arterial blood sample for measurement of blood gas tensions. The chest radiograph shows an enlarged heart, particularly the left ventricle. The lungs are diffusely more dense than normal, and the densities have a fluffy appearance, which suggests that that they are in the alveoli. There is also increased density along the walls of the major airways.

Arterial oxygen tension (Pa_{O_2}) is 70 mm Hg, and arterial carbon dioxide tension (Pa_{CO_2}) is 30 mm Hg. The radiographs confirm your suspicion of a heart problem. The left side of the heart is enlarged, which suggests that there is left-sided heart failure.

Comment Left-sided heart failure is accompanied by insufficiency of the mitral valve, and so blood leaking back into the left atrium during systole creates a murmur. The elevation in left atrial pressure as a result of mitral regurgitation is leading to an increased pressure in the pulmonary veins and capillaries. The increased pulmonary capillary hydrostatic pressure causes fluid filtration into the interstitium and now into the alveolar air spaces. It is likely that this condition has been progressing for some time, and only when it became severe enough for fluid to accumulate in the air spaces of the lung did the owner notice the deterioration in the dog's condition.

The hypoxemia is a result of ventilation-perfusion mismatching because of accumulation of fluids within the alveolar spaces. These fluid-filled spaces are still perfused, but the blood passing through this region does not pick up a sufficient amount of oxygen. This results in hypoxemia. The hypoxemia stimulates ventilation, and the increase in total ventilation to the lung is sufficient to eliminate more carbon dioxide than normal, so Pa_{CO_2} is 30 mm Hg, rather than the normal level of 40 mm Hg.

Treatment The dog is treated with a diuretic and a digitalis glycoside. The diuretic causes fluid elimination by the kidneys, which reduces vascular volume and intravascular pressures and, therefore, reduces the amount of fluid being filtered into the lung. In time, this causes resolution of the edema. The digitalis glycoside increases the contractility of the heart and, therefore, the dog's cardiac output, which improves the ability of the dog to exercise.

Bibliography

Guyton AC, Hall JE: Pulmonary circulation; pulmonary edema; pleural fluid. In Textbook of Medical Physiology, 9th ed. Philadelphia: WB Saunders, 1996, pp 491–499.
Leff AR, Schumacker PT: Respiratory Physiology: Basics and Applications. Philadelphia: WB Saunders, 1993, pp 66–68, 155–164.
Lekeux P, Art T: The respiratory system: Anatomy, physiology and adaptations to exercise and training. In Hodgson DR, Rose RJ (eds): The Athletic Horse. Philadelphia: WB Saunders, 1994, pp 79–127.
Murray JF: The Normal Lung. Philadelphia: WB Saunders, 1986, pp 283–337.

PRACTICE QUESTIONS

1. Particles greater than 5 µm in diameter are deposited in the respiratory tract by
    a. inertial deposition in small airways.
    b. sedimentation in airways.
    c. diffusion in the alveoli.
    d. inertial deposition in large airways.
    e. sedimentation in the alveoli.

2. The mucociliary system
    a. consists of a gel layer in which cilia beat, overlain by a sol layer that entraps particles.
    b. is restricted to the nasal cavity and trachea and does not extend into the bronchi.
    c. consists in part of mucus produced by goblet cells in the respiratory bronchioles and by Clara cells in the trachea.
    d. has a more rapid transport rate in the trachea than in the bronchioles.
    e. lacks ciliated cells in the bronchioles, so mucus must be pulled into the larger airways by viscous drag.

3. Phagocytosis of inhaled particles
    a. is generally by type II alveolar cells.
    b. can always be accomplished by alveolar macrophages.
    c. sometimes requires both macrophages and neutrophils.
    d. is accentuated by alveolar hypoxia.
    e. Both c and d.

4. Movement of fluid between the pulmonary capillaries and lung lymphatic vessels
    a. does not occur in a normal animal.
    b. is accentuated by an increase in capillary hydrostatic pressure.
    c. is accentuated by an increase in capillary oncotic pressure.
    d. occurs by way of the alveolar surface.
    e. Both b and d.

5. Which of the following occurs as a result of enzymes localized on the pulmonary endothelium?
    a. Conversion of angiotensin I to angiotensin II.
    b. Conversion of angiotensinogen to angiotensin I.
    c. Release of renin.
    d. Conversion of renin to angiotensin II.
    e. None of the above.

PRACTICE ANSWERS

1. d   2. d   3. c   4. b   5. a

HOMEOSTASIS

N. Edward Robinson

50

Fetal and neonatal
oxygen transport

1 The fetus depends on the placenta for exchange of gas, nutrients, and metabolic byproducts

2 The efficiency of gas exchange at the placenta depends on the arrangement of fetal and maternal blood vessels, which varies with species

3 The fetal circulation mixes oxygenated and deoxygenated blood at several points, and so the fetus exists in a state of hypoxemia

4 Fetal oxygen transport is assisted by fetal hemoglobin, which has a high affinity for oxygen

5 The lung, which is an outgrowth of the foregut, develops in three stages, and surfactant must be present at the time of birth

6 At the time of birth or shortly thereafter, umbilical vessels rupture, pulmonary vascular resistance decreases, and the foramen ovale and ductus arteriosus close

The fetus depends on the placenta for exchange of gas, nutrients, and metabolic byproducts

From conception until birth, the *embryo* and *fetus* depend on the mother for a supply of oxygen and nutrients and for removal of carbon dioxide and other metabolic byproducts. The embryo exchanges these substances by diffusion through the uterine fluids. As the *conceptus* increases in size, the specialized exchange organ, known as the *placenta*, becomes essential. The placenta brings maternal and fetal blood into close apposition over a large surface area that is provided by a network of capillaries.

The gross appearance of the placenta of different species varies widely. In horses and pigs, the placenta is *diffuse* and covers most of the uterine epithelium. In ruminants, the placenta has rows of discrete circular-to-oval *cotyledons* that are attached to approximately 100 highly vascularized *caruncles* in the uterine epithelium. In dogs, the placenta is *zonary,* forming a circular band around the *allantochorion* of the puppy. A complete listing of types of placentation of different species is provided in Table 50–1.

In addition to differing in the amount of uterine surface to which they are attached, placentas also differ in the number of layers of cells that separate the maternal and fetal blood (see Table 50–1). In horses, pigs, sheep, and cows, the fetal *chorion* is applied to the maternal uterine epithelium (*epitheliochorial* placentation), whereas in cats and dogs, the chorion is applied to the endothelium of maternal vessels (*endotheliochorial* placentation); in rodents and most primates, the chorion invades the uterine mucosa and erodes the maternal capillaries, so it becomes bathed by maternal blood (*hemochorial* placentation).

The efficiency of gas exchange at the placenta depends on the arrangement of fetal and maternal blood vessels, which varies with species

The exchange of gases and other substances across the placenta is determined by several factors, including the amount of surface apposition between fetal and maternal tissues and the number of layers of cells separating fetal and maternal blood. However, a major factor determining exchange is the arrangement of fetal and maternal blood vessels within the small interdigitating villi of the placenta. Figure 50–1 is a schematic representation of the possible arrangements

TABLE 50–1. **Placentation in domestic mammals**

| Species | Classification | |
	GROSS	HISTOLOGIC
Horse	Diffuse	Epitheliochorial
Pig	Diffuse	Epitheliochorial
Cow	Cotyledonary	Epitheliochorial
Sheep	Cotyledonary	Epitheliochorial
Goat	Cotyledonary	Epitheliochorial
Dog	Zonary	Endotheliochorial
Cat	Zonary	Endotheliochorial
Rabbit	Discoid	Hemochorial
Guinea pig	Discoid	Hemochorial

A. Countercurrent

Maternal

Fetal

B. Concurrent

Maternal

Fetal

C. Crosscurrent

Maternal

Fetal

D. Pool

Maternal

Fetal

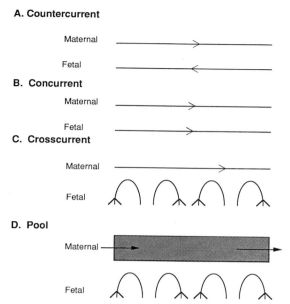

FIGURE 50–1. Schematic representation of possible arrangements of fetal and maternal blood vessels. (From Dawes GS: Foetal and Neonatal Physiology. Chicago: Year Book Medical, 1968.)

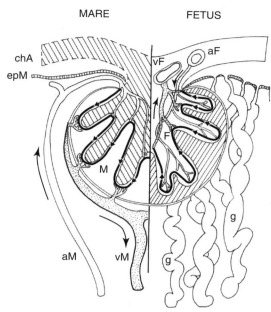

FIGURE 50–2. Diagram showing the arrangement of maternal and fetal blood vessels in the microcotyledons of the equine placenta. *Small open arrows* demonstrate the postulated countercurrent directions of maternal and fetal blood flows. aF, fetal artery; aM, maternal artery; chA, chorioallantois; epM, uterine epithelium; F, fetal; g, endometrial glands; M, maternal; vF, fetal vein; vM, maternal vein. (Based on data in Tsutsumi Y: Journal of Agriculture, Hokkaido Imperial University 52:372–482, 1962; reproduced with permission from Comline KS, Cross GS, Dawes GS, et al [eds]: Foetal and Neonatal Physiology. Proceedings of the Sir Joseph Barcroft Centenary Symposium. Cambridge, United Kingdom: Cambridge University Press, 1973, pp 245–271.)

of vessels. *Countercurrent* flow of maternal and fetal blood provides the most efficient exchange and allows equilibration of fetal and maternal arterial gas tensions. *Concurrent* flow of fetal and maternal blood allows fetal vessels to equilibrate with the maternal venous gas tensions. In *crosscurrent* and *pool* types of *equilibrators,* fetal capillaries loop down to maternal vessels or into a pool of maternal blood. These types of exchangers are not easily described by any simple model. It is likely that several different arrangements of vessels are found in the placentas of all species, but some seem to have more of the characteristics of countercurrent exchangers, and others have those of venous equilibrators.

Figure 50–2 shows the arrangement of vessels in the *microcotyledon* of the horse, a species in which fetal and maternal blood flow is primarily countercurrent. The cotyledonary placenta of sheep functions as a venous equilibrator, whereas the hemochorial placenta of the rabbit seems to be a countercurrent exchanger.

Placental gas exchange has been best studied in the sheep and is summarized in Figure 50–3. Maternal blood enters the uterus via the uterine artery with an oxygen tension (Po_2) of 80 mm Hg and leaves through the uterine vein with a Po_2 of 50 mm Hg. Some of the blood entering the uterus supplies the myometrium and endometrium, but most participates in gas exchange in the cotyledon. Fetal arterial blood reaches the placenta through the umbilical artery and enters the cotyledon with a Po_2 of 24 mm Hg. Placental gas exchange occurs, and the blood leaving the placenta in the umbilical veins has a Po_2 of only 32 mm Hg. This is because the sheep placenta is a venous equilibrator, and so the maximal possible Po_2 would be

50 mm Hg. However, this maximum is not reached, because venous blood, which has provided nutrient blood flow to the chorion, dilutes the better oxygenated blood draining from the cotyledon. The countercurrent exchanger of the horse is apparently more

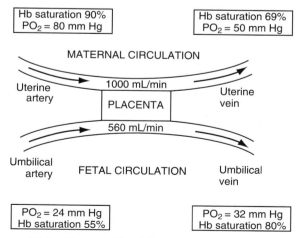

FIGURE 50–3. Placental blood flow, oxygen tension (Po_2), and hemoglobin (Hb) saturation in the uterine and umbilical circulation of the sheep. (From Battaglia FC, Meschia G: An Introduction to Fetal Physiology. Orlando, Fla.: Academic Press, 1986, p 157.)

efficient, because umbilical venous Po₂ averages 48 mm Hg.

The amount of placenta available for exchange in part determines the ultimate size of the fetus. If uterine caruncles are surgically removed from sheep so there are fewer sites for formation of fetal cotyledons, the full-term weight of lambs is reduced. The diffuse placenta of the horse apparently can support only one full-size fetus. One foal in a set of twins usually dies in utero or is very small. It is rare for twins to survive to term and be of equal size.

The fetal circulation mixes oxygenated and deoxygenated blood at several points, and so the fetus exists in a state of hypoxemia

In the adult, the cardiac output of the right and left ventricles is separated and perfuses the pulmonary and systemic circulations, respectively. In the fetus, the output of the two sides of the heart mixes at several points, so it is convenient to use the term cardiac output to refer to the combined output of the right and left ventricles. The combined cardiac output averages 500 mL/min/kg in fetal sheep; the output of the right ventricle exceeds that of the left. Figure 50–4 is a diagram of the fetal circulation showing the percentage of the cardiac output traversing the major vessels and the Po₂ within these vessels.

The placenta, which has a low vascular resistance, receives 45% of the cardiac output through the *umbilical arteries*. The *umbilical veins* drain the placenta toward the liver. In species such as the sheep, most of the umbilical venous blood passes through the liver through a low-resistance channel known as the *ductus venosus*; in other species, such as the pig and horse, the ductus venosus disappears early in gestation, and umbilical venous blood flows through the liver capillaries. Within the liver, the oxygenated blood from the placenta is mixed with a small amount of more poorly oxygenated blood draining the liver sinusoids. The hepatic venous blood enters the posterior vena cava, where it mixes with poorly oxygenated blood, draining the hind end of the fetus, so the blood returning to the right atrium has a Po₂ of 25 mm Hg.

A low-resistance pathway, the *foramen ovale*, connects the right and left atria, and a structure known as the *crista dividens* directs the better oxygenated blood from the posterior vena cava through the foramen ovale to the left atrium. The poorly oxygenated blood returning to the right atrium in the cranial vena cava is directed into the right atrium and right ventricle. Most of the output of the right ventricle does not go through the lungs, however, because in the fetus the lungs have a high vascular resistance. Another low-resistance channel, the *ductus arteriosus*, connects the *pulmonary artery* with the *aorta* and allows blood to bypass the lungs. It is important to note that the arrangement of the fetal circulation allows the better oxygenated blood to enter the left ventricle, from which it reaches the brachycephalic

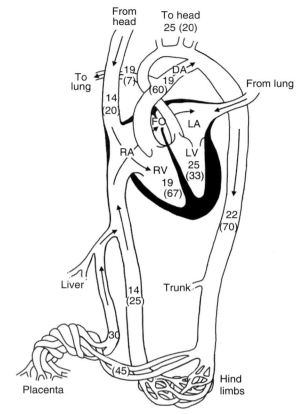

FIGURE 50–4. Diagrammatic representation of the fetal circulation showing the oxygen tension in millimeters of mercury and percentage of cardiac output (in parentheses) in different parts of the circulation. DA, ductus arteriosus; FO, foramen ovale; LA, left atrium; LV, left ventricle; RA, right atrium; RV, right ventricle.

vessels and the front of the animal. The more poorly oxygenated blood from the ductus arteriosus enters the aorta downstream from the brachycephalic vessels. The tissues of the hind end of the animal and the placenta receive blood with a Po₂ of approximately 22 mm Hg.

Flow of blood from the right atrium to the left atrium through the foramen ovale and from the pulmonary artery to the aorta through the ductus arteriosus requires that the pressure in the right side of the fetal circulation be greater than that in the left side. This pressure difference occurs because the left side of the circulation provides most of its output to the *low-resistance* placenta, whereas the right side of the fetal circulation is opposed by the *high-resistance* pulmonary circulation. At term, systemic arterial pressure in the lamb is about 42 mm Hg.

The fetal circulation is not a passive system but is capable of considerable regulation, particularly as the fetus matures. *Fetal hypoxia* can stimulate vasodilation in the heart and brain, and vasoconstriction in the gut, kidneys, and skeletal tissues. The fetal pulmonary circulation constricts vigorously when the fetus is hypoxic. This constriction diverts more blood through the ductus arteriosus to the systemic tissues.

Fetal oxygen transport is assisted by fetal hemoglobin, which has a high affinity for oxygen

Fetal arterial blood has a low P_{O_2} because the placenta is not a highly efficient gas exchanger and because oxygenated and venous blood mix at several points in the fetal circulation. The fetus is adapted to this state of chronic hypoxia in two ways. First, it has a high cardiac output that delivers a large volume of blood per minute to the tissues. Second, the fetus produces erythrocytes containing hemoglobin with a high *affinity* for oxygen.

The production of erythrocytes initially occurs in the *yolk sac*. These embryonic erythrocytes are nucleated and contain embryonic hemoglobin, the oxygen affinity of which has not been clearly defined. At the termination of the embryonic period, erythrocyte production shifts to the liver and spleen. Depending on the species, fetal erythrocytes contain either *fetal* or *adult hemoglobin* (see later discussion). Simultaneously, there are changes in glycolytic enzymes to provide the fetal concentrations of *2,3-diphosphoglycerate* (2,3-DPG). Fetal erythrocytes have a higher affinity (lower partial pressure at which hemoglobin is 50% saturated with oxygen [P_{50}]) for oxygen than do maternal erythrocytes; that is, the fetal blood oxyhemoglobin dissociation curve lies to the left of the adult curve (Fig. 50–5). In some species, such as the cat, the difference in the P_{50} between fetus and adult is small, whereas in ruminants, the difference is 10 to 20 mm Hg.

Three mechanisms account for the position of the fetal oxyhemoglobin dissociation curve. In ruminants, the higher oxygen affinity results from the synthesis of fetal hemoglobin with a high intrinsic oxygen affinity. Fetal hemoglobin of these species is unresponsive to 2,3-DPG. After birth there is gradual replacement of fetal hemoglobin by adult hemoglobin. In primates, there is little intrinsic difference in the oxygen affinity of fetal and maternal hemoglobin, but fetal hemoglobin has a decreased interaction with 2,3-DPG. In horses and pigs, there is no fetal hemoglobin; embryonic hemoglobin is replaced immediately by adult hemoglobin. The fetal erythrocytes of these species have a low concentration of 2,3-DPG. After birth, there is an increase in the concentration of 2,3-DPG, which gives the hemoglobin its adult dissociation curve.

The high affinity of fetal hemoglobin for oxygen allows the hemoglobin in the umbilical veins, with a P_{O_2} of 30 mm Hg, to be 80% saturated with oxygen and allows the hemoglobin in the aorta, with a P_{O_2} of 22 mm Hg, to be 56% saturated. The high affinity of fetal hemoglobin for oxygen not only allows the transport of oxygen at the low P_{O_2} existing in fetal arteries but also makes it necessary for fetal tissues to have very low oxygen tensions. The low tissue oxygen tensions provide an oxygen concentration gradient in order to unload oxygen from the fetal hemoglobin. Therefore, the fetus exists in a state of tissue hypoxia in comparison with the adult.

The lung, which is an outgrowth of the foregut, develops in three stages, and surfactant must be present at the time of birth

By the time of birth, the lung must be ready to assume the gas exchange functions of the placenta. The lung develops in three stages of equivalent duration. Beginning as an outgrowth of the foregut, the lung bud invades the *mesenchyme* of the thorax and divides into all the major airway branches during the first third of gestation. Because these *primordial airways* are lined with a *cuboidal epithelium* and look like a gland in cross section, this stage of development is known as the *glandular stage*. In the second phase of development, the lung is invaded by blood vessels (the *canalicular stage*). In the final, or *alveolar sac stage*, alveolar sacs and, in some species, *alveoli*, develop. The stage of maturity of the lung at birth in general matches the maturity of the fetus. Lambs and piglets have well-developed alveoli, but humans, and especially rodents, have thicker-walled alveolar sacs. In these latter species, alveoli develop as the animal grows postnatally.

Pulmonary surfactant is essential if the lung is to remain inflated after birth (see Chapter 44). Beginning at about mid-gestation, there is an increase in the synthesis of surfactant components, such as lecithin, within the lung. This increase in lecithin synthesis coincides with the appearance of type II alveolar cells (the source of surfactant) and with an increase in pulmonary blood flow. Some of this lecithin is secreted into the alveolar lumens and appears in the amniotic fluid, where it can be measured as an indicator of the state of lung maturity. Lung maturity coincides with an increase in *serum cortisol* levels in the fetus.

Until the time of birth, the vascular resistance of the fetal pulmonary circulation is high, for several reasons. The fetal lung is not inflated; therefore, the large vessels are not pulled open by the surrounding

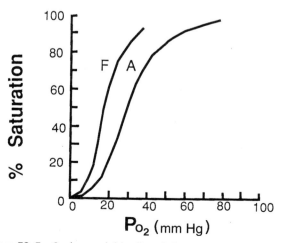

FIGURE 50–5. Oxyhemoglobin dissociation curves of fetal (F) and adult (A) sheep.

alveolar septa. In addition, the hypoxia of the fetus maintains the pulmonary vascular smooth muscle in a state of contraction that narrows the arteries. Both these conditions are alleviated by the first few breaths.

The fetal lung continuously secretes fluid until about 2 days before birth. This fluid, which is rich in chloride and low in bicarbonate and protein, travels up the trachea and through the fetus's mouth into the amniotic cavity. The fluid in the alveolar spaces and airways is in part squeezed out of the lung as the thorax is compressed during birth. The majority is reabsorbed by lymphatic and blood vessels shortly after birth.

In late gestation, the fetus makes *breathing movements,* although it moves little of the viscous fluid to and fro in the airways. These movements apparently prepare the respiratory muscles for their postnatal function.

At the time of birth or shortly thereafter, umbilical vessels rupture, pulmonary vascular resistance decreases, and the foramen ovale and ductus arteriosus close

At term, the fetus is dependent on the placenta and the mother for exchange with the environment, but the lung and other organs must be ready to assume their postnatal functions. During a normal birth, the newborn emerges from the birth canal at about the time the placenta is detaching from the uterine wall. Placental gas exchange probably continues well into third-stage *labor.* If labor is prolonged, the placenta may detach before the newborn is delivered. This is a medical emergency.

Normally, the newborn takes the first breath immediately after delivery. The stimuli for this include (1) hypoxia and hypercarbia, which result from the loss of the placental gas exchanger; (2) cooling of the fetus as the fetal fluids evaporate from the skin; and (3) a generalized increase in sensory input to the fetus as it is licked and nuzzled by its dam. Moving the first air into the lungs requires a considerable effort as viscous fluids must be inhaled down the airways before air can enter the alveoli. The critical opening pressures of the fluid-filled small airways and alveoli must also be exceeded. Not all alveoli may inflate during the first breath, but subsequent inhalations will inflate the entire lung and distribute surfactant over the alveolar surface. This surfactant makes the alveoli stable and prevents their collapse, so that a stable end-expiratory lung volume, known as *functional residual capacity,* can be established. After the first few breaths, arterial oxygen tension is much higher than it was before birth, and yet breathing continues. It therefore appears that breathing is inhibited in utero, and the chemoreceptors are insensitive to hypoxia. This inhibition is removed after birth.

Inflation and oxygenation of the lung reduce the pulmonary vascular resistance, which leads to a decreased pressure in the pulmonary artery, right ventri-cle, and right atrium. At about the same time, the umbilical vessels rupture, because the animal struggles to stand or the umbilical cord is torn by the mother. Umbilical blood flow is arrested by local vasoconstriction in the umbilical vessels. The loss of the low-resistance placental circulation increases systemic vascular resistance, which results in an increased pressure in the aorta, left ventricle, and left atrium. As a result of these changes, aortic pressure exceeds pulmonary arterial pressure, and left atrial pressure exceeds right atrial pressure. Therefore, blood flow through the ductus arteriosus and foramen ovale reverses. Flow reversal in the foramen ovale causes a flap valve to close and occlude the foramen. Over succeeding days to weeks, this valve becomes adherent to the wall of the atrium, thus permanently closing the foramen.

Reversal of flow in the ductus arteriosus exposes the ductus wall to well-oxygenated blood. This causes constriction of smooth muscle in the wall of the ductus, thus arresting blood flow. Ductus closure involves a change in *prostaglandin* levels. Administration of drugs, such as indomethacin, that inhibit prostaglandin synthesis constricts the ductus in fetal sheep, and administration of prostaglandin E_2 dilates it. Once the ductus has constricted and flow has been arrested, the ductus is gradually converted into a fibrous band of scar tissue.

The changes just described convert the fetal circulation into the adult circulation able to support the gas exchange function of the lung. What is amazing is that these changes happen routinely and without medical assistance in almost all animal births.

CLINICAL CORRELATIONS

Patent ductus arteriosus in a Pomeranian

History   A 7-week-old female Pomeranian puppy is presented to you because it is not growing as fast as its littermates. The breeder says it is lethargic and prefers to sleep, whereas the other puppies play.

Clinical examination   Clinical examination reveals a small puppy with a rapid heart rate. The mucous membranes of its gums are pink, and its temperature is normal. While holding the puppy around the thorax, you notice a vibration in the region of the heart. When you listen with a stethoscope, you hear a loud murmur that is almost continuous through systole and diastole, and you recall that this is called a *machinery murmur.* It is difficult to listen to the breath sounds because the murmur is audible all over the thorax. A radiograph reveals an enlarged heart, but the lungs appear normal, although a little compressed by the heart.

Comment   The clinical and radiographic findings in a puppy of this age are characteristic of a patent ductus arteriosus. In some animals, the ductus fails to close after birth, and blood continues to flow through it, usually from the aorta to the pulmonary artery. This presents the animal with two problems. First, the left ventricle must increase its output to supply the systemic tissues because so much blood is passing through the ductus. Second, the pulmonary circulation has a volume overload that increases the pressure against which the right ventricle must work. These extra loads result in dilation of the ventricles and sometimes in hypertrophy of the myocardium, which is seen on radiographs as an enlarged heart. The puppy is not growing and is listless because the tissues are not receiving a normal blood flow. It would be unwise to breed this animal in the future, because the condition is inherited.

Treatment   The patent ductus must be closed surgically.

Bibliography

Battaglia FC, Meschia G: An Introduction to Fetal Physiology. Orlando, Fla.: Academic Press, 1986, pp 1–48, 154–211.

Dawes GS: Foetal and Neonatal Physiology. Chicago: Year Book Medical, 1968.

Faber JJ, Thornburg KL: Placental Physiology: Structure and Function of Fetomaternal Exchange. New York: Raven Press, 1983, pp 1–32.

Leff AR, Schumacker PT: Respiratory Physiology: Basics and Applications. Philadelphia: WB Saunders, 1993, pp 137–154.

Murray JF: The Normal Lung: The Basis for Diagnosis and Treatment of Pulmonary Disease, 2nd ed. Philadelphia: WB Saunders, 1986, pp 1–21.

Silver M, Steven DH, Comline KS: Placental exchange and morphology in ruminants and the mare. *In* Comline KS, Cross KW, Dawes GS, et al (eds): Foetal and Neonatal Physiology. Proceedings of the Sir Joseph Barcroft Centenary Symposium. Cambridge, United Kingdom: Cambridge University Press, 1973, pp 245–271.

PRACTICE QUESTIONS

1. The vascular channel that allows fetal blood to pass from the pulmonary artery to the aorta is known as the
 a. foramen ovale.
 b. ductus arteriosus.
 c. ductus venosus.
 d. fetal cotyledon.
 e. allantois.

2. Which of the following fetal blood vessels contains blood with the highest PO_2?
 a. Aorta.
 b. Ductus arteriosus.
 c. Pulmonary artery.
 d. Left ventricle.
 e. Umbilical artery.

3. Which of the following statements about the fetal circulation is true?
 a. Right atrial pressure is higher than left atrial pressure.
 b. Pulmonary vascular resistance is high.
 c. The placenta receives about 45% of the combined output of both ventricles.

 d. The output of the right ventricle is greater than that of the left ventricle.
 e. All of the above.

4. Which of the following does *not* correctly describe the lung in utero?
 a. Type II cells, which produce surfactant, are present within the first few days of gestation in sheep.
 b. Chloride-rich fluid is secreted into the airways and flows into the amniotic cavity.
 c. Components of surfactant can be detected in the amniotic fluid when the lung approaches maturity.
 d. All the major branches of the tracheobronchial tree are present at birth, but alveoli continue to multiply after birth in some species.
 e. Breathing movements occur in utero, but the volume of fluid moved in and out of the lungs is small.

5. Which of the following lists in the correct sequence the events that follow birth?
 a. Closure of foramen ovale, first breath, rupture of umbilical vessels.
 b. Decrease in right atrial pressure, first breath, closure of the ductus arteriosus.
 c. First breath, closure of the ductus arteriosus, decrease in pulmonary arterial pressure.
 d. First breath, decrease in pulmonary arterial pressure, closure of the foramen ovale.
 e. Closure of the foramen ovale, closure of the ductus arteriosus, first breath.

6. Fetal oxygen transport is assisted by
 a. fetal hemoglobin, which has a lower oxygen capacity than adult hemoglobin.
 b. fetal hemoglobin, which has a lower P_{50} than adult hemoglobin.
 c. a cardiac output that is less per kilogram of body weight than in the adult.
 d. a cardiac output that preferentially delivers the blood with the highest PO_2 to the placenta.
 e. a fetal lung, which is an efficient gas exchanger.

7. Which of the following domestic mammals has a diffuse, epitheliochorial placenta in which fetal and maternal blood flow is countercurrent in the microcotyledons?
 a. Dog.
 b. Cow.
 c. Horse.
 d. Rabbit.
 e. Sheep.

PRACTICE ANSWERS

1. b   2. d   3. e   4. a   5. d   6. b   7. c

51

Acid-base homeostasis

Acid-base regulation

1 Relative constancy of the body's pH is essential, because metabolism requires enzymes that operate at an optimal pH

2 Hydrogen ion concentration is measured as pH

3 An acid can donate a hydrogen ion, and a base can accept a hydrogen ion

4 Buffers are combinations of salts and weak acids that prevent major changes in pH

5 Hemoglobin and bicarbonate are the most important blood buffers

6 Intracellular buffering is provided by proteins and organic phosphates

7 The first defense against a change in blood pH is provided by the blood buffers, but it is the lungs and the kidneys that must ultimately correct the hydrogen ion load

8 Changes in ventilation can rapidly change P_{CO_2} and therefore alter the pH

9 Metabolic production of fixed acids requires that the kidneys eliminate hydrogen ions and conserve HCO_3^-

Acid-base disturbances

1 Acid-base abnormalities accompany many diseases, and the restoration of normal blood pH should be a consideration in the treatment of any disease

2 Respiratory acidosis is caused by the accumulation of carbon dioxide, which decreases blood pH

3 Respiratory alkalosis is caused by the loss of carbon dioxide, which increases blood pH

4 Metabolic acidosis is caused by the accumulation of fixed acids or the loss of buffer base, which decreases blood pH

5 Metabolic alkalosis is caused by the excessive elimination of hydrogen ions or by the intake of base, such as HCO_3^-, which increases blood pH

6 Respiratory compensations for acid-base abnormalities occur rapidly; renal compensations occur over several hours

7 Hydrogen and potassium ions are interrelated in acid-base homeostasis

8 The diagnosis of acid-base disturbances depends on interpretation of measurements of arterial blood pH and P_{CO_2}, from which the HCO_3^- concentration and total buffer base are calculated

9 Over the years, a large number of terms have been used to explain acid-base balance

ACID-BASE REGULATION

Relative constancy of the body's pH is essential, because metabolism requires enzymes that operate at an optimal pH

For optimal functioning of the cells constituting the animal, the ionic composition of body fluids is maintained within fairly narrow limits. Hydrogen is one of the ions that determines the *acidity* or *alkalinity,* or *pH,* of the body fluids. Serious deviations of pH outside the normal range can drastically disrupt cell metabolism and, therefore, body function.

When veterinarians use the terms *acidosis* and *alkalosis,* they are comparing the pH of an animal's arterial blood with the normal value of 7.4. A pH below 7.4 is referred to as *acidosis;* a pH above 7.4 is referred to as *alkalosis.* The range of pH compatible with life is 6.85 to 7.8, but rarely are these extremes ap-

proached. The body buffers, lungs, and kidneys all defend the body from onslaught of hydrogen ions from a variety of sources.

The biggest daily load of hydrogen ions (*protons*) arises during the transport of carbon dioxide from the tissues to the lungs. If the lungs eliminate carbon dioxide as fast as it is produced in the tissues, there is no net hydrogen ion gain by the body. However, the balance between carbon dioxide production and its elimination may be disturbed during exercise or in respiratory disease, thus threatening the acid-base homeostasis of the body.

Hydrogen ions are also a product of protein metabolism, which produces sulfuric and phosphoric acids, fat metabolism, and the incomplete oxidation of glucose to lactic acid. Hydrogen ions from these sources, although normally few in comparison with those produced in carbon dioxide transport, must be eliminated continuously by the kidneys. In a disease state, the hydrogen ion load imposed on the body is frequently increased because of an increase in tissue breakdown (catabolism) or because the kidneys fail to eliminate hydrogen ion. On more rare occasions, such as in vomit, hydrogen ion is lost from the body. To understand how the body regulates pH and how acid-base disorders are diagnosed, it is necessary to first review acids, bases, and buffering.

Hydrogen ion concentration is measured as pH

Only 1 in 550 million molecules of water is *ionized*; thus, the concentration of hydrogen and hydroxyl ions in water is 1×10^{-7} mol/L. The *chemical potential* of the hydrogen ions is known as the *acidity* and is expressed in pH units. pH is the *negative logarithm* of the hydrogen ion concentration. Water with 1×10^{-7} mol/L of hydrogen ion and an equal concentration of hydroxyl ions has a pH of 7.0: that is, a neutral pH. A decrease in pH indicates increasing acidity, caused by an increase in the concentration of hydrogen ions. For example, a decrease of 1.0 pH unit represents a 10-fold increase in hydrogen ion concentration. Doubling hydrogen ion concentration decreases pH by only 0.3 unit.

The normal range of blood pH, 6.85 to 7.80, represents a hydrogen ion concentration of 1.4×10^{-7} to 1.6×10^{-8} Eq/L. Thus, although the hydrogen ion concentration is regulated, changes up to 10-fold in magnitude can occur, much greater than the fluctuations observed in the concentration of other ions, such as sodium or potassium.

An acid can donate a hydrogen ion, and a base can accept a hydrogen ion

Hydrochloric acid (HCl) is a *strong acid*, because it dissociates completely in water into H^+ and Cl^-. Chloride ion is a base, because it has the potential to accept a hydrogen ion, but it is a *weak base*, because HCl is so completely dissociated. Carbonic acid, in contrast, is a *weak acid*, because it is incompletely dissociated in solution to hydrogen and bicarbonate ions. Bicarbonate, however, is a relatively *strong base* that can accept a hydrogen ion and form undissociated carbonic acid. The latter reaction removes hydrogen ions from solution, and the concentration of free hydrogen ions decreases, causing the pH to rise. Bases do not have to be ions; for example, ammonia (NH_3) is a base because it can accept a proton and become ammonium ion (NH_4^+). This reaction is of little importance in the blood, but it is important in the distal renal tubule. In addition, proteins also act as buffers by virtue of the terminal amino and carboxyl groups, which can accept and donate protons, respectively.

Buffers are combinations of salts and weak acids that prevent major changes in pH

Buffers "soak up" free hydrogen ions and prevent their accumulation in body fluids. By so doing, buff-

ers prevent drastic changes in pH. Buffers are usually mixtures of weak acids and their salts. For example, sodium bicarbonate dissociates completely into sodium and bicarbonate ions; carbonic acid dissociates incompletely into hydrogen and bicarbonate ions. Thus, in a solution containing sodium bicarbonate and carbonic acid, there are sodium, hydrogen, and bicarbonate ions, and undissociated carbonic acid. If a strong acid such as hydrochloric acid is added to the solution, the added hydrogen ions upset the dissociation equilibrium of carbonic acid. Hydrogen ions combine with bicarbonate ion to form carbonic acid, thus reducing the concentration of hydrogen ions: that is, preventing a major change in pH.

If, in contrast, sodium hydroxide is added to the solution, the hydroxyl ions, formed by dissociation of sodium hydroxide, combine with hydrogen ion to form water. The decrease in hydrogen ion causes dissociation of more carbonic acid and liberation of hydrogen ions, again preventing a large change in pH.

The dissociation of a weak acid and, therefore, the concentration of hydrogen ion, base, and undissociated acid are determined by the *dissociation constant* (K_a) and can be described by the *law of mass action*. For carbonic acid,

$$K_a = [H^+][HCO_3^-]/[H_2CO_3].$$

Taking logarithms of both sides of this equation results in

$$\log K_a = \log[H^+] + \log[HCO_3^-]/[H_2CO_3].$$

Rearrangement of this equation yields

$$-\log[H^+] = -\log K_a + \log[HCO_3^-]/[H_2CO_3],$$

but $-\log[H^+]$ is pH and $-\log K_a$ is called pKa. Therefore,

$$pH = pKa + \log[HCO_3^-]/[H_2CO_3].$$

This is the *Henderson-Hasselbalch equation* written for the bicarbonate, carbonic acid system. It can be written for any buffering system in the generic form

$$pH = pKa + \log[base]/[acid].$$

This equation shows that the pH of a solution is determined by the ratio of the concentration of base (the hydrogen ion acceptor) to that of undissociated acid (the hydrogen ion donor) and by the pKa of the buffering system.

Figure 51–1 shows the change in pH that results when acid is added to a phosphate buffer with a pKa of 6.8. This is a graphic presentation of the Henderson-Hasselbalch equation. Initially, as acid is added, there is a large decrease in pH. As considerably more acid is added to the solution, the pH changes little. Hydrogen ions combine with HPO_4^{2-} and form $H_2PO_4^-$. Finally, the pH decreases considerably. The zone over which the pH changes little as acid is added (i.e., where buffering capacity is optimal) is within ± 1 pH unit of the pKa. Note that when the pH equals the pKa, 50% of the buffer has been consumed. From this buffer curve, it is obvious that an effective buffer must have a pKa within ± 1 pH unit

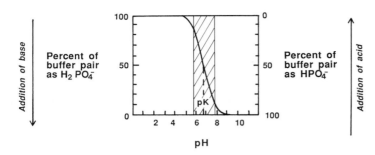

FIGURE 51–1. Titration curve for the phosphate buffer system. The pK is 6.8. The shaded area represents the range of pH over which this buffer is effective.

of the solution in which it operates. Thus, the optimal blood buffers should have a pKa between 6.4 and 8.4. In addition, buffers must be sufficiently plentiful to be effective.

Hemoglobin and bicarbonate are the most important blood buffers

Hemoglobin is an important blood buffer because it is plentiful and because the *imidazole residues* of globin *histidine* have a pKa close to the blood pH. In actuality, the pKa of hemoglobin changes with the degree of oxygenation. Because deoxyhemoglobin has a pKa (7.93) closer to blood pH than does oxyhemoglobin (pKa = 6.68), deoxyhemoglobin provides more buffering capacity. When arterial blood enters the tissue capillaries, oxygen leaves hemoglobin, so the resulting deoxyhemoglobin is an excellent buffer for the hydrogen ions produced when carbon dioxide is added to the blood.

The other blood buffer with an optimal pKa is the HPO_4^{2-}-$H_2PO_4^-$ system with a pKa of 6.8 (see Fig. 51–1). The normally low phosphate concentration in the blood makes this buffering system quantitatively unimportant; however, it is important in the renal tubules, where phosphate is concentrated. *Plasma proteins* also provide a small amount of blood buffering.

Although a pKa of 6.1 seems to make the HCO_3^--H_2CO_3 buffer unimportant for blood buffering, this is not so for two reasons. First, there is a large amount (24 mEq/L) of HCO_3^- in the blood, making it readily available for buffering. Second, the kidneys can regulate the concentration of HCO_3^-, and the lungs can regulate the concentration of H_2CO_3. Because the salt and acid concentration can be regulated, the HCO_3^--H_2CO_3 system is said to be an *open system*. Figure 51–2 shows the value of this open system in maintaining body pH.

The HCO_3^--H_2CO_3 buffering system is also of great value to clinicians, because its components can be readily measured in the clinical laboratory and used to diagnose acid-base disturbances. It is not necessary to measure the components of every buffering system to diagnose acid-base disturbances. If one system is known, changes in other systems can be predicted.

Of convenience is that the concentration of H_2CO_3 in solution is directly proportional to the carbon dioxide tension (P_{CO_2}); 1 molecule of H_2CO_3 is in equilibrium with 340 molecules of CO_2. Therefore, the con-

centration of H_2CO_3 is calculated as $0.03 \times P_{CO_2}$. According to the HCO_3^--H_2CO_3 system, it is standard to measure the pH and the concentration of H_2CO_3 (P_{CO_2}) and, using the Henderson-Hasselbalch equation, derive the concentration of HCO_3^-. For clinical use, the Henderson-Hasselbalch equation for the HCO_3^--H_2CO_3 system is written

$$pH = pK + \log[HCO_3^-]/[0.03 \cdot P_{CO_2}].$$

Under normal conditions, the pH of arterial blood is 7.4, the concentration of HCO_3^- is 24 mEq/L, and the arterial carbon dioxide tension (Pa_{CO_2}) is equal to 40 mm Hg:

$$7.4 = 6.1 + (\log 24)/(0.03 \cdot 40) = 6.1 + \log 20.$$

This equation demonstrates that a normal blood pH requires a $[HCO_3^-]/[0.03 \cdot P_{CO_2}]$ ratio of 20:1. An increase or decrease in this ratio increases or decreases pH, respectively.

Intracellular buffering is provided by proteins and organic phosphates

Whereas the hemoglobin and bicarbonate provide the most immediately available source of buffers to prevent drastic changes in blood pH, *intracellular buffers* within the body tissues, other than blood, provide another large reserve of buffering capacity. In order to enter cells, hydrogen ion must be exchanged with other cations, such as sodium or potassium. Once inside the cell, hydrogen ion is buffered by *amino acids*, *peptides*, *proteins*, and *organic phosphates*. These buffers provide approximately five times the buffering capacity of the extracellular fluid.

The first defense against a change in blood pH is provided by the blood buffers, but it is the lungs and the kidneys that must ultimately correct the hydrogen ion load

When body pH is threatened by a change in the production or elimination of hydrogen ions, the first line of defense is provided by buffers within the blood and tissues. However, buffers only prevent drastic changes in pH; they cannot correct the problem by increasing or decreasing the elimination of hydrogen ions or by replacing lost buffering capacity.

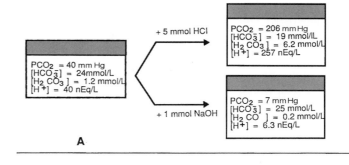

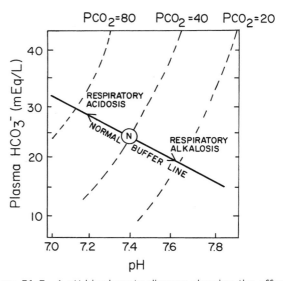

FIGURE 51–2. Buffer function of the carbonic acid-bicarbonate system under closed and open conditions. Under closed conditions *(A)*, the total quantity of the buffer (acid plus base components) remains constant. Under open conditions *(B)*, the carbon dioxide tension (P_{CO_2}) of the system, and thus the concentration of H_2CO_3, is maintained at a fixed level by continuous equilibration of the liquid phase with a gas reservoir of constant P_{CO_2}. The term $[H_2CO_3]$ denotes the combined concentration of carbonic acid and dissolved carbon dioxide. (From Madias NE, Cohen JJ: Acid-base chemistry and buffering. In Cohen JJ, Kassirer JP [eds]: Acid-Base. Boston: Little, Brown, 1982, p 14.)

Ultimately, pH must be corrected by adjustments in ventilation or by changes in renal function. Because the lungs can alter Pa_{CO_2} and the kidneys can regulate the concentration of HCO_3^-, the Henderson-Hasselbalch equation has been written as

$$pH = pK + \log \frac{\text{renal function}}{\text{ventilation}}.$$

Changes in ventilation can rapidly change P_{CO_2} and therefore alter the pH

As blood flows through the tissues, carbon dioxide diffuses into the plasma and the erythrocytes, where carbonic acid forms and then *dissociates* into hydrogen and bicarbonate ions:

$$H_2O + CO_2 \rightarrow H_2CO_3 \rightarrow H^+ + HCO_3^-.$$

Because the initial concentration of HCO_3^- in the blood is greater than that of H_2CO_3, the relative increase in the concentration of H_2CO_3 is greater than the increase in the concentration of HCO_3^-, and so the $[HCO_3^-]/[H_2CO_3]$ ratio (i.e., $[HCO_3^-/0.03 \cdot P_{CO_2}]$) is decreased; consequently, pH decreases. In the lungs, CO_2 leaves the blood, and the pH increases again. For these reasons, venous blood is more acidic than arterial blood. Normally, the lungs eliminate CO_2 as fast as it is produced by the tissues, and so the Pa_{CO_2} and pH of arterial blood remain relatively constant.

The lungs can cause rapid changes in blood pH by increasing or decreasing the elimination of CO_2. When ventilation increases in relation to CO_2 production

(hyperventilation), Pa_{CO_2} decreases, the $[HCO_3^-/0.03 \cdot Pa_{CO_2}]$ ratio increases, and pH increases. Conversely, when ventilation decreases in relation to CO_2 production *(hypoventilation)*, Pa_{CO_2} increases, the $[HCO_3^-/0.03 \cdot Pa_{CO_2}]$ ratio decreases, and pH decreases. Figure 51–3, a pH-bicarbonate diagram, shows how the concentration of HCO_3^- and the pH change as the P_{CO_2} of the blood increases or decreases.

FIGURE 51–3. A pH-bicarbonate diagram showing the effect of increasing and decreasing P_{CO_2} on pH and bicarbonate (HCO_3^-) concentration. N represents the normal arterial blood composition. As P_{CO_2} increases or decreases, the changes in pH and bicarbonate concentration are predicted by the normal buffer line.

Metabolic production of fixed acids requires that the kidneys eliminate hydrogen ions and conserve HCO_3^-

When fixed acids are added to the blood, for example, from protein metabolism, the hydrogen ions are buffered in part by HCO_3^-. Buffering results in the conversion of HCO_3^- to H_2CO_3 and CO_2, which is eliminated from the lungs. Fixed acids are produced continuously and would consume the body's HCO_3^- if the kidneys were not continually regenerating HCO_3^-.

The role of the kidneys in acid-base balance is described in Chapter 43. Large amounts of HCO_3^- are filtered daily through the glomerulus and subsequently reabsorbed in the renal tubule. The amount of HCO_3^- reabsorbed depends on the amount filtered, which is determined by the plasma concentration of HCO_3^-, the *glomerular filtration rate,* and the rate of hydrogen ion secretion by renal tubular cells. This last rate is controlled in part by the acid-base status of the body.

When P_{CO_2} is high, the reaction

$$H_2O + CO_2 \rightarrow H_2CO_3 \rightarrow H^+ + HCO_3^-$$

within the *renal tubules* is driven to the right, producing more hydrogen ions for secretion into the *tubular lumen* and HCO_3^- for return to the blood. When P_{CO_2} is low, hydrogen ion elimination and, therefore, HCO_3^- reabsorption decrease.

Ammonia, an important buffer in the distal renal tubule, is produced by the action of *glutaminase* on *glutamine.* In acidosis, the activity of glutaminase increases, resulting in increased ammonia production, an increased buffering capacity of the renal tubular fluid and, therefore, increased ability to eliminate hydrogen ions.

ACID-BASE DISTURBANCES

Acid-base abnormalities accompany many diseases, and the restoration of normal blood pH should be a consideration in the treatment of any disease

In most diseases, the buffering systems, lungs, and kidneys keep pH within tolerable limits, but in severe disease, these homeostatic mechanisms may be inadequate, and life-threatening changes in pH can occur. In the diagnosis and treatment of acid-base abnormalities, it is important to realize that a primary abnormality causes the change in blood pH, which is followed by compensatory changes. Because of the body's attempt to correct the abnormality, the clinician often must disentangle the data to differentiate the primary cause of the problem from the compensatory changes. The primary problems are excessive accumulation or elimination of carbon dioxide (respiratory abnormalities) or the excessive accumulation or elimination of fixed acids (metabolic abnormalities).

Respiratory acidosis is caused by the accumulation of carbon dioxide, which decreases blood pH

Respiratory acidosis is caused by *alveolar hypoventilation,* which can result from damage to or depression of the respiratory control centers, injury to the respiratory pump (e.g., fractured ribs or bloated abdomen), or severe respiratory disease that either obstructs the airways or excessively stiffens the lungs. When alveolar hypoventilation occurs, carbon dioxide is incompletely eliminated by the lungs, causing blood P_{CO_2} to increase. In the absence of other buffers, such as hemoglobin, the reaction

$$H_2O + CO_2 \rightarrow H_2CO_3 \rightarrow H^+ + HCO_3^-$$

is driven to the right by the accumulating CO_2; H^+ accumulates, and pH decreases. Bicarbonate accumulates simultaneously, but the amount is too small to keep the $[HCO_3^-/0.03 \cdot P_{CO_2}]$ ratio at a normal value of 20:1.

In the blood, other nonbicarbonate buffers not only take up H^+ produced by the accumulation of CO_2 but also assist in the accumulation of HCO_3^-, as follows:

$$H_2O + CO_2 \rightarrow H_2CO_3 \rightarrow H^+ + HCO_3^-$$
$$\downarrow$$
$$H^+ + Hb^- \rightarrow HHb.$$

By buffering H^+, hemoglobin (Hb^-) pulls the first reaction to the right and produces HCO_3^-. This accumulation of bicarbonate, shown on the *normal buffer line* in the pH-HCO_3^- diagram (see Fig. 51-3), is still insufficient to maintain a normal $[HCO_3^-/0.03 \cdot P_{CO_2}]$ ratio, and therefore the pH decreases. As a result of these various reactions, the characteristic findings in acute respiratory acidosis are an elevated Pa_{CO_2}, a decreased pH, and a minor increase in the concentration of HCO_3^-.

To facilitate the clinical interpretation of acid-base status, clinicians use the terms *total buffer base, base excess,* and *base deficit.* Total buffer base is the sum of the concentrations of available blood buffers. *Base excess* and *base deficit* refer to an increase or decrease, respectively, in total buffer base. In acute respiratory acidosis, total buffer base does not change, because the accumulation of HCO_3^- is accompanied by an equivalent decrease in the concentration of other buffers such as Hb^-. Therefore, there is no base excess or base deficit.

The ideal way to correct respiratory acidosis is to restore alveolar ventilation. However, because the respiratory acidosis is caused by disease processes that impede ventilation, this option is not open to the animal, and other means to correct pH, primarily renal mechanisms, must be used. The elevated P_{CO_2} and decreased pH increase H^+ and NH_3 production in the kidney. This increases the elimination of H^+ in the urine and generates new HCO_3^-, and so the plasma concentration of HCO_3^- increases; the $[HCO_3^-/0.03 \cdot P_{CO_2}]$ ratio and pH are adjusted toward normal. The newly generated HCO_3^- adds to

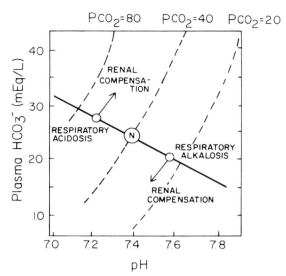

FIGURE 51–4. A pH-bicarbonate diagram showing the effects of respiratory acidosis and alkalosis on pH, bicarbonate (HCO_3^-) concentration, and P_{CO_2} of arterial blood. In acute respiratory acidosis, as P_{CO_2} increases the changes in pH and bicarbonate concentration are predicted by the normal buffer line. Renal compensation leads to an accumulation of bicarbonate, which increases the pH, whereas P_{CO_2} remains constant. In respiratory alkalosis, Pa_{CO_2} and bicarbonate decrease and pH increases. The kidneys compensate by increasing bicarbonate resorption, which decreases pH. N, normal arterial blood composition.

the total buffer base and therefore causes a base excess. Figure 51–4 shows how this accumulating HCO_3^- adjusts the pH toward normal during respiratory acidosis, even though P_{CO_2} remains constant.

Respiratory alkalosis is caused by the loss of carbon dioxide, which increases blood pH

Respiratory alkalosis is caused by *alveolar hyperventilation*, which results from stimulation of the chemoreceptors by hypoxia or from stimulation of intrapulmonary receptors by lung injury or inflammation. Overly vigorous use of a ventilator can cause hyperventilation in an anesthetized animal. Carbon dioxide is eliminated faster than it is produced by the tissues, and so blood P_{CO_2} decreases. The changes in blood chemistry are the inverse of those in respiratory acidosis:

$$H_2O + CO_2 \leftarrow H_2CO_3 \leftarrow H^+ + HCO_3^-$$
$$\uparrow$$
$$H^+ + Hb^- \leftarrow HHb.$$

As CO_2 is eliminated, H_2CO_3 is formed from H^+ and HCO_3^-, and so the pH increases and the concentration of HCO_3^- decreases. Hydrogen ion is supplied by release from nonbicarbonate buffers, such as hemoglobin. The net result of these processes is that Pa_{CO_2} decreases, the pH increases, and the concentration of HCO_3^- decreases and is replaced by other buffers. There is no change in total buffer base. The

increase in the [$HCO_3^-/0.03 \cdot P_{CO_2}$] ratio increases pH.

Figure 51–4 shows the increase in pH and decrease in the concentration of HCO_3^- as P_{CO_2} decreases. In order to adjust the pH toward normal, hyperventilation must be stopped, or the kidneys must eliminate HCO_3^-. The latter occurs because the low P_{CO_2} and alkalosis reduce H^+ and NH_3 production by the kidney. When H^+ is not produced in sufficient amounts to capture all the filtered HCO_3^-, the latter spills into the urine.

Metabolic acidosis is caused by the accumulation of fixed acids or the loss of buffer base, which decreases blood pH

Metabolic acidosis is the most common acid-base abnormality. During metabolism, there is a continuous production of fixed acids. An increase in their production, or failure of hydrogen ion elimination by the kidneys, is the cause of metabolic acidosis. Increased production of fixed acids occurs as a result of protein catabolism or ketone production during starvation or as a result of anaerobic metabolism that leads to lactic acidosis. *Diarrhea* can also cause metabolic acidosis, because excessive amounts of HCO_3^- (buffer) are lost in the feces. In ruminants, excessive feeding of carbohydrates can lead to increased hydrogen ion production in the rumen *(rumen acidosis)*. The hydrogen ions that are absorbed cause metabolic acidosis.

The accumulation of H^+ in the blood is combined with HCO_3^- and other buffers. The CO_2 produced by the combination of H^+ and HCO_3^- is lost through the lungs. The loss of buffer base gives rise to a base deficit, and the HCO_3^- depletion decreases the [$HCO_3^-/0.03 \cdot P_{CO_2}$] ratio; therefore, the pH decreases (Fig. 51–5).

The decrease in pH accompanying metabolic acidosis stimulates ventilation. This increase in alveolar ventilation has a compensatory effect on metabolic acidosis by eliminating CO_2, leading to a decreased P_{CO_2}, which ultimately adjusts the [$HCO_3^-/0.03 \times P_{CO_2}$] ratio and pH toward normal. This sequence is shown in Figure 51–5. As the P_{CO_2} decreases, the pH and HCO_3^- concentration decrease along a line that parallels the normal buffer line. Complete restoration of normal acid-base balance requires the restoration of the depleted base by the kidney or by therapy with intravenous fluid that contains buffers, such as bicarbonate.

Metabolic alkalosis is caused by the excessive elimination of hydrogen ions or by the intake of base, such as HCO_3^-, which increases blood pH

The most common cause of metabolic alkalosis is *vomiting*, during which gastric contents rich in hydrogen ion are lost from the body. In ruminants, torsion

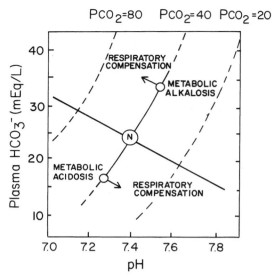

FIGURE 51–5. A pH-bicarbonate diagram showing the effects of metabolic acidosis and alkalosis on pH, bicarbonate concentration, and Pco_2 of arterial blood. In uncompensated metabolic acidosis, there is a decrease in the bicarbonate concentration, which leads to a decrease in pH, whereas Pco_2 remains constant. Respiratory compensation results in a decrease in Pco_2, with a subsequent increase in pH and movement of data points parallel to the normal buffer line. In metabolic alkalosis, the bicarbonate increases and causes an increase in pH. Respiratory compensation is by alveolar hypoventilation, which leads to an increase in $Paco_2$ and a return of pH toward normal. N, normal arterial blood composition.

and dilation of the *abomasum* cause metabolic alkalosis, because hydrogen ions are trapped in the abomasum. Low levels of potassium in the blood *(hypokalemia)* can also cause metabolic alkalosis. When extracellular fluid potassium levels are low, potassium moves from the intracellular to the extracellular fluid and is replaced in part by hydrogen ions that are lost from the plasma, resulting in alkalosis. In addition, hydrogen ions instead of potassium are lost into the urine.

The loss of hydrogen ion from the body frees buffer, and so the plasma concentration of HCO_3^- and total buffer base increase. The $[HCO_3^-/0.03 \cdot Pco_2]$ ratio, pH, and base excess all increase (see Fig. 51–5). The increase in pH reduces the drive to ventilate; alveolar ventilation decreases, and so Pco_2 increases. This adjusts the $[HCO_3^-/0.03 \cdot Pco_2]$ ratio toward normal, and hence the pH decreases toward normal (see Fig. 51–5).

Respiratory compensations for acid-base abnormalities occur rapidly; renal compensations occur over several hours

The discussion of acid-base disturbances has shown that the lungs compensate for metabolic problems, and the kidneys compensate for respiratory problems. Because the *chemoreceptors* respond almost immediately to changes in blood pH, and because changes in

ventilation rapidly change Pco_2, respiratory compensation for metabolic acid-base problems occurs almost immediately. For this reason, it is rare to observe "pure" metabolic acidosis or alkalosis without a respiratory compensation. The response of the kidneys to a respiratory acid-base disturbance is less rapid, and changes in NH_3 and HCO_3^- production occur over about 24 hours.

As compensatory mechanisms adjust the pH toward normal, there is less "error signal" to drive the compensation; thus, it is rare for these mechanisms alone to return the pH to normal. For example, in metabolic acidosis, the low pH drives ventilation to decrease Pco_2. However, as the pH returns to normal, the respiratory drive to compensate is reduced; therefore, restoration of normal pH is rarely complete.

Hydrogen and potassium ions are interrelated in acid-base homeostasis

As previously mentioned, the interrelationship between potassium and hydrogen is a factor in metabolic alkalosis. In this situation, a lack of intracellular potassium causes the movement of hydrogen ions into the cells, making the blood more alkaline. In the kidney, the lack of potassium for secretion is made up by hydrogen ions, and so the urine can be acidic when the blood is alkaline. This is, however, not the only example of potassium–hydrogen ion interaction. When there is an excess of hydrogen ion in the blood, such as occurs in metabolic acidosis, hydrogen ion replaces potassium in the cells. The potassium that spills from the cells into the extracellular space would cause life-threatening *hyperkalemia* if it were not lost through the kidneys. When the acidosis is subsequently corrected, hydrogen ion leaves the cells and must be replaced by potassium from the extracellular fluid. The intracellular potassium deficit is frequently much greater than the amount of potassium that can be supplied by the extracellular pool, so it may be necessary to supply potassium to prevent hypokalemia in the treatment of metabolic acidosis.

The diagnosis of acid-base disturbances depends on interpretation of measurements of arterial blood pH and Pco_2, from which the HCO_3^- concentration and total buffer base are calculated

Arterial samples must be used to determine the respiratory component of an acid-base abnormality, and samples must be obtained anaerobically to prevent the loss of CO_2 from the blood. The $Paco_2$ and pH are measured with specific electrodes in a blood-gas machine. The plasma concentration of HCO_3^- and total buffer base are determined from nomograms or, frequently, from a built-in program in the blood-gas analyzer.

When blood-gas data are analyzed, it is useful to ask the following questions:

1. Is the sample acidotic (pH < 7.4) or alkalotic (pH > 7.4)?
2. What is the respiratory component (is Pa_{CO_2} high, low, or normal), and will it explain the pH?
3. What is the metabolic component (is there a base excess or deficit), and will it explain the pH?
4. How can items 1, 2 and 3 be combined to explain the data, in view of the fact that compensations rarely return the pH toward normal?

Examples are provided in Table 51–1.

━ **Over the years, a large number of terms have been used to explain acid-base balance**

Some of the terms used to explain acid-base balance are as follows.

Anion gap: In the blood, the total cation concentration (the concentration of Na^+ + K^+ + Mg^{2+} + Ca^{2+}) should approximately equal the total anion concentration (the concentration of HCO_3^- + Cl^-). Usually, the total cations exceed the total anions; the difference is called the *anion gap*. This gap results from the presence of unaccounted-for anions from fixed acids, such as lactate. In metabolic acidosis, the anion gap increases because of increased production of fixed acids.

Standard bicarbonate: The plasma concentration of HCO_3^- when P_{CO_2} is equal to 40 mm Hg is known as *standard bicarbonate*. The plasma concentration of HCO_3^- can change as a result of respiratory and metabolic disturbances. An increase or decrease in the concentration of HCO_3^-, measured when P_{CO_2} is normal (i.e., 40 mm Hg), results only from metabolic disturbances.

Total carbon dioxide (T_{CO_2}): Carbon dioxide is present in the blood in solution and as carbamino compounds, but largely as HCO_3^-. T_{CO_2} can be measured by adding an acid to the blood and collecting the evolved CO_2, which comes primarily from HCO_3^-. Changes in T_{CO_2} should be interpreted as changes in the concentration of HCO_3^-.

CLINICAL CORRELATIONS

Upper airway obstruction in a Boston terrier (Fig. 51–6)

History A Boston terrier exhibits signs of severe respiratory distress. It has difficulty inhaling and makes a snoring sound during inhalation. The effort of walking magnifies the distress. An arterial blood sample reveals that Pa_{CO_2} is 80 mm Hg, pH is 7.3, HCO_3^- concentration is 39 mEq/L, and base excess equals 10 mEq/L.

Clinical examination Examination reveals excessively narrowed (stenotic) nares and excessive folds of tissue in the soft palate, the latter occluding the glottis. The larynx and trachea appear normal.

Treatment Reconstructive surgery is performed on the dog to enlarge the nares and remove the excessive tissues from the palate. Two weeks after surgery, respiratory distress is much less. Blood gas analysis reveals that Pa_{CO_2} is 45 mm Hg, pH is 7.39, HCO_3^- concentration is 27 mEq/L, and base excess is 2 mEq/L.

Comment Before surgery, the animal is acidotic with an elevated Pa_{CO_2} and base excess. Only the high Pa_{CO_2} explains the acidosis; therefore, the dog has respiratory acidosis. The increase in the concentration of HCO_3^- (normal, 24 mEq/L) is caused primarily by creation of new HCO_3^- (a base excess) by the kidneys and indicates the condition is of at least several days' duration. Respiratory acidosis is caused by alveolar hypoventilation resulting from the upper airway obstruction. Surgery corrects the obstruction and alleviates the hypoventilation. This returns the pH to a more normal value. Two weeks after surgery, the base excess has been virtually eliminated.

Torsion of the abomasum in a cow (see Fig. 51–6)

History A Holstein cow gave birth 2 weeks ago and became inappetent 2 days ago. Over the past 12 hours she has become lethargic, and her right flank is distended. Examination shows she is depressed and dehydrated. Her extremities are cold. Rectal examination reveals a large fluid-filled organ between the rumen and the right abdominal wall. A fluid sample obtained percutaneously from the distended organ is chloride-rich and very acidic. An arterial blood sample shows that Pa_{CO_2} is 50 mm Hg, pH is 7.6, HCO_3^- concentration is 50 mEq/L, and base excess is 24 mEq/L.

Comment The history and physical findings are typical

TABLE 51–1. **Examples of blood gas abnormalities**

pH	Pa_{CO_2}	HCO_3^-	Base excess	Base deficit	Diagnosis
7.4	40	24	0	0	Normal
7.26	60	27	0	0	Uncompensated respiratory acidosis
7.38	60	36	9	0	Partially compensated respiratory acidosis
7.2	40	15	0	12	Uncompensated metabolic acidosis
7.35	22	11	0	12	Partially compensated metabolic acidosis
7.45	20	13	0	11	Partially compensated respiratory alkalosis
7.55	40	34	11	0	Uncompensated metabolic alkalosis
7.2	50	19	0	9	Combined metabolic and respiratory acidosis
7.6	20	20	0	0	Uncompensated respiratory alkalosis
7.3	20	9	0	15	Partially compensated metabolic acidosis

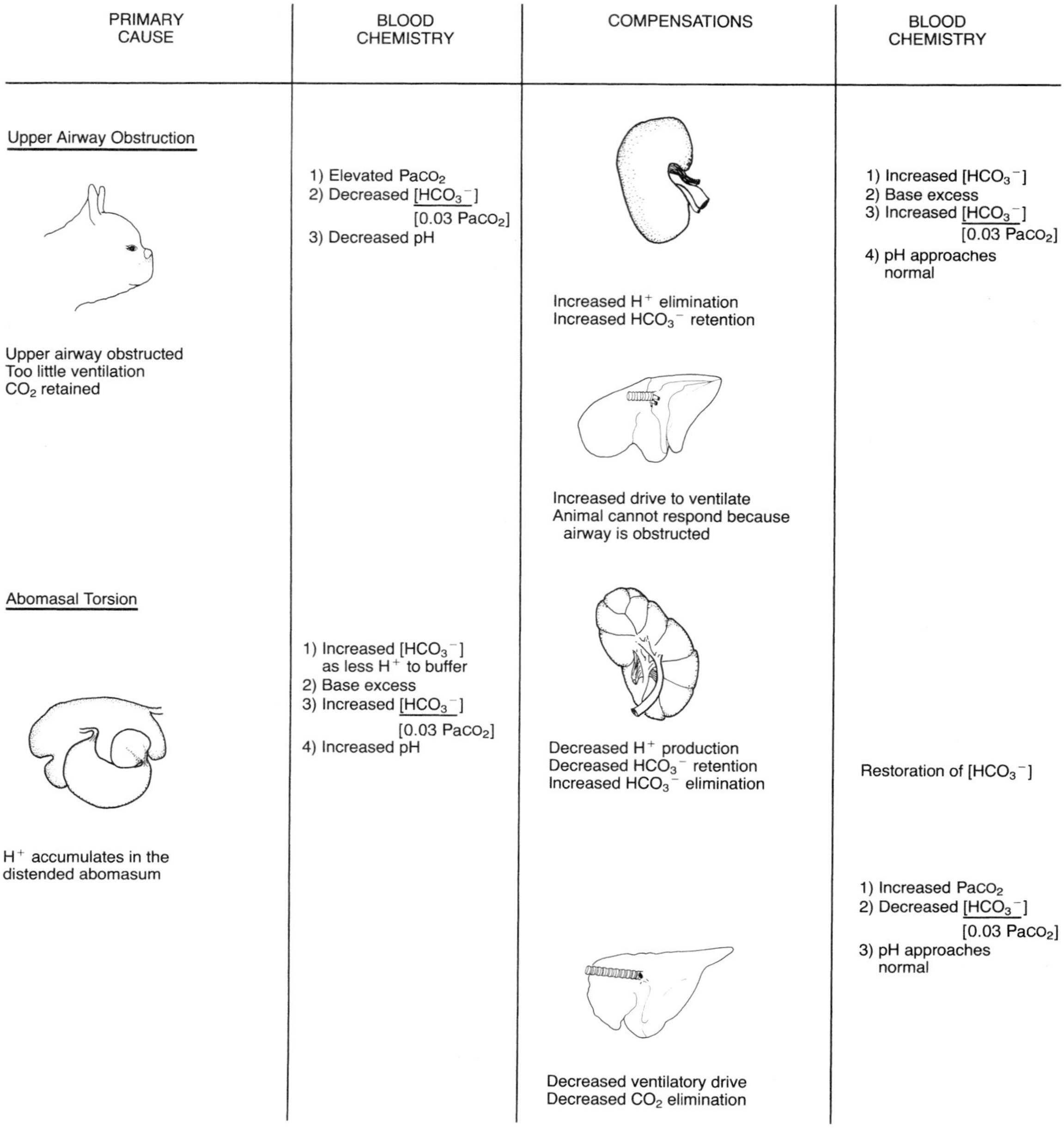

PRIMARY CAUSE	BLOOD CHEMISTRY	COMPENSATIONS	BLOOD CHEMISTRY
Upper Airway Obstruction	1) Elevated $Paco_2$ 2) Decreased $[HCO_3^-]$ $\qquad [0.03\ Paco_2]$ 3) Decreased pH	Increased H^+ elimination Increased HCO_3^- retention Increased drive to ventilate Animal cannot respond because airway is obstructed	1) Increased $[HCO_3^-]$ 2) Base excess 3) Increased $[HCO_3^-]$ $\qquad [0.03\ Paco_2]$ 4) pH approaches $\quad$ normal
Upper airway obstructed Too little ventilation CO_2 retained			
Abomasal Torsion	1) Increased $[HCO_3^-]$ $\quad$ as less H^+ to buffer 2) Base excess 3) Increased $[HCO_3^-]$ $\qquad [0.03\ Paco_2]$ 4) Increased pH	Decreased H^+ production Decreased HCO_3^- retention Increased HCO_3^- elimination Decreased ventilatory drive Decreased CO_2 elimination	Restoration of $[HCO_3^-]$ 1) Increased $Paco_2$ 2) Decreased $[HCO_3^-]$ $\qquad [0.03\ Paco_2]$ 3) pH approaches $\quad$ normal
H^+ accumulates in the distended abomasum			

FIGURE 51–6. *See legend on opposite page*

of a dilatation or torsion of the abomasum. This condition occasionally occurs shortly after parturition in dairy cows fed high levels of concentrates and chopped feeds. The abomasum distends and may rotate, so that its inlet and outlet are obstructed. Fluid rich in chloride and hydrogen ion continues to be secreted into and is trapped within the abomasum. The loss of hydrogen ion from the blood results in a base excess and causes the metabolic alkalosis. The alkalosis depresses ventilation, which elevates $Paco_2$. This is a compensation to restore pH toward normal.

Treatment The torsion on the abomasum must be surgically corrected. However, the metabolic alkalosis and any fluid deficits should be treated first in order to provide the best chance of recovery. The alkalosis is enhanced by loss of chloride ion into the abomasum along with hydrogen ion. Repletion of chloride ion allows the

kidneys to eliminate the excess bicarbonate and restores normal pH. In practicality, this is accomplished by treating the cow intravenously with large volumes of 0.9% sodium chloride solution.

Neonatal diarrhea in a foal
(see Fig. 51–6)

History A 2-week-old foal has profuse diarrhea. It is lethargic and cold to the touch, its eyes are sunken and dull, and it lies in a pool of feces. The foal's hematocrit is 65, pH is 7.2, $Paco_2$ is 30 mm Hg, HCO_3^- concentration is 12 mEq/L, and base deficit is 15 mEq/L.

Comment The foal shows typical clinical signs of severe dehydration as a result of excessive fluid loss in the feces. Fluid loss from the intravascular compartment re-

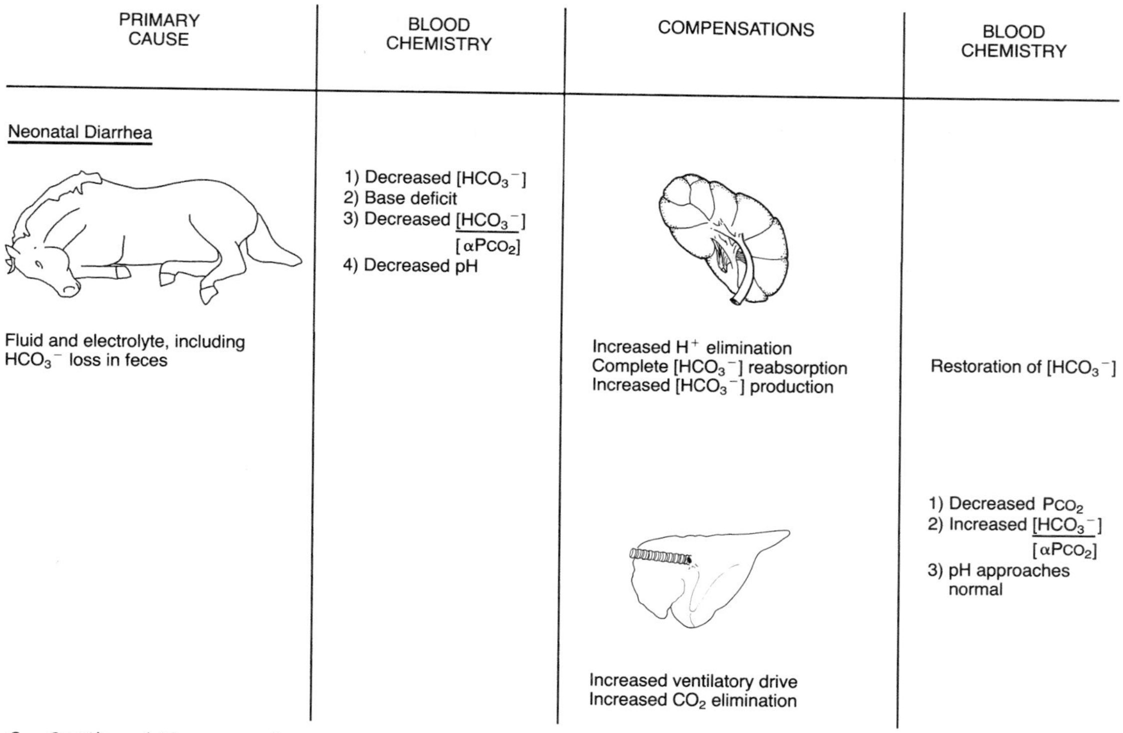

PRIMARY CAUSE	BLOOD CHEMISTRY	COMPENSATIONS	BLOOD CHEMISTRY
Neonatal Diarrhea Fluid and electrolyte, including HCO_3^- loss in feces	1) Decreased $[HCO_3^-]$ 2) Base deficit 3) Decreased $[HCO_3^-]$ $[\alpha P_{CO_2}]$ 4) Decreased pH	Increased H^+ elimination Complete $[HCO_3^-]$ reabsorption Increased $[HCO_3^-]$ production Increased ventilatory drive Increased CO_2 elimination	Restoration of $[HCO_3^-]$ 1) Decreased P_{CO_2} 2) Increased $[HCO_3^-]$ $[\alpha P_{CO_2}]$ 3) pH approaches normal

FIGURE 51–6. *Continued* Diagrammatic representation of the acid-base changes initiated by upper airway obstruction, abomasal torsion, and neonatal foal diarrhea.

duces blood volume and cardiac output. To maintain blood pressure, vasoconstriction occurs in the extremities, which therefore have less blood flow and become cold. The loss of fluid from the interstitial space causes the dryness of the eyes and muzzle, the sunken appearance of the eyes, and inelastic skin. The increased hematocrit of 65 (normal, 45) confirms the dehydration.

Feces contain HCO_3^-, and its excessive loss causes a base deficit and a decrease in pH. In addition, poor tissue perfusion results in lactic acidosis. The acidosis results from loss of buffer base and accumulation of lactic acid. It is a metabolic acidosis. The acidosis stimulates ventilation, which reduces Pa_{CO_2} in an attempt to correct pH.

Treatment This foal needs fluid replacement to increase plasma volume, raise cardiac output, and restore circulatory perfusion. The fluid should contain electrolytes, to replace those lost in diarrhea, and a source of buffer, such as bicarbonate. A good choice would be lactated Ringer's solution supplemented with additional bicarbonate. If the foal's respiratory and acid-base homeostasis can be maintained until the diarrhea ceases, it has a good chance of recovery.

Bibliography

Cohen JJ, Kassirer JP (eds): Acid-Base. Boston: Little, Brown, 1982, pp 3–94.
Davenport HW: The ABC of Acid-Base Chemistry, 6th ed. Chicago: University of Chicago Press, 1974.
Gamble JL: Acid-Base Physiology: A Direct Approach. Baltimore: Johns Hopkins University Press, 1982, pp 1–54.
Guyton AC, Hall JE: Regulation of acid-base balance. In *Textbook of Medical Physiology*, 9th ed. Philadelphia: WB Saunders, 1996, pp 385–403.
Stubbs DW: The physiology of acid-base balance. In Brown AM, Stubbs DW (eds): Medical Physiology. New York: Wiley, 1983, pp 567–597.

PRACTICE QUESTIONS

1. Elevated Pa_{CO_2}, low pH, and no base excess or deficit are characteristic of
   a. acute respiratory acidosis.
   b. acute respiratory alkalosis.
   c. metabolic acidosis.
   d. metabolic alkalosis.
   e. none of the above.

2. Elevated Pa_{CO_2}, alkaline pH, and base excess are characteristic of
   a. chronic respiratory acidosis.
   b. chronic respiratory alkalosis.
   c. metabolic acidosis.
   d. metabolic alkalosis.
   e. none of the above.

3. Low Pa_{CO_2}, acid pH, and base deficit are characteristic of
   a. chronic respiratory acidosis.
   b. acute respiratory alkalosis.
   c. metabolic acidosis.
   d. metabolic alkalosis.
   e. none of the above.

4. The most likely acid-base disturbance to be found in a dog at the top of Mount McKinley (Denali) in Alaska (height, 20,320 feet, or 6353 m) is

a. respiratory acidosis.
b. respiratory alkalosis.
c. metabolic acidosis.
d. metabolic alkalosis.
e. none of the above.

5. The distal tubule of the kidney affects acid-base balance by
a. altering the pK of the HCO_3^--H_2CO_3 buffer.
b. concentrating carbon dioxide in the renal tubular cell.
c. generating new HCO_3^-.
d. producing ammonia to buffer H^+.
e. both c and d.

6. Which of the following buffers will be most effective in blood (pH = 7.4)?
a. HX/X^-, pK = 4.2, plentiful.
b. HY/Y^-, pK = 7.2, scarce.
c. HZ/Z^-, pK = 9.6, scarce.
d. HW/W^-, pK = 7.6, plentiful.
e. HA/A^-, pK = 10.2, plentiful.

PRACTICE ANSWERS

1. a   2. d   3. c   4. b   5. e   6. d

52

Thermoregulation

1 Temperature is a major factor affecting tissue function

2 Homeotherms and poikilotherms use different strategies to regulate body temperature

3 Body temperature depends on the balance between heat input and output

Heat exchange with the environment

1 Heat loss by convection occurs when air or water is warmed by the body

2 Heat loss by conduction occurs when the body is in contact with a cooler surface

3 Heat loss by emission of infrared radiation and its absorption by cooler objects can be significant

4 Heat loss by evaporation occurs when the water in sweat, saliva, and respiratory secretions is converted into water vapor

Heat production

1 Heat is a byproduct of all metabolic processes

2 Shivering produces heat by muscle contraction

3 Nonshivering thermogenesis is an increase in basal metabolic rate, caused especially by the oxidation of fats, to produce heat

Heat transfer in the body

1 Because tissues are poor conductors, heat is most effectively transferred in the blood

2 Countercurrent heat exchange conserves body heat

Temperature regulation

1 Mammals and birds normally regulate the input and output of heat to maintain body temperature within a narrow limit

2 Temperature-sensitive receptors are located in the central nervous system, in the skin, and in some internal organs

3 Information from central and peripheral heat-sensitive neurons is integrated in the hypothalamus to regulate heat-losing or heat-conserving mechanisms

Integrated responses

1 The responses to heat stress are peripheral vasodilation and increased evaporative cooling

2 The responses to cold stress are peripheral vasoconstriction, piloerection, and increased metabolic heat production by shivering and nonshivering thermogenesis

3 Fever is an elevation of body temperature that results from an increase in the thermoregulatory set-point

Heat stroke, hypothermia, and frostbite

1 Heat stroke occurs when heat production or input exceeds heat output, so body temperature rises to dangerous levels

2 Hypothermia occurs when heat output exceeds heat production, so body temperature decreases to dangerous levels

3 Frostbite occurs when ice crystals form in the tissues of the extremities

Temperature is a major factor affecting tissue function

Because body function is the result of chemical and physical processes that are sensitive to changes in temperature, animals use a variety of strategies to regulate the temperature of their tissues. If *body temperature* is allowed to decrease too far, metabolic processes are slowed to such an extent that body function ceases. Conversely, an increase in temperature beyond the normal value of about 38°C to 45°C can denature proteins and also be fatal.

Homeotherms and poikilotherms use different strategies to regulate body temperature

Fish, reptiles, and amphibians are called *cold-blooded animals*, or *poikilotherms*, because their body temperature varies with the temperature of the environment. However, this does not mean that these animals have no control over their body temperature. They use behavioral methods to prevent major changes in their temperature. For example, the lizard basks on a sun-baked rock to increase its temperature early in the morning and hides beneath the rock later in the day to prevent overheating. Veterinarians are sometimes asked to advise on the management of captive poikilotherms; it is important to remind owners to provide supplemental heat if they want their animals to be active at the cooler times of the year.

Mammals and birds are *homeotherms*; they maintain a constant body temperature in the presence of considerable changes in environmental temperature. Although the maintenance of a constant temperature allows mammals to live in a wide variety of environments and to remain active during the cold times of the year, it is not without cost. Homeotherms must maintain a high metabolic rate just to provide the heat necessary to maintain body temperature. This requires a high energy intake and, therefore, almost constant foraging for food. Poikilotherms require much less energy and are better able to survive times of food shortage. Because most veterinarians are primarily concerned with mammals and birds, this chapter focuses on the maintenance of a normal body temperature by homeotherms.

Body temperature depends on the balance between heat input and output

Heat inputs to the body are from metabolism and from external sources (Fig. 52–1). Once food energy is ingested, heat is produced at all stages of the metabolic process. Eventually, all food energy is converted into heat, which is dissipated into the environment and radiated into space. Some of the conversion of food energy into heat occurs during metabolism, and some occurs when external work is performed. When the running horse pulls a cart, the leg muscles work to overcome the effects of gravity and to oppose the friction in the muscles and joints and in the cart wheels. The heat produced in this process must be dissipated to the environment if body temperature is to remain constant.

Animals gain heat from the environment when ambient temperature exceeds body temperature and when they are exposed to *radiant heat* sources. The latter occurs when an animal is exposed to sunlight or is placed close to solid objects that are warmer than its body temperature.

Heat is lost to the environment by *radiation* from the body surface to a cooler object; by *convection* as the surrounding air or water is warmed by the body; by *evaporation* of respiratory secretions, sweat, or saliva; and by *conduction* to cooler surfaces with which the animal is in contact. A small amount of heat is also lost with urine and feces.

Many of the metabolic heat sources, such as the liver, heart, and limb muscles, are remote from the skin, which is the site of heat loss. Therefore, it is necessary to transfer heat among these sites. Body tissues are poor conductors, and so heat is transferred mainly by convection in the circulation.

HEAT EXCHANGE WITH THE ENVIRONMENT

Heat loss by convection occurs when air or water is warmed by the body

When the air or water in contact with the skin is heated, it flows away, thereby exposing the skin to cooler fluids. Because it takes more heat to warm water than it does to warm an equivalent mass of air, water-dwelling animals lose more heat by convection than do terrestrial mammals. The amount of heat lost by convection depends on the *thermal gradient* (temperature difference) between the skin of the animal and the fluid overlying the skin; a bigger thermal gradient results in more heat loss. In *natural convection*, the warmed air or water rises from the surface of the animal, because it is less dense than the cooler fluid. In *forced convection*, cooler fluid is moved over the skin surface by a breeze or current or simply because the limbs and animal are moving. Forced convection is more effective than natural convection as a mode of heat loss because the thermal gradient is maintained by the constant renewal of the cooler air or water that blankets the surface of the skin. Young or small animals left in a cool draft can quickly lose a lot of body heat by convection and should be protected from such situations.

The thermal gradient for heat loss can be altered by changes in skin blood flow and the amount of *insulation* separating the animal from the environment. Increasing blood flow to the skin raises skin temperature and, therefore, heat loss, whereas a reduction in skin blood flow reduces heat loss. Hair traps air and impairs convection. The thickness of the

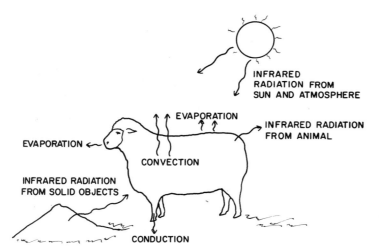

FIGURE 52–1. Diagrammatic representation of the heat input and output between a mammal and the environment.

INFRARED RADIATION FROM SUN AND ATMOSPHERE

EVAPORATION

INFRARED RADIATION FROM ANIMAL

EVAPORATION

CONVECTION

INFRARED RADIATION FROM SOLID OBJECTS

CONDUCTION

layer of hair can be altered by *piloerection* (making the hair stand up) and by growing a thicker hair coat in preparation for winter. The thick layer of blubber in sea mammals also provides a layer of insulation. Reducing exposed body surface area by curling up in a ball or by huddling with other animals also reduces convective heat loss.

Heat loss by conduction occurs when the body is in contact with a cooler surface

Because animals usually do not lie on cool surfaces for long periods, conduction is not usually a major form of heat loss. There are, however, some situations in which conductive heat loss can lead to hypothermia. A cold stainless steel surgery table can form a heat sink for a small anesthetized bird or mammal. Insulation or a heat source should be provided for such animals. Similarly, newborn piglets can lose a lot of heat by lying on a cold concrete floor. Adult pigs cool themselves by conduction when they wallow in cool mud puddles.

Heat loss by emission of infrared radiation and its absorption by cooler objects can be significant

All solid objects emit invisible *electromagnetic radiation* in the *infrared* range. Warm objects emit on a shorter *wavelength* and more emissions per unit time than do cool objects. When these emissions strike another object, some are absorbed and thus transfer heat. Although all objects emit radiant heat, the net heat transfer is from warm to cool objects. It is important to realize that radiant heat loss can occur even when the animal is surrounded by a thermally neutral or warm environment. Heat can be lost from an animal to the uninsulated walls of a building even though the intervening air is warm.

Heat loss by evaporation occurs when the water in sweat, saliva, and respiratory secretions is converted into water vapor

The evaporation of 1 L of water into water vapor requires 580 kilocalories (kcal) of work. If the body provides this heat, evaporation can be a major form of heat loss. Evaporative heat loss occurs continuously by the diffusion of water through the skin and by loss of water vapor from the respiratory tract. This water loss is obligatory, but under thermal stress, evaporative cooling can increase greatly, because *sweat glands* are activated or the animal begins to *pant*. Evaporative heat loss becomes increasingly important

as the ambient temperature approaches body temperature; it is the only form of heat loss available once ambient temperature exceeds body temperature. The effectiveness of evaporation is reduced as the *relative humidity* increases—that is, as the air becomes more saturated with water vapor.

Sweating occurs from two types of coiled, tubular *sweat glands* located in the dermis. *Apocrine* glands produce a protein-containing secretion, whereas *eccrine* glands produce an aqueous secretion. All placental mammals except rodents and lagomorphs have sweat glands, but in the dog and pig they are poorly developed and of little use in thermoregulation. The thermoregulatory sweat from hoofed animals is produced by the apocrine glands, whereas in primates, sweat is produced by the eccrine glands. Secreted sweat has an ionic composition similar to that of plasma. As it passes to the skin surface along the duct, its composition is altered by the reabsorption of ions. If secretion rates are low, almost all the sodium and chloride, along with water, is absorbed. Therefore, the sweat reaching the skin is a concentrated solution of urea, lactic acid, potassium ions, and, in the case of hoofed mammals, protein. When secretion rates are high, less sodium and chloride are absorbed, more water is lost, and the other constituents are consequently diluted. In hot environments, acclimatization increases the sweating rates, and, because of increased secretion of *aldosterone,* most of the sodium and chloride is reabsorbed before the sweat reaches the skin.

In most species, sweating is under the control of *sympathetic cholinergic* nerve fibers, but in the horse, control seems to be through *sympathetic adrenergic* fibers. Apocrine glands also are stimulated to secrete by an increase in levels of circulating *catecholamines.*

Panting is one mode of increasing evaporation from the respiratory tract. Small tidal volumes are moved at rapid frequency (200 breaths per minute) over the respiratory dead-space. The rate of panting is close to the resonant frequency of the respiratory system, and so the work of breathing is minimized and does not add to the heat load. In the panting animal, two mechanisms act to elevate heat loss through evaporation: (1) vascular engorgement of the respiratory and oral mucosa and (2) increased salivation. By ventilating primarily dead-space, severe hyperventilation and respiratory alkalosis are avoided. In birds, *gular flutter* is another method of increasing air flow over the respiratory dead-space. Even in mammals that do not pant, such as the horse, evaporative heat loss from the respiratory tract probably increases during prolonged exercise, because dead-space ventilation increases.

Mammals vary in the relative importance of different modes of evaporative heat loss. In horses and cattle, sweating is the major form of evaporative heat loss. Sheep sweat, but panting is also of considerable importance. The dog relies almost totally on panting. Even small rodents, which neither pant nor sweat, increase evaporative heat loss by smearing saliva or water on their fur.

TABLE 52–1. Amount of heat produced by metabolism of major food types

Food Types	Heat Production (kcal/g)		
	PER GRAM OF FOOD	PER LITER OF O₂ CONSUMED	PER LITER OF CO₂ PRODUCED
Carbohydrates	4.1	5.05	5.05
Fat	9.6	4.75	6.67
Proteins (to urea)	4.2	4.46	5.57

HEAT PRODUCTION

Heat is a byproduct of all metabolic processes

Table 52–1 shows the amount of heat produced by the metabolism of carbohydrates, fats, and proteins. The *basal metabolic rate* is the rate of energy metabolism measured under minimal stress while the animal is fasting. Basal metabolic rate is greater in homeotherms than in poikilotherms, because homeotherms need to generate heat to maintain body temperature. The metabolic rate per kilogram of body weight is greater in smaller than in larger mammals (Fig. 52–2). This is in part necessitated by the greater surface/volume ratio of smaller animals. The relatively greater surface area per kilogram of body weight of small animals provides a bigger area for heat loss.

An increase in metabolic rate—as occurs, for example, during exercise—results in increased heat production and therefore necessitates increased heat loss from the animal. In addition to exercise, an increase in body temperature also elevates the metabolic rate.

Shivering produces heat by muscle contraction

Shivering is one method of increasing the metabolic production of heat. Antagonistic groups of limb mus-

cles are activated so that they produce no useful work. The chemical energy used in shivering is transferred to the body core as heat.

Nonshivering thermogenesis is an increase in basal metabolic rate, caused especially by the oxidation of fats, to produce heat

When animals are chronically exposed to cold, they develop the ability to increase metabolic heat production without shivering (nonshivering thermogenesis). This increase in metabolism is mediated through an increase in thyroxine secretion and the calorigenic effects of catecholamines on lipids. Brown fat is a specialized vascular, mitochondria-rich fat found between the scapulae of newborn small mammals. Catecholamines increase metabolism in all fats, but particularly in brown fat, and the heat produced is distributed around the body via the blood stream.

HEAT TRANSFER IN THE BODY

Because tissues are poor conductors, heat is most effectively transferred in the blood

Because heat is produced primarily in muscles of the limbs and in the liver and is eliminated through the skin and in the respiratory tract, it is necessary to distribute heat around the body. Tissues have a *thermal conductivity* similar to that of cork; therefore, conduction is not an efficient means of heat redistribution.

The blood perfusing a metabolically active organ collects heat and transfers it to cooler parts of the body. Redistribution of blood flow can deliver heat preferentially to certain body regions or can allow regions to cool when the maintenance of the temperature of the brain and major viscera (*core temperature*) is threatened. First, the *arterioles* of skin vascular beds dilate, which results in increased capillary blood flow. Second, *arteriovenous anastomoses* open in the limbs, ears, and muzzles. These two actions greatly increase the total blood flow to the periphery, and the increased heat delivery warms the peripheral tissues toward the core temperature. Conversely, under cold stress, skin vascular beds vasoconstrict and arteriovenous anastomoses close, so that skin and limb temperatures decrease. This results in reduced heat loss from

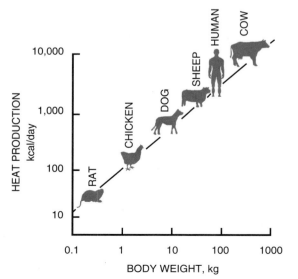

FIGURE 52–2. The relationship between body weight and heat production.

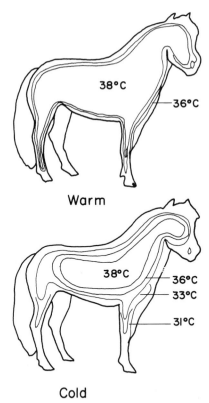

38°C

36°C

Warm

38°C

36°C
33°C

31°C

Cold

FIGURE 52–3. Diagrammatic representation of the distribution of temperatures in a pony under warm and cold environmental conditions. Under warm conditions, the core body temperature extends into the limbs and close to the skin surface of the animal. Under cold conditions, vasoconstriction in the peripheral blood vessels results in a gradient of temperatures between the core and the extremities. The core temperature is maintained only in the abdomen, thorax, and brain of the animal. The more peripheral tissues are allowed to cool considerably.

the skin and in a gradient of temperatures along the limb (Fig. 52–3). Under severe cold stress, the skin temperature of the extremities can approach ambient temperature. Interestingly, the lipids in the limb extremities have a lower melting point than those in the core, and so fats do not solidify in extreme cold stress.

Countercurrent heat exchange conserves body heat

When the environmental temperature is high, the blood perfusing the skin vascular beds returns to the core through superficial veins from which heat is lost to the skin and air. Under cold conditions, limb blood flow returns to the core through deep veins that accompany arteries (Fig. 52–4). Heat is transferred by countercurrent exchange from the warm arterial blood to the cooler venous blood and thereby returned to the core of the body.

A similar countercurrent exchange of heat occurs in a *carotid rete* in sheep and some other ungulates. In this system, the carotid artery forms a rete bathed in a sinus of venous blood that has drained the nasal

cavity. The colder venous blood from the nose cools the arterial blood supplying the brain and protects the temperature of the brain. This mechanism becomes important during exercise, when the increase in ventilation aids in cooling the blood that drains from the nose. As a result, the arterial blood carrying heat from the exercising muscles is cooled before it enters the brain.

Some mammals, including humans and horses, do not possess a carotid rete and must rely on other thermoregulatory mechanisms to cool their brains during exercise. In the case of the horse, the *guttural pouches* may serve as such a mechanism. The guttural pouches contain air that is cooler than the arterial blood carried in the internal carotid artery. Because, anatomically, these guttural pouches surround the internal carotid arteries, heat is transferred from the blood being carried to the brain to the guttural pouches, thus protecting the brain from hyperthermia (Fig. 52–5). In addition, the *intracranial cavernous venous sinuses* may also act in the cooling of the horse's brain during exercise. This mechanism is thought to function in the same manner as the carotid rete but is believed to be less efficient.

TEMPERATURE REGULATION

Mammals and birds normally regulate the input and output of heat to maintain body temperature within a narrow limit

It is customary to measure body temperature as a first part of the clinical examination of mammals. This is because body temperature is maintained within fairly narrow limits despite large variations in ambient conditions. In diseased animals, the ability to regulate temperature can be impaired by, for example, dehydration. In addition, infectious and other agents produce pyrogens that can increase body temperature. Table 52–2 lists the normal ranges of *rectal temperatures* in some common domestic mammals. The rectal temperature is somewhat lower than the core temperature of the animal, and changes in rectal temperature lag behind changes in core temperature. However, rectal temperature is a convenient measure

TABLE 52–2. Rectal temperature (in °C) of domestic mammals

Species	Average	Range
Cat	38.6	38.1–39.2
Cattle (beef)	38.3	36.7–39.1
Cattle (dairy)	38.6	38.0–39.3
Dog	38.9	37.9–39.9
Donkey	37.4	36.4–38.4
Goat	39.1	38.5–39.7
Horse	37.7	37.2–38.2
Pig	39.2	38.7–39.8
Sheep	39.1	38.5–39.9

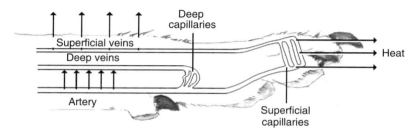

FIGURE 52–4. Diagrammatic representation of a limb showing the arterial supply and venous drainage by deep and superficial veins. Under warm conditions, blood perfuses the more superficial capillary beds and heat is lost to the environment through the skin. Blood returns from these superficial vascular beds through the superficial veins, and this provides an additional source of heat loss. Under cold conditions, peripheral vasoconstriction occurs, and the blood flow to the limb is directed to the deeper vascular beds and returns to the trunk through the deep veins. Countercurrent heat exchange between the arteries and veins conserves body heat.

in domestic mammals and provides a useful indication of core temperature.

In well-hydrated animals living in temperate climates, the range of normal temperature is quite narrow. Mammals living in hot, arid climates tolerate a wider range of temperature, allowing body temperature to decrease during the cool nights, so that more heat can be absorbed during the ensuing hot day.

In order to maintain temperature within narrow limits, the animal must regulate its heat inputs and outputs. The inputs and outputs clearly cannot be equal at all times. During exercise, for example, heat production exceeds heat loss. Heat is stored in the body and then dissipated when exercise ceases. The specific heat of body tissues is similar to that of water; therefore, large amounts of heat can be stored without a potentially lethal increase in temperature.

Temperature-sensitive receptors are located in the central nervous system, in the skin, and in some internal organs

To regulate body temperature, the animal has a variety of *temperature sensors* at various locations within the body. These sensors relay information to the brain, which then initiates mechanisms to either increase or decrease heat loss or production.

Numerous heat-sensitive neurons are located in the preoptic area of the hypothalamus. These neurons increase their firing rate in response to minor increases in local temperature. In addition, experimentally warming this area immediately initiates heat-losing mechanisms, such as peripheral vasodilation and sweating. These observations suggest that this region of the brain may be the main center for temperature regulation. Other hypothalamic and midbrain neurons decrease their firing in response to heat, and still others increase firing in response to cold. All of these temperature-sensitive neurons are monitoring brain or core temperature.

When an animal is exposed to cold, there can be considerable heat loss before a change in core temperature occurs. Therefore, it is advantageous to have temperature-sensitive neurons located in the skin, so that environmental temperature changes are detected before they threaten core temperature. The most numerous temperature-sensitive neurons in the skin respond to cold, so chilling of the skin can initiate heat conservation before the core temperature decreases.

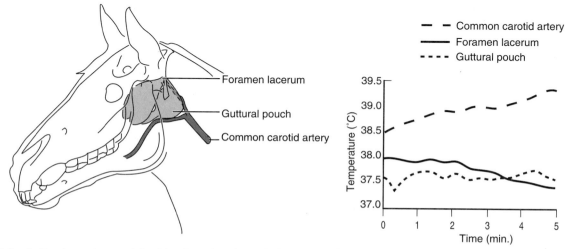

FIGURE 52–5. Guttural pouches cool the blood passing through the internal carotid artery on its way to the brain. *Left,* The anatomic arrangement of the guttural pouches and internal carotid arteries (ICA) in the skull and the position of the temperature probes used to measure blood temperature. *Right,* Graph of blood and guttural pouch temperatures during a period of cantering. Note that even though the temperature of blood entering the guttural pouch in the common carotid artery increases with the duration of exercise, temperature at the foramen lacerum (where the artery enters the cranium) decreases slightly.

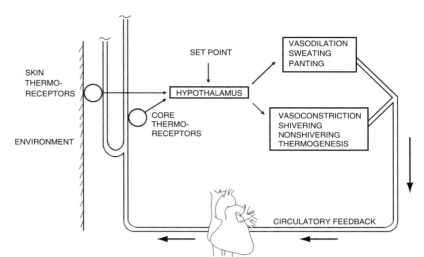

FIGURE 52–6. Feedback control mechanisms for the regulation of body temperature. Temperature receptors in the skin and the core relay information to the hypothalamus, which adjusts the responses to either conserve and produce or to lose heat. The results of these responses are relayed to the receptors through the circulatory feedback.

Skin cold receptors are particularly sensitive to the rate of decrease in temperature. For this reason, shivering can occur after exercise as the skin is rapidly cooled by sweat evaporation, despite the fact that the core temperature may be normal or slightly elevated. Skin receptors sensitive to heat also exist and can initiate heat loss when the skin temperature rises.

Temperature-sensitive neurons also exist at various locations in the viscera. Drinking large volumes of cold fluids may stimulate cold receptors in the gastrointestinal system, so that body heat-conserving mechanisms are initiated.

Information from central and peripheral heat-sensitive neurons is integrated in the hypothalamus to regulate heat-losing or heat-conserving mechanisms

Figure 52–6 shows the *feedback control* mechanisms for the regulation of body temperature. Central integration of the information from various receptors occurs in the anterior hypothalamus. Information from central temperature receptors seems to predominate over information from skin and visceral receptors, and so a rise in core temperature of only 0.5°C causes a sevenfold increase in the amount of skin blood flow; a modest decrease in core temperature initiates vasoconstriction and shivering. The effect of central receptors is about 20-fold greater than the effect of peripheral receptors.

In the regulation of body temperature, the hypothalamus behaves as if it has a normal *set-point*. When the core temperature rises above the set-point, heat-losing mechanisms are initiated; when temperature decreases, heat conservation or production begins. This thermoregulatory set-point is believed to be determined by the firing frequency of two groups of neurons located in the hypothalamus: *warm-sensitive neurons* and *temperature-insensitive neurons*. When an animal's body temperature increases, the warm-sensi-

tive neurons fire more frequently, which leads to heat loss by thermoregulatory reactions such as sweating. However, temperature-insensitive neurons do not respond to an increase in body temperature, and thus they maintain a consistent firing rate. The thermoregulatory set-point occurs when the firing rates of these two groups of neurons overlap (Fig. 52–7). Information from peripheral receptors modifies the set-point, and so shivering begins at a higher core temperature when the skin is cool than when the skin is warm. Similarly, sweating is initiated at a higher core temperature when the skin is cool than when the skin is warm.

INTEGRATED RESPONSES

The responses to heat stress are peripheral vasodilation and increased evaporative cooling

For all mammals and birds, there exists an environmental temperature at which body temperature can

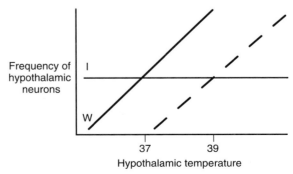

FIGURE 52–7. Graphic representation of the overlap between firing rates of temperature insensitive neurons (I) and warm-sensitive neurons (W). The point of intersection is the hypothalamic set-point. In the presence of pyrogens (broken line), firing of warm sensitive neurons is suppressed, and the intersection of firing rates between the two sets of neurons occurs at a higher temperature, the new set-point.

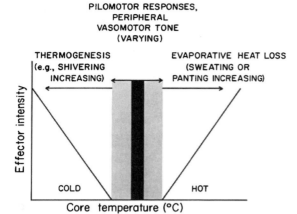

FIGURE 52-8. Relationship between the intensity of thermoregulatory responses and core temperature. The set-point for temperature regulation is indicated by the black shaded zone. On either side of this set-point there exists a zone in which temperature can be maintained by vasomotor responses (gray areas). As the core temperature deviates more dramatically from the set-point, there is a need either to increase thermogenesis during cold stress or to increase evaporative heat loss during heat stress. (Modified with permission from Bligh J: Temperature regulation in environmental physiology of animals. In Bligh J, Cloudsley-Thompson JL, MacDonald AG [eds]: Environmental Physiology of Animals. Oxford, United Kingdom: Blackwell Scientific, 1976, p 426.)

be maintained in a normal range primarily by vasomotor mechanisms (Fig. 52–8). This *zone of thermoneutrality* varies with the metabolic rate and the amount of insulation. The pig, which lacks fur, clearly has a higher thermoneutral temperature than does the sheep, which has thick wool. Dairy cattle that have high milk production produce so much metabolic heat that their thermoneutral zone is surprisingly low: 4°C to 15°C (40°F to 60°F). In the thermoneutral zone, body temperature can be regulated by vasomotor mechanisms that increase or decrease skin blood flow and therefore change the amount of heat loss by convection and radiation.

When a homeotherm is exposed to heat stress, the initial response is vasodilation, which increases skin and limb blood flow. The resulting increase in skin temperature and the extension of core temperature down the limbs increase the temperature gradient between the skin and the environment, resulting in more heat loss by radiation and convection (see Fig. 52–3).

If vasodilation alone is ineffective in maintaining a normal temperature, evaporative cooling is increased by sweating, panting, or both. Evaporative cooling is the only method of heat loss available once the environmental temperature exceeds the skin temperature and is most effective when relative humidity is low. Figure 52–9 shows that at −10°C (14°F) cows lose about 10% of their heat by evaporation, but as the ambient temperature rises to 30°C (90°F), they lose 80% by evaporation. As relative humidity rises, animals have increasing difficulty losing heat; therefore, exercise in hot humid conditions is likely to cause heat exhaustion. This was a major concern for

horses competing in the 1996 Olympics in Athens, Georgia, where the high July temperatures were combined with high humidity.

Animals also use behavioral methods to resist heat stress. These methods, which include seeking shade, standing in water, or wallowing in mud, are not available to intensively managed livestock. The producer must assume increased responsibility for the animals' comfort and survival. Because high-producing dairy cattle have such a low thermoneutral temperature, their primary requirement is shade in hot climates, which is more of a concern than is a source of heat or insulation in cold climates.

The responses to cold stress are peripheral vasoconstriction, piloerection, and increased metabolic heat production by shivering and nonshivering thermogenesis

As the ambient temperature decreases, homeotherms initially conserve heat by peripheral vasoconstriction. This sets up a temperature gradient along the limbs and reduces skin temperature, so that there is only a narrow temperature gradient for radiation and convective heat loss (see Fig. 52–3). Piloerection provides insulation and also decreases heat loss. Further cold stress initiates increases in metabolic heat production by shivering or nonshivering thermogenesis. All adult mammals can shiver, and neonates born in an advanced state of development, such as lambs and foals, can also shiver. Puppies and other less-developed neonates cannot shiver and rely on the warmth of mother and the nest to protect them from cooling. *Brown fat* is present in some of the latter neonates and in other small mammals and provides a source of nonshivering thermogenesis.

Chronic exposure of animals to cold results in increased secretion of *thyroxine* and an increase in basal metabolism, which increases basal heat production. When animals are housed where they receive natural light, the thickness of the hair coat increases at cold times of the year. Hair growth is the result of decreasing daylight as cold weather approaches.

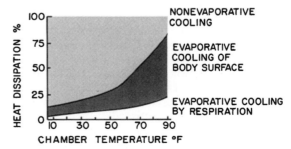

FIGURE 52-9. Methods of heat loss used by a cow as the environmental temperature increases. At low temperatures, the majority of heat loss is by nonevaporative cooling (gray shading), but as the environmental temperature increases, the cow becomes increasingly dependent on evaporation (black shading).

Fever is an elevation of body temperature that results from an increase in the thermoregulatory set-point

Fever, also known as *pyrexia*, occurs in response to the elevation of an animal's thermoregulatory set-point and most commonly occurs with the onset of infectious and other diseases. The phenomenon known as fever is believed to be an evolutionary adaptation to fight off infection and can be induced in some of the oldest species, such as reptiles and amphibians. Studies indicate that during infection, an increase in body temperature enhances leukocyte activity. This results in a decrease in animal morbidity and mortality from infections.

Throughout this chapter, the various ways in which an animal's body maintains a temperature within its normal range have been discussed. As previously mentioned, to maintain this normal range, the hypothalamus acts as if it has a thermal set-point. To raise this thermoregulatory set-point, and thus induce fever, a number of steps must occur. Initially, potent substances known as *pyrogens* begin the cascade that leads to fever. There are two categories of pyrogens: exogenous and endogenous. Exogenous pyrogens, such as toxins and the lipopolysaccharide complex in gram-negative bacteria, originate outside of the body; endogenous pyrogens, such as interleukin-1 (IL-1) (considered to be the most important pyrogen), tumor necrosis factor (TNF), interleukin-6 (IL-6), interferon (IFN), and platelet-activating factor, originate inside of the body. In addition, prostaglandins (PG), products of the arachidonic acid cascade, are produced by endothelial cells and are known to be major participants in the pathogenesis of fever. Exogenous pyrogens enter the body and induce endothelial cells, macrophages, lymphocytes, and various other cells of the immune system to release endogenous pyrogens and prostaglandins, notably prostaglandin E_2 (PGE$_2$), into the blood stream. When the endogenous pyrogens IL-1 and TNF, in addition to other cytokines, monokines, and lymphokines, are released, they act to signal additional cells to respond (Fig. 52–10). The endogenous pyrogens then travel to areas of the hypothalamus called the *organa vasculosum of the lamina terminalis* (OVLT). These areas of the hypothalamus are near large numbers of neurons and are highly vascularized. Also, the blood-brain barrier is almost nonexistent in the OVLT, and so endogenous pyrogens and PGs enter the brain easily from the blood stream. Once in the hypothalamus, the endogenous pyrogens act on the endothelial cells to produce additional PGE$_2$ and other arachidonic metabolites. Finally, these substances inhibit the warm-sensitive neurons, causing their firing rate to decrease and, consequently, the set-point to rise (see Fig. 52–7).

When the set-point increases, the animal initiates responses to conserve and produce heat until the body temperature reaches the new set-point (Fig. 52–11). Shivering, peripheral vasoconstriction, piloerection, and huddling behavior are all characteristic of the onset of fever. Once the new set-point is reached, the animal maintains its body at the new temperature until the pyrogen is metabolized and production ceases. When this occurs, the set-point decreases back to normal, and the animal initiates heat-losing mechanisms to decrease body temperature. Because the local production of PGE$_2$ in the hypothalamus is involved in increasing the set-point, cyclooxygenase-blocking drugs, such as aspirin, flunixin, or ibuprofen, are used to treat fever. These antipyretic drugs act to block the enzyme cyclooxygenase, an integral enzyme in the arachidonic acid cascade, thus blocking prostaglandin production (see Fig. 52–10). In addition to drugs, the body naturally controls endogenous pyrogens by using specific cytokines such as IFN-γ, IL-4, and interleukin-6. These cytokines work by reducing the amount of IL-1 and TNF produced by cells involved in inducing fever.

HEAT STROKE, HYPOTHERMIA, AND FROSTBITE

Heat stroke occurs when heat production or input exceeds heat output, so body temperature rises to dangerous levels

In hot, humid weather it is difficult for animals to lose heat, because evaporative cooling cannot occur effectively. Strenuous exercise under these conditions can lead to a dangerous increase in body temperature. Similarly, when dogs are closed in cars in the sun, their panting saturates the air with water vapor, and so further heat loss is impossible. As the body temperature rises, the metabolic rate increases, and more heat is produced. In addition, panting, sweating, or both leads to dehydration and circulatory collapse, so it is more difficult to transfer heat to the skin. Once the body temperature exceeds 41.5°C to 42.5°C, cellular function is seriously impaired and consciousness is lost.

Hypothermia occurs when heat output exceeds heat production, so body temperature decreases to dangerous levels

Small or sick animals exposed to a cold environment may lose more heat than they can generate, and body temperature may decrease to a point at which heat-regulating mechanisms no longer work. The ability of the hypothalamus to regulate body temperature is greatly impaired below a temperature of 29°C. Cardiac arrest occurs at around 20°C. Neonates seem to be able to withstand cooling more than adults, and apparently comatose lambs, piglets, and puppies can be revived through warming.

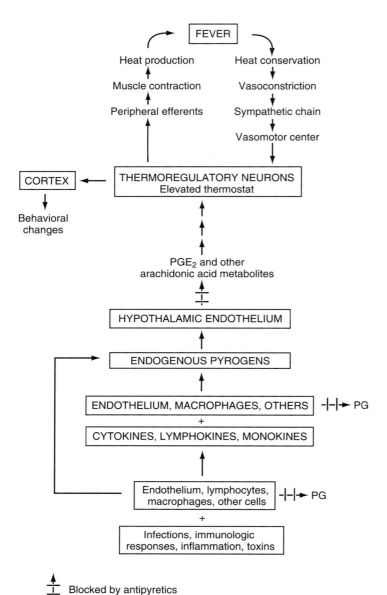

FEVER

Heat production   Heat conservation

Muscle contraction   Vasoconstriction

Peripheral efferents   Sympathetic chain

Vasomotor center

CORTEX ← THERMOREGULATORY NEURONS
Elevated thermostat

Behavioral
changes

PGE_2 and other
arachidonic acid metabolites

HYPOTHALAMIC ENDOTHELIUM

ENDOGENOUS PYROGENS

ENDOTHELIUM, MACROPHAGES, OTHERS ‑|‑|‑► PG
+
CYTOKINES, LYMPHOKINES, MONOKINES

Endothelium, lymphocytes,
macrophages, other cells ‑|‑|‑► PG
+
Infections, immunologic
responses, inflammation, toxins

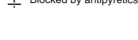 Blocked by antipyretics

FIGURE 52–10. Peripheral and central mechanisms involved in the pathogenesis of fever.

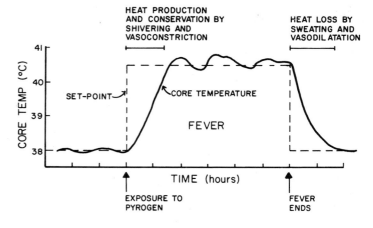

HEAT PRODUCTION
AND CONSERVATION BY
SHIVERING AND
VASOCONSTRICTION

HEAT LOSS BY
SWEATING AND
VASODILATION

SET-POINT   CORE TEMPERATURE

FEVER

CORE TEMP (°C)

TIME (hours)

EXPOSURE TO
PYROGEN

FEVER
ENDS

IGURE 52–11. The events involved in fever. Exposure to a pyrogen increases the set-point of the temperature-regulating system. This results in heat production and conservation to elevate body temperature, which in turn results in fever. When the fever ends, the set-point decreases, and heat must be lost from the body through sweating and vasodilation.

Frostbite occurs when ice crystals form in the tissues of the extremities

In extremely cold conditions, when the extremities are vasoconstricted to conserve heat, the tissues may cool below the freezing point of tissue water. Ice crystals disrupt the tissue integrity, and gangrene can result. Normally, frostbite is prevented by the fact that vascular smooth muscle dilates in extreme cold, causing an inflow of warm blood. The latter mechanism apparently works adequately in animals that winter outdoors in northern climates.

CLINICAL CORRELATIONS

Influenza in pigs

History   You are called to examine a group of 3-month-old pigs in an intensively managed fattening house. The group of 20 pigs is in a pen, and there are multiple similar pens within the barn. In the last 2 days in this particular pen of pigs, the animals have been reluctant to eat and have started huddling together. The owner has observed that the outer pigs in the huddle continually try to burrow toward the center of the pile of pigs and that they appear to be trembling. At this time the remaining pigs in the barn are not affected. When you enter the barn and the pigs are disturbed, they begin sneezing and coughing, and some are reluctant to move.

Clinical examination   Three pigs are caught, and the rectal temperature is found to be 41°C (normal, 39.2°C). There is a nasal discharge, and the conjunctiva and nasal mucosa are congested. You treat the pigs with antibiotics, and over a period of several days, the pigs recover; however, the disease spreads progressively through the remaining pens in the fattening house. All pigs show the same clinical signs, and no pigs die from the disease. Blood samples are taken for virus neutralization tests from the acutely affected pigs 2 weeks after they have recovered.

  The diagnosis from the viral neutralization test is swine influenza, which has a high morbidity rate but a low mortality rate.

Comment   The clinical signs produced by this disease are caused largely by the development of fever. The pigs that were examined had an elevated body temperature, because the infection had adjusted the set-point of their thermoregulatory centers to a high value. In order to raise body temperature to this new value, the pigs huddled together, and the pigs on the outside shivered in order to generate metabolic body heat. Once the infection is overcome and pyrogen is metabolized, the behavior of the pigs changes; they need to lose heat, so they separate and move around the pens more freely.

Heat stroke in a Boston terrier

History   At 3:00 PM on a 95°F (35°C) day in August, you receive a frantic phone call from a client. The client went to a shopping mall and left her car parked in the lot. She had her Boston terrier with her, but because she thought she would only be a few minutes, she left the dog in the car. While in the mall, she was delayed by an uncooperative clerk at a store. When she came out of

the store, her dog was prostrate with its tongue hanging out of its mouth, and it was unresponsive to the owner's attentions. You instruct the owner to bring the dog over to your practice immediately and to drive with the windows open for the half-mile trip.

Clinical examination   On arrival at the clinic, the dog is laid on the examining table, where it fails to respond to its name. Its mouth is open, its tongue is distended, and its mucous membranes are dry. Body temperature is 42.2°C (normal, 38.5°C).

  From the history, the animal's body temperature, and its lack of response, you diagnose heat stroke. The dog is placed in a bath of cool water, and fluids are administered intravenously. Within 5 to 10 minutes, the dog begins to look around and recognizes its owner. The water bath treatments are continued for 2 hours, at which time the body temperature is close to normal. The dog remains in the hospital overnight and is then discharged to a delighted owner the next day.

Comment   The temperature inside a car parked in the hot sun rises rapidly to above body temperature. At this time, the only mechanism available for losing heat is evaporation of water from the respiratory tract, which the dog attempts by panting and salivating. For a while this is an effective means of losing heat, but water vapor is transferred to the air in the car and progressively saturates the atmosphere with water. As the percentage saturation of the air increases, the animal has more and more difficulty achieving evaporation and therefore heat loss. Eventually the animal cannot lose heat, and the body temperature begins to rise. Once the body temperature exceeds 41.5°C to 42.5°C, the animal loses consciousness. In addition, the panting results in dehydration and reduces the ability of the dog to deliver heat from the core of the body to the extremities. Brachycephalic dogs, such as Boston terriers, have an added disadvantage in temperature regulation: the short nose and convolutions in the wall of the pharynx increase the work of breathing, especially when the dogs pant. This increased work is an additional source of body heat, and the anatomy of the upper airway probably makes evaporative cooling less effective.

  Therapy for this condition is to reduce body temperature and to restore circulatory function as rapidly as possible. For this reason, the dog is placed in a cool water bath to reduce body temperature and also receives intravenous fluids to rehydrate it by expanding its circulatory volume and restoring the ability of the circulation to redistribute heat within the body.

Bibliography

Eckert R, Randall D: Animal Physiology: Mechanisms and Adaptations. New York: WH Freeman, 1983, pp 689–744.
Hales JRS: The partition of respiratory ventilation of the panting ox. J Physiol 188:45–68, 1966.
Heller HC, Crawshaw LI, Hammel HT: The thermostat of vertebrate animals. Sci Am 239:102–113, 1978.
Mackowiak, Philip A (ed): Fever: Basic Mechanisms and Management. New York: Raven Press, 1991.
Maugham RJ, Lindinger MI: Preparing for and competing in the heat: The human perspective. Equine Vet J Suppl 20:8–15, 1995.
Schmidt-Nielsen K: Animal Physiology: Adaptation and Environment. Cambridge, United Kingdom: New York: Cambridge University Press, 1997, pp 217–297.

PRACTICE QUESTIONS

1. Sweating is an effective cooling mechanism because
   a. sweat secretion produces heat, which is carried to the skin surface in the sweat.
   b. conversion of sweat into water vapor requires heat, which is supplied to the skin by blood flow.
   c. sweat dripping from the body carries away large amounts of heat.
   d. the ions in sweat carry large amounts of heat from the body.

2. In the cold, animals both conserve and produce heat. Which of the following is a method of heat conservation?
   a. Shivering.
   b. Brown fat metabolism.
   c. Increased thyroxine secretion.
   d. Countercurrent heat exchange in the limbs.
   e. All of the above.

3. Which of the following methods of heat loss can occur in an animal (body temperature = 38°C) standing in a room (temperature = 40°C) with relative humidity of zero? The walls of the room have a temperature of 30°C.
   a. Convection and evaporation.
   b. Convection and radiation.
   c. Evaporation and radiation.
   d. Radiation alone.
   e. Convection, evaporation, and radiation.

4. Which of the following describes thermoregulation?
   a. Temperature receptors in both the brain and skin can initiate thermoregulatory responses.
   b. The brain temperature receptors have a greater influence on thermoregulation than do skin receptors.
   c. The core temperature at which shivering begins is higher if the skin is cold than if the skin is warm.
   d. Skin cooling can initiate shivering even if core temperature is normal.
   e. All of the above.

5. Which of the following correctly describes fever?
   a. It results when the set-point for body temperature decreases.
   b. It is accompanied by sweating to lose heat as body temperature rises.
   c. It is accompanied by shivering to gain heat as body temperature decreases once pyrogens are metabolized.
   d. It can be initiated by pyrogens from bacteria or leukocytes.
   e. All of the above.

PRACTICE ANSWERS

1. b   2. d   3. c   4. e   5. d

Note: Page numbers followed by the letter f refer to figures and those followed by t refer to tables.

A

A band, of cardiac myofibril, 124, 124f
AaDo$_2$ (alveolar-arterial oxygen tension difference), 491, 492–493
Abdominal muscles, expiration and, 470
Abductor muscles, of upper airway, 470, 475
Abomasum, 295, 298
  microbial protein in, 287
  torsion of, 465–466, 527–528, 529–530, 530f
ABP (androgen-binding protein), 425, 426f
Absolute refractory period, cardiac, 129–130, 130f
Absorption, intestinal, 255, 255f, 262–276. See also Enterocyte(s).
  metabolic needs and, 305
  metabolism during, 307, 308f
    amino acids in, 308–312, 308f, 309t, 310f–311f, 313f
    fatty acids in, 307–308, 309f, 313
    glucose in, 307–308, 308f
    insulin in, 307, 312, 312f
  of amino acids, 264, 265, 266f, 270, 309–310, 310f
  of calcium, 367, 370–371, 370f
  of carbohydrates, 263–264, 263f–264f, 265
    thyroid hormones and, 345
  of electrolytes, 265–269, 266f–268f, 268t
  of fats, 271–272, 273f–275f, 275–276
  of proteins, in neonate, 276
  of water, 265, 268–269, 270–271, 270f
    diarrhea and, 276–277, 277f
  transport systems in, 13–14, 13f, 262–265, 263f–266f
Acclimatization, to altitude, 505
Accommodation, 88–89, 89f
ACE (angiotensin-converting enzyme), 355, 435, 435f, 512
Acetate, ruminal, 284, 284f–286f, 285, 285t
  absorption of, 296
  dilution rate and, 294
  fatty acid synthesis from, 320
  Krebs cycle and, 320
Acetazolamide, carbonic anhydrase and, 504
Acetoacetate, 307f, 362f, 363
Acetone, 307f, 362f, 363
Acetyl coenzyme A
  fatty acid synthesis from, 308, 309f
  from fatty acid β-oxidation, 319, 319f
  insulin and, 362, 362f, 363
  ketone body synthesis from, 318f, 319
Acetylcholine, 82–83, 83f
  at neuromuscular synapse, 15, 41, 42, 43
  at sympathetic nerve terminals, 201–202
  bronchoconstriction and, 474, 475f
  cardiovascular effects of, 132, 132f, 135, 200, 201–202, 201t
  enteric nervous system and, 224, 249
  gastric motility and, 236
  in adrenal medulla, 82, 83f, 357, 357f
  insulin secretion and, 363
  pulmonary vascular response to, 482, 483t

Acetylcholine (Continued)
  pupillary diameter and, 92
Acetylcholine receptors, 21, 41, 42, 83, 83f
  in myasthenia gravis, 43
  of gastric secretory cells, 249
  of pancreatic secretory cells, 250
Acetylcholinesterase, 42, 43, 83
Acetylcholinesterase inhibitor, for myasthenia gravis, 43
Acid, definition of, 523
Acid-base balance
  abnormalities of, 526, 528–529, 529t. See also Acidosis; Alkalosis.
  basic principles of, 522–523
  buffers in. See Buffers.
  renal regulation of, 459–465, 524–525, 526, 528
    ammonium ion in, 460–461, 461f
    bicarbonate secretion in, 462, 464, 464f–465f
    buffers in, 459–460, 460f, 462, 464, 524
    hydrogen ion excretion in, 459–460, 461–462, 462f–463f, 522–523
    in respiratory acidosis, 526–527, 527f
    in respiratory alkalosis, 527, 527f
  respiratory regulation of, 459, 522, 524–525, 525f, 527–528, 528f
  terminology about, 526, 529
Acidosis, 522. See also Acid-base balance; pH.
  ammoniagenesis in, 460, 526
  in calf diarrhea, 278
  in ruminants, carbohydrate feeding and, 527
  ketone bodies in, 363
  metabolic, 505, 505f, 527, 528, 528f
    anion gap in, 529
    blood gas abnormalities in, 529t
    buffering by bone in, 459
    in hypoadrenocorticism, 355, 450
  renal proton pump and, 462, 463f, 465
  respiratory, 463f, 465, 526–527, 527f, 529t
Aciduria, paradoxic, 465
Acini
  bile canaliculi as, 250, 251f
  of pancreas, 249, 250
  of salivary glands, 246, 246f
Acromegaly, 338
Acrosin, 398
Acrosome, 423, 424
Acrosome reaction, 398
ACTH. See Corticotropin (ACTH).
Actin
  in non-muscle cells, 6
  molecular mechanism of, 6–8, 6f–7f, 21
  of cardiac muscle, 49, 124, 124f, 129, 130, 134
  of skeletal muscle, 45, 48, 48f
  of smooth muscle, 21, 22f, 23, 49
  uterine, 403
Action potential(s), 35, 37–39, 37f–39f
  at neuromuscular synapse, 41–43, 45
  cardiac. See Cardiac action potential(s).
  conduction velocity of, 38–39
  of sensory nerve, 51

Action potential(s) (Continued)
  of skeletal muscle, 45, 48
    duration of, 130
    vs. cardiac muscle, 123, 124t, 126–128, 128f, 130
  of smooth muscle, 49
    gastrointestinal, 232–233, 232f
    voltage-gated channels and, 15
Action tremor, 68, 78, 79
Active hyperemia, 192, 193f, 195
Active transport, 10, 12–14, 12f
  in intestinal absorption, 263
  in proximal tubule, 442–444, 442f–443f
  of calcium
    in cardiac muscle, 129, 130
    in intestinal mucosa, 367, 370f, 371
  of iodide, 342
  secondary
    definition of, 13
    in intestinal absorption, 13, 13f, 263–264, 263f–264f
    in renal tubular reabsorption, 442–443, 442f, 445, 447f
  tertiary, 263, 264
  vs. diffusion, 113
Activin, 425
Adaptive relaxation, of stomach, 235, 235f, 236
Adenohypophysis (anterior pituitary)
  cortisol secretion and, 352, 352f
    in Cushing's syndrome, 353, 354
  fetal, parturition and, 402, 404
  gonadal regulation by, 376–379, 377f, 384
  hormones of, 335–336, 335t, 336f. See also specific hormones.
  hypothalamic control of, 116, 330–331, 331f, 335–338, 336f–337f, 337f
  male reproductive system and, 425, 426, 426f, 427
  thyroid hormones and, 346, 346f
Adenosine monophosphate. See Cyclic adenosine-3',5'-monophosphate (cAMP)
Adenosine triphosphate (ATP). See also H$^+$,K$^+$-ATPase pump; Na$^+$,K$^+$-ATPase pump.
  cyclic AMP and, 20, 23, 23f
  in active transport, 10, 12–13, 12f, 14
  in enteric nervous system, 224
  in fermentative digestion, 283, 284, 284f, 288f
    microbial yield and, 287, 294
  in gastric HCl secretion, 248
  in muscle contraction, 6, 7f
    of cardiac muscle, 49, 124
    of skeletal muscle, 45
    of smooth muscle, 49
  in nervous system, 36, 39
  in protein hormone secretion, 326
  oxyhemoglobin dissociation curve and, 496
  protein kinases and, 21, 23
Adenyl cyclase, 23, 24, 24f
  chloride channels and, 269–270, 277

Adenyl cyclase *(Continued)*
 glucagon and, 313
 hormone action and, 329, 330f
 insulin secretion and, 363
ADH. *See* Vasopressin (antidiuretic
  hormone [ADH]).
Adipose tissue
 epinephrine and, 359
 fatty acid mobilization from, 317
 fatty acid storage in, 306–307, 312, 313
 fatty acid synthesis in, 308
  in ruminants, 320
 glucocorticoids and, 351
 insulin and, 313, 362, 362t
 VLDLs derived from, 319
Adrenal cortex
 fetal, 401, 402, 402f
 histology of, 348–349, 349f
 hormones of. *See also* Glucocorticoids;
   Mineralocorticoids.
  biosynthesis of, 348–350, 350f
  deficiency of, 356
  metabolism of, 351
  overlapping activities of, 351, 351t
  transport of, in blood, 350–351
 hypophysectomy and, 349f
 sex steroids produced by, 350
  mammary development and, 409,
    410f
 tumors of, 353, 354
Adrenal medulla, 82, 83, 83f, 356–357. *See
  also* Catecholamines.
 cardiovascular effects of, 200, 201
 histology of, 348, 349f
 in defense-alarm reaction, 206
 neural control of, 325, 359, 360
 stressful stimuli and, 24
Adrenaline. *See* Epinephrine.
β-Adrenergic agonists, 135
 cardiac contractility and, 159
 for AV node block, 136, 140
 for sick sinus syndrome, 136
β-Adrenergic antagonists, 135
 antiarrhythmic effects of, 139
 cardiac contractility and, 159
 for pulmonic stenosis effects of, 166
Adrenergic neurons, 82, 83, 83f, 84t, 85
α-Adrenergic receptors
 cardiovascular, 200, 201t, 202, 482
 catecholamines and, 358, 359, 359f
 cyclic AMP and, 23
 of pancreatic β cells, 363
 renal vascular, 436
β-Adrenergic receptors
 bronchodilation and, 474–475, 475f
 catecholamines and, 358–359, 359f
 cyclic AMP and, 23, 24
 of arterioles, 200–201, 201t
 of cardiac muscle, 24, 134–135, 200,
   201t, 202
  drug effects on, 139, 159
  of pacemaker, 132
 of salivary glands, 246
 renin-angiotensin system and, 436
 thyroid hormones and, 345
Adrenocorticotropic hormone. *See*
  Corticotropin (ACTH).
Aerobic conditioning, pulse pressure and,
  178
Aerobic species, 468
Aerosols, 508
Afferent arteriole, glomerular, 432, 432f,
  435, 436
 of reptilian-type nephron, 432, 432f, 435,
   436
Afferent (sensory) nerves, 32t, 33

Afferent (sensory) nerves *(Continued)*
 disease of, 59
 of muscle spindle, 53f–54f, 54
 reflex arc and, 51, 51f, 52, 62
 visceral, 32t, 33, 85
Afterload, cardiac, 159, 160
Airflow rate, 471, 471f, 474
 particle deposition and, 508
Airway(s). *See also* Bronchi.
 abductor muscles of, 470, 475
 anatomy of, 473–474
 as dead-space, 469
 blood supply to, 484
 conducting, 469
 dynamic compression of, 475
 lymphoid tissue of, 508, 510
 particle deposition in, 508–509, 509f
 receptors in, 503
 smooth muscle of, 474–475, 475f
  epinephrine and, 359
  stretch receptors in, 503
Airway obstruction
 acid-base changes in, 529, 530f
 alveolar hypoventilation caused by, 487
 chronic, in horse, 477
 collateral ventilation and, 476
 distribution of ventilation and, 475, 476f
 in brachycephalic syndrome, 492
 inflammatory mediators of, 474
 right-to-left shunt caused by, 491
Airway resistance, 471, 473–474, 473f–474f
Alanine, 309–310, 309t, 310f, 312, 315–316,
  316f
Albumin
 in colostrum, 410, 410t
 in milk, 416
 in plasma, 118, 119t, 120. *See also*
   Plasma proteins.
  aldosterone transport by, 350
  cortisol transport by, 350
  edema and, 12
  fatty acid transport by, 317, 319
  glomerular filtration of, 434, 435,
    438
  loss of, in enteropathy, 190
  steroid transport by, 328
  thyroid hormone transport by, 343
 synthesis of, in liver, 310
Aldosterone, 349. *See also*
  Mineralocorticoids.
 angiotensin II and, 355, 355f, 435, 435f,
   436
  atrial volume receptor reflex and, 205
  hemorrhage and, 215
 deficiency of, 449–450
 in atrial volume receptor reflex, 205
 potassium secretion and, 447, 448, 448f
 regulation of, 355f
 sodium reabsorption and, 354f, 447–448,
   448f
  from sweat, 535
 synthesis of, 350
 transport of, in blood, 350, 351
Alkaline tide, 248
Alkalosis, 522. *See also* Acid-base balance;
  pH.
 bicarbonate secretion in, 464
 metabolic, 505, 505f, 527–528, 528f
  abomasal torsion causing, 465–466,
    527–528, 529–530
  blood gas abnormalities in, 529t
  mineralocorticoid hypersecretion caus-
    ing, 355
  with paradoxic aciduria, 465–466
 respiratory, 527, 527f, 529t
Allantochorion, 516

Allergy
 cytokines in, 511
 edema associated with, 189–190, 190f
 glucocorticoids for, 353
 heaves caused by, 477
Allostery, 4–5, 4f
 in catecholamine biosynthesis, 5
 in gated channels, 15
 in muscle contraction, 6, 7f, 8
 in receptor-mediated signaling, 19
α cells, 360, 361f, 363, 364, 365, 365f
Altitude. *See* High altitude.
Alveolar carbon dioxide tension (PA_{CO_2}),
  487, 488
Alveolar dead-space, 469, 491
Alveolar gas equation, 487
Alveolar hyperventilation, 487, 491, 527
Alveolar hypoventilation, 487, 487f, 491
 in anesthetized horse, 492
 in anesthetized Saint Bernard, 506
 in brachycephalic syndrome, 492
 pH of blood and, 525
 respiratory acidosis caused by, 526–527,
   527f
Alveolar hypoxia, 479, 482, 482f, 483
Alveolar macrophages, 510, 510f
Alveolar oxygen tension (PA_{O_2}), 487, 488,
  489f, 491
 in brachycephalic syndrome, 492
 with oxygen supplementation, 492
 with ventilation/perfusion mismatch,
   490f, 491
Alveolar sacs, 519
Alveolar septum(a), 479, 480, 480f
 airway resistance and, 473, 474, 474f
 fluid movement through, 511–512, 511f
 pulmonary vascular resistance and, 482,
   482f
Alveolar ventilation, 487, 491
 definition of, 469
 in cold-stressed animals, 470
 regulation of, 469, 501
Alveolar vessels, 479, 480f, 482
 resistance in, 482, 482f
Alveolar-arterial oxygen tension difference
  (AaD_{O_2}), 491, 492–493
Alveolus(i), mammary, 407, 407f, 409,
  409f, 411f
 hormonal stimulation of, 417
 involution of, 416
 myoepithelial cells and, 407f, 413f, 414
 nutrients synthesized by, 412, 413f, 414
Alveolus(i), pulmonary, 469
 capillary gas exchange with, 113, 114f,
   488, 488f–490f, 489–491
 collapsed, 491
 fetal development of, 519
 fluid accumulation in, 511–512
 in neonate, 520
 particle deposition in, 508, 509f
 surface area of, 113
 surfactant in, 472, 473f, 503, 519, 520
  in edema, 511
 type II cells of, 472, 473f, 519
  IL-8 produced by, 511
Amacrine cells, 89, 89f, 90, 91
Amino acids
 absorption of, 13, 13f, 264, 265, 266f, 270
  modification during, 309–310, 310f
 as fuels, 306
 buffering by, 524
 carbohydrates derived from, 311–312,
   311f, 315, 351
 classification of, metabolic, 308–309,
   309t
 deamination of, 311, 312, 315, 316

Amino acids (Continued)
  fatty acids derived from, 313
  from luminal-phase digestion, 260
  from membranous-phase digestion, 262, 262f
  gluconeogenesis from, 306, 311–312, 311f, 315–316, 316f
    in ruminants, 320
  hepatic metabolism of, 310–312, 310f–311f
  in skeletal muscle, 306, 312, 315–316, 316f, 317
  insulin and, 361, 362, 362f, 362t, 363
  intracellular pool of, 312, 313f, 315
  keto-analogues of, 309–310, 310f, 311
  microbial metabolism of, 286–287, 286f, 288f
  reabsorption of, in kidney, 442, 442f, 443, 444
γ-Aminobutyric acid (GABA)
  prolactin and, 379
  Purkinje neurons and, 76
p-Aminohippurate, 444
Ammonia
  as base, 523
  in microbial metabolism, 286, 286f, 287, 288
  in renal medullary interstitium, 460–461, 461f
  urea derived from, 316, 316f
Ammoniagenesis, renal, 460–461, 461f, 526, 527, 528
Ammonium ion, 523
  excretion of, 460–461, 461f
cAMP. See Cyclic adenosine-3′,5′-monophosphate (cAMP).
cAMP-dependent protein kinase, 23
Ampulla(e)
  of deferent duct, 421, 422, 422t, 423
  of semicircular canal, 70f–72f, 72
  of uterine tube, fertilization and, 398, 399
α-Amylase, 259, 262f
  salivary, 245, 246
Amylopectin, 259–260, 259f
Amylose, 259, 259f
Anabolic nervous system, 85
Anabolic steroids, 427–428
  for anemia, 438
Anaerobic threshold, 505
Anal sphincter, 241, 241f
Anatomic dead-space, 469, 470f
Androgen insensitivity, 380
Androgen-binding protein (ABP), 425, 426f
Androgens. See also Anabolic steroids; Testosterone.
  as pheromones, 395
  biosynthesis of, 327f, 328
    in adrenal cortex, 350
  genital development and, 374–375
  in pregnancy, 401
  libido and, 393
  testicular production of, 425, 426f
  thecal production of, 380, 393
Androstenedione, 380, 393
Anemia, 121
  in chronic renal failure, 437, 438
  in flea infestation, 499
  in hypoadrenocorticism, 356
  oxygen transport in, 495, 495f, 499
  ventilatory response to, 504
Anesthesia
  alveolar hypoventilation during, 506
  alveolar-arterial oxygen difference in, 491

Anesthesia (Continued)
  cardiovascular effects of, 112
  equipment dead-space during, 470
  hypoxemia during, in large animals, 492–493
  overdose during, 112
  oxygen administration with, 491
Anestrus, 389, 390f
  photoperiod and, 394, 394f
Angiotensin I, 355, 355f, 435, 435f
Angiotensin II, 355, 355f, 435, 435f, 436
  atrial volume receptor reflex and, 205
  hemorrhage and, 215
  pulmonary vascular response to, 483t, 512
Angiotensin-converting enzyme (ACE), 355, 435, 435f, 512
Angiotensinogen, 355, 355f, 435, 435f
Anion gap, 529
Anterior pituitary. See Adenohypophysis (anterior pituitary).
Antiarrhythmic drugs, 138–139
Antibiotics
  glucocorticoids with, 353
  renal excretion of, 444
Antibodies. See Immunoglobulins.
Anticoagulant, 118, 119
Antidiuretic hormone. See Vasopressin (antidiuretic hormone [ADH]).
Antigen-presenting cells, 510
Antigravity muscle tone, 62, 67–68
Anti-insulin effect, 351
Antioxidants, as lung protectants, 510
Antiperistalsis, 240, 240f, 241
  in birds, 243
  in horses, 299, 300
Antiports, 14, 264, 266
  calcium reabsorption by, 449
  in proximal tubule, 443
Antithyroglobulin autoantibody test (ATAA), 347
α₁-Antitrypsin, as lung protectant, 510
Antral follicle(s), 378, 380, 382, 384, 387
  sexual receptivity and, 392–393
Antrum, gastric, 236, 237, 238
Aorta, 115, 115f, 117, 117t
  hepatic artery and, 116
Aortic arch baroreceptors, 202–203, 202f
  vasopressin and, 333
Aortic blood pressure, 116, 176–177, 176f
  determinants of, 172–173
  vascular resistance and, 169–170, 170f
Aortic bodies, 503
Aortic depressor nerve, 203
Aortic insufficiency (regurgitation), 161t, 162, 162f, 165
  pulse pressure and, 178f, 179
Aortic pulse pressure, 176, 176f
Aortic stenosis, 161f, 161t, 162, 165
Aortic valve, 154, 155, 156
Apnea, airway receptors and, 503
Apocrine glands, 535
Appendix testis, 376f
Aquaporins, renal, 14–15, 456
Aqueduct of Sylvius, 94, 96
Aqueous humor, 87, 88, 92
Arachidonic acid
  fever and, 541
  glucocorticoids and, 353
  prostaglandins and, 329–330
    in parturition, 403
  pulmonary vascular response to, 483t
Arachnoid, 33, 33f
Arachnoid villi, 95–96, 95f
Archicerebellum, 77
Arcuate nucleus, 377, 379, 379f

Arginine vasopressin (AVP), 333, 437. See also Vasopressin (antidiuretic hormone [ADH]).
Arginine vasotocin, 333, 456
Aromatic-L-amino acid decarboxylase, 5, 5f, 357–358, 358f
Aromatization, of androgens, 375
Arousal
  EEG and, 99
  emotional, 206, 206f
  reticular formation and, 67
Arrhythmias. See Cardiac arrhythmias.
Arterial baroreceptor reflex. See Baroreceptor reflex.
Arteries, 117, 117t, 118f
  as pressure reservoirs, 170
  cholinergic muscarinic receptors of, 202
  compliance of, 170, 171f
    pulse pressure and, 178–179, 178f–179f
  elasticity of, 181
  pressure profile in, 169, 170f
  wall properties of, 182f
Arterioles, 117, 117t, 118f
  adrenergic receptors of, 200–201, 201t, 202
  cholinergic muscarinic receptors of, 201t, 202
  glomerular, 432, 432f, 435, 436
  in human hypertension, 173
  of exercising muscle, 174f, 175, 183–184, 192, 216
  of skin, heat transfer and, 536
  precapillary sphincters and, 181–182, 193
  resistance of, 169, 170, 170f, 171–172, 172f–173f
    autonomic control of, 200–202, 201t, 204
    blood flow to organs and, 175, 192
    capillary hydrostatic pressure and, 185
    during exercise, 173, 174f, 216
    factors affecting, 192
    histamine and, 190, 192
    metabolic control of, 193
  wall properties of, 181, 182f
Arteriovenous anastomoses, heat transfer and, 536
Arteriovenous fistulas, 162
Arteriovenous oxygen difference, during exercise, 498
Ascites, 188
Aspartate, 309, 309t
Asthma
  edema in, 189–190
  hypoxic vasoconstriction in, 176
  in cats, 474
Astrocytes, 98
ATAA (antithyroglobulin autoantibody test), 347
Ataxia, 78, 79
Atelectasis
  blood flow reduction in, 483
  right-to-left shunt in, 491
  thoracic compliance and, 473
Atenolol, 135
  cardiac contractility and, 159
ATP. See Adenosine triphosphate (ATP).
ATPases. See also H⁺,K⁺-ATPase pump; Na⁺,K⁺-ATPase pump.
  in active transport, 12–14, 12f–13f
Atrial fibrillation, 137
  AV node refractory period and, 133, 137
  calcium channel blockers for, 139
  ECG in, 151

Atrial fibrillation *(Continued)*
  in horse, 499
  mitral stenosis causing, 165
  ventricular filling and, 155
Atrial flutter, 137
  AV node refractory period and, 133
  calcium channel blockers for, 139
Atrial natriuretic peptide, 356, 436, 447
Atrial systole, 155
Atrial tachycardia, 137
  paroxysmal, 151–152, 160
Atrial volume receptor reflex, 202f, 204–205, 205f
  hemorrhage and, 213, 213f, 214, 215
  vasopressin secretion and, 333, 334f
Atrioventricular (AV) bundle, 126, 126f–127f, 133
  tachycardia associated with, 137
Atrioventricular (AV) junction, 126
Atrioventricular (AV) node, 126, 126f–127f, 133–134, 133f, 134t
  calcium channel blockers and, 139
  parasympathetic effects on, 135, 201
  tachycardias associated with, 137
Atrioventricular (AV) node block, 136, 140
  ECG in, 150, 150f
Atrioventricular (AV) valves. *See* Mitral valve; Tricuspid valve.
Atrophy, muscle, 58–59
Atropine
  for AV node block, 136, 140
  for bronchospasm, 477
  for sick sinus syndrome, 136
  muscarinic receptors and, 83
Auditory bones (ossicles), 104, 105, 105f–106f
Auditory (eustachian) tube, 104, 105f
Auerbach (myenteric) plexus, 222
  of esophagus, 234
  of stomach, 236
Augmented unipolar limb leads, 147
Autocrine effectors, 325, 325f
  gastrointestinal, 226
Autonomic nervous system, 80–86. *See also* Parasympathetic nervous system; Sympathetic nervous system.
  cardiovascular system and, 134–135, 200–202, 201t
  central control of, 85, 85f
  gastrointestinal system and, 84t, 85, 224, 225f
  glucagon secretion and, 365, 365f
  insulin secretion and, 363, 365f
  major divisions of, 81–82, 81f–82f
  neuron loss in, postganglionic, 85–86
  neurotransmitters in, 82–83, 83f
    biosynthesis of, 5, 5f
  peripheral nerves of, 32t, 33, 80–81, 81f
  pulmonary arteries and, 482
  reflexes of, 85
  response of organs to, 83, 84t, 85
  vs. somatic motor system, 80–81, 81f
Auxiliary pacemaker, 133–134, 136
AV (atrioventricular) bundle, 126, 126f–127f, 133
  tachycardia associated with, 137
AV (atrioventricular) junction, 126
AV (atrioventricular) node, 126, 126f–127f, 133–134, 133f, 134t
  calcium channel blockers and, 139
  parasympathetic effects on, 135, 201
  tachycardias associated with, 137
AV (atrioventricular) node block, 136, 140
  ECG in, 150, 150f
AV (atrioventricular) valves. *See* Mitral valve; Tricuspid valve.

AVP (arginine vasopressin), 333, 437. *See also* Vasopressin (antidiuretic hormone [ADH]).
Axon, 32, 34, 35f
Axoplasmic transport, 34
Azotemia. *See also* Uremia.
  in hypoadrenocorticism, 356, 450
  prerenal, 450
Azygos vein, bronchial circulation and, 484

B

B vitamins, rumen microbes and, 282
Backward heart failure, 28, 213
Bacteremia, shock caused by, 111
Balance. *See also* Posture.
  vestibulocerebellum and, 77
Barbiturates, cardiac contractility and, 159
Barometric pressure, 486, 491
Baroreceptor reflex, 202–204, 202f–204f, 205
  during exercise, 216
  hemorrhage and, 213–214, 213f, 215
  in defense-alarm reaction, 206
  in heart failure, 210, 212
  vasopressin secretion and, 333
Basal ganglia, 33, 63, 66, 68
  lesions of, 68
  reticular activating system and, 67, 67f
Basal metabolism, 468, 536. *See also* Metabolic rate.
  cold stress and, 536, 540
  thyroid hormones and, 344–346
Base, definition of, 523
Base deficit
  definition of, 526
  diagnostic significance of, 529t
  in hypoadrenocorticism, 450
  in metabolic acidosis, 527
Base excess
  definition of, 526
  diagnostic significance of, 529t
  in respiratory acidosis, 527
Basic electrical rhythm. *See* Slow waves.
Basket cells, 76, 76f
BCAAs (branch-chain amino acids), 309, 309t, 312
  as muscle energy source, 315–316, 316f
  in fermentative digestion, 286, 287
β cells, 360, 361f, 363, 365, 365f
Betaine, in renal medulla, 457
Betamethasone, 353f
Bicarbonate. *See also* Acidosis; Alkalosis.
  as strong base, 523
  buffering by, 523–526, 525f
    in kidney, 460, 460f, 462, 524, 525, 526
  central chemoreceptor and, 504–505, 504f–505f
  chloride absorption and, 267, 267f
  diagnostic measurement of, 528–529, 529t
  from glutamine metabolism, 460
  gastric acid secretion and, 248, 248f
  in bile, 251, 252
  in carbon dioxide transport, 497, 497f, 498
  in equine hindgut, 301
  in ruminant
    omasum and, 295
    salivary concentration of, 246, 247f
    VFA absorption and, 296, 297f
  intestinal absorption of, 267–268, 267f, 268t
  pancreatic secretion and, 250
  renal secretion of, 462, 464, 464f–465f

Bicarbonate *(Continued)*
  renal tubular reabsorption of, 443, 443f, 461–462, 462f, 464, 526
    impaired, 450
  sodium absorption and, 266, 266f
  standard plasma concentration of, 529
Bile, 250–252, 251f–252f
Bile acids, 251, 251f, 252, 272, 273f
  in blood, 321
  intestinal reabsorption of, 272, 274f, 275
Bile pigments, 252
Bile salts, renal secretion of, 444
Bilirubin, 252
Biomembrane(s). *See* Membrane(s).
Bipolar cells, 89, 89f, 90, 91
Birds
  acid-base balance in, 459, 460
  carbohydrate metabolism in, 365
  dead-space ventilation in, 535
  digestive tracts in
    anatomy of, 241–243, 242f
    motility of, 241, 242–243
    saliva of, 246
  kidneys in, 432, 436–437
    concentrating ability of, 453
    portal circulation of, 441
    salt balance and, 447, 457
    tubular secretion in, 444
    water balance and, 457
Birth. *See* Neonate; Parturition.
Bites, lower motor neuron disease caused by, 59
Bladder
  autonomic regulation of, 84t
  infection of, in spayed bitch, 396
  smooth muscle of, catecholamines and, 359
Blastocyst, 399
Blind spot, 90
Blood
  constituents of, 118–119, 118f, 119t, 120t, 121, 121f
  pH of. *See* pH, of blood.
  substances transported by, 112
  viscosity of, 120–121, 120f, 498
Blood cell counts, 119, 120t
Blood flow. *See also* Vascular resistance.
  autoregulation of, 194–195, 194f, 199
  control mechanisms of, 192, 199
  coronary, control of, 195–196, 199
    autonomic, 200, 201, 201t, 202
  determinants of, 173, 175
  during exercise. *See* Exercise.
  gastrointestinal, 270–271, 270f–271f
  heat transfer by, 534, 536–537, 537f, 540
  mechanical compression and, 195–197, 195f–196f
  metabolic control of, 192–195, 193f–194f
    during exercise, 216
    in coronary circulation, 199
  neurohumoral control of, 199–200
  renal, 435–436, 435f
  resistance to. *See* Vascular resistance.
  skin, heat loss and, 534, 540
  velocity of, 117, 118f
Blood gases. *See also* Carbon dioxide tension (P_{CO_2}); Oxygen tension (P_{O_2}).
  chemoreceptors in control of, 501, 501f
  measurement of, 491, 528–529, 529t
Blood pressure, 116–117. *See also* Baroreceptor reflex; Hypertension; Hypotension.
  afterload and, 159, 160
  aortic, 116, 176–177, 176f
    determinants of, 172–173
    vascular resistance and, 169–170, 170f

Blood pressure *(Continued)*
  arterial
    atrial volume receptor reflex and, 205, 205f
    capillary hydrostatic pressure and, 185
    determinants of, 172–173
    in heart failure, 210
    neurohormonal control of, 200, 201
  atrial natriuretic peptide and, 356
  autonomic control of, 83, 85
  catecholamines and, 360
  central venous, 157
    autonomic control of, 200
    during exercise, 217, 217f
    hemorrhage and, 207
  glomerular filtration rate and, 435, 436
  mineralocorticoids and, 354–355
  profile of, 169–170, 171f
  pulmonary arterial, 176–177, 176f, 480
    at high altitude, 483, 484f
    during exercise, 483
    low, dead-space and, 491
    resistance and, 175
  pulmonary venous, 480
    resistance and, 175
  thyroid hormones and, 345
  vasopressin (ADH) and, 205, 333, 456
Blood vessels, 117, 117t, 118f. *See also* Arteries; Capillaries; Veins.
  walls of, 181, 182f
Blood volume
  atrial volume receptor reflex and, 202f, 204–205, 205f
    hemorrhage and, 213, 213f, 214, 215
    vasopressin secretion and, 333, 334f
  distribution of, 117, 117t, 169, 170
  glomerular filtration rate and, 435, 436
  hemorrhage and, 214–216, 214f–215f
  in heart failure, 212
  vasopressin secretion and, 333, 334f
Blood-brain barrier, 96, 96f, 183
  central chemoreceptor and, 504–505, 504f
  ketone bodies and, 307
  pyrogens and, 541
Blood-testis barrier, 422
Bloodworms, equine colic caused by, 111, 121–122
Body weight, metabolic rate and, 468, 536, 536f
Bohr shift, 496, 496f
Boldenone undecylenate, 427
Bone
  buffering by, in acidosis, 459
  calcitonin and, 369, 369f
  calcium exchange with, 367, 371
  hydroxyapatite of, 366, 367
  osteon structure of, 367f
  parathyroid hormone and, 368, 369f
  vitamin D and, 371
Bony labyrinth, 70, 70f, 104–105
Bowman's capsule, 432, 432f, 434f
Bowman's space, 432, 432f, 433
Brachycephalic syndrome, 492
Bradycardia, in sick sinus syndrome, 135
Bradykinin, pulmonary vascular response to, 482, 483t, 512
Brain, 32, 33. *See also* Central nervous system (CNS); Cerebellum; Cerebral cortex; Cerebrospinal fluid (CSF).
  anatomic regions of, 33, 63, 63f
  blood flow in, autoregulation of, 194, 194f
  capillaries of, 96, 96f, 113, 114f, 182–183
  cerebrospinal fluid and, 94, 95f

Brain *(Continued)*
  cooling of, during exercise, 537
  glucose for, 39, 96, 183
  meninges and, 33
  movement disorders and, 59
Brain tumor
  EEG pattern and, 103
  homonymous hemianopia caused by, 92–93
Brainstem, 63, 63f. *See also* Medulla; Midbrain; Pons.
  autonomic control centers of, 85, 85f
  cochlear nucleus of, 105
  deglutition and, 234
  extrapyramidal system and, 67
  pupillary reflex and, 92
  pyramidal system and, 64, 66
  reflex arc and, 52
  respiratory control by, 502, 502f, 504–505, 504f
  vomiting and, 238
Brainstem auditory evoked response (BSAER), 100, 103f, 106
Branch-chain amino acids (BCAAs), 309, 309t, 312
  as muscle energy source, 315–316, 316f
  in fermentative digestion, 286, 287
Breathing pattern. *See also* Ventilation.
  regulation of, 501–503, 502f
Brisket disease, 483, 484–485
Bromocriptine, for hyperprolactinemia, 379
Bronchi, 469, 473, 474. *See also* Airway(s).
  frictional resistance of, 473f, 474
  irritant receptors in, 503
  mucociliary clearance in, 509, 509f
  smooth muscle of, 474–475, 475f
    epinephrine and, 359
    stretch receptors in, 503, 510
Bronchial circulation, 479, 484
Bronchial glands, 473, 509, 509f
Bronchioles, 469, 473, 474
  frictional resistance of, 473f, 474
  mucociliary clearance in, 509, 509f
  smooth muscle of, 474–475, 475f
Bronchoconstriction
  airway receptors and, 503, 510
  parasympathetic nervous system and, 474
  particle deposition and, 509
Bronchodilation, 474–475
  particle deposition and, 509
Bronchoesophageal artery, 484
Bronchospasm, in heaves, 477
Bronchovascular bundle, 479–480, 480f, 481–482
Brown fat, 536, 540
Bruce effect, 395
Brush border
  intestinal, 255, 256f–257f
  renal tubular, 440, 440f–441f, 443, 444, 445f
  water reabsorption in, 452
BSAER (brainstem auditory evoked response), 100, 103f, 106
Buffers, 523–526, 524f–525f
  clinical terminology for, 526
  in respiratory acidosis, 526, 527f
  intracellular, 524
  protein, 497, 498, 523, 524
    hemoglobin as, 459, 497, 497f, 524, 526, 527
  renal, 459–460, 460f, 462, 464, 524
Buffy coat, 118f, 119
Bulbospinal pathways, respiratory, 502
Bulbourethral (Cowper) glands, 421, 422t, 423

Bulk flow, 112–115, 114f
  through capillary pores, 184
Bulldogs, brachycephalic syndrome in, 492
Bundle branches, 126, 126f–127f
Bundle of His, 126, 126f–127f
Burns, plasma protein loss from, 188–189
Butyrate, 284, 284f–286f, 285, 285t
  absorption of, 296, 297
  Krebs cycle and, 320

C

C cells, thyroid, 342, 368
C fibers, pulmonary, 503
C17-20 lyase, placental, 402
Cabergoline, as prolactin inhibitor, 379
Cajal, interstitial cells of, 231–232
Calbindin 28k, 449
Calcitonin, 368–369, 369f
  calcium excretion and, 449
  thyroid histology and, 342
Calcium. *See also* Hypercalcemia; Hypocalcemia.
  as second messenger, 20, 21, 22f, 23
    in hormone action, 329
  dietary deficiency of, 371
  distribution of, in body, 366–367, 371
  in cardiac muscle contraction, 7–8, 7f, 49
  in hypoxic vasoconstriction, 483
  in lactation, 418–419
  in parturition, 403
  in protein hormone secretion, 326, 326f
  in skeletal muscle contraction, 7–8, 7f, 15, 21, 45, 48, 49
  in smooth muscle contraction, 21, 22f, 23, 49
  intestinal absorption of, 367, 370–371, 370f
  physiologic roles of, 366
  regulation of, 367
    calcitonin and, 368–369, 369f
    parathyroid hormone and, 368, 368f–369f
    vitamin D and, 369–371, 370f
  renal excretion of, 369
  renal reabsorption of, 367, 443, 445, 447, 447f, 448–449
  supplementation of, inappropriate, 418–419
Calcium channel blockers, 49
  antiarrhythmic effects of, 139
  cardiac contractility and, 159
Calcium ion channels, 4f, 20, 21
  of cardiac muscle, 24, 127, 128–129, 129f, 130, 131
    β-adrenergic receptors and, 134
    in pacemaker cells, 131–132, 131f
  of presynaptic membrane, 41–42
  PIP$_2$ pathway and, 25
Calcium-phosphorus product, 371
Calcium-triggered calcium release, 129
Calf diarrhea, 278
Calmodulin, 21, 22f, 23, 25
  hormone action and, 329
Calorigenic effect, of thyroid hormones, 345
Canaliculi, bile, 250, 251, 251f
Capacitation of sperm, 398
Capillaries, 117, 117t, 118f, 181–182, 182f
  cerebral, 96, 96f, 113, 114f, 182–183
  endothelial cells of. *See* Endothelial cells.
  fenestrated, 182, 182f
    glomerular, 432, 433f

Capillaries *(Continued)*
  peritubular, 442f
  gas exchange with, 113–114, 114f, 183–184, 488–489, 489f
  glomerular, 116, 432–433, 432f–434f
    selective permeability of, 433–435
  hydrostatic pressure in, 11–12, 28, 184–188, 190
    glomerular, 433, 434f, 435
  intestinal, 257, 257f, 271
    nutrient diffusion into, 265, 270
    water transport from, 269
    water transport into, 270, 270f, 271
  metabolic control of flow in, 193, 193f
  of liver, 182, 182f, 271
  of portal systems, 115–116, 115f
  of skeletal muscle, 114, 114f, 183–184
  peritubular, 440–441, 440f, 442f, 452
  pores in, 182–183, 182f, 184, 186
  pressure decrease in, 169, 170f
  pulmonary. *See* Pulmonary capillaries.
  recruitment of, 489
  resistance of, 171, 172f
  surface area of, 117
  transport across walls of, 9, 11–12, 182–188, 182f–183f, 190
    in gas exchange, 113–114, 114f, 183–184, 488–489, 489f
  tubular, 116
Capillary filtration, 12, 28, 184–188, 189, 190
Capillary filtration coefficient, 185, 511
Capillary oxygen tension (PcapO₂), 488
Capillary reabsorption, 12, 28
Carbamino compounds, 118, 497, 497f
Carbohydrates. *See also* Glucose; Glycogen.
  absorption of, 263–264, 263f–264f, 265
  digestion of, 258–260, 258f–259f, 261–262, 261f–262f
  fatty acids derived from, 307–308, 309f, 313
  fermentative digestion of, 281–282, 283–285, 284f–286f, 285t, 287, 288f
    in equine hindgut, 298
  from amino acids, 311–312, 311f, 315, 351
  in colostrum, 410, 410t
  in milk, 320, 412, 415t, 416
  metabolism of
    heat produced by, 536, 536t
      in birds, 365
    insulin and, 361–362, 362f–363f, 362t
    thyroid hormones and, 345
  of plant cell walls, 282–283, 298
Carbon dioxide
  in fermentative digestion, 283, 284, 284f, 285t, 286, 287, 288f
  eructation of, 290
  VFA absorption and, 296, 297f
  production of, 468, 487
    in cold-stressed animals, 470
  total (TcO₂), 529
  transport of, 468, 488, 497–498, 497f–498f
    from interstitial fluid, 183, 184
  ventilatory response to, 504–505, 504f–505f
    anesthesia and, 506
Carbon dioxide content, 498, 498f
Carbon dioxide equilibration curves, 498, 498f
Carbon dioxide tension (PcO₂)
  alveolar, 487, 488
  arterial, 487, 488, 491
    bicarbonate reabsorption and, 526

Carbon dioxide tension (PcO₂) *(Continued)*
  chemoreceptors and, 503, 504–505, 504f–505f
    in anesthetized horse, 492
    in brachycephalic syndrome, 492
    in lung disease, 491
    in respiratory acidosis, 526–527, 527f
    measurement of, 528–529, 529t
    pH of blood and, 524, 525
  blood content of carbon dioxide and, 498, 498f
  oxyhemoglobin dissociation curve and, 496
  tissue, 488–489
  venous, 488
Carbon monoxide poisoning, 497, 504
Carbonic acid, 497, 497f, 498
  as weak acid, 523
  buffering and, 523, 524, 525–526, 525f
  central chemoreceptor and, 504
  gastric acid secretion and, 248, 248f
  pancreatic secretions and, 250
Carbonic anhydrase, 497, 497f
  acid-base balance and, 459, 460, 461, 462, 462f
    bicarbonate secretion and, 464, 465f
  gastric acid secretion and, 248, 248f
  inhibitor of, 504
  of proximal tubule, 443, 443f, 461
  pancreatic secretions and, 250
  sodium absorption and, 266
Carboxypeptidase A, 260t, 261f
Carboxypeptidase B, 260t, 261f
Cardiac. *See also* Heart.
Cardiac action potential(s), 49, 123, 124t, 125, 126, 127f
  β-adrenergic receptors and, 134–135
  atrial vs. ventricular, 130–131
  duration of, 126–128, 128f, 129–131, 130f, 132
  of pacemaker cells, 131–132, 131f–133f, 133–134, 134t
  reentrant, 137–138, 138f
Cardiac afterload, 159, 160
Cardiac arrhythmias, 135–140
  drug treatment of, 138–139
  electrolyte imbalance causing, 111
  in AV node block, 136
  in sick sinus syndrome, 135–136, 135t
  myocardial ischemia causing, 115
  reentrant, 138
  tachyarrhythmias as, 137–138, 138f, 139
Cardiac contractility
  β-adrenergic activation and, 134–135
  antiarrhythmic drugs and, 139
  in heart failure, 209, 210, 212–213
  neurohumoral control of, 199
  thyroid hormones and, 345, 346
  ventricular, 158–159, 159f, 160–161
Cardiac cycle, 154–156, 155f
Cardiac decompensation, 212–213
Cardiac glycosides, 139, 159
Cardiac hypertrophy, 162, 163–165
Cardiac mucosa, 247
Cardiac murmurs, 161–163, 161f–162f, 161t
  grading of, 166
  pulse pressure and, 179
Cardiac muscle, 5–6, 7, 44, 49. *See also* Cardiac action potential(s).
  β-adrenergic receptors of, 24, 134–135, 200, 201t, 202
    drug effects on, 139, 159
    on pacemaker cells, 132
  autonomic nervous system and, 32t, 33, 134–135, 201, 201t
  contraction mechanism of, 5–8, 6f–7f, 21, 123–125, 124t, 134

Cardiac muscle *(Continued)*
  cyclic AMP and, 23–24
  ketone bodies used by, 307
  muscarinic receptors of, 201, 202
  neurohumoral control of, 199
  oxygen transport to, 114–115
  pacemaker cells of, 125, 131–134, 131f–133f
    ectopic, 137
  refractory period of, 129–130, 130f
    β-adrenergic activation and, 134, 135
    atrial vs. ventricular, 131
    of AV node, 133, 134, 134t, 136, 137
    parasympathetic effects on, 135
  sodium ion channels of, 127–128, 129f, 130–131
    in pacemaker cells, 131, 131f
  structure of, 123–125, 124f
Cardiac output, 116, 156
  aortic blood pressure and, 172–173
  baroreceptor reflex and, 202, 203, 203f, 204
  control of, 156–161, 156f–160f, 199–200
  during exercise, 160, 160f, 160t, 483, 498, 498f
    metabolic control and, 216
    muscle pump and, 217
    respiratory pump and, 217
    vascular resistance and, 173, 174f
    with atrial fibrillation, 499
  epinephrine and, 359
  in anemia, 121, 484, 499
  in heart failure, 209, 210
  of fetus, 518, 519
  pulmonary vascular resistance and, 175, 480
  thyroid hormones and, 345
Cardiac pacemaker, artificial, 136
Cardiac tamponade, ECG in, 148
Cardiac valve defects, 111, 115, 161–163, 161f–162f, 161t
Cardiogenic shock, 111
Cardiomyopathy
  dilative
    exercise intolerance in, 217–218
    paroxysmal atrial tachycardia in, 151–152
  hypertrophic, in feline hyperthyroidism, 348
Cardiovascular system. *See also* Blood vessels; Heart.
  dysfunctions of, 111–112, 113–114, 115
  general layout of, 115–116, 115f
  neurohumoral control of, 199–200
    autonomic nervous system in, 134–135, 200–202, 201t
    psychogenic effects in, 205–206, 206f–207f
    reflexes in, 202–205, 202f–205f
Carnitine, 318
Carnitine palmitoyltransferase I (CPT I), 318, 318f, 319
Carotid artery, cooling of, in horse, 537, 538f
Carotid bodies, 503–504, 504f
Carotid rete, 537
Carotid sinus baroreceptors, 202, 202f, 203
  vasopressin and, 333
Carrier-mediated transport, 14, 14f
Caruncles, uterine, 400, 516, 518
Caseins
  in colostrum, 410, 410t
  in milk, 412, 416
Castration, libido and, 393
Cat
  cerebellar hypoplasia in, 79

Cat (*Continued*)
  Cushing's syndrome in, 353, 354
  estrous cycle in, 417
  flea infestation in, 499
  hepatic lipidosis in, 321
  hyperthyroidism in, 348
  hypertrophic cardiomyopathy in, 348
Catalysis, 3. *See also* Enzymes.
Cataracts, 89
Catecholamines. *See also specific*
    catecholamines.
  biosynthesis of, 5, 5f, 357–358, 357f–358f
  bronchodilation and, 474–475, 475f
  cold stress and, 536
  effects of, 358–359, 359f, 360t
  endocytosis of, 18
  glomerular filtration rate and, 436
  in carotid bodies, 503
  insulin secretion and, 363
  metabolism of, 358
  pulmonary vasoconstriction and, 482–
    483, 483t
  regulation of secretion of, 359–360
  sweating and, 535
  thyroid hormones and, 345, 348
Cauda equina, 95
Caudate nucleus, 68
Caveolae, 512
Cavernous venous sinuses, 537
CCK. *See* Cholecystokinin (CCK).
Cecum(a)
  avian, 242, 242f, 243
  fermentative digestion in, 281
    in horse, 298–300, 299f–301f, 301
Cell membrane. *See* Membrane(s).
Cell walls, plant, 282–283, 298
Cellulase, 283
Cellulose, 283
Central chemoreceptor, 504–505, 504f–505f
Central circulation, 115, 115f
  blood volume in, 117, 117t
Central command, 216
Central nervous system (CNS). *See also*
    Brain; Cerebrospinal fluid (CSF);
    Spinal cord.
  anatomic regions of, 32–33, 33f, 62–63,
    63f
  catecholamines and, 359
  fuel for
    glucose as, 305
    ketone bodies as, 307
  meninges and, 33, 33f
  muscle spindle receptors and, 53, 54, 55,
    55f, 56
  reflex arc and, 51, 51f, 52
  thyroid hormones and, 345
  upper motor neurons of, 59, 60
Central venous catheter, 157
Central venous pressure, 157
  autonomic control of, 200
  during exercise, 217, 217f
  hemorrhage and, 207
Centroacinar cells, pancreatic, 249–250
Cephalic phase of digestion, 236, 249, 250
  in ruminant, 298
Cerebellar cortex, 76, 76f
Cerebellum, 33, 62, 75–79, 75f–77f
  disease of, 78–79
  hypoplasia of, 78–79
  in coordination of movement, 66, 67, 68
  pons and, 63, 64
  vestibular system and, 73
Cerebral aqueduct, 94, 95f, 96
Cerebral cortex, 33, 63, 63f
  anatomic divisions of, 64, 64f
  autonomic nervous system and, 85

Cerebral cortex (*Continued*)
  extrapyramidal system and, 67, 67f, 68
  functional divisions of, 64
  histology of, 98, 99f
  pyramidal system and, 63–64, 64f, 66
  reflex arc and, 52
  sound perception in, 105
  visual pathway and, 91–92, 92f, 93
Cerebral hemorrhage, hydrocephalus
    secondary to, 96
Cerebral infarction, 113–114
Cerebral vascular disease, 115
Cerebrocerebellum, 77, 77f, 78
Cerebrospinal fluid (CSF), 33, 94–97, 95f
  pH of, ventilation and, 504–505, 504f–
    505f
  pressure of, 96–97
Cervical ganglion, 92
Cervix, uterine
  fertilization and, 398
  in parturition, 402, 403, 404
  in pregnancy, 401, 402
  oxytocin release and, 414
CG (chorionic gonadotropin)
  equine, 335, 401–402, 401f
  primate, 335, 400, 400f, 402
Channels. *See* Ion channels.
Chemical energy, 3
Chemical potential, 10, 523
Chemical synapses, 41
Chemokines, in lung defense, 510–511
Chemoreceptor trigger zone, 238
Chemoreceptors, 503–505, 504f–505f
  acid-base balance and, 528
  of gastrointestinal system, 222, 224f
  of reticulorumen, 295
Chest wall, compliance of, 472–473
Chewing. *See* Mastication.
Chief cells
  gastric, 247, 248, 248f
  parathyroid, 368
Chloride
  gastric acid secretion and, 248, 248f
  in erythrocytes, 497, 497f
  in renal bicarbonate exchangers, 462,
    462f, 464, 465f
  intestinal absorption of, 264, 266–267,
    266f–267f, 268t
  intestinal water secretion and, 269, 269f
    in diarrhea, 277, 278
  membrane potential and, 36
  renal reabsorption of
    in collecting ducts, 446–447
    in tubules, 442f, 443, 445–446, 447f
  renin-angiotensin system and, 355
Chloride gates, of crypt enterocytes, 269,
    277, 278
Chloride-bicarbonate exchanger, 264, 266,
    267f
Cholecystokinin (CCK), 226, 227t, 228, 250
  bile secretion and, 252
  calcitonin and, 369
  gastric emptying and, 237, 237f
  gastric motility and, 236
  insulin secretion and, 363
  pancreatic polypeptide and, 366
Cholera, G proteins and, 23
Cholesterol, 272, 273f, 275, 275f
  bile acid synthesis from, 251, 251f
  hormone synthesis from, 326–327, 327f
    in adrenal cortex, 349–350, 350f
  in bile, 251
  in plasma membrane, 17
  in VLDL, 308, 309f
  structure of, 326f
  thyroid hormones and, 345, 347, 348

Cholesterol (*Continued*)
  transport of, 17–18, 18f
Cholesterol esterase, 272
Cholesterol esters, 272, 273f, 275, 275f
  in adrenal cortex, 349, 350f
  storage of, 326, 328
Cholic acid, 251, 251f, 273f
Cholinergic neurons, 82–83, 83f, 84t, 85
  of enteric nervous system, 224
Cholinergic receptors. *See* Muscarinic
    cholinergic receptors; Nicotinic
    cholinergic receptors.
Chorea, in distemper, 68
Chorion, 516, 517
Chorionic girdle, 401
Chorionic gonadotropin (CG)
  equine, 335, 401–402, 401f
  primate, 335, 400, 400f, 402
Choroid, 87, 87f, 88
Choroid plexuses, 94, 95f, 96, 505
Chromaffin cells, 357, 357f, 358, 360
Chronic obstructive pulmonary disease
  hypoxic vasoconstriction in, 176
  in horse, 477
Chylomicrons, 275–276, 275f, 312, 313
Chymosin (rennin), 260t
Chymosinogen, 260
Chymotrypsin, 260t, 261f
Chymotrypsinogen, 260t, 261f
Cilia, of respiratory epithelium, 509, 509f,
    510, 512–513
Ciliary body, 87f, 88, 89, 92
Ciliary ganglion, 92
Ciliary muscle, 87f, 88–89, 89f
  epinephrine and, 359
Ciliary process, 92
Circadian rhythms, 331
  in glucocorticoid secretion, 352, 352f
Circling, compulsive, 70, 73
Circulation
  bronchial, 479, 484
  central, 115, 115f
    blood volume in, 117, 117t
  enterohepatic, 252, 252f
    iodide in, 344
  fetal, 404, 518, 518f, 520
  pulmonary. *See* Pulmonary circulation.
  splanchnic, 115, 115f, 116
    vasoconstriction in
      exercise-induced, 174f, 175
      in heart failure, 212
  systemic, 115–116, 115f
    blood volume distribution in, 117,
      117t
    perfusion pressure of, 116
    pressure profile in, 169–170,
      170f
    resistance of, 172–173
    vessels of, 117, 117t, 118f
Circus movement, 138
Cisterna magna, 95, 97
Cisterns, mammary, 407, 409f, 414
Citrate
  as anticoagulant, 118
  in fatty acid synthesis, 308, 309f
Civetone, 395
CL. *See* Corpus luteum (CL).
Clara cells, 509, 509f
Clearance equation, 437
Climbing fibers, 76, 76f, 78
Clitoris, 375
Cloaca, 242, 242f, 243
  salt reabsorption and, 447, 457
  water reabsorption and, 457
Coactivation, of α and γ lower motor
    neurons, 66

Coagulation
  of blood, 118, 119
  of milk, 416
Coated pits, 18, 18f
  of proximal tubules, 441f, 444f
Cochlea, 70, 70f, 104–106, 105f–106f
  congenital defect of, 106
Coelomic epithelium, 374
Cold adaptation, gastrointestinal, 228
Cold stress, 540. *See also* Hypothermia;
    Temperature.
  blood flow in, 536–537, 537f
  catecholamine response to, 360
  frostbite in, 543
  respiratory response to, 470
  skin receptors and, 538–539
Cold-blooded animals, 533, 534
Colic, equine
  impaction causing, 300–301, 302
  Strongylus causing, 111, 121–122
Co-lipase, 272, 274f
Collateral ventilation, 476
Colligative properties, 11
Colloid, of thyroid gland, 342–343, 342f
Colloid osmotic (oncotic) pressure, 11–12,
    184–186. *See also* Osmotic pressure.
  edema and, 28, 188, 189, 190
  in glomerular capillary, 433, 434f
  in pulmonary fluid exchange, 511–512,
    511f
Colloid reflection coefficient, 511
Colon
  bicarbonate reabsorption in, 267–268,
    267f
  electrolyte absorption mechanisms in,
    268t
  fermentation in, 281, 282, 283, 289
    in horse, 298–302, 299f–301f
    species differences and, 239, 239f
  functions of, 239
  impaction of, in horse, 300–301, 302
  in carnivores, 239f–240f, 240
  in horse, 239f, 240–241
    fermentation and, 298–302, 299f–301f
  in ruminants and swine, 239f, 241
  motility of, 231, 233, 240–241, 240f–241f
    in horse, 298–301
  potassium absorption in, 268
  species differences in, 239, 239f, 240,
    241, 301–302
Color blindness, 91
Color vision, 89, 91
Colostral milk, 416
Colostrum, 409–410, 410t
  antibodies in, 276, 410
    neonatal isoerythrolysis and, 418, 419
  changeover from, to milk, 416
  delayed, fetal defect causing, 404
Common bile duct
  pancreatic secretions in, 250
  sphincter of Oddi and, 252
Complement, in respiratory secretions,
    510
Compliance
  of arteries, 170, 171f
    definition of, 170
    pulse pressure and, 178–179, 178f–
    179f
  of lungs
    alveolar hypoventilation and, 487,
    487f
    decreased, 475, 476–477, 476f
    definition of, 472
    pleural pressure and, 471
  of veins, 170, 171f, 181
  of ventricles, 158, 158f, 160

Concentration gradient
  membrane potential and, 16–17
  molecular transport and, 9, 10, 11, 183–
    184
Conduction deafness, 106
Conduction system, cardiac, 126,
    126f–127f
  dysfunction in, 135–136, 135t
Conduction velocity, cardiac, 133, 134,
    134t, 135
Conductive heat loss, 534, 534f, 535
Cones, 89, 89f, 90, 91, 91f
Congestive heart failure. *See* Heart failure.
Connecting segment, renal, 446–447, 448
  bicarbonate secretion by, 464
  calcium reabsorption in, 449
  H⁺ concentration in, 462
Conscious proprioception, 52, 66–67, 69
  lower motor neuron disease and, 59
  upper motor neuron disease and, 60
Consciousness, 63
Continuous murmurs, 161, 162, 197
Contractility. *See* Cardiac contractility.
Convective heat loss, 534–535, 534f, 540
Cooling. *See* Heat.
Coonhound paralysis, 59–60
Copulation
  luteal phase and, 385, 387
  ovulation induced by, 387, 387f, 399
Cor pulmonale, 483
Core temperature, 536, 537–538, 539
Cornea, 87, 87f, 88
  electroretinogram and, 91
Coronary arteries, 114–115
Coronary arterioles, 174f, 175
Coronary artery disease, 115
  exercise in, 196
  hypertension with, 164
  ventricular ischemia in, 196
Coronary blood flow, control of, 195–196,
    199
  autonomic, 200, 201, 201t, 202
Coronary veins, 491
Corpus cavernosum penis, 423
Corpus luteum (CL), 384–387. *See also*
    Luteal phase.
  at puberty, 391, 392
  estrous cycle and, 389, 390, 393, 393f
  in pregnancy, 399, 400, 400f–401f, 401–
    402
  persistent in mare, 387–388
  regression of, 382, 383f, 385–386, 385f–
    386f
    before delivery, 403
    induced, 388
  relaxin produced by, 404
Corpus spongiosum penis, 423
Corti, organ of, 105, 106f
Corticobulbar tract, 64, 65, 66
Corticopontine-cerebellar tract, 64, 66, 78
Corticospinal tract, 63–64, 64f, 65, 66
  lesions of, 66–67
Corticosteroid-binding globulin, 350
Corticosteroids. *See* Glucocorticoids.
Corticosterone, 350
  negative feedback by, 352
  transport of, in blood, 328
Corticotropin (ACTH), 335, 336f, 337, 376
  deficiency of, 356
  fetal, 402, 402f, 404
  in Cushing's disease, 339
  mechanism of action of, 350f, 351–352
  mineralocorticoid secretion and, 356
Corticotropin stimulation test, 354, 356
Corticotropin-like intermediate lobe
  peptide, 335, 336f

Corticotropin-releasing hormone, 336–337,
    337t, 352, 352f
Cortisol, 349, 350. *See also* Glucocorticoids.
  circadian rhythm of, 352f
  deficiency of, 356
  excess of, 353–354
  fetal, 401, 402, 402f
    deficient, 404
    lung maturity and, 472, 519
  glucose mobilization by, 316–317
  mineralocorticoid activity of, 351, 351t
  negative feedback by, 352, 352f
  phenylethanolamine-N-
    methyltransferase and, 358
  stress and, 352, 352f
  transport of, in blood, 328, 350, 351
Cosyntropin, 356
Co-transport proteins, 13–14, 13f, 263,
    263f–264f, 265–266. *See also* Sodium
    co-transport.
Cotyledonary placenta, 516, 516t, 517,
    517f, 518
Coughing, 475, 503, 510
Countercurrent exchange
  in loop of Henle, 431f, 460–461
  in placenta, 517–518, 517f
  of heat, 537, 538f
  of PGF₂α, 385
  urine osmolality and, 453–455, 454f–455f
Cow, lactation in, 396, 417, 417f
Cowper (bulbourethral) glands, 421, 422t,
    423
CPT I (carnitine palmitoyltransferase I),
    318, 318f, 319
Cranial nerves. *See also* Glossopharyngeal
    nerve; Vagus nerve.
  eighth, 73, 105
  parasympathetic nervous system and,
    81f–82f, 82
  pupillary light reflex and, 92
Craniosacral system, 82
Creatine phosphokinase, in
    hypothyroidism, 347
Creatinine
  fractional excretion rate of, 440
  proximal tubular secretion of, 444
Creatinine clearance, 437
Cremaster muscles, 421
Cricopharyngeal muscle, 234
Crista dividens, 518
Critical organs, 192, 195, 199, 200
  baroreceptor reflex and, 204
  defense-alarm reaction and, 206
Crop, 242–243, 242f
  salivary amylase and, 245
Crotalaria spp., 512
Cryptorchidism, 393, 422
Crypts of Lieberkühn, 223f, 255, 256f
  replication of enterocytes in, 276
  secretion by, 269–270, 269f
    in diarrhea, 277, 278
CSF (cerebrospinal fluid), 33, 94–97, 95f
  pH of, ventilation and, 504–505, 504f–
    505f
  pressure of, 96–97
Cud chewing, 293
Cumulus oophorus, 380
Cupula, 71f–72f, 72
Curare, nicotinic receptors and, 83
Curdling, 416
Cushing's disease, equine, 338–339, 352f
Cushing's syndrome
  canine, 353–354
  feline, 353, 354
Cyanosis, 120, 496
  congenital cardiac defect causing, 507

Cyanosis *(Continued)*
    in brachycephalic syndrome, 492
Cyclic adenosine-3',5'-monophosphate
    (cAMP), 20, 23–24, 24f, 25
    chloride channels and, 269–270, 277
    glucagon and, 364, 364f
    hormone activity and, 325, 329, 330f
        parathyroid, 368, 449
        thyroid, 346
Cyclic guanosine monophosphate (cGMP),
    24
Cyclic nucleotide phosphodiesterase, 23,
    24
Cyclooxygenase, fever and, 541
Cytokines
    fever and, 541, 542f
    in gastrointestinal system, 227
    in lung defense, 510–511

D

D cells, 360, 361f, 365, 366f
DAG (diacylglycerol), 20, 25, 25f, 26
    hormone action and, 329
Dead-space, 469, 470f
Dead-space ventilation, 469–470, 491
    in panting, 535
Dead-space/tidal volume ratio (VD/VT),
    469
Deafness, 106
Deamination of amino acids, 311–312,
    311f, 315, 316
Death, rigor mortis in, 6, 8
Decerebrate rigidity, 68
Decibel scale, 104
Decremental conduction, 136, 140
Defecation, 241, 241f
    in birds, 243
    respiratory system and, 503
Defense-alarm reaction, 83, 133, 201, 202,
    206, 206f, 356–357, 359. *See also*
    Stressful stimuli.
Deferent ducts (vasa deferentia), 421, 422,
    423
    embryonic development of, 374, 375f–
    376f
Defibrillation, 138
Deglutition. *See* Swallowing (deglutition).
Dehydration
    ADH release in, 456
    arterial pressure reduction in, 173
    in calf diarrhea, 278
    in diabetes insipidus, 335
7-Dehydrocholesterol, 370, 370f
Dehydroepiandrosterone, 401
Dendrites, 32, 34, 35f
11-Deoxycorticosterone, 350
Deoxyhemoglobin, buffering by, 497, 498,
    524
Depolarization
    by action potential, 37, 37f–38f, 38
    by excitatory potential, 36
Desynchronized EEG, 100
Detergent action, 251, 272
Dexamethasone, 353f
Dexamethasone suppression test, 354
Dextrins, 259, 259f, 260
Diabetes insipidus, 333–335, 456, 457
Diabetes mellitus, 360, 363, 371–372. *See
    also* Insulin.
    acromegaly with, 338
    glucagon in, 364
    glucosuria in, 449
    hyperadrenocorticism with, 353–354
    ketone bodies in, 318–319
Diacylglycerol (DAG), 20, 25, 25f, 26

Diacylglycerol (DAG) *(Continued)*
    hormone action and, 329
Diaphragm, 470
    neural control of, 502
    stretch receptors of, 503
Diarrhea, 276–278, 277f
    metabolic acidosis caused by, 527
    neonatal, 530–531, 531f
    potassium and, 268
Diastasis, 155
Diastole, ventricular, 154, 155, 155f
Diastolic filling time, 158, 160, 160f, 161
Diastolic murmurs, 161, 161t, 162, 162f
Diastolic pressures, 116, 176–177, 176f
Dictyate stage, 379
Diencephalon, 33, 63, 63f
Diestrus, 389, 390f
Differential white blood cell count, 119
Diffusion
    across capillary walls, 182–185, 182f–
    183f
    facilitated, 14–15, 14f, 183
        in glucose absorption, 265
        in proximal tubule, 443
    Fick's law of, 183–184, 183f
    free energy and, 9
    in intestinal absorption, 264–265, 265f,
        270
    in proximal tubule, 440, 442, 443
    in secondary active transport, 13
    of gases
        between alveolus and capillary, 468,
            488, 488f–489f
        between blood and tissues, 113, 114f,
            117, 183–184, 468, 469f, 488–489,
            489f
    of particles in airways, 508, 509f
    of water, 184–187
Diffusion coefficient, 183
Digestion, 257–262
    cephalic phase of, 236, 249, 250
        in ruminant, 298
    definition of, 255, 255f
    fermentative. *See* Fermentative diges-
        tion.
    hydrolysis in, 258, 258f
    in neonate, 276
    luminal phase of, 258–260, 259f, 260t,
        262f
    membranous phase of, 258, 259f, 260–
        262, 261f–262f
        absorption and, 265, 266f
    of carbohydrates, 258–260, 258f–259f,
        261–262, 261f–262f
    of fats, 258, 258f, 271–272, 273f–274f
        bile acids and, 251, 252
        pancreatic enzymes in, 250
    of proteins, 258, 258f, 260, 260t, 261f–
        262f, 262
        pancreatic enzymes in, 249, 250
        pancreatic polypeptide and, 366
    particle size reduction in, 257–258
Digestive enzymes
    amylase as, 245, 246, 259, 262f
    gastric, 247, 248–249, 257, 260, 260t
    membranous-phase, 260–262, 261f–262f
    microbial, 283, 286
    pancreatic. *See* Pancreas, exocrine secre-
        tions of.
    two general classes of, 258
Dihydrotestosterone, 330, 375, 425
Dihydroxyphenylalanine (DOPA), 5, 5f,
    357, 357f–358f
Diiodotyrosine, 342, 343, 343f
Dilative cardiomyopathy
    exercise intolerance in, 217–218

Dilative cardiomyopathy *(Continued)*
    paroxysmal atrial tachycardia in, 151–
    152
Diluting segments, of nephron, 446, 455
Dilution rate, in rumen, 293–294
Dipalmitoyl phosphatidylcholine, 472
Dipeptides, absorption of, 262, 262f, 265,
    266f
Diphosphoglycerate (DPG)
    in fetus, 519
    oxyhemoglobin dissociation curve and,
    496
Diplotene stage, 379
Direct pupillary light reflex, 92
Dirofilaria immitis. See Heartworm disease.
Disaccharides, 258–259, 260
    digestion of, 261–262, 261f–262f
Dissociation constant, 523
Distal tubule, 431f, 444–446, 446f–447f
    calcium reabsorption in, 449
    connecting segment and, 446–447
    tubuloglomerular feedback and, 436
    water balance and, 453, 455
Distemper, chorea in, 68
Distending pressure, 112–113
Diuretics
    loop of Henle and, 445
    renal excretion of, 444
Diurnal rhythms, 331
DNA, transcription factors and, 26, 27f, 28
Dog
    acromegaly in, progesterone and, 338
    bladder infection in, in spayed bitch,
        396
    brachycephalic syndrome in, 492
    Cushing's syndrome in, 353–354
    heartworm disease in, 111
        pulmonary embolism and, 179–180
        tricuspid stenosis and, 162
    hypothyroidism in, 417
    lactational induction in, 417
    mitral insufficiency in, 513
    ovariectomy in, mammary neoplasia
        and, 418
    panting in, 469–470
    pituitary dwarfism in, 338
    pregnancy diagnosis in, 404
    pulmonary fibrosis in, 476–477
    sexual receptivity in, 385
DOPA (dihydroxyphenylalanine), 5, 5f,
    357, 357f–358f
Dopamine
    biosynthesis of, 5, 5f, 357–358, 357f–358f
    hypothalamic production of, 337, 337t,
        377
    in carotid bodies, 503
    in sympathetic ganglia, 82
    nonintention tremor and, 68
    prolactin secretion and, 379, 379f, 395,
        412, 412f
Dopamine-β-hydroxylase, 5, 5f, 358, 358f
Dormitory effect, 395
Dorsal nerve roots, 33, 33f, 51, 62
Dorsal respiratory group, 502, 502f
Dorsal root ganglia, 81
DPG (diphosphoglycerate)
    in fetus, 519
    oxyhemoglobin dissociation curve and,
    496
Ductus arteriosus, 404, 518, 518f, 520
    patent, 161f–162f, 162, 164f, 165
        case studies of, 197–198, 520–521
        pulse pressure and, 178f, 179
Ductus deferens. *See* Deferent ducts (vasa
    deferentia).
Ductus venosus, 404, 518

Duodenum
  bile in, 252, 274f
  electrolyte absorption in, 268t
  gastric acid secretion and, 249
  gastric emptying and, 237, 237f, 238
  motility of, 231, 238–239
  pancreatic secretions and, 250, 260
Dura mater, 33, 33f
  venous sinuses in, 95, 95f
Dwarfism, pituitary, in dogs, 338
Dysmetria, 78, 79

E

Ear
  external, 104, 105f
  inner, 70–71, 70f. *See also* Cochlea; Vestibular system.
  middle, 104, 105, 105f–106f
Eardrum (tympanic membrane), 104, 105, 105f–106f
Eccentric implantation, 400
Eccrine glands, 535
ECG (electrocardiogram), 142–151
  abnormal patterns in, 147–151, 147f–151f
  basic principles of, 142–144, 143f–144f
  leads used for, 146–147, 146f
  normal trace in, 144–146, 145f–146f
eCG (equine chorionic gonadotropin), 335, 401–402, 401f
Ectopic pacemaker, 137, 138, 139
  ECG and, 149
  paroxysmal atrial tachycardia and, 160
Edema, 184, 185, 187–190, 188f–190f
  capillary filtration and, 12
  fluid therapy causing, 111
  in brisket disease, 483, 484–485
  in heart failure, 28, 188, 211–212, 211f
  pulmonary. *See* Pulmonary edema.
Edrophonium, myasthenia gravis and, 43
EEG (electroencephalogram), 98, 99–100, 100f–102f
  brain tumor and, 103
Effector (target) organ, 51, 51f, 52
Efferent arteriole, glomerular, 432, 432f, 433, 435, 436
Efferent (motor) nerves, 32t, 33. *See also* Motor neuron(s).
Egestion, 243
Einthoven's triangle, 146f, 147
Ejaculation, 422, 423
Ejection fraction, 154
  during exercise, 160t
Ejection zone, 292, 292f
Elastase, 260t, 261f
Elastic force, respiratory, 470
Elastic lamina, of pulmonary arterioles, 479
Elastic vessels, 181
Elasticity, of lung, 471–472, 471f–472f
Electrical dipole, 142, 143f
Electrical potential. *See* Action potential(s); Electrochemical potential; Resting membrane potential.
Electrical synapses, 41
Electrocardiogram (ECG), 142–151
  abnormal patterns in, 147–151, 147f–151f
  basic principles of, 142–144, 143f–144f
  leads used for, 146–147, 146f
  normal trace in, 144–146, 145f–146f
Electrochemical potential, 9–10
  across gut surface, 267
  active transport and, 12
  facilitated diffusion and, 14

Electrochemical potential *(Continued)*
  sodium co-transport and, 263–264, 263f–264f
Electroencephalogram (EEG), 98, 99–100, 100f–102f
  brain tumor and, 103
Electrolytes
  cardiovascular function and, 111
  in plasma, 118, 119t
  intestinal absorption of, 265–269, 266f–268f, 268t
  intestinal secretion of, 269–270, 269f
  mineralocorticoids and, 354–355, 354t
Electromagnetic radiation, infrared, 534f, 535
Electromyogram, 48
Electrophysiologic procedures, 98
Electroretinogram, 91
Elephantiasis, 189
Embden-Meyerhof pathway. *See* Glycolysis.
Embryo, 399. *See also* Fetus.
  implantation of, 400–401
Emission, 423
Emotional arousal, 206, 206f
Emulsification, 272, 274f
End product inhibition, 5
End-diastolic ventricular pressure. *See* Preload.
End-diastolic ventricular volume, 154, 156–158, 157f–159f, 159–160
Endocrine activity, definition of, 225
Endocrine system. *See also* Hormone(s).
  amplification of signal from, 325
  gastrointestinal, 224–226, 226f, 227t, 228t
    cytokines and, 227
    enterogastric reflex and, 237
  nervous system and, 325
Endocytosis, 17–18, 17f–18f
  in capillary endothelium, 186
  in renal tubular reabsorption, 441f, 444, 444f
  of receptor-hormone complex, 329
  of receptors, 18, 18f, 21
Endolymph, 71, 72, 73, 105
Endometrial cups, 401f, 402
Endometrial glands, fertilization and, 399
Endometrium, implantation in, 400–401
Endopeptidases, 260, 260t
  microbial, 286
Endoplasmic reticulum
  calcium channels in, 25
  in hormone synthesis, 326, 326f
  milk proteins synthesized on, 412, 413f
  of muscle fiber, 45
  of neuron, 34
β-Endorphin, 335, 336f, 339
  gonadotropin secretion and, 379
Endosome, 18, 18f
Endothelial cells
  of arterioles
    muscarinic receptors of, 201t, 202
    pulmonary, 479
  of capillaries, 181
    diffusion through, 182, 182f, 183
    glomerular, 432, 433f, 435
    lipoprotein lipase of, 313
    oncotic pressure and, 11
    pinocytosis by, 186, 188
    pores in, 182–183, 182f
    pulmonary, 511, 511f, 512
Endothelin, 436
Endotheliochorial placentation, 516, 516t
Endothelium-derived relaxing factor. *See* Nitric oxide.
Endotoxic shock, 111–112

Endotoxic shock *(Continued)*
  in *Strongylus* infestation, 121–122
Endotracheal tube, dead-space and, 470, 470f
End-systolic ventricular volume, 154, 156, 158–159, 160
Energy deficiency, 317–320, 317f–319f
Enteric nervous system, 81, 82, 222, 223f–225f, 224
  colonic pacemaker and, 240
  cytokines and, 227
  gastric acid secretion and, 249
  gastric emptying and, 237, 237f
  pancreatic secretions and, 250
  smooth muscle contraction and, 232–233
    in esophagus, 234
Enterochromaffin-like cells, 249
Enterocyte(s), 255–257, 256f–257f. *See also* Absorption, intestinal; Villus(i).
  basolateral membrane of, 256, 257f, 263
  chloride transport through, 266–267, 269, 269f
  glucose transport through, 265
  digestive enzymes of, 261–262, 261f–262f
  in neonate, 276
  infectious injury to, 277, 277f
  lateral spaces of, 256–257, 257f, 265f
    chloride absorption through, 267, 267f
    chylomicrons in, 275
    glucose diffusion through, 265
    nutrient absorption from, 270
    water in, 270, 270f
    water secretion and, 269
  of crypts, 269, 269f, 276
  replication of, 276
  transport systems of, 263–265, 263f–266f
Enterogastric reflex, 237, 237f
Enteroglucagon, 226, 228
Enterohepatic circulation, 252, 252f
  iodide in, 344
Enterokinase, 260, 261f
Enteropathy, protein-losing, 190–191
Enterotoxins, 277–278
Entropy of solution, 11
Enzymes, 3
  digestive. *See* Digestive enzymes.
  in catecholamine biosynthesis, 5, 5f, 357–358, 357f–358f
  ligand-dependent, 19–20, 20f, 23, 24f
Epididymis, 421, 422
  androgens in, 425
  embryonic development of, 374, 376f
  fertilization and, 398
Epinephrine, 82, 83
  actions of, 358–359, 359f
  adipose tissue and, 317
  adrenal medulla and, 357
  biosynthesis of, 5, 5f, 357–358, 357f–358f
  cardiovascular effects of, 135, 200, 201, 201t
  cyclic AMP and, 23, 24
  discovery of, 356
  glucocorticoids and, 351
  hypoglycemia and, 359–360
  in defense-alarm reaction, 206
  insulin secretion and, 363
  parathyroid hormone secretion and, 368
  pulmonary vascular response to, 483t
  renal excretion of, 444
  smooth muscle effects of, 359
  stressful stimuli and, 24
Epitheliochorial placentation, 516, 516t
Epoöphoron, 376f
EPSP (excitatory postsynaptic potential), 36, 37, 37f

EPSP (excitatory postsynaptic potential) (Continued)
  EEG and, 99
Equilibrium, electrochemical, 9–10
Equilibrium potential, of ion, 16
Equipment dead-space, 470, 470f
Eructation contractions, 290, 291f
Erythrocyte sedimentation rate (ESR), 119
Erythrocytes, 119–121, 121f
  carbon dioxide in, 497–498, 497f
  diphosphoglycerate in, 496
  fetal, 519
  from splenic contraction, 495, 498
  oxygen capacity and, 113, 495
  pentose-phosphate pathway in, 306
Erythropoietin, chronic renal failure and, 437, 438
Escherichia coli, enterotoxigenic, 277–278
Esophageal groove, 297–298
Esophagus, motility of, 234–235
ESR (erythrocyte sedimentation rate), 119
Ester bond, hydrolysis of, 258, 258f
Estradiol-17
  follicular synthesis of, 380
  metabolism of, 330
  sexual behavior and, 392
Estriol, 401
Estrogen(s)
  biosynthesis of, 327f, 328
    embryonic, 399
    follicular, 380, 384
    in adrenal cortex, 350
  fertilization and, 398
  gonadotropin secretion and, 378–379, 391
  in induced ovulators, 387
  hypothalamic development and, 392
  in male, 375
  in mammary development, 409, 410f
  in parturition, 402, 402f, 403
  in pregnancy, 399, 401, 401f
  lactation and, 409, 417
  luteinization and, 331, 385
  luteolysis and, 386
  mammary neoplasia and, 418
  menopause and, 392
  metabolism of, 330
  ovalbumin expression and, 26, 27f
  prolactin secretion and, 379
  sexual receptivity and, 392–393
  testicular, 425, 426f
  thyroid hormone binding and, 344
Estrogen receptor, 26, 27f
Estrogen response element, 26, 27f
Estrogen-binding proteins, 328
Estrone, 330
Estrous cycle, 389–390, 390f. *See also* Ovarian cycle(s).
  photoperiod and, in cat, 417
  uterine infection and, 386
Estrus, 389, 390, 390f, 392–394, 393f. *See also* Sexual receptivity.
  lactation and, 395
  pheromones and, 395
  photoperiod and, 394
Eupnea, 502
Eustachian tube, 104, 105f
Euthyroid sick syndrome, 347, 348
  with hyperadrenocorticism, 347, 353
Evaporative heat loss, 534, 534f, 535, 540, 540f
Evoked potentials, 100, 103, 103f, 106
Exchange vessels, 181
Exchangers. *See* Antiports.
Excitation-contraction coupling, 7
  in cardiac muscle, 49

Excitation-contraction coupling (Continued)
  in skeletal muscle, 48
  in smooth muscle, 21, 22f, 23, 49
Excitatory postsynaptic potential (EPSP), 36, 37, 37f
  EEG and, 99
Exercise
  brain cooling during, 537
  cardiac output during, 160, 160f, 160t, 483, 498, 498f
    metabolic control and, 216
    muscle pump and, 217
    respiratory pump and, 217
    vascular resistance and, 173, 174f
    with atrial fibrillation, 499
  cardiovascular response to, 216–217, 216f–217f
  gas exchange during, 468, 469f, 487, 488, 489, 489f
  heat production during, 536
  laryngeal hemiplegia and, in horses, 470
  oxygen demands of, 498–499, 498f
  pulmonary circulation during, 175, 479, 481, 481f, 482, 483
  pulmonary fluid exchange and, 511
  pulmonary hemorrhage during, in horse, 483
  respiratory muscles and, 470, 471f
  skeletal muscle changes in
    arteriolar vasodilation and, 174f, 175, 183–184, 192, 216
    capillary blood flow and, 183–184
    gas transport and, 498–499
  splenic contraction during, 495
  ventilatory response to, 469, 505
Exercise intolerance
  aortic stenosis with, 165
  atrial fibrillation with, 155
  coronary artery disease with, 196
  heart failure with, 111, 175, 209, 211, 217–218
  mitral regurgitation with, 164–165
  patent ductus arteriosus with, 165
  pulmonic stenosis with, 166
  ventricular septal defect with, 165
Exercise reflex, 216
Exhalation, 470, 471f
  central regulation of, 502
  forced, 475
  functional residual capacity and, 470–471
  muscle contraction in, 470
  residual volume and, 472
Exocrine effectors, 325
Exocytosis, 17, 17f, 18
  in capillary endothelium, 186
  in mammary gland, 412, 413f
  in pancreas, 25–26
  of protein hormones, 326, 326f
    in neurohypophysis, 333
Exopeptidases, 260, 260t
Extension, 44
Extensor antigravity muscles, 62, 67–68
Extra-alveolar vessels, 479–480, 480f
  resistance in, 482, 482f
Extracellular fluid. *See* Interstitial fluid; Plasma.
Extrafusal muscle fibers, 54, 62
Extragonadal sperm reserves, 422
Extraocular muscles, vestibular reflexes and, 73
Extrapyramidal system, 62, 63, 67–68
  cerebellum and, 75, 76, 77f, 78
  lesions of, 68
Eye. *See also* Retina; Visual system.

Eye (Continued)
  anatomy of, 87–88, 87f–88f
  autonomic control of, 83, 84t, 85
  catecholamines and, 359
  movement of, 73
    vestibulocerebellum and, 77
Eyelid, innervation of, 92

F

F cells, 360, 361f, 365
Facilitated diffusion, 14–15, 14f, 183
  in glucose absorption, 265
  in proximal tubule, 443
F-actin, 6, 6f
FAD (flavin adenine dinucleotide), microbial, 283, 284f
Faraday constant, 16
Far-field potentials, 100
Fast action potentials, 132
Fast sodium channels, 129, 130–131
Fasting, 317–320, 317f–319f
Fast-twitch fibers, 48–49
  myoglobin in, 498
Fats (lipids). *See also* Phospholipids.
  absorption of, 271–272, 273f–275f, 275–276
  digestion of, 258, 258f, 271–272, 273f–274f
    bile acids and, 251, 252
    pancreatic enzymes for, 250
  emulsification of, 272, 274f
  in colostrum, 410, 410t
  in milk, 412, 413f, 415–416, 415t
  insulin and, 361, 362, 362f, 362t
  malabsorption of, 278
  metabolism of
    glucocorticoids and, 351
    heat produced by, 536, 536t
    hydrogen ions from, 522
    thyroid hormones and, 345
Fatty acid–binding proteins, 272
Fatty acids
  chemical structures of, 273f
  epinephrine and, 359
  from adipose tissue, 317
  from triglyceride hydrolysis, 272, 313
  glucagon and, 364
  hepatic metabolism of, 317–319, 317f–318f
  in biomembranes, 8, 8f
  in milk, 415
  insulin and, 361, 362, 362f, 363
  ketone bodies derived from, 318–319, 318f
  nonesterified, 317, 319, 320
  β-oxidation of, 305, 306f, 319
  storage function of, 306–307, 313
  sympathetic discharge and, 83
  synthesis of
    by ruminants, 320
    in adipose tissue, 308, 313
    in liver, 307–308, 309f, 312, 318, 318f
  transport of
    in blood, 317
    out of liver, 308, 309f
  VLDL formation from, 308, 309f, 319
  volatile. *See* Volatile fatty acids (VFA).
Fatty liver, in cat, 321
Fear, fight, or flight reaction. *See* Defense-alarm reaction.
Feces. *See also* Defecation.
  equine, 301
Feline panleukopenia virus, cerebellar hypoplasia and, 79
Femoral arterial pressure, 176f, 177

Femoral nerve, mononeuropathy of, 56
Fenestrated capillaries, 182, 182f
  glomerular, 432, 433f
  peritubular, 442f
Ferguson reflex
  milk removal and, 414
  parturition and, 403, 403f
Fermentative digestion, 281. See also
      Rumen; Ruminant(s).
  efficiency of, 287, 288f
  grain engorgement toxemia and, 302
  in colon, 281, 282, 283, 289. See also
      Hindgut.
  of horse, 298–302, 299f–301f
    species differences and, 239, 239f
  in equine hindgut, 298–302, 299f–301f
  microbial ecosystem of, 281–282, 282t
    establishment of, 297
  of carbohydrates, 283–285, 284f–286f,
      285t, 287, 288f
    in equine hindgut, 298
  omasal function in, 295
  overall reaction in, 287
  protein in, 281, 283, 285–288, 286f, 288f
    in equine hindgut, 298
  sites of, 281
  substrates of, 282–283
  VFAs in. See Volatile fatty acids (VFAs).
Fertilization, 398–399
Fetal zone, of adrenal cortex, 349
Fetus
  adrenal medullary hormones in, 357
  aortic bodies in, 503
  circulation in, 404, 518, 518f, 520
  cortisol in, 401, 402, 402f
    deficient, 404
    lung maturity and, 472, 519
  energy sources for, 320–321
  gonadal development in, 374–375, 375f–
      376f, 401, 401f
  hemoglobin of, 495, 519, 519f
  hypoxia in, 518, 519, 520
  labor and, 402, 402f, 404
  lung development in, 472, 519–520
  mammary glands of, 407, 408
  oxygen transport in, 516–520, 517f–519f
  red blood cell–agglutinating antibodies
      against, 418, 419
  steroid metabolism of, 401, 401f
Fever, 541, 542f
Fiber, dietary, 258
  for diabetic animal, 372
Fibrin, 118, 119
Fibrinogen, 118, 119, 119t, 120, 121f
Fick's law of diffusion, 183–184, 183f
Fight or flight reaction. See Defense-alarm
      reaction.
Filarial parasites, lymphedema caused by,
      189
Filtration, of water, 12, 28, 184–188, 189,
      190
Filtration coefficient, 185, 511
Fimbria, 374, 376f
FIO₂ (fraction of inspired oxygen), 486,
      487, 491
First polar body, 384
Fistulas, arteriovenous, 162
Flaccid paralysis, 58
Flavin adenine dinucleotide (FAD),
      microbial, 283, 284f
Flea infestation, in cat, 499
Flexion, 44
Flexor muscles, 62, 66
Flexor reflex, 52
Flocculonodular lobe, 73, 77
Fludrocortisone, 353f

Fludrocortisone (Continued)
  for hypoadrenocorticism, 450
Fluid mosaic model, 8, 8f, 9
Fluid therapy
  for calf diarrhea, 278
  incorrect, 111
FO₂ (fraction of oxygen), 486
Follicle. See Ovarian follicle(s).
Follicle cells, 374, 375f
Follicle-stimulating hormone (FSH), 335,
      376–377, 377f. See also Gonadotropins.
  in male, 425, 426, 426f, 427
  inhibin and, 379, 382, 384
  ovarian receptors for, 329, 380, 384
Follicular atresia, 384
Follicular phase, 377f, 378, 379, 386–387
  estrous cycle and, 389, 390
Food deprivation, 317–320, 317f–319f
Foot processes, 433, 434f
Foramen of Magendie, 95
Foramen of Monro, 94
Foramen ovale, 404, 518, 518f, 520
  patent, 506
Forced convection, 534
Forestomach(s), 281, 283. See also Rumen.
  epithelium of, 294, 295–296, 296f
  VFA absorption in, 295–297, 296f–297f
Forward heart failure, 213
Fourth ventricle, 94, 95f, 96
Fovea, 90, 90f, 91
Foveola, 90, 90f
Fraction of inspired oxygen (FIO₂), 486,
      487, 491
Fraction of oxygen (FO₂), 486
Fractional excretion rate, 439–440
Fractional reabsorption rate, 440
FRC (functional residual capacity), 471
  in newborn, 520
  pulmonary vascular resistance and, 482,
      482f
Free energy, molecular transport and,
      9–10, 11
Frequency, of sound wave, 104, 104f, 105
Frequency coding, of action potentials, 51
Friction
  in airways. See Airway resistance.
  in systemic circulation, 169, 177
Frontal lobe, 64, 64f
Frostbite, 543
Fructose, 258, 259, 262, 262f
  spermatozoa and, 398
Fructose-1,6-bisphosphatase, 314, 314f, 315
FSH (follicle-stimulating hormone), 335,
      376–377, 377f. See also Gonadotropins.
  in male, 425, 426, 426f, 427
  inhibin and, 379, 382, 384
  ovarian receptors for, 329, 380, 384
Fuel homeostasis, 305, 306, 313
Functional residual capacity (FRC), 471
  in newborn, 520
  pulmonary vascular resistance and, 482,
      482f
Fusion, of muscle contractions, 130

G

G cells, 249
G proteins, 23, 24, 24f, 25
GABA (γ-aminobutyric acid)
  prolactin and, 379
  Purkinje neurons and, 76
G-actin, 6f
Gait
  respiratory frequency and, 470, 471f,
      505
  wide-based, 78, 79

Galactose, 258, 262, 262f
  absorption of, 261f, 265
  in lactose, 416
Galactosyl transferase, 416
Gallbladder, 252, 252f
  pancreatic polypeptide and, 366
γ loop, 55, 66, 67, 67f, 68
Ganglion (ganglia), 80–81, 81f
Ganglion cells, of retina, 88, 89, 89f, 90, 91
GAP (GnRH-associated peptide), 377–378,
      379, 395
Gap junctions
  of granulosa, 380
  of intercalated disks, 125
  of visceral smooth muscle, 49
    gastrointestinal, 231
    uterine, 402
Gartner's cyst, 376f
Gas exchange, 113–114, 114f, 183–184,
      488–491, 488f–490f
  abbreviations used for, 486t
  processes involved in, 468, 469f
Gases, toxic, 509
Gastric. See also Stomach.
Gastric inhibitory peptide (GIP), 227t
  gastric emptying and, 237
  gastric motility and, 236
  insulin secretion and, 307, 363
Gastric phase, 249, 250
Gastric pits, 247, 248f
Gastric secretions, 247–249, 248f, 258. See
      also Hydrochloric acid (HCl).
Gastrin, 226, 227t, 228, 228f, 249
  calcitonin and, 369
  gastric motility and, 236
  insulin secretion and, 363
  pancreatic polypeptide and, 366
Gastrointestinal motility, 230
  action potentials in, 232–233, 232f
  functions of, 230
  in birds, 241, 242–243
  in swallow reflex, 233–234, 233f
  of colon, 231, 233, 240–241, 240f–241f
    equine, 299
  of esophagus, 234–235
  of rumen, 289–290, 291f–292f, 292
    control of, 294–295
  of small intestine, 238–239, 238f
  of stomach, 231, 232, 233, 235–238, 235f–
      237f
  pancreatic polypeptide and, 366
  slow waves in, 231–233, 231f–232f
  somatostatin and, 365
Gastrointestinal system. See also Digestion;
      "Intestinal" entries.
  blood flow in, 270–271, 270f–271f
  blood vessels of, 115–116, 115f
  cross-sectional anatomy of, 222, 223f
  epithelium of. See Enterocyte(s); Vil-
      lus(i).
  lymphatic vessels of, 271f
    chylomicrons in, 275
  motility of. See Gastrointestinal motility.
  regulation of, 222, 223f
    autonomic, 84t, 85, 224, 225f
    by immune system, 227–228
    by intrinsic endocrine system, 224–
        226, 226f, 227t, 228t
      cytokines and, 227
      enterogastric reflex and, 237
    by intrinsic nervous system. See En-
        teric nervous system.
    by peptides, 226–227, 227t, 228, 228t
  smooth muscle of
    electrical properties of, 231–233, 231f–
        232f

Gastrointestinal system (Continued)
  epinephrine and, 359
  innervation of, 222, 224f
Gated channels, 14f, 15, 19–20, 20f. See also
  Ion channels.
Gel, of mucociliary system, 509, 509f, 510
Gene expression, steroid receptors and,
  26, 27f, 28
Genital ridge, 374
Genitalia
  development of, 375, 375f–376f
  vasodilation in, 201t, 202
Germ cells, primordial, 374, 375f
Germinal epithelium, 374
Gestation. See Pregnancy.
GFR. See Glomerular filtration rate (GFR).
GH. See Growth hormone (GH).
Gibbs-Donnan equilibrium, 497
GIP (gastric inhibitory peptide), 227t
  gastric emptying and, 237
  gastric motility and, 236
  insulin secretion and, 307, 363
Gizzard, 242, 242f, 243
Glaucoma, 92
Glial cells, 32, 34
  blood-brain barrier and, 96, 96f
  of cerebral cortex, 98
Glicentin, 364
Globulin, 118, 119t, 120, 121f
  corticosteroid-binding, 350
Globus pallidus, 68
Glomerular arterioles, 432, 432f, 435, 436
Glomerular basement membrane, 432,
  433f, 435
Glomerular capillaries, 116, 432–433,
  432f–434f
  selective permeability of, 433–435
Glomerular filtrate, 430, 431f–432f, 432,
  433
Glomerular filtration pressure, 433, 434f,
  435
Glomerular filtration rate (GFR), 430, 433
  acid-base balance and, 526
  factors affecting, 435–437, 435f
  glucocorticoids and, 351
  in birds, 436–437
  in feline hyperthyroidism, 348
  measurement of, 437
Glomerular tuft. See Glomerular
  capillaries.
Glomerulonephritis, 438
Glomerulus(i), 430, 431f–434f, 432–433. See
  also Nephron(s).
Glomus cells, 503–504
Glossopharyngeal nerve
  carotid baroreceptors and, 202f, 203
  carotid bodies and, 503
  salivary glands and, 246
Glucagon, 361f, 363–365, 364f–366f
  adipose tissue and, 317
  calcitonin and, 369
  cyclic AMP and, 23
  epinephrine and, 359
  glucocorticoids and, 351
  hepatic enzymes and, 313–315
  in birds, 365
  insulin secretion and, 311–312, 312f, 363
  ketone bodies and, in diabetes, 318–319
  somatostatin and, 365, 366f
Glucocorticoids. See also Cortisol.
  biosynthesis of, 327f, 328, 350
  circadian rhythm of, 352, 352f
  corticotropin and, 350f, 351–352, 352f
  deficiency of, 356
  effects of, 351, 352t
  excess of, 351, 353–354

Glucocorticoids (Continued)
  for delayed parturition, 404
  for hypoadrenocorticism, 450
  for inflammation, 352–353
  in Cushing's disease, 339
  lung defenses and, 510, 513
  metabolism of, 351
  mineralocorticoid activity of, 351, 351t
  synthetic analogues of, 353f
  thyroid hormones and, 346, 347
  transport of, plasma proteins in, 350–
    351
  zona fasciculata and, 349, 349f, 350
  zona reticularis and, 349, 349f, 350
Gluconeogenesis, 306, 311–312, 311f
  epinephrine and, 358
  from amino acids, 306, 311–312, 311f,
    315–316, 316f
  in ruminants, 320
  glucagon and, 364, 364f
  glucocorticoids and, 316–317, 351
  hepatic enzymes in, 314, 314f, 315
  in ruminants, 320–321, 320f
  insulin and, 362, 363
  muscle glycogen and, 312
Glucose
  absorption of, 13–14, 13f, 261f, 263–264,
    263f–264f, 265
    thyroid hormones and, 345
    water secretion and, 270
  as fuel, 305–306
  epinephrine and, 358–359
  fatty acids derived from, 307–308, 309f,
    312, 313
  for calf diarrhea, 278
  for nervous system, 36, 39
    blood-brain barrier and, 96, 183
  from carbohydrate digestion, 258–259,
    262, 262f
  glucagon and, 364
  glucocorticoids and, 351
  hepatic metabolism of, 306, 307, 313–
    315, 314f, 316, 316f. See also Gluco-
    neogenesis.
  in fermentative digestion, 283, 284f,
    285t, 287, 288f
  in lactose, 416
  in skeletal muscle, 312, 315, 316f
  insulin and, 345, 361–362, 361f–363f,
    362t
  reabsorption of, in kidney, 439, 442,
    442f, 443
  ruminant metabolic diseases and, 320–
    321
  storage of, 307–308, 308f. See also Glyco-
    gen.
  sympathetic discharge and, 83
Glucosuria, 449
Glutamate, 309, 309t, 310f
Glutamine, ammonium ion from, 460,
  461f, 526
Glutathione peroxidase, as lung
  protectant, 510
Glycerol, 306
  in ruminants, 320
Glycerophosphorylcholine, in renal
  medulla, 457
Glycocalyx, 255, 257, 261, 272
Glycogen, 306, 307
  glucagon and, 364, 364f
  glucocorticoids and, 351
  hepatic synthesis of, 314, 315
  in muscle, 312
  insulin and, 307, 361, 362, 362f, 362t
  thyroid hormones and, 345
Glycogen phosphatase, 314, 314f, 315

Glycogen synthase, 314, 314f, 315
Glycogenolysis, 306, 314–315, 314f
  epinephrine and, 358
  glucagon and, 364, 364f
  in diabetes, 363
Glycolysis, 305, 306, 306f
  fatty acid synthesis and, 307–308, 309f
  in microbial cells, 283–284, 284f
  insulin and, 362, 362f
  regulation of, 314, 314f, 315
Glycoproteins
  gonadotropins as, 377
  of spermatozoa, 398
Glycosaminoglycans, cervical, 403
Glycosidic bond, hydrolysis of, 258, 258f
GM-CSF (granulocyte-macrophage colony-
  stimulating factor), 511
cGMP (cyclic guanosine monophosphate),
  24
GnRH. See Gonadotropin-releasing
  hormone (GnRH).
GnRH stimulation test, 393
GnRH-associated peptide (GAP), 377–378,
  379, 395
Goblet cells
  of airways, 509, 509f
  of intestine, 257
Goiter, 346
Goitrogens, 346
Golgi apparatus
  lactose and, 412
  milk proteins and, 412, 413f
  of neuron, 34
  protein hormones and, 326, 326f
Golgi cells, 76, 76f
Golgi tendon organ(s), 53, 53f, 55–56, 56f
  intercostal muscles and, 503
Gonadotropin-releasing hormone (GnRH),
  337, 337t, 377–378, 377f
  at puberty, 391
  in male, 379, 425–426, 426f
  pulsatile secretion of, 378, 378f
  sexual receptivity and, 393–394
Gonadotropins, 376–377, 377f. See also
  Chorionic gonadotropin (CG);
  Follicle-stimulating hormone (FSH);
  Luteinizing hormone (LH).
  follicle development and, 384
  in spontaneous vs. induced ovulators,
    387
  lactation and, 395
  menopause and, 392
  negative feedback inhibition of, 378–
    379, 391, 392
  ovarian receptors for, 329, 380, 384
  pheromones and, 395
  preovulatory surge of, 380, 384, 384f,
    385
    at puberty, 391, 391f
    sexual receptivity and, 393–394, 393f
  puberty and, 391–392
  secretory patterns of, 337–338, 378–379,
    378f, 382
Gonads, fetal development of, 374–375,
  375f–376f, 401, 401f
Grain engorgement toxemia, 302
Granular cell layer, 76, 76f, 79
Granule cells, 76, 76f, 79
Granulocyte-macrophage colony-
  stimulating factor (GM-CSF), 511
Granulosa cells, 374, 380, 384
  fertilization and, 398
  gonadotropin receptors of, 329
  inhibin produced by, 379, 382
  of corpus luteum, 384–385
  progesterone derived from, 393

Gravity
  blood pressure and, 116–117
  cardiovascular response to, 215–216
  muscle stretch receptors and, 53, 54, 56
  otoliths and, 73
  postural muscle tone and, 62, 67–68
  pulmonary blood flow and, 175, 176f
  ventilation-perfusion mismatch and, 175
Grit, 243
Growth, endocrine control of, 325
Growth hormone (GH), 335, 376
  deficiency of, 338
  fat mobilization and, 320
  for lactational enhancement, 417, 417f
  hypersecretion of, 338
  in mammary development, 409, 410f
  lactation and, 412
  somatomedins and, 337, 338
  thyroid hormones and, 345
  vitamin D and, 371
Growth hormone–inhibiting hormone, 337, 337t
Growth hormone–releasing hormone, 337, 337t
Growth-factors, receptors for, 19, 20, 25, 26
GTP-binding proteins. See G proteins.
Guanosine monophosphate (GMP), cyclic, 24
Guanosine triphosphate (GTP), 23, 24f
Gular flutter, 535
Gut closure, 276
Gut glucagon, 364
Guttural pouches, 537, 538f
Gynecomastia, in dogs, hypothyroidism causing, 417

H

Hair, heat loss and, 534–535, 540
Hair cells
  of cochlea, 105, 106
  of vestibular system, 71, 71f, 72, 73
Haldane effect, 498
Hardware disease, 28
Haustrum(a), 240, 299
HCl. See Hydrochloric acid (HCl).
Head movement, vestibular system and, 72–73, 72f, 77
Hearing, 104–107, 104f–106f
  brainstem evoked response and, 100, 103f, 106
  mechanosensitive protein in, 4
Heart. See also "Cardiac" entries; Cardiovascular system.
  autonomic regulation of, 83, 84t, 85, 125, 134–135, 200–202, 201t
  conduction system of, 126, 126f–127f
  dysfunction in, 135–136, 135t
  workload of, 163–164
Heart failure, 111–112, 159, 209–213, 210f–211f
  afterload and, 159
  backward, 28, 213
  baroreflex in, 204
  causes of, 209
  compensatory mechanisms in, 209–210, 210f
  complications of, 210–213, 211f
  consequences of, 209, 210f
  definition of, 209
  edema in, 28, 188, 211–212, 211f
  exercise intolerance in, 111, 175, 209, 211, 217–218
  forward, 213
  pulmonary fluid exchange and, 188, 511, 513

Heart failure (Continued)
  right-sided, 209, 483, 485–486
    GI blood flow and, 271
    pulmonary hypertension and, 176
    systemic edema in, 188, 212
Heart rate
  autonomic regulation of, 132–133, 132f, 134–135, 134t
    baroreceptor reflex in, 203–204, 203f
  cardiac output and, 156, 156f, 158, 159–161, 160f
  catecholamines and, 359
  diastolic filling time and, 158
  exercise and, 160, 160f, 160t
  in anemic animal, 499
  intrinsic, 132, 133
  neurohumoral control of, 199
  pulse pressure and, 177, 178f
  thyroid hormones and, 345
  with AV node as pacemaker, 133
Heart sounds, 155–156, 155f, 161
  abnormal, 161–163, 161f–162f, 161t
Heartbeat, 126, 154–156, 155f
Heartworm disease, 111
  pulmonary embolism in, 179–180
  tricuspid stenosis in, 162
Heat. See also Temperature.
  loss of, 534–535, 534f
    evaporative, 534, 534f, 535, 540, 540f
    through cardiovascular system, 112
    through respiratory system, 469–470
  sources of, 534, 534f, 536, 536f, 536t
  transfer of, in body, 536–537, 537f
Heat stress, 539–540, 540f
  respiratory response to, 470
Heat stroke, 541, 543
Heaves, 474, 477, 508
Hematocrit, 118f, 119, 120–121, 120t
  exercise-induced increase in, 498, 499
  hemorrhage and, 214, 214f, 215
  low. See Anemia.
Hematologic values, normal, 119, 120t
Heme
  bile pigments and, 252
  of hemoglobin, 495
  of myoglobin, 498
Heme-heme interactions, 495
Hemianopia, homonymous, 92–93
Hemicellulose, 283
Hemiparesis, 66
Hemochorial placentation, 516, 516t, 517
Hemoglobin, 113, 119–121, 494, 495–497, 495f–496f
  buffering by, 459, 497, 497f, 524
    in respiratory acidosis, 526
    in respiratory alkalosis, 527
  carbamino compound of, 118, 497, 497f
  diffusion driving pressure and, 488
  embryonic, 519
  exercise-induced increase in, 498, 498f
  fetal, 495, 519, 519f
  glycosylated, 372
  in anemia, 495, 495f, 499
  in venous blood, oxygenation of, 498
  percent saturation of, 495–496, 496f
Hemoglobinopathies, 120
Hemorrhage, 110
  cardiovascular responses to, 173, 213–216, 213f–215f
  intraoperative, 207
Hemorrhagic shock, 111
Hemostasis, 119
Henderson-Hasselbalch equation, 523, 524, 525
Henle's loop. See Loop of Henle.
Heparin, 118

Hepatic artery, 116
Hepatic lipidosis, in cat, 321
Hepatocytes, bile secretion by, 250, 251, 252
Hering-Breuer reflex, 503
Hering's nerves, 203
Herniated intervertebral disk, 60
Heterometric autoregulation, 158
High altitude
  hypoxic vasoconstriction at, 483, 484f, 485
  oxygen tension at, 486, 491
  ventilatory response to, 505
High-pressure, high-resistance side, 116
Hindgut, 281, 289
  equine, 298–301, 299f–301f, 302
  species variations in, 301–302
Histamine
  airway irritant receptors and, 503
  arteriolar resistance and, 192
  bronchoconstriction and, 474
  edema caused by, 190, 190f
  gastric acid secretion and, 249
  glucocorticoids and, 353
  pulmonary vascular response to, 483t
H^+,K^+-ATPase pump
  of distal colon, 268
  of renal collecting duct, 462
  of renal tubule, 460
  of stomach, 248
Homeostasis, 96
  of fuels, 305, 306, 313
Homeotherms, 533–534, 536
Homonymous hemianopia, 92–93
Horizontal cells, 89, 89f, 90, 91
Hormone(s). See also specific hormones.
  cell responses to, 329–330, 329f–330f
  circadian rhythms and, 331
  definition of, 324
  feedback control of, 330–331, 331f
  major classes of, 326
  metabolism of, 330
  receptors for, 19–21, 20f, 328–329
    cyclic AMP and, 23
    for steroid hormones, 26, 27f, 28, 328–329
    PIP_2 pathway and, 25, 26
  synthesis of, 326–328, 326f–327f
  transport of, in blood, 112, 328
Hormone-sensitive lipase (HSL), 317
  in diabetes, 319
Horner's syndrome, 86
Horse
  airway obstruction in, chronic, 477
  anesthetized, hypoxemia in, 492–493
  atrial fibrillation in, 499
  chorionic gonadotropin of, 335, 401–402, 401f
  colic in
    impaction causing, 300–301, 302
    Strongylus causing, 111, 121–122
  colon impaction in, 300–301, 302
  Cushing's disease in, 338–339, 352f
  feces of, 301
  fermentative digestion in, 298–302, 299f–301f
  laryngeal hemiplegia in, 470
  mucociliary clearance in, 509, 513
  persistent luteal phase in, 387–388
  placenta of, 517, 517f
  pulmonary hemorrhage in, during exercise, 483
  rabies in, 243
  thermoregulation in, 537, 538f
Huddling behavior, fever and, 541, 543
Humidified gas, 486–487

Humidity, relative, 535, 540
Hyaluronic acid, fertilization and, 398
Hyaluronidase, fertilization and, 398
Hydrocephalus, 94, 96
Hydrochloric acid (HCl), 247–248, 249, 257
  calcitonin and, 369
  in bicarbonate neutralization, 267
  neonatal delay in secretion of, 276
  protein digestion and, 260
Hydrogen bonding
  in protein structures, 3, 4
  of membrane with water, 8
Hydrogen ions. *See also* pH.
  chemoreceptors and, 503, 504–505, 504f
  from exercising muscle, 498
  H^+,K^+-ATPase pump and
    in distal colon, 268
    in kidney, 460, 462
    in stomach, 248
  in erythrocyte, 497, 497f, 498
  Na^+/H^+ exchanger and, 264, 266, 266f
    in proximal tubule, 443, 443f, 460, 461
  potassium ions and, 528
  renal excretion of, 459–460, 461–462,
    462f–463f, 526
    mineralocorticoids and, 354t, 355
  sources of, 522–523
Hydrogen peroxide, in thyroid hormone
  synthesis, 342
Hydrolysis, 258, 258f
  by microbial enzymes, 283
  of lipids, 272
Hydrophilic amino acids, 3
Hydrophobic interaction, 3
Hydrostatic pressure, 10, 10f, 11
  bulk flow and, 112
  in Bowman's space, 433, 434f
  in capillaries, 11–12, 28, 184–188, 190
    glomerular, 433, 434f, 435
  in intestinal epithelium, 270, 270f
  in pulmonary fluid exchange, 511, 511f
  of interstitial fluid, 184–188
Hydroxyapatite, 366, 367
β-Hydroxybutyrate, 296–297, 307f, 362f,
  363
  in ruminants, 307
17-Hydroxylase
  adrenal, 350
  placental, 402
21-Hydroxylase, 350
Hyperadrenocorticism, 351, 353–354
Hypercalcemia, 371
  calcitonin and, 369
Hypercapnia
  diffusion of carbon dioxide and, 183
  lung disease and, 491
  peripheral chemoreceptors and, 504
Hypercarbia. *See* Hypercapnia.
Hypercholesterolemia, in hypothyroidism,
  345, 347
Hyperemia
  active, 192, 193f, 195
  reactive, 193, 193f, 195
Hyperkalemia
  aldosterone stimulated by, 448
  in hypoadrenocorticism, 356, 450
Hypermetria, 78
Hyperparathyroidism, primary, 371
Hyperphosphatemia
  in hypoadrenocorticism, 356
  in hypoparathyroidism, 371
Hyperpnea, 503
Hyperpolarization, 36–37
Hyperprolactinemia, 379, 379f
Hypersecretory diarrhea, 277–278, 277f
Hypersomatotropism, 338

Hypertension
  baroreflex in, 204
  human, 164, 173, 179
  mineralocorticoid excess causing, 355
Hyperthyroidism
  drug treatment of, 346
  feline, 348
Hyperventilation
  alveolar, 487, 491, 527
  at high altitude, 505
  congenital cardiac defect causing, 506–
    507
  pH of blood and, 525, 527, 527f
Hypoadrenocorticism, 356, 449–450
Hypocalcemia
  calcitonin and, 369
  causes of, 371
  parathyroid hormone and, 369, 369f,
    371, 449
  parturient, 369f, 418–419
  renal response to, 449
  signs of, 371
Hypochloremia, in hypoadrenocorticism,
  356
Hypoglycemia
  catecholamine response to, 359–360
  glucagon and, 364, 365f
  in hypoadrenocorticism, 356
  insulinoma causing, 39
Hypogonadotropic hypogonadism,
  anabolic steroids and, 427
Hypokalemia
  from metabolic acidosis treatment, 528
  metabolic alkalosis caused by, 528
  renal proton pump in, 462
Hyponatremia
  in hypoadrenocorticism, 356, 450
  in hypothyroidism, 347
Hypoparathyroidism, 371
Hypophosphatemia
  calcitonin causing, 369
  in primary hyperparathyroidism, 371
Hypopolarization
  by action potential, 38
  by excitatory potential, 36
Hypoproteinemia
  edema in, 188–189, 189f
  pulmonary edema in, 511–512
Hypotension
  in mineralocorticoid deficiency, 355
  in shock, 111–112
  renin release caused by, 435
Hypothalamic-hypophyseal portal system,
  116, 335–336, 336f, 377, 377f
Hypothalamic-pituitary-testicular axis,
  425, 426f
  anabolic steroids and, 427, 428
Hypothalamus, 63, 331
  adenohypophysis and, 116, 330–331,
    331f, 335–338, 336f–337f, 337t
  atrial volume receptor reflex and, 205,
    205f
  autonomic nervous system and, 85
  blood-brain barrier and, 96
  cortisol regulation by, 352, 352f
  feedback control of, 330–331, 331f
  fetal, parturition and, 402, 402f
  fever and, 541, 542f
  gonadal control by, 376, 377–379, 377f
  male reproductive system and, 425, 426f
  neurohypophysis and, 332–333, 332f–
    333f, 377
  nuclei of, 376, 377
  ovulation and, 384
  oxytocin release and, 403, 403f, 414, 414f
  prolactin release and, 412, 412f

Hypothalamus (*Continued*)
  puberty and, 391
  releasing hormones of, 336–337, 337t
  sexual differentiation of, 375, 381, 392
  sexual receptivity and, 394
  temperature regulation by, 538, 539,
    539f, 541, 542f
  thyroid hormones and, 346, 346f
Hypothermia, 541. *See also* Cold stress.
  conductive heat loss causing, 535
  oxyhemoglobin dissociation curve and,
    496
Hypothyroidism, 345, 346–348, 347t
  canine gynecomastia in, 417
Hypoventilation. *See* Alveolar
  hypoventilation.
Hypovolemia, ADH release in, 456
Hypovolemic shock
  in calf diarrhea, 278
  in grain engorgement toxemia, 302
Hypoxemia, 490, 491
  chemoreceptors and, 503, 504, 505
  congenital cardiac defect causing, 506–
    507
  exercise-associated, 488, 489f
  in anesthetized horse, 492–493
  in brachycephalic syndrome, 492
  in lung diseases, 491
  pulmonary edema with, 513
Hypoxia
  alveolar, 479, 482, 482f, 483
  diffusion of oxygen and, 183
  in fetus, 518, 519, 520
  macrocyte function and, 510
  pulmonary edema causing, 211, 212
  ventilatory response to, 503–504, 504f
    at high altitude, 505
Hypoxic vasoconstriction, 175–176, 483,
  484f, 485
Hysteresis, pressure-volume, 472, 472f

I

I band, of cardiac myofibril, 124, 124f
IGF-1 (insulin-like growth factor 1)
  glomerular filtration rate and, 436
  in pituitary dwarfism, 338
Ileocecal sphincter, 239
Ileum
  bile acid reabsorption in, 272, 274f
  electrolyte absorption in, 268t
  equine, secretions of, 301, 301f
Immune system
  alveolar macrophages in, 510, 510f
  gastrointestinal, 227–228
Immunoglobulins
  in colostrum, 276, 410
    fetal red blood cells and, 418, 419
  placental transfer of, 410
Impaction, in tracheobronchial tree, 508,
  509, 509f
Impaction colic, 300–301, 302
Incus, 104, 105f
Indirect pupillary light reflex, 92
Induced ovulators, 387, 399
Inertial impaction, in tracheobronchial
  tree, 508, 509, 509f
Infarction, 110, 113
  cerebral, 113–114
  myocardial, 115
    ECG associated with, 148
  pressure-induced, 195
Inferior colliculus, 105
Infertility, anabolic steroids causing,
  427–428
Inflammatory mediators,
  bronchoconstriction and, 474

Inflammatory response
glucocorticoids for, 352–353
in lung defense, 510–511
Influenza, in pigs, 543
Information. *See also* Signaling.
definition of, 3
gated channels and, 15
in receptor-ligand complex, 20–21
proteins and, 3, 8, 9
Infrared radiation, 534f, 535
Ingestion, 233
Inhalation, 470, 471f
central regulation of, 502
upper airway compression during, 475
Inhibin, 379, 382, 425
Inhibitory postsynaptic potential (IPSP),
37, 37f
EEG and, 99
Injury
adrenocortical response to, 348
edema associated with, 189, 190, 190f
Inner ear, 70–71, 70f. *See also* Cochlea;
Vestibular system.
Inositol, in renal medulla, 457
Inositol-1,4,5-triphosphate (IP$_3$), 20, 25,
25f, 26
hormone action and, 329
Insulation, thermal, 534–535
Insulin, 360–363. *See also* Diabetes
mellitus.
adipose tissue and, 313
administration of, 372
amino acid metabolism and, 311–312,
312f
control of secretion of, 362–363, 363f,
363t, 365f
epinephrine and, 358, 359
functions of, 361–362, 362f, 362t
glucagon and, 364, 365f–366f
glucocorticoids and, 351
hepatic enzymes and, 314–315
in absorptive phase, 307, 308, 311, 312,
312f
in postabsorptive phase, 315, 316
metabolism of, 361
somatostatin and, 365, 366f
species differences in, 360–361
synthesis of, 361, 361f
Insulin resistance
acromegaly with, 338
hyperadrenocorticism with, 354
Insulin-like growth factor 1 (IG-1)
glomerular filtration rate and, 436
in pituitary dwarfism, 338
Insulinoma, hypoglycemia caused by, 39
Intention tremor, 68, 78, 79
Intercalated cells of collecting ducts, 447,
448f
bicarbonate secretion by, 464, 464f–465f
proton pumps of, 460, 462, 462f–463f
Intercalated disks, of cardiac muscle, 49,
124f, 125
Intercostal muscles, 470
stretch receptors of, 503
Interdigestive motility complex, 238
Interferon, 541
Interleukin-1 (IL-1)
as pyrogen, 541
in lung, 510–511
Interleukin-6 (IL-6)
as pyrogen, 541
in lung, 511
Interleukin-8 (IL-8), in lung, 511
Intermediary metabolism, 305, 306f. *See
also* Glycolysis; Krebs cycle;
Metabolism.

Intermediary metabolism *(Continued)*
catecholamines and, 358
enzymes of, 313–315, 314f
glucocorticoids and, 351
Interpubic ligament, relaxin and, 403
Intersegmental reflex, 52
loss of, 59, 60
Interstitial cells of Cajal, 231–232
Interstitial fluid. *See also* Edema.
calcium in, 367
central chemoreceptor and, 504–505,
504f
composition of, 12t
electrolytes in, 118
in edema, 28, 184, 185, 187–190, 188f–
190f
lymphatic system and, 185, 186f–187f
membrane potential and, 16
of lungs, 186–187
pressure of, 184, 185–188, 189, 190
proteins in, 184, 186, 188, 189
reabsorption of, after hemorrhage, 214–
215, 214f
transport between capillaries and, 11–
12, 113, 114f, 117, 182–187, 182f–
183f
Interstitial implantation, 400
Interventricular foramen, 94, 95f
Intestinal absorption. *See* Absorption,
intestinal.
Intestinal ischemia
in heart failure, 212
in *Strongylus* infestation, 111, 121–122
Intestinal phase, of pancreatic secretion,
250
Intestinal secretion
of electrolytes, 269–270, 269f
of water, 269–270, 269f
diarrhea and, 277–278, 277f
Intestines. *See* Colon; Gastrointestinal
system; Small intestine.
Intracellular fluid, composition of, 12t
Intracranial pressure, 94
increased, 96–97
Intrafusal muscle fibers, 53–54
Intraocular pressure, 92
Intravenous fluids, pulmonary edema
and, 511–512
Inulin clearance, 437, 439f, 440
Iodinated casein, 417
Iodine
dietary, 346
in thyroid hormone synthesis, 342
Iodotyrosine dehalogenase, 343
Ion channels, 14–15, 14f. *See also* Calcium
ion channels; Potassium ion channels;
Sodium ion channels.
action potential and, 37
allosteric changes in, 4f
in intestinal absorption, 264
ligand-gated, 14f, 15, 19–20, 20f
in postsynaptic muscle membrane, 42
PIP$_2$ pathway and, 25
resting membrane potential and, 35
Ions. *See also* Calcium; Potassium; Sodium.
diffusion through lipid bilayer, 9
osmotic pressure and, 10, 10f, 11
IP$_3$ (inositol-1,4,5-triphosphate), 20, 25, 25f,
26
hormone action and, 329
IPSP (inhibitory postsynaptic potential),
37, 37f
EEG and, 99
Iris, 87–88, 87f, 89f, 92
epinephrine and, 359
Irritant receptors, in airways, 474, 503, 510

Ischemia, 110, 111–112, 113
intestinal
in heart failure, 212
in *Strongylus* infestation, 111, 121–122
myocardial, 115
ECG associated with, 148
in coronary artery disease, 196
of skeletal muscle, 196
pressure causing, 195
Islets of Langerhans, 360, 360f–361f, 362
regulation of, 365, 366f
Isobutyric acid, 284, 285f, 286
Isoerythrolysis, neonatal, 418, 419
Isoleucine, 309, 309t
microbial degradation of, 286
Isomaltase, 262, 262f
Isomaltose, 259, 259f, 260
digestion of, 261, 262f
Isoproterenol, 135
for AV node block, 136, 140
for sick sinus syndrome, 136
pulmonary vascular response to, 483t
Isovaleric acid, 284, 285f, 286
Isovolumetric contraction, 154
Isovolumetric relaxation, 155

J

Jejunum
electrolyte absorption in, 268t
lactase in, 416
micelle formation in, 274f
Joints, muscle contraction across, 44, 45f
Junctional folds, 41, 42, 42f
in myasthenia gravis, 43
Junctional tachycardias, 137
Juxtacapillary receptors, pulmonary, 503
Juxtaglomerular apparatus, 355, 355f, 431f,
436
avian, 437
epinephrine and, 359
Juxtaglomerular cells, 435
Juxtamedullary nephrons, 431f, 453, 454

K

α-Keto-acids, of BCAAs, 315, 316f
α-Ketoglutarate, 309, 310f
Ketone bodies, 307, 307f
growth hormone and, 320
hepatic formation of, 307, 318, 318f, 319
in diabetes mellitus, 318–319, 363, 372
in ruminants, 297, 307, 320
urinary excretion of, 318
Ketosis, lactational, 321
K$_f$ (ultrafiltration coefficient), 433, 435, 436
Kidney(s). *See also* "Glomerular" entries;
"Renal" entries.
acid-base regulation by, 459–465, 524–
525, 526, 528
ammonium ion in, 460–461, 461f
bicarbonate secretion in, 462, 464,
464f–465f
buffers in, 459–460, 460f, 462, 464, 524
hydrogen ion excretion in, 459–460,
461–462, 462f–463f, 522–523
in respiratory acidosis, 526–527, 527f
in respiratory alkalosis, 527, 527f
aquaporins in, 14–15, 456
atrial volume receptor reflex and, 205,
205f
blood flow in, 435–436, 435f
calcium homeostasis and, 367, 368, 371
collecting ducts of, 430, 431f, 445, 446–
448, 447f
aldosterone activity in, 435

Kidney(s) *(Continued)*
  ammonium formation in, 461, 461f
  bicarbonate secretion by, 462, 464,
    464f–465f
  calcium transport in, 449
  hydrogen ion secretion by, 459, 460f,
    462, 462f–463f
  pH of urine determined in, 459, 462
  urea reabsorption in, 435, 453, 454f
  vasopressin (ADH) and, 435, 456–457,
    456f–457f
    water permeability of, 453
    water reabsorption in, 435
  functions of, 430
  glomeruli of, 430, 431f–434f, 432–433
  gluconeogenesis in, 306
  heart failure and, 212–213
  mineralocorticoids and, 354t, 355, 355f
  nephrons of, 430, 431f
    juxtamedullary, 431f, 453, 454
    reptilian-type, 432, 436–437, 441
      concentrating ability and, 453
      salt balance and, 447
      uric acid secretion by, 444
    superficial, 431f, 453
    tubuloglomerular feedback in, 436
  of birds, 432, 436–437
    concentrating ability of, 453
    portal circulation of, 441
    salt balance and, 447
    tubular secretion in, 444
    water balance and, 457
  phosphate reabsorption by, 368
  transcellular transport in, 17
  tubules of, 430, 431f. *See also* Distal tu-
    bule; Loop of Henle; Proximal tu-
    bule.
    acid secretion by, 459–460, 462–463
    fractional excretion rate and, 439–440
    fractional reabsorption rate and, 440
    function of, 439
    organic ion secretion by, 444
    reabsorption in, 440–444, 440f–444f,
      445–446, 447f
      in birds, 441
      in medulla, 453–455, 455f
      water balance and, 452–457, 454f–457f
    vasoconstriction in, exercise-induced,
      174f, 175
    vasopressin (ADH) and, 23, 333, 334f,
      435, 456–457, 456f–457f
    vitamin D metabolism in, 370
Knee jerk reflex, 52, 55, 55f
Koilin, 243
Krebs cycle, 305, 306, 306f
  fatty acid β-oxidation and, 319, 319f
  gluconeogenesis and, 315
    in ruminants, 320, 320f
  in muscle, 315
  vs. fatty acid synthesis, 308, 309f
Kwashiorkor, 188

L

Labia, development of, 375
Labyrinth. *See* Inner ear.
Labyrinthitis, 74
Lacrimal gland, 88
α-Lactalbumin, 416
Lactase, 261f, 262, 262f, 416
  waning activity of, 276
Lactate, from glycogenolysis, 358–359
Lactation, 410, 411f–415f, 412, 414–415. *See
  also* Milk; Prolactin.
  cycle of, 416–417, 416f–417f
  delayed, fetal defect causing, 404

Lactation *(Continued)*
  glucose homeostasis and, 320
  hormonal induction of
    in bitches, 417
    in cows, 417, 417f
  hypocalcemia caused by, 418–419
  ovarian activity and, 395
    in dairy cattle, 396
  photoperiod and, 417, 418f
Lactational ketosis, 321
Lactic acid
  acid-base regulation and, 522
  ventilatory response to, in exercise, 505
Lactic acidosis, 527
Lactoferrin, 410
Lactogen, placental, 402
Lactoperoxidase system, 410
Lactose, 258
  digestion of, 261, 261f–262f, 262
  in colostrum, 410, 410t
  in milk, 412, 415t, 416
    synthesized from glucose, 320
Lactose synthetase, 416
Lamina densa, 432, 433f
Laminae rarae, 432, 433f
Laminar flow
  of air, 474
  of blood, 161
Laryngeal hemiplegia, 470, 475
  hypoventilation caused by, 487
Larynx, 469
  dynamic compression of, 475
  frictional resistance of, 473, 473f
  inhalation and, 470
  receptors of, 503
Lateral geniculate nucleus, 91, 92f
Lateral ventricles, 94, 95f
Law of mass action, 523
LDDS (low-dose dexamethasone
  suppression) test, 354
LDL (low-density lipoproteins)
  in cholesterol transport, 18, 18f, 326
  thyroid hormones and, 345
Leak channels, 14f, 15, 16, 17
Leaves, of omasum, 295
Lecithin, in pulmonary surfactant, 519
Left atrial pressure, 480
  in exercising horse, 483
Left atrium, 115, 115f, 479
Left ventricle, 115, 115f, 479
  work done by, 163–164
Left ventricular hypertrophy, 163–165
Left-sided heart failure, 209. *See also* Heart
  failure.
  pulmonary fluid exchange and, 188,
    511, 513
Lens, 87f, 88, 89, 89f
  diabetes and, 372
  epinephrine and, 359
Letdown of milk, 414, 415
Leucine, 309, 309t
  microbial degradation of, 286
Leukocytes, 119
Leukotrienes
  bronchoconstriction and, 474
  glucocorticoid inhibition of, 353
  neutrophil metabolism of, 512
  pulmonary vascular response to, 483t
Leydig cells, 374, 375f, 421, 425, 426f, 427
LH. *See* Luteinizing hormone (LH).
Ligand binding, to proteins, 3, 4, 4f
Ligand-gated channels, 14f, 15, 19–20, 20f
  in postsynaptic muscle membrane, 42
  PIP₂ pathway and, 25
Light. *See* Photoperiod.
Lignin, 283

Limit dextrins, 259f, 260
Lingual glands, 246
Lingual lipase, 245
Lipase, 272, 274f
  insufficiency of, 278
  lingual, 245
Lipemia, 276
Lipid bilayer. *See* Membrane(s).
Lipidosis, hepatic, in cat, 321
Lipids. *See* Fats (lipids).
Lipolysis
  epinephrine and, 359
  glucagon and, 364
  insulin and, 362, 363
Lipoprotein lipase (LPL), 313
  in muscle, 319–320
  insulin and, 362
β-Lipotropin, 335, 336f
Liver
  amino acid metabolism in, 310–312,
    310f–311f
  autonomic regulation of, 84t
  bile secretion by, 250–252, 251f–252f
  blood supply to, 115–116, 115f
  capillaries of, 182, 182f, 271
  excretion of lipid-soluble substances by,
    252
  fatty acid metabolism in, 317–319, 317f–
    318f
  fatty acid synthesis in, 307–308, 309f,
    312, 318, 318f
  fatty acid uptake by, 317
  GI blood flow and, 271, 271f
  glucagon action on, 364
  glucose metabolism in, 306, 307, 313–
    315, 314f, 316, 316f
  insulin action on, 362, 362t
  ketone body formation in, 307, 318–319,
    318f
  of fetus, 518
  of ruminant
    nitrogen cycling and, 288, 289f
    propionate extraction and, 320
  portal system of, 271, 271f
    amino acids in, 309, 310, 310f
    bile acids in, 252, 252f, 272
    propionate in, 320
  protein synthesis in, 310, 310f
    of plasma proteins, 118
  steroid metabolism in, 330
  vitamin D metabolism in, 370
  VLDL formation in, 308, 309f, 319
Liver disease
  chronic, edema in, 12
  lipidosis as, 321
Lobar bronchus, 474
Local anesthetics, antiarrhythmic effect of,
  138, 139
Long-loop feedback system, 337, 337f
Loop diuretics, 445
Loop of Henle, 431f, 436, 444–446,
  445f–446f
  ammonium reabsorption in, 460, 461f
  calcium reabsorption in, 448–449
  diuretic site of action in, 444
  medullary hypertonicity and, 453, 454,
    455f
  of juxtamedullary nephrons, 453, 454
Loudness, 104, 104f, 105
Low-density lipoproteins (LDL)
  in cholesterol transport, 18, 18f, 326
  thyroid hormones and, 345
Low-dose dexamethasone suppression
  (LDDS) test, 354
Lower brain, 33
Lower motor neurons, 58

Lower motor neurons *(Continued)*
α, 48, 54, 54f–55f, 55
disease of, 58–60
γ, 54, 54f–55f, 55
pyramidal system and, 66
Low-pressure, low-resistance side, 116
LPL (lipoprotein lipase), 313
in muscle, 319–320
insulin and, 362
Luminal-phase digestion, 258–260, 259f, 260t, 262f
Lung(s). *See also* "Alveolar" *entries;* "Pulmonary" *entries;* "Respiratory" *entries.*
acid-base regulation by, 459, 522, 524–525, 525f, 527–528, 528f
airways in, 473–474, 474f. *See also* Airway(s).
angiotensin-converting enzyme in, 435
autonomic regulation of, 84t
compliance of
alveolar hypoventilation and, 487, 487f
decreased, 475, 476–477, 476f
definition of, 472
pleural pressure and, 471
distribution of gas in, 468, 469f
elasticity of, 471–472, 471f–472f
fetal development of, 472, 519–520
fibrosis of, in dog, 476–477
interlobular septa of, 484
interstitial fluid in, 186–187
lymphatic vessels of, 186–187, 511
metabolic functions of, 512
secondary lobules of, 475–476
viral infection of
epithelial damage by, 512–513
macrophages and, 510, 510f, 512
Lung sounds, 474
Luschka, foramen of, 95
Luteal phase, 378, 386–387. *See also* Corpus luteum (CL).
copulation and, 387
duration of, 385, 386
estrous cycle and, 389, 390
estrus and, 393
follicular growth during, 382
in pregnancy, 400
menstruation and, 389
persistent in mare, 387–388
Luteinization, 385
at puberty, 391
Luteinizing hormone (LH), 335, 376–377, 377f. *See also* Gonadotropins.
corpus luteum and, 385
β-endorphin and, 379
in male, 425, 426, 426f, 427
in pregnancy, 400, 400f
ovarian receptors for, 329, 380
preovulatory surge of, 384, 384f, 385
as positive feedback, 331
at puberty, 391f
sexual receptivity and, 393–394, 393f
secretion patterns of, 378, 378f
Luteinizing-inhibiting factor, 384
Luteolysis, 385–386, 385f–386f, 387, 393
in parturition, 403, 404
in pregnancy, 401
Luteotropins, 385
in pregnancy, 400
Lymphatic vessels, 185, 186, 186f–187f
edema and, 187, 188, 189
obstruction of, 189, 189f
of GI tract, 271
chylomicrons in, 275
of lungs, 186–187, 511

Lymphatic vessels *(Continued)*
pleural space and, 512
pulmonary, 511
Lymphedema, 189, 189f
Lymphocytic thyroiditis, 346
Lymphoid tissue, of airways, 508, 510
Lysine vasopressin, 333
Lysophospholipids, 272, 273f
Lysosome, 8
hormone degradation by, 329
in prostaglandin synthesis, 353, 403
in thyroid hormone synthesis, 343, 343f
LDL digestion by, 18
reabsorbed proteins degraded in, 444, 444f
receptor digestion by, 21
Lysozyme
in milk, 410
in respiratory secretions, 510
in saliva, 245

M

Machinery murmur, 162, 520
Macrophages, alveolar, 510, 510f
Macula, hair cells of, 71f, 72
Macula densa, 355, 355f, 431f, 436
Magendie, foramen of, 95
Magnesium
parathyroid hormone and, 368
renal reabsorption of, 445, 447f
Magnocellular nuclei, 332
Malabsorption diarrhea, 277, 277f
Male reproductive system. *See also* Spermatogenesis; Spermatozoa.
functional anatomy of, 421–423, 422t
hypothalamic-pituitary regulation of, 425, 426f, 427, 428
Malleus, 104, 105f
Malnutrition, 317–320, 317f–319f
Malonyl CoA, 318, 318f, 319
Maltase, 261f, 262, 262f, 276
Maltose, 259, 259f
digestion of, 261–262, 261f–262f
Maltotriose, 259, 259f, 262f
Mammary buds, 407, 408
Mammary cord, 407
Mammary ducts
anatomy of, 407–408, 407f–408f
involution of, 416
myoepithelial cells and, 407f, 414
proliferation of, 409, 410f–411f
Mammary gland
anatomy of, 407–408, 407f–408f, 409, 411f
development of
fetal, 407, 408
postfetal, 409, 410f–411f
infection of, 417–418
inflammation of, 353
male, 407
mammalian reproductive strategy and, 406–407
neoplasia of, 418
number of pairs of, 408
of neonate, 408
Mandibular glands, 246
Mass action, law of, 523
Mass movements
in cecum, equine, 299
in colon, 240
avian, 243
Mast cells. *See also* Histamine.
in gastric mucosa, 249
Mastication, 233, 234, 246, 257
by ruminant, 292, 293, 294

Mastitis, 417–418
MCHC (mean cell hemoglobin concentration), 120
Mean aortic pressure, 116
Mean arterial pressure, 176–177, 176f
determinants of, 177–179, 178f–179f
Mean cell hemoglobin concentration (MCHC), 120
Mean circulatory filling pressure, 170, 170f–171f
Mean hemoglobin per red cell (MHC), 120
Mechanoreceptors
of gastrointestinal system, 222, 224f, 249
of respiratory system, 501, 503, 510
Mechanosensitive proteins, 4
Media, of pulmonary arteries, 479, 482f, 483
Medial geniculate body, 105
Medial longitudinal fasciculus, 73
Medial preoptic nucleus, 377, 392
Median eminence, 377, 379
oxytocin release and, 414
Medulla, 33, 63, 63f. *See also* Brainstem.
cochlear nuclei in, 105
corticospinal tract and, 63, 64, 64f
extrapyramidal system and, 67, 68
pyramids of, 64, 64f, 65
respiratory control by, 502, 502f, 504–505, 504f
vestibular nuclei in, 73
Megakaryocytes, 119
Meiosis
in ovary, 379, 384
fertilization and, 399
in testis, 422, 423, 424, 424f, 425
Meiosis-inhibiting factor, 379
Meissner (submucosal) plexus, 222, 224f
α-Melanocyte–stimulating hormone (α-MSH), 335, 336f, 339
Melatonin, 394, 395, 417
Membrana propria, of ovarian follicle, 380, 384
Membrane(s), 8–9, 8f
cholesterol component of, 17
of muscle fiber (sarcolemma), 44
action potential on, 45, 48, 49
transverse tubules and, 45, 47f
proteins of, 8–9, 8f
in active transport, 10, 12–14, 12f–13f
in facilitated diffusion, 14–15, 14f
in signal transduction, 19–20, 20f
spatial organization of, 17, 23
transport through. *See also* Active transport; Diffusion; Osmosis.
by membrane fusion, 17–18, 17f–18f
energetics of, 9–10
unaided, 9
Membrane potential. *See* Action potential(s); Postsynaptic potentials; Resting membrane potential.
Membranous labyrinth, 70–71, 70f, 105
Membranous-phase digestion, 258, 259f, 260–262, 261f–262f
absorption and, 265, 266f
Menarche, 392
Meninges, 33, 33f
Meningitis, hydrocephalus secondary to, 96
Menopause, 392
Menstrual cycle, 389, 390f
Menstruation, 389, 391, 392
Mesangial cells, 435, 436
Mesencephalon, 33, 63
Mesonephros, in gonadal development, 374, 375f–376f

Messenger RNA (mRNA)
  steroid receptors and, 26, 27f, 325, 329, 329f
  thyroid hormones and, 344–345, 345f
Metabolic acidosis, 505, 505f, 527, 528, 528f
  anion gap in, 529
  blood gas abnormalities in, 529t
  buffering by bone in, 459
  in hypoadrenocorticism, 355, 450
Metabolic alkalosis, 505, 505f, 527–528, 528f
  abomasal torsion causing, 465–466, 527–528, 529–530
  blood gas abnormalities in, 529t
  mineralocorticoid hypersecretion causing, 355
  with paradoxic aciduria, 465–466
Metabolic fuels, 305–307, 307f
Metabolic rate
  basal, 468, 536
    cold stress and, 536, 540
    thyroid hormones and, 344–346
  blood flow and, 192–195, 193f–194f
    coronary, 199
    during exercise, 216
  body weight and, 468, 536, 536f
  capillary blood flow and, 181–182
  in cold-stressed animals, 470, 536
  of homeotherms vs. poikilotherms, 534, 536
  oxygen consumption and, 468, 469
    during exercise, 498
  oxyhemoglobin dissociation curve and, 496
Metabolism
  absorptive phase of, 307, 308f
    amino acids in, 308–312, 308f, 309t, 310f–311f, 313f
    fatty acids in, 307–308, 309f, 313
    glucose in, 307–308, 308f
    insulin in, 307, 312, 312f
  catecholamines and, 358
  glucagon and, 364
  glucocorticoids and, 351
  heat produced by, 534, 536, 536f, 536t
  hormonal control of, 325
  hydrogen ions from, 522–523
  in birds, 365
  insulin and, 361–362, 362f–363f, 362t, 363
  postabsorptive phase of, 313–317, 314f, 316f
  thyroid hormones and, 345
Metestrus, 389, 390f
Methane, 283, 284, 284f, 285, 285t, 287, 288f
  eructation of, 290
Methemoglobin, 497
2-Methylbutyric acid, 284, 285f, 286
Methyl-*p*-hydroxybenzoate, 395
6α-Methylprednisol, 353f
Metoclopramide, for lactational enhancement, in bitches, 417
MHC (mean hemoglobin per red cell), 120
Micelles, 272, 274f–275f
Microbial yield, 287, 294
Microcirculation, 181
Microcotyledon, of equine placenta, 517, 517f
Microfilaments, 6, 6f
Microglial cells, 98
Micropedici, 441f
Micropuncture studies, of pulmonary circulation, 481, 481f

Microvilli
  of intestinal epithelium, 255, 256f–257f
  of renal tubular epithelium, 440, 440f–441f
  of respiratory epithelium, 510
Midbrain, 63, 63f
  extrapyramidal system in, 67, 68
Middle ear, 104, 105, 105f–106f
Migrating motility complex (MMC), 238–239
Milk. *See also* Lactation.
  composition of, 415–416, 415t
  fatty acid synthesis for, 320
  secretion of, 410, 412, 412f–415f, 414–415
  storage of, 407–408
  suppression of, 414
Milking, 414–415, 415f
  mastitis associated with, 417–418
  stopping of, 416
Mineral metabolism, 325
Mineralocorticoids. *See also* Aldosterone.
  acidification of urine and, 462
  biosynthesis of, 327f, 328, 350
  deficiency of, 356, 449–450
  effects of, 354–355, 354t
  glucocorticoid activity of, 351t
  hypersecretion of, 355
  hyposecretion of, 355
  metabolism of, 351
  regulation of secretion of, 355–356, 355f
  zona glomerulosa and, 348–349, 349f, 350
Minute ventilation, 469
  during exercise, 470
Minute work, by left ventricle, 163
Mitochondria
  fatty acid synthesis and, 308, 309f
  ketone body formation in, 318, 318f, 319
  of muscle fibers, 44, 47f, 49, 468
  of presynaptic nerve terminal, 41
  steroid synthesis in, 327, 327f
    in adrenal cortex, 350, 350f
  thyroid hormones and, 345
Mitral insufficiency (regurgitation), 161–162, 161f, 161t
  in dog, 513
  pathologic consequences of, 164–165, 164f
Mitral stenosis, 155, 161t, 162, 162f, 163
  pathologic consequences of, 164f, 165
Mitral valve
  first heart sound and, 156
  in cardiac cycle, 154, 155
Mixed venous blood
  definition of, 488
  oxygen tension of, 488, 489f
  percentage saturation of, 495
MMC (migrating motility complex), 238–239
Molecular layer, of cerebellum, 76, 76f
Monoamine oxidase, of pulmonary endothelium, 512
Monocytes, lung defenses and, 510
5′-Monodeiodinase, 343, 344, 344f
Monoglycerides, 272, 273f
Monoiodotyrosine, 342, 343, 343f
Monopodial branching, of bronchi, 474
Monosaccharides, 258, 262. *See also* Glucose.
Monosynaptic reflex, 51, 54, 55
Monro, foramen of, 94
Morula, 399
Mossy fibers, 76, 76f, 78
Motilin, 227t
Motor cortex, 64, 65, 65f
  basal ganglia and, 68

Motor cortex (*Continued*)
  cerebrocerebellum and, 78
  focal lesion of, 69
Motor learning, 78
Motor memory, 76
Motor (efferent) nerves, 32t, 33
Motor neuron(s)
  autonomic, 80–81, 81f
  enteric, 222, 224f
  neuromuscular synapse of, 41–43, 42f
    action potential at, 41–43, 45
    nicotinic receptors at, 15, 83, 83f
  reflex arc and, 51, 51f, 52
  respiratory, 502
  somatic, 32t, 33, 80–81, 81f
α Motor neuron(s), 48
  as final common pathway, 62
  as lower motor neuron, 58
  disease of, 56, 58–59
  extrapyramidal system and, 67, 68, 73
  Golgi tendon organ and, 56
  muscle spindle and, 54, 54f–55f, 55
  pyramidal system and, 66
γ Motor neuron(s), 54, 54f–55f, 55
  as lower motor neuron, 58
  extrapyramidal system and, 67–68, 73
  pyramidal system and, 66
Motor unit, 48
Mouth breathing, 473, 476
Movement
  central control of, 53
  skeletal muscle contraction and, 44, 45f
  voluntary vs. involuntary, 62
Movement disorders
  extrapyramidal lesions causing, 68
  in cerebellar disease, 78–79
  in upper motor neuron disease, 59
α-MSH (α-melanocyte–stimulating hormone), 335, 336f, 339
Mucociliary system, 509–510, 509f
  macrophages in, 510
  transportation of horses and, 509, 513
  viral impairment of, 512–513
Mucous neck cells, gastric, 247, 248f
Mucus
  airway irritant receptors and, 503
  intestinal, 257, 261
Müllerian duct, 374, 375, 375f–376f
Müllerian tubercle, 376f
Müllerian-inhibiting factor, 375, 381
Multiunit smooth muscle, 49
Murmurs, cardiac, 161–163, 161f–162f, 161t
  grading of, 166
  pulse pressure and, 179
Muscarine, 83
Muscarinic cholinergic agonist, 135
Muscarinic cholinergic antagonist, 135
  for AV node block, 136, 140
  for sick sinus syndrome, 135–136, 135t
Muscarinic cholinergic receptors, 21, 83, 83f
  cardiovascular, 200, 201–202, 201t
    on sympathetic terminals, 202
  on airway smooth muscle, 474, 475f
  on cardiac muscle cells, 135
    of pacemaker, 132
  PIP$_2$ pathway and, 25
Muscle. *See also* Cardiac muscle; Skeletal muscle; Smooth muscle.
  lipoprotein lipase in, 319–320
  types of, 5–6, 44
Muscle cells. *See* Muscle fibers.
Muscle fibers, 44–45, 46f
  cardiac, 124–125, 124f
  extrafusal, 54, 62

Muscle fibers (Continued)
  fast-twitch vs. slow-twitch, 48–49, 498
  innervation of, 48
  intrafusal, 53–54
  myoglobin in, 498
  of muscle spindle, 53–54
Muscle pump, 217, 217f
Muscle spindle stretch receptors, 51,
    53–55, 53f–55f, 56
  cerebellum and, 75
  of respiratory muscles, 503
  voluntary movement and, 66
Muscle stretch reflex, 52, 54–55, 55f, 56
  lower motor neuron disease and, 59
Muscle tension, detection of, 53, 56
Muscle tone
  postural, 62, 67–68
  spinocerebellum and, 78
Muscular vessels, 181
Myasthenia gravis, 43
Myelin, 34
  glial cells and, 32
Myelinated axons
  in autonomic nervous system, 81
  saltatory conduction in, 39, 39f
Myelography, 94
Myenteric (Auerbach) plexus, 222
  of esophagus, 234
  of stomach, 236
Myocardial infarction, 115
  ECG associated with, 148
Myocardial ischemia, 115
  ECG associated with, 148
  in coronary artery disease, 196
Myocarditis, 110
Myoepithelial cells, mammary, 333, 407f,
    413f, 414
Myofibrils
  of cardiac muscle, 49, 124, 124f
  of skeletal muscle, 44–45, 46f–47f
Myogenic hypothesis, 195
Myogenic reflex, 435, 436
Myoglobin, 49, 498–499
Myosin, 6–8, 6f–7f, 21
  of cardiac muscle, 49, 124, 124f, 129,
    130, 134
  of skeletal muscle, 45, 48, 48f
  of smooth muscle, 21, 22f, 23, 49
  uterine, 403
Myosin ATPase, 6, 21
Myosin kinase, 21, 22f, 23
Myosin phosphatase, 21
Myotatic reflex, 55, 55f

N

NAD (nicotinamide adenine dinucleotide),
    microbial, 283, 284, 284f
Na⁺/H⁺ exchanger
  of intestine, 264, 266, 266f
  of proximal tubule, 443, 443f, 460, 461
Na⁺,K⁺-ATPase pump, 12–14, 12f–13f, 36
  of cardiac cells, 139
  of intestines, 13, 13f, 14, 263, 263f, 264,
    266
    water secretion and, 269
  of renal collecting ducts, 447, 448, 448f
  of renal tubules, 17, 442, 442f–443f, 443
    distal, 445, 447f
    sodium reabsorption and, 354f, 355
    water reabsorption and, 452
  resting membrane potential and, 15–17,
    35, 36
Nares, 469
  dilation of, 470, 473, 477
  dynamic compression of, 475

Nasal cavity, 469
  dynamic compression of, 475
  frictional resistance of, 473, 473f
  receptors in, 503
Nasal retina, 91
Nasolacrimal duct, 88
Necrosis, 110, 113
NEFAs (nonesterified fatty acids), 317,
    319, 320
Neocerebellum, 78
Neonatal isoerythrolysis, 418, 419
Neonate. See also Suckling.
  arterial oxygen tension in, 491
  breathing by, 520
  brown fat in, 536, 540
  carbohydrate stores of, 415
  circulation in, 404, 520
  colostrum for. See Colostrum.
  compliant thorax of, 473
  diarrhea in, 530–531, 531f
  digestion in, 276
  heat loss by, 535, 540, 541
  mammary gland of, 408
Nephrogenic diabetes insipidus, 333–335,
    456, 457
Nephron(s), 430, 431f
  juxtamedullary, 431f, 453, 454
  reptilian-type, 432, 436–437, 441
    concentrating ability and, 453
    salt balance and, 447
    uric acid secretion by, 444
  superficial, 431f, 453
  tubuloglomerular feedback in, 436
Nephrotic syndrome, 188
Nernst equation, 16
Nerve deafness, 106
Nervous system. See also Autonomic
    nervous system; Central nervous
    system (CNS); Enteric nervous
    system; Peripheral nervous system.
  endocrine system and, 325
  subsections of, 32–33, 32t, 33f
Net hydrostatic pressure difference,
    184–185
Net oncotic pressure difference, 184–185
Neural stalk, 377
Neurocrine peptides, gastrointestinal,
    226–227, 228t
Neuroglial cell, 34
Neurohypophysis (posterior pituitary),
    331, 332–335, 332f–334f, 376, 377. See
    also Oxytocin; Vasopressin
    (antidiuretic hormone [ADH]).
Neurologic examination, reflexes in, 52
Neuromuscular synapse, 41–43, 42f
  action potential at, 41–43, 45
  nicotinic receptors at, 15, 83, 83f
Neuron(s), 32, 34–40. See also Action
    potential(s); Motor neuron(s).
  anatomic regions of, 34, 35f
  neurosecretory, 332
  number of, in nervous system, 34
  oxygen transport to, 113–114, 114f
  postganglionic, 80, 81f, 85–86
    enteric nervous system and, 224, 225f
  preganglionic, 80, 81f, 85, 85f
    enteric nervous system and, 224, 225f
  resting membrane potential of, 34–37,
    36f–37f
Neurophysins, 333, 333f, 377
Neurotransmitter(s), 41, 325, 325f. See also
    specific neurotransmitters.
  at neuromuscular synapse, 15, 41, 42,
    43, 83, 83f
  in autonomic nervous system, 82–83,
    83f

Neurotransmitter(s) (Continued)
  in receptor-mediated signaling, 19–21,
    20f
    cyclic AMP and, 23
    PIP₂ pathway and, 25, 26
    postsynaptic potentials and, 36, 37f
Neutrophils, in lung, 510, 512, 513
Nexus(i). See Gap junctions.
Nicotinamide adenine dinucleotide
    (NAD), microbial, 283, 284, 284f
Nicotine, 83
Nicotinic cholinergic receptors, 15, 21, 83,
    83f
Nipple, 407. See also Teat.
Nitrate poisoning, 120
Nitrates, in rumen, 288, 497
Nitric oxide
  glomerular filtration rate and, 436
  in enteric nervous system, 224
  of nonadrenergic noncholinergic inhibi-
    tory nervous system, 475, 475f
  vasodilation by, 201t, 202
    pulmonary, 482, 483
Nitrite poisoning, 497
Nitrogen, diffusion of, through lipid
    bilayer, 9
Nitrogen balance
  glucocorticoids and, 351
  insulin and, 362
Nociceptive reflex, 59
Nodes of Ranvier, 34
  saltatory conduction and, 39
Nonadrenergic noncholinergic inhibitory
    nervous system, 475, 475f
Nonesterified fatty acids (NEFAs), 317,
    319, 320
Nonintention tremor, 68
Nonshivering thermogenesis, 536, 540
Noradrenergic neurons, 83, 83f, 84t
Norepinephrine, 82, 83, 83f, 85
  actions of, 358, 359
  adipose tissue and, 317
  adrenal medulla and, 357
  biosynthesis of, 5, 5f, 357, 357f–358f, 358
  bronchodilation and, 475
  cardiac contractility and, 159
  cardiac muscle cells and, 24, 132, 132f,
    134, 135
  cardiovascular effects of, 200, 201, 201t,
    202
  cyclic AMP and, 23
  in defense-alarm reaction, 206
  insulin secretion and, 363
  of GI sympathetic fibers, 224
  pulmonary vascular response to, 483t,
    512
  smooth muscle effects of, 359
  vasoconstriction and, 482
Nostrils. See Nares.
Nuclear receptors, 26, 27f, 28
Nucleic acids, digestion of, 258, 258f
Nucleus ambiguus, 502
Nucleus retroambiguus, 502
Nucleus tractus solitarius, 502, 504
Nystagmus, 70, 73
  cerebellum and, 78

O

Occipital lobe, 64, 64f
Oculomotor cranial nerve, 92
Oddi, sphincter of, 252
Olfactory system, pheromones and, 395
Oligodendrocytes, 98
Oligosaccharides, 258, 260
  in fermentative digestion, 283

Omasal transport failure, 295
Omasum, 292, 293, 295
    esophageal groove and, 298
Oncotic (colloid osmotic) pressure, 11–12, 184–186. *See also* Osmotic pressure.
    edema and, 28, 188, 189, 190
    in glomerular capillary, 433, 434f
    in pulmonary fluid exchange, 511–512, 511f
Oocyte(s), 374, 379–380, 384
    depletion of, at menopause, 392
    fertilization of, 398–399
Oocyte-inhibiting factor, 384
Ophthalmoscope, 88, 88f
Opioids
    G proteins and, 23
    renal excretion of, 444
Opsins, 90, 91
Opsonins, in respiratory secretions, 510
Optic chiasm, 91, 92f
Optic disk, 87f–88f, 88, 90, 90f
Optic nerve
    origin of, 87f, 88, 89, 90, 90f
    visual pathway and, 91, 92f
Optic radiations, 91
Organ of Corti, 105, 106f
Organa vasculosum of lamina terminalis, 541
Osmolality
    of plasma
        renal water balance and, 452, 456
        vasopressin and, 333, 334f, 335
    of rumen fluid, 289, 294, 295
    of urine, 452, 453, 454–455, 455f–456f, 456–457
Osmolar concentration, 11
Osmoreceptors, hypothalamic, 333
Osmosis, 10, 10f
    water absorption by, 268–269
    water secretion by, 269
Osmotic coefficient, 11
Osmotic pressure, 9, 10–11, 10f. *See also* Oncotic (colloid osmotic) pressure.
    in capillaries, 11–12, 184–185
    in intestinal lateral spaces, 270
    in intestinal lumen, 269
    in pulmonary fluid exchange, 511–512, 511f
Osmotic-multiplier system, villous, 270–271
Ossicles, 104, 105, 105f–106f
Osteoblasts, 367, 367f, 368, 369
Osteoclasts, 367, 368, 369
Osteocytes, 367, 367f, 368, 369
Osteon, 367f
Otoliths, 71, 71f, 72–73
Oval window, 104, 105, 106f
Ovalbumin, estrogen and, 26, 27f
Ovarian cycle(s), 386–387. *See also* Estrous cycle; Ovulation.
    definition of, 389
    establishment of, 392
    nutrition and, 396
    photoperiod and, 394–395, 394f
Ovarian follicle(s), 374, 377, 377f, 379–380. *See also* Follicular phase.
    development of, 382, 383f, 384
    menopause and, 392
    puberty and, 391
    rupture of, 384
Ovariectomy
    gonadotropins after, 378, 378f
    mammary neoplasia and, in dogs, 418
Ovariohysterectomy, lactation after, 379
Ovary
    embryonic development of, 374, 375f–376f

Ovary (*Continued*)
    gonadotropin receptors of, 329, 380, 384
    gonadotropin secretion modified by, 378, 379
    nutrition and, 396
Oviduct
    embryonic development of, 374, 375, 376f
    fertilization in, 398–399
Ovulation, 374, 377, 378, 380, 382, 383f–384f, 384
    at puberty, 391, 391f, 392
    fertilization and, 398, 399
    sexual receptivity and, 393, 393f
    spontaneous vs. induced, 386–387, 387f
    timing of, 389
Oxaloacetate, 308, 309f
    aspartate and, 309
    from fatty acid β-oxidation, 319, 319f
    in ruminant gluconeogenesis, 320
Oxygen
    administration of, 488, 491
        with anesthesia, 491, 492–493
    diffusion of
        between capillaries and alveoli, 488, 489f
        between capillaries and interstitial fluid, 183–184
        through lipid bilayer, 9
    fraction of, inspired, 486, 487
    myoglobin binding of, 498–499
    neuronal dependence on, 36, 39
    plasma solubility of, 119–120, 494, 494f
Oxygen affinity, of heme, 495
Oxygen capacity, 113, 120, 495
    exercise-induced increase in, 498
    in anemia, 499
Oxygen consumption, 468, 469
    blood flow and, 192–193, 193f
    during exercise, 498–499, 498f
    in cold-stressed animals, 470
    maximal, 468
    thyroid hormones and, 345
Oxygen content, 495, 504
Oxygen radicals, in lung, 510, 512
Oxygen tension (P_{O_2}), 486–487
    alveolar, 487, 488, 489f, 491
        in brachycephalic syndrome, 492
        with oxygen supplementation, 492
        with ventilation/perfusion mismatch, 490f, 491
    arterial, 488, 489f, 491. *See also* Hypoxemia.
        chemoreceptors and, 503, 504, 504f
        during exercise, 488, 489f
        in anesthetized horse, 492–493
        in brachycephalic syndrome, 492
        in tissue capillaries, 488
        with ventilation/perfusion mismatch, 491
    capillary, 488
    inspired, 491
    mixed venous, 488, 489f, 495
    oxyhemoglobin dissociation curve and, 495, 495f
    solubility in plasma and, 494, 494f
    tissue, 488–489, 489f, 495
Oxygen transport, 113–115, 114f, 468, 494–497, 494f–496f
    during exercise, 498–499
    in fetus, 516–520, 517f–519f
Oxyhemoglobin dissociation curve, 495–496, 495f–496f
    carbon monoxide and, 497
    fetal, 519, 519f
Oxyphil cells, 368

Oxytocin, 332–333, 332f, 377
    lactation and, 325, 414–415, 414f–415f, 417
    luteal, 386
    parturition and, 402–403, 403f
Oxytocin receptors, 403

P

P wave, 144, 145f–146f, 147
    in atrial fibrillation, 499
Pacemaker
    artificial cardiac, 136, 140
    gastrointestinal, 231–232
        in colon, 240, 240f, 241
        of horse, 299
Pacemaker cells, cardiac, 125, 131–134, 131f–133f
    ectopic, 137
Pacemaker potential, 131–132, 131f–133f
Packed cell volume, 119
Paleocerebellum, 78
Pampiniform plexus, 421
Pancreas
    autonomic regulation of, 84t
    exocrine secretions of, 249–250, 258
        insufficiency of, 278
        lipid-digesting, 272
        neonatal delay in, 276
        pancreatic polypeptide and, 366
        PIP_2 pathway and, 25–26
        proteolytic, 260, 260t, 261f
    hormones of, 360, 360f–361f. *See also specific hormones.*
    insulinoma of, 39
Pancreatic atrophy, juvenile, 278
Pancreatic polypeptide, 361f, 365–366
Panting
    evaporative cooling by, 535, 540, 541
    in dogs, 469–470
Papillae, of rumen, 297
Paracellular absorption, 264–265, 265f
    of chloride, 267, 267f
    of potassium, 268, 268f
Paracrine effectors, 192, 325, 325f
    gastrointestinal, 225, 226, 228t
Parafollicular cells, thyroid, 342, 368
Parallel fibers, 76, 76f
Paralysis, 58
Paramethasone, 353f
Parasympathetic nervous system, 81, 81f–82f, 82, 83, 85. *See also* Autonomic nervous system.
    airway smooth muscle and, 474, 475f, 477
    anal sphincter and, 241
    cardiac regulation by, 125, 132, 132f, 133, 135, 201–202, 201t
        AV node and, 133–134, 134t, 136
    chemoreceptors and, 503
    exercise and, 216
    gastrointestinal regulation by, 224, 225f
        gastric acid and, 249
        pancreatic secretions and, 250
        smooth muscle and, 233
    in atrial volume receptor reflex, 205, 205f
    in baroreceptor reflex, 203–204, 203f
    in defense-alarm reaction, 206
    in vasovagal syncope, 206, 207f
    pulmonary arteries and, 482
    pupillary constriction and, 92
    salivary glands and, 246
    vascular regulation by, 201t, 202
Parathyroid glands, 367–368, 368f
    lactation and, 418–419

Parathyroid hormone (PTH), 368, 368f–369f, 369
  calcium excretion and, 449
  deficiency of, 371
  excess of, 371
  vitamin D and, 368, 370, 370f, 371
Paraventricular nucleus, 332, 332f, 377
  oxytocin release and, 414, 414f
  prolactin release and, 412, 412f
Paravertebral sympathetic ganglion chain, 81–82, 82f
Parietal cells, gastric, 247, 248, 248f, 249
Parietal lobe, 64, 64f
Parietal pleura, 472, 512
Parietal sensory cortex, 64
Parkinson's tremor, 68
Paroöphoron, 376f
Parotid glands, 246
Paroxysmal atrial tachycardia, 151–152, 160
Pars distalis. *See* Adenohypophysis (anterior pituitary).
Pars intermedia, 335, 336f, 376
  Cushing's disease and, 339
Pars nervosa. *See* Neurohypophysis (posterior pituitary).
Partial pressure, 486
Partial thromboplastin time (PTT), 119
Parturition, 402–404, 402f–403f
  delayed, 404
  hypocalcemia associated with, 418–419
  respiratory system and, 503
  stages of, 404
Passive immunity, 409–410
Passive transport. *See* Diffusion.
Patent ductus arteriosus (PDA), 161f–162f, 162, 164f, 165
  case studies of, 197–198, 520–521
  pulse pressure and, 178f, 179
PCO_2. *See* Carbon dioxide tension (PCO_2).
Pectin, 283
Pelvic flexure, 299, 300
Pelvic nerve, colon and, 224, 225f
Pelvic urethra, 422, 423
Penis, 421, 423
  development of, 375
  ejaculation and, 376
  erection of, 423
    cyclic GMP in, 24
    parasympathetic nervous system and, 202
    sympathetic nervous system and, 359
  species differences in, 422t
Pentose-phosphate pathway, 306
Pepsin, 247, 248–249, 257, 260, 260t
Pepsinogen, 247, 248–249, 260, 260t
Peptidases
  of enterocytes, 262
  of proximal tubule, 443
Peptide bond, hydrolysis of, 258, 258f
Peptide hormones. *See also specific hormones.*
  cell responses to, 329–330, 330f
  feedback control of, 330–331, 331f
  hypothalamic, 376, 377–378, 377f
  receptors for, 328–329
  synthesis of, 326, 326f
  transport of, 328
Peptides
  buffering by, 524
  in protein digestion, 260, 261, 262, 262f
    fermentative, 286–287, 286f, 288f
  renal tubular reabsorption of, 443
Perfusion. *See* Blood flow; Ventilation/perfusion ratio.
Perfusion pressure, 112, 116–117, 169

Perfusion pressure *(Continued)*
  blood flow and, 175, 192
  renal, 435
  resistance and, 171, 172, 172f–173f, 177
Peribronchial plexus, 484
Pericarditis, in hardware disease, 28
Perikaryon, of neuron, 32, 35f
Perilymph, 71, 105, 106f
Peripheral chemoreceptors, 503–504, 504f, 505
Peripheral nervous system, 32t, 33, 34. *See also* Autonomic nervous system; Motor neuron(s); Sensory (afferent) nerves.
Peripheral receptors, 33
Peristalsis, 234, 234f. *See also* Gastrointestinal motility.
  of colon, 240, 240f, 241
    equine, 299
  of esophagus, 234
  of rectum, 241, 241f
  of small intestine, 238–239
  of stomach, 236, 236f
Peritubular capillary(ies), 440–441, 440f, 442f, 452
Persistent luteal-phase syndrome, 387–388
Pertussis toxin, G proteins and, 23
Petrous temporal bone, 70, 70f, 105
PG. *See* Prostaglandin(s).
pH, 523. *See also* Acid-base balance; Acidosis; Alkalosis; Buffers; Hydrogen ions.
  in rumen, 295, 296
  in stomach, 226
  of blood
    chemoreceptors and, 501, 501f, 504–505
    gastric acid production and, 248
    lactic acid and, 505
    measurement of, 528–529, 529t
    normal, 522, 523
    oxyhemoglobin dissociation curve and, 496, 496f, 498
    regulation of, 459, 524–526, 525f
  of cerebrospinal fluid, 504–505, 504f–505f
  of urine, 459, 462
    in paradoxic aciduria, 465–466
    species differences in, 464–465
Pharynx, 469
  dynamic compression of, 475
  frictional resistance of, 473, 473f
  inhalation and, 470
  receptors in, 503
Phenylephrine, pulmonary vascular response to, 483t
Phenylethanolamine-*N*-methyltransferase, 5, 5f, 358, 358f
Pheromones, 395
Phorbol esters, 26
Phosphate
  buffering by, 523–524, 524f
    intracellular, 524
    renal, 460, 460f
  calcitonin and, 369
  in membrane bilayer, 8, 8f
  in muscle contraction, 6, 7f
  in saliva, 246, 247f
  oxyhemoglobin dissociation curve and, 496
  parathyroid hormone and, 368
  physiologic roles of, 366
  renal excretion of, 369
  renal tubular reabsorption of, 442
  vitamin D and, 370, 371
Phosphatidyl inositol-4,5-bisphosphate (PIP$_2$), 20, 24f–25f, 25, 329

Phosphodiester bond, hydrolysis of, 258, 258f
Phosphodiesterase, 23
  hormone action and, 329, 330f
Phosphofructokinase, 314, 314f, 315
Phospholipase, pancreatic, 272
Phospholipase A
  in parturition, 403
  prostaglandins and, 329–330, 353
Phospholipase C, 25, 25f, 26
Phospholipid bilayer. *See* Membrane(s).
Phospholipids
  digestion and absorption of, 272, 273f, 275, 275f
  in bile, 251, 272
  in milk, 415
  in prostaglandin synthesis, 403
  in VLDL, 308, 309f
Phosphoric acid, from protein metabolism, 522
Phosphorylation
  of hepatic enzymes, 313–315, 314f
  of proteins, 4, 4f
  of tyrosine hydroxylase, 5
Photoperiod
  endocrine secretion and, 331
  lactation and, 417, 418f
  puberty and, 391–392
  refractoriness to, 392, 394
  reproductive cycles and, 394–395, 394f, 417
Photoreceptor cells, 89, 89f, 90–91, 91f
Photorefractoriness, 394
Phrenic nerve, 470
Physiologic dead-space, 469
Physiology, definition of, 2
Pia mater, 33, 33f
Piloerection, 535, 540
  epinephrine and, 359
  fever and, 541
Pineal gland, 394
Pinocytosis, 186, 188
PIP$_2$ (phosphatidyl inositol-4,5-bisphosphate), 20, 24f–25f, 25, 329
Pitch, 104, 104f, 105
Pitting edema, 28
Pituitary dwarfism, in dogs, 338
Pituitary gland, 331–332, 332f, 376. *See also* Adenohypophysis (anterior pituitary); Neurohypophysis (posterior pituitary).
  intermediate lobe of, 335, 336f, 376
    Cushing's disease and, 339
pK$_a$, 523–524, 525
PKC (protein kinase C), 26
Placenta, 400, 401–402, 516–518, 517f–518f
  antibodies transferred by, 410
  chorionic gonadotropin produced by, 335
  delivery of, 404
  detachment of, 520
  estrogen produced by, 349
  lactogen produced by, 402
  relaxin produced by, 404
  species differences in, 516, 516t
  vitamin A transferred by, 410
Plasma
  calcium in, 367
  composition of, 12t, 118, 118f, 119t
  osmolality of
    renal water balance and, 452, 456
    vasopressin and, 333, 334f, 335
Plasma cells, in mammary gland, 410
Plasma membrane. *See* Membrane(s).
Plasma oncotic pressure. *See* Oncotic (colloid osmotic) pressure.

Plasma proteins, 118, 119t, 120, 121, 121f
  buffering by, 524
  edema and, 188–189, 189f
  enteropathy and, 190
  fenestrated capillaries and, 182
  glomerular filtration of, 434–435, 438
  hemorrhage and, 215
  histamine and, 190
  hormone transport by, 112, 328
    adrenocortical, 350–351
    thyroid, 343–344
  lung capillaries and, 186
  lymphatic transport of, 186, 188
  oncotic pressure and, 11, 12, 184, 185–186
  renal tubular reabsorption of, 443–444
  synthesis of, in liver, 310, 310f
  vitamin D transport by, 370
Platelets, 119
"Playing dead reaction," 206, 207f
Pleura, blood supply to, 484
Pleural effusion, in heart failure, 212
Pleural fluid, 472, 512
Pleural pressure, 471, 471f
  elevated, 476, 477
Pleural space, 512
Pleuritis, 512–513
Pleuropneumonia, 512–513
Plicae circulares, 255
Pluripotent stem cells, 119
PMSG (pregnant mare serum
  gonadotropin), 335, 401–402, 401f
Pneumonia. *See also* Pleuropneumonia.
  mucociliary clearance and, in horses,
    509
  right-to-left shunt in, 490f, 491
  vascular permeability in, 511–512
Pneumotaxic center, 502, 502f
Po₂. *See* Oxygen tension (Po₂).
Podocytes, 433, 434f
Poikilotherms, 533, 534, 536
Poiseuille's law, 171, 172
Polycythemia, 121, 495, 495f
Polymorphonuclear leukocytes, in lung,
  510
Polyradiculoneuritis, 59–60
Polysaccharides, 258, 261. *See also*
  Carbohydrates.
Pons, 33, 63, 63f. *See also* Brainstem.
  corticopontine-cerebellar tract and, 64
  respiratory control by, 502, 502f
  reticular activating system in, 67
Pontine respiratory group, 502, 502f
Portal system
  definition of, 115
  hepatic, 271, 271f
    amino acids in, 309, 310, 310f
    bile acids and, 252, 252f, 272
    propionate in, 320
  hypothalamic-hypophyseal, 116, 335–336, 336f, 377, 377f
  renal, 115f, 116
  splanchnic, 115–116, 115f
Portal vein, 115, 115f
Postabsorptive metabolism, 313–317, 314f,
  316f
Posterior pituitary. *See* Neurohypophysis
  (posterior pituitary).
Postganglionic neurons, 80, 81f, 85–86
  enteric nervous system and, 224, 225f
Postpartum period, ovarian activity in,
  396
Postsynaptic cell, 34
Postsynaptic membrane, of neuromuscular
  synapse, 41, 42f
Postsynaptic potentials, 36–37, 37f, 99

Posture, 62, 67–68
Potassium. *See also* H⁺,K⁺-ATPase pump;
  Hyperkalemia; Hypokalemia; Na⁺,K⁺-
  ATPase pump.
  acid-base homeostasis and, 528
  active transport and, 12–14, 12f
  intestinal absorption of, 268, 268f, 268t
  neurologic deficits and, 36
  renal reabsorption of, 442, 442f–443f,
    443
    in collecting duct, 447
    in distal tubule, 445, 447f
  renal secretion of
    in collecting duct, 447, 448, 448f
    mineralocorticoids and, 354t, 355–356,
      448, 448f
  resting membrane potential and, 9, 15–
    17, 35–36
Potassium ion channels
  action potential and, 37
  in pulmonary artery smooth muscle,
    483
  inhibitory potential and, 36–37
  leak channels as, 15, 16
  of cardiac muscle, 127–128, 129f, 131
    β-adrenergic receptors and, 134
    calcium channel blockers and, 139
    in pacemaker cells, 131, 131f
  of glomus cells, 504, 504f
PP interval, 146, 146f
PR interval, 145–146, 146f
Prealbumin, thyroxine-binding, 343
Preantral follicles, 380
Precapillary sphincters, 181–182, 193
Precentral gyrus, 64
Precontraction, 137, 138
Precordial leads, 147
Prednisolone, 353f
Prednisone, 353f
Preganglionic neurons, 80, 81f, 85, 85f
  enteric nervous system and, 224, 225f
Pregnancy, 399–402, 399f–401f
  diagnosis of, in dog, 404
  glucose homeostasis in, 320–321
  hypocalcemia in, 418
  mammary development in, 409, 411f
  prolonged, 404
  steroid-binding proteins in, 350
  toxemia of, in ewes, 321
  vitamin D production in, 371
Pregnant mare serum gonadotropin
  (PMSG), 335, 401–402, 401f
Pregnenolone, 327, 327f, 328, 401
  in adrenal cortex, 350, 350f
Prehension of food, 233, 234
Preload, ventricular, 156–158, 157f–158f,
  160
  abnormal reduction in, 173
  during exercise, 217
  in heart failure, 209, 210, 210f
Premature beat, 137, 138
Premature ventricular contractions, 149,
  149f
Premotor cortex, 64, 66, 68
  cerebrocerebellum and, 78
Preprohormones, 326, 326f
Prepro-oxyphysin, 332
Prepropressophysin, 332, 333f
Prerenal azotemia, 450
Pressure. *See also* Hydrostatic pressure;
  Oncotic (colloid osmotic) pressure;
  Osmotic pressure.
  barometric, 486, 491
  free energy and, 9, 10
Pressure sores, 195
Pressure-volume hysteresis, 472, 472f

Presynaptic cell, 34
Presynaptic membrane, of neuromuscular
  synapse, 41, 42f
Presynaptic terminals, 34, 35f
Pretectal region, 92
Prevertebral ganglia, 82
Primary follicles, 380
Principal cells, of collecting ducts, 447,
  448, 448f, 464f
Procarboxypeptidase A, 260t, 261f
Procarboxypeptidase B, 260t, 261f
Proelastase, 260t, 261f
Proestrus, 389, 390f, 392
  sexual receptivity and, 395
Progesterone
  biosynthesis of, 327f, 328
  exogenous, canine acromegaly and,
    338
  follicular secretion of, 384
  gonadotropin secretion and, 378–379
  in pregnancy, 399, 400, 400f–401f, 401,
    402
  lactation and, 409, 416, 417
  luteal secretion of, 384–385, 388
  luteinization and, 385
  luteolysis and, 386
  mammary development and, 409, 410f
  mammary neoplasia and, 418
  ovarian status and, 390
  parturition and, 402, 402f, 403, 404
  placental production of, 401
  sexual receptivity and, 392, 393, 393f,
    394
  transport of, in blood, 328
Progoitrin, 346
Prohormones, 326, 326f
Prolactin, 335, 376, 378, 379
  as luteotropin, 385
  dopamine and, 337, 337t
  estrus cycle and, in cat, 417
  hypothalamic releasing factors and, 337,
    337t
  in lactogenesis, 410, 412, 412f, 414–415
  in mammary development, postfetal,
    409, 410f
  in pregnancy, 400, 402
  lactose synthetase and, 416
  light exposure and, 417
  pheromones and, 395
  pseudopregnancy and, 387
  suckling and, 395
  thyrotropin-releasing hormone and, 417
  vitamin D and, 371
Pro-opiomelanocortin, 335, 336f, 337, 379
  Cushing's disease and, 339
Propionate, 284, 284f–286f, 285, 285t, 416
  absorption of, 296, 297
  dilution rate and, 294
  gluconeogenesis and, 320–321, 320f
Propranolol, 135
  cardiac contractility and, 159
Proprioception, conscious, 52, 66–67, 69
  lower motor neuron disease and, 59
  upper motor neuron disease and, 60
Prostacyclin (prostaglandin I₂ [PGI₂])
  pulmonary vasodilation by, 483t
  renal release of, 435, 436
Prostaglandin(s), 329–330
  ductus arteriosus closure and, 520
  fever and, 541
  glucocorticoid inhibition of, 353
  renal excretion of, 444
  vasodilation caused by, 482–483
Prostaglandin E, 385
  degradation of, by lung, 512
  in parturition, 403

Prostaglandin E₂
  ductus arteriosus and, 520
  fever and, 541
  renal release of, 435, 436
Prostaglandin F₂ₐ (PGF₂ₐ), 384, 385–386, 385f–386f
  degradation of, in lung, 512
  in parturition, 402–403, 402f, 404
  in postpartum period, 404
  in pregnancy, 399–400, 399f
    inadequate, 387–388
Prostaglandin I₂ (PGI₂)
  pulmonary vasodilation by, 483t
  renal release of, 435, 436
Prostate gland, 421, 422t, 423
Protease inhibitors, as lung protectants, 510
Protein(s), 2–5. See also Enzymes.
  allosteric properties of, 4–5, 4f
    in catecholamine biosynthesis, 5
    in gated channels, 15
    in muscle contraction, 6, 7f, 8
    in receptor-mediated signaling, 19
  buffering by, 497, 498, 523, 524
    hemoglobin in, 459, 497, 497f, 524, 526, 527
  dietary, glomerular filtration rate and, 436
  digestion of, 258, 258f, 260, 260t, 261f–262f, 262
    pancreatic enzymes in, 249, 250
    pancreatic polypeptide and, 366
  functions of, 2–3
  in colostrum, 410, 410t
  in fermentative digestion, 281, 283, 285–288, 286f, 288f
    in equine hindgut, 298
  in interstitial fluid, 184, 186, 188, 189
  in milk, 412, 413f, 415t, 416
  in muscle contraction, 5–8, 6f–7f
  in plasma. See Plasma proteins.
  intestinal absorption of, in neonate, 276
  metabolism of
    glucagon and, 364
    glucocorticoids and, 351
    heat produced by, 536, 536t
    hydrogen ions from, 522–523
    insulin and, 361, 362, 362f, 362t, 363
  of cell membrane, 8–9, 8f
    in active transport, 10, 12–14, 12f–13f
    in facilitated diffusion, 14–15, 14f
    in signal transduction, 19–20, 20f
    spatial organization of, 17, 23
  phosphorylation of, 4, 4f, 5, 313–315, 314f
  synthesis of
    in liver, 118, 310, 310f, 312
    in muscle, 312, 313f
    in nonhepatic tissue, 310, 312
Protein hormones
  cell responses to, 329–330, 330f
  metabolism of, 330
  receptors for, 328–329
  synthesis of, 326, 326f
  transport of, 328
Protein kinase A, 23, 24
Protein kinase C (PKC), 26
Protein kinases, 21
  cyclic AMP and, 23, 24
  in hormone action, 329, 330f
  with thyroid hormones, 346
  in smooth muscle contraction, 21
  PIP₂ pathway and, 25, 26
Protein-losing enteropathy, 190–191
Proteinuria, in glomerulonephritis, 438

Proteolytic enzymes
  of pulmonary phagocytic cells, 510
  pancreatic, 260, 260t, 261f
Prothrombin time (PT), 119
Proton pumps
  gastric, 248, 248f
  renal, 460, 461, 462, 462f–463f
    bicarbonate secretion and, 464, 465f
Protons. See Hydrogen ions.
Proventriculus, 242, 242f, 243
Proximal tubule, 431f, 432
  ammoniagenesis in, 460, 461f
  anatomy of, 440, 440f–442f
  reabsorption in, 440–444, 440f–444f
    of bicarbonate, 462, 464
    of calcium, 448
    of water, 452
  secretion of H⁺ by, 459, 460f, 461–462
  secretion of organic ions by, 444
PT (prothrombin time), 119
PTH. See Parathyroid hormone (PTH).
PTH-related protein, 371
PTT (partial thromboplastin time), 119
Puberty, 390–392, 391f
  in males, 392, 425–426
  mammary development at, 409
  Whitten effect and, 395
Pubic symphysis, relaxin and, 403
Pulmonary. See also Lung(s); "Respiratory" entries.
Pulmonary arterial pressure, 176–177, 176f, 480
  at high altitude, 483, 484f
  during exercise, 483
  low, dead-space and, 491
  resistance and, 175
Pulmonary arterioles, 479, 481
Pulmonary artery(ies), 115, 115f
  cardiac cycle and, 155
  hypoxic vasoconstriction of, 483
  resistance in, 481f
  smooth muscle of, 479, 482–483, 482f
    Crotalaria toxicity to, 512
    in hypoxia, 483, 484f, 485
  species differences in, 479, 482, 482f, 483
Pulmonary artery pulse pressure, 176, 176f
Pulmonary capillaries, 113, 114f, 479, 480f
  C fibers and, 503
  endothelial cells of, 511, 511f, 512
  fluid exchange with, 511–512, 511f
  gas exchange with, 488, 488f–489f
  in exercising horse, 483
  metabolic functions of, 512
  pulsatile flow in, 481
  resistance in, 481, 481f, 482
Pulmonary circulation, 115, 115f, 479–483.
    See also Pulmonary artery(ies);
    Pulmonary capillaries; Pulmonary veins.
  alveolar pressure and, 196–197, 196f
  blood vessels in, 479–480, 480f
  bronchial circulation and, 484, 491
  chemical mediators and, 482–483, 483t
  distribution of, in lung, 481, 481f
  exercise and, 175, 479, 481, 481f, 482, 483
  perfusion pressure in, 116
  pressures in, 480
  resistance in. See Pulmonary vascular resistance (PVR).
  species differences in, 479, 482, 482f, 483
Pulmonary edema, 111, 511–512
  aortic regurgitation with, 165
  heart failure with, 188, 211–212
  mitral insufficiency with, 164, 165, 513

Pulmonary edema (Continued)
  mitral stenosis with, 165
  patent ductus arteriosus with, 165
  ventricular septal defect with, 165
Pulmonary embolism, in canine heartworm disease, 179–180
Pulmonary hemorrhage, exercise-induced, 483
Pulmonary hypertension, 176, 483
  in Crotalaria poisoning, 512
  ventilation/perfusion ratio in, 490
Pulmonary stretch receptors, 502, 503, 510
Pulmonary surfactant, 472, 473f, 503, 519, 520
  in edema, 511
Pulmonary vascular resistance (PVR), 175–176, 176f, 177, 480–481, 481f
  at high altitude, 484f
  during exercise, 483
  humoral factors affecting, 482–483, 483t
  lung inflation and, 481–482, 482f
  neural factors affecting, 482
Pulmonary veins, 115, 115f, 479, 480f, 481
  resistance in, 175, 481f
Pulmonary venous pressure, 480
  resistance and, 175
Pulmonary venules, 479
Pulmonary wedge pressure, 480
Pulmonic regurgitation, 161t, 162, 162f
Pulmonic stenosis, 161f, 161t, 162, 165, 166
  in heartworm disease, 179
Pulmonic valve
  in cardiac cycle, 155
  second heart sound and, 156
Pulse, palpation of, 177
Pulse pressure, 176–177, 176f
  aging and, 178–179
  determinants of, 177–179, 178f–179f
  hemorrhage and, 214
Pump failure, 209
Pupil, 87f, 88, 92
Pupillary diameter
  autonomic control of, 83, 84t, 85, 92
  epinephrine and, 359
Pupillary light reflex, 52, 85, 92
Purkinje cells, 76, 76f–77f, 78
  in cerebellar hypoplasia, 79
Purkinje's fibers, 126, 126f–127f
Putamen, 68
PVR. See Pulmonary vascular resistance (PVR).
Pyloric mucosa, 247
Pyramidal cells, 98, 99f
  EEG and, 100
Pyramidal system, 62, 63–67, 64f
  basal ganglia and, 68
  cerebellum and, 75, 76, 77f, 78
  lesions in, 66–67
Pyrexia, 541, 542f
Pyrogens, 541, 542f
Pyruvate
  alanine derived from, 309–310, 310f, 315–316, 316f
  in fatty acid synthesis, 308, 309f
  in gluconeogenesis, 315
  in microbial metabolism, 283, 284, 284f
  in muscle, 315, 316f

Q

Q wave, 144, 145f–146f
QRS complex, 145, 146, 146f
QT interval, 146, 146f
Quadriceps muscle, 56
  knee jerk reflex and, 54–55, 55f
Quinidine sulfate, for atrial fibrillation, 499

R

R wave, 144–145, 145f–146f, 147
Rabies, equine, 243
Radiant heat loss, 534, 534f, 535, 540
Radiant heat sources, 534, 534f
Rathke's pouch, 332, 332f, 376
  cystic, dwarfism and, 338
Reabsorption, capillary, 184
Reaction coupling, 3
  in active transport, 10, 12
Reactive hyperemia, 193, 193f, 195
Receptor-mediated endocytosis, 18, 18f
Receptors
  cell-surface, 19–21, 20f
    desensitization of, 21
    down-regulation of, 21, 329
    endocytosis of, 18, 18f, 21
    hypersensitization of, 21
  chemoreceptors as, 503–505, 504f–505f
    acid-base balance and, 528
    of gastrointestinal system, 222, 224f
    of reticulorumen, 295
  hormone receptors as, 19–21, 20f, 328–329
    cyclic AMP and, 23
    for steroid hormones, 26, 27f, 28, 328–329
    PIP$_2$ pathway and, 25, 26
  mechanoreceptors as
    gastrointestinal, 222, 224f, 249
    respiratory, 501, 503, 510
  peripheral, 33. See also Muscle spindle
    stretch receptors.
    of vestibular system, 71, 71f
  reflex arc and, 51, 51f
  postsynaptic, 41
Rectal temperature, 537–538, 537t
Rectosphincteric reflex, 241, 241f
Red blood cell count, 120, 120t
Red blood cell–agglutinating antibodies, 418, 419
Red blood cells. See Erythrocytes.
Red muscle, 49
5α-Reductase, 375
5α-Reductase inhibitors, 375
Reentry, 137–138, 138f
Reflex arc, 51–52, 51f
  motor neuron disease and, 59
  muscle spindles and, 54–55, 55f
Reflexes
  autonomic, 85
  vestibular, 73
  vs. responses, 69
Refractory period
  of cardiac muscle, 129–130, 130f
    β-adrenergic activation and, 134, 135
    atrial vs. ventricular, 131
    of AV node, 133, 134, 134t, 136, 137
    parasympathetic effects on, 135
  of skeletal muscle, 130
Reissner's membrane, 105, 106f
Relative humidity, 535, 540
Relaxin, 384, 400, 401, 403–404
Renal. See also Kidney(s).
Renal artery(ies), 115f, 116
  blood pressure in, 436
  of birds vs. mammals, 432
Renal blood flow, 435–436, 435f
Renal failure
  chronic, 437–438
  heart failure causing, 212–213
  hypercalcemia in, 371
  vs. hypoadrenocorticism, 356
Renal insufficiency
  chronic, 457–458
  in feline hyperthyroidism, 348

Renal portal system, 115f, 116
Renal tubules. See Kidney(s), tubules of.
Renin, 435, 435f
  arterial baroreceptor reflex and, 205
  atrial volume receptor reflex and, 205, 205f
  epinephrine and, 359
Renin-angiotensin-aldosterone system, 355, 355f, 435–436, 435f. See also
    Angiotensin II.
  atrial volume receptor reflex and, 205
  hemorrhage and, 215
Rennin (chymosin), 260t
Repolarization, 37
Reproductive cycles, 389–390, 390f. See
    also Ovarian cycle(s).
  lactation and, 395
  nutrition and, 396
  pheromones and, 395
  photoperiod and, 394–395, 394f
Reproductive senescence, 392
RER (rough endoplasmic reticulum). See
    also Endoplasmic reticulum.
  in hormone synthesis, 326, 326f
Residual volume (RV), 472
  pulmonary vascular resistance and, 482, 482f
Resistance. See Airway resistance;
    Vascular resistance.
Respiration. See Ventilation.
Respiratory acidosis, 463f, 465, 526–527, 527f, 529t
Respiratory alkalosis, 527, 527f, 529t
Respiratory epithelium, 509–510, 509f
  cytokines and chemokines of, 510–511
  viral injury to, 512–513
Respiratory exchange ratio, 487
Respiratory frequency, 469–470
  brainstem control of, 502
  gait frequency and, 470, 471f, 505
Respiratory muscles, 470–471
  control of, 501, 501f, 502
  stretch receptors of, 503
Respiratory pump, 217
Respiratory system. See also Lung(s);
    "Pulmonary" entries.
  defense mechanisms of, 508–511, 509f–510f
  functions of, 468
Resting membrane potential, 15–17
  ligand-gated channels and, 20
  of GI smooth muscle, 231, 231f, 233
  of neuron, 34–37, 36f–37f
  of skeletal muscle, 45
  voltage-gated channels and, 14f, 15
Resting tremor, 68
Rete ovarii, 375f, 379
Rete testis, 375, 375f–376f, 422
Reticular activating system, 63, 67, 67f
  EEG and, 100
Reticular groove, 297–298
Reticulo-omasal orifice, 290f, 292, 293, 298
Reticulorumen. See Rumen.
Reticulospinal tract, 67
  in decerebrate rigidity, 68
Retina, 87, 87f–88f, 88
  as extension of brain, 89
  blood vessels of, 88, 88f
  cell types in, 89, 89f
  cyclic GMP in, 24
  electroretinogram and, 91
  focusing on, 88–89
  fovea of, 90, 90f
  nasal, 91
  photoperiod and, 394
  pupillary reflex test and, 92

Retina (Continued)
  temporal, 91–92
Retinal, in photopigments, 90
Reverse T$_3$, 343, 344, 344f
  in euthyroid sick syndrome, 347
Rhodopsin, 90
Rhythmic extrapyramidal disorders, 68
Ribosomes, preprohormone synthesis in, 326
Right atrium, 115, 115f
Right ventricle, 115, 115f, 479
Right ventricular hypertrophy
  ECG associated with, 147–148, 147f
  patent ductus arteriosus with, 164f, 165
  pulmonic stenosis with, 165, 166
  ventricular septal defect with, 165
Right-sided heart failure, 209, 483, 485–486. See also Heart failure.
  GI blood flow and, 271
  pulmonary hypertension and, 176
  systemic edema in, 188, 212
Right-to-left shunt, 491
  in anesthetized horse, 493
  through cardiac defect, 506
Rigor mortis, 6, 8
RNA. See also Messenger RNA (mRNA).
  in ovarian follicle, 380
Roaring, 470
Rods, 89, 89f, 90, 91, 91f
  cyclic GMP in, 24
Rolling, compulsive, 70, 73
Rough endoplasmic reticulum (RER). See
    also Endoplasmic reticulum.
  in hormone synthesis, 326, 326f
RR interval, 146, 146f
Rumen. See also Fermentative digestion.
  anatomy of, 289, 290f
  development of, 297–298
  epithelium of, 295–296, 296f, 297
  feed characteristics and, 292–293, 294–295, 297
  grain engorgement toxemia and, 302
  ketone bodies formed in, 297, 307, 310
  motility of, 289–290, 291f–292f, 292
    control of, 294–295
  movement of material through, 292–293, 292f
  movement of water through, 293–294
  mucosa of, 294
  necessary characteristics of, 289
  papillae of, 297
  pH in, 295, 296
  stratification in, 290, 292, 292f
  VFA absorption in, 295–297, 296f–297f
Rumen acidosis, 527
Rumen mat, 290, 294–295
Ruminant(s). See also Fermentative
    digestion; Rumen.
  gluconeogenesis in, 320–321, 320f
  glucose homeostasis in, 320–321
  glucose sources for, 311
  liver of
    nitrogen cycling and, 288, 289f
    propionate extraction and, 320
  saliva of, 246, 247f
    flow rate of, 294
    urea in, 288, 289t
  urine pH in, 465
Rumination, 293, 294
  in calves, 297
RV (residual volume), 472
  pulmonary vascular resistance and, 482, 482f

S

S wave, 145, 145f–146f
SA (sinoatrial) node, 125, 126, 126f–127f

SA (sinoatrial) node (*Continued*)
  action potentials at, 131–132, 131f–133f
  autonomic regulation of, 132, 132f, 135,
    201, 204
  calcium channel blockers and, 139
  tachycardia associated with, 137
Saccharides, 258–259, 259f. *See also*
    Carbohydrates.
Saccule, 70f–71f, 71, 72–73
Saliva, 245–246
  electrolyte composition of, 246, 247f
  heat loss and, 535
  of ruminants, 246, 247f
    flow rate of, 294
    urea in, 288, 289t
Salivary glands, 246–247, 246f, 258
Saltatory conduction, 39, 39f
Sarcolemma, 44
  action potential on, 45, 48, 49
  transverse tubules and, 45, 47f
Sarcomeres
  of cardiac muscle, 124–125, 124f
  of skeletal muscle, 45, 46f–48f, 48
Sarcoplasmic reticulum(a)
  of cardiac muscle, 49, 129, 130
    β-adrenergic activation and, 134
  of skeletal muscle, 21, 45, 47f, 48, 128,
    130
  of smooth muscle, 49
Scala media, 105
Scala tympani, 106f
Scala vestibuli, 105, 106f
Schwann cells, 34
Sclera, 87, 87f, 88
Scrotum, 421, 422
  development of, 375
Sebaceous glands, pheromones secreted
    by, 395
Second messengers, 20, 20f
  calcium ions as, 20, 21, 22f, 23, 329
  cyclic AMP as, 20, 23–24, 24f, 25
  for hormones, 329, 330f
  PIP₂ and, 20, 24f–25f, 25
Secondary active transport
  definition of, 13
  in intestinal absorption, 13, 13f, 263–
    264, 263f–264f
  in renal tubular reabsorption, 442–443,
    442f, 445, 447f
Secretin, 227t
  bile secretion and, 252
  calcitonin and, 369
  gastric acid secretion and, 249
  gastric emptying and, 237
  gastric motility and, 236
  insulin secretion and, 363
  pancreatic polypeptide and, 366
  pancreatic secretions and, 250
Secretory diarrhea, 277–278, 277f
Secretory granules, of GI endocrine cells,
    225, 226f
Sedimentation, of particles in airways,
    508, 509f
Segmental reflex, 52
  loss of, 59
Segmentation
  in colon, 240, 241
    equine, 299, 301
  in small intestine, 238, 238f
Seizures
  EEG pattern and, 103
  serum glucose and, 39
Selective transport, 8
Semen
  composition of, 422–423
  deposition of, in different species, 422t

Semen (*Continued*)
  ejaculation of, 423
Semicircular canals, 70f, 71, 72, 72f, 73
  vomiting and, 238
Seminal vesicles, 421, 422t, 423
Seminiferous cords, 375f–376f
Seminiferous tubules, 421–422, 423, 425,
    426f
Semipermeable membrane, 10, 184
Senescence, reproductive, 392
Sensory cortex, voluntary movement and,
    66
Sensory evoked potentials, 100, 103, 103f,
    106
Sensory (afferent) nerves, 32t, 33
  disease of, 59
  of muscle spindle, 53f–54f, 54
  reflex arc and, 51, 51f, 52, 62
  visceral, 32t, 33, 85
Septic shock, 111
  in heart failure, 212
Serine, phosphorylation of, 4, 4f
Serotonin, pulmonary vascular response
    to, 483t, 512
Sertoli cells, 374, 375f, 422, 425, 426f
Serum, 119
Sex cords, 374, 375f
Sex glands, accessory, 421, 422t, 423
Sex pheromones, 395
Sexual receptivity, 389, 392–394, 393f. *See
    also* Estrus.
  fertilization and, 399
  in dog, 385
  persistent luteal phase and, 387, 388
  pheromones and, 395
Shivering, 536, 539, 540
  fever and, 541
Shock, 111–112
  in calf diarrhea, 278
  in grain engorgement toxemia, 302
  in heart failure, 212
  in *Strongylus* infestation, 121–122
Shock-lung syndrome, 111
Short-loop feedback system, 337, 337f
Sick sinus syndrome, 135–136, 135t
Sighs, pulmonary surfactant and, 503
Signaling, 3, 18–19, 19f. *See also*
    Information; Neurotransmitter(s);
    Receptors; Second messengers.
Sildenafil (Viagra), 24
Sinoatrial (SA) node, 125, 126, 126f–127f
  action potentials at, 131–132, 131f–133f
  autonomic regulation of, 132, 132f, 135,
    201, 204
  calcium channel blockers and, 139
  tachycardia associated with, 137
Sinus arrest, 135
Sinus bradycardia, 149f, 150
Sinus tachycardia, 137, 149f, 150
Sinusoids, of liver, 271
Skeletal muscle, 5–6, 7, 44
  amino acid metabolism in, 306, 312,
    315–316, 316f, 317
  atrophy of, 58–59
  capillaries of, 114, 114f, 183–184
  classification of fibers in, 48–49
  contraction mechanism of, 5–8, 6f–7f,
    21, 45, 48, 48f
    vs. cardiac mechanism, 123–124, 124t,
      126–128, 128f, 130
  electromyogram of, 48
  exercise-induced changes in
    arteriolar vasodilation as, 174f, 175,
      183–184, 192, 216
    capillary blood flow as, 183–184
    gas transport and, 498–499

Skeletal muscle (*Continued*)
  glucose in, 312, 315, 316f
  glycogen synthesis in, 312
  Golgi tendon organs and, 53, 53f, 55–56,
    56f
  intercostal muscles and, 503
  heat produced in, 534
  insulin effects on, 312, 362, 362t
  ischemia of, 196
  length of, detection of, 53, 54, 56
  mitochondria in, 44, 47f, 49, 468
  motor neurons and, 32t, 33
  movement and, 44, 45f
  neuromuscular synapse of, 41–43, 42f
    action potential at, 41–43, 45
    nicotinic receptors at, 15, 83, 83f
  oxygen transport to, 114, 114f
  protein synthesis in, 312, 313f
  reflex arc and, 51–52, 51f
    in motor neuron disease, 59
    muscle spindles and, 54–55, 55f
  respiratory, 470–471
    control of, 501, 501f, 502
    stretch receptors of, 503
  sparing of, in undernutrition, 317
  stretch receptors of, 51, 53–55, 53f–55f,
    56
    cerebellum and, 75
    of respiratory muscles, 503
    voluntary movement and, 66
  structural organization of, 44–45, 46f–
    47f
  vasodilation in
    β₂-adrenergic receptors and, 200, 201,
      201t, 202
    cholinergic neurons and, 82
    exercise-induced, 174f, 175, 192
    M₃ receptors and, 201t, 202
Skin
  autonomic innervation of, 84t
  blood flow in, 534, 540
  receptors in, 51
    for temperature, 538–539, 539f
Sleep. *See also* Circadian rhythms.
  EEG and, 99
  parathyroid hormone and, 368
Slit diaphragm, 433, 433f
Slow action potentials, 132, 133
Slow calcium channels, 129, 131
Slow waves, 231–233, 231f–232f
  in colon, 231, 233, 240, 240f
Slow-twitch fibers, 49
  myoglobin in, 498
Slow-wave focus, 103
Small intestine. *See also* Absorption,
    intestinal; Digestion.
  equine, 298, 299, 299f
  glicentin produced by, 364
  lipid emulsification in, 272, 274f
  microbial protein in, 287
  motility of, 238–239, 238f
    slow waves and, 231, 233
  mucosa of, 223f, 255–257, 256f–257f
  of birds, 242, 242f, 243
Smooth muscle, 6, 44, 49
  autonomic nervous system and, 32t, 33,
    80, 85
  catecholamines and, 359
  contraction mechanism of, 21, 22f, 23
  of airways, 474–475, 475f
    epinephrine and, 359
    stretch receptors in, 503, 510
  of bladder, catecholamines and, 359
  of esophagus, 234
  of gut
    electrical properties of, 231–233, 231f–
      232f

Smooth muscle (*Continued*)
  epinephrine and, 359
  innervation of, 222, 224f
  of pulmonary arteries, 479, 482–483, 482f
    Crotalaria toxicity to, 512
    in hypoxia, 483, 484f, 485
  oxytocin and, 333
  reflex arc and, 52
  uterine, catecholamines and, 359
  vascular. *See* Vascular smooth muscle.
Sneezing, 503
Sodium. *See also* Hyponatremia; Na⁺/H⁺ exchanger; Na⁺,K⁺-ATPase pump.
  atrial volume receptor reflex and, 205, 205f
  intestinal absorption of, 265–267, 266f, 268t
  neurologic deficits and, 36
  reabsorption of, in kidney, 17, 439, 442, 442f–443f, 443
    aldosterone and, 435, 447–448, 448f
    atrial natriuretic peptide and, 356
    in collecting duct, 447–448, 448f
    in distal tubule, 445–446, 446f–447f
    mineralocorticoids and, 354f, 354t, 355
  resting membrane potential and, 9, 35–36
  VFA absorption and
    in horse, 301
    in ruminants, 296, 297f
Sodium channel blockers, for arrhythmias, 138
Sodium chloride transport, coupled, 266–267, 266f–267f
Sodium co-transport, 13–14, 13f, 263–264, 263f–264f, 265–266, 266f
  crypt secretion and, 270, 278
  distribution of, in gut, 268t
  in bile acid reabsorption, 272, 274f
  in renal tubular reabsorption, 442, 442f
  with paracellular chloride transport, 267, 267f
Sodium ion channels
  action potential and, 37, 38
  at nodes of Ranvier, 39
  excitatory potential and, 36
  intestinal absorption through, 267
  of cardiac muscle, 127–128, 129f, 130–131
    in pacemaker cells, 131, 131f
  of neuromuscular synapse, 15, 42
  of renal tubules, 17
  of retinal rods, 90
Sol, of mucociliary system, 509, 509f, 510
Solvent drag, 440, 442, 443
Somatic motor neurons, 32t, 33, 80–81, 81f
Somatic sensory peripheral nerves, 32t, 33
Somatomedins, 337, 338
Somatostatin, 224, 337, 337t, 361f, 365, 366f
  glucagon secretion and, 364–365
  insulin secretion and, 363
  pancreatic polypeptide and, 366
Somatotropin. *See* Growth hormone (GH).
Sorbitol, in renal medulla, 457
Sound waves, 104, 104f, 105
Spatial summation, 48
Spermatic cord, 421
Spermatids, 422, 423, 424f
Spermatocytes, 422, 423, 424, 424f, 425
Spermatocytogenesis, 423
Spermatogenesis, 423–425, 424f
  anabolic steroids and, 427
  androgen dependence of, 425
  at puberty, 392

Spermatogenesis (*Continued*)
  temperature dependence of, 422
Spermatogonia, 422, 423, 424, 424f
Spermatozoa, 398–399, 422
  anabolic steroids and, 427
  daily production of, 424–425
  development of. *See* Spermatogenesis.
  emission of, 423
  extragonadal reserves of, 422
Spermiation, 423, 425
Spermiogenesis, 423
Sphincter of Oddi, 252
Spinal cord, 32–33, 33f, 62–63, 63f. *See also* Cerebrospinal fluid (CSF).
  corticospinal tract and, 63–64, 64f, 65
  disease of, 59
  reflex arc and, 51, 51f, 52
Spinal interneurons, locomotion and, 68
Spinal tap, 94, 95
Spinocerebellum, 77, 77f, 78
Splanchnic circulation, 115, 115f, 116
  vasoconstriction in
    exercise-induced, 174f, 175
    in heart failure, 212
Spleen
  autonomic regulation of, 84t
  exercise-induced contraction of, 495, 498
  hemorrhage and, 214
Split second heart sound, 156
Spontaneous ovulators, 386–387
ST segment changes, 148, 148f, 150
Standard bicarbonate, 529
Stanozolol, 427
Stapes, 104, 105f
Star thistle poisoning, 68
Starch, 259–260, 259f, 262f, 265. *See also* Glycogen.
  fermentative digestion of, 281–282, 285, 286f
    in horse, 298
  intestinal osmotic pressure and, 269
  weaning and, 276
Starling forces, 185–187
  edema and, 188, 189
  in lung, 186–187
  intestinal absorption and, 270
  pleural fluid and, 512
  proximal tubular reabsorption and, 441
Starling's equation, 185, 511
Starling's hypothesis, 11–12
Starling's law of the heart, 157–158
Starling's mechanism, 210
Stellate cells, 76, 76f, 98, 99f
Stem cells, 119
  of seminiferous tubules, 423
Steroid diabetes, 351
Steroid hormones. *See also* Androgens; Estrogen(s); Glucocorticoids; Mineralocorticoids; Progesterone.
  categories of, 326
  cell responses to, 329, 329f
  metabolism of, 330
  receptors for, 26, 27f, 28, 328–329
  secretion of, 328
  structure of, 326
  synthesis of, 326–328, 327f
    adrenal, 349–350, 350f
  transport of, 328
Stimulus-secretion coupling, 357, 357f
Stomach. *See also* "Gastric" entries.
  emptying of, 236–238, 237f
    pancreatic polypeptide and, 366
  glucagon produced by, 364
  lipid emulsification in, 272, 274f
  motility of, 231, 232, 233, 235–238, 235f–237f

Stomach (*Continued*)
  mucosal types in, 247
  particle size reduction in, 235–236, 236f, 257
  pH regulation in, 226
  protein digestion in, 260
  secretions of, 247–249, 248f, 257, 260, 260t
Stress leukogram, in hyperadrenocorticism, 353
Stressful stimuli. *See also* Defense-alarm reaction.
  adrenocortical response to, 348, 352, 352f
  cardiac contraction and, 23–24
  catecholamine response to, 360
  lung defenses and, 510, 513
Stretch receptors
  atrial. *See* Atrial volume receptor reflex.
  muscle spindle, 51, 53–55, 53f–55f, 56
    cerebellum and, 75
    of respiratory muscles, 501, 503
    voluntary movement and, 66
  of reticulorumen, 294, 295
  pulmonary, 502, 503, 510
Striated muscle. *See* Skeletal muscle.
Striatum, 68
Stroke, 114
Stroke volume, 154
  cardiac output and, 156–161, 156f–157f, 159f
  during exercise, 160, 160t
  in heart failure, 209, 210, 210f
  pulse pressure and, 177, 178, 178f
  work and, 163
Stroke work, 163
Strongylus vulgaris infestation, 111, 121–122
Subarachnoid space, 33, 94–95, 95f
Subclavian veins, 185, 186
Subendocardial layers, 126
Submucosal (Meissner) plexus, 222, 224f
Substance K, 224
Substance P, 224
Substantia nigra, 68
Subthalamus, 68
Succinate, in ruminant gluconeogenesis, 320, 320f
Suckling
  absence of, milk suppression in, 414
  in mammalian reproductive strategy, 407
  oxytocin release and, 325, 414, 414f
  prolactin release and, 395, 412, 412f
  timing of, 415
Sucrase, 262, 262f
Sucrose, 258, 261, 262f
Sudden cardiac death, 137
Sugars, 258–259, 259f. *See also* Carbohydrates.
Sulfuric acid, from protein metabolism, 522
Superior cervical ganglion, photoperiod and, 394
Superior colliculus, 68
Supplementary motor cortex, 64, 66
Suprachiasmatic nucleus, photoperiod and, 394
Supraoptic nucleus, 332, 332f, 377
  oxytocin release and, 414, 414f
Supraventricular tachycardia, 137
Surface tension, lung elasticity and, 471–472, 472f
Surfactant, pulmonary, 472, 473f, 503, 519, 520
  in edema, 511

Suspensory ligaments
  of eye, 87f, 88, 89
  of udder, 408
Sustentacular cells, of carotid bodies, 504
Swallowing (deglutition), 233–234, 233f,
    235, 503
  rabies and, 243
Sweat, composition of, 535
Sweat glands
  epinephrine and, 359
  evaporative cooling and, 535, 540, 541
  neural control of, 82, 92, 539
Swine
  colon anatomy in, 239f, 241
  influenza in, 543
Sylvius, aqueduct of, 94
Sympathetic nervous system, 81–82,
    81f–82f, 83, 85. See also Autonomic
    nervous system.
  adipose tissue and, 317
  anal sphincter and, 241
  cardiac regulation by, 24, 125, 132–133,
    132f, 134–135, 200, 201t, 202
    AV node and, 133–134, 134t
    contractility and, 159, 160
    diastolic filling time and, 160, 160f,
      161
    in heart failure, 210, 210f
    in hemorrhage, 213–214
  chemoreceptors and, 503
  cholinergic muscarinic receptors in,
    201–202
  exercise and, 216, 217
  gastrointestinal regulation by, 224, 225f,
    233
  Horner's syndrome and, 86
  in atrial volume receptor reflex, 205,
    205f
  in baroreceptor reflex, 203–204, 203f
  in defense-alarm reaction, 206
  in vasovagal syncope, 206, 207f
  pulmonary arteries and, 482
  pupillary dilation and, 92
  salivary glands and, 246
  sweating and, 535
  thyroid hormones and, 345, 348
  vascular regulation by, 200–201, 201t,
    202
Symports, 13–14, 263, 263f. See also Co-
    transport proteins; Sodium co-
    transport.
Synapse(s), 34, 35f, 41
  neuromuscular, 41–43, 42f
    action potential at, 45
    nicotinic receptors at, 15, 83, 83f
  of reflex arc, 51, 51f
  postsynaptic potentials and, 36–37, 37f,
    99
Synaptic cleft, 34
  of neuromuscular synapse, 41, 42, 42f
Synaptic vesicles, 34
  of neuromuscular synapse, 41, 42, 42f
Synchronized EEG, 100
Syncope, vasovagal, 206, 207f
Syncytiotrophoblasts, embryonic, 400
Syncytium
  of cardiac muscle, 125
  of GI smooth muscle, 231
Syndrome of inappropriate antidiuretic
    hormone secretion, 335
Systemic circulation, 115–116, 115f
  blood volume distribution in, 117, 117t
  perfusion pressure of, 116
  pressure profile in, 169–170, 170f
  resistance of, 172–173
  vessels of, 117, 117t, 118f

Systole
  atrial, 155
  ventricular, 154–155, 155f, 156
Systolic murmurs, 161–162, 161f, 161t
Systolic pressures, 116, 176–177, 176f

T

T_3 (triiodothyronine), 342, 342f–346f,
    343–345. See also Thyroid hormones.
  in hypothyroidism, 347–348
  reverse, 343, 344, 344f
    in euthyroid sick syndrome, 347
  serum values of, 347t
T_4 (tetraiodothyronine), 342, 342f–346f,
    343–344. See also Thyroid hormones.
  in hypothyroidism, 346, 347–348
  serum values of, 347, 347t
T tubules, 49
T wave, 145, 145f–146f, 147
  abnormal, 149
Tachyarrhythmias, 137–138, 138f
  drug treatment for, 139
  paroxysmal atrial tachycardia as, 151–
    152, 160
  ventricular tachycardia as, 137, 150, 151f
Tapetum, 88f, 90
Target (effector) organ, 51, 51f, 52
TBG (thyroxine-binding globulin), 342,
    343, 343f, 344
Tears, 88
Teat, 407, 409f
  injury to, 417–418
  prolactin release and, 410, 412, 412f
Tectospinal tract, 67, 68
Temperature, body. See also Heat.
  climate and, 538
  core, 536, 537–538, 539
  elevation of, 541, 542f
  metabolic rate and, 536
  normal, 537–538, 537t
  of homeotherms, 533–534, 536
  of poikilotherms, 533, 534, 536
  oxyhemoglobin dissociation curve and,
    496, 498
  rectal, 537–538, 537t
  regulation of, 538–540, 539f–540f
    by respiratory system, 469–470
    in testes, 421
  set-point of, 539, 541, 542f
  tissue function and, 533
Temperature sensors, 538
Temporal bone, 104
  petrous, 70, 70f, 105
Temporal lobe, 64, 64f
Temporal retina, 91–92
Temporal summation, 48, 130
Tendon(s), 44, 48
  Golgi tendon organ(s) of, 53, 53f, 55–56,
    56f
    intercostal muscles and, 503
  intrafusal muscle fibers and, 54
Teniae, 240
Tension (partial pressure), 486
Tertiary active transport, 263, 264
Testis(es), 421–422
  anabolic steroids and, 427–428
  descent of, 422
  embryonic development of, 374, 375f–
    376f
  hypothalamic-pituitary regulation of,
    425, 426f, 427
  species differences in, 422, 422t
Testosterone
  anabolic steroids and, 427
  genital development and, 374–375

Testosterone (Continued)
  gonadotropins and, 379
  hypothalamic development and, 392
  in androgen insensitivity, 381
  libido and, 393
  metabolism of, 330
  testicular production of, 425, 426f
  thecal production of, 380, 393
Tetany, 48
Tetraiodothyronine (T_4), 342, 342f–346f,
    343–344. See also Thyroid hormones.
  in hypothyroidism, 346, 347–348
  serum values of, 347, 347t
Tetralogy of Fallot, 491
Thalamus, 63
  cerebrocerebellum and, 78
  cortical projections from, 98
  EEG and, 100, 102f
Theca cells, 374, 380, 384–385
  androgens secreted by, 380, 393
Thermal conductivity, 536
Thermal gradient, 534
Thermoneutral zone, 540
Thermoregulation, 538–540, 539f–540f. See
    also Heat; Temperature.
  by respiratory system, 469–470
  of testes, 421
Thiazide diuretics, 446
Thick filaments, 6, 6f
  of cardiac muscle, 124, 124f
  of smooth muscle, 22f
Thin filaments, 6, 6f–7f, 7
  of cardiac muscle, 124, 124f
  of smooth muscle, 21, 22f
Thiocyanates, iodine and, 346
Third eyelid, innervation of, 92
Third ventricle, 94, 95f
  chemoreceptor trigger zone and, 238
  hypothalamus and, 376
  neurohypophysis and, 332, 332f
Thoracic duct, 275
Thoracolumbar system, 81
Thorax, compliance of, 472–473
Threonine, phosphorylation of, 4, 4f
Threshold potential, 15, 37, 37f, 38
Thrombin, 119
Thrombocytes, 119
Thromboxane
  glucocorticoid inhibition of, 353
  pulmonary vasoconstriction by, 483t
  renal vascular tone and, 436
Thrombus(i)
  bloodworm infestation causing, 121–122
  ischemia and, 113, 115
Thymus, myasthenia gravis and, 43
Thyroglobulin, 342, 343, 343f
Thyroid function tests, 347–348
Thyroid gland, histology of, 342, 342f
Thyroid hormones. See also Calcitonin;
    Tetraiodothyronine (T_4);
    Triiodothyronine (T_3).
  carrier proteins for, 328
  cold stress and, 536, 540
  deficiency of, 345, 346–348, 347t
    canine gynecomastia in, 417
  excess of
    drug treatment for, 346
    in cats, 348
  functions of, 344–346, 345f
  histology of thyroid gland and, 342,
    342f
  metabolism of, 330, 344
  plasma transport of, 343–344
  receptors for, 26
  release of, 343, 343f
  storage of, 342–343

Thyroid hormones (*Continued*)
  synthesis of, 342, 342f
Thyroiditis
  autoimmune, 347
  lymphocytic, 346
Thyroid-stimulating hormone (TSH), 335, 344, 346, 346f, 376
  in hypothyroidism, 347, 348
Thyroperoxidase, 342
Thyroprotein, for lactational enhancement, 417
Thyrotropin. *See* Thyroid-stimulating hormone (TSH).
Thyrotropin-releasing hormone (TRH), 337, 337t, 346, 346f
  prolactin secretion and, 379, 417
Thyroxine. *See* Tetraiodothyronine (T$_4$).
Thyroxine-binding globulin (TBG), 342, 343, 343f, 344
Thyroxine-binding prealbumin, 343
TIDA (tuberoinfundibular dopamine) neurons, 379f, 412f
Tidal volume (VT), 469–470, 471f
  neural regulation of, 502, 503
Tight junctions, 17, 256, 257, 257f
  of rumen epithelium, 296, 296f
  passive transport through, 264–265, 265f
  of chloride, 267, 267f
Tissue pressure hypothesis, 195
Titan, 45
TNF (tumor necrosis factor)
  as pyrogen, 541
  in lung, 510–511
Toe-pinch withdrawal reflex, 59
Tonsils, particle impaction on, 508
Total buffer base, 526, 527, 528
Total carbon dioxide (TCO$_2$), 529
Total lung capacity (TLC)
  definition of, 472
  pulmonary vascular resistance and, 482f
Total peripheral resistance (TPR), 172–173, 177
  epinephrine and, 359
  pulse pressure and, 178f, 179
  vasoconstriction and, 200, 204
  in heart failure, 210
Toxic substances
  gaseous, 509
  pulmonary removal of, 512
Trachea, 469, 473
  collapsing, 475
  frictional resistance of, 473f
  irritant receptors in, 503
  mucociliary clearance in, 509, 509f
  stretch receptors in, 503
Trachealis muscle, 474
Tracheobronchial tree, 473–474. *See also* Bronchi.
  irritant receptors of, 474, 503
  particle deposition in, 508–509, 509f
Transcalciferin, 370
Transcellular absorption, 265, 265f
Transcellular transport, 17
Transcortin. *See* Corticosteroid-binding globulin.
Transcription factors, 26, 27f, 28
Transduction
  by cell-surface receptors. *See* Signaling.
  by peripheral receptors, 51
Transit time, in gut, 230
Transmural pressure, 112–113
  of pulmonary blood vessels, 481–482, 483f
Transport, 3. *See also* Active transport; Diffusion; Osmosis.
Transport amino acids, 309, 309t

Transpulmonary pressure, 471–472, 472f
Transverse tubules
  of cardiac muscle, 49
  of skeletal muscle, 45, 47f, 48
Tremor
  action, 68, 78, 79
  resting, 68
TRH (thyrotropin-releasing hormone), 337, 337t, 346, 346f
  prolactin secretion and, 379, 417
TRH stimulation test, 347, 348
Triacylglycerols. *See* Triglycerides.
Triamcinolone, 353f
Tricarboxylic acid cycle. *See* Krebs cycle.
Tricuspid stenosis, 161t, 162, 162f
Tricuspid valve
  congenital defect of, 506
  first heart sound and, 156
  in cardiac cycle, 155
Triglycerides, 272, 273f, 275, 275f
  hepatic synthesis of, 318, 319
  in milk, 415
  in VLDL, 308, 309f, 312
  insulin and, 361, 362, 363
  release of, from adipose tissue, 317
  storage function of, 306–307, 313
Triiodothyronine (T$_3$), 342, 342f–346f, 343–345. *See also* Thyroid hormones.
  in hypothyroidism, 347–348
  reverse, 343, 344, 344f
    in euthyroid sick syndrome, 347
  serum values of, 347t
Tripeptides, absorption of, 262, 262f, 265, 266f
Trisaccharides, 258, 259, 260
Trophoblastin, 399
Tropomyosin, 6, 7–8, 7f, 21, 45, 48
  in cardiac muscle, 24
Troponin, 6, 7–8, 7f, 21, 45, 128
  in cardiac muscle, 24, 129, 130, 134
Trypsin, 260, 260t, 261f
Trypsinogen, 260, 260t, 261f
TSH (thyroid-stimulating hormone), 335, 344, 346, 346f, 376
  in hypothyroidism, 347, 348
TSH assay, endogenous, 347, 348
TSH stimulation test, 347, 348
  in hyperadrenocorticism, 353
Tuberoinfundibular dopamine (TIDA) neurons, 379f, 412f
Tubuloglomerular feedback, 435, 436, 437
Tumor necrosis factor (TNF)
  as pyrogen, 541
  in lung, 510–511
Tunica albuginea, 375f–376f, 423
Tunica dartos, 421
Turbulent flow
  of air, 474
  of blood, 161
Tympanic membrane (eardrum), 104, 105, 105f–106f
Tyrosine
  in catecholamine synthesis, 5, 5f, 357, 357f–358f
  in thyroid hormone synthesis, 342
  phosphorylation of, 4, 4f
Tyrosine hydroxylase, 5, 5f, 357, 357f–358f

U

Udder, 408, 409f. *See also* Mammary gland.
  development of, in pregnancy, 409
  flushing of colostrum from, 416
  letdown of milk and, 414, 415
  mastitis and, 418
Ultimobranchial glands, 369

Ultradian rhythms, 331
Ultrafiltrate, glomerular, 433, 439
Ultrafiltration coefficient (K$_f$), 433, 435, 436
Umbilical arteries, 517, 518
Umbilical veins, 518, 519
Unipolar limb leads, augmented, 147
Uniports, 14
Unstirred water layer, 257, 261
  lipid absorption from, 272
Upper brain, 33
Upper motor neuron(s), 59. *See also* Cerebellum; Extrapyramidal system; Pyramidal system.
  autonomic coordination by, 85
  movement and, 62
Upper motor neuron disease, 59, 60
Urea
  diffusion of, through lipid bilayer, 9
  hepatic synthesis of, 316, 316f
  in fermentative digestion
    equine, 298
    ruminant, 288, 289f
  reabsorption of, in kidney, 435, 453, 454f
Uremia. *See also* Azotemia.
  in heart failure, 212–213
Uric acid, avian excretion of, 444, 460
Urinary bladder. *See* Bladder.
Urine
  dilute, 455, 456, 456f, 457
  discharge of, 447
  osmolality of, 452, 453, 454–455, 455f–456f, 456–457
  pH of, 459, 462
    in paradoxic aciduria, 465–466
    species differences in, 464–465
  pheromones in, 395
Uterus. *See also* Cervix, uterine.
  catecholamines and, 359
  contraction of, 402, 403, 404
  embryonic development of, 375, 376f
  fertilization and, 399
  in pregnancy, 402
  infection of, estrous cycle and, 386
  luteolysis and, 385, 385f, 386
  PGF$_{2\alpha}$ synthesized by, 385–386, 385f–386f, 399–400, 399f
  postpartum size reduction in, 404
  progesterone and, 384
Utricle, 70f–71f, 71, 72–73
Utriculus prostaticus, 376f

V

Vagal indigestion, 295
Vagina, development of, 375, 376f
Vagosympathetic trunk, 92
Vagovagal reflex, pancreatic secretion and, 250
Vagus nerve
  airway smooth muscle and, 474, 475, 475f
  aortic baroreceptors and, 202f, 203
  aortic bodies and, 503
  esophageal striated muscle and, 234
  gastric acid secretion and, 249
  gastric emptying and, 237, 237f
  gastric motility and, 236
  gastrointestinal innervation by, 224, 225f
    in birds, 242
  in ruminants
    esophageal groove closure and, 298
    forestomach motility and, 294, 295
  in vasovagal syncope, 206, 207f
  pancreatic secretions and, 250, 366
  pulmonary receptors and, 503
  respiratory pattern and, 502, 502f

Vagus nerve (Continued)
  vasopressin secretion and, 333
Valeric acid, 284
Valine, 309, 309t
  microbial degradation of, 286
Van't Hoff's equation, 11
Varicosities, of enteric nervous system, 222, 224f
Vas deferens (vasa deferentia), 421, 422, 423
  embryonic development of, 374, 375f–376f
Vasa efferentia, 375f–376f
Vasa recta, 453, 454, 454f, 455, 456f
Vasa vasorum, 484
Vascular resistance, 170–172, 172f–173f. See also Arterioles, resistance of; Vasoconstriction; Vasodilation.
  angiotensin II and, 355
  blood flow and, 173, 174f, 175, 192
  coronary, 195–196
  definition of, 171, 177
  factors affecting, 192
  friction and, 169, 177
  glomerular, 436
  pulmonary. See Pulmonary vascular resistance (PVR).
  systemic pressure profile and, 169–170, 170f
  total peripheral, 172–173, 177
    epinephrine and, 359
    pulse pressure and, 178f, 179
    vasoconstriction and, 200, 204, 210
Vascular smooth muscle, 181, 182f
  adrenergic receptors of, 200–201, 201t
  cholinergic receptors of, 202
  cyclic GMP in, 24
  sympathetic innervation of, 92
  vasopressin and, 333
Vasoactive intestinal peptide, 224, 236
  crypt secretion and, 270
  prolactin secretion and, 379, 412, 412f
Vasoconstriction, 172, 175. See also Vascular resistance.
  adrenergic neurons and, 85
  adrenergic receptors and, 200, 201t, 202
  angiotensin II and, 355, 435–436, 435f
  cholinergic muscarinic receptors and, 202
  hypoxic, 175–176, 483, 484f, 485
  in autoregulation of blood flow, 195
  in baroreceptor reflex, 204
  in cold stress, 536–537, 537f, 539, 540
  in dehydration, 173
  in heart failure, 212
  in hemorrhage, 173
  in noncritical organs, 200, 204, 205, 206
    during exercise, 216
  pulmonary, 482, 483, 483t
  pulse pressure and, 179
Vasodilation, 172, 173f, 175. See also Vascular resistance.
  β₂-adrenergic receptors and, 200, 201, 201t, 202
  atrial natriuretic peptide and, 356
  cholinergic muscarinic receptors and, 201t, 202
  in heat stress, 540
  in skeletal muscle
    β₂-adrenergic receptors and, 200, 201, 201t, 202
    cholinergic neurons and, 82
    exercise-induced, 174f, 175, 192
    M₃ receptors and, 201t, 202
  metabolic control of, 193, 193f–194f, 195
    during exercise, 216

Vasodilation (Continued)
  pulmonary, 482–483, 483t
  renal prostaglandins and, 435–436
Vasopressin (antidiuretic hormone [ADH]), 332–335, 332f–334f, 377
  angiotensin II and, 435, 436
  arterial baroreceptor reflex and, 205
  atrial volume receptor reflex and, 205, 205f
  cyclic AMP and, 23
  deficiency of
    in Cushing's disease, 339
    in diabetes insipidus, 457
  glucocorticoids and, 351
  hypersecretion of, 335
  renal tubular reabsorption and, 446, 447
  reticular groove reflex and, 298
  urea reabsorption and, 453
  urine osmolality and, 453, 456–457, 456f–457f
Vasovagal syncope, 206, 207f
VD/VT (dead-space/tidal volume ratio), 469
Vegetative nervous system, 85
Veins, 117, 117t, 118f
  abdominal
    adrenergic receptors of, 200, 201t
    hemorrhage and, 214
    respiratory pump and, 217
  as volume reservoirs, 170, 181, 200
  low resistance of, 169, 170f
  wall properties of, 181, 182f
Venae cavae, 115, 115f
  hepatic veins and, 271
  pressure in, 169–170, 170f, 172
  thoracic duct and, 275
Venoconstriction, 200, 201t
Venous carbon dioxide tension, 488
Venous pressure, edema and, 185, 187, 188, 188f
Venous sinuses, cavernous, 537
Ventilation, 468–470, 469f
  alveolar, 487, 491
    definition of, 469
    in cold-stressed animals, 470
    regulation of, 469, 501
  blood pH and, 525
  collateral, 476
  control of, 501, 501f
    airway receptors in, 503
    at high altitude, 505
    central, 501–503, 502f
    chemoreceptors in, 503–505, 504f–505f
    during exercise, 505
    pulmonary receptors in, 503
  distribution of, 475, 476f
  energy cost of, 468
  mechanical, pressure elevation in, 196–197
  muscular energy required for, 470, 471f
Ventilation/perfusion mismatching, 489–491, 490f
  gravity and, 175
  hypoxic vasoconstriction and, 175–176
  in anesthetized horse, 492–493
Ventilation/perfusion ratio, 489–491, 490f
  of alveolar dead-space, 491
  with right-to-left shunt, 491
Ventral nerve roots, 33, 33f, 51, 63
Ventral respiratory group, 502, 502f, 504
Ventricles
  cardiac, 115, 115f, 479
    work done by, 163–164
  cerebral, 63
    cerebrospinal fluid and, 33, 94, 95f, 96
Ventricular compliance, 158, 158f, 160

Ventricular contractility, 158–159, 159f, 160–161
Ventricular diastole, 154, 155, 155f
Ventricular end-diastolic pressure. See Ventricular preload.
Ventricular end-diastolic volume, 156–158, 157f–159f, 159–160
  during exercise, 160t
Ventricular end-systolic volume, 154, 156, 158–159, 160
  during exercise, 160t
Ventricular fibrillation, 137, 138
  ECG in, 150–151, 151f
Ventricular function curve(s), 156, 157f
  hemorrhage and, 213, 213f
  in heart failure, 209–210, 210f
Ventricular preload, 156–158, 157f–158f, 160
  abnormal reduction in, 173
  during exercise, 217
  in heart failure, 209, 210, 210f
Ventricular septal defect (VSD), 161f, 162–163, 165
Ventricular systole, 154–155, 155f, 156
Ventricular tachycardia, 137
  ECG in, 150, 151f
Ventriculus, 242, 242f
Venules, 117, 117t, 118f
  pressure decrease in, 169, 170f
  pulmonary, 479
  wall properties of, 181, 182f
Very low density lipoprotein (VLDL), 308, 309f, 312, 313
  distribution of, 319–320
  from adipose tissue, 319
Vestibular nuclei, 67, 68, 73
  cerebellar input to, 77
Vestibular reflexes, 73
Vestibular syndrome, 73–74
Vestibular system, 70–74, 70f–72f
  cerebellum and, 75, 77
  lesions of, 70
  vestibulospinal tract and, 68
Vestibulocerebellum, 77, 77f, 78
Vestibulospinal tract, 67, 68, 73, 77
VFA. See Volatile fatty acids (VFA).
Vibrio cholerae, G proteins and, 23
Villus(i), intestinal, 223f, 255, 256f. See also Enterocyte(s); Microvilli.
  growth and development of, 276
  infectious injury to, 277, 277f
  of neonate, 276
  osmotic-multiplier system of, 270–271
  trophic regulatory peptides and, 228
Visceral afferent (sensory) nerves, 32t, 33, 85
Visceral pleura, 472, 512
  blood supply to, 484
Visceral smooth muscle. See Smooth muscle.
Viscosity, 171
  of blood, 120–121, 120f, 498
Visual cortex, 91–92, 92f
Visual pathway, 91–92, 92f
Visual system, 87–93. See also Eye; Retina.
  accommodation by, 88–89, 89f
  anatomy of, 87–88, 87f–88f, 89–90, 90f
  cerebellum and, 75, 77
  cerebral cortex in, 91–92, 92f, 93
  intraocular pressure in, 92
  of nocturnal animals, 90
  ophthalmoscope view of, 88, 88f
  photoreceptors of, 89, 89f, 90–91, 91f
  pupillary diameter in
    autonomic control of, 83, 84t, 85, 92
    epinephrine and, 359

Visual system (*Continued*)
  pupillary light reflex in, 52, 85, 92
Visual tectum, 67, 68
Vitamin A
  in colostrum, 410, 410t
  intestinal absorption of, 272
  photopigments and, 90
  placental transfer of, 410
  signaling by, 26
Vitamin D, 369–371, 370f
  calcium excretion and, 449
Vitamins
  lipid-soluble, 272
  rumen microbes and, 282
Vitreous humor, 87f, 88
VLDL (very low density lipoprotein), 308,
    309f, 312, 313
  distribution of, 319–320
  from adipose tissue, 319
Vocalization, 503
Volatile fatty acids (VFA)
  absorption of, 295–297, 296f–297f
  as energy substrates, 285, 289, 295
  gluconeogenesis from, 320, 320f
  in equine hindgut, 299, 301
  microbial production of, 283–285, 284f–
      286f, 285t, 286, 287, 288f
  motility of forestomach and, 294, 295
  omasum and, 295
  papillary growth and, 297
Voltage, molecular transport and, 9, 10
Voltage-dependent proteins, 4, 4f
Voltage-gated channels, 14f, 15
  in cardiac muscle, 24
  in pulmonary artery smooth muscle,
      483
Volume condition, 98
Volume receptor reflex, atrial, 202f,
    204–205, 205f
  hemorrhage and, 213, 213f, 214, 215
  vasopressin secretion and, 333, 334f

Voluntary movement, 62, 65, 66, 67
Vomiting, 238
  metabolic alkalosis caused by, 527–528
VP. *See* Vasopressin (antidiuretic hormone
    [ADH]).
VSD (ventricular septal defect), 161f,
    162–163, 165
VT (tidal volume), 469–470, 471f
  neural regulation of, 502, 503
Vulva, development of, 375

W

Water
  aquaporin channels for, 14–15, 456
  capillary filtration of, 184–188, 189, 190
  capillary reabsorption of, 184
  capillary wall transport of, 182, 182f,
      184–188
  diffusion through lipid bilayer, 9
  evaporation of
    from respiratory system, 470
    heat loss by, 534, 534f, 535
  in equine hindgut, 301, 301f
  in rumen, 293–294
  intake of
    after hemorrhage, 215
    arterial baroreceptor reflex and, 205
    atrial volume receptor reflex and,
        205
    in diabetes insipidus, 334, 335
  intestinal
    absorption of, 265, 268–269, 270–271,
        270f
    diarrhea and, 276–278, 277f
    secretion of, 269–270, 269f
  osmosis and, 10–11, 10f
  pH of, 523
  renal excretion of
    glucocorticoids and, 351
    hypothyroidism and, 347

Water (*Continued*)
  renal reabsorption of, 435, 439, 439f,
      452, 455
Water balance, 452–457, 454f–457f
Water deprivation test, 335, 457
Water vapor, 486–487
Wedge pressure, pulmonary, 480
Weight, metabolic rate and, 468, 536, 536f
Whey, 416
White blood cells, 119
White coat, congenital deafness and, 106
White muscle, 49
Whitten effect, 395
Wolffian duct, 374, 375, 375f–376f

X

X zone, of adrenal cortex, 349

Y

Yolk sac, 374
  embryonic erythrocytes in, 519
Young-Helmholtz theory, 91

Z

Z disk
  of cardiac muscle, 124, 124f
  of skeletal muscle, 45, 46f–48f
Zinc fingers, 26, 28
Zona fasciculata, 349, 349f, 350, 351
Zona glomerulosa, 348–349, 349f, 350
  regulation of, 355, 356
Zona pellucida, 380, 398
Zona reticularis, 349, 349f, 350, 351
Zonary placenta, 516, 516t
Zone of potential escape, 292, 292f, 293
Zonula occludens, 440, 441f–442f, 443
Zymogens, 249, 260, 261f